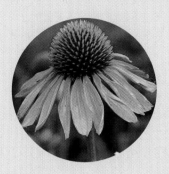

Core Concepts
in Health

Preface

Now in its ninth edition, *Core Concepts in Health* has maintained its leadership in the field of health education for more than 25 years. Since we pioneered the concept of self-responsibility for personal health in 1976, hundreds of thousands of students have used our book to become active, informed participants in their own health care. Each edition of *Core Concepts* has brought improvements and refinements, but the principles underlying the book have remained the same. Our commitment to these principles has never been stronger than it is today.

OUR GOALS

Our goals in writing this book can be stated simply:

- To present scientifically based, accurate, up-to-date information in an accessible format
- To involve students in taking responsibility for their health and well-being
- To instill a sense of competence and personal power in students

The first of these goals means making expert knowledge about health and health care available to the individual. *Core Concepts* brings scientifically based, accurate, up-to-date information to students about topics and issues that concern them—exercise, stress, nutrition, weight management, contraception, intimate relationships, HIV infection, drugs, alcohol, and a multitude of others. Current, complete, and straightforward coverage is balanced with "user-friendly" features designed to make the text appealing. Written in an engaging, easy-to-read style and presented in a colorful, open format, *Core Concepts* invites the student to read, learn, and remember. Boxes, tables, artwork, photographs, and many other features highlight areas of special interest throughout the book.

The second of our goals is to involve students in taking responsibility for their health. *Core Concepts* uses innovative pedagogy and unique interactive features to get students thinking about how the material they're reading relates to their own lives. We invite them to examine their emotions about the issues under discussion, to consider their personal values and beliefs, and to analyze their health-related behaviors. Beyond this, for students who want to change behaviors that detract from a healthy lifestyle, we offer guidelines and tools, ranging from samples of health journals and personal contracts to detailed assessments and behavior change strategies.

Perhaps our third goal in writing *Core Concepts in Health* is the most important: to instill a sense of competence and personal power in the students who read the book. Everyone has the ability to monitor, understand, and affect his or her own health. Although medical and health professionals possess impressive skills and have access to a huge body of knowledge that benefits everyone in our society, people can help to minimize the amount of professional care they actually require in their lifetime by taking care of themselves—taking charge of their health—from an early age. Our hope is that *Core Concepts* will continue to help young people make this exciting discovery—that they have the power to shape their own futures.

ORGANIZATION AND CONTENT OF THE NINTH EDITION

The organization of the book as a whole remains essentially the same as in the eighth edition, with some improvements. The book is divided into eight parts. Part One, Establishing a Basis for Wellness, includes chapters on taking charge of your health (Chapter 1), stress (Chapter 2), and psychological health (Chapter 3). Part Two, Understanding Sexuality, opens with an exploration of communication and intimate relationships, including friendship, intimate partnerships, marriage, and family (Chapter 4), and then moves on to discuss physical sexuality (Chapter 5), contraception (Chapter 6), abortion (Chapter 7), and pregnancy and childbirth (Chapter 8). As in previous editions of *Core Concepts,* we devote a separate chapter to abortion to reflect both the importance of this issue and our belief that abortion is not a form of contraception and should not be included in the chapter on that topic.

Part Three, Making Responsible Decisions: Substance Use and Abuse, opens with a discussion of addictive behavior and the different classes of psychoactive drugs (Chapter 9), followed by chapters on alcohol (Chapter 10) and tobacco (Chapter 11). Part Four, Getting Fit, includes a detailed discussion of nutrition (Chapter 12), exercise (Chapter 13), and weight management (Chapter 14).

Part Five, Protecting Yourself Against Disease, deals with the most serious health threats facing Americans today—cardiovascular disease (Chapter 15), cancer (Chapter 16), infectious diseases (Chapter 17), and sexually transmitted diseases (Chapter 18). Part Six, Accepting

Physical Limits, explores aging (Chapter 19) and dying and death (Chapter 20).

The order of topics in Part Seven, Making Choices in Health Care, has been revised for the ninth edition. The part opens with expanded coverage of both conventional and complementary medicine (Chapter 21), followed by information about medical self-care and use of the health care system (Chapter 22). And finally, Part Eight, Improving Your Chances: Personal Safety and Environmental Health, expands the boundaries of health to include injury prevention (Chapter 23) and the effects of environment on wellness (Chapter 24). Taken together, the chapters of the book provide students with a complete guide to promoting and protecting their health, now and through their entire lives, as individuals, as participants in a health care community and system, and as citizens of a planet that also needs to be protected if it is to continue providing human beings with the means to live healthy lives.

For the ninth edition, all chapters were carefully reviewed, revised, and updated. The latest information from scientific and health-related research is incorporated in the text, and newly emerging topics and issues are discussed. The following list gives a sample of some of the current concerns addressed in the ninth edition:

- Healthy People 2010 objectives
- Dietary Guidelines for Americans, 2000 Edition, and Dietary Reference Intakes
- Complementary and alternative medicine
- Causes and prevention of violence
- Ecstasy, GHB, and other "club drugs"
- West Nile virus and other emerging infections
- Emergency contraception and other new methods of contraception
- Mifepristone (RU-486)
- Dietary supplement labeling and safety issues
- Health and safety effects of cell phone use
- Implications of the Human Genome Project
- Women's health issues
- Effective communication
- Genetically modified foods, organic foods, food irradiation, food safety, and other nutrition issues
- Campus safety
- Spiritual wellness
- Carpal tunnel syndrome
- Health risks of cigars, bidis, and spit tobacco

For the ninth edition, the coverage of health care has been substantially revised. An all-new Chapter 21, "Health Care: Conventional and Complementary Medicine," provides consumer-oriented coverage of both conventional Western medicine and widely used comple-

mentary and alternative practices. Topics include the basic premises of conventional medicine; the scientific method and the U.S. drug-approval process; guidelines for choosing a primary care physician; general characteristics of complementary and alternative medicine (CAM); descriptions of such CAM practices as acupuncture, chiropractic, homeopathy, and herbal remedies; and consumer guidelines for evaluating CAM practitioners and therapies. In addition, coverage of dietary supplements has been expanded throughout the text; topics new to the ninth edition include dietary supplement labeling (Chapter 12) and the use of specific supplements for depression (Chapter 3), premenstrual syndrome (Chapter 5), athletic performance (Chapter 13), weight loss (Chapter 14), and elevated cholesterol levels (Chapter 15).

The ninth edition includes a greater emphasis on the development of total wellness, with expanded coverage of spiritual wellness and the close connections between mind and body. New and updated topics include paths to spiritual wellness; global religious views on tobacco use; the effects of stress on the brain, the immune system, and the course of pregnancy; and the benefits of close connections with others. Chapter 4 has been expanded to include more information on the benefits of intimate relationships and additional strategies for building and maintaining healthy interpersonal relationships. Suggested journal writing activities throughout the book help students to further explore their feelings and values.

Many other areas of special concern to students have also been expanded and updated in the ninth edition. The discussion of violence in Chapter 23 includes new material on stalking, cyberstalking, and date-rape drugs; the coverage of unintentional injuries has been updated with new material on the link between cell phone use and car crashes, the dangers of sleepy driving, scooter injuries, and repetitive stress injuries such as carpal tunnel syndrome. Chapter 12 on nutrition has been thoroughly updated to include the most recent dietary recommendations as well as new information on special topics such as food irradiation, genetically modified foods, organic foods, functional foods, and foodborne illness. Chapter 15 presents the latest research on cardiovascular disease, the leading killer of Americans; it reports on the effects of diet, exercise, tobacco use, genetics, infectious agents, and other recently discovered factors on an individual's risk of developing cardiovascular disease.

Core Concepts also takes care to address the health issues and concerns of an increasingly diverse student population. While most health concerns are universal—we all need to eat well, exercise, and manage stress, for example—certain differences among people have important implications for health. These differences can be genetic or cultural, based on factors such as gender, socioeconomic status, age, and ethnicity. Where such differences are important for health, they are discussed in the text or in a type of highlight box called Dimensions of Diversity (discussed in greater detail below). Examples of these discussions include the links between ethnicity and genetic diseases, the relationship between poverty and environmental health, and the effects of gender and ethnicity on body image. Topics in women's health receive special attention; the ninth edition includes discussions of how contraceptive use varies among U.S. women, the special risks faced by women who smoke or drink, hormonal influences on cardiovascular health and disease, the increased risk women face for depression and autoimmune disorders, and special dietary challenges faced by women.

The health field is dynamic, with new discoveries, advances, trends, and theories reported every week. Ongoing research—on the role of diet in cancer prevention, for example, or on new treatments for HIV infection —continually changes our understanding of the human body and how it works in health and disease. For this reason, no health book can claim to have the final word on every topic. Yet within these limits, *Core Concepts* does present the latest available information and scientific thinking on innumerable topics.

To aid students in keeping up with rapidly advancing knowledge about health issues, the ninth edition of *Core Concepts* also includes coverage of a key source of up-to-date information—the Internet. Each chapter includes an annotated list of World Wide Web sites that students can use as a launching point for further exploration of important topics. Appendix C, Resources for Self-Care, provides a brief introduction to the Internet, including guidelines for performing Web searches, using newsgroups and mailing lists, and evaluating health information from the Web.

WWw. Each chapter in the ninth edition is also closely tied to the Web site developed as a companion to the text. Boxes, illustrations, tables, and sections of text marked with the special new World Wide Web icon have corresponding links and activities on the *Core Concepts in Health* Online Learning Center (http://www.mhhe.com/ insel9). The Web site and other online supplements are described below in greater detail.

FEATURES OF THE NINTH EDITION

This edition of *Core Concepts in Health* builds on the features that attracted and held our readers' interest in the previous editions. One of the most popular features has always been the **boxes,** which allow us to explore a wide range of current topics in greater detail than is possible in the text itself. More than one-third of the boxes are new to the ninth edition, and many others have been significantly revised or updated. The boxes are divided into seven categories, each marked with a unique icon and label.

New to the ninth edition, **In the News** boxes focus on current health issues that have recently been highlighted in the media. Topics covered include the Human Genome Project, same-sex marriage and civil unions, cybersex, club drugs, genetically modified foods, medical errors, cell phones and distracted driving, mifepristone (RU-486), and emerging infectious diseases. Each In the News box is accompanied by the new World Wide Web icon, indicating that the *Core Concepts* Online Learning Center has links to Internet resources students can use to learn more about the topic of the box.

Mind/Body/Spirit boxes are an expanded version of the Sound Mind, Sound Body boxes that appeared in previous editions of *Core Concepts*. The new label reflects their broader focus and greater emphasis on spiritual wellness and the close connections between people's feelings and states of mind and their physical health. Included in Mind/Body/Spirit boxes are topics such as paths to spiritual wellness, religious views of tobacco use, benefits of being a volunteer, sexual decision making and personal values, the placebo effect, how exercise fosters emotional wellness, and how stress affects pregnancy and the immune system. Mind/Body/Spirit boxes emphasize that all the dimensions of wellness must be developed in order for an individual to achieve optimal health and well-being.

Take Charge boxes distill from each chapter the practical advice students need in order to apply information to their own lives. By referring to these boxes, students can easily find ways to foster friendships, for example; to become more physically active; to enhance support in their relationships; to reduce the amount of fat in their diets; and to help a friend who has a problem with tobacco or drugs or has an eating disorder.

Critical Consumer boxes emphasize the key theme of critical thinking by helping students develop and apply critical thinking skills, thereby allowing them to make sound choices related to health and well-being. Critical Consumer boxes provide specific guidelines for evaluating health news and advertising, using food labels to make dietary choices, choosing a bicycle helmet, avoiding quackery, selecting exercise footwear, making environmentally friendly shopping choices, and so on.

Dimensions of Diversity boxes are part of our commitment to reflect and respond to the diversity of the student population. These boxes give students the opportunity to identify any special health risks that affect them because of who they are as individuals or as members of a group. The boxes also broaden students' perspectives by exposing them to a wide variety of viewpoints on health-related issues. The different dimensions these boxes reflect include gender, ethnicity, socioeconomic status, and age. The principles embodied by these boxes are described in Chapter 1; topics covered in later chapters include special cardiovascular disease risks for African Americans, exercise for people with disabilities, suicide among older men, drug use in rural America, ethnic foods, links between poverty and poor environmental health, and attitudes toward aging.

In addition, some Dimensions of Diversity boxes highlight health issues and practices in other parts of the world, allowing students to see what Americans share with people in other societies and how they differ. Students have the opportunity to learn about laws and attitudes toward abortion in other countries, tobacco control around the world, the global pattern of HIV infection, health care systems around the world, and other topics of interest.

Assess Yourself boxes give students the opportunity to examine their behavior and identify ways that they can change their habits and improve their health. By referring to these boxes, students can examine their eating habits, for example; evaluate their fitness level; discover if they are at increased risk for cancer or cardiovascular disease; evaluate their driving habits; determine what triggers their eating; and examine their drinking and drug-taking behavior. These self-assessments are included on the student CD-ROM in an interactive format; see below for more on the CD-ROM.

In Focus boxes highlight current wellness topics of particular interest. Topics include diabetes, headaches, injection drug use, asthma, genetic testing for cancer, carpal tunnel syndrome, and shyness.

In addition to the box program, many new and refined features are included in the ninth edition of *Core Concepts.* Each chapter opens with **Test Your Knowledge**—a series of 4–6 multiple choice and true-false questions, with answers. These self-quizzes facilitate learning by getting students involved in a variety of wellness-related issues. The questions emphasize important points, highlight common misconceptions, and spark debate. Many questions are new to the ninth edition.

Vital Statistics tables and figures highlight important facts and figures in a memorable format that often reveals surprising contrasts and connections. From tables and figures marked with the Vital Statistics label, students can learn about drinking and drug use among college students, alternative medicine use in the United States, world population growth, prevalence of psychological disorders, trends in public opinion about abortion, and a wealth of other information. For students who grasp a subject best when it is displayed graphically, numerically, or in a table, the Vital Statistics feature provides alternative ways of approaching and understanding the text. In addition, for each Vital Statistics table and figure, the *Core Concepts* Online Learning Center has links to sites where students can find the latest statistics and information.

Core Concepts features a wealth of attractive and helpful **illustrations,** more than 30 of which are new to the ninth edition. The anatomical art, which has been prepared by medical illustrators, is both visually appealing and highly informative. These illustrations help students understand such important information as how blood flows through the heart, how the process of conception occurs, and how to use a condom. New topics illustrated for the ninth edition include diabetes, the effects of cocaine use on brain chemistry, the allergic response, the process of tumor development, osteoarthritis, and the vegetarian food pyramid. These lively and abundant illustrations will particularly benefit those students who learn best from visual images

Many of the illustrations in the ninth edition are marked with the new CD icon, indicating that they appear in an enhanced format on *Core Concepts Interactive,* the student CD-ROM that accompanies the text. From self-guided mini-tutorials on the CD-ROM, students can learn more about the stress response, the effects of alcohol and tobacco use, physical processes of aging, immediate and long-term effects of physical activity, the development of cancerous tumors, the greenhouse effect, and many other topics. The CD-ROM is described in more detail below.

New to the ninth edition, **Communicate!** exercises suggest strategies and activities for improving communication skills in ways that will enhance wellness. Communicate! covers all aspects of communication, from interpersonal communication and communication with oneself to mass communication, from assertive speaking to empathic listening, and from methods of persuasion to critical evaluation of public messages. These exercises appear at appropriate points throughout each chapter.

Also new to the ninth edition are chapter-ending **Tips for Today** sections. These provide a very brief distillation of the major message of each chapter, followed by suggestions for a few simple things that students can try right away. Tips for Today are designed to encourage students and to build their confidence by giving them easy steps they can take immediately to improve their wellness.

Take Action, appearing at the end of every chapter, suggests hands-on exercises and projects that students can undertake to extend and deepen their grasp of the material. Suggested projects include interviews, investigations of campus or community resources, and experimentation with some of the behavior change techniques suggested in the text. Special care has been taken to ensure that the projects are both feasible and worthwhile.

Journal Entry also appears at the end of each chapter. These entries suggest ways for students to use their Health Journal (which we recommend they keep while using *Core Concepts*) to think about topics and issues, explore and formulate their own views, and express their thoughts in written form. They are designed to help students deepen their understanding of their own health-related behaviors. (Journal Entry questions also appear on the *Core Concepts Online Learning Center* in a format that enables students to e-mail their responses to their instructors.)

Making wise choices about health requires students to sort through and evaluate health information. To help students become skilled evaluators, each chapter contains at least one **Critical Thinking Journal Entry.** These entries help students develop their critical thinking skills, including finding relevant information, separating fact from opinion, recognizing faulty reasoning, evaluating information, and assessing the credibility of sources. Critical Thinking Journal Entry questions do not have right or wrong answers; rather, they ask students to analyze, evaluate, or take a stand on a particular issue.

The **Behavior Change Strategies** that conclude many chapters offer specific behavior management/modification plans relating to the chapter's topic. Based on the principles of behavior management that are carefully explained in Chapter 1, these strategies will help students change unhealthy or counterproductive behaviors. Included are strategies for dealing with test anxiety, quitting smoking, developing responsible drinking habits, planning a personal exercise program, phasing in a healthier diet, and many other practical plans for change.

Three quick-reference appendixes provide students with resources they can keep and use for years to come:

- Appendix A, "Nutritional Content of Popular Items from Fast-Food Restaurants," provides information on commonly ordered menu items.

- Appendix B, "Self-Care Guide for Common Medical Problems," provides information to help students manage common symptoms, including fever, sore throat, indigestion, headache, and cuts and scrapes.

- Appendix C, "Resources for Self-Care," lists books, information centers, hotlines, and electronic sources of wellness-related materials. Guidelines for using the Internet—how to perform searches, how to evaluate online information, and how to use newsgroups, mailing lists, and chat rooms—are also provided.

"First Aid at a Glance" from the Red Cross appears inside the back cover of the text, providing information that can save lives.

LEARNING AIDS

Although all the features of *Core Concepts in Health* are designed to facilitate learning, several specific learning aids have also been incorporated in the text. Learning objectives labeled **Looking Ahead** appear on the opening page of each chapter, identifying major concepts and helping to guide students in their reading and review of the text. Important terms appear in boldface type in the text and are defined in a **running glossary,** helping students handle a large and complex new vocabulary. A pronunciation guide to all the key terms appears on the student CD-ROM.

Chapter summaries offer students a concise review and a way to make sure they have grasped the most important concepts in the chapter. Also found at the end of every chapter are **Selected Bibliographies** and sections called For More Information. **For More Information** sections contain annotated lists of books, newsletters, hotlines, organizations, and Web sites that students can use to extend and broaden their knowledge or pursue subjects of interest to them. A complete **Index** at the end of the book includes references to glossary terms in boldface type.

TEACHING TOOLS

Available to qualified adopters of the ninth edition of *Core Concepts in Health* is a comprehensive package of supplementary materials that enhance teaching and learning. Included in the package are the following items:

- Instructor's Resource Binder
- Transparency Acetates
- Instructor's CD-ROM
- Students on Health Custom Video and McGraw-Hill Health and Wellness Custom Video
- Computerized Test Bank
- *Core Concepts in Health* Online Learning Center
- *Core Concepts Interactive* Student CD-ROM
- Wellness Worksheets
- *Mayfield's Quick View Guide to the Internet for Students of Health, Physical Education, and Exercise Science, Version 2.0*
- Nutrition and Weight Management Journal
- Additional videos, software, and other multimedia
- PageOut, PowerWeb, and other distance learning and online instruction options

The **Instructor's Resource Binder,** contains a variety of helpful teaching materials in an easy-to-use form.

- The **Instructor's Resource Guide,** prepared for the ninth edition by Cathy Kennedy, Colorado State University, includes learning objectives, extended chapter outlines, classroom activities, Internet resources, selected Healthy People 2010 objectives, and health crossword puzzles.

- **Transparency masters and handouts**—157 in all—are provided as additional lecture resources. The transparency masters include tables, graphs, and key points from the text; illustrations of many body systems are also provided.

- The **examination questions** have been completely revised and updated for the ninth edition by Kathy McGinnis, San Diego City College. The test bank contains nearly 3000 multiple choice and true-false questions. The answer key lists the page number in the text where each answer is found.

- A complete set of **Wellness Worksheets,** a student learning aid described below, is also included in the Instructor's Resource Binder.

Expanded for the ninth edition, the set of 80 **transparency acetates** provides material suitable for lecture and discussion. The acetates do not duplicate the transparency masters in the Instructor's Resource Binder, and many of them are from sources other than the text.

The **Instructor's CD-ROM,** expanded for the ninth edition, contains annotated PowerPoint® lecture outlines, an image set, transparency acetates, and an electronic version of the Instructor's Resource Guide, including the transparency masters and handouts. Also available on the CD-ROM is a new **Integrated Teaching Solutions** tool, which allows the user to create customized chapter lecture outlines keyed to all the supplements available with the text.

Two **customized videos** are available with the ninth edition. The **McGraw-Hill Health and Wellness Custom Video,** new for the ninth edition, includes brief video segments with additional information on health topics such as nutrition, exercise, and heart disease. **Students on Health** was filmed exclusively for *Core Concepts* with students at college campuses across the country. The 8–10-minute segments focus on key wellness concerns and are designed to stimulate critical thinking and class discussion. The accompanying Instructor's Video Guide provides summaries of each segment and discussion questions.

A **computerized test bank** is available to qualified adopters. Diploma, developed by Brownstone Research Group, allows instructors to design tests using the examination questions included with *Core Concepts in Health* and/or incorporating their own questions. It is available in both Windows and Macintosh formats.

Updated and expanded for the ninth edition, the *Core Concepts in Health* **Online Learning Center** includes a variety of tools for both instructors and students. Password-protected instructor's resources include links to professional resources and downloadable versions of the PowerPoint slides, acetates, image set, wellness worksheets, and Instructor's Resource Guide. The Integrated Teaching Solutions tool is also available online. Student resources include a wide variety of elements keyed to each chapter in the text: chapter outlines and learning objectives, interactive study guide questions, glossary flashcards with a pronunciation guide, interactive crossword puzzles, Journal Entry exercises, Internet activities that guide students in locating and evaluating health-related Web sites, In the News and Vital Statistics Web links, and extensive sets of health and wellness Web links. In addition, the Online Learning Center

includes a Behavior Change Workbook and information on career opportunities in health. All of the resources in the Online Learning Center can also be used with PageOut, Web CT, Blackboard, PowerWeb, and other options for online courses.

The *Core Concepts Interactive* **Student CD-ROM** is also expanded and updated for the ninth edition. Packaged with each copy of the text, this interactive CD-ROM provides many helpful learning aids and wellness tools. Resources include chapter objectives and summaries, interactive quizzes and wellness self-assessments, self-guided tutorials on special topics, a pronunciation guide to key terms, an electronic fitness log, and a guide to using the Internet.

The more than 100 **Wellness Worksheets** available with the ninth edition help students become more involved in their own wellness and better prepared to implement successful behavior change. The worksheets include assessment tools, Internet activities, and knowledge-based reviews of key concepts. They are available shrink-wrapped with the text in an easy-to-use pad.

Other practical items for the student can also be shrink-wrapped with the text:

- The **Nutrition and Weight Management Journal** guides students in assessing their current diet and making appropriate changes.

- Available in a new edition is *Mayfield's Quick View Guide to the Internet for Students of Health, Physical Education, and Exercise Science, Version 2.0,* by Jennifer Campbell Koella and Michael Keene, University of Tennessee, Knoxville. In addition to listing useful Web links, it provides step-by-step instructions on how to access the Internet; how to find, evaluate, and use online information about wellness; and many other topics.

Additional videos, software, and other multimedia are available to qualified adopters. The video library includes tapes on topics such as stress, AIDS, violence, nutrition, alcohol use, and many more. DINE Healthy software provides an easy way for students to evaluate their diets and track the energy expenditure of their activities. HealthQuest software contains interactive assessments, behavior change activities, current articles, video clips, Web links, and many other resources.

McGraw-Hill also offers a wide variety of **digital solutions** to help instructors put courses online. **PageOut** is a simple program that enables instructors to easily develop Web sites for their courses. PageOut can be used to create a course home page, an instructor home page, an interactive syllabus that can be linked to elements in the Online Learning Center, Web links, online discussion areas, an online grade book, and much more. The Online Learning Center can also be customized to work with products like WebCT and Blackboard. **PowerWeb** is a student Internet resource that includes articles from the Annual Editions series, weekly updates with assessments, informative and timely world news, Web links, research and study tools, and interactive exercises. For more information on these and other digital solutions offered by McGraw-Hill, contact your local representative or visit our Web site (http://www.mhhe.com/solutions).

A NOTE OF THANKS

The efforts of innumerable people have gone into producing this ninth edition of *Core Concepts in Health*. The book has benefited immensely from their thoughtful commentaries, expert knowledge and opinions, and many helpful suggestions. We are deeply grateful for their participation in the project.

Academic Contributors

David Antonuccio, Ph.D., Department of Psychiatry and Behavioral Sciences, University of Nevada School of Medicine
Toward a Tobacco-Free Society

Roger Baxter, M.D., Internist and Infectious Disease Specialist, Kaiser Permanente Medical Center, Oakland, California; Associate Clinical Professor, University of California, San Francisco
Immunity and Infection

Andrea T. Borchers, Ph.D., Carl L. Keen, Ph.D., and M. Eric Gershwin, M.D., Division of Rheumatology, Allergy, and Clinical Immunology, University of California at Davis School of Medicine
Health Care: Conventional and Complementary Medicine

Virginia Brooke, Ph.D., University of Texas Medical Branch at Galveston
Aging: A Vital Process

Boyce Burge, Ph.D., *Institute for Human Nutrition Cancer*

Theodore C. Dumas, Ph.D., Stanford University
Stress: The Constant Challenge

Thomas Fahey, Ed.D., California State University, Chico
Exercise for Health and Fitness

Michael R. Hoadley, Ph.D., University of South Dakota
Personal Safety: Protecting Yourself from Unintentional Injuries and Violence

Paul M. Insel, Ph.D., Stanford University
Taking Charge of Your Health

Shepard A. Insel, Ed.D.
Intimate Relationships and Commmunication

Nancy Kemp, M.D.
Abortion; The Responsible Use of Alcohol; Cardiovascular Health; Sexually Transmitted Diseases

Charles Ksir, Ph.D., University of Wyoming
The Use and Abuse of Psychoactive Drugs

Jessica McAlpine, M.D., Department of Gynecology and Obstetrics, Stanford University Medical Center
Pregnancy and Childbirth

Joyce D. Nash, Ph.D., Clinical Psychologist in private practice (San Francisco and Palo Alto)
Weight Management

David Quadagno, Ph.D., Florida State University
Sex and Your Body

Walton T. Roth, M.D., Stanford University
Psychological Health

James H. Rothenberger, M.P.H., and Lynn C. Faust, M.P.H., University of Minnesota
Environmental Health

David S. Sobel, M.D., M.P.H., Director of Patient Education and Health Promotion, Kaiser Permanente Northern California
Self-Care: Skills for the Health Care Consumer

Albert Lee Strickland and Lynne Ann DeSpelder, Cabrillo College
Dying and Death

Mae V. Tinklenberg, R.N., N.P., M.S.
Contraception

R. Elaine Turner, Ph.D., R.D., University of Florida
Nutrition Basics

Academic Advisers and Reviewers

Rick Barnes, East Carolina University

Lois Beach, State University of New York at Plattsburgh

M. Betsy Bergen, Kansas State University

Penny J. Brynildson, Bethel College

Sandra Minor Bulmer, Southern Connecticut State University

Patricia A. Cost, Weber State University

Claire B. Elkins, Saddleback Community College

Natalie Erlich, Oklahoma State University

Sally J. Ford, Pima Community College

Marianne Frauenknecht, Western Michigan University

Kathy French, University of Central Arkansas

Daniel S. Gerber, University of Massachusetts at Amherst

Roger B. Imbrogno, Merced College

Richard Madson, Palm Beach Community College

Bobby C. Martin, Hampton University

La Tonya D. Mouzon, Southern Illinois University at Carbondale

Miguel A. Pérez, California State University Fresno

Kerry J. Redican, Virginia Polytechnical Institute and State University

Connie Reynolds, Utah Valley State

Jan S. Richter, University of Central Oklahoma

Thea Siria Spatz, University of Arkansas at Little Rock

Ladona Tornabene, University of South Dakota

Beatrice G. Wallace, Southside Virginia Community College

Helen Welle-Graf, Georgia Southern University

Scott D. Winnail, University of Wyoming

Kristin Jacoby Yusko, University of Maryland College Park

Finally, we would like to thank the staff at Mayfield Publishing Company, particularly the members of the *Core Concepts* book team. First, we are indebted to Kirstan Price for her dedication and her extraordinary creative energies, which have helped to make this book such a success.

Thanks also go to Reid Hester, Sponsoring Editor; Kate Engelberg, Susan Shook Malloy, Star MacKenzie, and Elisa Adams, Developmental Editors; Jennifer Hardy, Developmental Editing Assistant; Kara Indelli, Editorial Assistant; Linda Toy, Production Director; Melissa Williams, Senior Production Editor; Jeanne M. Schreiber, Art Director; Violeta Diaz, Design Manager; Robin Mouat, Art Editor; Marty Granahan, Permissions Editor; Brian Pecko, Photo Editor; Randy Hurst, Manufacturing Manager; Matthew Ballantine, Production Assistant; Kristin Davis, Marketing Manager; and Jay Bauer, Marketing Communications Specialist. To all we express our deep appreciation.

Paul M. Insel
Walton T. Roth

Brief Contents

Contents

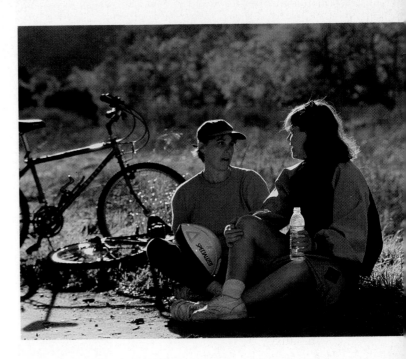

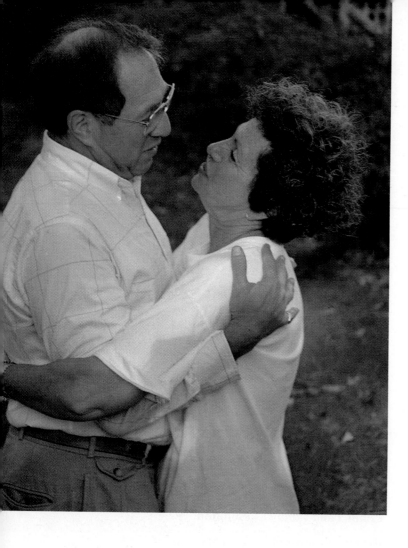

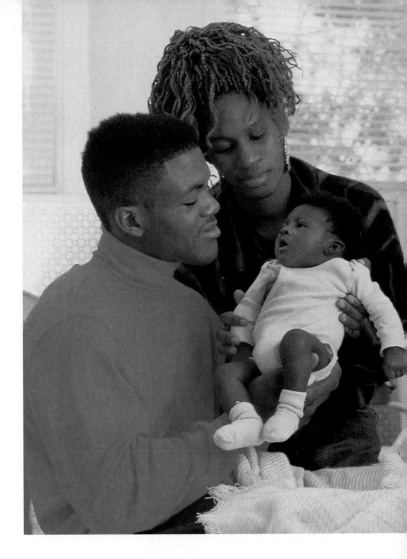

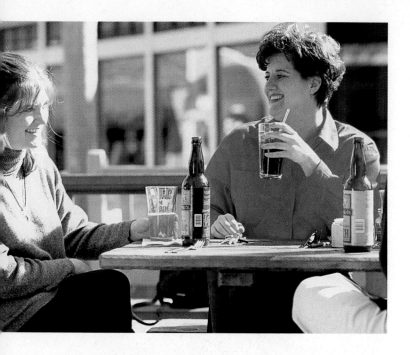

PART FOUR
Getting Fit

Chapter 12
NUTRITION BASICS   313

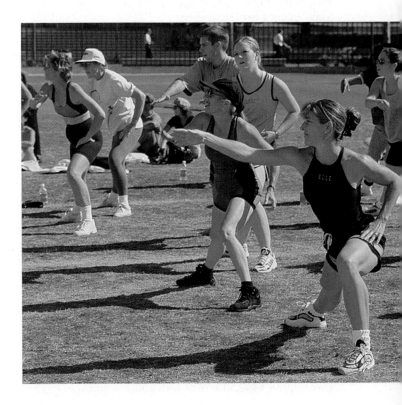

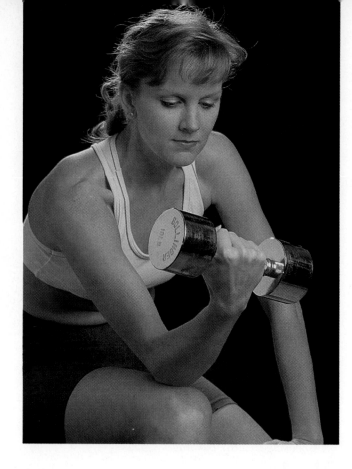

Chapter 14

WEIGHT MANAGEMENT 393

Chapter 13

EXERCISE FOR HEALTH AND FITNESS 361

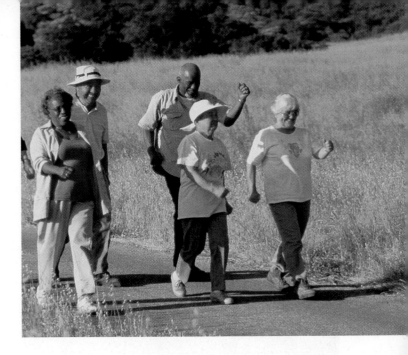

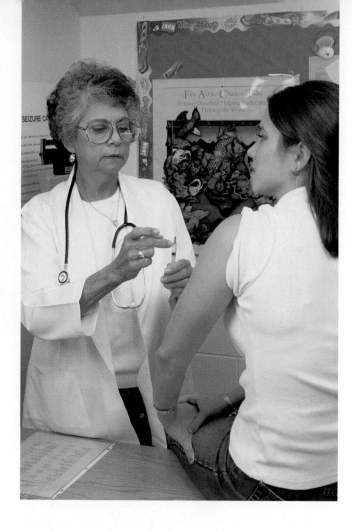

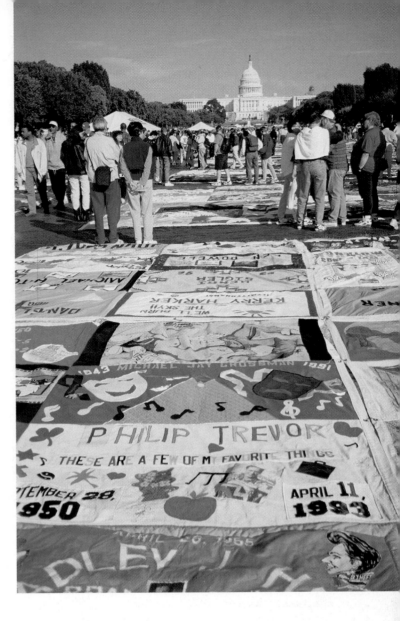

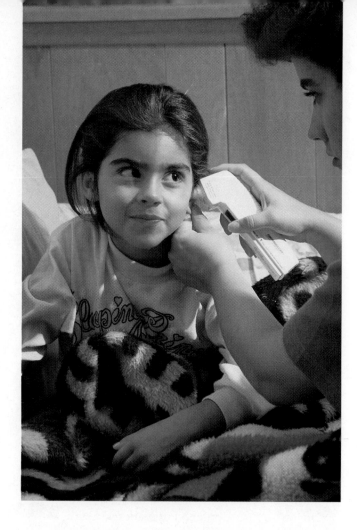

PART SEVEN
Making Choices in Health Care

Chapter 21
HEALTH CARE: CONVENTIONAL AND
COMPLEMENTARY MEDICINE   601

Chapter 22
SELF-CARE: SKILLS FOR THE HEALTH CARE
CONSUMER   625

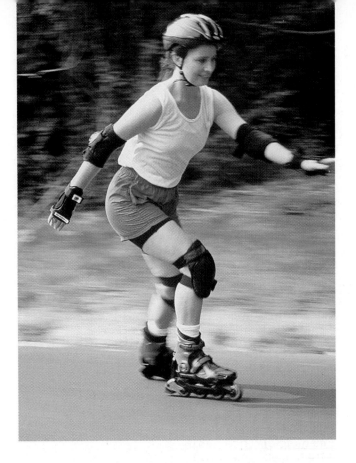

BOXES

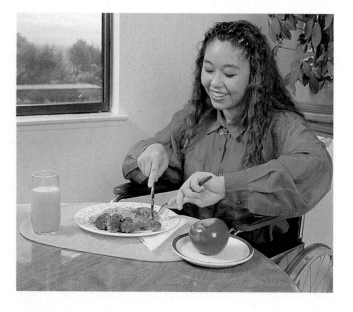

Critical Consumer

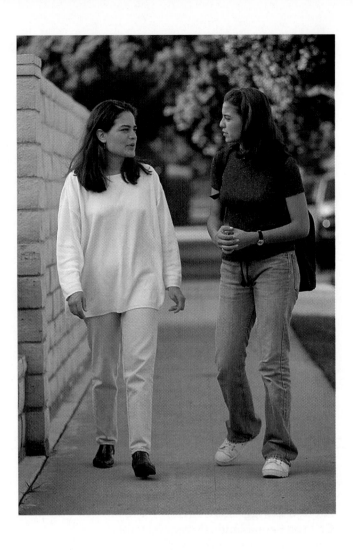

Dimensions of Diversity

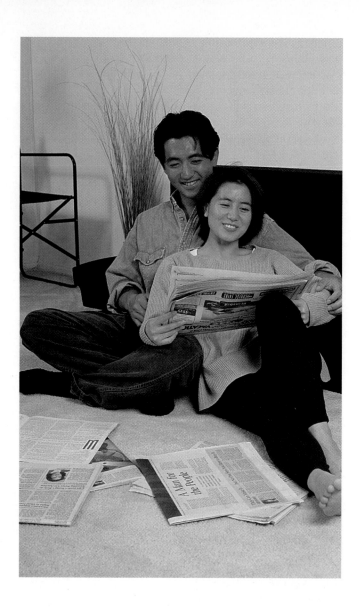

TOPICS OF SPECIAL CONCERN TO WOMEN

TOPICS OF SPECIAL CONCERN TO MEN

Note: The health issues and conditions listed here include those that disproportionately influence or affect women or men, For more information, See the index under gender, women, men, and any of the special topics listed here.

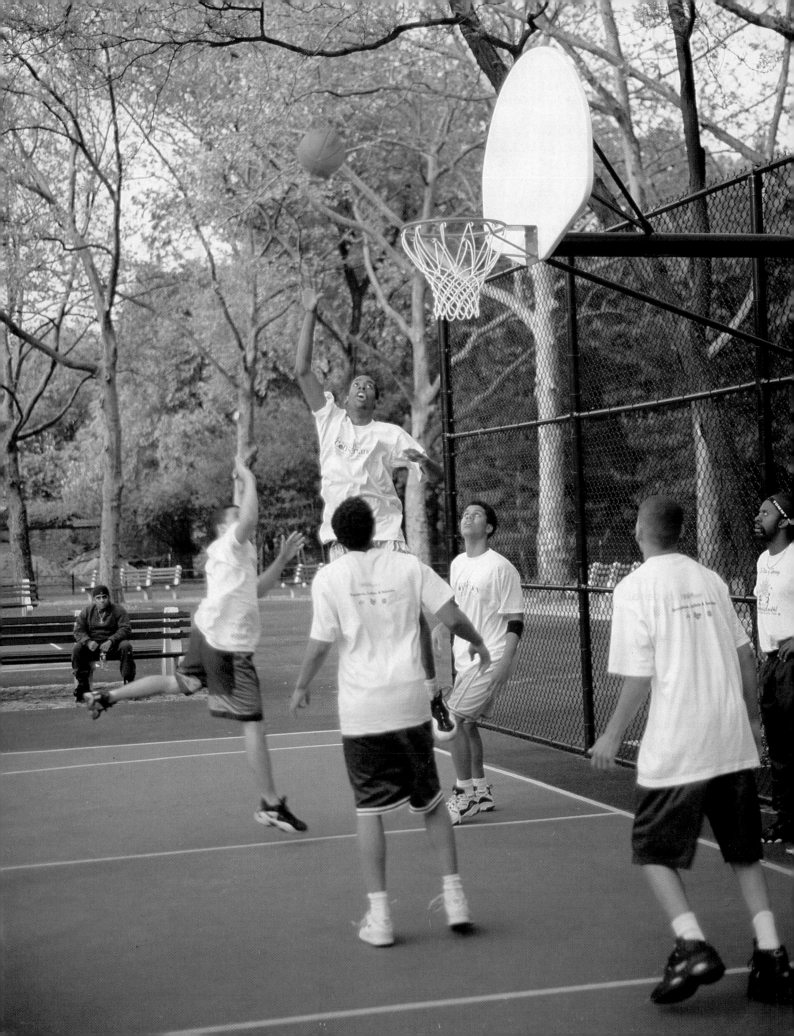

After reading this chapter, you should be able to

- Describe the six dimensions of wellness and a wellness lifestyle

- Identify major goals of the national Healthy People initiative

- Explain the importance of personal decision making and behavior change in achieving a wellness lifestyle

- Describe the steps in creating a behavior management plan to change a health-related behavior

- Describe the influence of gender, ethnicity, income, and disability on health

- Discuss the available sources of health information and how to think critically about them

Taking Charge of Your Health

1

TEST YOUR KNOWLEDGE

1. In 1900, infectious diseases such as pneumonia and tuberculosis were responsible for more than one-third of all deaths in the United States.
   True or false?

2. The leading cause of death among Americans age 15–25 years is unintentional injuries (accidents).
   True or false?

3. Which of the following lifestyle factors is the leading preventable cause of death for Americans?
   a. alcohol abuse
   b. cigarette smoking
   c. poor dietary habits and lack of exercise

4. If you have a family history of heart disease or cancer, there's not much you can do to lower your risk of getting these diseases.
   True or false?

5. More than two-thirds of all college students make which of the following positive lifestyle choices?
   a. using safety belts
   b. not drinking and driving
   c. using contraception (if sexually active)
   d. eating two or fewer high-fat foods per day
   e. not using tobacco

A first-year college student resolves to meet the challenge of making new friends. A long-sedentary senior starts riding her bike to school every day instead of taking the bus. A busy graduate student volunteers to plant trees in a blighted inner-city neighborhood. What do these people have in common? Each is striving for optimal health and well-being. Not satisfied to be merely free of major illness, these individuals want more. They want to live life actively, energetically, and fully, in a state of optimal personal, interpersonal, and environmental well-being. They have taken charge of their health and are on the path to wellness.

WELLNESS: THE NEW HEALTH GOAL

Wellness is an expanded idea of health. Many people think of health as being just the absence of physical disease. But wellness transcends this concept of health—for example, when individuals with serious illnesses or disabilities rise above their physical or mental limitations to live rich, meaningful, vital lives. Some aspects of health are determined by your genes, your age, and other factors that may be beyond your control. But true wellness is largely determined by the decisions you make about how to live your life. In this book, we will use the terms *health* and *wellness* interchangeably to mean the ability to live life fully—with vitality and meaning.

The Dimensions of Wellness

No matter what your age or health status, you can optimize your health in each of the following six interrelated dimensions. Wellness in any dimension is not a static goal but a dynamic process of change and growth (Figure 1-1).

Physical Wellness Optimal physical health requires eating well, exercising, avoiding harmful habits, making responsible decisions about sex, learning about and recognizing the symptoms of disease, getting regular medical and dental checkups, and taking steps to prevent injuries at home, on the road, and on the job. The habits you develop and the decisions you make today will largely determine not only how many years you will live, but also the quality of your life during those years.

Emotional Wellness Optimism, trust, self-esteem, self-acceptance, self-confidence, self-control, satisfying relationships, and an ability to share feelings are just some of the qualities and aspects of emotional wellness. Emotional health is a dynamic state that fluctuates with your physical, intellectual, spiritual, interpersonal and social, and environmental health. Maintaining emotional wellness requires monitoring and exploring your thoughts and feelings, identifying obstacles to emotional well-being, and finding solutions to emotional problems, with the help of a therapist if necessary.

Intellectual Wellness The hallmarks of intellectual health include an openness to new ideas, a capacity to question and think critically, and the motivation to master new skills, as well as a sense of humor, creativity, and curiosity. An active mind is essential to overall wellness, for learning about, evaluating, and storing health-related information. Your mind detects problems, finds solutions, and directs behavior. People who enjoy intellectual wellness never stop learning. They relish new experiences and challenges and actively seek them out.

Spiritual Wellness To enjoy spiritual health is to possess a set of guiding beliefs, principles, or values that give meaning and purpose to your life, especially during difficult times. Spiritual wellness involves the capacity for love, compassion, forgiveness, altruism, joy, and fulfillment. It is an antidote to cynicism, anger, fear, anxiety, self-absorption, and pessimism. Spirituality transcends

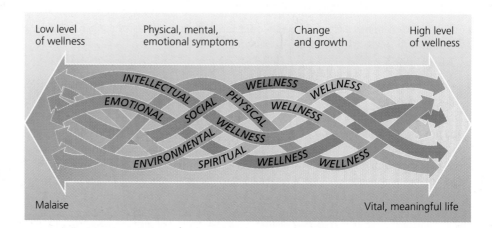

Figure 1-1 The wellness continuum. Wellness is composed of six interrelated dimensions, all of which must be developed in order to achieve overall wellness.

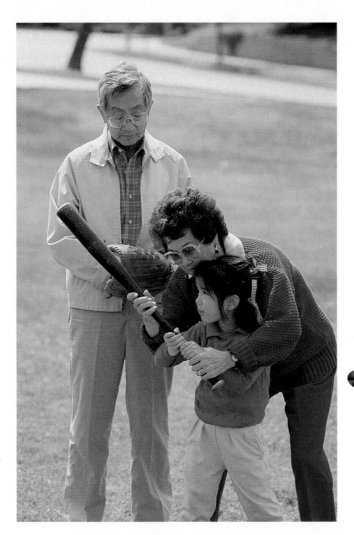

With wellness come health and vitality throughout the life span.

from the safety of the food supply to the degree of violence in a society. Other examples of environmental threats to health are ultraviolet radiation in sunlight, air and water pollution, lead in old house paint, and secondhand tobacco smoke in indoor air. Wellness requires learning about and protecting yourself against such hazards—and doing what you can to reduce or eliminate them, either on your own or with others.

The six dimensions of wellness interact continuously, influencing and being influenced by one another. Making a change in one dimension often affects some or all of the others. For example, regular exercise (developing the physical dimension of wellness) can increase feelings of well-being and self-esteem (emotional wellness), which in turn can increase feelings of confidence in social interactions and your achievements at work or school (interpersonal and social wellness). Maintaining good health is a dynamic process, and increasing your level of wellness in one area of life often influences many others (see the box "Ten Warning Signs of Wellness").

New Opportunities, New Responsibilities

Wellness is a relatively recent concept. A century ago, people considered themselves lucky just to survive to adulthood. A child born in 1900, for example, could expect to live only about 47 years. Many people died as a result of common **infectious diseases** and poor environmental conditions (unrefrigerated food, poor sanitation, air and water pollution). However, over the past 100 years, the average life span has nearly doubled, thanks largely to the development of vaccines and antibiotics to prevent and fight infectious diseases and to public health campaigns to improve environmental conditions (Figure 1-2).

But a different set of diseases has emerged as our major health threat, and heart disease, cancer, and stroke are now the top three causes of death in the United States (Table 1-1). Treating these and other **chronic diseases** has proved enormously expensive and extremely difficult. It has become clear that the best treatment for these diseases is prevention—people having a greater awareness about their own health and about taking care of their bodies.

the individual and can be a common bond among people. Organized religions help many people develop spiritual health. Many others find meaning and purpose in their lives on their own—through nature, art, meditation, political action, or good works.

Interpersonal and Social Wellness Satisfying relationships are basic to both physical and emotional health. We need to have mutually loving, supportive people in our lives. Developing interpersonal wellness means learning good communication skills, developing the capacity for intimacy, and cultivating a support network of caring friends and/or family members. Social wellness requires participating in and contributing to your community, country, and world.

Environmental or Planetary Wellness Increasingly, personal health depends on the health of the planet—

wellness Optimal health and vitality, encompassing physical, emotional, intellectual, spiritual, interpersonal, social, and environmental well-being.

infectious disease A disease that is communicable from one person to another; caused by invading microorganisms such as bacteria and viruses.

√**chronic disease** A disease that develops and continues over a long period of time; usually caused by a variety of factors, including lifestyle factors.

Terms

1. The persistent presence of a support network
2. Chronic positive expectations; the tendency to frame events in a constructive light
3. Episodic outbreaks of joyful, happy experiences
4. A sense of spiritual involvement
5. A tendency to adapt to changing conditions
6. Rapid response and recovery of stress response systems to repeated challenges

7. An increased appetite for physical activity
8. A tendency to identify and communicate feelings
9. Repeated episodes of gratitude and generosity
10. A persistent sense of humor

SOURCE: Ten warning signs of good health. 1996. *Mind/Body Health Newsletter* 5(1). Reprinted by permission.

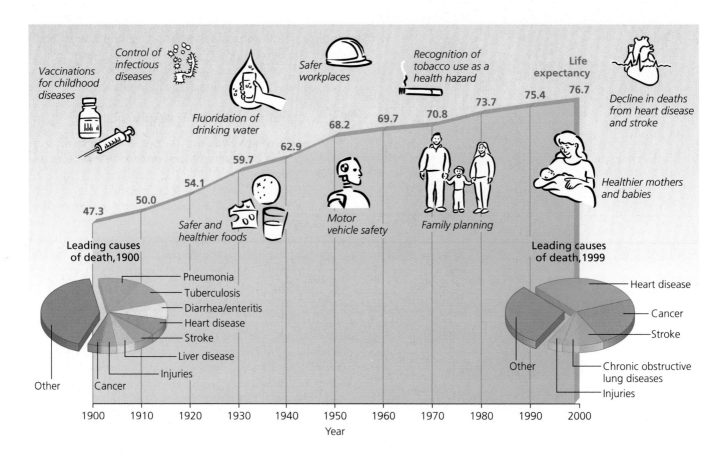

Figure 1-2   Public health achievements of the twentieth century.   During the twentieth century, public health achievements greatly improved the quality of life for Americans, and life expectancy rose from 47 to 77. A dramatic shift in the leading causes of death also occurred, with deaths from infectious diseases declining from over 33% of all deaths to just 2.2%. Heart disease, cancer, and stroke are now responsible for over 50% of all deaths among Americans.   SOURCES: National Center for Health Statistics. 2000. *Health, United States, 2000, with Adolescent Health Chartbook.* Hyattsville, Md.: National Center for Health Statistics. Centers for Disease Control and Prevention. 1999. Ten great public health achievements—United States, 1900–1999. *Morbidity and Mortality Weekly Report* 48(50): 1141. National Center for Health Statistics. 2001. United States life tables, 1998. *National Vital Statistics Reports* 48(18): 29–34.

Table 1-1   Leading Causes of Death in the United States

Rank	Cause of Death	Number of Deaths	Percent of Total Deaths	Female/Male Ratio*	Lifestyle Factors
1	Heart disease	724,859	31.0	51/49	D I S A
2	Cancer	541,532	23.2	48/52	D I S A
3	Stroke	158,448	6.8	61/39	D I S
4	Chronic obstructive lung diseases	112,584	4.8	49/51	S
5	Unintentional injuries	97,835	4.2	36/64	S A
	Motor-vehicle-related	(43,501)	(1.9)	33/67	
	All others	(54,334)	(2.3)	37/63	
6	Pneumonia and influenza	91,871	3.9	55/45	S
7	Diabetes mellitus	64,751	2.8	54/46	D I S
8	Suicide	30,575	1.3	20/80	A
9	Kidney diseases	26,182	1.1	52/48	D
10	Chronic liver disease and cirrhosis	25,192	1.1	35/65	A
	All causes	2,337,256			

Key: D Cause of death in which diet plays a part.   I Cause of death in which an inactive lifestyle plays a part.

  S Cause of death in which smoking plays a part.   A Cause of death in which excessive alcohol consumption plays a part.

*Ratio of females to males who died of each cause. For example, an equal number of women and men died of heart disease, but only about half as many women as men died of motor-vehicle-related injuries.

SOURCE: National Center for Health Statistics. 2000. Deaths: Final data for 1998. *National Vital Statistics Reports* 48(11).

The good news is that people do have some control over whether they develop heart disease, cancer, and other chronic diseases. People make choices every day that either increase or decrease their risks for these diseases—lifestyle choices involving such behaviors as exercise, diet, smoking, and drinking. When researchers look at the lifestyle factors that contribute to death in the United States, it becomes clear that individuals can profoundly influence their own health risks (see the last column in Table 1-1). Smoking is the leading preventable cause of death among Americans, responsible for over 400,000 deaths each year; it is followed by poor diet and inactivity (over 300,000 deaths per year) and alcohol use (over 100,000 deaths per year). From these figures, it is clear that wellness cannot be prescribed; physicians and other health care professionals can provide information, advice, and encouragement—but the rest is up to each of us.

National Wellness Goals: The Healthy People Initiative

You may think of health and wellness as personal concerns, goals that you strive for on your own for your own benefit. But the U.S. government also has a vital interest in the health of all Americans. A healthy population is the nation's greatest resource, the source of its vitality, creativ-ity, and wealth. Poor health, in contrast, drains the nation's resources and raises national health care costs. As the embodiment of our society's values, the federal government also has a humane interest in people's health.

The U.S. government's national Healthy People initiative seeks to prevent unnecessary disease and disability and to achieve a better quality of life for all Americans. Healthy People reports, published first in 1980 and revised every decade, set national health goals based on 10-year agendas. Each report includes both broad goals and specific targets in many different areas of wellness. The latest report, *Healthy People 2010,* proposes two broad national goals:

- *Increase quality and years of healthy life.* The life expectancy of Americans has increased significantly in the past century; however, people can expect poor health to limit their activities and cause distress during the last 15% of their lives (Figure 1-3). Health-related quality of life reflects a personal sense of physical and mental health and the ability to react to factors in the physical and social environments. It calls for a full range of functional capacity to enable people to work, play, and maintain satisfying relationships. This national goal stresses the importance of health status and quality of life, not just longevity.

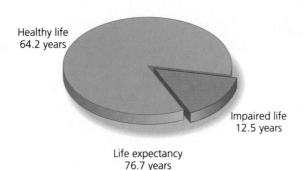

Healthy life
64.2 years

Impaired life
12.5 years

Life expectancy
76.7 years

WW. VITAL STATISTICS

Figure 1-3 Quantity of life versus quality of life. Years of healthy life as a proportion of life expectancy in the U.S. population. SOURCES: U.S. Department of Health and Human Services. 2000. *Healthy People 2010.* 2nd ed. Washington, D.C.: DHHS. National Center for Health Statistics. 2000. Deaths: Final data for 1998. *National Vital Statistics Reports* 48(11).

• *Eliminate health disparities among Americans.* Many health problems today disproportionately affect certain American populations—for example, ethnic minorities, people of low socioeconomic status or educational attainment, and people with disabilities. *Healthy People 2010* calls for eliminating disparities in health status, health risks, and use of preventive services among all population groups within the next decade.

Giving substance to these broad goals are hundreds of specific objectives—measurable targets for the year 2010—in many different focus areas that relate to wellness, including fitness, nutrition, safety, substance abuse, health care, and chronic and infectious diseases. Specific Healthy People targets serve as the basis for national monitoring and tracking of the health status and health risks of Americans and our use of health services. They encompass individual actions as well as larger-scale changes in environment and medical services. Examples of health promotion objectives from *Healthy People 2010,* as well as estimates of our progress toward these targets, appear in Table 1-2.

Healthy People 2010 reflects the changing attitude of Americans: an emerging sense of personal responsibility as the key to good health. This new perspective is seen in our concern about smoking and drug abuse, for example; in our emphasis on physical and emotional fitness; in our interest in good nutrition; and in our concern about the environment. The primary concerns of *Healthy People 2010* are the principal topics covered in this book. In many ways, personal wellness goals are not different from the national aspirations.

WW. Health Issues for Diverse Populations

Americans are a diverse people. Our ancestry is European, African, Asian, Pacific Islander, Latin American, and Native American. We live in cities, suburbs, and rural areas and work at every imaginable occupation. In no other country in the world do so many diverse people live and work together every day. And in no other country is the understanding and tolerance of differences so much a part of the political and cultural ideal. We are at heart a nation of diversity, and, though we often fall short of our goal, we strive for justice and equality among all.

When it comes to health, most differences among people are insignificant; most health issues concern us all equally. We all need to eat well, exercise, manage stress, and cultivate satisfying personal relationships. We need to know how to protect ourselves from heart disease, cancer, sexually transmitted diseases, and injuries. We need to know how to use the health care system.

But some of our differences, as individuals and as members of groups, do have important implications for health. Some of us, for example, have a genetic predisposition for developing certain health problems, such as high cholesterol. Some of us have grown up eating foods that raise our risk of heart disease or obesity. Some of us live in an environment that increases the chance that we will smoke cigarettes or abuse alcohol. These health-related differences among individuals and groups can be biological—determined genetically—or cultural—acquired as patterns of behavior through daily interactions with our families, communities, and society. Many health conditions are a function of biology and culture combined. A person can have a genetic predisposition for a disease, for example, but won't actually develop the disease itself unless certain lifestyle factors are present, such as stress or a poor diet.

When we talk about health issues for diverse populations, we face two related dangers. The first is the danger of stereotyping, of talking about people as groups rather than as individuals. It's certainly true that every person is an individual with a unique genetic endowment and unique life experiences. But many of these influences are shared with others of similar genetic and cultural background. Statements about these group similarities can be useful; for example, they can alert people to areas that may be of special concern for them and their families.

The second danger is that of overgeneralizing, of ignoring the extensive biological and cultural diversity that exists among peoples who are grouped together. Groups labeled Latino or Hispanic, for example, include Mexican Americans, Puerto Ricans, people from South and Central America, and other Spanish-speaking peoples. Similarly, the population labeled American Indian includes hundreds of recognized tribal nations, each with its own genetic and cultural heritage. It's important to keep these considerations in mind whenever you read about culturally diverse populations.

Health-related differences among groups can be identified and described in the context of several different

Table 1-2   Selected *Healthy People 2010* Objectives

Objective	Estimate of Current Status (%)	Goal (%)
Increase the proportion of people age 18 and older who engage regularly, preferably daily, in moderate physical activity for at least 30 minutes per day.	15	30
Increase the proportion of people age 2 and older who consume at least three daily servings of vegetables, with at least one-third being dark-green or orange vegetables.	3	50
Increase the prevalence of healthy weight among all people age 20 and older.	42	60
Reduce the proportion of adults 18 and older who use cigarettes.	24	12
Reduce the proportion of college students reporting binge drinking during the past 2 weeks.	39	20
Increase the proportion of sexually active persons who use condoms.	23	50
Increase the proportion of adults who take protective measures to reduce the risk of skin cancer (sunscreens, sun-protective clothing, and so on).	47	75
Increase the use of safety belts by motor vehicle occupants.	69	92
Increase the number of residences with a functioning smoke alarm on every floor.	87	100
Increase the proportion of persons with health insurance.	83	100

SOURCE: U.S. Department of Health and Human Services. 2000. *Healthy People 2010*. 2nd ed. Washington, D.C.: DHHS.

dimensions. Those highlighted in *Healthy People 2010* are gender, ethnicity, income and education, disability, geographic location, and sexual orientation.

Gender   Men and women have different life expectancies, different reproductive concerns, and different incidences of many diseases, including heart disease, cancer, stroke, and cirrhosis of the liver. Men are more likely to develop heart disease in middle age. They have higher rates of deaths from injuries, suicide, homicide, and HIV/AIDS. Women are more affected by issues involving contraception and reproductive choices. They are at greater risk for Alzheimer's disease and for major depression. They live longer than men, and they are more likely to be poor.

Ethnicity   Some genetic diseases are concentrated in certain gene pools, the result of each ethnic group's relatively distinct history. Sickle-cell disease occurs almost exclusively among people of African ancestry. Tay-Sachs disease afflicts people of Eastern European Jewish heritage. Cystic fibrosis is more common among Northern Europeans. In addition to biological differences, many cultural differences occur along ethnic lines. Ethnic groups may vary in their traditional diets; their patterns of family and interpersonal relationships; their attitudes toward tobacco, alcohol, and other drugs; and their health

beliefs and practices. For more on the health concerns of specific ethnic groups, see the box "Health Disparities Among Ethnic Minorities."

Income and Education   Inequalities in income and education underlie many of the health disparities among Americans. Income and education are closely related, and groups with the highest poverty rates and least education have the worst health status. People with low incomes and less education have higher rates of infant mortality, traumatic injury and violent death, and many diseases, including heart disease, diabetes, tuberculosis, and HIV infection. They are more likely to eat poorly, be overweight, smoke, drink, and use drugs. They are exposed to more stressors and have less access to health care services. Poverty and low educational attainment are far more important predictors of poor health than any ethnic factor. However, they are often mixed with other factors in a way that makes it difficult to distinguish what causes what.

Disability   People with disabilities are those who have activity limitations, need assistance, or perceive themselves as having a disability. About one in five people in the United States has some level of disability, and the rate is rising, especially among younger segments of the population. People with disabilities are more likely to be inactive and overweight. They report more days of

Compared to the U.S. population as a whole, American ethnic minorities have higher rates of death and disability from many causes. These disparities result from a complex mix of genetic variations, environmental factors, and health behaviors, and it is often difficult to separate factors related to ethnicity from those associated with socioeconomic status and educational attainment. Achieving the *Healthy People 2010* goal of eliminating all health disparities will require a national effort to identify and address the underlying causes of these disparities, including poverty, lack of access to quality health care, environmental hazards in homes and neighborhoods, and the need for disease prevention programs tailored to specific community needs.

The federal government collects population and health information on five broad ethnic minority groups in American society: blacks, or African Americans; Hispanics, or Latinos; Asian Americans; American Indians and Alaska Natives; and Native Hawaiian and other Pacific Islander Americans. Each group has some specific health concerns.

Blacks, or African Americans

On the 2000 census, about 12.9% of the population reported that they were either African American or African American *and* one or more other races. (Census 2000 allowed respondents to choose more than one race, so percentages reflect both those who reported only one race and those who reported two or more races.) Although African Americans are represented in every socioeconomic group, nearly 30% live below the poverty line. The health status of blacks lags behind that of the total population in several areas, including life expectancy and incidence of chronic and infectious diseases.

The leading causes of death among African Americans are the same as for the general population, but blacks have a higher infant mortality rate and a lower suicide rate. The death rate for HIV infection and homicide among blacks is about six to eight times the rate for whites. African Americans also die from stroke at almost twice the rate of whites. Strokes are related to high blood pressure, which is much more common among blacks than in the general population. Diabetes, another risk factor for cardiovascular disease, is a special concern for black women, especially those who are overweight. African American men face a 60% greater risk of prostate cancer than whites, giving them the highest prostate cancer risk of any group in the world.

Hispanics, or Latinos

About 12.5% of the population reported that they were of Spanish/Hispanic/Latino origin on Census 2000. They are a diverse group, with roots in Mexico, Puerto Rico, Cuba, and South and Central America. Many Latinos are of mixed Spanish and American Indian descent or of mixed Spanish, Indian, and African American descent.

Overall, the leading causes of death for Latinos are the same as those for the general population—heart disease and cancer—but Latinos tend to have lower rates of death from heart disease and cancer than non-Hispanic whites and African Americans. Hispanics have higher rates of death from diabetes, homicide, HIV infection, and infant mortality than non-Hispanic whites, but they have lower rates of death from suicide and lung cancer. Some special concerns are diabetes, gallbladder disease, and obesity, all probably related to American Indian

descent. The birth rate among Latinos is higher than that of the general population, and contraceptive use is relatively low.

Asian Americans

About 4.2% of the population reported that they were Asian American, alone or in combination with one or more other races. They include people who trace their ancestry to countries in the Far East, Southeast Asia, or the Indian subcontinent, including Japan, China, Vietnam, Laos, Cambodia, Korea, the Philippines, India, and Pakistan. Numbering 11.8 million people, they speak more than 30 different languages and represent a similar number of distinct cultures.

Asian Americans have lower death rates overall than does the general population. For example, the death rate for coronary heart disease is 40% lower for Asian American men than for white men. However, health differences exist among these groups. For example, Southeast Asian men have higher rates of lung cancer, smoking, and liver cancer than the rest of the population; Vietnamese American women have higher rates of cervical cancer. Among recent immigrants from Southeast Asia, tuberculosis and hepatitis B are serious health problems. Many Asian Americans lack health insurance, and more than 20% have no regular source of health care.

American Indians and Alaska Natives

American Indians and Alaska Natives, alone or in combination with one or more other races, represent about 1.5% of the population. Most embrace a tribal identity, such as Sioux, Navaho, or Hopi, rather than the identity of American Indian or Alaska Native. American Indians and Alaska Natives have lower rates of death from heart disease, stroke, and cancer than the general population, but they also have high rates of early death. For those under 45, leading causes of death include unintentional injuries, homicide, suicide, and cirrhosis; many of these problems are linked to alcohol abuse. Smoking rates are also high. Diabetes is prevalent, occurring at twice the rate for the general population; in some tribes, more than 20% of all adults are affected, and the Pimas of Arizona have the highest known prevalence of diabetes of any population in the world. American Indians and Alaska Natives have a high teen birth rate and a high infant mortality rate; more than 10% of children and 20% of adults have no regular source of health care.

Native Hawaiian and Other Pacific Islander Americans

Native Hawaiians and other Pacific Islander Americans trace their ancestry to the original peoples of Hawaii, Guam, Samoa, or other Pacific Islands; they represent less than 1% of the total population. Native Hawaiians have a higher overall death rate than whites and higher rates of many diseases, including hypertension, diabetes, lung cancer, stroke, and asthma. The high rate of smoking and high prevalence of overweight and obesity among Native Hawaiians and other Pacific Islander Americans may contribute to these conditions. In addition, many Native Hawaiians and other Pacific Islander Americans lack health insurance and access to regular health care. Among some Pacific Islander populations, the rate of infant mortality is more than double that of the general population.

depression and fewer days of vitality than people without activity limitations. Many people with disabilities also lack access to health care services.

Geographic Location About one in four Americans currently lives in a rural area—a place with fewer than 2500 residents. People living in rural areas are less likely to be physically active, to use safety belts, or to obtain screening tests for preventive health care. They have less access to timely emergency services and much higher rates of injury-related death than people living in urban areas. They are also more likely to lack health insurance.

Sexual Orientation The 1–5% of Americans who identify themselves as homosexual or bisexual make up a diverse community with varied health concerns. Their emotional wellness and personal safety are affected by factors relating to personal, family, and social acceptance of their sexual orientation. Gay, lesbian, and bisexual teens are more likely to engage in risky behaviors such as unsafe sex and drug use; they are also more likely to be depressed and to attempt suicide. HIV/AIDS is a major concern for gay men, and gay men and lesbians may have higher rates of substance abuse, depression, and suicide.

In this book, topics and issues in health that affect different American populations are given special consideration. Look for these discussions in the text and in boxes labeled Dimensions of Diversity. Also discussed in Dimensions of Diversity boxes are health issues and practices in other parts of the world. Explorations beyond the borders of the United States broaden our view, showing us both what we share with people in other societies and how we differ—our common concerns and our divergent solutions. All these discussions are designed to deepen our understanding of the core concepts of wellness in the context of ever-growing diversity.

CHOOSING WELLNESS

Each of us has the option and the responsibility to decide what kind of future we want—one characterized by zestful living or one marked by symptoms and declining energy. The message of this book is that wellness is something everyone can have. Achieving it requires knowledge, self-awareness, motivation, and effort—but the benefits last a lifetime. Optimal health comes mostly from a healthy lifestyle, patterns of behavior that promote and support your health now and as you get older. In the pages that follow, you'll find current information and suggestions you can use to build a better lifestyle. You'll also find tools for assessing yourself, for improving your communication skills, and for planning and carrying out specific behavior changes. You can use this book as a guide for taking charge of your health and improving the quality of your life.

Factors That Influence Wellness

Scientific research is continuously revealing new connections between our habits and emotions and the level of health we enjoy. For example, heart disease, the nation's number one killer, is associated with cigarette smoking, high levels of stress, habitually hostile and suspicious attitudes toward people and the world, a diet high in fat and low in fiber, and a sedentary way of life. Other habits are beneficial. Regular exercise, for example, can help prevent heart disease, high blood pressure, diabetes, osteoporosis, and depression and may reduce the risk of colon cancer, stroke, and back injury. A balanced and varied diet provides the energy and nutrients we need to live a vital life and also helps prevent many chronic diseases. As we learn more about how our actions affect our bodies and minds, we can make informed choices for a healthier life.

Of course, behavior isn't the only factor involved in wellness. Our heredity, the environment we live in, and whether we have access to adequate health care are other important influences. These factors, which vary for both individuals and groups, can interact in ways that produce either health or disease. For example, a sedentary lifestyle combined with a genetic predisposition for diabetes can greatly increase a person's risk of developing the disease. If this person also lacks adequate health care, he or she is much more likely to suffer dangerous complications from diabetes and have a lower quality of life.

But in many cases, behavior can tip the balance toward good health, even when heredity or environment is a negative factor. For example, breast cancer can run in families, but it also may be associated with being overweight and inactive. A woman with a family history of breast cancer is less likely to develop and die from the disease if she controls her weight, exercises regularly, performs breast self-exams, and has regular mammograms.

Similarly, a young man with a family history of obesity can maintain a normal weight by being careful to balance calorie intake against activities that burn calories. If your life is highly stressful, you can lessen the chances of heart disease and stroke by learning ways to manage and cope with stress. If you live in an area with severe air pollution, you can reduce the risk of lung disease by not smoking. You can also take an active role in improving your environment. Behaviors like these enable you to make a difference in how great an impact heredity and environment will have on your health. (For more about the effects of heredity on health risks, see the box "Deciphering the Human Genome.")

A Wellness Profile

What does it mean to be healthy today? A basic list of important behaviors and habits includes the following:

- Having a sense of responsibility for your own health and taking an active rather than a passive stance toward your life

In June 2000, government and private-sector researchers announced that they had completed a rough draft of the human genome. Their findings pave the way for many potential health benefits but also raise many difficult ethical issues.

Genome Basics

Your genome consists of the complete set of genetic material in your cells—the master blueprint for all cellular structures and activities. The nucleus of each cell contains 23 pairs of chromosomes, which are made up of tightly packed coils of deoxyribonucleic acid (DNA). DNA consists of two long strands wound around each other in a spiral, ladderlike structure referred to as a double helix. The rungs of the ladder are made from pairings of four different nucleotide bases: adenine, thymine, cytosine, and guanine, or A, T, C, and G. When researchers say they have mapped the genome, they mean they have sequenced the entire string of billions of A's, T's, C's, and G's.

A gene is a smaller unit of DNA made up of a specific sequence of hundreds or thousands of nucleotide base pairs. You have two copies of each gene—one inherited from each parent. Each of the estimated 30,000–40,000 genes in your DNA controls the production of a particular protein. Proteins serve both as the structural material for your body and as the regulators of all chemical reactions and metabolic processes. Many diseases are thought to be caused or promoted by an absence or excess of particular proteins. About 3% of the total human genome is made of genes; the function of the other 97%, called "junk" DNA, isn't completely understood.

Further work is needed to transform the draft of the genome into information useful for improving human health. Once the sequence is completed and checked, the next step will be to locate genes and identify the structure and function of the proteins they make. Researchers will also look closely at variations among individuals. Humans differ from one another at the rate of only about one base in every thousand (0.1%). Most of these differences occur in junk DNA and have no effect on health. However, some variations occur at critical spots that cause a gene to make the wrong protein. By sequencing the genomes of many individuals, it should be possible to identify the specific gene variations linked to increased risk for particular diseases.

Vast Promise

Researchers hope to use the deciphered human genome to improve health and quality of life for all people. Some likely developments include the following:

- *Personalized risk assessment:* A study of your genes could replace family history and other indirect clues as a means of determining your risk of particular diseases. Individualized lifestyle and medical screening advice may someday replace blanket public health recommendations.

- *Pharmacogenomics:* Genetic information could help physicians prescribe medications based on individual drug sensitivities and the likelihood that a particular disorder will respond to a particular drug.

- *Gene therapy and other new treatments:* Gene research will help develop new therapies that will directly affect the underlying biological mechanisms—genes and proteins—of serious disorders such as asthma, diabetes, and cancer.

Limitations and Troubling Questions

Despite the many potential benefits of knowledge of the genome, there are limitations to what this information can do for human health. Errors in our genes are responsible for an estimated 3000 to 4000 clearly hereditary conditions, including sickle-cell disease, Huntington's disease, and cystic fibrosis. Altered genes also play a part in heart disease, cancer, stroke, diabetes, and many other common conditions. However, in these more common and complex disorders, genetic alterations serve only to increase an individual's risk. The disease itself results from the interaction of many genes with environmental and behavioral factors. It will be much more difficult to develop tests and therapies for disorders with complex causes.

In addition, access to information about the human genome and the genes of individuals raises many difficult ethical issues. Privacy and discrimination are key concerns. If genetic testing can identify years in advance who will get sick and who will not, employers and health insurance companies could save millions of dollars by not hiring or enrolling people whose genes show them to be at increased risk for disease. This is especially troubling because it is likely that tests for genetic susceptibility to many conditions will be available years, perhaps decades, before any gene-based treatments are developed. Chapter 16 has more information on genetic testing.

Other questions relate to potential uses of tools for altering the genome. Do we have enough information to know how knocking out "bad" genes will affect our species? For example, the gene alteration that causes sickle-cell disease must be present in both copies of the gene for a person to develop the disorder; people with only one copy of the altered gene have an increased resistance to malaria. If the gene for sickle-cell disease were eliminated, would many more people succumb to malaria? What other unknown effects might we cause by tinkering with the genome? In addition, if it becomes easy to change ourselves and our children, will we become less tolerant of people who have such "conditions" as short stature or baldness?

The Role of Behavior and Environmental Factors

Most common disorders result from the complex interaction of many different genes, environmental factors, and lifestyle choices. For example, researchers have identified genes that increase a woman's risk for breast cancer, but these genes explain only a small proportion of cases. Behavior and environment exert a powerful influence on health and the risk of disease. This power can be seen in the 33% increase in the incidence of diabetes that has occurred among Americans since 1990. This huge increase is not due to any sudden change in our genes; it is the result of increasing rates of obesity due to poor dietary choices and lack of physical activity.

It's important not to adopt a position of biological determinism—a belief that your genes inevitably completely control your future health. Genomics research will certainly lead to a better understanding of the underlying causes of disease and to new techniques for diagnosis and treatment. However, your health, both in terms of your lifestyle choices and your use of genetic information, is still in your own hands.

- Learning to manage stress in effective ways
- Maintaining high self-esteem and mentally healthy ways of interacting with other people
- Understanding your sexuality and having satisfying intimate relationships
- Avoiding tobacco and other drugs; using alcohol responsibly, if at all
- Eating well, exercising, and maintaining healthy weight
- Knowing the facts about cardiovascular disease, cancer, infections, sexually transmitted diseases, and injuries and using your knowledge to protect yourself against them
- Understanding the health care system and using it intelligently
- Knowing when to treat your illnesses yourself and when to seek help
- Understanding the natural processes of aging and dying and accepting the limits of human existence
- Understanding how the environment affects your health and taking appropriate action to improve it

Incorporating these behaviors into your daily life may seem like a tall order, and in a sense it is the work of a lifetime. But the habits you establish now are crucial: They tend to set lifelong patterns. Some behaviors do more than set up patterns—they produce permanent changes in your health. If you become addicted to drugs or alcohol at age 20, for example, you may be able to kick the habit, but you will always face the struggle of a recovering addict. If you contract gonorrhea, you may discover later that your reproductive organs were damaged without your realizing it, making you infertile or sterile. If you ruin your knees doing the wrong exercises or hurt your back in an automobile crash, you won't have them to count on when you're older. Some things just can't be reversed or corrected.

COMMUNICATE! To get started thinking and talking about health behaviors, ask some of your close family members what they think wellness is. Are they aware of its many dimensions? Do they know, for example, that spending time with friends, having a spiritual practice, and keeping an active mind all contribute to wellness? Do they have some ideas about wellness that haven't occurred to you? What can you learn from them, and what can they learn from you?

Ww. HOW DO YOU REACH WELLNESS?

Your life may not resemble the one described by the wellness profile at all. You probably have a number of healthy habits and some others that place your health at risk. Maybe your life is more like this:

It's Tuesday. Simon wakes up feeling blue, not really wanting to get out of bed. He wishes he knew what he wanted to do with his life. He wishes he'd meet someone new and fall in love. No time for breakfast, so he grabs a cup of coffee to drink during his first class. He hasn't done the reading and stares blankly at the teacher during the lecture. Later he goes to the student union and has a sugary doughnut and some more coffee; he lights up his first cigarette of the day. Lunch is a fast-food cheeseburger, french fries, and a shake. He spends the afternoon at the library desperately researching a paper that's due the next day, finally quitting at 6:00 and heading to the student union for a beer. He meets up with some buddies and joins them for pizza instead of having dinner at the dorm. By 11:00 he's tired, but he's written only one page of his paper, so he takes an "upper" to keep going. It makes his heart race and floods his head with so many ideas he has difficulty sorting them all out. He works feverishly and finally finishes at 4:00 the next morning. Exhausted, he falls asleep in his clothes. The next thing he knows, it's Wednesday morning, time to start a new day.

This is hardly an ideal lifestyle, but it's not unusual. Simon functions OK, meets his commitments, and shows some self-discipline. On the other hand, time gets away from him, and he doesn't get much exercise, doesn't eat as well as he could, and flirts with the dangers of taking drugs. Overall, he is low on energy and has little control over his life. He could be living a lot better.

Simon isn't alone in neglecting or abusing his health; many people fall into a lifestyle that puts their health at risk. Some aren't aware of the damage they're doing to themselves; others are aware but aren't motivated or don't know how to change; still others want to change but can't seem to get started. All of these are very real problems, but they're not insurmountable. If they were, there would be no ex-smokers, recovering alcoholics, or successful graduates of weight-loss programs. People can and do make difficult changes in their lives.

Taking big steps toward wellness may at first seem like too much work, but as you make progress, it gets easier. At first you'll be rewarded with a greater sense of control over your life, a feeling of empowerment, higher self-esteem, and more joy. These benefits will encourage you to make further improvements. Over time, you'll come to know what wellness feels like—more energy; greater vitality; deeper feelings of curiosity, interest, and enjoyment; and a higher quality of life.

Ww. Getting Serious About Your Health

Before you can start changing a health-related behavior, you have to know that the behavior is problematic and that you *can* change it. To make good decisions, you need information about relevant topics and issues, including what resources are available to help you change your behavior. You also need knowledge about yourself—how you relate to the wellness profile and what strengths you can draw on to change your behavior and improve your health.

Examining Your Current Health Habits   Have you considered how your current lifestyle is affecting your health today and how it will affect your health in the future? Do you know which of your current habits enhance your health and which detract from it? Begin your journey toward wellness with self-assessment: Think about your own behavior and talk with friends and family members about what they've noticed about your lifestyle and your health.

Many people start to consider changing a behavior when they get help from others. An observation from a friend, family member, or physician can help you see yourself as others do and may get you thinking about your behavior in a new way. For example, Jason has been getting a lot of stomachaches lately. His girlfriend Anna notices other changes as well and suggests that the stress of classes plus a part-time job and serving as president of the school radio station might be causing some of Jason's problems. Jason never thought much about trying to control the stressors in his life, but with encouragement from Anna, he starts noticing what events trigger stress for him.

Landmark events can also get you thinking about behavior change. A birthday, the birth of a child, or the death of someone close to you can be powerful motivators for thinking seriously about behaviors that affect wellness. New information can also help you get started. As you read this text, you may find yourself reevaluating some of your health-related behaviors. This could be a great opportunity to make healthful changes that will stay with you for the rest of your life. To help determine whether your current health habits promote wellness, take the quiz in the box "Wellness: Evaluate Your Lifestyle." Use the results to identify behaviors you could change to improve your health and well-being.

Choosing a Target Behavior   A careful examination of your current lifestyle may reveal a number of habits that are candidates for change. To maximize your chances of success, don't try to change all your problem behaviors at once—to quit smoking, give up high-fat foods, start jogging, avoid drugs, get more sleep. Working on even one behavior change will make high demands on your energy. Concentrate on one behavior that you want to change, your **target behavior,** and work on it systematically. Start with something simple, like snacking on candy between afternoon classes or always driving to a particular class instead of walking or biking.

Obtaining Information About Your Target Behavior
Once you've chosen a target behavior, you need to find out more about it. You need to know its risks and benefits for you—both now and in the future. How is your target behavior affecting your level of wellness today? What diseases or conditions does this behavior place you at risk for? What effect would changing your behavior have on your health?

You also need enough information to set an overall target for change. For some behaviors, this is simple. For example, if your target behavior is smoking, your goal will be to quit. But if your target behavior is something like a poor diet or an inactive lifestyle, you may need additional information to set an appropriate goal. Further investigation can help you determine that you should consume five servings of fruits and vegetables each day, for example, or that you should add 30 minutes of brisk walking to your daily routine.

To evaluate your target behavior and set an appropriate target for change, you'll need accurate information. As a starting point, use material from this text and from the resources listed in the For More Information section at the end of each chapter. See the box "Evaluating Sources of Health Information" for tips on becoming a critical consumer of health information from a wide variety of sources.

Finding Outside Help   Have you identified a particularly challenging target behavior, something like alcohol addiction, excessive overeating, or depression that interferes with your ability to function or places you at a serious health risk? Outside help is often needed for changing behaviors or conditions that may be too deeply rooted or too serious for a self-management approach. If this is the case, don't be stopped by the seriousness of the problem—there are many resources available to help you solve it. On campus, the student health center or campus counseling center may be a source of assistance. Many communities offer a variety of services through adult education, health departments, and private agencies. Consult the yellow pages, your physician, your local health department, or the United Way; the latter often sponsors local referral services.

Building Motivation for Change

Knowledge is a necessary ingredient for behavior change, but it isn't usually enough to make people act. Millions of people smoke or have sedentary lifestyles, for example, even though they know it's bad for their health. To succeed at behavior change, you need strong motivation. Strategies for building motivation include examining the pros and cons of change, boosting self-efficacy, and overcoming key barriers to change.

Examining the Pros and Cons of Change   Health behaviors have short-term and long-term benefits and costs associated with them. For example, in the short

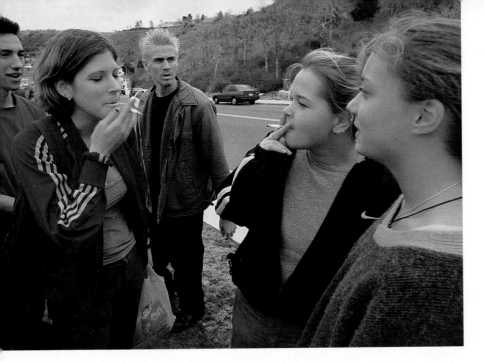

Changing powerful, long-standing habits requires motivation, commitment, and a belief that we are in control of our own behavior. To quit smoking, these young women must overcome a habit that is supported by their addiction to nicotine and by their social environment.

term, an inactive lifestyle allows for more time to watch TV and hang out with friends but leaves a person less able to participate in recreational activities. In the long term, it increases risk for heart disease, cancer, stroke, and premature death. For successful behavior change, you must believe that the benefits of changing outweigh the costs. Do a careful analysis of the short-term and long-term benefits and costs of continuing your current (target) behavior and of changing to a new, healthier behavior. Focus on the effects that are most meaningful to you, including those that are tied to your personal identity and values. For example, if you see yourself as an active person who is a good role model for others, then adopting behaviors such as regular physical activity and adequate sleep would support your personal identity. If you value independence and control over your life, then quitting smoking would be consistent with your values and goals. To complete your analysis, ask friends and family members about the effects of your behavior on them. For example, a roommate may tell you that he never ate candy in the evening until he started living with you, or a younger sister may tell you that your smoking habit influenced her decision to take up smoking.

Pay special attention to the short-term benefits of behavior change, as these can be an important motivating force. Although some people are motivated by long-term goals, such as avoiding a disease that may hit them in 30 years, most are more likely to be moved to action by shorter-term, more personal goals. Feeling better, doing better in school, improving at a sport, reducing stress, and increasing self-esteem are common short-term benefits of health behavior change.

You can further strengthen your motivation by engaging your emotions and raising your consciousness about your problem behavior. This will enable you to focus on the current negatives of the behavior and to imagine the consequences if you don't make a change. Ask yourself: What do I want for myself, now and in the future?

For example, Ruby has never worried much about her smoking because the problems associated with it seem so far away. But lately she's noticed her performance on the volleyball team isn't as good as it used to be. Over the summer she visited her aunt, who has emphysema from smoking and can barely leave her bed. Ruby knows she wants to have children and a career as a teacher, and seeing her aunt makes her wonder if her smoking habit could make it difficult for her to reach these goals. She starts to wonder whether her smoking habit is worth the short- and long-term sacrifices.

Social pressures can also increase the motivation to make changes. In Ruby's case, anti-smoking ordinances keep her from smoking in her dorm and in many public places. The inconvenience of finding a place to smoke—and pressure from her roommate, who doesn't like the smoky smell of Ruby's clothes in their room—are among the short-term costs of Ruby's smoking habit that can add to her motivation to quit.

target behavior An isolated behavior selected as the object of a behavior change plan.

Terms

All of us want optimal health. But many of us do not know how to achieve it. Taking this quiz, adapted from one created by the U.S. Public Health Service, is a good place to start. The behaviors covered in the test are recommended for most Americans. (Some of them may not apply to people with certain diseases or disabilities or to pregnant women, who may require special advice from their physician.) After you take the quiz, add up your score for each section.

Tobacco Use

If you never use tobacco, enter a score of 10 for this section and go to the next section.

	Almost Always	Sometimes	Never
1. I avoid using tobacco.	2	1	0
2. I smoke only low-tar/nicotine cigarettes *or* I smoke a pipe or cigars *or* I use smokeless tobacco.	2	1	0

Tobacco Score: _____

Alcohol and Other Drugs

	Almost Always	Sometimes	Never
1. I avoid alcohol *or* I drink no more than 1 (women) or 2 (men) drinks a day.	4	1	0
2. I avoid using alcohol or other drugs as a way of handling stressful situations or problems in my life.	2	1	0
3. I am careful not to drink alcohol when taking medications, such as for colds or allergies, or when pregnant.	2	1	0
4. I read and follow the label directions when using prescribed and over-the-counter drugs.	2	1	0

Alcohol and Other Drugs Score: _____

Nutrition

	Almost Always	Sometimes	Never
1. I eat a variety of foods each day, including five or more servings of fruits and vegetables.	3	1	0
2. I limit the amount of fat and saturated fat in my diet.	3	1	0
3. I avoid skipping meals.	2	1	0
4. I limit the amount of salt and sugar I eat.	2	1	0

Nutrition Score: _____

Exercise/Fitness

	Almost Always	Sometimes	Never
1. I engage in moderate exercise for 20–60 minutes, 3–5 times a week.	4	1	0
2. I maintain a healthy weight, avoiding overweight and underweight.	2	1	0
3. I do exercises to develop muscular strength and endurance at least twice a week.	2	1	0
4. I spend some of my leisure time participating in physical activities such as gardening, bowling, golf, or baseball.	2	1	0

Exercise/Fitness Score: _____

Emotional Health

	Almost Always	Sometimes	Never
1. I enjoy being a student, and I have a job or do other work that I like.	2	1	0
2. I find it easy to relax and express my feelings freely.	2	1	0

Boosting Self-Efficacy   When you start thinking about changing a health behavior, a big factor in your eventual success is whether you have confidence in yourself and in your ability to change. **Self-efficacy** refers to your belief in your ability to successfully take action and perform a specific task. Self-efficacy varies with each behavior and depends on many factors, including your level of self-esteem and your past experiences with your target behavior. Strategies for boosting self-efficacy include developing an internal locus of control, using visualization and self-talk, and obtaining encouragement from supportive people. Developing specific skills for change, discussed

	Almost Always	Sometimes	Never
3. I manage stress well.	2	1	0
4. I have close friends, relatives, or others I can talk to about personal matters and call on for help.	2	1	0
5. I participate in group activities (such as church and community organizations) or hobbies that I enjoy.	2	1	0

Emotional Health Score: _____

Safety

	Almost Always	Sometimes	Never
1. I wear a safety belt while riding in a car.	2	1	0
2. I avoid driving while under the influence of alcohol or other drugs.	2	1	0
3. I obey traffic rules and the speed limit when driving.	2	1	0
4. I read and follow instructions on the labels of potentially harmful products or substances, such as household cleaners, poisons, and electrical appliances.	2	1	0
5. I avoid smoking in bed.	2	1	0

Safety Score: _____

Disease Prevention

	Almost Always	Sometimes	Never
1. I know the warning signs of cancer, diabetes, heart attack, and stroke.	2	1	0
2. I avoid overexposure to the sun and use a sunscreen.	2	1	0
3. I get recommended medical screening tests (such as blood pressure checks and Pap tests), immunizations, and booster shots.	2	1	0
4. I practice monthly breast/testicle self-exams.	2	1	0
5. I am not sexually active *or* I have sex with only one mutually faithful, uninfected partner *or* I always engage in safer sex (using condoms) *and* I do not share needles to inject drugs.	2	1	0

Disease Prevention Score: _____

What Your Scores Mean

Scores of 9 and 10 Excellent! Your answers show that you're aware of the importance of this area to wellness. More important, you are putting your knowledge to work for you by practicing good health habits. As long as you continue to do so, this area should not pose a serious health risk. It's likely that you are setting an example for your family and friends to follow. Since you scored high on this part of the quiz, you may want to focus on other areas where your scores indicate room for improvement.

Scores of 6–8 Your health practices in this area are good, but there is room for improvement. Look again at the items you answered with "Sometimes" or "Never." What changes can you make to improve your score? Even a small change can often help you achieve better health.

Scores of 3–5 Your health risks are showing! You may need more information about the risks you're facing and about why it's important for you to change these behaviors. Perhaps you need help in deciding how to successfully make the changes you want.

Scores of 0–2 Your answers show that you may be taking serious and unnecessary risks with your health. Perhaps you are not aware of the risks and what to do about them. You can easily get the information and help you need to improve, if you wish. The next step is up to you.

later in this chapter, is also critical for improving self-efficacy.

LOCUS OF CONTROL   Who do you believe is controlling your life? Is it your parents, friends, or school? Is it "fate"? Or is it you? **Locus of control** refers to the figurative

self-efficacy The belief in one's ability to take action and perform a specific behavior.

locus of control The figurative "place" a person designates as the source of responsibility for the events in his or her life.

Terms

Making sound choices about your own wellness requires critical thinking. In order to choose and implement healthy behaviors, you must be able to identify accurate information about health in general and your own personal risk factors in particular. You must be able to evaluate health-related products and services such as exercise shoes, fast food, health insurance, and medical treatments. Thinking critically is crucial if you are to take advantage of all the opportunities you have to optimize your health and well-being.

General Strategies

A key first step in sharpening your critical thinking skills is to look carefully at your sources of health information. Critical thinking involves knowing where and how to find relevant information, how to separate fact from opinion, how to recognize faulty reasoning, how to evaluate information, and how to assess the credibility of sources. The following strategies can help you sort through the health information you receive from common sources, including television, newspapers, magazines, books, advertisements, Web sites, and friends and family members.

- *Go to the original source.* Media reports often simplify the results of medical research. Find out for yourself what a study really reported, and determine whether it was based on good science. What type of study was it? Was it published in a recognized medical journal? Was it an animal study or did it involve people? Did the study include a large number of people? What did the authors of the study actually report in their findings? (You'll find additional strategies for evaluating research studies in Chapter 21.)

- *Watch for misleading language.* Reports that feature "breakthroughs" or "dramatic proof" are probably hype. Some studies will find that a behavior "contributes to" or is "associated with" an outcome; this does not imply a proven cause-and-effect relationship. Information may also be distorted by an author's point of view. Carefully read or listen to information in order to understand its implications.

- *Distinguish between research reports and public health advice.* If a study finds a link between a particular vitamin and cancer, that should not necessarily lead you to change your behavior. But if the Surgeon General or the American Cancer Society advises you to eat less fat or quit smoking, you can assume that many studies point in this direction and that this is advice you should follow.

- *Remember that anecdotes are not facts.* Sometimes we do get helpful health information from our friends and family. But just because your cousin Bertha lost 10 pounds on Dr. Amazing's new protein diet doesn't mean it's a safe, effective way for you to lose weight. Before you make a big change in your lifestyle, verify the information with your physician, this text, or other reliable sources.

- *Be skeptical, and use your common sense.* If a report seems too good to be true, it probably is. Be especially wary of information contained in advertisements. The goal of an ad is to sell you something, to create a feeling of need for a product where no real need exists. Evaluate "scientific" claims carefully, and beware of quackery (see Chapter 21).

- *Make choices that are right for you.* Your roommate swears by swimming; you prefer aerobics. Your sister takes a yoga class to help her manage stress; your brother unwinds by walking in the woods. Friends and family members can be a great source of ideas and inspiration, but each of us needs to find a wellness lifestyle that works for us.

Internet Resources

More than half of all Internet users report having surfed for health information. Evaluating health information from online sources poses special challenges and requires additional critical thinking skills. When reviewing a health-related Web site, ask the following questions:

- *What is the source of the information? Who is the author or sponsor of the Web page?* Web sites maintained by government agencies, professional associations, or established academic or medical institutions are likely to present trustworthy information. Many other groups and individuals post accurate information, but it is important to look at the qualifications of the people who are behind the site. (Check the home page or click on an "about us" or "who we are" link.)

- *How often is the site updated?* Look for sites that are updated frequently. Also check the "last modified" date of any specific Web page on a site.

- *What is the purpose of the page? Does the site promote particular products or procedures? Are there obvious reasons for bias?* Be wary of information from sites that sell specific products, use testimonials as evidence, appear to have a social or political agenda, or ask for money.

- *What do other sources say about a topic?* Be cautious of claims or information that appears at only one site or comes from a chat room or bulletin board.

- *Does the site conform to any set of guidelines or criteria for quality and accuracy?* Look for sites that identify themselves as conforming to some code or set of principles, such as those set forth by the Health on the Net Foundation or the American Medical Association. These codes include criteria such as use of information from respected sources and disclosure of the site's sponsors.

Additional strategies for locating and assessing health-related information from the Internet can be found in Appendix C and on the *Core Concepts in Health* Web site (http://www.mhhe.com/insel9).

You will find boxes labeled Critical Consumer throughout the text to help you develop and apply your critical thinking skills. In addition, be sure to work through the Critical Thinking Journal Entry activities at the end of each chapter. Developing the ability to think critically and independently about health issues will serve you well throughout your life.

"place" a person designates as the source of responsibility for the events in his or her life. People who believe they are in control of their own lives are said to have an internal locus of control. Those who believe that factors beyond their control—heredity, friends and family, the environment, fate, luck, or other outside forces—are more important in determining the events of their lives are said to have an external locus of control. Most people are not purely "internalizers" or "externalizers"; their locus of control changes in response to the situation.

For lifestyle management, an internal locus of control is an advantage because it reinforces motivation and commitment. An external locus of control can actually sabotage efforts to change behavior. For example, if you believe you are destined to die of breast cancer because your mother died from the disease, you may view monthly breast self-exams and regular checkups as a waste of time. In contrast, an internal locus of control is an advantage. If you believe you can take action to reduce your hereditary risk of breast cancer, you will be motivated to follow guidelines for early detection of the disease.

People who tend to have an external locus of control can learn to view the events in their lives differently and increase their feelings of self-efficacy. If you find yourself attributing too much influence to outside forces, gather more information about your target behavior. Make a list of all the ways that behavior change will improve your health. If you recognize and accept that you are in charge of your life, you're well on your way to wellness.

VISUALIZATION AND SELF-TALK One of the best ways to boost your confidence and self-efficacy is to visualize yourself successfully engaging in a new, healthier behavior. Imagine yourself turning down cigarettes, going for a regular after-dinner walk, or choosing healthier snacks. Also visualize yourself enjoying all the short-term and long-term benefits that behavior change will bring. Create a new self-image: What will you and your life be like when you become a nonsmoker, a regular exerciser, or a healthy eater?

You can also use self-talk, the internal dialogue you carry on with yourself, to increase your confidence in your ability to change. Counter any self-defeating patterns of thought with more positive or realistic thoughts: "Behavior change is difficult, but if I work at it, I will succeed," or "I am a strong, capable person, and I can maintain my commitment to change." Refer to Chapter 3 for more on self-talk.

ROLE MODELS AND OTHER SUPPORTIVE INDIVIDUALS Social support can also make a big difference in your level of motivation and your chances of success. Perhaps you know people who have reached the goal you are striving for; they could be role models or mentors for you, providing information and support for your efforts. Talk to

them about how they did it. What were the most difficult parts of changing their behavior? What strategies worked for them? Gain strength from their experiences, and tell yourself, "If they can do it, so can I."

In addition, find a buddy who wants to make the same changes you do and who can take an active role in your behavior change program. For example, an exercise buddy can provide companionship and encouragement for times when you might be tempted to skip that morning jog. Or you and a friend can watch to be sure that you both have only one alcoholic beverage at a party. If necessary, look beyond your current social network at possible new sources of help, such as a support group. Later in this chapter, you'll learn some specific strategies for involving other people in your behavior change program.

Identifying and Overcoming Key Barriers to Change

Have you tried and failed to change your target behavior in the past? Don't let past failures discourage you; they can be a great source of information you can use to boost your chances of future success. Make a list of the problems and challenges you faced in your previous behavior change attempts; to this, add the short-term costs of behavior change that you identified in your analysis of the pros and cons of change. Once you've listed these key barriers to change, develop a practical plan for overcoming each one. For example, if one of your key barriers for physical activity is that you believe you can't make time for a 40-minute workout, look for ways to incorporate shorter bouts of physical activity into your daily routine. If you always smoke when you're with certain friends, practice in advance how you will turn down the next cigarette you are offered. Developing strategies to cope with difficult situations is one of the most important factors in successful behavior change. You'll find additional advice and examples later in the chapter in the section "Developing Skills for Change."

Self-talk can also help overcome barriers. Make behavior change a priority in your life, and plan to commit the necessary time and effort. Ask yourself: How much time and energy will behavior change *really* require? Isn't the effort worth all the short- and long-term benefits?

Enhancing Your Readiness to Change

The transtheoretical, or "stages of change," model, developed by psychologists James Prochaska and Carlo DiClemente, has been shown to be an effective approach to lifestyle self-management. According to this model, you move through six well-defined stages as you work to change your target behavior. It is important to determine what stage you are in now so that you can choose appropriate strategies for progressing through the cycle of change (see the box "What Stage of Change Are You In?"). Using this approach can help you enhance your readiness and intention to change.

To determine your stage, circle true or false for each of the following statements:

T   F   **1.**   I changed my target behavior more than 6 months ago.

T   F   **2.**   I changed my target behavior within the past 6 months.

T   F   **3.**   I intend to take action within the next month and have already made a few small changes in my behavior.

T   F   **4.**   I intend to take action on my target behavior within the next 6 months.

Find the stage that corresponds to your responses:

False for all four statements = Precontemplation

True for statement 4, false for statements 1–3 = Contemplation

True for statements 3 and 4, false for statements 1 and 2 = Preparation

True for statement 2, false for statement 1 = Action

True for statement 1 = Maintenance

SOURCE: Prochaska, J. O., C. A. Redding, and K. E. Evers. 1997. The transtheoretical model and stages of change. In *Health Behavior and Health Education: Theory, Research, and Practice*, 2nd ed. San Francisco: Jossey-Bass.

Precontemplation   People at this stage have no intention of changing their behavior. They may be unaware of the risks associated with their behavior, or they may deny that their behavior will have any serious consequences for them. They may have tried unsuccessfully to change in the past and may now feel demoralized and think the situation is hopeless. They may also blame others for their problems.

If you are in the precontemplation stage, begin to move forward by raising your consciousness of your target behavior and its effects on you and those around you. Obtain accurate information about your behavior, and ask yourself what has prevented you from changing in the past. Enlist friends and family members to help you become more aware of your behavior and your reasons for continuing an unhealthy habit. Also find out more about the campus and community resources available to help you with behavior change.

Contemplation   People at this stage are aware that they have a problem and have started to think and learn about it. They acknowledge the benefits that behavior change will have for them but are also very aware of the costs of changing. They wonder about possible courses of action but may feel stuck and unsure of how best to proceed.

At this stage, it's a good idea to begin keeping a written record of your target behavior—to learn more about it and to use when you begin to plan the specifics of your behavior change program. Work on your analysis of the pros and cons of change: Expand your list of the benefits, and problem-solve to overcome the key barriers on your list of the costs of changing. To be successful, you must believe that the benefits of change outweigh the costs. Engage your emotions and boost self-efficacy through visualization, self-talk, and the support of other people.

Preparation   People at this stage plan to take action within a month and may have already begun to make small changes in their behavior. If you are in the preparation stage, your next step is to create a specific plan for change that includes a start date, realistic goals, rewards, and information on exactly how you will go about changing your behavior. You'll also want to prepare yourself emotionally and socially by practicing visualization and self-talk and by involving the people around you in your efforts at change. A step-by-step plan for developing a successful behavior change program is included in the next section of the chapter.

Action   During the action stage, people outwardly modify their behavior and their environment. The action stage requires the greatest commitment of time and energy, and people in this stage are at risk for reverting to old, unhealthy patterns of behavior. If you are in the action stage, you'll need to use all the plans and strategies that you developed during earlier stages. In particular, be sure to plan ahead to overcome temptations and deal with problem situations.

Maintenance   People at this stage have maintained their new, healthier lifestyle for at least 6 months. To guard against slips and relapses, they continue with all the positive strategies they used in earlier stages. Their confidence and self-efficacy increase. The maintenance stage typically lasts from 6 months to about 5 years.

Termination   People at this stage have exited the cycle of change and are no longer tempted to lapse back into their old behavior. They have a new self-image and total self-efficacy with regard to their target behavior. This stage applies to some behaviors, such as addictions, but may not be appropriate for others.

Lapses are a natural part of the process at all stages of change. Many people lapse and must recycle through earlier stages, although most don't go back to the first stage. If you lapse, use what you learn about yourself and the process of change to help you in your next attempt at behavior change.

Next, we'll take a closer look at the specific steps and skills involved in creating and implementing a plan for change.

> **COMMUNICATE!**   As you begin your study of wellness, it's natural to think about the health behaviors of your friends and family members, especially if someone smokes, drinks irresponsibly, or engages in other behaviors that detract from wellness. If this is the case for you, are you in a position to talk to your friend or relative about the problematic behavior? Can you determine what "stage of change" he or she is at in relation to the behavior (precontemplation, contemplation, and so on)? How do you feel about offering facts or information about the behavior or supporting the person in behavior change?

Developing Skills for Change: Creating a Personalized Plan

Once you are committed to making a change, it's time to put together a detailed plan of action. Your key to success is a well-thought-out plan that sets goals, anticipates problems, and includes rewards.

1. Monitor Your Behavior and Gather Data

Begin by keeping careful records of the behavior you wish to change (your target behavior) and the circumstances surrounding it. Keep these records in a health journal, a notebook in which you write the details of your behavior along with observations and comments. Note exactly what the activity was, when and where it happened, what you were doing, and what your feelings were at the time. In a journal for a weight-loss or dietary-change plan, for example, you would typically record how much food you ate, the time of day, the situation, the location, your feelings, and how hungry you were (Figure 1-4). If your goal is to start an exercise program, use your journal to track your daily activities to determine how best to make time for your workouts. Keep your journal for a week or two to get some solid information about the behavior you want to change.

2. Analyze the Data and Identify Patterns

After you have collected data on the behavior, analyze the data to identify patterns. When are you most hungry? When are you most likely to overeat? What events seem to trigger your appetite? Perhaps you are especially hungry at mid-morning or when you put off eating dinner until 9:00. Perhaps you overindulge in food and drink when you go to a particular restaurant or when you're with certain friends. Be sure to note the connections between your feelings and such external cues as time of day, location, situation, and the actions of others around you. Do you always think of having a cigarette when you read the newspaper? Do you always bite your fingernails when you're studying?

3. Set Realistic, Specific Goals

Don't set an impossibly difficult overall goal for your program—going from a sedentary lifestyle to running a marathon within 2 months, for example. Working toward more realistic, achievable goals will greatly increase your chances of success. Your goal should also be specific and measurable, something you can easily track. Instead of a vague general goal such as improving eating habits or being more physically active, set a specific target—eating five servings of fruits and vegetables each day or walking or biking for 30 minutes at least 5 days per week.

Whatever your ultimate goal, it's a good idea to break it down into a few small steps. Your plan will seem less overwhelming and more manageable, increasing the chances that you'll stick to it. You'll also build in more opportunities to reward yourself (discussed in step 4), as well as milestones you can use to measure your progress. If you plan to lose 15 pounds, for example, you'll find it easier to take off 5 pounds at a time. If you want to start an exercise program, begin by taking 10- to 15-minute walks a few times per week. Take the easier steps first and work up to the harder steps. With each small success, you'll build your confidence and self-efficacy.

4. Devise a Strategy or Plan of Action

Next, you need to develop specific strategies and techniques that will support your day-to-day efforts at behavior change.

OBTAIN INFORMATION AND SUPPLIES   Identify campus and community resources that can provide practical help—for example, a stop-smoking course or a walking club. Take any necessary preparatory steps, such as signing up for a stress-management workshop or purchasing walking shoes, nicotine replacement patches, or a special calendar to track your progress.

Date __November 5__   Day   M (TU) W TH F SA SU

Time of day	M/S	Food eaten	Cals.	H	Where did you eat?	What else were you doing?	How did someone else influence you?	What made you want to eat what you did?	Emotions and feelings?	Thoughts and concerns?
7:30	M	1 C Crispix cereal	110	3	dorm cafeteria	reading newspaper	eating w/ friends, but I ate what I usually eat	I always eat cereal in the morning	a little keyed up & worried	thinking about quiz in class today
		1/2 C skim milk	40							
		coffee, black	—							
		1 C orange juice	120							
10:30	S	1 apple	90	1	library	studying	alone	felt tired & wanted to wake up	tired	worried about next class
12:30	M	1 C chili	290	2	cafeteria terrace	talking	eating w/ friends; we decided to eat at the cafeteria	wanted to be part of group	excited and happy	interested in hearing everyone's plans for the weekend
		1 roll	120							
		1 pat butter	35							
		1 orange	60							
		2 oatmeal cookies	120							
		1 soda	150							

M/S = Meal or snack   H = Hunger rating (0–3)

Figure 1-4   Sample health journal entries.

MODIFY YOUR ENVIRONMENT   As you write in your health journal, you gather quite a lot of information about your target behavior—the times it typically occurs; the situations in which it usually happens; the ways sight, smell, mood, situation, and accessibility trigger it. You can probably trace the chain of events that leads to the behavior and perhaps also identify points along the way where making a different choice would mean changing the behavior.

You can be more effective in changing behavior if you control the environmental cues that provoke it. This might mean not having cigarettes or certain foods or drinks in the house, not going to parties where you're tempted to overindulge, or not spending time with particular people, at least for a while. If you always get a candy bar at a certain vending machine, change your route so you don't pass by it. If you always end up taking a coffee break and chatting with friends when you go to the library to study, choose a different place to study, such as your room.

It's also helpful to control other behaviors or habits that seem to be linked to the target behavior. You may give in to an urge to eat when you have a beer (alcohol increases the appetite) or when you watch TV. Try substituting some other activities for habits that seem to be linked with your target behavior, such as exercising to music instead of plopping down in front of the TV. Or, if possible, put an exercise bicycle in front of the set and burn calories while you watch your favorite show.

You can change the cues in your environment so they trigger the new behavior you want instead of the old one. Tape a picture of a cyclist speeding down a hill on your TV screen. Leave your exercise shoes in plain view. Put a chart of your progress in a special place at home to make your goals highly visible and inspire you to keep going. When you're trying to change an ingrained habit, small cues can play an important part in keeping you on track.

REWARD YOURSELF   Another very powerful way to affect your target behavior is to set up a reward system that will reinforce your efforts. Most people find it difficult to change long-standing habits for rewards they can't see right away. Giving yourself instant, real rewards for good behavior along the way will help you stick with a plan to change your behavior.

Carefully plan your reward payoffs and what they will be. In most cases, rewards should be collected when you reach specific objectives or subgoals in your plan. For example, you might treat yourself to a movie after a week of avoiding extra snacks. Don't forget to reward yourself for good behavior that is consistent and persistent—such as simply sticking with your program week after week. Decide on a reward after you reach a certain goal, or mark off the sixth week or month of a valiant effort. Write it down in your health journal and remember it as you follow your plan—especially when the going gets rough.

Make a list of your activities and favorite events to use as rewards. They should be special, inexpensive, and

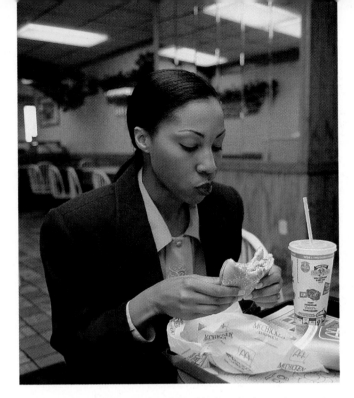

Many actions and behaviors are shaped by cues in the environment. Fast food is quick and widely available, making it a more likely lunch choice for this busy woman than the many healthier alternatives.

preferably unrelated to food or alcohol. Depending on what you like to do, you might treat yourself to a concert, a ball game, a new CD, a long-distance phone call to a friend, a day off from studying for a long hike in the woods—whatever is rewarding to you.

INVOLVE THE PEOPLE AROUND YOU   Rewards and support can also come from family and friends. Tell them about your plan, and ask for their help. Encourage them to be active, interested participants. Ask them to support you when you set aside time to go running or avoid second helpings at Thanksgiving dinner. You may have to remind them not to do things that make you "break training" and not to be hurt if you have to refuse something when they forget. To help friends and family members who will be involved in your program respond appropriately, you may want to create a specific list of dos and don'ts. Getting encouragement, support, and praise from important people in your life can powerfully reinforce the new behavior you're trying to adopt.

PLAN AHEAD FOR CHALLENGING SITUATIONS   Take time out now to list situations and people that have the potential to derail your program and to develop possible coping mechanisms. For example, if you think that you'll have trouble exercising during finals week, schedule short bouts of physical activity as stress-reducing study breaks. If a visit to a friend who smokes is likely to tempt you to lapse, plan to bring nicotine patches, chewing gum, and a copy of your behavior change contract to strengthen your resolve.

5. Make a Commitment by Signing a Personal Contract   Once you have set your goals and developed a plan of action, make your plan into a personal contract. A serious personal contract—one that commits your word—can result in a higher chance of follow-through than will a casual, offhand promise. Your contract can help prevent procrastination by specifying the important dates and can also serve as a reminder of your personal commitment to change.

Your contract should include a statement of your goal and your commitment to reaching it. Include details of your plan: the date you'll begin, the steps you'll use to measure your progress, the concrete strategies you've developed for promoting change, and the date you expect to reach your final goal. Have someone—preferably someone who will be actively helping you with your program—sign your contract as a witness.

A Sample Behavior Change Plan   Let's take the example of Michael, who wants to improve his diet. By monitoring his eating habits in his health journal for several weeks, he gets a good sense of his typical diet—what he eats and where he eats it. Through self-assessment and investigation, he discovers that he currently consumes only about one serving of fruit per week, much less than the recommended two to four servings per day. He also finds out that fruit is a major source of fiber, vitamins, minerals, and other substances important for good health. He sets the target of eating three servings of fruit per day as the overall goal for his behavior change plan. Next, he sets a start date and decides to break his plan into three parts. He'll begin by adding a serving of fruit to his breakfast. Once he successfully reaches this goal, he'll add other servings of fruit, first as part of his lunch and then in place of one of the sodas he typically consumes as a snack.

To help increase his chances of success, Michael decides to make several changes in his behavior and his environment. Since he often eats breakfast and lunch on the run, he decides to stock his small dorm-room refrigerator with a supply of easy-to-carry items such as oranges, apples, and small containers of juice. He empties one of the outside pockets of his book backpack so he has a special place to carry fruit. He also places reminders in several locations so that he remembers to keep both his refrigerator and his backpack stocked. He checks out the places he typically buys meals on campus and makes note of several that sell fruit juice and fruit salad. Finally, Michael decides on some rewards he'll give himself when he meets his goals, choosing things he likes that aren't too expensive.

After Michael has thought through his plan to eat three servings of fruit each day, he's ready to create and sign a behavior change contract. He decides to enlist one of his lab partners as a witness to his contract; he also asks her to check

My Personal Contract for Eating Three Servings of Fruit per Day

I agree to increase my consumption of fruit from one serving per week to three servings per day. I will begin my program on ___10/5___ and plan to reach my final goal by___12/7___. I have divided my program into three parts, with three separate goals. For each step in my program, I will give myself the reward listed.

1. I will begin to have a serving of fruit with breakfast on ___10/5___.
   (Reward: _baseball game_____)
2. I will begin to have a serving of fruit with lunch on ___10/26___.
   (Reward: _music CD_____)
3. I will begin to substitute fruit juice for soda for one snack each day on ___11/16___.
   (Reward: _Concert_____)

My plan for increasing fruit consumption includes the following strategies:

1. _Keeping my dorm room refrigerator stocked with easy-to-carry fruit and fruit juice._
2. _Packing fruit in my book backpack every day._
3. _Placing reminders to buy, carry, and eat fruit in my dorm room, backpack, and wallet._
4. _Buying lunch at a place that serves fruit or fruit juice._

I understand that it is important for me to make a strong personal effort to make the change in my behavior. I sign this contract as an indication of my personal commitment to reach my goal.

Michael Cook   9/28

Witness: _____Katie Lim_____   9/28

Figure 1-5   A sample behavior change contract.

on his progress and offer encouragement (Figure 1-5). Once Michael has signed his contract, he's ready to take action.

You can apply the general behavior change planning framework presented in this chapter to any target behavior. Additional examples of behavior change plans are presented in the Behavior Change Strategy sections that appear at the end of many chapters. In these, you'll find specific plans and advice for overcoming test anxiety (Chapter 2), reducing caffeine consumption (Chapter 9), quitting smoking (Chapter 11), beginning an exercise program (Chapter 13), eating more fruits and vegetables (Chapter 16), and many other positive lifestyle changes.

Putting Your Plan into Action

The starting date has arrived, and you are ready to put your plan into action. This stage requires commitment, the resolve to stick with the plan no matter what temptations you encounter. Remember all the good reasons you have to make the change—and remember that *you* are the boss.

Use all your strategies to make your plan work. Substituting behaviors are often very important—go for a walk after class instead of eating a bag of chips. Make sure your environment is change-friendly by keeping cues that trigger the problem behavior to a minimum. Be sure to also obtain as much support and encouragement from others as possible.

Use your health journal to keep track of how well you are doing in achieving your ultimate goal. Record your daily activities and any relevant details, such as how far you walked or how many calories you ate. Each week, chart your progress on a graph and see how it compares to the subgoals on your contract. You may want to track more than one behavior, such as the time you spend exercising each week and your weight.

If you don't seem to be making progress, analyze your plan to see what might be causing the problem. Possible barriers to success are listed in the section "Staying with It," along with suggestions for addressing them. Once you've identified the problem, revise your plan.

Be sure to reward yourself for your successes by treating yourself as specified in your contract. And don't forget to give yourself a pat on the back—congratulate yourself, notice how much better you look or feel, and feel good about how far you've come and how you've gained control of your behavior.

Changing behavior takes motivation. But how do you get motivated? The following strategies may help:

- Write down the potential benefits of the change. If you want to lose weight, your list might include increased ease of movement, energy, and self-confidence.

- Now write down the costs of not changing.

- Frequently visualize yourself achieving your goal and enjoying its benefits. If you want to manage time more effectively, picture yourself as a confident, organized person who systematically tackles important tasks and sets aside time each day for relaxation, exercise, and friends.

- Discount obstacles to change. Counter thoughts such as "I'll never have time to shop for and prepare healthy foods" with thoughts such as "Lots of other people have done it and so can I."

- Bombard yourself with propaganda. Subscribe to a self-improvement magazine. Take a class dealing with the change you want to make. Read books and watch talk shows on the subject. Post motivational phrases or pictures on your refrigerator or over your desk. Listen to motiva-

tional tapes in the car. Talk to people who have already made the change you want to make.

- Build up your confidence. Remind yourself of other goals you've achieved. At the end of each day, mentally review your good decisions and actions. See yourself as a capable person, one who is in charge of his or her health.

- Create choices. You will be more likely to exercise every day if you have two or three types of exercise to choose from, and more likely to quit smoking if you've identified more than one way to distract yourself when you crave a cigarette. Get ideas from people who have been successful, and adapt some of their strategies to suit you.

- If you slip, keep trying. Research suggests that four out of five people will experience some degree of backsliding when they try to change a behavior. Only one in four succeeds the first time around. If you retain your commitment to change even when you lapse, you are still farther along the path to change than before you made the commitment. Try again. And again, if necessary.

Staying with It

As you continue with your program, don't be surprised when you run up against obstacles; they're inevitable. In fact, it's a good idea to expect problems and give yourself time to step back, see how you're doing, and make some changes before going on again. If you find your program is grinding to a halt, try to identify what is blocking your progress. It may come from one of these sources.

Social Influences   Take a hard look at the reactions of the people you're counting on, and see if they're really supporting you. If they come up short, try connecting and networking with others who will be more supportive.

A related trap is trying to get your friends or family members to change *their* behaviors. The decision to make a major behavior change is something people come to only after intensive self-examination. You may be able to influence someone by tactfully providing facts or support, but that's all. Focus on yourself. If you succeed, you may become a role model for others.

Levels of Motivation and Commitment   You won't make real progress until an inner drive leads you to the stage of change at which you are ready to make a personal commitment to the goal. If commitment is your problem, you may need to wait until the short-term costs of your target behavior make your life more unhappy or unhealthy; then your desire to change it will be stronger. Or

you may find that changing your goal will inspire you to keep going. If you really want to change but your motivation comes and goes, look at your support system and at your own level of confidence. Building these up may be the key to pushing past a barrier. For more ideas, refer to the box "Motivation Boosters."

Choice of Techniques and Level of Effort   Your plan may not be working as well as you thought it would. Make changes where you're having the most trouble. If you've lagged on your running schedule, for example, maybe it's because you really don't like running. A group exercise class might suit you better. There are many ways to move toward your goal. Or you may not be trying hard enough. You do have to push toward your goal. If it were easy, you wouldn't need to have a plan.

Stress Barriers   If you've hit a wall in your program, look at the sources of stress in your life. If the stress is temporary, such as catching a cold or having a term paper due, you may want to wait until it passes before strengthening your efforts. If the stress is ongoing, try to find healthy ways to manage it. For example, taking a half-hour walk after lunch may help. You may even want to make stress management your highest priority for behavior change (see Chapter 2).

Games People Play   Procrastinating, rationalizing, and blaming; even when they want to change, people hold on

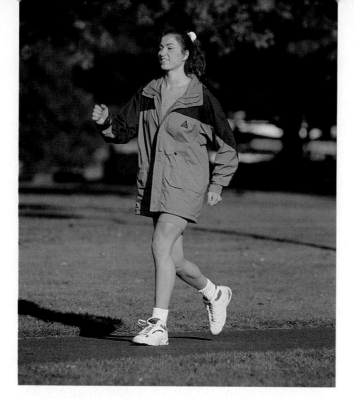

A beautiful day and a spectacular setting contribute to making exercise a satisfying and pleasurable experience. Choosing the right activity and doing it the right way are important elements in a successful health behavior change program.

fiercely to what they know and love (or know and hate). You may have very mixed feelings about the change you're trying to make, and your underlying motives may sabotage your conscious ones if you keep them hidden from yourself. Try to detect the games you might be playing with yourself so that you can stop them.

If you're procrastinating ("It's Friday already; I might as well wait until Monday to begin"), try breaking your plan down into still smaller steps that you can accomplish one day at a time. If you're rationalizing or making excuses ("I wanted to go swimming today, but I wouldn't have had time to wash my hair afterward"), remember that the only one you're fooling is yourself, and that when you "win" by deceiving yourself, it's not much of a victory. If you're wasting time blaming yourself or others ("Everyone in that class talks so much that I don't get a chance to speak"), recognize that blaming is a way of taking your focus off the real problem and denying responsibility for your actions. Try refocusing by taking a positive attitude and renewing your determination to succeed.

COMMUNICATE! How do others see your future? Ask a couple of close friends how they see you 5, 10, and 20 years from now. Which of their predictions do you like? For instance, do they see you as happy, healthy, successful? Which predictions do you hope won't come true? What can you do now to control these outcomes?

BEING HEALTHY FOR LIFE

Your first few behavior change projects may never go beyond the planning stage. Those that do may not all succeed. But as you taste success by beginning to see progress and changes, you'll start to experience new and surprising positive feelings about yourself. You'll probably find that you're less likely to buckle under stress. You may accomplish things you never thought possible—winning a race, climbing a mountain, quitting smoking. Being healthy takes extra effort, but the paybacks in energy and vitality are priceless.

Once you've started, don't stop. Remember that maintaining good health is an ongoing process. Tackle one area at a time, but make a careful inventory of your health strengths and weaknesses and lay out a long-range plan. Take on the easier problems first, and then use what you have learned to attack more difficult areas. Keep informed about the latest health news and trends; research is constantly providing new information that directly affects daily choices and habits.

Making Changes in Your World

You can't completely control every aspect of your health. At least three other factors—heredity, health care, and environment—play important roles in your well-being. After you quit smoking, for example, you may still be inhaling smoke from other people's cigarettes. Your resolve to eat better foods may suffer a setback when you can't find any healthy choices in vending machines.

But you can make a difference—you can help create an environment around you that supports wellness for everyone. You can help support nonsmoking areas in public places. You can speak up in favor of more nutritious foods and better physical fitness facilities. You can include nonalcoholic drinks at your parties.

You can also work on larger environmental challenges: air and water pollution, traffic congestion, overcrowding and overpopulation, depletion of the atmosphere's ozone layer, toxic and nuclear waste, and many others. These difficult issues need the attention and energy of people who are informed and who care about good health. On every level, from personal to planetary, we can all take an active role in shaping our environment.

What Does the Future Hold?

Sweeping changes in lifestyle have resulted in healthier Americans in recent years and could have even greater effects in the years to come. In your lifetime, you can choose to take an active role in the movement toward increased awareness, greater individual responsibility and control, healthier lifestyles, and a healthier planet. Your choices and actions will have a tremendous impact on your present and future wellness. The door is open, and the time is now—you simply have to begin.

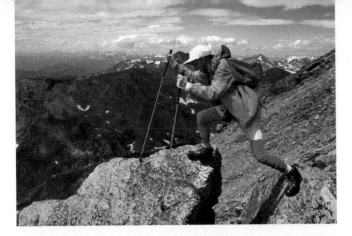

This retiree spends leisure time hiking and climbing mountains. If you want to enjoy vigor and health in *your* middle and old age, begin now to make the choices that will give you lifelong vitality.

SUMMARY

- Wellness is the ability to live life fully, with vitality and meaning. Wellness is dynamic and multidimensional; it incorporates physical, emotional, intellectual, spiritual, interpersonal and social, and environmental dimensions.

- As chronic diseases have become the leading cause of death in the United States, people have recognized that they have greater control over, and greater responsibility for, their health than ever before.

- The Healthy People initiative seeks to achieve a better quality of life for all Americans. The broad goals of the *Healthy People 2010* report are to increase quality and years of healthy life and to eliminate health disparities among Americans.

- Health-related differences among people that have implications for wellness can be described in the context of gender, ethnicity, income and education, disability, geographic location, and sexual orientation.

- Although heredity, environment, and health care all play roles in wellness and disease, behavior can mitigate their effects.

- Behaviors and habits that reinforce wellness include (1) taking an active, responsible role in your health; (2) managing stress; (3) maintaining self-esteem and good interpersonal relationships; (4) understanding sexuality and having satisfying intimate relationships; (5) avoiding tobacco and other drugs and restricting alcohol intake; (6) eating well, exercising, and maintaining healthy weight; (7) knowing about diseases and injuries and protecting yourself against them; (8) understanding and wisely using the health care system; (9) knowing when to seek treatment for an illness; (10) understanding and accepting the processes of aging and dying; and (11) understanding how the environment affects your health and working to improve the environment.

- To make lifestyle changes, you need information about yourself, your health habits, and resources available to help you change.

- You can increase your motivation for behavior change by examining the benefits and costs of change, boosting self-efficacy, and identifying and overcoming key barriers to change.

- The stages of change model describes six stages that people move through as they try to change their behavior: precontemplation, contemplation, preparation, action, maintenance, and termination.

- A specific plan for change can be developed by (1) monitoring behavior by keeping a journal, (2) analyzing the recorded data, (3) setting specific goals, (4) devising strategies for modifying the environment, rewarding yourself, and involving others, and (5) making a personal contract.

- To start and maintain a behavior change program you need commitment, a well-developed plan, social support, and a system of rewards.

- Although we cannot control every aspect of our health, we can make a difference in helping create an environment that supports wellness for everyone.

1.   Ask some older members of your family (parents and grandparents) what they recall about patterns of health and disease when they were young. Do they remember any large outbreaks of infectious disease? Did any of their friends or relatives die while very young or die of a disease that can now be treated? How have health concerns changed during their lifetime?

2.   Choose a person you consider a role model, and interview him or her. What do you admire about this person? What can you borrow from his or her experiences and strategies for success?

JOURNAL ENTRY

1.   Purchase a small notebook to use as your health journal throughout this course. At the end of each chapter, we include suggestions for journal entries—opportunities to think about topics and issues, explore and formulate your own views, and express your thoughts in written form. These exercises are intended to help you deepen your understanding of health topics and your own behaviors in relation to them. For your first journal entry, make a list of the positive behaviors that enhance your health (such as jogging and getting enough sleep). Consider what additions you can make to the list or how you can strengthen or reinforce these behaviors. (Don't forget to congratulate yourself for these positive aspects of your life.) Next, list the behaviors that detract from wellness (such as smoking and eating a lot of candy). Consider which of these behaviors you might be able to change. Use these lists as the basis for self-evaluation as you proceed through this book.

2.   Think of the last time you did something you knew to be unhealthy primarily because those around you were doing it. How could you have restructured the situation or changed the environmental cues so that you could have avoided the behavior? In your health journal, describe several possible actions that will help you avoid the behavior the next time you're in a similar situation.

3.   Make a list in your health journal of rewards that are meaningful to you. Add to the list as you think of new things to use. Refer to this list of rewards when you're developing plans for behavior change.

4.   *Critical Thinking*   In this book, several Journal Entry items are designed to help you sharpen your critical thinking skills. For your first Critical Thinking journal entry, write a short essay describing your sources of health information. Do you rely on newspaper or magazine articles? On television? On a particular Web site? On friends and family? What criteria do you use to evaluate this information, to assess its credibility, and to make decisions about your health?

FOR MORE INFORMATION

Books

Columbia University's Health Education Program. 1998. *The "Go Ask Alice" Book of Answers.* New York: Henry Holt. *Presents answers to a variety of student-oriented health questions from the popular "Go Ask Alice" Web site.*

Prochaska, J. O., J. C. Norcross, and C. C. DiClemente. 1994. *Changing for Good: The Revolutionary Program That Explains the Six Stages of Change and Teaches You How to Free Yourself from Bad Habits.* New York: Morrow. *Outlines the authors' model of behavior change and offers suggestions and advice for each stage of change.*

Ridley, M. 2000. *Genome: The Autobiography of a Species in 23 Chapters.* New York: HarperCollins. *Describes the findings from the Human Genome Project and their implications for individuals and society as a whole.*

Swartzberg, J. E., and S. Margen. 2001. *The Complete Home Wellness Handbook.* New York: Rebus. *Provides information and strategies for promoting health and well-being throughout the life span.*

Newsletters

Consumer Reports on Health (800-234-2188; http://www. ConsumerReports.org)

Harvard Health Letter (800-829-9045; http://www.health.harvard. edu/newsletters)

Harvard Men's Health Watch (800-829-3341)

Harvard Women's Health Watch (800-829-5921)

HealthNews (800-848-9155)

Mayo Clinic Health Letter (800-333-9037)

University of California at Berkeley Wellness Letter (904-445-6414; http://www.wellnessletter.com)

Organizations, Hotlines, and Web Sites

The Internet addresses (also called uniform resource locators, or URLs) listed here were accurate at the time of publication. Up-to-date links to these and many other wellness-oriented Web sites are provided on the links page of the *Core Concepts in Health* Web site (http://www.mhhe.com/insel9). Refer to Appendix C for tips on how to search for and evaluate information from the Internet.

Centers for Disease Control and Prevention. Through phone, fax, and the Internet, the CDC provides a wide variety of health information.

404-332-4555 (CDC Infoline); 888-CDC-FAXX (CDC FAX)
http://www.cdc.gov

Many other government Web sites provide access to health-related materials:

Agency for Healthcare Research and Quality: http://www.ahrq.gov/consumer
National Institutes of Health: http://www.nih.gov
National Library of Medicine, MedlinePlus: http://www.nlm.nih.gov/medlineplus
U.S. Consumer Gateway—Health: http://www.consumer.gov/health.htm

Go Ask Alice. Sponsored by the Columbia University Health Service, this site provides answers to student questions about stress, sexuality, fitness, and many other wellness topics.

http://www.goaskalice.columbia.edu

Healthfinder. A gateway to online publications, Web sites, support and self-help groups, and agencies and organizations that produce reliable health information.

http://www.healthfinder.gov

Healthy People 2010. Provides information on Healthy People objectives and priority areas.

202-205-8583; 301-468-5960
http://web.health.gov/healthypeople

National Health Information Center (NHIC). Puts consumers in touch with the organizations that are best able to provide answers to health-related questions.

800-336-4797
http://nhic-nt.health.org

National Women's Health Information Center. Provides information and answers to frequently asked questions.

800-994-WOMAN
http://www.4woman.org

NOAH: New York Online Access to Health. Provides consumer health information in both English and Spanish.

http://www.noah-health.org

The following are just a few of the many sites that provide consumer-oriented information on a variety of health issues:

InteliHealth: http://www.intelihealth.com
Mayo Health Oasis: http://www.mayohealth.org
Medscape Healthwatch: http://healthwatch.medscape.com
OnHealth: http://www.onhealth.com
WebMD: http://webmd.com

The following sites provide daily health news updates:

HealthScout: http://www.healthscout.com
Yahoo Health News: http://dailynews.yahoo.com/h/hl
Your Health Daily: http://www.yourhealthdaily.com

See also the listings in Appendix C.

SELECTED BIBLIOGRAPHY

American Cancer Society. 2001. *Cancer Facts and Figures—2001.* Atlanta: American Cancer Society.

American Heart Association. 2001. *2001 Heart and Stroke Statistical Update.* Dallas: American Heart Association.

Baker, C. 1999. *Your Genes, Your Choices: Exploring the Issues Raised by Genetic Research.* Washington, D.C.: American Association for the Advancement of Science.

Centers for Disease Control and Prevention. 1999. Achievements in public health, 1900–1999: Tobacco use, United States. *Morbidity and Mortality Weekly Report* 48(43): 986–993.

Centers for Disease Control and Prevention. 1999. Ten great public health achievements—United States, 1900–1999. *Morbidity and Mortality Weekly Report* 48(50): 1141.

Centers for Disease Control and Prevention. 2000. State- and sex-specific prevalence of selected characteristics—Behavioral Risk Factor Surveillance System. *MMWR Surveillance Summaries* 49(SS-6).

Centers for Disease Control and Prevention, Division of Nutrition and Physical Activity. 1999. *Promoting Physical Activity: A Guide for Community Action.* Champaign, Ill.: Human Kinetics.

Collins, F.S., and V. A. McKusick. 2001. Implications of the Human Genome Project for medical science. *Journal of the American Medical Association* 285(5): 540–544.

Cubbin, C., F. B. LeClere, and G. S. Smith. 2000. Socioeconomic status and the occurrence of fatal and nonfatal injury in the United States. *American Journal of Public Health* 90(1): 70–77.

Glanz, K., F. M. Lewis, and B. K. Rimer, eds. 1997. *Health Behavior and Health Education: Theory, Research, and Practice,* 2nd ed. San Francisco: Jossey-Bass.

Holtzman, N. A., and T. M. Marteau. 2000. Will genetics revolutionize medicine? *New England Journal of Medicine* 343(2): 141–144.

Martin, G., and J. Pear. 1999. *Behaviour Modification: What It Is and How to Do It,* 6th ed. Upper Saddle River, N.J.: Prentice-Hall.

Nathan, D. G., P. B. Fontanarosa, and J. D. Wilson. 2001. Opportunities for medical research in the 21st century. *Journal of the American Medical Association* 285(5): 533–534.

National Center for Health Statistics. 2000. *Health, United States, 2000, with Adolescent Health Chartbook.* Hyattsville, Md.: National Center for Health Statistics.

Office of Hawaiian Affairs. 1998. *Native Hawaiian Databook 1998* (http://oha.org/databook; retrieved July 21, 2000).

Pink slip in your genes. 2001. *Scientific American,* January.

Schank, M. J. 1999. Self-health appraisal: Learning the difficulties of lifestyle change. *Journal of Nursing Education* 38(1): 10–12.

Schlicht, J., J. Godin, and D. C. Camaione. 1999. How to help your clients stick with an exercise program: Build self-efficacy to promote exercise adherence. *ACSM's Health and Fitness Journal* 3(6): 27–31.

U.S. Bureau of the Census. 1999. *Poverty 1998* (http://www.census.gov/hhes/poverty/poverty98/pv98est1.html; retrieved August 1, 2000).

U. S. Bureau of the Census. 2001. *Census 2000 Brief: Overview of Race and Hispanic Origin.* Washington, D.C.: U.S. Bureau of the Census.

U.S. Department of Health and Human Services. 1999. *Eliminating Racial and Ethnic Disparities in Health* (http://raceandhealth.hhs.gov/sidebars/sbinitOver.htm; retrieved July 31, 2000).

U.S. Department of Health and Human Services. 2000. *Healthy People 2010.* 2nd ed. Washington, D.C.: DHHS.

U.S. Department of Health and Human Services, Office of Minority Health. 1998. *Asian Americans and Pacific Islanders: Executive Overview* (http://www.omhrc.gov/overview2.htm; retrieved July 31, 2000).

Zimmerman, G. L., C. G. Olsen, and M. F. Bosworth. 2000. A "stages of change" approach to helping patients change behavior. *American Family Physician* 61(5): 1409–1416.

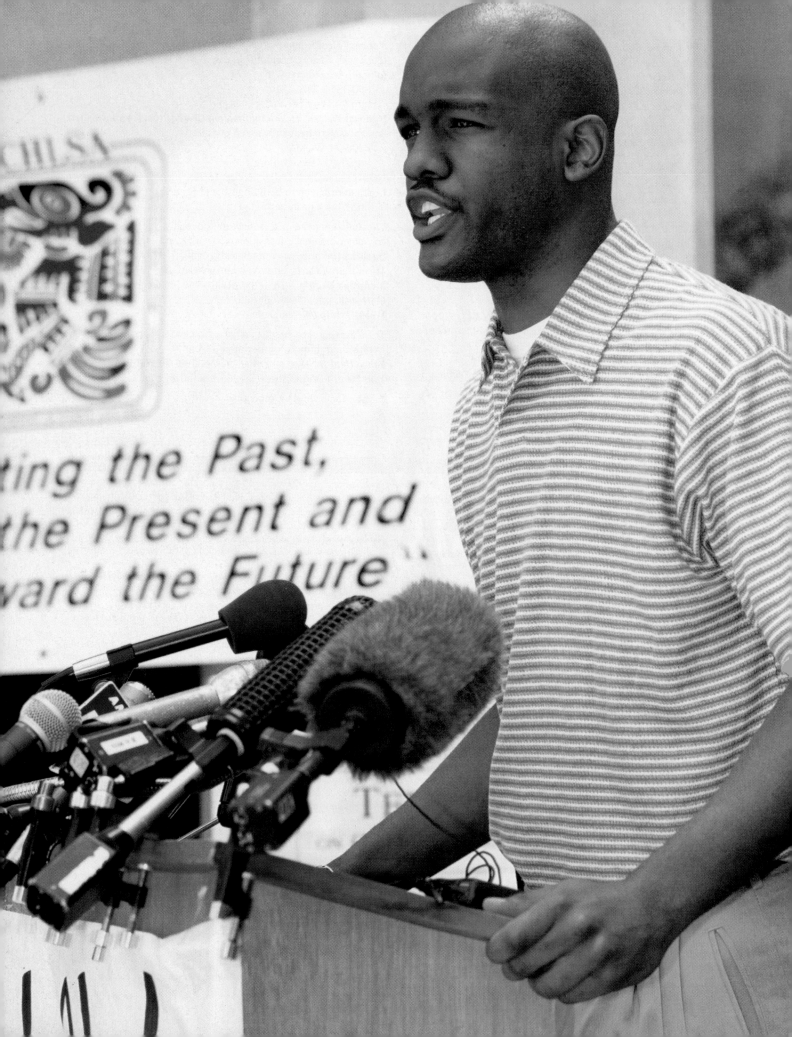

After reading this chapter, you should be able to

- Explain what stress is and how people react to it—physically, emotionally, and behaviorally

- Describe the relationship between stress and disease

- List common sources of stress

- Describe techniques for preventing and managing stress

- Put together a step-by-step plan for successfully managing the stress in your life

Stress: The Constant Challenge

2

TEST YOUR KNOWLEDGE

1. Which of the following events can cause stress?
   a. taking out a loan
   b. failing a test
   c. graduating from college
   d. watching a hockey game

2. About twice as many male college students as female college students report feeling frequently overwhelmed.
   True or false?

3. High levels of stress can impair memory and cause physical changes in the brain.
   True or false?

4. Which of the following may be caused or aggravated by stress?
   a. headaches
   b. irritable bowel syndrome
   c. insomnia
   d. high blood pressure

5. About how many car crashes each year are caused by drowsy driving?
   a. 10,000
   b. 100,000
   c. 200,000

ANSWERS

1. **ALL FOUR.** Stress-producing factors can be pleasant or unpleasant and can include physical challenges and the achievement of personal goals as well as what would commonly be perceived as negative events.

2. **FALSE.** In recent surveys, about 20% of male and 40% of female college students report feeling frequently overwhelmed. Female college students are more likely to report financial worries, and they spend more time in potentially stress-producing activities such as volunteer work, housework, and child care.

3. **TRUE.** Low levels of stress may improve memory, but high stress levels impair learning and memory and, over the long term, may shrink an area of the brain called the hippocampus.

4. **ALL FOUR.** Stress—interacting with heredity, personality, social environment, and behavior—increases one's vulnerability to many health problems.

5. **C.** Among drivers age 18–29, 60% report driving while drowsy, and nearly 25% say they have fallen asleep at the wheel. Driving while drowsy is nearly as dangerous as driving while intoxicated.

Everybody talks about stress. People say they're "overstressed" or "stressed out." They may blame stress for headaches or ulcers, and they may try to combat stress with aerobics classes—or drugs. But what is stress? And why is it important to manage it wisely?

Most people associate stress with negative events: the death of a close relative or friend, financial problems, or other unpleasant life changes that create nervous tension. But stress isn't merely nervous tension. And it isn't something to be avoided at all costs. In fact, only death brings complete freedom from stress. Before we explore more fully what stress is, consider this list of common stressful situations or events:

- Interviewing for a job
- Running in a race
- Being accepted to college
- Going out on a date
- Watching a basketball game
- Getting a promotion

Obviously, stress doesn't arise just from unpleasant situations. Stress can also be associated with physical challenges and the achievement of personal goals. Physical and psychological stress-producing factors can be pleasant or unpleasant. The actions you take in response to stress are influenced by your biological predispositions, past experiences, and current circumstances. While you cannot change who you are or what you've been through in the past, you *can* modify your current behavior and seek out people, places, and experiences that will improve your ability to deal with stress. In other words, what is crucial is how you respond, whether in positive, life-enhancing ways or in negative, counterproductive ways.

Terms

stressor Any physical or psychological event or condition that produces stress.

stress response The physiological changes associated with stress.

stress The collective physiological and emotional responses to any stimulus that disturbs an individual's homeostasis.

autonomic nervous system The branch of the peripheral nervous system that, largely without conscious thought, controls basic body processes; consists of the sympathetic and parasympathetic divisions.

parasympathetic division A division of the autonomic system that moderates the excitatory effect of the sympathetic division, slowing metabolism and restoring energy supplies.

sympathetic division A division of the autonomic nervous system that reacts to danger or other challenges by almost instantly accelerating body processes.

endocrine system The system of glands, tissues, and cells that secrete hormones into the bloodstream to influence metabolism and other body processes.

hormone A chemical messenger produced in the body and transported by the bloodstream to target cells or organs for specific regulation of their activities.

As a college student, you may be in one of the most stressful periods of your life (see the box "How High Is Your Stress Level?"). You may be on your own for the first time, or you may be juggling the demands of college with the responsibilities of a job, a family, or both. Financial pressures may be intense. Housing and transportation may be sources of additional hassles. You're also meeting new people, engaging in new activities, learning new information and skills, and setting a new course for your life. Good and bad, all these changes and challenges are likely to have a powerful effect on you, both physically and psychologically. Respond ineffectively to stress, and eventually it will take a toll on your sense of wellness. Learn effective responses, however, and you will enhance your health and gain a feeling of control over your life.

How do you know when your stress level is getting dangerously high? How can you develop techniques to cope positively with the stress that is part of your life? This chapter will help you discover answers to these questions.

WHAT IS STRESS?

Just what is stress, if such vastly different situations can cause it? In common usage, "stress" refers to two different things: situations that trigger physical and emotional reactions *and* the reactions themselves. In this text, we'll use the more precise term **stressor** for situations that trigger physical and emotional reactions and the term **stress response** for those reactions. A date and a final exam, then, are stressors; sweaty palms and a pounding heart are symptoms of the stress response. We'll use the term **stress** to describe the general physical and emotional state that accompanies the stress response. A person on a date or taking a final exam experiences stress.

Each individual's experience of stress depends on many factors, including the nature of the stressor and how the stressor is perceived. Responses to stressors include physical changes and emotional and behavioral responses.

Physical Responses to Stressors

Imagine you are waiting to cross a street, perhaps daydreaming about a movie you saw last week. The light turns green and you step off the curb. Almost before you see it, you feel a car speeding toward you. With just a fraction of a second to spare, you leap safely out of harm's way. In that split second of danger and in the moments following it, you have experienced a predictable series of physical reactions. Your body has gone from a relaxed state to one prepared for physical action to cope with a threat to your life.

Two major control systems in your body are responsible for your physical response to stressors: the nervous

Many symptoms of excess stress are easy to self-diagnose. To help determine how much stress you experience on a daily basis, answer the following questions.

1. How many of the symptoms of excess stress listed in the table below do you experience frequently?

2. Are you easily startled or irritated?

3. Are you increasingly forgetful?

4. Do you have trouble falling or staying asleep?

5. Do you continually worry about events in your future?

6. Do you feel as if you are constantly under pressure to produce?

7. Do you frequently use tobacco, alcohol, or other drugs to help you relax?

8. Do you often feel as if you have less energy than you need to finish the day?

9. Do you have recurrent stomachaches or headaches?

10. Is it difficult for you to find satisfaction in simple life pleasures?

11. Are you often disappointed in yourself and others?

12. Are you overly concerned with being liked or accepted by others?

13. Have you lost interest in intimacy or sex?

14. Are you concerned that you do not have enough money?

Experiencing some of the stress-related symptoms or answering "yes" to a few questions is normal. However, if you experience a large number of stress symptoms or you answered "yes" to a majority of the questions, you are likely experiencing a high level of stress. Take time out to develop effective stress-management techniques. Many coping strategies that can aid you in dealing with your college stressors are described in this chapter. Additionally, your school's counseling center can provide valuable support.

Symptoms of Excess Stress

Physical Symptoms	Emotional Symptoms	Behavioral Symptoms
Dry mouth	Anxiety or edginess	Crying
Excessive perspiration	Depression	Disrupted eating habits
Frequent illnesses	Fatigue	Disrupted sleeping habits
Gastrointestinal problems	Hypervigilance	Harsh treatment of others
Grinding of teeth	Impulsiveness	Increased use of tobacco, alcohol, or other drugs
Headaches	Inability to concentrate	
High blood pressure	Irritability	Problems communicating
Pounding heart	Trouble remembering things	Sexual problems
Stiff neck or aching lower back		Social isolation

system and the endocrine system. Through a variety of rapid chemical reactions affecting almost every part of your body, you are primed to act quickly and appropriately in time of danger.

Actions of the Nervous System The nervous system consists primarily of the brain, spinal cord, and nerves. Part of the nervous system is under voluntary control: commanding your arm to reach for a chocolate, for instance. The part that is not under conscious supervision, such as what controls the digestion of the chocolate, is known as the **autonomic nervous system.** In addition to digestion, it controls heart rate, breathing, blood pressure, and hundreds of other functions you normally take for granted.

The autonomic nervous system consists of two divisions. The **parasympathetic division** is in control when you are relaxed; it aids in digesting food, storing energy, and promoting growth. In contrast, the **sympathetic division** is activated during arousal or when there is an emergency, such as severe pain, anger, or fear. Sympathetic nerves act on many targets—on nearly every organ, sweat gland, blood vessel, and muscle, in fact—to enable your body to handle an emergency. In general, it commands your body to stop storing energy and instead to mobilize all energy resources to respond to the crisis.

Actions of the Endocrine System One important target of the sympathetic nervous system is the **endocrine system.** This system of glands, tissues, and cells helps control body functions by releasing **hormones** and other chemical messengers into the bloodstream. Chemicals released into the blood are relatively free to travel throughout the body. The sites of action for circulating stress

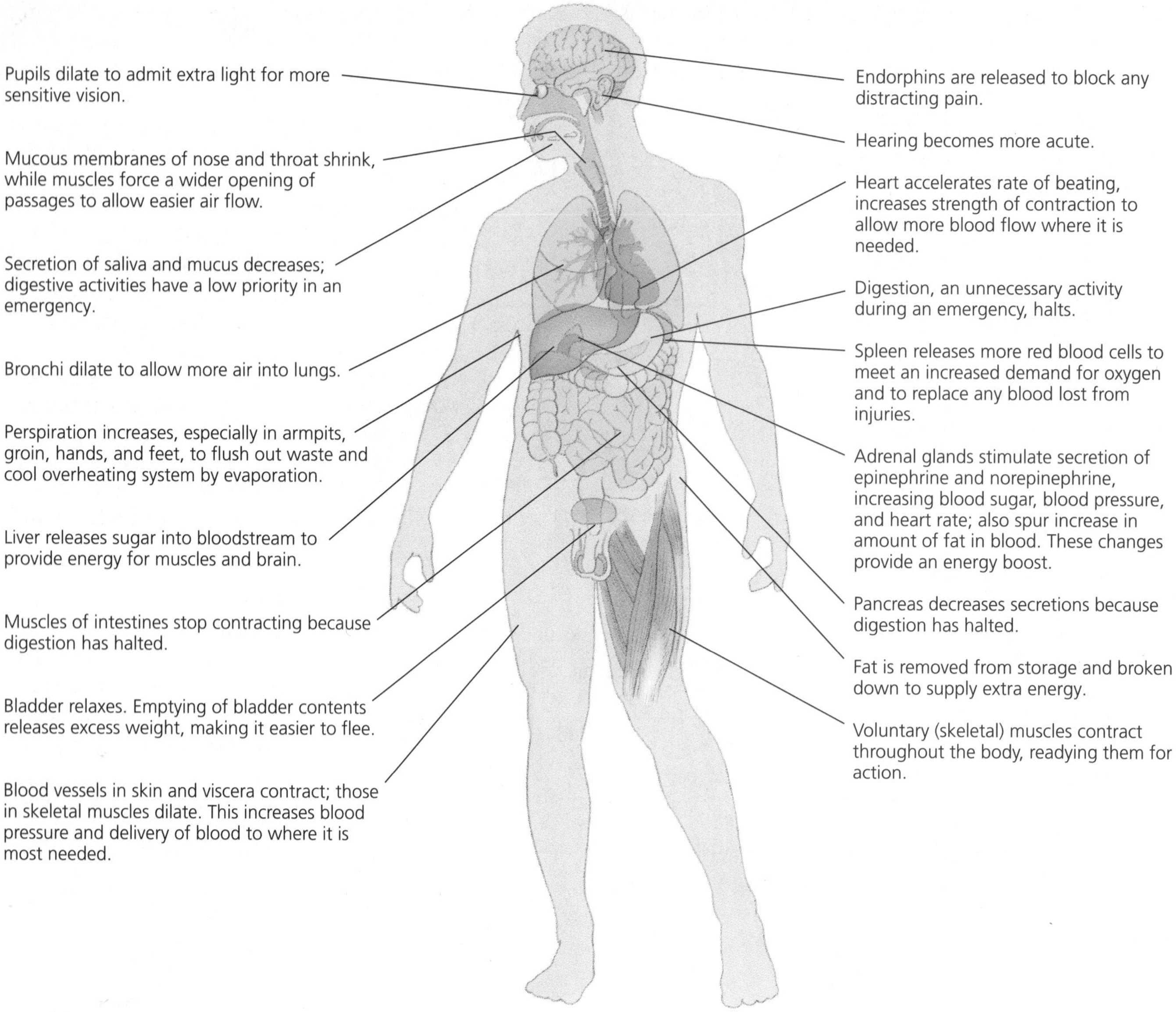

Pupils dilate to admit extra light for more sensitive vision.

Mucous membranes of nose and throat shrink, while muscles force a wider opening of passages to allow easier air flow.

Secretion of saliva and mucus decreases; digestive activities have a low priority in an emergency.

Bronchi dilate to allow more air into lungs.

Perspiration increases, especially in armpits, groin, hands, and feet, to flush out waste and cool overheating system by evaporation.

Liver releases sugar into bloodstream to provide energy for muscles and brain.

Muscles of intestines stop contracting because digestion has halted.

Bladder relaxes. Emptying of bladder contents releases excess weight, making it easier to flee.

Blood vessels in skin and viscera contract; those in skeletal muscles dilate. This increases blood pressure and delivery of blood to where it is most needed.

Endorphins are released to block any distracting pain.

Hearing becomes more acute.

Heart accelerates rate of beating, increases strength of contraction to allow more blood flow where it is needed.

Digestion, an unnecessary activity during an emergency, halts.

Spleen releases more red blood cells to meet an increased demand for oxygen and to replace any blood lost from injuries.

Adrenal glands stimulate secretion of epinephrine and norepinephrine, increasing blood sugar, blood pressure, and heart rate; also spur increase in amount of fat in blood. These changes provide an energy boost.

Pancreas decreases secretions because digestion has halted.

Fat is removed from storage and broken down to supply extra energy.

Voluntary (skeletal) muscles contract throughout the body, readying them for action.

Figure 2-1 The fight-or-flight reaction. In response to a stressor, the autonomic nervous system and the endocrine system cause physical changes that prepare the body to deal with an emergency.

hormones are determined by specialized receptors in target tissues. Thus, stress hormones will act only on those organs that have stress hormone receptors. Along with the nervous system with which it closely interacts, the endocrine system helps prepare the body to respond to a stressor.

The Two Systems Together   How do both systems work together in an emergency? Let's go back to your close call with that car. As you first sense the car speeding toward you, your sympathetic nervous system prompts the **hypothalamus,** a control center in the brain, to release a chemical messenger to the nearby **pituitary gland.** In turn, the pituitary gland releases **adrenocorticotropic hormone**

(ACTH) into the bloodstream. When ACTH reaches the **adrenal glands,** located just above the kidneys, it stimulates them to release **cortisol** and other key hormones into the bloodstream. Simultaneously, sympathetic nerves instruct your adrenal glands to release the hormones **epinephrine,** or adrenaline, and **norepinephrine,** which in turn trigger a series of profound changes as they circulate throughout your body (Figure 2-1). Your hearing and vision become more acute. Bronchi dilate to allow more air into your lungs. Your heart rate accelerates and blood pressure increases to ensure that your blood—and the oxygen, nutrients, and hormones it carries—will be rapidly distributed where needed. Your liver releases extra sugar into your bloodstream to provide an energy boost for your muscles and brain. Your digestion halts. You perspire more to cool your skin. **Endorphins** are released to relieve pain in case of injury. Blood cell production increases.

Taken together, these almost-instantaneous physical changes are called the **fight-or-flight reaction.** They give you the heightened reflexes and strength you need to dodge the car or deal with other stressors. Although these physical changes may vary in intensity, the same basic set of physical reactions occurs in response to any type of stressor, positive or negative.

The Return to Homeostasis Why doesn't your body remain in a hypervigilant state, perpetually ready for action? Why shouldn't your body always be prepared for a crisis? As you have probably guessed, it would be too exhausting. Your body actually resists dramatic changes. Whenever normal functioning is disrupted, such as during the fight-or-flight reaction, your body strives for **homeostasis,** a state in which blood pressure, heart rate, hormone levels, and other vital functions are maintained within a narrow range of normal.

Once a stressful situation ends, the parasympathetic division of your autonomic nervous system takes command and halts the reaction. It initiates the adjustments necessary to restore homeostasis. Your parasympathetic nervous system calms your body down, slowing a rapid heartbeat, drying sweaty palms, and returning breathing to normal. Gradually, your body resumes its normal "housekeeping" functions, such as digestion and temperature regulation. Damage that may have been sustained during the fight-or-flight reaction is repaired. The day after you narrowly dodge the car, you wake up feeling fine. In this way, your body can grow, repair itself, and acquire reserves of energy. When the next crisis comes, you'll be ready to respond—instantly—again.

The Fight-or-Flight Reaction in Modern Life The fight-or-flight reaction is a part of our biological heritage, a survival mechanism that has served humankind well. It enables our bodies to quickly prepare to escape from an injury or to engage in a physical battle. In modern life, however, the fight-or-flight reaction is often absurdly inappropriate. Many of the stressors we face in everyday life do not require a physical response—for example, an exam, a mess left by a roommate, or a red traffic light. The fight-or-flight reaction prepares the body for physical action regardless of whether such action is a necessary or appropriate response to a particular stressor.

Emotional and Behavioral Responses to Stressors

The physical response to a stressor may vary in intensity from person to person and situation to situation, but we all experience a similar set of physical changes—the fight-or-flight reaction. However, there is a great deal of variation in how people view potential stressors and how people respond to them. For example, you may feel confident about taking exams but be nervous about talking to people don't know, while your roommate may love challenging social situations but be very nervous about taking tests. Many factors, some external and some internal, help explain these differences. Your cognitive appraisal of a potential stressor will influence how a particular stressor is viewed. Two factors that can reduce the magnitude of the stress response are successful prediction and the perception of having some control over the stressor. For instance, obtaining course syllabi at the beginning of the term allows you to predict the timing of major deadlines and exams. Having this predictive knowledge also allows you to exert some control over your study and recreation plans and can thus help reduce the stress caused by exams.

Emotional and behavioral responses to stressors also vary among individuals. A poor grade on a group project may prompt you to go for a 10-mile jog, while other members of your project team respond by eating chocolate or getting drunk. Let's take a closer look at the effects and causes of these differing patterns of emotional and behavioral responses.

Effective and Ineffective Responses Our emotional and behavioral responses to stressors are as critical to our overall experience of stress as are our physical responses. Common emotional responses to stressors include anxiety, depression, and fear. Although emotional responses are determined in part by inborn personality, we often can

Terms

hypothalamus A part of the brain that activates, controls, and integrates the autonomic mechanisms, endocrine activities, and many body functions.

pituitary gland The "master gland," closely linked with the hypothalamus, that controls other endocrine glands and secretes hormones that regulate growth, maturation, and reproduction.

adrenocorticotropic hormone (ACTH) A hormone, formed in the pituitary gland, that stimulates the outer layer of the adrenal gland to secrete its hormones.

adrenal glands Two glands, one lying atop each kidney, their outer layer (cortex) producing steroid hormones such as cortisol, and their inner core (medulla) producing the hormones epinephrine and norepinephrine.

cortisol A steroid hormone secreted by the cortex (outer layer) of the adrenal gland; also called *hydrocortisone.*

epinephrine A hormone secreted by the medulla (inner core) of the adrenal gland; also called *adrenaline,* the "fear hormone."

norepinephrine A hormone secreted by the medulla (inner core) of the adrenal gland; also called *noradrenaline,* the "anger hormone."

endorphins Brain secretions that have pain-inhibiting effects.

fight-or-flight reaction A defense reaction that prepares an individual for conflict or escape by triggering hormonal, cardiovascular, metabolic, and other changes.

homeostasis A state of stability and consistency in an individual's physiological functioning.

learn to control them. Coping techniques are
detail later in the chapter.
...ioral responses—controlled by the **somatic**
...tem, which manages our conscious actions
...our control. Effective behavioral responses
...wellness and enable us to function at our
best. Ineffective behavioral responses to stressors can impair wellness and can even become stressors themselves. Depending on the stressor involved, effective behavioral responses may include talking, laughing, exercising, meditating, learning time-management skills, or finding a more compatible roommate. Inappropriate behavioral responses include overeating and using tobacco, alcohol, or other drugs.

Let's consider the different emotional and behavioral responses of two students, Amelia and David, to a common stressor: the first exam of the semester. Both students feel anxious as the exam is passed out. Amelia relaxes her muscles and starts by writing the answers she knows. On a second pass through the exam, she concentrates carefully on the wording of each question. Some material comes back to her, and she makes educated guesses on the remaining items. She spends the whole hour writing as much as she can and checking her answers. She leaves the room feeling calm, relaxed, and confident that she has done well on the exam.

David responds to his initial anxiety with more anxiety. He finds that he doesn't know some of the answers, and he becomes more worried. The more upset he gets, the less he can remember; and the more he blanks out, the more anxious he gets. He begins to imagine the consequences of failing the course and berates himself for not having studied more. David turns in his paper before the hour is up, without checking his answers or going back to the questions he skipped. He leaves feeling depressed and angry at himself.

As you can see, although both Amelia and David experienced the physical stress response as the exam was passed out, their emotional and behavioral responses were quite different—and led to very different outcomes. What determines these differences? Emotional and behavioral responses to stressors depend on a complex set of factors that includes personality, cultural background, gender, and past experiences.

Personality and Stress Some people seem to be nervous, irritable, and easily upset by minor annoyances; others are calm and composed even in difficult situations.

Scientists remain unsure just why this is or how the brain's complex emotional mechanisms work. But personality, the sum of behavioral and emotional tendencies, clearly affects how an individual perceives and reacts to stressors. To investigate the links among personality, stress, and overall wellness, researchers have looked at different constellations of characteristics, or "personality types."

TYPE A AND B PERSONALITIES   The potential link between stress and heart disease has been the subject of research for many years. Cardiologists Meyer Friedman and Ray Rosenman reported that people with certain personality characteristics had a higher incidence of heart disease than people with other characteristics. They describe people with "Type A personalities" as ultracompetitive, controlling, impatient, aggressive, and hostile. Type A people tend to react more explosively to stressors, and they are upset by events that others would consider only mild annoyances. On the other hand, Type B individuals are relaxed, contemplative, and much less hurried. They tend to be less frustrated by the flow of daily events and more tolerant of the behavior of others.

Early studies indicated that Type A people have a greater risk of heart disease. However, recent evidence suggests that only particular characteristics of the Type A pattern—anger, cynicism, and hostility—increase the heart disease risk. (The link between hostility and heart disease is discussed further in Chapter 15.) What about Type A traits and other aspects of health? Studies indicate that Type A people may have a higher perceived stress level and more problems coping with stress.

THE HARDY PERSONALITY   Researchers have also looked at personality traits that seem to enable people to deal more successfully with stress. Psychologist Suzanne Kobasa examined "hardiness," a particular form of optimism. She found that people with a hardy personality view potential stressors as challenges and opportunities for growth and learning, rather than as burdens. Hardy people tend to perceive fewer situations as stressful, and their reaction to stressors tends to be less intense. They are committed to their activities, have a sense of inner purpose, and feel at least partly in control of events in their lives.

People with a hardy personality typically have an internal locus of control. As described in Chapter 1, this means that they feel responsible for their own actions and in control of many of the events in their lives. This sense of control helps them cope with stress in a more positive way and put setbacks in proper perspective. People with an external locus of control—a belief that the events in their lives are controlled by outside factors—typically have more difficulties with stress. A person with an external locus of control may feel helpless in a stressful situation

Terms   **somatic nervous system** The branch of the peripheral nervous system that governs motor functions and sensory information; largely under our conscious control.

gender role A culturally expected pattern of behavior and attitudes determined by whether a person is male or female.

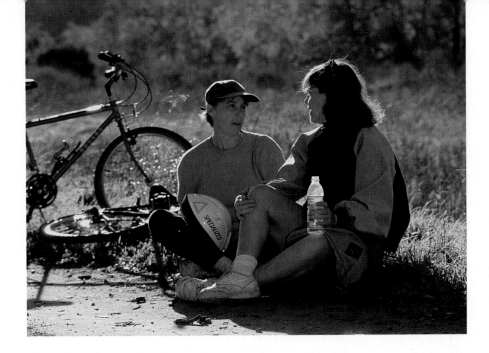

A person's emotional and behavioral responses to stressors depend on many different factors, including personality, gender, and cultural background. Research suggests that women are more likely than men to respond to stressors by seeking social support.

and believe it's pointless to make constructive attempts to deal with stressors.

Is there anything people can do to change their personality and become more stress-resistant? It is unlikely that you can change your basic personality. However, you can change your typical behaviors and patterns of thinking and develop positive techniques for coping with stressors. Strategies for successful stress management are described later in the chapter.

Cultural Background   We all know that cultural stereotypes are exaggerations and that a variety of personalities exist within every ethnic group. However, people of various cultures do differ in their values, lifestyles, and what they consider to be acceptable behavior. It's not surprising that dealing with stress is also influenced by the family and the culture in which you are brought up. Even whether you perceive a situation to be stressful or not will depend on your upbringing. Suppose you go out on a date with someone who doesn't say much. You might worry that the person is behaving this way because he or she doesn't like you, and you may experience stress as a result. If you are quiet by nature and because of your cultural background, you'll probably feel things are going just fine.

Gender   Like cultural background, our **gender role**—the activities, abilities, and behaviors our culture expects of us based on whether we're male or female—also affects our experience of stress. Some behavioral responses to stressors, such as crying or openly expressing anger, may be deemed more appropriate for one gender than the other. Strict adherence to gender roles can thus place limits on how a person responds to stress and can itself become a source of stress. Adherence to traditional gender roles can also affect the perception of a potential stressor. For example, if a man derives most of his sense of self-worth from his work, retirement may be a more stressful life change for him than for a woman whose self-image is based on several different roles.

Oxytocin, a hormone involved in social interaction and the regulation of mood, may underlie some of the gender differences in behavioral responses to stressors. Women produce more oxytocin than men, and the female hormone estrogen enhances its effects. Although both men and women experience the fight-or-flight physiological response to stress, women are more likely to respond behaviorally with a pattern of "tend-and-befriend"— nurturing friends and family and seeking social support and social contacts. Rather than becoming aggressive or withdrawing from difficult situations, women are more likely to act to create and enhance their social networks in ways that reduce stress.

Past Experiences   Your past experiences significantly influence your response to stressors. For example, if you were unprepared for the first speech you gave in your speech class and performed poorly, you will probably experience greater anxiety in response to future assignments. If you had performed better, your confidence and sense of control would increase, and you would probably experience less stress with future speeches. Effective behavioral responses, such as careful preparation and visualizing yourself giving a successful speech, can help overcome the effects of negative past experiences.

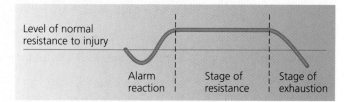

Figure 2-2   The general adaptation syndrome.   Selye observed a predictable sequence of responses to stress. During the alarm phase, a lower resistance to injury is evident. With continued stress, resistance to injury is actually enhanced. With prolonged exposure to repeated stressors, exhaustion sets in, with a return of low resistance levels seen during acute stress.

The Stress Experience as a Whole

Physical, emotional, and behavioral responses to stressors are intimately interrelated. The more intense the emotional response, the stronger the physical response. Effective behavioral responses can reduce stress; ineffective ones only worsen it. Sometimes people have such intense emotional responses and such ineffective or counterproductive behavioral responses to stressors that they need professional help for learning to cope. More often, however, people can learn to handle stressors on their own. Actions you can take to successfully deal with the stress in your life are described later in the chapter.

STRESS AND DISEASE

The role of stress in health and disease is complex, and much remains to be learned about the exact mechanisms by which stress influences health. However, mounting evidence suggests that stress—interacting with a person's genetic predisposition, personality, social environment, and health-related behaviors—can increase vulnerability to numerous ailments. A variety of related theories have been proposed to explain the relationship between stress and disease.

The General Adaptation Syndrome

Biologist Hans Selye, working in the 1930s and 1940s, was one of the first scientists to develop a comprehensive theory of stress and disease. Selye coined the term **general adaptation syndrome (GAS)** to describe what he believed was a universal and predictable response pattern to all stressors. He recognized that stressors could be pleasant, such as attending a party, or unpleasant, such as getting a flat tire or a bad grade. He called stress triggered by a pleasant stressor **eustress** and stress triggered by an unpleasant stressor **distress.** The sequence of physical responses associated with GAS is the same for both eustress and distress and occurs in three stages: alarm, resistance, and exhaustion (Figure 2-2).

Alarm   This stage includes the complex sequence of events brought on by the activation of the sympathetic nervous system and the endocrine system—the fight-or-flight

reaction. During this stage, the body is more susceptible to disease or injury because it is geared up to deal with a crisis. A person in this phase may experience headaches, indigestion, and anxiety. Sleeping and eating patterns may also be disrupted.

Resistance   With continued stress, Selye theorized that the body developed a new level of homeostasis in which it was more resistant to disease and injury than it normally would be. During the resistance stage, a person can cope with normal life and added stress.

Exhaustion   As you might imagine, both the mobilization of forces during the alarm reaction and the maintenance of homeostasis during the resistance stage require a considerable amount of energy. If a stressor persists or if several stressors occur in succession, general exhaustion results. This is not the sort of exhaustion people complain of after a long, busy day. It's a life-threatening type of physiological exhaustion characterized by such symptoms as distorted perceptions and disorganized thinking.

Allostatic Load

While Selye's model of GAS is still viewed as a key contribution to modern stress theory, some aspects of it are now discounted. For example, increased susceptibility to disease after repeated or prolonged stress is now thought to be due to the effects of the stress response itself rather than to a depletion of resources (Selye's exhaustion state). In particular, long-term overexposure to stress hormones such as cortisol has been linked with health problems. Researchers have termed the long-term wear and tear of the stress response the *allostatic load.* An individual's allostatic load is dependent on many factors, including genetics, life experiences, and emotional and behavioral responses to stressors. A high allostatic load may be due to frequent stressors, poor adaptation to common stressors, an inability to shut down the stress response, or imbalances in the stress response of different body systems.

Researchers have linked high allostatic load with heart disease, hypertension, obesity, and reduced brain and immune system functioning. In other words, when your allostatic load exceeds your ability to cope, you are more likely to get sick.

Psychoneuroimmunology

One of the most fruitful areas of current research into the relationship between stress and disease is **psychoneuroimmunology (PNI)**. PNI is the study of the interactions among the nervous system, the endocrine system, and the immune system. The underlying premise of PNI is that stress, through the actions of the nervous and endocrine systems, impairs the immune system and thereby affects health.

Researchers have discovered a complex network of nerve and chemical connections between the nervous and endocrine systems and the immune system. We have already seen that the hormones and other chemical messengers released during the stress response produce profound physical changes to prepare the body to deal with a stressor. These compounds also affect the immune system. For example, increased levels of cortisol are linked to a decreased number of immune system cells, or lymphocytes. Epinephrine and norepinephrine appear to promote the release of lymphocytes but at the same time reduce their efficiency. Activation of the sympathetic nervous system during the stress response also affects the immune system because certain nervous system fibers directly connect the brain to tissues and organs that produce lymphocytes.

The nervous, endocrine, and immune systems share other connections. Scientists have identified hormone-like substances called neuropeptides that appear to translate emotions into physiological events. Neuropeptides are produced and received by both brain and immune cells, so that the brain and the immune system share a biochemical "language," which is also the language of emotions. The biochemical changes that accompany particular emotions can strongly influence the functioning of the immune system; some emotions may suppress lymphocyte function, while others promote it.

Why would you want a system in your body that decreases immune function? One reason might be that an overactive immune system can produce autoimmune diseases such as lupus. Autoimmune diseases occur when your immune system mistakenly identifies your body's own cells as foreign intruders and begins to attack them as it would viruses or bacteria. The stress response helps prevent the immune system from becoming overzealous: When levels of interleukins, chemical messengers used by immune cells, become too high, the stress response is activated, tempering immune function. However, when stress levels are too high, immune suppression may not only prevent autoimmune disorders but also reduce the immune system's ability to fight infection and retard disease progression. (See Chapter 17 for more on immune function and autoimmune diseases.)

The degree to which stress affects the immune system and the way in which immune system changes influence health are still being investigated. However, research indicates that stress does affect immunity and health in both the short and long term. Studies of students have found that concentrations of immune cells drop during the period of final exams. Investigators have also found that the long-term stress of caring for someone with Alzheimer's disease is associated with reduced immune function.

Links Between Stress and Specific Conditions

Although much remains to be learned, it is clear that people who have unresolved chronic stress in their lives or who handle stressors poorly are at risk for a wide range of health problems. In the short term, the problem might just be a cold, a stiff neck, or a stomachache. Over the long term, the problems can be more severe—cardiovascular disease, high blood pressure, or impairment of the immune system.

Cardiovascular Disease During the stress response, heart rate increases and blood vessels constrict, causing blood pressure to rise. Chronic high blood pressure is a major cause of **atherosclerosis,** a disease in which the lining of the blood vessels becomes damaged and caked with fatty deposits. These deposits can block arteries, causing heart attacks and strokes.

Recent research suggests that certain types of emotional responses increase a person's risk of cardiovascular disease. So-called hot reactors, people who exhibit extreme increases in heart rate and blood pressure in response to emotional stressors, may face an increased risk of cardiovascular problems. As described earlier in the section on Type A personality, people who tend to react to situations with anger and hostility are more likely to have heart attacks than are people with a less explosive, more trusting personality. (For further discussion of heart disease and trust, see Chapter 15.)

general adaptation syndrome (GAS) A pattern of stress responses consisting of three stages: alarm, resistance, and exhaustion.

eustress Stress resulting from a pleasant stressor.

distress Stress resulting from an unpleasant stressor.

psychoneuroimmunology (PNI) The study of the interactions among the brain, the endocrine system, and the immune system.

atherosclerosis The buildup of hard yellow plaques of fatty material in the lining of arteries that have become damaged from advancing age or high blood pressure; a leading cause of heart disease and stroke.

Terms

Like a computer that registers information in response to typing on a keyboard, your brain is able to respond to and store information about changes in your environment. Unlike a computer, your brain has the attribute of plasticity—it physically changes its structure and function in response to experience. Also unlike a computer, your brain is altered by psychological stress. Moderate stress enhances the ability to acquire information and remember daily events, while high levels of acute stress can impair learning. For example, people can often remember minute details following a fender bender but can't recall the events surrounding a major car crash. Thus, it is good to be a little bit nervous before an exam—but not highly anxious.

The effects of stress on brain form and function are apparent in a structure called the hippocampus, which is involved in learning and memory. High levels of chronic stress cause brain cells (neurons) in the hippocampus to shrink in size or die, thus impairing learning and memory. Exciting new research in neuroscience has revealed that the hippocampus actually grows new neurons during adulthood. However, stress acts to reduce new cell birth in the hippocampus, reducing the replacement of lost neurons. Together, these effects of stress result in fewer neurons and fewer connections between neurons in the hippocampus, thus decreasing the capacity for information processing. People who are depressed or who suffer from post-traumatic stress disorder have higher levels of stress hormones in their bloodstream and smaller hippocampi than others. Even in the absence of a serious disorder, it is thought that the accumulation of stress effects across the life span can contribute to brain aging. Thus, the way you cope with stress can affect the way your brain works both immediately and over the long term.

Altered Functioning of the Immune System   Sometimes you seem to get sick when you can least afford it—during exam week, when you're going on vacation, or when you have a big job interview. As research in PNI suggests, this is more than mere coincidence. Some of the health problems linked to stress-related changes in immune function include the following:

- *Colds and other infections.* Stress can leave people more vulnerable to contracting a cold and less able to fight one off.

- *Asthma and allergies.* Stress is a trigger or aggravator of asthma, hives, eczema, and other allergies.

- *Cancer.* One of the functions of the immune system is recognizing and destroying any abnormal cells produced in the body; left unchecked, such cells can develop into cancerous tumors. Stress does not cause cancer, but by compromising the immune system, it may increase a person's chance of developing cancer and decrease her or his chance of surviving it.

- *Chronic disease flare-ups.* Symptoms of chronic diseases such as genital herpes, HIV infection, and diabetes may flare up during episodes of stress. In addition to decreasing the effectiveness of the immune system, stress may also distract people from their commitment to important disease-management behaviors like eating a healthy diet, exercising, and taking medications.

Psychological Problems   The hormones and other chemicals released during the stress response cause emotional as well as physical changes (see the box "Stress and Your Brain"). Moreover, many stressors—a hurricane, for example, or the death of a loved one—are inherently anxiety-producing, depressing, or both. Stress has been found to contribute to such psychological problems as depression, panic attacks, anxiety, eating disorders, and post-traumatic stress disorder (PTSD). PTSD, which afflicts war veterans, rape and child abuse survivors, and others who have suffered or witnessed severe trauma, is characterized by nightmares, flashbacks, and a diminished capacity to experience or express emotion. (For more information on psychological problems, see Chapter 3.)

Other Health Problems   Many other health problems may be caused or worsened by uncontrolled stress, including the following:

- *Digestive problems.* Stress is associated with stomachaches, diarrhea, and constipation, and it may aggravate problems such as irritable bowel syndrome and ulcers.

- *Headaches.* Muscle contractions and changes in blood vessels associated with the stress response can cause tension headaches and trigger migraines (see the box "Headaches: A Common Symptom of Stress").

- *Insomnia and fatigue.* Chemical messengers produced during the fight-or-flight reaction promote alertness and ward off sleep. Sleep disruption in turn can produce fatigue.

- *Injuries.* Stress may distract people and cause them to become less vigilant about key injury prevention behaviors such as wearing a safety belt or bicycle helmet. On-the-job injuries, including repetitive-strain injury (RSI), are also linked to job stress.

Are you among the more than 45 million Americans who have chronic, recurrent headaches? Headaches come in various types but are often grouped into three major categories: tension headaches, migraines, and cluster headaches. Other types of headaches have underlying organic causes, such as sinus congestion or infection.

Tension Headaches

Approximately 90% of all headaches are tension headaches, characterized by a dull, steady pain, usually on both sides of the head. It may feel as though a band of pressure is tightening around the head, and the pain may extend to the neck and shoulders. Acute tension headaches may last from hours to days, while chronic tension headaches may occur almost every day for months or even years. Psychological stress, poor posture, and immobility are the leading causes of tension headaches. There is no cure, but the pain can be relieved with over-the-counter painkillers and with therapies such as massage, relaxation, hot or cold showers, and rest.

If your headaches are frequent, keep a diary with details about the events surrounding each one. Are your headaches associated with late nights, academic deadlines, or long periods spent sitting at a computer? If you can identify the stressors that are consistently associated with your headaches, you can begin to gain more control over the situation. If you suffer persistent tension headaches, you should consult your physician.

Migraines

Migraines typically progress through a series of stages lasting from several minutes to several days. They may produce a variety of symptoms, including throbbing pain that starts on one side of the head and may spread; heightened sensitivity to light; visual disturbances such as flashing lights; nausea; and fatigue. About 70% of migraine sufferers are women, and migraine headaches may have a genetic component. Research suggests that people who get migraines may have abnormally excitable nerve cells in their brains. When triggered, these nerve cells send a wave of electrical activity throughout the brain, which in turn causes migraine symptoms. Potential triggers include menstruation, stress, fatigue, atmospheric changes, specific sounds or odors, and certain foods. The frequency of attacks varies from a few in a lifetime to several per week.

Keeping a headache journal can help a migraine sufferer identify headache triggers—the first step to avoiding them. In addition, many new treatments can help reduce the frequency, severity, and duration of migraines.

Cluster Headaches

Cluster headaches are extremely severe headaches that cause intense pain in and around one eye. They usually occur in clusters of one to three headaches each day over a period of weeks or months, alternating with periods of remission in which no headaches occur. About 90% of people with cluster headaches are male. There is no known cause or cure for cluster headaches, but a number of treatments are available. During cluster periods, it is important to refrain from smoking cigarettes and drinking alcohol, because these activities can trigger attacks.

For more on treating headaches, as well as warning signs for when a headache may signal a serious illness, refer to the self-care guide in Appendix B.

- *Endocrine effects and pregnancy complications.* Menstrual irregularities and impotence are both associated with periods of unusual stress. Women who experience significant stress before or during pregnancy may have an increased risk of delivering a premature or low-birth-weight infant.

COMMON SOURCES OF STRESS

We are surrounded by stressors—at home, at school, on the job, and within ourselves. Being able to recognize potential sources of stress is an important step in successfully managing the stress in our lives.

Major Life Changes

Any major change in your life that requires adjustment and accommodation can be a source of stress. Early adulthood and the college years are typically associated with many significant changes, such as moving out of the family home, establishing new relationships, setting educational and career goals, and developing a sense of identity and purpose. Even changes typically thought of as positive—graduation, job promotion, marriage—can be stressful.

Clusters of major life changes may be linked to the development of health problems in some people. Research indicates that some life changes, particularly those that are perceived negatively, can affect health. However, personality and coping skills are important moderating influences. People with a strong support network and a stress-resistant personality are less likely to become ill in response to major life changes than people with fewer internal and external resources.

Daily Hassles

Have you done any of the following in the past week?
- Misplaced your keys, wallet, or an assignment

The college experience has the potential, and the intention, of making you a more mature individual with the capacity to function successfully in the real world. Any experience with so much influence over your immediate state of mind and long-term behavior is bound to be stressful. The fact that college is stressful is not a new discovery. UCLA's Higher Education Research Institute has been surveying first-year college students since 1966. The 1999 survey revealed that, more than ever, college students feel overwhelmed with responsibility and under immense pressure to excel. These feelings stem from increased demands in college (more college students report that they will work full-time while in college), a highly competitive job market, and, on average, a decreased preparedness on the part of incoming students compared to past years (high school grade inflation is greater than ever). Interestingly, many stressors associated with the college experience have little to do with scholastics directly. These stressors include things like relationship difficulties, adjusting to a stranger as a roommate, leaving home, financial worries, and lack of privacy.

Twice as many female as male students report they frequently feel overwhelmed. This could be due to a real difference in stress perception between genders or to a gender-related difference in the likelihood of honestly reporting stress levels. However, more women than men are concerned that they will not have enough money to finish their schooling. Female students also report that they spend more time studying, doing volunteer work, and tending to housework or child-care responsibilities; male students report more time exercising, playing sports, watching television, and playing computer and video games. These survey results suggest that women spend more time than men on goal-oriented activities, which may contribute to the gender difference in perceived stress.

Irrespective of gender, college is stressful. For you to fully realize your college expectations, you will need to evaluate your stress levels, identify the common stressors that you experience, and learn successful coping techniques.

SOURCES: UCLA Higher Education Research Institute. 2001. An Overview of the 2000 Freshman Norms (http://www.gseis.ucla.edu/heri/00_exec_summary.htm; retrieved January 22, 2001). UCLA Higher Education Research Institute. 2000. *An Overview of the 1999 Freshman Norms* (http://www.gseis.ucla.edu/heri/test/executive.htm; retrieved February 1, 2000)

- Had an argument with a troublesome neighbor, coworker, or customer
- Waited in a long line
- Been stuck in traffic or had another problem with transportation
- Worried about money
- Been upset about the weather

While major life changes are undoubtedly stressful, they seldom occur regularly. Psychologist Richard Lazarus has proposed that minor problems—life's daily hassles—can be an even greater source of stress because they occur much more often. People who perceive hassles negatively are likely to experience a moderate stress response every time they are faced with one. Over time, this can take a significant toll on health. Researchers have found that for some people, daily hassles contribute to a general decrease in overall wellness.

College Stressors

College is a time of major life changes and abundant minor hassles (see the box "College Students and Stress"). You will be learning new information and skills and making major decisions about your future. You may be away from home for the first time, or you may be adding extra responsibilities to a life already filled with job and family.

Academic Stressors   Exams, grades, and choosing a major are among the many academic stressors faced by college students. In addition to an increased workload compared to that in high school, many students are unpleasantly surprised by a more rigorous evaluation of their work in college. Higher-quality efforts are expected of college students, so earning good grades takes more effort and dedication. Careful planning and preparation can help make academic stressors more predictable and manageable. Techniques for overcoming test anxiety, a common stress-related academic problem, are described in the Behavior Change Strategy at the end of the chapter.

Students close to graduation may find themselves faced with the need to plan for life after college—a potentially daunting task. Remember that you'll have many opportunities to change career paths in the future, and the training and life experience gained from one path can often be transferred to other endeavors.

Interpersonal Stressors   The college years often involve such potential stressors as establishing new relationships and balancing multiple roles—student, employee, friend, spouse, parent, and so on. You'll have the opportunity to meet new people and make new friends at the start of every term and in every new class and activity. Social engagements may be exhilarating for some and painful for others. Viewed as an exciting challenge or an odious necessity, interacting with others involves attention, on-the-spot decision making, and energy expenditure—and is stressful. Be yourself, go with the flow, and try not to be overly concerned with being liked by everyone you meet.

Time-Related Pressures Do you accept too many responsibilities or manage your time poorly? Time pressures are a problem for most students, but they may be particularly acute for those who also have job and family responsibilities. Most people do have enough time to fulfill all of their responsibilities, but they don't manage their time or their priorities effectively. For these people, it's important to make a plan and *stick to it*. Strategies for more effective time management are described in the next section.

Financial Concerns As young adults leave home and become independent, financial responsibilities such as paying tuition, taking out loans, and managing living expenses are likely to arise. A few college students have personal or family resources that allow them freedom from financial worries during college. However, most students live off savings from full-time summer jobs and part-time jobs during the school year, and many take out loans in order to pay tuition. Some students work full-time and support a family while taking college courses. Regardless of your situation, try to avoid extravagant spending and excessive worry about finances. Instead, use your resources to pursue academic achievements that will help enhance your future financial picture.

Job-Related Stressors

In recent surveys, Americans rate their jobs as one of the key sources of stress in their lives. Tight schedules and overtime contribute to time-related pressures. More than one-third of Americans report that they always feel rushed, and nearly half say they would give up a day's pay for a day off. Worries about job performance, salary, and job security are a source of stress for some people. Interactions with bosses, coworkers, and customers can also contribute to stress. High levels of job stress are also common for people who are left out of important decisions relating to their jobs. When workers are given the opportunity to shape how their jobs are performed, job satisfaction goes up and stress levels go down.

If job-related (or college-related) stress is severe or chronic, the result can be **burnout,** a state of physical, mental, and emotional exhaustion. Burnout occurs most often in highly motivated and driven individuals who come to feel that their work is not recognized or that they are not accomplishing their goals. People in the helping professions—teachers, social workers, caregivers, police officers, and so on—are also prone to burnout. For some

people who suffer from burnout, a vacation or leave of absence may be appropriate. For others, a reduced work schedule, better communication with superiors, or a change in job goals may be necessary. Improving time-management skills can also help.

Social Stressors

Although social support is a key buffer against stress, your interactions with others can also be a source of stress themselves. As mentioned earlier, the college years are a time of great change in interpersonal relationships. The community and society in which you live can also be major sources of stress. Social stressors include prejudice and discrimination. You may feel stress as you try to relate to people of other ethnic or socioeconomic groups. As a member of a particular ethnic group, you may feel pressure to assimilate into mainstream society. If English is not your first language, you face the added burden of conducting many daily activities in a language with which you may not be completely comfortable. All of these pressures can become significant sources of stress. (For more information on stressors that disproportionately affect people in particular groups, refer to the box "Stress and Diverse Populations.")

Environmental Stressors

Claire loves the food at a certain restaurant, but she always feels "on edge" when eating there because of continuous loud background music. This is an example of an environmental stressor—some condition or event in the physical environment that causes stress. Environmental stressors include things like natural disasters, industrial accidents, and intrusive noises, smells, or sights. Like the loud music that bothers Claire, some environmental stressors are mere inconveniences that are easy to avoid. Others, such as pollen season for a hayfever sufferer or living next to a construction site, may be an unavoidable daily source of stress. For those who live in poor or violent neighborhoods or in a war-torn country, environmental stressors can be major life stressors.

Internal Stressors

Some stressors are found not in our interactions with our environment but within ourselves. We put pressure on ourselves to reach personal goals, and we continuously evaluate our progress and performance. Setting high goals and then striving to reach them can enhance self-esteem if the goals are reasonable. However, unrealistic expectations can be a significant source of stress and a serious

burnout A state of physical, mental, and emotional exhaustion.

Terms

Stress is universal, but some groups within the United States face unique stressors and have higher-than-average rates of stress-related physical and emotional problems. These include women, ethnic minorities, the economically disadvantaged, and people with disabilities. Many of the unique stressors that affect special populations stem from prejudice—biased, negative attitudes toward a group of people.

Discrimination occurs when people act according to their prejudices; it can be blatant or subtle. Blatant examples of discrimination are not common, but they are major stressors, akin to significant life changes. Examples include a swastika painted on a Jewish studies house, the defacement of a sculpture honoring the achievements of gay men, and sexual harassment during a fraternity party. More subtle acts may occur much more frequently. For example, an African American student in a mostly white college town feels that shopkeepers are keeping an eye on him, a student using a wheelchair has difficulty with narrow aisles and high counters at local stores, and a female business executive finds that restaurants always assume the lunch check should go to her male clients. Some of these social stressors are unique to certain groups, and it may be difficult for other people to understand how serious such stressors can be.

Women and minorities also often face additional job-related stressors because of stereotypes and discrimination. They make less money than white males in comparable jobs and with comparable levels of education. Women are more likely to face sexual harassment on the job. As employment opportunities have expanded, women also find themselves balancing multiple roles—employee, parent, spouse, caregiver to aging parents, and so on. Women who work outside the home still do most of the housework, and time-related stress can be severe. All these types of stressors can contribute to higher levels of stress-related health problems.

blow to self-esteem. Other internal stressors are physical and emotional states such as illness and exhaustion; these can be both a cause and an effect of unmanaged stress.

> **COMMUNICATE!**   Many speakers suffer from the stress of performance anxiety, yet it can be a positive force if channeled effectively. Identify one or more individuals whose public speaking style you admire, such as an instructor, a boss, or a local community or group leader. Ask them whether they experience stress before giving a talk or presentation and, if so, how they turn it into a positive force. Would any of their strategies be effective for you the next time you have to give a class presentation or a speech?

TECHNIQUES FOR MANAGING STRESS

What can you do about all this stress? A great deal. By shoring up your social support systems; improving your communication skills; developing and maintaining healthy exercise, eating, and sleeping habits; and mastering simple techniques to identify and moderate individual stressors, you can learn to control the stress in your life—instead of allowing it to control you. The effort is well worth the time: People who manage stress effectively not only are healthier but also have more time to enjoy life and accomplish their goals.

Social Support

People need people. Sharing fears, frustrations, and joys not only makes life richer but also seems to contribute to the well-being of body and mind. Research supports this conclusion: One study of college students living in overcrowded apartments, for example, found that those with a strong social support system were less distressed by their cramped quarters than were the "loners" who navigated life's challenges on their own. Participation in a support group has been shown to extend the lives of cancer patients and improve their emotional health. Other studies have shown that married people live longer than single people and have lower death rates from a wide range of conditions. People with a strong social support system are also better able to withstand the stress of major life changes. The crucial common denominator in all these findings is meaningful connections with others.

Allow yourself time to nourish and maintain a network of people at home, at work, at school, or in your community that you can count on for emotional support, feedback, and nurturance. To evaluate your current social support system and to find strategies for strengthening your social ties, refer to the box "Healthy Connections."

Communication

Do you find yourself often angry at others? Some people express their anger directly by yelling or being aggressive; others indirectly express anger by excessively criticizing others or making cynical comments. A person who is angry with others often has difficulty forming and maintaining successful social relationships. Better communication skills can help: Learn to listen to others and to express your needs and desires nonaggressively. Increase your communication skills in order to decrease stress in your relationships—at school, at work, and at home.

At the other extreme, you may suppress your feelings and needs entirely. You may have trouble saying no and

Meaningful connections with others can play a key role in stress management and overall wellness. A sense of isolation can lead to chronic stress, which in turn can increase one's susceptibility to temporary illnesses like colds and to chronic illnesses like heart disease. Although the mechanism isn't clear, social isolation can be as significant to mortality rates as factors like smoking, high blood pressure, and obesity.

There is no single best pattern of social support that works for everyone. However, research suggests that having a variety of types of relationships may be important for wellness. To help determine whether your social network measures up, circle whether each of the following statements is true or false for you.

T   F   1.   If I needed an emergency loan of $100, there is someone I could get it from.

T   F   2.   There is someone who takes pride in my accomplishments.

T   F   3.   I often meet or talk with family or friends.

T   F   4.   Most people I know think highly of me.

T   F   5.   If I needed an early morning ride to the airport, there's no one I would feel comfortable asking to take me.

T   F   6.   I feel there is no one with whom I can share my most private worries and fears.

T   F   7.   Most of my friends are more successful making changes in their lives than I am.

T   F   8.   I would have a hard time finding someone to go with me on a day trip to the beach or country.

To calculate your score, add the number of true answers to questions 1–4 and the number of false answers to questions 5–8. If your score is 4 or more, you should have enough support to protect your health. If your score is 3 or less, you may need to reach out. There are a variety of things you can do to strengthen your social ties:

- *Foster friendships.* Keep in regular contact with your friends. Offer respect, trust, and acceptance, and provide help and support in times of need. Express appreciation for your friends.

- *Keep your family ties strong.* Stay in touch with the family members you feel close to. Participate in family activities and celebrations. If your family doesn't function well as a support system for its members, create a second "family" of people with whom you have built meaningful ties.

- *Get involved with a group.* Do volunteer work, take a class, attend a lecture series, join a religious group. These types of activities can give you a sense of security, a place to talk about your feelings or concerns, and a way to build new friendships. Choose activities that are meaningful to you and that include direct involvement with other people.

- *Build your communication skills.* The more you share your feelings with others, the closer the bonds between you will become. When others are speaking, be a considerate and attentive listener. (Chapters 3 and 4 include more information on effective communication.)

Individual relationships change over the course of your life, but it's never too late to build friendships or become more involved in your community. Your investment of time and energy in your social network will pay off—in a brighter outlook now, and in better health and well-being for the future.

SOURCE: Friends can be good medicine. 1998. *Mind/Body Newsletter* 7(1): 3–6. QUIZ SOURCE: Japenga, A. 1995. A family of friends. *Health,* November/December, 94. Adapted with permission. Copyright © 1995 Health.

---

allow people to take advantage of you. Many businesses encourage employees to take assertiveness training workshops to help them overcome shyness and resistance to communicating their needs. Such communication skills are also valuable in social relationships. (For a fuller discussion of how to enhance communication and resolve interpersonal conflicts, see Chapters 3 and 4.)

Exercise

Exercise helps manitain a healthy body and mind. Accumulating research results indicate that regular physical activity can reduce various aspects of stress as well. One recent study from the National Academy of Sciences found that taking a long walk can help decrease anxiety and blood pressure. Another study found that just a brisk 10-minute walk leaves people feeling more relaxed and energetic for up to 2 hours. Researchers have also found that people who exercise regularly react with milder physical stress responses before, during, and after exposure to stressors. People who took three brisk 45-minute walks a week for 3 months reported that they perceived fewer daily hassles. Their sense of wellness also increased.

These findings are not surprising since, as stated earlier, the stress response mobilizes energy resources and readies the body for physical emergencies. If you experience stress and do not physically exert yourself, you are not completing the energy cycle. You may not be able to exercise while your daily stressors occur—during class, for example, or while sitting in a traffic jam—but you can be active later in the day. Physical activity allows you to expend the nervous energy you have built up and trains your body to more readily achieve homeostasis following future disturbances in normal functioning.

It's not hard to incorporate light to moderate exercise into your day. Walk to class or bike to the store instead of

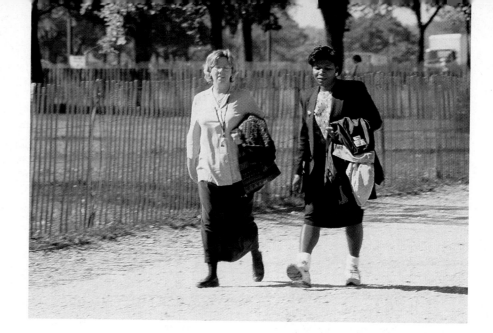

Exercise is a particularly effective antidote to stress. A lunchtime walk gives these coworkers a chance to both exercise and foster a friendship.

driving. Use the stairs instead of the elevator. Take a walk with a friend instead of getting a cup of coffee. Go bowling, play tennis, or roller-skate instead of seeing a movie. Make a habit of taking a brisk after-dinner stroll. Plan hikes and easy bike outings for the weekends.

Consider taking a class in a kind of exercise you've always wanted to try, such as yoga, t'ai chi, square dancing, or fencing. The important thing is to find an activity that you enjoy, so it can become a habit and thereby an effective stress reducer. Chapter 13 presents guidelines for creating an exercise program to fit your individual needs and preferences.

Nutrition

A healthy diet will give you an energy bank to draw on whenever you experience stress. Eating wisely also will enhance your feelings of self-control and self-esteem. Learning the principles of sound nutrition is easy, and sensible eating habits rapidly become second nature when practiced regularly. (For more on sound nutrition, see Chapter 12.)

Avoiding or limiting caffeine is also important in stress management. Although one or two cups of coffee a day probably won't hurt you, caffeine is a mildly addictive stimulant that leaves some people jittery, irritable, and unable to sleep. Consuming caffeine during stressful situations can raise blood pressure and increase levels of cortisol. Tea, cola, some other soft drinks, chocolate, and more than a thousand over-the-counter drugs, including cold remedies, aspirin, and weight-loss preparations, also contain caffeine, sometimes in high doses.

WW. Sleep

Lack of sleep can be both a cause and an effect of excess stress. Without sufficient sleep, our mental and physical processes steadily deteriorate. We get headaches, feel irritable, are unable to concentrate, forget things, and may be more susceptible to illness. Levels of the stress hormones in the bloodstream vary throughout the day and are related to sleep patterns. Peak concentrations occur in the early morning, followed by a slow decline during the day and evening. Concentrations return to peak during the final stages of sleep and in the early morning hours. Acute sleep deprivation slows the daytime decline in stress hormones, so evening levels are higher than normal. In addition, a decrease in total sleep time causes an increase in the release of stress hormones. Together, these changes may cause an increase in stress hormone levels throughout the day and may contribute to the mental and physical effects associated with acute sleep deprivation. Fatigue and sleep deprivation are major factors in many fatal car, truck, and train crashes. Extreme sleep deprivation can lead to hallucinations and other psychotic symptoms.

Adequate sleep, on the other hand, improves mood, fosters feelings of competence and self-worth, and supports optimal mental and emotional functioning. If you are sleep-deprived, sleeping extra hours may significantly improve your daytime alertness and mental abilities. Sleep requirements vary considerably among individuals; some adults need only 5 hours of sleep, while others need 9 hours or more to feel fully refreshed and alert.

Sleep occurs in two phases: rapid eye movement (REM) and non-REM. Non-REM sleep consists of four stages of successively deeper sleep, during which blood pressure, heart rate, temperature, and breathing rate drop; growth hormone is released; and brain wave patterns become slow and even. REM sleep, during which dreams occur, is characterized by the rapid back-and- forth movement of the eyes under closed eyelids. Heart rate, blood pressure, and breathing rate increase; brain activity increases to levels equal to or greater than during waking.

Most people can overcome insomnia by discovering the cause of poor sleep and taking steps to remedy it. Insomnia that lasts for more than 6 months and interferes with daytime functioning requires consultation with a physician. Sleeping pills are not recommended for chronic insomnia because they can be habit-forming; they also lose their effectiveness over time.

If you're bothered by insomnia, here are some tips for getting a better night's sleep:

- Determine how much sleep you need to feel refreshed the next day, and don't sleep longer than that (but do make sure you get enough).

- Go to bed at the same time every night and, more important, get up at the same time every morning, 7 days a week, regardless of how much sleep you got. Don't nap during the day.

- Exercise every day, but not too close to bedtime. Your metabolism takes up to 6 hours to slow down after exercise.

- Avoid tobacco (nicotine is a stimulant), caffeine in the later part of the day, and alcohol before bedtime (it causes disturbed, fragmented sleep).

- Have a light snack before bedtime; you'll sleep better if you're not hungry.

- Deal with worries before bedtime. Try writing them down, along with some possible solutions, and then allow yourself to forget about them until the next day.

- Use your bed only for sleep. Don't eat, read, study, or watch television in bed.

- Relax before bedtime with a warm bath (again, not too close to bedtime—allow about 2 hours for your metabolism to slow down afterward), a book, music, or some relaxation exercises. Don't lie down in bed until you're sleepy.

- If you don't fall asleep in 15–20 minutes, or if you wake up and can't fall asleep again, get out of bed, leave the room if possible, and do something monotonous until you feel sleepy.

- Keep a perspective on your plight. Losing a night's sleep isn't the end of the world. Getting upset only makes it harder to fall asleep. Relax, and trust in your body's natural ability to drift off to sleep.

Muscles in the limbs relax completely, causing temporary paralysis and preventing the sleeper from acting out her or his dreams. A sleeper goes through several cycles of non-REM and REM sleep each night. Stress hormone levels are low during deep sleep and increase during REM sleep. The increase in REM sleep duration with each sleep cycle may underlie the progressive increase in circulating stress hormones during the final stages of sleep.

Nearly everyone, at some time in life, has trouble falling asleep or staying asleep—a condition known as insomnia. The most common causes of insomnia are lifestyle factors, such as high caffeine or alcohol intake before bedtime; medical problems, such as a breathing disorder; and psychological stress. About 75% of people who suffer chronic insomnia report some stressful life event at the onset of their sleep problem. Due to the emotional stress that accompanies sleep disorders, stress-management techniques are often recommended. If you suffer from sleeping problems, try some of the strategies in the box "Overcoming Insomnia."

Time Management

A surprising number of the stressors in most people's lives relate to time. Many people never seem to have enough time, and they always seem to feel overwhelmed by the pace of their lives. Others have too much time on their hands and are often bored. Learning to manage your time successfully is crucial to coping with the stressors you face every day. Three common factors that negatively impact time management for college students are perfectionism, overcommitment, and procrastination.

Perfectionism is the need to constantly improve a project, situation, or personal trait. It is frequently based on a self-deprecating fear of failure or harsh judgment by friends or family. Student perfectionists often spend an inordinate amount of time rewriting papers, reorganizing notes, and rearranging their work space to the point that they sacrifice social interaction and sleep. Perfectionists will torture themselves for getting an A− instead of an A on a test rather than congratulate themselves on a job well done. They will appraise the situation negatively using "should" statements: "I should have studied an hour more each night," "I shouldn't have taken so much time off last weekend," and so on. There is no such thing as perfection, so perfectionists are striving for unreachable goals. This unfulfilled effort increases stress and compromises time spent on other academic projects and social functions that are integral to a fulfilling college experience. If perfectionism is a problem for you, try not to put so much pressure on yourself. Focus on doing your best rather than trying to be the best. College is not a competition; it is a setting for personal growth. Accept your limits and try not to expect so much of yourself or others.

Overcommitters are less concerned with the quality of their efforts. Instead, they take on project after project

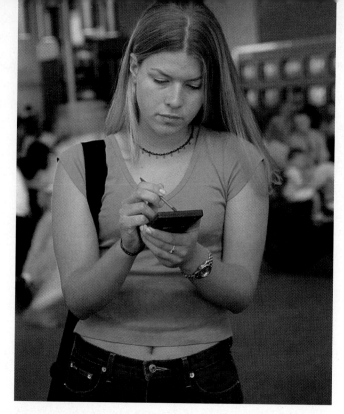

Managing the many commitments of adult life—including work, school, and parenthood—can sometimes feel overwhelming and produce a great deal of stress. Time-management skills, including careful scheduling with a date book or handheld computer, can help people cope with busy days.

and activity after activity because they find it difficult to say no or to accurately assess their current workload. Being well-rounded is admirable, but there are only so many sports one can play, so many committees one can serve on, and so many social functions one can attend and still perform well academically. Overcommitters often feel they are missing out when they say no to something, and they often don't fully experience many college activities because they don't take the time to fully immerse themselves in any one thing.

Procrastination—putting something off until later—is a problem for many people. People who put off key tasks and decisions may sabotage personal relationships, college life, careers, and health. Although reasons for procrastination vary, it often camouflages self-doubt, an unreasonable desire for perfection, or a reluctance to make changes. People who set impossibly high standards for themselves may actually protect their self-esteem by procrastinating; if they fail to complete a project, for example, their work will never be evaluated.

If procrastination or another time-related stressor is a problem for you, try some or all of the following strategies for managing your time more productively and creatively:

- *Set priorities.* Divide your tasks into three groups: essential, important, and trivial. Focus on the first two. Ignore the third.

- *Schedule tasks for peak efficiency.* You've undoubtedly noticed you're most productive at certain times of the day (or night). Schedule as many of your tasks for those hours as you can, and stick to your schedule.

- *Set realistic goals, and write them down.* Attainable goals spur you on. Impossible goals, by definition, cause frustration and failure. Fully commit yourself to achieving your goals by putting them in writing.

- *Budget enough time.* For each project you undertake, calculate how long it will take to complete. Then tack on another 10–15%, or even 25%, as a buffer against mistakes, interruptions, or unanticipated problems.

- *Break down long-term goals into short-term ones.* Instead of waiting for or relying on large blocks of time, use short amounts of time to start a project or keep it moving. Say you have a 50-page report due and are about to panic. Divide the assignment into three tasks: research, outlining, and writing. Then budget enough time slots (half an hour or an hour) to complete each task. Your steady progress will make you feel so much better that you'll be encouraged to continue.

- *Visualize the achievement of your goals.* By mentally rehearsing your performance of a task, you will be able to reach your goal more smoothly.

- *Keep track of the tasks you put off.* Analyze the reasons why you procrastinate. If the task is difficult or unpleasant, look for ways to make it easier or more fun. If you hate cleaning up your room, break the work into 10-minute tasks and do a little at a time. If you find the readings for one of your classes particularly difficult, choose an especially nice setting for your reading, and then reward yourself each time you complete a section or chapter.

- *Consider doing your least favorite tasks first.* Once you have the most unpleasant ones out of the way, you can work on the projects you enjoy more.

- *Consolidate tasks when possible.* For example, try walking to the store so that you run your errands and exercise in the same block of time.

- *Identify quick transitional tasks.* Keep a list of 5-minute tasks you can do while waiting or between other tasks, such as watering your plants, doing the dishes, or checking a homework assignment.

- *Delegate responsibility.* Asking for help when you have too much to do is no cop-out; it's good time management. Just don't delegate to others the jobs you know you should do yourself, such as researching a paper.

- *Say no when necessary.* If the demands made on you don't seem reasonable, say no—tactfully, but without guilt or apology.

- *Give yourself a break.* Allow time for play—free, unstructured time when you ignore the clock. Don't consider this a waste of time. Play renews you and enables you to work more efficiently.

• *Stop thinking or talking about what you're going to do, and just do it!* Sometimes the best solution for procrastination is to stop waiting for the right moment and just get started. You will probably find that things are not as bad as you feared, and your momentum will keep you going.

COMMUNICATE! Learning to say no—whether to extra work or extra play—is an important part of effective time management. If you don't have enough time for something that your friends are pressuring you to do, you may need to use assertive communication to maintain control of your own time. Begin by knowing your priorities and believing in your right to decide what you will do. Remain calm in the face of pressure and don't feel guilty about saying no. For example, "I'd like to go to the club with you, but I have to get started on my English paper. I have only this week to work on it, and it's important to me. I'm sorry you don't have anyone else to go with right now—I could go on Friday if you're available then."

Cognitive Techniques

Some stressors arise in our own minds. Ideas, beliefs, perceptions, and patterns of thinking can add to our stress level. Each of the techniques described below can help you change unhealthy thought patterns to ones that will help you cope with stress. As with any skill, mastering these techniques takes practice and patience.

Think and Act Constructively Worrying, someone once said, is like shoveling smoke. Think back to the worries you had last week. How many of them were needless? Think about things you *can* control. Try to stand aside from the problem, consider the positive steps you can take to solve it, and then carry them out. Remember, successful prediction of a stressful event is a major factor determining the magnitude of the stress response. In the evening, try to predict stressful events you might encounter the following day. Will you see someone who makes you feel uncomfortable? If so, decide now how you will interact with that person. Will you attend a class that doesn't hold your attention? Develop a strategy now that will help you maintain focus. Will you have to wait in line to register or buy tickets? If so, plan to pass the time by listening to music to relax or by catching up on some reading.

Take Control A situation often feels more stressful if you feel you're not in control of it. Time may seem to be slipping away before a big exam, for example. Unexpected obstacles may appear in your path, throwing you off course. When you feel your environment is controlling you instead of the other way around, take charge! Concentrate on what is possible to control, and set realistic goals. Be confident of your ability to succeed.

Problem-Solve When you find yourself stewing over a problem, take a moment to sit down with a piece of paper and go through a formal process of problem solving. Within a few minutes you can generate a plan. Try this approach:

1. Define the problem in one or two sentences.
2. Identify the causes of the problem.
3. Consider alternative solutions; don't just stop with the most obvious one.
4. Weigh positive and negative consequences for each alternative.
5. Make a decision—choose a solution.
6. Make a list of what you will need to do to carry out your decision.
7. Begin to act on your list; if you're unable to do that, temporarily turn to other things.
8. Evaluate the outcome and revise your approach if necessary.

Modify Your Expectations Expectations are exhausting and restricting. The fewer expectations you have, the more you can live spontaneously and joyfully. The more you expect from others, the more often you will feel let down. And trying to meet the expectations others have of you is often futile.

Maintain Positivity If you catch your mind beating up on you—"Late for class again! You can't even cope with college! How do you expect to ever hold down a professional job?"—change your inner dialogue. Talk to yourself as you would to a child you love: "You're a smart, capable person. You've solved other problems; you'll handle this one. Tomorrow you'll simply schedule things so you get to class with a few minutes to spare." (Chapter 3 has more information on self-talk.)

Cultivate Your Sense of Humor When it comes to stress, laughter may be the best medicine. Even a fleeting smile produces changes in your autonomic nervous system that can lift your spirits. And a few minutes of belly laughing can be as invigorating as brisk exercise. Hearty laughter elevates your heart rate, aids digestion, eases pain, and triggers the release of endorphins and other pleasurable and stimulating chemicals in the brain. After a good laugh, your muscles go slack; your pulse and blood pressure dip below normal. You are relaxed. Cultivate the ability to laugh at yourself, and you'll have a handy and instantly effective stress reliever. Try some of the following strategies:

- Keep a humor journal. Write down funny things that you and others say, including unintentional slips of the tongue. Collect funny and clever sayings that make you smile.

- Look at newspaper and magazine cartoons. Cut out those you find particularly funny and add them to your humor journal.

- Collect some funny props—clown noses, "arrow" headbands, Groucho glasses—that you can put on the next time you feel stressed or anxious. Or simply try making funny faces in front of a mirror.

- Watch funny films and television programs. In a study of college students, those who watched an episode of *Seinfeld* prior to giving an impromptu speech were less anxious and had a lower heart rate than those who didn't watch the program.

Weed Out Trivia You can burden your memory with too much information. A major source of stress is trying to "store" too much data. Forget unimportant details (they will usually be self-evident) and organize important information. One technique you can try is to "chunk" the important material into categories. If your next exam covers three chapters from your textbook, consider each chapter a chunk of information. Then, break down each chunk into its three or four most important features. Create a mental outline that allows you to trace your way from the most general category down to the most specific details. This technique can be applied to managing daily responsibilities as well. Break your daily tasks down into three or four categories, such as academics, family and friends, fitness, and daily living. For each, list the three most important items for the day. Items on the family and friends list might include caring for a child, calling home, and helping a classmate; your daily living items might be going to the dentist, buying gas, and shopping for dinner. Cross items off your mental outline as you complete them to free up memory and attention for the unexpected.

Live in the Present Do you clog your mind by reliving past events? Clinging to experiences and emotions, particularly unpleasant ones, can be a deadly business. Clear your mind of the old debris; let it go. Free yourself to enjoy life today.

Go with the Flow Remember that the branch that bends in the storm doesn't break. Try to flow with your life, accepting the things you can't change. Be forgiving of faults, your own and those of others. Instead of anticipating happiness at some indefinite point in the future, realize that pleasure is integral to being alive. You can create it every day of your life. View challenges as an opportunity to learn and grow. Be flexible. In this way, you can make stress work for you rather than against you, enhancing your overall wellness.

 Relaxation Techniques

First identified and described by Herbert Benson of the Harvard Medical School, the **relaxation response** is a physiological state characterized by a feeling of warmth and quiet mental alertness. This is the opposite of the fight-or-flight reaction. When the relaxation response is triggered by a relaxation technique, heart rate, breathing, and metabolism slow down. Blood pressure and oxygen consumption decrease. At the same time, blood flow to the brain and skin increases, and brain waves shift from an alert beta rhythm to a relaxed alpha rhythm. Practiced regularly, relaxation techniques can counteract the debilitating effects of stress.

If you decide to try a relaxation technique, practice it daily until it becomes natural to you, and then use it whenever you feel the need. You may feel calmer and more refreshed after each session. If one technique doesn't seem to work well enough for you after you've given it a good try, try another one. You'll know you've mastered a deep relaxation technique when you start to see subtle changes in other areas of your life: You may notice you've been encountering fewer hassles, working more efficiently, or enjoying more free time. None of the techniques takes long to do—for instance, just a few minutes away from the TV should do the trick.

Progressive Relaxation Unlike most of the others, this simple method requires no imagination, willpower, or self-suggestion. You simply tense, and then relax, the muscles in your body, group by group. The technique, also known as deep muscle relaxation, helps you become aware of the muscle tension that occurs when you're under stress. When you consciously relax those muscles, other systems of the body get the message and ease up on the stress response.

Start, for example, with your right fist. Inhale as you tense it. Exhale as you relax it. Repeat. Next, contract and relax your right upper arm. Repeat. Do the same with your left arm. Then, beginning at your forehead and ending at your feet, contract and relax your other muscle groups. Repeat each contraction at least once, breathing in as you tense, breathing out as you relax. To speed up the process, tense and relax more muscles at one time—both arms simultaneously, for instance. With practice, you'll be able to relax very quickly and effectively by clenching and releasing only your fists.

Visualization Also known as using imagery, **visualization** lets you daydream without guilt. Athletes find that the technique enhances sports performance, and visualization is even part of the curriculum at U.S. Olympic training camps. You can use visualization to help you relax, change your habits, or perform well—whether on an exam, a stage, or a playing field.

Next time you feel stressed, close your eyes. Imagine

Dr. Herbert Benson developed a simple, practical technique for eliciting the relaxation response.

The Basic Technique

1. Pick a word, phrase, or object to focus on. If you like, you can choose a word or phrase that has a deep meaning for you, but any word or phrase will work. Some meditators prefer to focus on their breathing.

2. Take a comfortable position in a quiet environment, and close your eyes if you're not focusing on an object.

3. Relax your muscles.

4. Breathe slowly and naturally. If you're using a focus word or phrase, silently repeat it each time you exhale. If you're using an object, focus on it as you breathe.

5. Keep a passive attitude. Disregard thoughts that drift in.

6. Continue for 10–20 minutes, once or twice a day.

7. After you've finished, sit quietly for a few minutes with your eyes first closed and then open. Then stand up.

Suggestions

• Allow relaxation to occur at its own pace; don't try to force it. Don't be surprised if you can't tune your mind out for more than a few seconds at a time; it's not a reason for anger or frustration. The more you ignore the intrusions, the easier doing so will get.

• If you want to time your session, peek at a watch or clock occasionally, but don't set a jarring alarm.

• The technique works best on an empty stomach, before a meal or about 2 hours after eating. Avoid times of day when you're tired—unless you want to fall asleep.

• Although you'll feel refreshed even after the first session, it may take a month or more to get noticeable results. Be patient. Eventually the relaxation response will become so natural that it will occur spontaneously, or on demand, when you sit quietly for a few moments.

---

yourself floating on a cloud, sitting on a mountaintop, or lying in a meadow. What do you see and hear? Is it cold out? Or damp? What do you smell? What do you taste? Involve all your senses. Your body will respond as if your imagery were real. An alternative: Close your eyes and imagine a deep purple light filling your body. Now change the color into a soothing gold. As the color lightens, so should your distress.

Visualization can also be used to rehearse for an upcoming event and enhance performance. By experiencing an event ahead of time in your mind, you can practice coping with any difficulties that may arise. Think positively, and you can "psych yourself up" for a successful experience.

Meditation The need to periodically stop our incessant mental chatter is so great that, from ancient times, hundreds of forms of **meditation** have developed in cultures all over the world. Meditation is a way of telling the mind to be quiet for a while. Because meditation has been at the core of many Eastern religions and philosophies, it has acquired an "Eastern" mystique that has caused some people to shy away from it. Yet meditation requires no special knowledge or background. Whatever philosophical, religious, or emotional reasons may be given for meditation, its power derives from its ability to elicit the relaxation response.

Meditation helps you tune out the world temporarily, removing you from both internal and external sources of stress. It allows you to transcend past conditioning, fixed expectations, and the trivial pursuits of the psyche; it clears out the mental smog. The "thinker" takes time out to become the "observer"—calmly attentive, without analyzing, judging, comparing, or rationalizing. Regular practice of this quiet awareness will subtly carry over into your daily life, encouraging physical and emotional balance no matter what confronts you. For a step-by-step description of a basic meditation technique, see the box "Meditation and the Relaxation Response."

Deep Breathing Your breathing pattern is closely tied to your stress level. Deep, slow breathing is associated with relaxation. Rapid, shallow, often irregular breathing occurs during the stress response. With practice, you can learn to slow and quiet your breathing pattern, thereby also quieting your mind and relaxing your body. Breathing techniques can be used for on-the-spot tension relief, as well as for long-term stress reduction.

The primary goal of many breathing exercises is to change your breathing pattern from chest breathing to diaphragmatic ("belly") breathing. During the day, most adults breathe by expanding their chest and raising their

relaxation response A physiological state characterized by a feeling of warmth and quiet mental alertness.

visualization A technique for promoting relaxation or improving performance that involves creating or re-creating vivid mental pictures of a place or an experience; also called *imagery.*

meditation A technique for quieting the mind by focusing on a particular word, object (such as a candle flame), or process (such as breathing).

Terms

Diaphragmatic Breathing

1. Lie on your back with your body relaxed.

2. Place one hand on your chest and one on your abdomen. (You will use your hands to monitor the depth and location of your breathing.)

3. Inhale slowly and deeply through your nose into your abdomen. Your abdomen should push up as far as is comfortable. Your chest should expand only a little and only in conjunction with the movement of your abdomen.

4. Exhale gently through your mouth.

5. Continue diaphragmatic breathing for about 5–10 minutes per session. Focus on the sound and feel of your breathing.

Breathing In Relaxation, Breathing Out Tension

1. Assume a comfortable position, lying on your back or sitting in a chair.

2. Inhale slowly and deeply into your abdomen. Imagine the inhaled, warm air flowing to all parts of your body. Say to yourself, "Breathe in relaxation."

3. Exhale from your abdomen. Imagine tension flowing out of your body. Say to yourself, "Breathe out tension."

4. Pause before you inhale.

5. Continue for 5–10 minutes or until no tension remains in your body.

Chest Expansion

1. Sit in a comfortable chair, or stand.

2. Inhale slowly and deeply into your abdomen as you raise your arms out to the sides. Pull your shoulders and arms back and lift your chin slightly so that your chest opens up.

3. Exhale gradually as you lower your arms and chin, and return to the starting position.

4. Repeat 5–10 times or until your breathing is deep and regular and your body feels relaxed and energized.

Quick Tension Release

1. Inhale into your abdomen slowly and deeply as you count slowly to four.

2. Exhale slowly as you again count slowly to four. As you exhale, concentrate on relaxing your face, neck, shoulders, and chest.

3. Repeat several times. With each exhalation, feel more tension leaving your body.

SOURCES: Stop stress with a deep breath. 1996. *Health,* October, 53. Breathing for health and relaxation. 1995. *Mental Medicine Update* 4(2): 3–6. When you're stressed, catch your breath. 1995. *Mayo Clinic Health Letter,* December, 5.

---

shoulders rather than by expanding their abdomen. This pattern of chest breathing is associated with stress, a sedentary lifestyle, restrictive clothing, and cultural preferences for a large chest and a small waist. Diaphragmatic breathing, which involves free expansion of the diaphragm and lower abdomen, is the pattern of breathing characteristic of children and sleeping adults. (The diaphragm is a sheet of muscle and connective tissue that divides the chest and abdominal cavities.) Diaphragmatic breathing is slower and deeper than chest breathing. For instructions on how to perform diaphragmatic breathing, refer to the box "Breathing for Relaxation."

Hatha Yoga   *Yoga* is an ancient Sanskrit word referring to the union of mind, body, and soul. The development and practice of yoga are rooted in the Hindu philosophy of spiritual enlightenment. The founders of yoga developed a system of physical postures, called *asanas,* designed to cleanse the body of toxins, calm and clear the mind, bring energy into the body, and raise the level of consciousness.

Hatha yoga, the most common yoga style practiced in the United States, emphasizes physical balance and breathing control. It integrates components of flexibility, muscular strength and endurance, and muscle relaxation; it also sometimes serves as a preliminary to meditation.

A session of hatha yoga typically involves a series of *asanas,* held for a few seconds to several minutes, that stretch and relax different parts of the body. The emphasis is on breathing, stretching, and balance. There are hundreds of different *asanas,* and they must be performed correctly in order to be beneficial. For this reason, qualified instruction is recommended, particularly for beginners. Yoga classes are offered through many community recreation centers, YMCAs and YWCAs, and private clubs. Regardless of whether you accept the philosophy and symbolism of different *asanas,* the practice of yoga can induce the relaxation response as well as develop body awareness, flexibility, and muscular strength and endurance.

T'ai Chi Ch'uan   A martial art that developed in China, t'ai chi ch'uan is a system of self-defense that incorporates philosophical concepts from Taoism and Confucianism. An important part of this philosophy is *chi,* an energy force that surrounds and permeates all things. In addition to serving as a means of self-defense, the goal of t'ai chi ch'uan is to bring the body into balance and harmony with this universal energy, in order to promote health and spiritual growth. It teaches practitioners to remain calm and centered, to conserve and concentrate energy, and to harmonize with fear. T'ai chi ch'uan seeks to manipulate force by becoming part of it—"going with the flow," so to speak.

T'ai chi ch'uan is considered the gentlest of the martial arts. Instead of using quick and powerful movements, t'ai chi ch'uan consists of a series of slow, fluid, elegant movements, which reinforce the idea of moving *with* rather than *against* the stressors of everyday life. The practice of t'ai chi ch'uan promotes relaxation and concentration as well as the development of body awareness, balance, muscular strength, and flexibility. It usually takes some time and practice to reap the stress-management benefits of t'ai chi ch'uan, and, as with yoga, it's best to begin with some qualified instruction.

Listening to Music Listening to music is another method of inducing relaxation. It has been shown to influence pulse, blood pressure, and the electrical activity of muscles. Studies of newborns and hospitalized stroke patients have shown that listening to soothing, lyrical music can lessen depression, anxiety, and stress levels. Exposure to rhythmic music has been shown to help people with Parkinson's disease and other physical disabilities walk more steadily. Music therapy, which can involve both listening to music and creating music, has also been shown to be helpful in pain management, including lessening the need for anesthesia during labor. Although the effects of music are just beginning to be investigated, researchers have found that exposure to soothing music leads to reduced levels of the stress hormone cortisol and causes changes in the electrical activity in the brain.

To experience the stress-management benefits of music yourself, set aside a time to listen. Choose music that you enjoy and that makes you feel relaxed. If you are interested in learning more about formal music therapy, contact the American Music Therapy Association (see the For More Information section at the end of the chapter).

Biofeedback Using **biofeedback** helps people reduce the stress response by enabling them to become more aware of their level of physiological arousal. It involves mechanical monitoring of some measure of the physiological stress response such as perspiration, heart rate, skin temperature, or muscle tension. A person receives feedback about his or her condition through the use of sound (a tone or music), light, or a meter or dial. For example, as heart rate increases, the tone becomes louder; as it decreases, the tone softens. Through trial and error, people can learn to reduce their physiological stress response through conscious control.

The point of biofeedback training is to teach how re-

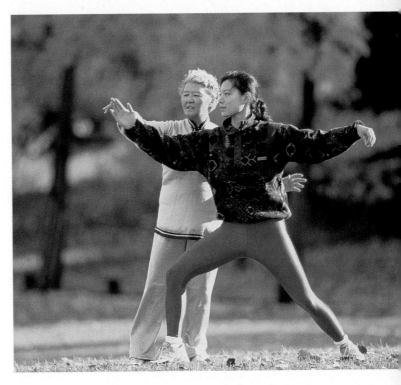

T'ai chi ch'uan is among the many techniques for inducing the relaxation response. In addition to helping this woman manage stress, regular practice of t'ai chi will also improve her balance and increase her muscular strength and flexibility.

laxation feels, how to induce relaxation, and how to transfer this skill to daily life (without the use of electronic equipment). In addition to monitoring equipment, biofeedback usually also requires the initial help of a therapist, stress counselor, or technician.

Other relaxation techniques include massage, hypnosis and self-hypnosis, and autogenic training. To learn more about these and other techniques for inducing the relaxation response, refer to For More Information at the end of the chapter.

Counterproductive Coping Strategies

College is a time when you'll learn to adapt to new and challenging situations and gain skills that will last a lifetime. It is also a time when many people develop habits, in response to stress, that are counterproductive and unhealthy and that may also last well beyond graduation.

Tobacco Use Many young adults who never smoked in high school—and who rebuked their parents for tobacco

biofeedback A technique in which monitoring devices are used to help a person become conscious of unconscious body processes, such as body temperature or blood pressure, in order to exert some control over them.

Terms

use—smoke their first cigarette in college, usually at a party or bar or in a dorm with friends. Cigarettes and other tobacco products contain nicotine, a chemical that enhances the actions of neurotransmitters. Nicotine can make you feel relaxed and even increase your ability to concentrate, but it is highly addictive. Cigarette smoke also contains many other substances that are harmful to your lungs and circulatory system and that cause heart disease, stroke, lung cancer, and emphysema. These negative consequences far outweigh any beneficial effects, and tobacco use should be avoided. The easiest thing to do is not to start. See Chapter 11 for more on the health effects of tobacco use and for tips on how to quit.

Use of Alcohol and Other Drugs

No college experience is complete without a party or two. Letting loose, dancing, laughing, and interacting with others—all are part of college parties and all can be very effective short-term coping strategies. However, partying in college is usually associated with drinking alcohol. Keg parties and drinking games can be fun, but they contribute to binge drinking and other forms of alcohol abuse. Like nicotine, alcohol is addictive, and many alcoholics find it hard to relax without a drink. Having a few drinks might make you feel temporarily at ease, and drinking until you're intoxicated may help you forget your current stressors. However, using alcohol to deal with stress places you at risk for all the short-term and long-term problems associated with alcohol abuse. It also does nothing to address the actual causes of stress in your life. Although moderate alcohol consumption may have potential health benefits for some people, many college students have patterns of drinking that detract from wellness. For more on the responsible use of alcohol, refer to Chapter 10.

Psychoactive drugs are ingested regularly by millions of Americans, often to help them to wake up when they are tired or to feel more relaxed when they are tense. However, using psychoactive drugs to cope with stress is usually counterproductive.

• Caffeine, found in coffee, tea, and many sodas, raises cortisol levels and blood pressure and can make you feel more stressed; caffeine also disrupts sleep.

• Marijuana is often used by people in an effort to induce relaxation. However, it can elicit panic attacks with repeated use, and some research has shown that the neuroactive chemicals in marijuana actually act to enhance the stress response. To compound this, withdrawal from marijuana may also be associated with an increase in circulating stress hormones.

• Opioids such as morphine and heroin can mimic the effects of your body's natural painkillers and act to reduce anxiety. However, tolerance to opioids develops quickly, and many users become dependent. What starts as a quick fix for anxiety may rapidly become a life-altering addiction.

In general, it's not a good idea to alter your body chemistry with drugs in order to cope with stress. In moderation, substances like caffeine and alcohol appear to have some positive attributes—but their use has many pitfalls and does not directly address the causes of stress in your life. Try some of the other coping strategies mentioned in this chapter instead. Use your natural ability to adapt.

Binge Eating

The nutrients in the food you eat provide energy and the substances needed to maintain your body. However, eating is also psychologically rewarding. We use food to end long days, to celebrate special events, and to enjoy the company of friends. The feelings of satiation and sedation that follow eating produce a relaxed state. However, regular use of eating as a means of coping with stress may lead to binge eating habits. Binge eating is defined as eating a large quantity of food in a discrete period of time, accompanied by a sense of lack of control over eating. Binge eating is a risky behavior associated with weight gain and serious eating disorders.

A good strategy to avoid unhealthy binge eating habits is to make sure you eat breakfast and lunch in the first half of your day—rather than waiting until the evening to consume a real meal. Eating early in the day increases your metabolism and gives you the energy to engage in all your activities. In addition, early meals will decrease feelings of hunger later in the day. See Chapters 12 and 14 for more on a healthy diet and on eating disorders.

CREATING A PERSONAL PLAN FOR MANAGING STRESS

What are the most important sources of stress in your life? Are you coping successfully with these stressors? No single strategy or program for managing stress will work for everyone, but you can use the principles of behavior management described in Chapter 1 to tailor a plan specifically to your needs. The most important starting point for a successful stress-management plan is to learn to listen to your body. When you learn to recognize the stress response and the emotions and thoughts that accompany it, you'll be in a position to take charge of that crucial moment and handle it in a healthy way.

Identifying Stressors

Before you can learn to manage the stressors in your life, you have to identify them. A strategy many experts recommend is keeping a stress journal for a week or two. Keep a log of your daily activities, and assign a rating to your stress level for every hour. Each time you feel or express a stress response, record the time and the circumstances in your journal. Note what you were doing at the time, what you were thinking or feeling, and the outcome of your response.

After keeping your journal for a few weeks, you should be able to identify your key stressors and spot patterns in how you respond to them. Take note of the people, places, events, and patterns of thought and behavior that cause you the most stress. You may notice, for example, that mornings are usually the most stressful part of your day. Or you may discover that when you're angry at your roommate, you're apt to respond with behaviors that only make matters worse. Once you've outlined the general pattern of stress in your life, you may want to focus on a particularly problematic stressor or on an inappropriate behavioral response you've identified. Keep a stress log for another week or two that focuses just on the early morning hours, for example, or just on your arguments with your roommate. The more information you gather, the easier it will be to develop effective strategies for coping with the stressors in your life.

Designing Your Plan

Earlier in this chapter, you learned about many different techniques for combating stress. Now that you've identified the key stressors in your life, it's time to choose the techniques that will work best for you and create an action plan for change. Finding a buddy to work with you can make the process more fun and increase your chances of success. Some experts recommend drawing up a formal contract with yourself.

Whether or not you complete a contract, it's important to design rewards into your plan. You might treat yourself to a special breakfast in a favorite restaurant on the weekend (as long as you eat a nutritious breakfast every weekday morning). If you practice your relaxation technique faithfully, you might reward yourself with a long bath or an hour of pleasure reading at the end of the day. It's also important to evaluate your plan regularly and redesign it as your needs change. Under times of increased stress, for example, you might want to focus on good eating, exercise, and relaxation habits. Over time, your new stress-management skills will become almost automatic. You'll feel better, accomplish more, and reduce your risk of disease.

Getting Help

If the techniques discussed so far don't provide you with enough relief from the stress in your life, you might want to read more about specific areas you wish to work on, consult a peer counselor, join a support group, or participate in a few psychotherapy sessions. Excellent self-help guides can be found in bookstores or the library. Additional resources are listed in the For More Information section at the end of the chapter.

Your student health center or student affairs office can tell you whether your campus has a peer counseling program. Such programs are usually staffed by volunteer students with special training that emphasizes maintaining confidentiality. Peer counselors can guide you to other campus or community resources or can simply provide understanding.

Support groups are typically organized around a particular issue or problem. In your area, you might find a support group for first-year students; for reentering students; for single parents; for students of your ethnicity, religion, or national origin; for people with eating disorders; or for rape survivors. The number of such groups has increased in recent years, as more and more people discover how therapeutic it can be to talk with others who share the same situation.

Short-term psychotherapy can also be tremendously helpful in dealing with stress-related problems. Your student health center may offer psychotherapy on a sliding-fee scale; the county mental health center in your area may do the same. If you belong to any type of religious organization, check to see whether pastoral counseling is available. Your physician can refer you to psychotherapists in your community. Not all therapists are right for all people, so be prepared to have initial sessions with several. Choose the one you feel most comfortable with.

Tips for Today

Some stress is unavoidable in life. How you respond to it is what determines whether you become "stressed out" or maintain your serenity. For the stress you can't avoid, develop a range of stress-management techniques and strategies.

Right now you can

- Sit in a comfortable chair and practice deep breathing for 5 to 10 minutes.

- Visualize a relaxing, peaceful place and imagine yourself experiencing it as vividly as possible; you might "feel" a gentle breeze on your skin or "hear" the soothing sound of a waterfall. Stay there as long as you can.

- Stand up and do some stretching exercises, such as gently rolling your head from side to side, stretching your arms out in front of your body and over your head, and slowly bending over and letting your arms hang toward the floor.

- Get out your date book and schedule what you'll be doing the rest of today and tomorrow. Pencil in a short walk and a conversation with a friend. Plan to go to bed 15 minutes earlier than usual.

SUMMARY

- When confronted with a stressor, the body undergoes a set of physical changes known as the fight-or-flight reaction. The sympathetic nervous system and endocrine system act on many targets in the body to prepare it for action—even if the situation does not require physical action.

Are you a person who doesn't perform as well as you should on tests? Do you find that anxiety interferes with your ability to study effectively before the test and to think clearly in the test situation? If so, you may be experiencing test anxiety. Two methods that have proven effective in helping people deal with test anxiety are systematic desensitization and success rehearsal.

Systematic Desensitization

Systematic desensitization is based on the premise that you can't feel anxiety and be relaxed at the same time. The method described here has three phases.

Phase I: Constructing an Anxiety Hierarchy   Begin the first phase by thinking of 10 or more situations related to your fear, such as hearing the announcement of the test date in class, studying for the test, sitting in the classroom waiting for the test to begin, reading the test questions, and so on. Write each situation on an index card, using a brief phrase to describe it on one side of the card. On the other side, list several realistic details or prompts that will help you vividly imagine yourself actually experiencing the situation. For example, if the situation is "hearing that 50% of the final grade will be based on the two exams," the prompts might include such details as "sitting in the big lecture auditorium in Baily Hall," "taking notes in my blue notebook," and "listening to Professor Smith's voice."

Next, arrange your cards in order, from least-tense to most-tense situation. Rate each situation to reflect the amount of anxiety you feel when you encounter it in real life, to confirm your anxiety hierarchy. Assign ratings on a scale of 0–100, and make sure the distances between items are fairly small and about equal. When you're sure your anxiety hierarchy is a true reflection of your feelings, number the cards.

Phase II: Learning and Practicing Muscle Relaxation   The second phase of the program involves learning to relax your muscles and to recognize when they are relaxed. A very effective way to do this is through progressive relaxation, which is described in this chapter. As you become proficient at this technique, you'll be able to go to a deeply relaxed state within just a few minutes. When you can do this, you're ready to go on to the next phase of the program.

Phase III: Implementing the Desensitization Program   Use the quiet place where you practiced your relaxation exercises. Sit comfortably and place your stack of numbered cards within reach. Take several minutes to relax completely, and then look at the first card, reading both the brief phrase and the descriptive prompts. Close your eyes and imagine yourself in that situation for about 10 seconds. Then put the card down and relax completely for about 30 seconds. Look at the card again, imagine the situation for 10 seconds, and relax again for 30 seconds.

At this point, evaluate your current level of anxiety about the situation on the card in terms of the rating scale you devised earlier. If your anxiety level is 10 or below, relax for 2 minutes and go on to the second card. If it's higher than 10, repeat the routine with the same card until the anxiety decreases. If you have difficulty with a particular item, go back to the previous item; then try it again. If you still can't visualize it without anxiety, try to construct three new items with smaller steps between them and insert them before the troublesome item. You should be able to move through one to four items per session. Sessions can be conducted anywhere from twice a day to twice a week and should last no longer than 20 minutes. It's helpful to graph your progress in a way that has meaning for you.

After you have successfully completed your program, you

- Emotional and behavioral responses to stressors vary among individuals. Ineffective responses increase stress but can be moderated or changed.

- Factors that influence emotional and behavioral responses to stressors include personality, cultural background, gender, and past experiences.

- Some personality characteristics, including impatience, hostility, and anger, make stress more difficult to handle. Other characteristics, such as optimism, commitment, and an inner locus of control, make an individual more stress-resistant.

- The general adaptation syndrome (GAS), an early model developed by Hans Selye to describe the relationship between stress and disease, has three stages: alarm, resistance, and exhaustion.

- A high allostatic load characterized by prolonged or repeated exposure to stress hormones can increase a person's risk of health problems.

- Psychoneuroimmunology (PNI) looks at how the physiological changes of the stress response affect the immune system and thereby increase the risk of illness.

- Health problems linked to stress include cardiovascular disease, colds and other infections, asthma and allergies, cancer, flare-ups of chronic diseases, psychological problems, digestive problems, headaches, insomnia, and injuries.

- A cluster of major life events that require adjustment and accommodation can lead to increased stress and an increased risk of health problems.

- Minor daily hassles increase stress if they are perceived negatively.

- Sources of stress associated with college may be academic, interpersonal, time-related, or financial pressures.

- Job-related stress is common, particularly for employees who have little control over decisions relating to their jobs. If stress is severe or prolonged, burnout may occur.

should be desensitized to the real-life situations that previously caused anxiety. If you find that you do experience some anxiety in the real situations, take 30 seconds or a minute to relax completely, just as you did when you were practicing. Remember: Fear and relaxation are incompatible; you have the ability to choose relaxation over fear.

Success Rehearsal

A variation on systematic desensitization is an approach called success rehearsal. To practice this method, take your hierarchy of anxiety-producing situations and vividly imagine yourself successfully dealing with each one. Create a detailed scenario for each situation, and use your imagination to experience genuine feelings of confidence. Recognize your negative thoughts ("I'll be so nervous I won't be able to think straight") and replace them with positive ones ("Anxiety will keep me alert so I can do a good job"). Proceed one step at a time, thinking of strategies for success as you go that you can later implement. These might include the following:

- Before the test, find out everything you can about it—its format, the material to be covered, the grading criteria. Ask the instructor for practice materials. Study in advance; don't just cram the night before. Avoid all-nighters.

- Devise a study plan. This might include forming a study group with one or more classmates or outlining what you will study, when, where, and for how long. Generate your own questions and answer them.

- Once in the test situation, sit away from possible distractions, listen carefully to instructions, and ask for clarification if you don't understand a direction.

- During the test, answer the easiest questions first. If you don't know an answer and there is no penalty for incorrect answers, guess. If there are several questions you have difficulty answering, review the ones you have already handled. Figure out approximately how much time you have to cover each question.

- For math problems, try to estimate the answer before doing the precise calculations.

- For true-false questions, look for qualifiers such as *always* and *never*. Such questions are likely to be false.

- For essay questions, look for key words in the question that indicate what the instructor is looking for in the answer. Develop a brief outline of your answer, sketching out what you will cover. Stick to your outline, and keep track of the time you're spending on your answer. Don't let yourself get caught with unanswered questions when time is up.

- Remain calm and focused throughout the test. Don't let negative thoughts rattle you. Avoid worrying about past performance, how others are doing, or the negative consequences of a poor test grade. If you start to become nervous, take some deep breaths and relax your muscles completely for a minute or so.

The best way to counter test anxiety is with successful test-taking experiences. The more times you succeed, the more your test anxiety will recede. If you find that these methods aren't sufficient to get your anxiety under control, you may want to seek professional help.

- New and changing relationships, prejudice, and discrimination are examples of interpersonal and social stressors.

- Other sources of stress include environmental stressors, such as natural disasters and noise, and internal stressors, such as illness, exhaustion, and unrealistically high expectations.

- Social support systems help buffer people against the effects of stress and make illness less likely. Good communication skills foster healthy relationships with others.

- Exercise, nutrition, and sleep are wellness behaviors that reduce stress and increase energy.

- Time management is an effective coping technique for those who tend to procrastinate, take on too many tasks, or organize their time poorly.

- Cognitive techniques for managing stress involve developing new and healthy patterns of thinking, such as practicing problem solving, monitoring self-talk, and cultivating a sense of humor.

- The relaxation response is the opposite of the fight-or-flight reaction. Techniques that trigger it, including progressive relaxation, imagery, meditation, deep breathing, hatha yoga, t'ai chi ch'uan, listening to music, and biofeedback, counteract the physiological effects of chronic stress. Counterproductive coping strategies include smoking, drinking, and binge eating.

- A successful individualized plan for coping with stress begins with the use of a stress journal or log to identify and study stressors and inappropriate behavioral responses. Completing a contract and recruiting a buddy can help your stress-management plan succeed.

- Additional help in dealing with stress is available from self-help books, peer counseling, support groups, and psychotherapy.

1. Choose a friend or family member who seems to deal particularly well with stress. Interview that person about his or her methods of managing stress. What strategies does he or she use? What can you learn from that person that can be applied to your own life?

2. Investigate the services available in your community—such as peer counseling, support groups, and time-management classes—to help people deal with stress. If possible, visit or gather information on one or more of them. Write a description and evaluation of their services, including your personal reactions.

3. Reread the stress-management techniques described in this chapter, and choose one to try for a week. If possible, select a behavior or strategy, such as regular exercise or systematic time management, that you've never tried before. After a trial period, evaluate the effectiveness of the strategy you chose. Did your stress level decrease during the week? Were you better able to deal with daily hassles and any more severe stressors that you encountered?

Ww. JOURNAL ENTRY

1. Watch for the physical changes of the stress response when you're in stressful situations. In your health journal, keep a stress log in which you note how many times in a day you experience the stress response to some degree. Also include a brief description of the circumstances surrounding your stress response. Is your life more or less stressful than you expected?

2. *Critical Thinking* Some techniques for stress management, including meditation and hypnosis, are considered strange or unscientific by some people. Find out more about one such technique through library or Internet research. What evidence can you find to support or oppose the idea that the technique can help people manage stress? Based on your research, write a brief essay in your health journal stating your opinion. As you consider the evidence, be sure to look closely at your sources of information.

3. Think about all the different environments in which you function, including your classrooms, the student union, the dorm, your house. Are some more stressful than others? Make a list of the environments in order from the most stressful to the least stressful. Indicate next to each environment the reasons you think it is stressful or nonstressful. Then start at the top of your list and record three or more ways to reduce the stressful impact these environments have on you.

4. Make a list of the daily hassles you commonly encounter, such as being awakened early by loud neighbors, standing in a long line for lunch, or repeatedly misplacing your keys. Divide your list into two groups: avoidable and unavoidable. For each stressor that is potentially avoidable, describe a strategy for eliminating it from your life. For stressors that are unavoidable, make a list of effective coping mechanisms.

FOR MORE INFORMATION

Books and Articles

Benson, H. 2000. *The Relaxation Response.* New York: Avon, Wholecare. *An expanded and updated edition of the 1975 classic on relaxation techniques and their physical benefits.*

Dement, W. C. 1999. *The Promise of Sleep.* New York: Delacorte. *An exploration of sleep and its effects on wellness by a prominent sleep researcher.*

Girdano, D. A., D. Dusek, and G. S. Everly. 2001. *Controlling Stress and Tension,* 6th ed. New York: Allyn & Bacon. *An easy-to-understand guide to identifying and combating stressors.*

Justice, B. 2000. *Who Gets Sick: How Beliefs, Moods, and Thoughts Affect Health.* Los Angeles: Jeremy Tarcher. *Explores what is known today about the role of thought and emotion in health and illness.*

Sapolsky, R. M. 1998. *Why Zebras Don't Get Ulcers: An Updated Guide to Stress-Related Diseases and Coping.* New York: W. H. Freeman. *An entertaining look at the effects of stress on the body and the relationship between stress and disease.*

Ww. Organizations and Web Sites

American Music Therapy Association. Provides information about music therapy and about how to find a certified therapist.
301-589-3300
http://www.musictherapy.org

American Psychological Association. Provides information on stress management and psychological disorders.
202-336-5500; 800-964-2000 (referrals)
http://www.apa.org; http://helping.apa.org

Association for Applied Psychophysiology and Biofeedback. Provides information about biofeedback and referrals to certified biofeedback practitioners.
800-477-8892
http://www.aapb.org

Center for Anxiety and Stress Treatment. A commercial site that also includes an anxiety symptom checklist and a list of stress-busting tips for work stress.
http://www.stressrelease.com

The Humor Project. A clearinghouse for information and practical ideas related to humor.

518-587-8770

http://www.humorproject.com

National Institute for Occupational Safety and Health (NIOSH). Provides information and links on job stress.

http://www.cdc.gov/niosh/stresshp.html

National Institute of Mental Health (NIMH). Publishes informative brochures about stress and stress management as well as other aspects of mental health.

800-421-4211; 301-443-4513

http://www.nimh.nih.gov

National Sleep Foundation. Provides information about sleep and how to overcome sleep problems such as insomnia and jet lag; brochures are available from the Web site or via fax.

202-347-3471; 202-347-3472 (fax)

877-BE-AWAKE (daytime sleepiness screening)

http://www.sleepfoundation.org

Student Counseling Virtual Pamphlet Collection. Links to online pamphlets from student counseling centers at colleges and universities across the country; topics include stress, sleep, and time management.

http://counseling.uchicago.edu/upc

See also the listings for Chapters 1 and 3.

SELECTED BIBLIOGRAPHY

Bowman, M. A., et al. 2000. Changes in functional status related to health maintenance visits to family physicians. *Journal of Family Practice* 49(5): 428–433.

Bremner, J. D. 1999. Does stress damage the brain? *Biological Psychiatry* 45(7): 797–805.

Bremner, J. D., et al. 2000. Hippocampal volume reduction in major depression. *American Journal of Psychiatry* 157(1): 115–118.

Brown, E. S., A. J. Rush, B. S. McEwen. 1999. Hippocampal remodeling and damage by corticosteroids: Implications for mood disorders. *Neuropsychopharmacology* 21(4): 474–484.

Cerbone, F. G., and C. L. Larison. 2000. A bibliographic essay: The relationship between stress and substance use. *Substance Use and Misuse* 35(5): 757–786.

Da Silva, J. A. P. 1999. Sex hormones and glucocorticoids: Interactions with the immune system. *Annals of the New York Academy of Sciences* 876: 102–117.

Daun, J. M., R. W. Ball, and J. G. Cannon. 2000. Glucocorticoid sensitivity of interleukin-1 agonist and antagonist secretion: The effects of age and gender. *American Journal of Physiological Regulation and Integrative and Comparative Physiology* 278(4): R855–862.

de Quervain, D. J., et al. 2000. Acute cortisone administration impairs retrieval of long-term declarative memory in humans. *Nature Neuroscience* 3(4): 313–314.

Gang, A., et al. 2001. Psychological stress perturbs epidermal permeability barrier homeostasis: Implications for the pathogenesis of stress-associated skin disorders. *Archives of Dermatology* 137(1): 53–59.

Jacobs, B. L., H. van Praag, and F. H. Gage. 2000. Adult brain neurogenesis and psychiatry: A novel theory of depression. *Molecular Psychiatry* 5(3): 262–269.

Kimata, H. 2001. Effect of humor on allergen-induced wheal reactions. *Journal of the American Medical Association* 285(6): 738.

Lacey, K., et al. 2000. A prospective study of neuroendocrine and immune alterations associated with the stress of an oral academic examination among graduate students. *Psychoneuroendocrinology* 25(4): 339–356.

Maes, M., et al. 1999. The effects of psychological stress on leukocyte subset distribution in humans: Evidence of immune activation. *Neuropsychobiology* 39(1): 1–9.

McEwen, B. S. 1998. Protective and damaging effects of stress mediators. *New England Journal of Medicine* 338(3): 171–179.

Nordstrom, C. K., et al. 2001. Work-related stress and early atherosclerosis. *Epidemiology* 12(2): 180–185.

Sapolsky, R. M., L. M. Romero, and A. U. Munck. 2000. How do glucocorticoids influence stress responses? Integrating permissive, suppressive, stimulatory, and preparative actions. *Endocrine Reviews* 21(1): 55–89.

Scheufele, P. M. 2000. Effects of progressive relaxation and classical music on measurements of attention, relaxation, and stress responses. *Journal of Behavioral Medicine* 23(2): 207–228.

Shepard, J. D., et al. 2000. Additive pressure effects of caffeine and stress in male medical students at risk for hypertension. *American Journal of Hypertension* 13(5 Pt. 1): 475–481.

Siegman, A. W., et al. 2000. Antagonistic behavior, dominance, hostility, and coronary heart disease. *Psychosomatic Medicine* 62(2): 248–257.

Skirka, N. 2000. The relationship of hardiness, sense of coherence, sports participation, and gender to perceived stress and psychological symptoms among college students. *Journal of Sports Medicine and Physical Fitness* 40(1): 63–70.

Taylor, S. E., et al. 2000. Biobehavioral responses to stress in females. Tend-and-befriend, not fight-or-flight. *Psychological Review* 107(3): 411–429.

Van Cauter, E., R. Leproult, and L. Plat. 2000. Age-related changes in slow wave sleep and REM sleep and relationship with growth hormone and cortisol levels in healthy men. *Journal of the American Medical Association* 284(7): 861–868.

Weber, B., et al. 2000. Increased diurnal plasma concentrations of cortisone in depressed patients. *Journal of Clinical Endocrinology and Metabolism* 85(3): 1133–1136.

Wolff, G. E., et al. 2000. Differences in daily stress, mood, coping, and eating behavior in binge eating and nonbinge eating college women. *Addictive Behaviors* 25(2): 205–216.

Young, D. R., et al. 1999. The effects of aerobic exercise and t'ai chi on blood pressure in older people. *Journal of the American Geriatrics Society* 47(3): 277–284.

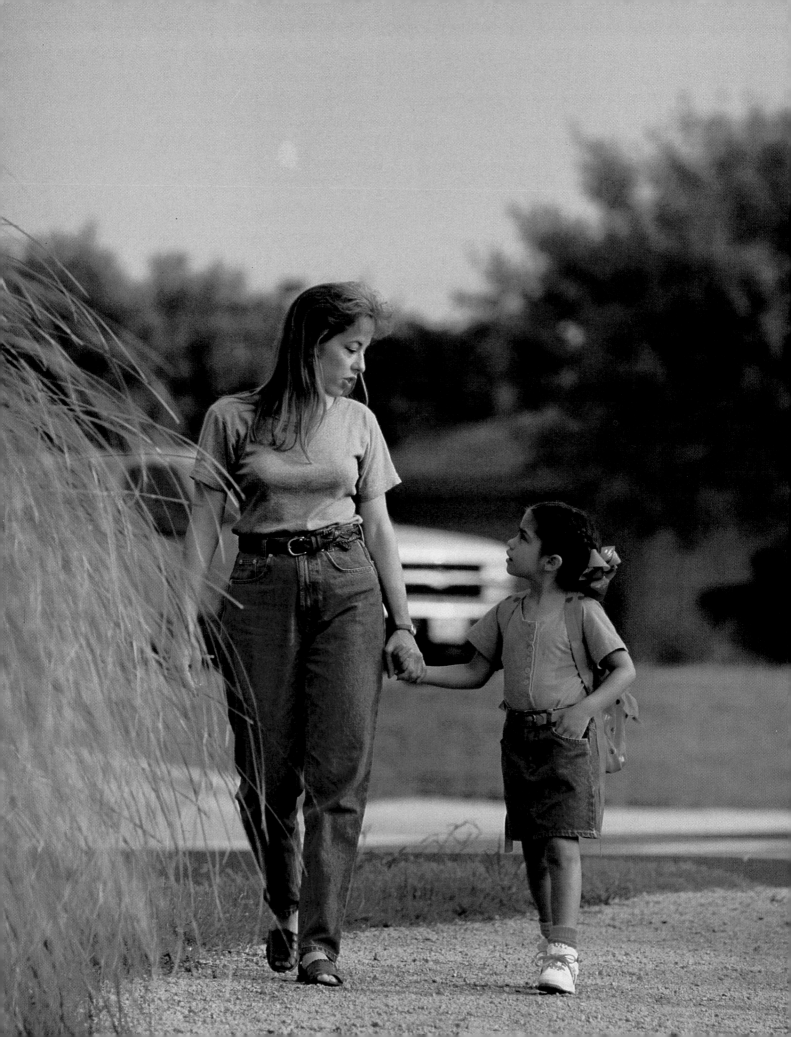

After reading this chapter, you should be able to

- Describe what it means to be psychologically healthy

- Explain how to develop and maintain a positive self-concept and healthy self-esteem

- Discuss the importance to psychological health of an optimistic outlook, good communication skills, and constructive approaches to dealing with loneliness and anger

- Describe common psychological disorders and list the warning signs of suicide

- Explain the different approaches and types of help available for psychological problems

Psychological Health

3

TEST YOUR KNOWLEDGE

1. Normality is a key component of psychological health.
   True or false?

2. People with an optimistic view of the events in their lives have better physical health and lower mortality rates than people who are more pessimistic.
   True or false?

3. About how many Americans have a diagnosable psychological disorder during the course of a year?
   a. 5%
   b. 10%
   c. 20%

4. On television, about 75% of mentally ill characters are depicted as violent. About what percentage of mentally ill people are actually violent?
   a. 7%
   b. 14%
   c. 21%
   d. 28%

5. People who really intend to commit suicide don't talk about it.
   True or false?

ANSWERS

1. FALSE. Normality simply means being close to average, and having unusual ideas or attitudes doesn't mean that a person is mentally ill. The fact that people's ideas are varied makes life interesting and helps people respond in creative ways to life's challenges.

2. TRUE. Although the reasons for this difference aren't entirely clear, pessimists may be more prone to depression or immune system impairment; because of an external locus of control, pessimists may also be more likely to engage in unhealthy lifestyle behaviors.

3. C. The most common types of disorders are simple phobias and depression. The majority of people with psychological disorders do not receive appropriate treatment.

4. A. The vast majority of violence is caused by people without psychological disorders. Targets of violence by people with a mental illness are much more likely to be family members or other caregivers than strangers.

5. FALSE. Most people who commit suicide have talked about doing it.

What exactly is psychological health? Many people over the centuries have expressed opinions about the nature of psychological (or mental) health. Some even claim that there is no such thing, that psychological health is just a myth. We disagree. We think there is such a thing as psychological health just as there is physical health—and the two are closely interrelated. Just as your body can work well or poorly, giving you pleasure or pain, your mind can also work well or poorly, resulting in happiness or unhappiness. Psychological health is a crucial component of overall wellness. (We are using "mental health" and "psychological health" interchangeably; the latter is the more current term, but it hasn't replaced "mental health" yet.)

If you feel pain and unhappiness rather than pleasure and happiness or if you sense that you could be functioning at a higher level, there may be ways you can help yourself—either on your own or with professional help. This chapter will explain how.

WHAT PSYCHOLOGICAL HEALTH IS NOT

Psychological health is not the same as psychological **normality**. Being mentally normal simply means being close to average. You can define normal body temperature because a few degrees above or below this temperature always means physical sickness. But your ideas and attitudes can vary tremendously without your losing efficiency or feeling emotional distress. And psychological diversity is valuable; living in a society of people with varied ideas and lifestyles makes life interesting and challenging.

Conforming to social demands is not necessarily a mark of psychological health. If you don't question what's going on around you, you're not fulfilling your potential as a thinking, questioning human being. For example, our society admires the framers of the U.S. Constitution and the abolitionists who rebelled against injustices. If conformity signified mental health, then political dissent would indicate mental illness by definition (and we have seen that definition used by dictators). If such a definition

were valid, Galileo would have been mad for insisting that the earth revolved around the sun.

Never seeking help for personal problems does not mean you are psychologically healthy, any more than seeking help proves you are mentally ill. Unhappy people may not want to seek professional help because they don't want to reveal their problems to others, may fear what their friends might think, or may not know whom to ask for help. People who are severely disturbed psychologically or emotionally may not even realize they need help, or they may become so suspicious of other people that they can only be treated without their consent.

We cannot say people are "mentally ill" or "mentally healthy" on the basis of symptoms alone. Life constantly presents problems. Time and life inevitably alter the environment as well as our minds and bodies, and changes present problems. The symptom of anxiety, for example, can help us face a problem and solve it before it gets too big. Someone who shows no anxiety may be refusing to recognize problems or do anything about them. A person who is anxious for good reason is likely to be judged more psychologically healthy in the long run than someone who is inappropriately calm.

Finally, we cannot judge psychological health from the way people look. All too often, a person who seems to be OK and even happy suddenly takes his or her own life. Usually such people lack close friends who might have known of their desperation. At an early age, we learn to conceal and "lie." We may believe that our complaints put unfair demands on others. While suffering in silence can sometimes be a virtue, it can also impede getting help.

DEFINING PSYCHOLOGICAL HEALTH

It is even harder to say what psychological health *is* than what it is *not*. Psychological health can be defined either negatively as the absence of sickness or positively as the presence of wellness. The narrower, negative definition has several advantages: It concentrates attention on the worst problems and on the people most in need, and it tends to avoid value judgments about the best way to lead our lives. However, if we consider everyone to be mentally healthy who is not severely mentally disturbed, we end up ignoring common problems that can be addressed.

A positive definition—psychological health as the presence of wellness—is a more ambitious outlook, one that encourages you to fulfill your own potential. Freedom from disorders is only one factor in psychological wellness. During the 1960s, Abraham Maslow eloquently described an ideal of mental health in his book *Toward a Psychology of Being*. He was convinced that psychologists were too preoccupied with people who had failed in some way. He also disliked the way psychologists tried to reduce human striving to physiological needs or drives.

Terms

normality The psychological characteristics attributed to the majority of people in a population at a given time.

self-actualization The highest level of growth in Maslow's hierarchy.

self-concept The ideas, feelings, and perceptions one has about oneself; also called *self-image*.

self-esteem Satisfaction and confidence in oneself; the valuing of oneself as a person.

autonomy Independence; the sense of being self-directed.

other-directed Guided in behavior by the values and expectations of others.

inner-directed Guided in behavior by an inner set of rules and values.

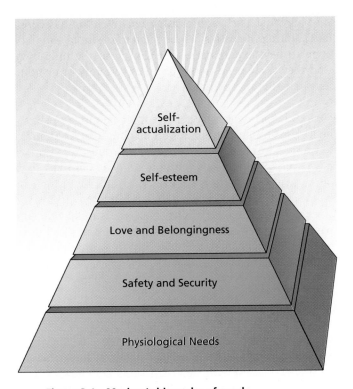

Figure 3-1   Maslow's hierarchy of needs.
 SOURCE: Maslow, A. 1970. *Motivation and Personality,* 2nd ed.
New York: Harper & Row.

According to Maslow, there is a *hierarchy of needs,* listed here in order of decreasing urgency: physiological needs, safety, being loved, maintaining self-esteem, and self-actualization (Figure 3-1). When urgent needs like the need for food, water, shelter, sleep, and safety are satisfied, less urgent needs take priority. Most of us are well fed and feel reasonably safe, so we are driven by higher motives. Maslow's conclusions were based on his study of a group of visibly successful people who seemed to have lived, or be living, at their fullest, including Abraham Lincoln, Henry David Thoreau, Ludwig van Beethoven, Eleanor Roosevelt, and Albert Einstein, as well as some of his own friends and acquaintances. He stated that these people had achieved **self-actualization;** he thought they had fulfilled a good measure of their human potential and suggested that self-actualized people all share certain qualities.

Realism

Self-actualized people are able to deal with the world as it is and not demand that it be otherwise. If you are realistic, you know the difference between what is and what you want. You also know what you can change and what you cannot. Unrealistic people often spend a great deal of time and energy trying to force the world and other people into their ideal picture. Realistic people accept evidence that contradicts what they want to believe, and if it is important evidence, they modify their beliefs.

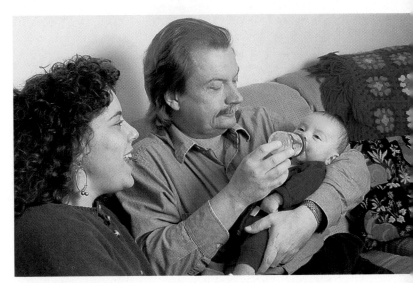

A positive self-concept begins in infancy. Knowing that he's loved and valued by his parents gives this baby a solid basis for lifelong psychological health.

Acceptance

Psychologically healthy people can largely accept themselves and others. Self-acceptance means having a positive **self-concept,** or self-image, or appropriately high **self-esteem.** They have a positive but realistic mental image of themselves and positive feelings about who they are, what they are capable of, and what roles they play. People who feel good about themselves are likely to live up to their positive self-image and enjoy successes that in turn reinforce these good feelings. A good self-concept is based on a realistic view of personal worth—it does not mean being egocentric or "stuck on yourself."

Being able to tolerate our own imperfections and still feel positive about ourselves helps us tolerate the imperfections of others. Psychologically healthy people tend to be optimistic about what they can expect from other people, until experience proves their optimism to be unrealistic. Acceptance means being willing to interact with people who are imperfect and unlikely to change.

Autonomy

Psychologically healthy people are able to direct themselves, acting independently of their social environment. **Autonomy** is more than freedom from physical control by something outside the self. Many people, for example, shrink from expressing their feelings because they fear disapproval and rejection. They respond only to what they feel as outside pressure. Behavior such as this is **other-directed.** In contrast, **inner-directed** people find guidance from within, from their own values and feelings. They are not afraid to be themselves. Psychologically free people act because they choose to, not because they are driven or pressured.

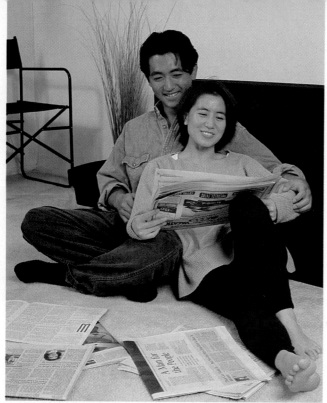

Self-actualized people respond in a genuine, spontaneous way to what happens around them. They are capable of maintaining close interpersonal relationships.

Autonomy can give healthy people certain childlike qualities. Very small children have a quality of being "real." They respond in a genuine, spontaneous way to whatever happens. Someone who is genuine has no pretenses. Being genuine means not having to plan words or actions to get approval or make an impression. It means being aware of feelings and being willing to express them—being unself-consciously oneself. This quality is sometimes called **authenticity**; such people are *authentic,* the "real thing."

A Capacity for Intimacy

Healthy people are capable of physical and emotional intimacy. They can expose their feelings and thoughts to other people. They are open to the pleasure of intimate physical contact and to the risks and satisfactions of being close to others in a caring, sensitive way. Intimate physical contact may mean "good sex," but it also means something more—intense awareness of both your partner and yourself in which contact becomes communication. Chapters 4 and 5 discuss intimacy in more detail.

Creativity

Psychologically healthy people are creative and have a continuing fresh appreciation for what goes on around them. They are not necessarily great poets, artists, or musicians, but they do live their everyday lives in creative

ways: "A first-rate soup is more creative than a second-rate painting." Creative people seem to see more and to be open to new experiences; they don't fear the unknown. And they don't need to minimize uncertainty or avoid it; they actually find it attractive.

How did Maslow's group achieve their exemplary psychological health, and (more important) how can *we* attain it? Maslow himself did not answer that question, but we have a few suggestions. Undoubtedly it helps to have been treated with respect, love, and understanding as a child, to have experienced stability and to have achieved a sense of mastery. As adults, since we cannot redo the past, we must concentrate on meeting current psychological challenges in ways that will lead to long-term mental wellness.

W. MEETING LIFE'S CHALLENGES

Life is full of challenges—large and small. Everyone, regardless of heredity and family influences, must learn to cope successfully with new situations and new people. For emotional and mental wellness, each of us must continue to grow psychologically, developing new and more sophisticated coping mechanisms to suit our current lives. We must develop an adult identity that enhances our self-esteem and autonomy. We must also learn to communicate honestly, handle anger and loneliness appropriately, and avoid being defensive.

Growing Up Psychologically

How we respond to the challenges of life influences the development of our personality and identity. Psychologist Erik Erikson proposed that development proceeds through a series of eight stages, extending throughout the life span. Each stage is characterized by a major crisis or turning point, a time of increased vulnerability as well as increased potential for psychological growth (Table 3-1).

The successful mastery of one stage is a basis for mastering the next, so early failures can have repercussions in later life. Fortunately, life provides ongoing opportunities for mastering these tasks. For example, although the development of trust begins in infancy, it is refined as we grow older. We learn to trust people outside our immediate family and to limit our trust by identifying people who are untrustworthy.

Developing an Adult Identity A primary task beginning in adolescence is the development of an adult identity: a unified sense of self, characterized by attitudes, beliefs, and ways of acting that are genuinely one's own. People with adult identities know who they are, what they are capable of, what roles they play, and their place among their peers. They have a sense of their own uniqueness but also appreciate what they have in com-

Table 3-1

Erikson's Stages of Development

Age	Conflict	Important People	Task
Birth–1 year	Trust vs. mistrust	Mother or other primary caregiver	In being fed and comforted, developing the trust that others will respond to your needs
1–3 years	Autonomy vs. shame and self-doubt	Parents	In toilet training, locomotion, and exploration, learning self-control without losing the capacity for assertiveness
3–6 years	Initiative vs. guilt	Family	In playful talking and locomotion, developing a conscience based on parental prohibitions that is not too inhibiting
6–12 years	Industry vs. inferiority	Neighborhood and school	In school and playing with peers, learning the value of accomplishment and perseverance without feeling inadequate
Adolescence	Identity vs. identity confusion	Peers	Developing a stable sense of who you are—your needs, abilities, interpersonal style, and values
Young adulthood	Intimacy vs. isolation	Close friends, sex partners	Learning to live and share intimately with others, often in sexual relationships
Middle adulthood	Generativity vs. self-absorption	Work associates, children, community	Doing things for others, including parenting and civic activities
Older adulthood	Integrity vs. despair	Humankind	Affirming the value of life and its ideals

SOURCE: Erikson, E. 1963. *Childhood and Society*. New York: Norton.

mon with others. They view themselves realistically and can assess their strengths and weaknesses without relying on the opinions of others. Achieving an identity also means that one can form intimate relationships with others while maintaining a strong sense of self.

Our identities evolve as we interact with the world and make choices about what we'd like to do and whom we'd like to model ourselves after. Developing an adult identity is particularly challenging in a heterogeneous, secular, and relatively affluent society like ours, in which many roles are possible, many choices are tolerated, and ample time is allowed for experimenting and making up one's mind.

Early identities are often modeled after parents—or the opposite of parents, in rebellion from what they represent. Later, peers, rock stars, sports heroes, and religious figures are added to the list of possible models. In high school and college, people often join cliques that assert a certain identity—the "jocks," the "brains," the "slackers." Although much of an identity is internal—a way of viewing oneself and the world—it can include such things as styles of talking and dressing, ornaments like earrings, and particular hairstyles.

Early identities are rarely permanent. A student who works for good grades and approval from parents and teachers one year can turn into a dropout devoted to hard rock and wild parties a year later. At some point, however, most of us adopt a more stable, individual identity that ties together the experiences of childhood and the expectations and aspirations of adulthood. Erikson's theory does not suggest that suddenly one day we assume our final identity and never change after that. Life is more interesting for people who continue to evolve into more distinct individuals, rather than being rigidly controlled by their pasts. Identity reflects a lifelong process, and it changes as a person develops new relationships and roles.

Developing an adult identity is an important part of psychological wellness. Without a personal identity, we begin to feel confused about who we are; Erikson called this situation an *identity crisis*. Until we have "found ourselves," we cannot have much self-esteem because a self is not firmly in place.

How far have you gotten in developing your adult identity? Write down a list of characteristics you think a friend who knows you well would use to describe you. Rank them from the most to the least important. Your list might include elements such as gender, socioeconomic status, ethnic and/or religious identification, choice of college or major, parents' occupations, interests and talents, attitudes toward drugs and alcohol, style of dress, the kinds of people with whom you typically associate,

authenticity Genuineness.

Terms

your expected role in society, and aspects of your personality. Which elements of your identity do you feel are permanent and which do you think may change over time? Are there any characteristics missing from your list that you'd like to add?

Another aid to developing an adult identity is to identify possible role models. Whom do you admire and want to be like? Which characteristics of that person do you want to emulate? How did that person acquire those characteristics, and how could you follow in her or his footsteps? Some role models might be willing to be mentors to you, spending time with you and sharing their wisdom.

Developing Intimacy   Erikson's developmental stages don't end with establishing an adult identity. Learning to live intimately with others and finding a productive role for yourself in society are other tasks of adulthood—to be able to love and work.

People with established identities can form intimate relationships and sexual unions characterized by sharing, open communication, long-term commitment, and love. Those who lack a firm sense of self may have difficulty establishing relationships because they feel overwhelmed by closeness and the needs of another person. As a result, they experience only short-term, superficial relationships with others and may remain isolated. As described in Chapter 2, a lack of social support can affect getting both physical and psychological help. (Chapter 4 has more information about intimate relationships.)

Developing Values and Purpose in Your Life   Erikson assigned his last two stages, generativity versus self-absorption and integrity versus despair, to middle adulthood and older adulthood. But these stages are concerned with values and purpose in life, issues that need to be addressed by young people and reexamined throughout life. Values are criteria for judging what is good and bad; they underlie our moral decisions and behavior. The first morality of the young child is to consider "good" to mean what brings immediate and tangible rewards, and "bad," whatever results in punishment. An older child will explain right and wrong in terms of authority figures and rules. But the final stage of moral development, one that not everyone attains, is being able to conceive of right and wrong in more abstract terms such as justice and virtue.

As adults we need to assess how far we have evolved morally and what values we actually have adopted, either explicitly or implicitly. Without an awareness of our personal values, our lives may be hurriedly driven forward by immediate desires and the passing demands of others. But are we doing things according to our principles? What are we striving for with our actions? Living according to values means considering your options carefully before making a choice, choosing between options without succumbing to outside pressures that oppose your values, and making a choice and acting on it rather than doing nothing. Your actions and how you justify them proclaim to others what you stand for.

A practical exercise for clarifying your values and goals is to write a draft of your obituary for a local newspaper. How would you like to be remembered? What would you like to have achieved? What will you have done to meet those goals? This obituary should not be a glorification, but an honest, realistic appraisal. End it by summarizing in a few sentences what was most important about your life. In reading what you have written, ask yourself, "How will I have to change to be the person I want to be?"

For more on developing meaning and purpose in your life, see the box "Paths to Spiritual Wellness."

COMMUNICATE!   One of the many challenges of adulthood is redefining your relationship with your parents, which is often most clearly expressed in the way you communicate with them. For example, do you resent their authority, or do you let them know you value their opinion even when you don't act on it? Listen carefully the next time you have a conversation with one or both of your parents. Do all of you sound like adults? If not, why not? What can you do to develop a more mature kind of communication?

Achieving Healthy Self-Esteem

Having a healthy level of self-esteem means regarding your self, which includes all aspects of your identity, as good, competent, and worthy of love. It is a critical component of wellness.

Developing a Positive Self-Concept   Ideally, a positive self-concept begins in childhood, based on experiences within the family and outside it. Children need to develop a sense of being loved and being able to give love and to accomplish their goals. If they feel rejected or neglected by their parents, they may fail to develop feelings of self-worth. They may grow to have a negative concept of themselves.

Another component of self-concept is integration. An integrated self-concept is one that you have made for yourself—not someone else's image of you or a mask that doesn't quite fit. Important building blocks of self-concept are the personality characteristics and mannerisms of parents, which children may adopt without realizing it. Later, they may be surprised to find themselves acting like one of their parents. Eventually, such building blocks should be reshaped and integrated into a new individual personality.

A further aspect of self-concept is stability. Stability depends on the integration of the self and its freedom from contradictions. People who have gotten mixed messages about themselves from parents and friends may

Spiritual wellness means different things to different people. For many, it involves developing a set of guiding beliefs, principles, or values that give meaning and purpose to life. It helps people achieve a sense of wholeness within themselves and in their relationships with others. Spiritual wellness influences people on an individual level, as well as on a community level, where it can bond people together through compassion, love, forgiveness, and self-sacrifice. For some, spirituality includes a belief in a higher power. Regardless of how it is defined, the development of spiritual wellness is critical for overall health and well-being. Its development is closely tied to the other components of wellness, particularly psychological health.

There are many paths to spiritual wellness. One of the most common in our society is organized religion. Some people object to the notion that organized religion can contribute to psychological health and overall wellness, asserting that it reinforces people's tendency to deny real difficulties and to accept what can and should be changed. Freud criticized religion as wishful thinking; Marx called it an opiate to make the poor accept social injustice. However, many elements of religious belief and practice can promote psychological health.

Organized religion usually involves its members in a community where social and material support is available. Religious organizations offer a social network to those who might otherwise be isolated. The major religions provide paths for transforming the self in ways that can lead to greater happiness and serenity and reduce feelings of anxiety and hopelessness. In Christianity, salvation follows turning away from the selfish ego to God's sovereignty and grace, where a joy is found that frees the believer from anxious self-concern and despair. Islam is the word for a kind of self-surrender leading to peace with God.

Buddhism teaches how to detach oneself from selfish desire, leading to compassion for the suffering of others and freedom from fear-engendering illusions. Judaism emphasizes the social and ethical redemption the Jewish community can experience if it follows the laws of God. Religions teach specific techniques for achieving these transformations of the self: prayer, both in groups and in private; meditation; the performance of rituals and ceremonies symbolizing religious truths; and good works and service to others. Christianity's faith and works are perhaps analogous to the cognitive and behavioral components of a program of behavior change.

Spiritual wellness does not require participation in organized religion. Many people find meaning and purpose in other ways. By spending time in nature or working on environmental issues, people can experience continuity with the natural world. Spiritual wellness can come through helping others in one's community or by promoting human rights, peace and harmony among people, and opportunities for human development on a global level. (The spiritual, psychological, and physical wellness benefits of helping others are discussed further in Chapter 19.) Other people develop spiritual wellness through art or through their personal relationships.

The search for meaning and purpose in life is reflected in Erikson's later stages of development. Particularly in the second half of life, people seem to have an urge to view their activities and consciousness from a transcendent perspective. Perhaps it is the approach of death that makes older people tend to take less interest in material possessions and to devote more time to interpersonal and altruistic pursuits. At every age, however, people seem to feel better if they have beliefs about the ultimate purpose of life and their own place in the universe.

---

have contradictory self-images, which defy integration and make them vulnerable to shifting levels of self-esteem. At times they regard themselves as entirely good, capable, and lovable—an ideal self—and at other times they see themselves as entirely bad, incompetent, and unworthy of love. While at the first pole, they may develop such an inflated ego that they totally ignore other people's needs and see others only as instruments for fulfilling their own desires. At the other pole, they may feel so small and weak that they run for protection to someone who seems powerful and caring. At neither extreme do such people see themselves or others realistically, and their relationships with other people are filled with misunderstandings and ultimately with conflict.

The concepts we have about ourselves and others are an important part of our personalities. And all the components of our self-concept profoundly influence our interpersonal relationships.

Meeting Challenges to Self-Esteem
As an adult, you sometimes run into situations that challenge your self-concept: People you care about may tell you they don't

love you or feel loved by you, or your attempts to accomplish a goal may end in failure. You can react to such challenges in several ways. The best approach is to acknowledge that something has gone wrong and try again, adjusting your goals to your abilities without radically revising your self-concept. Less productive responses are denying that anything went wrong and blaming someone else. While assuming these attitudes may preserve your self-concept temporarily, in the long run they keep you from meeting the challenge. The worst reaction is to develop a lasting negative self-concept in which you feel bad, unloved, and ineffective—in other words, to become demoralized. Instead of coping, the demoralized person gives up, reinforcing the negative self-concept and setting in motion a cycle of bad self-concept and failure. In people who are genetically predisposed to depression, demoralization can progress to additional symptoms, discussed later in the chapter.

NOTICE YOUR PATTERNS OF THINKING One method for fighting demoralization is to recognize and test your negative thoughts and assumptions about yourself and others.

The first step is to note exactly when an unpleasant emotion—feeling worthless, wanting to give up, feeling depressed—occurs or gets worse, to identify the events or daydreams that trigger that emotion, and to observe whatever thoughts come into your head just before or during the emotional experience. It is helpful to keep a daily journal about such events.

Let's consider the example of Jennifer, a student who went to the college counseling center because she'd been feeling "down" lately. Her social life had not been going well, and she had begun to think she was a boring, uninteresting person. Asked to keep a daily journal, she wrote that she felt let down and discouraged when a date who promised to meet her at 7:30 P.M. was 15 minutes late. The thoughts that occurred to her were: "He's not going to come. It's my fault. He has more important things to do. Maybe he's with someone else. He doesn't like me. Nobody likes me because I don't have anything interesting to say. What if he had a car accident?"

People who are demoralized tend to use all-or-nothing thinking. They overgeneralize from negative events. They overlook the positive and they jump to negative conclusions, minimize their own successes and magnify the successes of others. They take responsibility for unfortunate situations that are not their fault. The minute Jennifer's date was late, she jumped to the conclusion that he was not coming and blamed herself for it. From that point she jumped to more negative conclusions and more unfounded overgeneralizations. Patterns of thinking that make events seem worse than they are in reality are called **cognitive distortions**.

DEVELOP REALISTIC SELF-TALK   Jennifer needs to develop more rational responses. For Jennifer, more rational thinking could be "He's a little late so I'll reread the study questions." If he still hadn't come after 30 minutes, she might have called him to see if something was holding him up, without jumping to any conclusions about the meaning of his lateness.

In your own fight against demoralization, it may be hard to figure out a rational response until hours or days after the event that upset you. But once you get used to noticing the way your mind works, you may be able to catch yourself thinking negatively and change the thought process before it goes too far.

This approach is not the same as positive thinking—substituting a positive thought for a negative one. Instead, you simply try to make your thoughts as logical and accurate as possible. If Jennifer continues to think she's boring, she should try to collect evidence to prove or dis-

prove that. If she has exaggerated her dullness, as do many demoralized people, her investigations may prove her wrong. For example, she might ask her friends their candid opinions about her personality, and she can observe whether people seem interested in continuing a conversation with her.

Demoralized people can be so tenacious about their negative beliefs that they make them come true in a self-fulfilling prophecy. Jennifer might conclude that she is so boring no one will like her anyway, so she may as well not bother to be involved in what's going on around her. This behavior could help her negative belief become a reality. For additional tips on how to change distorted, negative ways of thinking, see the box "Realistic Self-Talk."

Being Less Defensive

Sometimes our wishes come into conflict with people around us or with our conscience, and we become frustrated and anxious. If we cannot resolve the conflict by changing the external situation, we try to resolve the conflict internally by rearranging our thoughts and feelings. Some standard **defense mechanisms** are listed in Table 3-2. The drawback of many of these coping mechanisms is that although they succeed temporarily, they are dead-ends that make finding ultimate solutions much harder. Some mechanisms, such as substitution and humor, can be very useful for coping, as long as they don't keep us from being who we want to be.

Recognizing your favorite defense mechanisms can be difficult, because they've probably become habits, occurring unconsciously. But we each have some inkling about how our mind operates. By remembering the details of conflict situations you have been in, you may be able to figure out which defense mechanisms you used in successful or unsuccessful attempts to cope. Try to look at yourself as an objective, outside observer would and analyze your thoughts and behavior in a psychologically stressful situation from the past. Having insight into what strategies you typically use can lead to new, less defensive and more effective ways of coping in the future.

Being Optimistic

Optimism and pessimism are abstract concepts that might seem to have more to do with philosophy than with psychological health. However, many psychologists believe that pessimism is not just a symptom of everyday depression but an important root cause as well. Pessimists not only expect repeated failure and rejection but also perversely accept it as deserved. Pessimists do not see themselves as capable of success, and they irrationally dismiss any evidence of their own accomplishments. This negative point of view is learned, typically at a young age from parents and other authority figures. But as an optimist would tell you, that means it also has the potential of being unlearned.

Terms   **cognitive distortion** A pattern of thinking that makes events seem worse than they are.

defense mechanism A mental mechanism for coping with conflict or anxiety.

Do your patterns of thinking make events seem worse than they truly are? Do negative beliefs about yourself become self-fulfilling prophecies? Substituting realistic self-talk for negative self-talk can help you build and maintain self-esteem and cope better with the challenges in your life. Here are some examples of common types of distorted negative self-talk, along with suggestions for more accurate and rational responses.

Cognitive Distortion	Negative Self-Talk	Realistic Self-Talk
Focusing on negatives	School is so discouraging—nothing but one hassle after another.	School is pretty challenging and has its difficulties, but there certainly are rewards. It's really a mixture of good and bad.
Expecting the worst	Why would my boss want to meet with me this afternoon if not to fire me?	I wonder why my boss wants to meet with me. I guess I'll just have to wait and see.
Overgeneralizing	(After getting a poor grade on a paper) Just as I thought—I'm incompetent at everything.	I'll start working on the next paper earlier. That way, if I run into problems, I'll have time to consult with the TA.
Minimizing	I won the speech contest, but none of the other speakers was very good. I wouldn't have done as well against stiffer competition.	It may not have been the best speech I'll ever give, but it was good enough to win the contest. I'm really improving as a speaker.
Blaming others	I wouldn't have eaten so much last night if my friends hadn't insisted on going to that restaurant.	I overdid it last night. Next time I'll make different choices
Expecting perfection	I should have scored 100% on this test. I can't believe I missed that one problem through a careless mistake.	Too bad I missed one problem through carelessness, but overall I did very well on this test. Next time I'll be more careful.
Believing you're the cause of everything	Sarah seems so depressed today. I wish I hadn't had that argument with her yesterday; it must have really upset her.	I wish I had handled the argument better, and in the future I'll try to. But I don't know if Sarah's behavior is related to what I said or even if she's depressed. In any case, I'm not responsible for how Sarah feels or acts; only she can take responsibility for that.
Thinking in black and white	I've got to score 10 points in the game today. Otherwise, I don't belong on the team.	I'm a good player or else I wouldn't be on the team. I'll play my best—that's all I can do.
Magnifying events	They went to a movie without me. I thought we were friends, but I guess I was wrong.	I'm disappointed they didn't ask me to the movie, but it doesn't mean our friendship is over. It's not that big a deal.

SOURCE: Adapted from Schafer, W. 1995. *Stress Management for Wellness,* 3rd ed. Copyright © 1996 by Holt, Rinehart, and Winston. Reprinted by permission of the publisher.

Psychologist Martin Seligman points out that we are more used to refuting negative statements, such as "The problem is going to last forever and ruin everything, and it's all my fault," when they come from a jealous rival rather than from our own mind. But refuting such negative self-statements is exactly what a pessimist must learn to do in order to avoid chronic unhappiness. Pessimists must first recognize and then dispute these false, negative predictions they generate about themselves. Seligman points out that learning to be optimistic is easier and more lasting than, for example, learning to eat less. Unlike refusing foods you love, disputing your own negative thoughts is fun—because doing so makes you feel better immediately.

Maintaining Honest Communication

Another important area of psychological functioning is communicating honestly with others. It can be very frustrating for us and for people around us if we cannot express what we want and feel. Others can hardly respond to our needs if they don't know what those needs are. We must recognize what we want to communicate and then express it clearly. For example, how do you feel about going to the party instead of to the movie? Do you care if your roommate talks on the phone late into the night? Some people know what they want others to do but don't state it clearly because they fear denial of the request,

	Table 3-2	Defense and Coping Mechanisms	

Mechanism	Description	Example
Projection	Reacting to unacceptable inner impulses as if they were from outside the self	A student who dislikes his roommate feels that the roommate dislikes him.
Repression	Expelling from awareness an unpleasant feeling, idea, or memory	The child of an alcoholic, neglectful father remembers him as a giving, loving person.
Denial	Refusing to acknowledge to yourself what you really know to be true	A person believes that smoking cigarettes won't harm her because she's young and healthy.
Passive-aggressive behavior	Expressing hostility toward someone by being covertly uncooperative or passive	A person tells a coworker, with whom she competes for project assignments, that she'll help him with a report but then never follows through.
Displacement	Shifting one's feelings about a person to another person	A student who is angry with one of his professors returns home and yells at one of his housemates.
Rationalization	Giving a false, acceptable reason when the real reason is unacceptable	A shy young man decides not to attend a dorm party, telling himself he'd be bored.
Substitution	Deliberately replacing a frustrating goal with one that is more attainable	A student having a difficult time passing courses in chemistry decides to change his major from biology to economics.
Humor	Finding something funny in unpleasant situations	A student whose bicycle has been stolen thinks how surprised the thief will be when he or she starts downhill and discovers the brakes don't work.

which they interpret as personal rejection. Such people might benefit from **assertiveness** training: learning to insist on their rights and to bargain for what they want. Assertiveness includes being able to say no or yes depending on the situation.

Because expressing feelings has become so central to popular psychology, many misconceptions have arisen. Neither "sharing" feelings with everyone on every occasion nor making important decisions based on feelings alone is a legitimate psychological health goal. But communicating your feelings appropriately and clearly is important. For example, if you tell people you feel sad, they may have various reactions. If they feel closer to you, they may express an intimate thought of their own. Or they may feel guilty because they think you're implying they have caused your sadness. They may even be angry because they feel obligated to help cheer you up.

Depending on your intention and prediction of how your statement will be taken, you may or may not wish to make it. For example, if you say you feel like staying home tonight, you may also be implying something different. You could really be saying "Don't bother me" or

opening a negotiation about what you would be willing to do that evening, given the right event or incentive.

Good communication means expressing yourself clearly. You don't need any special psychological jargon to communicate effectively. (For tips, see the box "Guidelines for Effective Communication" in Chapter 4, p. 98.)

Dealing with Loneliness

The right balance between being alone and being with others is often hard to achieve. Some people are motivated to socialize by a fear of being alone—not the best reason to spend time with others. If you discover how to be happy by yourself, you'll be better able to cope with periods when you're forced to be alone—for example, when you've just broken off a romantic relationship, when you've moved to a new town, or when your usual friends are away on vacation.

Unhappiness with being alone may come from interpreting it as a sign of rejection—that others are not interested in spending time with you. Before you conclude that, be sure that you give others a real chance to get to know you. Examine your patterns of thinking: You may harbor unrealistic expectations about other people—for example, that everyone you meet must like you and, if they don't, you must be terribly flawed. You might also consider the possibility that you expect too much from new acquaintances, and, sensing this, they start to draw

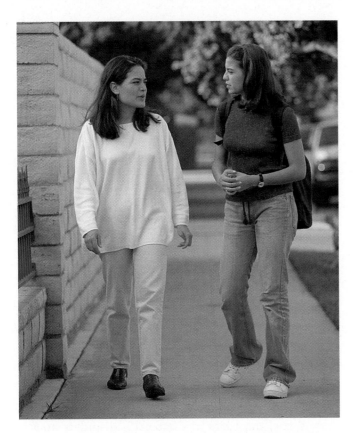

Communication is an important element in any interpersonal relationship. As these women express their thoughts and feelings to each other and listen attentively in response, they enhance their relationship, which in turn supports their psychological well-being.

Self-disclosure is essential to interpersonal relationships, but too much self-disclosure too soon can scare people off. You also want to make a good impression! When you're just getting to know someone, make sure you monitor and control how much you reveal about yourself, especially information that could be construed as negative. Pay attention to feedback from others—do they continue to be interested, or do they show signs of wanting to disengage from the conversation, such as looking around the room or moving away from you? Once you know people better and have begun to develop bonds of friendship, it is appropriate to disclose more personal and intimate information about yourself.

Dealing with Anger

Popular wisdom has said that you should express your anger rather than suppress it. Letting your anger out was thought to be beneficial for both psychological and physical health. However, recent studies have questioned this idea by showing that people who are overtly hostile seem to be at higher risk for heart attacks. Furthermore, angry words or actions won't contribute to psychological wellness if they damage important personal or professional relationships or produce feelings of guilt or loss of control. Perhaps the best way to resolve this contradiction is to look at the expression of anger in each situation and distinguish between a gratuitous expression of anger and a reasonable level of self-assertiveness.

At one extreme are people who never express anger or any opinion that might offend others, even when their own rights and needs are being jeopardized. They may find themselves in unhealthy relationships, which they can neither change nor escape from. They may be chronically deprived of satisfaction at work and at home. If you have trouble expressing your anger, you might explore training in assertiveness and appropriate expressions of anger to help you learn to express your needs, desires, and opinions constructively.

At the other extreme are people whose anger is explosive or misdirected. Explosive anger, or rage, like a child's tantrum, renders individuals temporarily unable to think straight or to act in their own best interest. In the long term, frequent expressions of rage can increase the risk for heart disease (see Chapter 15).

Managing Your Own Anger If you feel explosive anger coming on, consider the following two strategies to head it off. First, try to *reframe* what you're thinking at that moment. You'll be less angry at another person if there is a possibility that his or her behavior was not intentionally directed against you. Did the man who cut into your lane on the freeway do it deliberately to spite you, or did he simply fail to see you? Look for possible mitigating factors

back, triggering your feelings of rejection. Not everyone you meet is a suitable and willing person for a close or intimate relationship. Feeling pressure to have such a relationship may lead you to take up with someone whose interests and needs are remote from yours or whose need to be cared for leaves you with little time of your own. You will have traded loneliness for potentially worse problems.

Loneliness is a passive feeling state. If you decide that you're not spending enough time with people, take action to change the situation. College life provides many opportunities to meet people. In addition to classes and dorms, there are organizations of all kinds—hiking clubs, religious groups, advocacy groups, and so on—that offer a chance to meet others who share your interests. If you're shy, you may have to push yourself to join such groups. Look for something you've enjoyed in the past or in which you have a genuine interest. If your loneliness is the result of missing absent friends, remember that communication at a distance is cheaper and easier than ever before. For many people, e-mail and cell phones offer more immediate and satisfying contact than letters for keeping up with people in their lives.

that would make you less likely to blame him: Maybe he's late for a job interview and preoccupied with worries. If you're angry because you've just been criticized, avoid mentally replaying scenes from the past where you received similar unjust criticisms. Think about what is happening now, and try to act differently than in the past—less defensively and more analytically. What is it about me that makes it easy for this person to get my goat? Why am I taking it personally? Why am I acting like a jerk just because she did?

Second, until you're able to change your thinking, try do *distract* yourself. Use the old trick of counting to 10 before you respond, or start concentrating on your breathing. If needed, take a longer cooling-off period by leaving the situation until your anger has subsided. This does not mean that you should permanently avoid the issues and people who make you angry. When you've had a chance to think more clearly about the matter, return to it.

Dealing with Anger in Other People   Anger can be infectious and disruptive to cooperation and communication. If someone you're with becomes very angry, respond "asymmetrically" by reacting not with anger but with calm. Try to validate the other person by acknowledging that he or she had some reason to be angry. This does not mean apologizing, if you don't think you're to blame, or accepting verbal abuse, which is always inappropriate. Try to focus on solving the problem by allowing the individual to explain why he or she is so angry and what can be done to alleviate the situation. Finally, if the person cannot be calmed, it may be best to disengage, at least temporarily. After a time-out, a rational problem-solving approach may become more successful.

COMMUNICATE!   You have probably experienced someone else's anger, and perhaps you reacted by becoming angry yourself. But deflecting anger over a minor matter may be more helpful than responding to it directly. The next time someone is angry, see whether you can remain calm long enough to hear the real message behind the person's anger. Is there a way you can respond to what is said, instead of to the way it was said? For instance, instead of "Quit yelling at me!" you might say, "I realize you're upset because I erased your messages. Is there anything I can do to help you find out who called?"

PSYCHOLOGICAL DISORDERS

All of us have felt anxious at times, and in dealing with the anxiety we may have avoided doing something that we wanted to do or should have done. Most of us have had periods of feeling down when we became pessimistic, less energetic, and less able to enjoy life. Many of us have been bothered at times by irrational thoughts or odd feelings. Such feelings and thoughts can be normal responses to the ordinary challenges of life, but when emotions or irrational thoughts start to interfere with daily activities and rob us of our peace of mind, they can be considered symptoms of a psychological disorder.

Psychological disorders are generally the result of many factors. Genetic differences, which underlie differences in how the brain processes information and experiences, are known to play an important role. Learning and life events are important, too: Identical twins often don't have the same psychological disorders in spite of having identical genes. Some people have been exposed to more traumatic events than others, leading either to greater vulnerability to future traumas or, conversely, the development of better coping skills. Furthermore, what your parents, peers, and others have taught you strongly influences your level of self-esteem and how you deal with frightening or depressing life events.

In this section, we'll take a closer look at some of the more common psychological disorders, including anxiety disorders, mood disorders, and schizophrenia. (Table 3-3 shows the likelihood of these disorders occurring during one's lifetime and during the past year.) Elsewhere in this book you can learn about other disorders: sexual disorders in Chapter 5, disorders associated with drug and alcohol abuse in Chapters 9 and 10, eating disorders in Chapter 14, and Alzheimer's disease in Chapter 19.

Anxiety Disorders

Fear is a basic and useful emotion. Its value for our ancestors' survival cannot be overestimated; for modern humans, it provides motivation for self-protection and for learning to cope with new or potentially dangerous environmental or social situations. Only when fear is out of proportion to real danger can it be considered a problem. **Anxiety** is another word for fear, especially a feeling of fear that is not in response to any definite threat. Only when anxiety is experienced almost daily or in life situations that recur and cannot be avoided can anxiety be called a disorder. This section provides brief descriptions of the major types of anxiety disorders.

Simple Phobia   The most common and most understandable anxiety disorder, **simple,** or **specific, phobia** is a fear of something definite like lightning or a particular animal or location. Examples of commonly feared animals are snakes, spiders, and dogs; frightening locations are often high places or enclosed spaces. Sometimes, but not always, these fears originate in bad experiences, such as being bitten by a snake. A special kind of simple phobia is fear of blood, injections, or seeing injured people. These fears usually come from a tendency to faint or become nauseated in such situations.

Table 3-3	Prevalence of Selected Psychological Disorders Among Americans

| | Men | | Women | |
Disorder	Lifetime Prevalence (%)	Past Year Prevalence (%)	Lifetime Prevalence (%)	Past Year Prevalence (%)
Anxiety disorders				
Simple phobia	6.7	4.4	15.7	13.2
Social phobia	11.1	6.6	15.5	9.1
Panic disorder	2.0	1.3	5.0	3.2
Generalized anxiety disorder	3.6	2.0	6.6	4.3
Obsessive-compulsive disorder	1.7	0.5	2.8	0.8
Post-traumatic stress disorder	5.0	1.5	10.4	3.5
Mood disorders				
Major depressive episode	12.7	7.7	21.3	12.9
Manic episode	1.6	1.4	1.7	1.3
Schizophrenia and related disorders	1.0	0.8	0.5	0.4

SOURCES: U.S. Department of Health and Human Services. 1999. *Mental Health: A Report of the Surgeon General.* Rockville, Md.: DHHS. Weissman, M. M. 1998. Cross-national epidemiology of obsessive-compulsive disorder. *CNS Spectrums* 3(5 Suppl 1): 6–9. Kessler, R. C., et al. 1995. Posttraumatic stress disorder in the National Comorbidity Survey. *Archives of General Psychiatry* 52(12): 1048–1060. Kessler, R. C., et al. 1994. Lifetime and 12-month prevalence of DSM-III-R psychiatric disorders in the United States. *Archives of General Psychiatry* 51(1): 8–19.

Social Phobia   People with **social phobia** fear humiliation or embarrassment while being observed by others. Fear of speaking in public is perhaps the most common phobia of this kind. Extremely shy people can have social fears that extend to almost all social situations (see the box "Shyness"). People with these kinds of fears may not continue in school as far as they could and may restrict themselves to lower-paying jobs where they do not have to come into contact with new people.

Panic Disorder   People with **panic disorder** experience sudden unexpected surges in anxiety, accompanied by symptoms such as rapid and strong heartbeat, shortness of breath, loss of physical equilibrium, and a feeling of losing mental control. Such attacks usually begin in one's early twenties and can lead to a fear of being in crowds or closed places or of driving or flying. Sufferers fear that a panic attack will occur in a situation from which escape is difficult (such as while in an elevator), where the attack could be incapacitating and result in a dangerous or embarrassing loss of control (such as while driving a car or shopping), or where no medical help would be available if needed (as when a person is alone away from home). Fears such as these lead to avoidance of situations that might cause trouble. The fears and avoidance may spread to a large variety of situations until a person is virtually housebound, a condition called **agoraphobia.** People with panic disorder can often function normally in feared situations if someone they trust accompanies them.

Generalized Anxiety Disorder   A basic reaction to future threats is to worry about them. **Generalized anxiety disorder (GAD)** is a diagnosis given to people whose worries have taken on a life of their own, pushing out other thoughts and refusing banishment by any effort of will. The topics of the worrying are ordinary concerns: Will I be able to pass the exam next Friday? Where will I get money to get my car fixed? Is my boyfriend really interested in me? Furthermore, the worrying is not completely unjustified—after all, thinking about problems can result in solving them. But this kind of thinking seems to just go around in circles, and the more you try to stop it, the more you feel at its mercy. The end result is a

Terms

anxiety A feeling of fear that is not directed toward any definite threat.

simple (specific) phobia A persistent and excessive fear of a specific object, activity, or situation.

social phobia An excessive fear of performing in public; speaking in public is the most common example.

panic disorder A syndrome of severe anxiety attacks accompanied by physical symptoms.

agoraphobia An anxiety disorder characterized by fear of being alone away from help and avoidance of many different places and situations; in extreme cases, a fear of leaving home. From the Greek for "fear of the public market."

generalized anxiety disorder (GAD) An anxiety disorder characterized by excessive, uncontrollable worry about all kinds of things and anxiety in many situations.

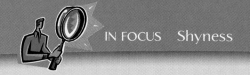

Shyness is a form of social anxiety, a fear of what others will think of one's behavior or appearance. Physical signs include a rapid heartbeat, a nervous stomach, sweating, cold and clammy hands, blushing, dry mouth, a lump in the throat, and trembling muscles. Shy people are often excessively self-critical, and they engage in very negative self-talk. The accompanying feelings of self-consciousness, embarrassment, and unworthiness can be overwhelming.

To avoid situations that make them anxious, shy people may refrain from making eye contact or speaking up in public. They may shun social gatherings. They may avoid college courses or job promotions that demand more interpersonal interaction or public speaking. Shyness is not the same thing as being introverted. Introverts prefer solitude to society. Shy people often long to be more outgoing, but their own negative thoughts prevent them from enjoying the social interaction they desire. The consequences of severe shyness can include social isolation, loneliness, and lost personal and professional opportunities. Very shy people also have higher than average rates of other anxiety and mood disorders and of substance abuse.

Shyness is very common, with 40–50% of Americans describing themselves as shy. However, only 5–10% of adults are so shy that their condition interferes seriously with work, school, daily life, or interpersonal relationships. Shyness is often hidden, and most shy people manage to appear reasonably outgoing, even though they suffer the physical and emotional symptoms of their anxiety. Many shy people do better in structured rather than spontaneous settings.

What causes people to be shy? Research indicates that for some, the trait may be partly inherited. But for shyness, as for many health concerns, biology is not destiny. Many shy children outgrow their shyness, just as others acquire it later in life. Clearly, other factors are involved. The type of attachment between a child and his or her caregiver is important, as are parenting styles. Shyness is more common in cultures where children's failures are attributed to their own actions but successes are attributed to other people or events. People's experiences during critical developmental transitions, such as starting school and entering adolescence, have also been linked to shyness. For adults, the precipitating factor may be an event such as divorce or the loss of a job.

Recent surveys indicate that shyness rates may be rising in the United States. With the advent of technologies such as ATM machines, video games, voice mail, faxes, and e-mail, the opportunities for face-to-face interaction are diminishing. Electronic media can be a wonderful way for shy people to communicate, but it can also allow them to hide from all social interaction. In fact, one study found that greater use of the Internet was associated with a decline in participants' communication with family members, a reduction in the size of their social circles, and an increase in levels of depression and loneliness. It remains to be seen whether the first generation to have cradle-to-grave access to home computers, faxes, and the Internet will experience higher rates of shyness.

Shyness is often undiagnosed, but help is available. Shyness classes, assertiveness training groups, and public speaking clinics are available (see the Behavior Change Strategy at the end of the chapter). For the seriously shy, effective treatments include cognitive-behavioral therapy and antidepressant drugs.

If you're shy, try to remember that shyness is widespread and that there are worse fates. Some degree of shyness has an up side. Shy people tend to be gentle, supportive, kind, and sensitive; they are often exceptional listeners. People who think carefully before they speak or act are less likely to hurt the feelings of others. Shyness may also facilitate cooperation. For any group or society to functon well, a variety of roles is required, and there is a place for quieter, more reflective individuals.

SOURCES: Carducci, B. J. 1999. *Shyness: A Bold New Approach.* New York: Perennial. Kraut, R., et al. 1998. Internet paradox: A social technology that reduces social involvement and psychological well-being? *American Psychologist* 53(9): 1017–1031. Lamberg, L. 1998. Social phobia—not just another name for shyness. *Journal of the American Medical Association* 280(8): 685–686.

persistent feeling of nervousness, often accompanied by depression, which impairs one's ability to enjoy life and to get things done.

Obsessive-Compulsive Disorder

The diagnosis of **obsessive-compulsive disorder (OCD)** is given to people with obsessions or compulsions or both. **Obsessions** are recurrent, unwanted thoughts or impulses. Unlike the worries of GAD, they are not ordinary concerns, but improbable fears such as of suddenly committing an antisocial act or of having been contaminated by germs. For example, a parent may have an impulse to kill a beloved child, or a person may brood over whether he or she got HIV from a handshake.

Compulsions are repetitive, difficult-to-resist actions usually associated with obsessions. A common compulsion is hand washing, associated with an obsessive fear of contamination by dirt. Other compulsions are counting and repeatedly checking if something has been done—for example, if a door has been locked or a stove turned off. People with OCD feel anxious, out of control, and embarrassed. Their rituals can occupy much of their time and make them inefficient at work and difficult to live with.

Post-Traumatic Stress Disorder

People who suffer from **post-traumatic stress disorder (PTSD)** are reacting to severely traumatic events (events that produce a sense of terror and helplessness) such as physical violence to oneself or loved ones. Trauma occurs in personal assaults (rape or military combat), natural disasters (floods, earthquakes), and tragedies like fires and airplane or car crashes. Symptoms include reexperiencing the trauma in dreams and in intrusive memories, trying to avoid anything associated with the trauma, and numbing of feelings. Sleep disturbances and other symptoms of anxiety and depression also commonly occur. Such symptoms can last months or even years.

Treating Anxiety Disorders Therapies for anxiety disorders range from medication to psychological interventions concentrating on a person's thoughts and behavior. As we discuss later, different models of human nature lead to different ideas of appropriate treatment. Both drug treatments and cognitive-behavioral therapies have proved effective in panic disorder, obsessive-compulsive disorder, and generalized anxiety disorder. Simple phobias are best treated without drugs.

Ⅶ. Mood Disorders

We all experience ups and downs in our mood in response to daily events. These temporary mood changes typically don't affect our overall emotional state or level of wellness. A person with a mood disorder, however, experiences emotional disturbances that are intense and persistent enough to affect normal functioning. The two most common mood disorders are depression and bipolar disorder.

Depression The most common mood disorder, **depression** has forms and degrees. It usually involves demoralization and can include the following:

- A feeling of sadness and hopelessness
- Loss of pleasure in doing usual activities
- Poor appetite and weight loss
- Insomnia or disturbed sleep
- Restlessness or, alternatively, fatigue
- Thoughts of worthlessness and guilt
- Trouble concentrating or making decisions
- Thoughts of death or suicide

Not all these features are present in every depressive episode. Sometimes instead of poor appetite and insomnia, the opposite occurs—eating too much and sleeping too long. Amazingly, people can have most of the symptoms of depression without feeling sad or hopeless or in a depressed mood, although they usually do experience a loss of interest or pleasure in things (see the box "Are You Suffering from a Mood Disorder?"). In some cases, depression is a clear-cut reaction to specific events, such as the loss of a loved one or failing in school or work, while in other cases no trigger event is obvious.

RECOGNIZING THE WARNING SIGNS OF SUICIDE One of the principal dangers of severe depression is suicide. Although a suicide attempt can occur unpredictably and unaccompanied by depression, the chances are greater if symptoms are numerous and severe. Additional warning signs of suicide include the following:

- Expressing the wish to be dead or revealing contemplated methods
- Increasing social withdrawal and isolation
- A sudden, inexplicable lightening of mood (which can mean the person has finally decided to commit suicide)

Certain risk factors increase the likelihood of suicide:

- A history of previous attempts
- A suicide by a family member or friend
- Readily available means, such as guns or pills
- A history of substance abuse or eating disorders
- Serious medical problems

The groups in the United States with the highest suicide rates are males age 20–34, Native American males, and white males over age 65. Women attempt three times as many suicides as men, yet men succeed at more than three times the rate of women.

HELPING YOURSELF OR A FRIEND If you are severely depressed or know someone who is, expert help from a mental health professional is essential. Don't try to do it all yourself. If you suspect one of your friends is suicidally depressed, try to get him or her to see a professional.

Don't be afraid to discuss the possibility of suicide with people you fear are suicidal. You won't give them an idea they haven't already thought of (see the box "Myths About Suicide"). And asking direct questions is the best way to determine whether someone seriously intends to commit suicide. Encourage your friend to talk and to take positive steps to improve his or her situation. If you feel there is an immediate danger of suicide, ensure that the person is not left alone, especially when he or she is emotionally upset

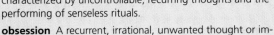

obsessive-compulsive disorder (OCD) An anxiety disorder characterized by uncontrollable, recurring thoughts and the performing of senseless rituals.

obsession A recurrent, irrational, unwanted thought or impulse.

compulsion An irrational, repetitive, forced action, usually associated with an obsession.

post-traumatic stress disorder (PTSD) An anxiety disorder characterized by reliving traumatic events through dreams, flashbacks, and hallucinations.

depression A mood disorder characterized by loss of interest, sadness, hopelessness, loss of appetite, disturbed sleep, and other physical symptoms.

Terms

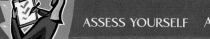

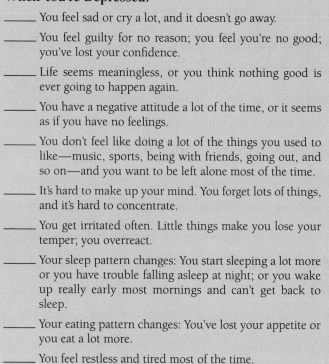

You should get evaluated by a professional if you've had five or more of the following symptoms for more than 2 weeks or if any of these symptoms cause such a big change that you can't keep up your usual routine.

When You're Depressed:

_____ You feel sad or cry a lot, and it doesn't go away.

_____ You feel guilty for no reason; you feel you're no good; you've lost your confidence.

_____ Life seems meaningless, or you think nothing good is ever going to happen again.

_____ You have a negative attitude a lot of the time, or it seems as if you have no feelings.

_____ You don't feel like doing a lot of the things you used to like—music, sports, being with friends, going out, and so on—and you want to be left alone most of the time.

_____ It's hard to make up your mind. You forget lots of things, and it's hard to concentrate.

_____ You get irritated often. Little things make you lose your temper; you overreact.

_____ Your sleep pattern changes: You start sleeping a lot more or you have trouble falling asleep at night; or you wake up really early most mornings and can't get back to sleep.

_____ Your eating pattern changes: You've lost your appetite or you eat a lot more.

_____ You feel restless and tired most of the time.

_____ You think about death or feel as if you're dying or have thoughts about committing suicide.

When You're Manic:

_____ You feel high as a kite . . . like you're "on top of the world."

_____ You get unrealistic ideas about the great things you can do . . . things that you really can't do.

_____ Thoughts go racing through your head, you jump from one subject to another, and you talk a lot.

_____ You're a nonstop party, constantly running around.

_____ You do too many wild or risky things—with driving, with spending money, with sex, and so on.

_____ You're so "up" that you don't need much sleep.

_____ You're rebellious or irritable and can't get along at home or school or with your friends.

If you are concerned about depression in yourself or a friend, or if you are thinking about hurting or killing yourself, talk to someone about it and get help immediately. There are many sources of help: a good friend; an academic or resident advisor; the staff at the student health or counseling center; a professor, coach, or advisor; a local suicide or emergency hotline (get the phone number from the operator or directory) or the 911 operator; or a hospital emergency room.

SOURCES: National Institute of Mental Health. 1999. *Let's Talk About Depression* (http://www.nimh.nih.gov/publicat/letstalk.cfm; retrieved August 31, 2000).

and more likely to act impulsively. If you must leave your friend alone, have your friend promise not to do anything to harm himself or herself without first calling you. Get qualified help as soon as possible.

If your friend refuses help, you might try to contact your friend's relatives and tell them that you are worried. If the depressed person is a college student, you may need to let someone in your health service or college administration know your concerns. Finally, most communities have emergency help available, often in the form of a hot-line telephone counseling service run by a suicide prevention agency (check the yellow pages).

TREATING DEPRESSION   Although treatments are highly effective, only about 35% of people who suffer from depression currently seek treatment. Treatment for depression depends on its severity and on whether the depressed person is suicidal. The best initial treatment for moderate to severe depression is probably a combination of drug therapy and some kind of psychotherapy. "Uppers" such as amphetamines are not good antidepres-

sants; much better are newer prescription antidepressants, although they may take several weeks to begin working. Therefore, when suicidal impulses are strong, hospitalization for a week or so may be necessary.

Antidepressants work by affecting the activity of key neurotransmitters in the brain, including serotonin (Figure 3-2). The over-the-counter herb St. John's wort may also affect serotonin levels, but because it is a dietary supplement, it is not subject to the same type of testing and regulation as prescription medications (see the box "Alternative Remedies for Depression" for more information). Anyone who may be suffering from depression should seek a medical evaluation rather than self-treating with supplements.

Electroconvulsive therapy (ECT) is effective for severe depression when other approaches have failed. In ECT, an epileptic-like seizure is induced by an electrical impulse transmitted through electrodes placed on the head. Patients are given an anesthetic and a muscle relaxant to reduce anxiety and prevent injuries associated with seizures. A typical course of ECT includes three treatments per week for 2 to 4 weeks.

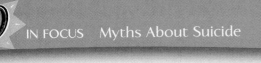
Myth People who really intend to kill themselves do not let anyone know about it.
Fact This belief can be an excuse for doing nothing when someone says he or she might commit suicide. In fact, most people who eventually commit suicide *have* talked about doing it.

Myth People who made a suicide attempt but survived did not really intend to die.
Fact This may be true for certain people, but people who seriously want to end their life may fail because they misjudge what it takes. Even a pharmacist may misjudge the lethal dose of a drug.

Myth People who succeed in suicide really wanted to die.
Fact We cannot be sure of that either. Some people are only trying to make a dramatic gesture or plea for help but miscalculate.

Myth People who really want to kill themselves will do it regardless of any attempts to prevent them.
Fact Few people are single-minded about suicide even at the moment of attempting it. People who are quite determined to take their life today may change their mind completely tomorrow.

Myth Suicide is proof of mental illness.
Fact Many suicides are committed by people who do not meet ordinary criteria for mental illness, although people with depression, schizophrenia, and other psychological disorders have a much higher than average suicide rate.

Myth People inherit suicidal tendencies.
Fact Certain kinds of depression that lead to suicide do have a genetic component. But many examples of suicide running in a family can be explained by factors such as psychologically identifying with a family member who committed suicide, often a parent.

Myth All suicides are irrational.
Fact By some standards all suicides may seem "irrational." But many people find it at least understandable that someone might want to commit suicide, for example, when approaching the end of a terminal illness or when facing a long prison term.

One type of depression is treated in a unique way—by having sufferers sit with eyes open in front of a bright light source for an hour or so early every morning. These patients have **seasonal affective disorder (SAD)**, in which depression worsens during winter months as the number of hours of daylight diminishes and then improves with the lengthening of daylight in the spring and summer. Seasonal depression is more common among people who live at higher latitudes, where there are fewer hours of light in winter. Light therapy may work by extending the perceived length of the day and thus convincing the brain that it is summertime even during the winter months.

Mania and Bipolar Disorder   People who experience **mania,** a less common feature of mood disorders, are restless, have a lot of energy, need little sleep, and often talk nonstop. They may devote themselves to fantastic projects and spend more money than they can afford. Many manic people swing between manic and depressive states, a syndrome called **bipolar disorder** because of the two opposite poles of mood. Tranquilizers are used to treat individual manic episodes, while special drugs like the salt lithium carbonate taken daily can prevent future mood swings.

Gender Differences   One of the mysteries about mood disorders is the gender gap in the incidence of depression. Although equal numbers of men and women suffer from bipolar disorder, women are nearly twice as likely as men to be clinically depressed. This gender gap starts in adolescence and continues until about age 65. Researchers have looked at both biological and social causative factors.

A genetic basis for depression linked to the female sex chromosome was investigated, but researchers failed to find a strong association. Studies have also not found any correlation between female hormone levels and depression. Neither contraceptive pills nor menopause, both of which modify hormone levels significantly, is clearly linked to depression.

What about social factors? Traditional gender roles make women generally less likely to deal directly and assertively with problems, resulting in stress, economic dependence, and low self-esteem. Researchers have theorized that people with "helpless/hopeless" personalities may be more prone to depression. They have an external locus of control combined with a pessimistic outlook: They expect bad things to happen, feel that negative events are their own fault, and believe there is

electroconvulsive therapy (ECT) The use of electric shock to induce brief, generalized seizures; used in the treatment of selected psychological disorders.

seasonal affective disorder (SAD) A mood disorder characterized by seasonal depression, usually occurring in winter, when there is less daylight.

mania A mood disorder characterized by excessive elation, irritability, talkativeness, inflated self-esteem, and expansiveness.

bipolar disorder A mental illness characterized by alternating periods of depression and mania.

Terms

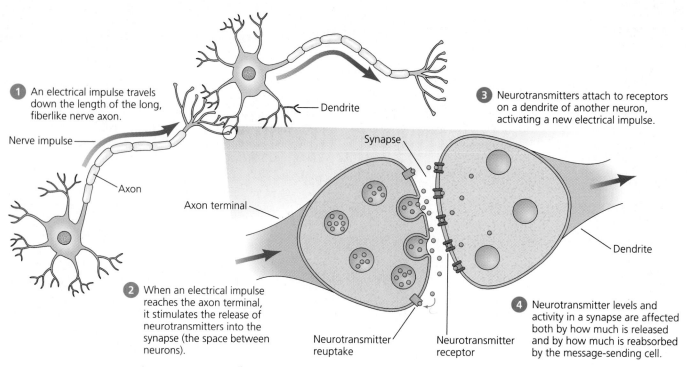

Figure 3-2 Nerve cell communication. Nerve cells (neurons) communicate through a combination of electrical impulses and chemical messages. Neurotransmitters such as serotonin and norepinephrine alter the overall responsiveness of the brain and are responsible for mood, level of attentiveness, and other psychological states. Many psychological disorders are related to problems with neurotransmitters and their receptors, and drug treatments frequently target them. For example, the antidepressant drug Prozac increases levels of serotonin by slowing the resorption (re-uptake) of serotonin.

① An electrical impulse travels down the length of the long, fiberlike nerve axon.

Nerve impulse

Axon

② When an electrical impulse reaches the axon terminal, it stimulates the release of neurotransmitters into the synapse (the space between neurons).

Dendrite

Synapse

Axon terminal

Neurotransmitter reuptake

Neurotransmitter receptor

③ Neurotransmitters attach to receptors on a dendrite of another neuron, activating a new electrical impulse.

Dendrite

④ Neurotransmitter levels and activity in a synapse are affected both by how much is released and by how much is reabsorbed by the message-sending cell.

nothing they can do to prevent them. Some psychologists have suggested that conditions related to women's social roles—discrimination in the workplace, lack of power in relationships, and role overload—may make women more prone to "learned helplessness," thereby predisposing them to depression. But no specific personality type has been clearly associated with depression, and it is possible that a helpless/hopeless personality is a result rather than a cause of depression.

Schizophrenia

Schizophrenia can be severe and debilitating or quite mild and hardly noticeable. Although people are capable of diagnosing their own depression, they usually don't diagnose their own schizophrenia, because they often can't see that anything is wrong. This disorder is not rare; in fact, 1 in every 100 people has a schizophrenic episode sometime in his or her lifetime, most commonly starting in adolescence. However, because people who are directly or indirectly affected do not like to talk about schizophrenia, its frequency is not generally appreciated. In addition, schizophrenic people tend to withdraw from society

when they are ill, another factor making it seem rarer than it is.

Some general characteristics of schizophrenia include the following:

- *Disorganized thoughts.* Thoughts may be expressed in a vague or confusing way.
- *Inappropriate emotions.* Emotions may be absent or strong but inappropriate.
- *Delusions.* People with delusions—firmly held false beliefs—may think that their minds are controlled by outside forces, that people can read their minds, that they are great personages like Jesus Christ or the president of the United States, or that they are being persecuted by a group like the CIA.
- *Auditory hallucinations.* Schizophrenic people may hear voices when no one is present.
- *Deteriorating social and work functioning.* Social withdrawal and increasingly poor performance at school or work may be so gradual that they are hardly noticed at first.

None of these characteristics is invariably present. Some schizophrenic people are quite logical except on the

Mainstream therapies for depression include medications accepted as safe and effective by government regulatory agencies, certain psychotherapies, and light therapy in the case of seasonal affective disorder. Yet, in surveys, 20% of people in the United States who suffer from depression report using unconventional therapies such as acupuncture, body movement therapy, homeopathy, qigong, faith healing, or herbs or other "natural" substances. With the exception of one herb, St. John's wort (*Hypericum perforatum*), these therapies have not been shown to be effective in double-blind placebo-controlled trials. Such trials are the only scientific way to show that a treatment has healing power beyond that of a **placebo.** (See Chapter 21 for more on different types of medical research studies.)

St. John's wort, a flowering plant that grows as a weed in the United States, has been reputed to have curative properties since the time of Hippocrates in ancient Greece. Modern pharmacological studies confirm that its active ingredients produce a number of biochemical and physiological changes in animals, although it's still unclear exactly how these changes might affect depression. Data from a number of studies demonstrate that St. John's wort can benefit some people with mild to moderate depression. St. John's wort may cause fewer adverse effects than conventional antidepressants, although the user may experience gastrointestinal disturbances, increased sensitivity to sunlight, dizziness, dry mouth, or other side effects; it should not be taken by pregnant women. In addition, St. John's wort may interact with, and reduce the effectiveness of, certain medications, including oral contraceptives and certain medications for treating heart disease, depression, HIV infection, and seizures.

One reason for the popularity of an herb for depression is that it doesn't require a prescription or any kind of contact with a physician or therapist; for those who are not members of a generous health care plan, an herbal remedy may also be less expensive than a prescription antidepressant. On the other hand, people suffering from depression *should* seek professional advice and not try to get along entirely with self-diagnosis and self-help. St. John's wort doesn't work for everyone, and it is not effective for severe depression. Also, because herbal products are classified as dietary supplements, they are not scrutinized by the regulatory agencies that oversee prescription drugs. Thus, customers have no guarantee that the product contains the herbs and dosages listed on the label (see Chapters 12 and 21 for more on dietary supplements).

Finally, although St. John's wort is more effective than a placebo for some people, it may not be as effective as newer prescription antidepressants. Research is currently underway to learn more about St. John's wort—its active ingredients, method of action, level of effectiveness, and possible side effects or drug interactions. Until more is known, caution may be the best approach.

SOURCES: Shelton, R. C. et al. 2001. Effectiveness of St. John's Wort in major depression. *Journal of the American Medical Association* 285 (15): 1978–1986. National Institute of Mental Health. 2000. *Questions and Answers About St. John's Wort* (http://www.nimh.nih.gov/publicat/stjohnqa.cfm; retrieved August 31, 2000); Ernst, E., J. I. Rand, and C. Stevinson. 1998. Complementary therapies for depression. An overview. *Archives of General Psychiatry* 55: 1026–1032; Wong, A. H., M. Smith, and H. S. Boon. 1998. Herbal remedies in psychiatric practice. *Archives of General Psychiatry* 55: 1033–1044.

subject of their delusions. Others show disorganized thoughts but no delusions or hallucinations.

A schizophrenic person needs help from a mental health professional. Suicide is a risk in schizophrenia, and expert treatment can reduce that risk and minimize the social consequences of the illness by shortening the period when symptoms are active. The key element in treatment is regular medication. At times medication is like insulin for diabetes—it makes the difference between being able to function or not. Sometimes hospitalization is temporarily required to relieve family and friends.

COMMUNICATE! The media portrayal of psychological problems and their treatment tends to be inaccurate at best and sometimes highly negative. How well can you interpret these messages? Select a book or film you've recently read or seen that deals with psychological illness and evaluate the author's or director's view of symptoms, causes, and treatment. How does he or she communicate this view, and how fair or biased is it? Does the book or film provide a counteropinion?

MODELS OF HUMAN NATURE AND THERAPEUTIC CHANGE

It is not surprising that beings as complicated as we humans cannot be satisfactorily encompassed by a single perspective. In fact, at least four different perspectives—biological, behavioral, cognitive, and psychodynamic—can be applied to human problems like the psychological disorders discussed in this chapter. Each perspective has a distinct view of human nature, and from those views of nature come distinct therapeutic approaches.

schizophrenia A psychological disorder that involves a disturbance in thinking and in perceiving reality.

placebo A chemically inactive substance that a patient believes is an effective medical therapy for his or her condition. To help evaluate a therapy, medical researchers compare the effects of a particular therapy with the effects of a placebo. The "placebo effect" occurs when a patient responds to a placebo as if it were an active drug.

Terms

The Biological Model

The biological model emphasizes that the mind's activity depends entirely on an organic structure, the brain, whose composition is genetically determined. The activity of neurons, mediated by complex chemical reactions, gives rise to our most complex thoughts, our most ardent desires, and our most pathological behavior. Of course, no one can assert that environment and learning have no influence. Even if the brain is nothing but a supercomputer, it still has to be programmed by experience.

Biological researchers have investigated all of the psychological disorders we have discussed and found genetic influences on anxiety and depression that cannot be accounted for by environment and learning. The fact that drugs can make anxiety and depression worse or better is evidence that chemicals in the brain influence our moods. Magnetic resonance imaging of the brain shows that the brain's structure is slightly different in people with schizophrenia.

Pharmacological Therapy The most important kind of therapy inspired by the biological model is pharmacological therapy. A list of some of the popular medications currently used for treating psychological disorders follows. All require a prescription from a psychiatrist or other medical doctor. All have received approval from the U.S. Food and Drug Administration (FDA) as being safe and more effective than a placebo. However, as with all pharmacological therapies, these drugs may cause side effects. For example, the side effects of widely used antidepressants range from diminished appetite to loss of sexual pleasure. In addition, an individual may have to try several drugs before finding one that is effective and has acceptable side effects.

1. *Antidepressants:* These include Prozac (fluoxetine), Paxil (paroxetine), Zoloft (sertraline), Luvox (fluvoxamine), Celexa (citalopram), Effexor (venlafaxine), Wellbutrin (bupropion), Serzone (nefazodone), Remeron (mirtazapine), Aventyl (nortriptyline), Elavil (amitriptyline), and Nardil (phenelzine). Surprisingly, these antidepressants are as effective in treating panic disorder and certain kinds of chronic anxiety as they are in depression, and they may also alleviate the symptoms of obsessive-compulsive disorder.

2. *Mood stabilizers:* Lithium carbonate and Depakote (valproic acid) are the most important mood stabilizers.

They are taken to prevent mood swings that occur in bipolar disorder and certain kinds of schizophrenia.

3. *Antipsychotics:* Older antipsychotics include Haldol (haloperidol) and Prolixin (fluphenazine); newer antipsychotics (sometimes called "atypical") are Clozaril (clozapine), Zyprexa (olanzapine), Risperdal (risperidone), and Seroquel (quetiapine). The drugs reduce hallucinations and disordered thinking in people with schizophrenia, bipolar disorder, and delirium, and they have a calming effect on agitated patients.

4. *Anxiolytics (anti-anxiety agents) and hypnotics (sleeping pills):* One of the largest and most prescribed classes of anxiolytics is the benzodiazepines, a group of drugs that includes Valium (diazepam), Librium (chlordiazepoxide), Xanax (alprazolam), and Ativan (lorazepam); Dalmane (flurazepam), Restoril (temazepam), and Halcion (triazolam) are benzodiazepines marketed as sleeping aids. Newer hypnotics are Sonata (zaleplon) and Ambien (zolpidem).

5. *Stimulants.* Ritalin (methylphenidate) and Dexedrine (dextroamphetamine) are most commonly used for **attention-deficit/hyperactivity disorder (ADHD)** in children, and for excessive daytime sleepiness in adults. Questions have been raised about the widespread use of Ritalin for treating ADHD; for more information, see the box "Attention-Deficit/Hyperactivity Disorder: A Controversial Diagnosis."

Issues in the Use of Pharmacological Therapy The discovery that many psychological disorders have a biological basis in disordered brain chemistry has led to a revolution in the treatment of many disorders, particularly depression. The new view of depression as based in brain chemistry has also lessened the stigma attached to the condition, leading more people to seek treatment, and antidepressants are now among the most widely prescribed drugs in the United States. The development of effective drugs has provided relief for many people, but wide use of antidepressants has also raised many questions.

Given the ability of antidepressants to affect brain chemistry and control symptoms, what role does psychotherapy have in treating depression? Research indicates that for mild cases of depression, psychotherapy and antidepressants are about equally effective. For major depression, combined therapy is significantly more effective than either type of treatment alone. Some mental health professionals worry that health insurance companies, in an effort to save money, will favor drug therapy over psychotherapy for all patients. Psychotherapy may be particularly important for people whose condition has a strong psychosocial component. Therapy can help provide insight into factors that precipitated the depression, such as high levels of stress, a history of abuse, unresolved grief, or relationship problems. A therapist can

Terms **attention-deficit/hyperactivity disorder (ADHD)** A disorder characterized by persistent, pervasive problems with inattention and/or hyperactivity to a degree that is not considered appropriate for a child's developmental stage and that causes significant difficulties in school, work, or relationships.

In May 2000, a class-action lawsuit was filed in Texas alleging that the American Psychiatric Association (APA) illegally conspired with the Novartis Pharmaceutical Corporation to boost profits for the company's stimulant drug Ritalin (methylphenidate). Ritalin is the most widely prescribed drug for treatment of attention-deficit/hyperactivity disorder (ADHD). The suit charges that the APA and Novartis have engaged in a concerted campaign to promote the diagnosis of ADHD and the usefulness of Ritalin for treating it and that the APA gained financially from this public relations initiative. According to the suit, the APA gave ADHD "an official-seeming imprimatur" to apply to behaviors that may in fact be normal. Among other demands, the plaintiffs' attorneys are asking for the court to order the refund of all money paid for Ritalin.

ADHD is among the most controversial of all psychiatric diagnoses. The APA describes ADHD as persistent, pervasive problems with inattention and/or hyperactivity to a degree that is not considered appropriate for a child's developmental stage and that causes significant difficulties in school, at home, and in peer relationships. Symptoms develop before a child is 7 years old and last at least 6 months; some symptoms may persist into adulthood, but the disorder always begins in childhood. The debate over ADHD arises because it is difficult to draw the line between normal degrees of inattention, hyperactivity, and impulsiveness and levels that are pathological and may benefit from treatment.

Some mental health professionals feel that the diagnosis of ADHD is applied too broadly and that large numbers of children who do not meet the criteria for ADHD are unnecessarily exposed to the potentially harmful side effects of Ritalin and other psychostimulants. (The use of stimulants to treat ADHD may appear counterintuitive, but it's believed they work by stimulating areas of the brain involved in planning and inhibiting activity, areas that may be less active in people with ADHD.) Concerned parents and physicians point to the large increase in the use of Ritalin in the past decade and the fact that U.S. children are much more likely than European children to be diagnosed with ADHD and treated with drugs. They feel that ADHD may sometimes be a conveniently simple diagnosis in cases where a child's difficulties are actually due to much more complex family, educational, or social problems. Other concerns relate to the use of medication in some very young children (under age 6) and the use of combinations of psychiatric medications that have not been tested in children and adolescents. In addition, the early and continued use of stimulants for ADHD may run counter to antidrug messages that ask children and adolescents to "just say no to drugs."

However, many mental health professionals feel that a strong case can be made for diagnosing some children with ADHD and treating them with medication. Many well-designed studies have found that treatment with psychostimulants reduces the core symptoms of ADHD and allows affected individuals to better focus their attention and control impulsive and aggressive behavior. Once treated, affected students do better at school both academically and socially. Without treatment, children with ADHD may be labeled absentminded, rude, and dumb; they may develop low self-esteem and more serious psychological and behavior problems as adolescents and adults. Medications may work best if combined with psychosocial treatments such as behavior modification, special teaching and parenting techniques, and family support services.

How many U.S. children have been diagnosed with ADHD and treated with medication? A widespread survey involving all public school children in Maryland found that about 3% of the students were receiving medication for ADHD. Boys were three to four times more likely than girls to be taking medication. White grade-school students were about twice as likely to be receiving medication as African American, Latino, and Asian American students; this disparity increased by high school, where the medication rate for white students was five times that of African American students. Ethnic differences in medication rates may reflect unequal access to health insurance and mental health care as well as differences in how physicians treat children of different ethnic groups.

What's unclear from these survey findings is how many of the children who are taking medication do not meet the criteria for ADHD and how many children who actually have ADHD remain undiagnosed and untreated. The American Academy of Pediatrics recently released a new set of physician guidelines for ADHD, and other major government and professional organizations are trying to raise awareness among teachers, parents, and health professionals about how best to identify children with ADHD. Despite these efforts, it is likely that the diagnosis and treatment of ADHD will remain controversial.

SOURCES: Safer, D. J., and M. Malever. 2000. Stimulant treatment in Maryland public schools. Pediatrics 106(3): 533–539. Angold, A., et al. 2000. Stimulant treatment for children: A community perspective. Journal of the American Academy of Child and Adolescent Psychiatry 39(8): 975–984. Hausman, K. 2000. Parents accuse APA, Novartis of conspiracy over Ritalin sales. Psychiatric News 35(15): 1 ff. Frances, A., and M. B. First. 1998. Your Mental Health. New York: Scribner.

also provide guidance in changing patterns of thinking and behavior that contribute to the problem.

What about the use of antidepressants to treat unwanted personality traits in psychologically healthy people? Anecdotal evidence suggests that Prozac and related drugs may help shy or pessimistic people become more outgoing and optimistic, for example. The potential use of antidepressants in this way has sparked ethical debate. Is some degree of vulnerability, anxiety, and sadness an essential part of being human? If antidepressants diminish or eliminate these feelings, will they rob people of the emotional experiences they need to grow and be creative? By masking mental pain, will they interfere with people's connection to reality and to their own emotional experience and expression? This ethical debate extends beyond the question of therapeutic benefits of antidepressants and other pharmacological treatments for psychological disorders.

The Behavioral Model

The behavioral model focuses on what people do—their overt behavior—rather than on brain structures and chemistry or on thoughts and consciousness. This model regards psychological problems as "maladaptive behavior" or bad habits. When and how a person learned bad behavior is less important than what makes it continue in the present. Behaviorists analyze behavior in terms of **stimulus, response,** and **reinforcement.** The essence of behavior therapy is to discover what reinforcements keep an undesirable behavior going and then to try to alter those reinforcements. For example, if people who fear speaking in class (the stimulus) remove themselves from that situation (the response), they experience immediate relief, which acts as reinforcement for future avoidance and escape.

To change their behavior, fearful people are taught to practice **exposure**—to deliberately and repeatedly enter the feared situation and remain in it until their fear begins to abate. Clients are often asked to keep a daily behavior journal to monitor the target behavior and the events that precede and follow it. A student who is afraid to speak in class might begin his behavioral therapy program by keeping a diary listing each time he makes a contribution to a classroom discussion, how long he speaks, and his anxiety levels before, during, and after speaking. He would then develop concrete but realistic goals for increasing his speaking frequency and contract with himself to reward his successes by spending more time in activities he finds enjoyable.

Although exposure to the real situation works best, exposure in one's imagination or through the virtual reality of computer simulation can also be effective. For example, in the case of someone afraid of flying, an imagined scenario would likely be vivid enough to elicit the fear necessary to practice exposure techniques. The Behavior Change Strategy at the end of Chapter 2 provides a model program for reducing test anxiety; refer to Chapter 1 for general strategies for behavior change.

Terms

stimulus Anything that causes a response.

response A reaction to a stimulus.

reinforcement Increasing the future probability of a response by following it with a reward.

exposure A therapeutic technique for treating fear, in which the subject learns to come into direct contact with a feared situation.

The Cognitive Model

The cognitive model emphasizes the effect of ideas on behavior and feeling. According to this model, behavior results from complicated attitudes, expectations, and motives rather than from simple, immediate reinforcements. When behavioral therapies such as exposure work, it is because they change the way a person thinks about the feared situation and his or her ability to cope with it.

According to one cognitive theory, recurring false ideas produce feelings such as anxiety and depression. Identifying and exposing these ideas as false should relieve the painful emotion. For example, people who are anxious are thinking, "Something bad is going to happen and I won't be able to handle it." The therapist challenges such ideas in three ways: showing that there isn't enough evidence for the idea, suggesting different ways of looking at the situation, and showing that no disaster is going to occur. The therapist does not just state his or her position but encourages clients to examine the logic of their own ideas and then to test their truth.

For example, a student afraid of speaking in class may harbor such thoughts as "If I begin to speak, I'll say something stupid; if I say something stupid, the teacher and my classmates will lose respect for me; then I'll get a low grade, my classmates will avoid me, and life will be hell." In cognitive therapy, these ideas will be examined critically. If the student prepares, will he or she really sound stupid? Does every sentence said have to be exactly correct and beautifully delivered, or is that an impossible perfection? Will classmates' opinions be completely transformed by one presentation? Do classmates even care that much? And why does the student care so much about what *they* think? People in cognitive therapy are taught to notice their unrealistic thoughts and to substitute more realistic ones, and they are advised to repeatedly test their assumptions.

The Psychodynamic Model

The psychodynamic model also emphasizes thoughts, but it asserts that false ideas cannot be fought directly because they are fed by other, unconscious, ideas and impulses. Symptoms are not isolated pieces of behavior but results of a complex system of secret wishes, emotions, and fantasies hidden by active defenses that keep them unconscious (see Table 3-2). The role of the past in shaping the present is often emphasized in psychodynamic therapy. By having the client speak as freely as possible in front of the therapist, the therapist can help the client achieve some insight into the reasons for his or her apparently irrational and self-defeating thoughts and actions. In essence, a trustworthy therapist helps clients become more honest with themselves. One contemporary version of this approach, interpersonal therapy, focuses on the relationship between the person and others. The therapist takes an active role in helping the client to understand and overcome self-isolation and to develop interpersonal skills.

Newer therapies referred to variously as humanistic, existential, or experiential are like psychodynamic therapies in encouraging self-awareness, but they focus more on the present and future than the past. Clients are encouraged to get in touch with their subjective experience (the here and now). The therapist acts as a guide to self-exploration and a facilitator for expanding the client's inherent human potential.

Evaluating the Models

Ignoring theoretical conflicts between psychological models, therapists have recently developed pragmatic *cognitive-behavioral therapies* that combine effective elements of both models in a single package. For example, the package for treating social anxiety emphasizes exposure as well as changing problematic patterns of thinking. Combined therapies have also been developed for panic disorder, obsessive-compulsive disorder, generalized anxiety disorder, and depression. These packages, involving ten or more individual or group sessions with a therapist and homework between sessions, have been shown to produce significant improvement.

Drug therapy and cognitive-behavioral therapies are also sometimes combined, especially in the case of depression. For anxiety disorders, both kinds of therapy are equally effective, but the effects of drug therapy last only as long as the drug is being taken, while cognitive-behavioral therapies produce longer-term improvement. For schizophrenia, drug therapy is a must, but a continuing relationship with therapists who give support and advice is also indispensable.

Psychodynamic therapies have been attacked as ineffective and endless. Of course, effectiveness is hard to demonstrate for therapies that do not focus on specific symptoms. But common sense tells us that being able to open yourself up and discuss your problems with a supportive but objective person who focuses on you and lets you speak freely can enhance your sense of self and reduce feelings of confusion and despair.

GETTING HELP

Knowing when self-help or professional help is required for mental health problems is usually not as difficult as knowing how to start or which professional to choose.

Self-Help

If you have a personal problem to solve, a smart way to begin is by finding out what you can do on your own. Some problems are specifically addressed in this book. Behavioral and some cognitive approaches are especially useful for helping yourself. They all involve becoming

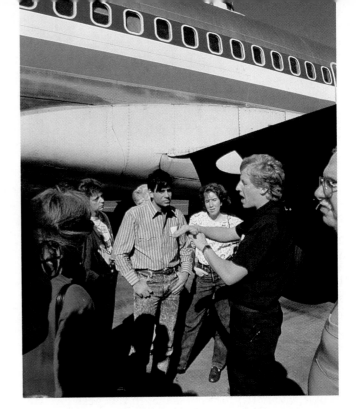

Cognitive-behavioral psychotherapy may be used to treat anxiety disorders such as simple phobias. During therapy, this group of people who are afraid to fly are encouraged to develop more realistic ideas about the risks of flying and to expose themselves to anxiety-provoking situations related to flying.

more aware of self-defeating actions and ideas and combating them in some way: by being more assertive; communicating honestly; raising your self-esteem by counteracting thoughts, people, and actions that undermine it; and confronting, rather than avoiding, the things you fear. Get more information by seeing what books are available in the psychology or self-help sections of libraries and bookstores. But be selective. Watch out for self-help books making fantastic claims that deviate from mainstream approaches.

Some people find it helpful to express their feelings in a journal. Grappling with a painful experience in this way provides an emotional release and can help you develop more constructive ways of dealing with similar situations in the future. Research indicates that using a journal this way can improve physical as well as emotional wellness.

For some people, religious belief and practice may promote psychological health. Religious organizations provide a social network and a supportive community, and religious practices, such as prayer and meditation, offer a path for personal change and transformation.

Peer Counseling and Support Groups

Sharing your concerns with others is another helpful way of dealing with psychological health challenges. Just being able to share what's troubling you with an accepting,

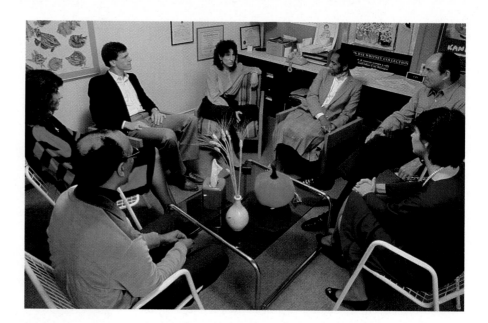

Group therapy is just one of many different approaches to psychological counseling. If you have concerns you would like to discuss with a mental health professional, shop around to find the approach that works for you.

empathetic person can bring relief. Comparing notes with people who have problems similar to yours can give you new ideas about coping.

Many colleges offer peer counseling through a health center or through the psychology or education department. Peer counseling is usually done by volunteer students who have received special training that emphasizes confidentiality. Peer counselors may steer you toward an appropriate campus or community resource or simply offer a sympathetic ear.

Many self-help groups work on the principle of bringing together people with similar problems to share their experiences and support each other. Support groups are typically organized around a specific problem, such as eating disorders or substance abuse. Self-help groups may be listed in the phone book or campus newspaper.

WWW. Professional Help

Sometimes self-help or talking to nonprofessionals is not enough. More objective, more expert, or more discreet help is needed. Many people have trouble accepting the need for professional help, and often those who most need help are the most unwilling to get it. You may someday find yourself having to overcome your own reluctance, or that of a friend, about seeking help.

Determining the Need for Professional Help   In some cases, professional help is optional. Some people are interested in improving their psychological health in a general way by going into individual or group therapy to learn more about themselves and how to interact with others. Clearly, seeking professional help for these reasons is a matter of individual choice. Interpersonal friction among family members or between partners often falls in the middle between necessary and optional. Successful

help with such problems can mean the difference between a painful divorce and a satisfying relationship.

It's sometimes difficult to determine whether someone needs professional help, but it is important to be aware of behaviors that may indicate a serious problem. Following are some strong indications that you or someone else needs professional help:

• If depression, anxiety, or other emotional problems begin to interfere seriously with school or work performance or in getting along with others

• If suicide is attempted or is seriously considered (refer to the warning signs earlier in the chapter)

• If symptoms such as hallucinations, delusions, incoherent speech, or loss of memory occur

• If alcohol or drugs are used to the extent that they impair normal functioning during much of the week, if finding or taking drugs occupies much of the week, or if reducing their dosage leads to psychological or physiological withdrawal symptoms

Choosing a Mental Health Professional   Mental health workers belong to several different professions and have different roles. Psychiatrists are medical doctors. They are experts in deciding whether a medical disease lies behind psychological symptoms, and they are usually involved in treatment if medication or hospitalization is required. Clinical psychologists typically hold a Ph.D. degree; they are often experts in behavioral and cognitive therapies. Other mental health workers include social workers, licensed counselors, and clergy with special training in pastoral counseling. In hospitals and clinics, various mental health professionals may join together in treatment teams. For more on finding appropriate help, see the box "Choosing and Evaluating Mental Health Professionals."

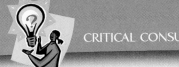

College students are usually in a good position to find convenient, affordable mental health care. Larger schools typically have both health services that employ psychiatrists and psychologists and counseling centers staffed by professionals and student peer counselors. Resources in the community may include a school of medicine, a hospital, and a variety of professionals who work independently. Although independent practitioners are listed in the telephone book, it's a good idea to get recommendations from physicians, clergy, friends who have been in therapy, or community agencies rather than pick a name at random.

Financial considerations are also important. Find out how much different services will cost and what your health insurance will cover. If you're not adequately covered by a health plan, don't let that stop you from getting help; investigate low-cost alternatives. City, county, and state governments often support mental health clinics for those who can afford to pay little or nothing for treatment. Some on-campus services may be free or offered at very little cost.

The cost of treatment is linked to how many therapy sessions will be needed, which in turn depends on the type of therapy and the nature of the problem. Psychological therapies focusing on specific problems may require eight or ten sessions at weekly intervals. Therapies aiming for psychological awareness and personality change can last months or years.

Deciding whether a therapist is right for you will require meeting the therapist in person. Before or during your first meeting, find out about the therapist's background and training:

- Does she or he have a degree from an appropriate professional school and a state license to practice?

- Has she or he had experience treating people with problems similar to yours?

- How much will therapy cost?

You have a right to know the answers to these questions and should not hesitate to ask them. After your initial meeting, evaluate your impressions:

- Does the therapist seem like a warm, intelligent person who would be able to help you and interested in doing so?

- Are you comfortable with the personality, values, and beliefs of the therapist?

- Is he or she willing to talk about the techniques in use? Do these techniques make sense to you?

If you answer yes to these questions, this therapist may be satisfactory for you. If you feel uncomfortable—and you're not in need of emergency care—it's worthwhile to set up one-time consultations with one or two others before you make up your mind. Take the time to find someone who feels right for you.

Later in your treatment, evaluate your progress:

- Are you being helped by the treatment?

- If you are displeased, is it because you aren't making progress or because therapy is raising difficult, painful issues you don't want to deal with?

- Can you express dissatisfaction to your therapist? Such feedback can improve your treatment.

If you're convinced your therapy isn't working or is harmful, thank your therapist for her or his efforts, and find another.

Tips for Today

Life inevitably brings change and challenge—they are a part of growth and development. Most of life's psychological challenges can be met with self-help and everyday skills—introspection and insight, honest communication, support from family and friends. Sometimes a psychological problem poses a greater challenge than we can handle on our own; for these situations, professional help is available.

Right now you can

- Consider the areas in your life where you can be creative (one of the qualities associated with self-actualization), whether in music, art, Web page design, party planning, or whatever you truly enjoy. With the knowledge that allowing your creative side to flourish is a valuable use of your time, plan a way to spend an hour or more on this activity this week.

- Sit down and write 100 positive adjectives that describe you (friendly, loyal, athletic, smart, musical, sensitive, and so on). If you can't think of 100 right now, write as many as you can and keep thinking about it over the next day or two until you reach 100.

- Take a serious look at how you've been feeling the past few weeks. If you have any feelings that are especially difficult to deal with, begin to think about how you can get help with them. Consider consulting the self-help section at the bookstore, talking to a trustworthy friend or peer counselor, or making an appointment with a staff person at the campus counseling center.

- Look at the list of defense mechanisms in Table 3-2. Do you recognize one you've used recently? Review the situation in your mind to see if there's a way you could have coped with it differently.

SUMMARY

- Psychological health encompasses more than a single particular state of normality. Psychological diversity is valuable among groups of people.

- Defining psychological health as the presence of wellness means that to be healthy you must strive to fulfill your potential.

- Maslow's definition of psychological health centered on self-actualization, the highest level in his hierarchy of needs. Self-actualized people have high self-esteem and are realistic, inner-directed, authentic, capable of emotional intimacy, and creative.

- Crucial parts of psychological wellness include developing an adult identity, establishing intimate relationships, and developing values and purpose in life.

- A sense of self-esteem develops during childhood as a result of giving and receiving love and learning to accomplish goals. Self-concept is challenged every day; healthy people adjust their goals to their abilities.

- Using defense mechanisms to cope with problems can make finding solutions harder. Analyzing thoughts and behavior can help people develop less defensive and more effective ways of coping.

- A pessimistic outlook can be damaging; it can be overcome by developing more realistic self-talk.

- Honest communication requires recognizing what needs to be said and saying it clearly. Assertiveness enables people to insist on their rights and to participate in the give-and-take of good communication.

- People may be lonely if they haven't developed ways to be happy on their own or if they interpret being alone as a sign of rejection. Lonely people can take action to expand their social contacts.

- Dealing successfully with anger involves distinguishing between a reasonable level of assertiveness and gratuitous expressions of anger, heading off rage by reframing thoughts and distracting oneself, and responding to the anger of others with an asymmetrical, problem-solving orientation.

- People with psychological disorders have symptoms severe enough to interfere with daily living.

- Anxiety is a fear that is not directed toward any definite threat. Anxiety disorders include simple phobias, social phobias, panic disorder, generalized anxiety disorder, obsessive-compulsive disorder, and post-traumatic stress disorder.

- Depression is a common mood disorder; loss of interest or pleasure in things seems to be its most universal symptom. Severe depression carries a high risk of suicide, and suicidally depressed people need professional help.

- Symptoms of mania include exalted moods with unrealistically high self-esteem, little need for sleep, and rapid speech. Mood swings between mania and depression characterize bipolar disorder.

- Schizophrenia is characterized by disorganized thoughts, inappropriate emotions, delusions, auditory hallucinations, and deteriorating social and work performance.

- The biological model emphasizes that the mind's activity depends on the brain, whose composition is genetically determined. Therapy based on the biological model is primarily pharmacological.

- The behavioral model focuses on overt behavior and treats psychological problems as bad habits. Behavior change is the focus of therapy.

- The cognitive model considers how ideas affect behavior and feelings; behavior results from complicated attitudes, expectations, and motives, not just from simple reinforcements. Cognitive therapy focuses on changing one's thinking.

- The psychodynamic model asserts that false ideas are fed by unconscious ideas and cannot be addressed directly. Treatment is based on psychotherapy.

- Help is available in a variety of forms, including self-help, peer counseling, support groups, and therapy with a mental health professional. For serious problems, professional help may be the most appropriate.

TAKE ACTION

1. Investigate the mental health services on your campus and in your community. What services are available? Think about which ones you would feel comfortable using, for either yourself or someone else, should the need ever arise.

2. Many colleges and communities have peer counseling programs, hotline services (for both general problems and specific issues such as rape, suicide, and drug abuse), and other kinds of emergency counseling services. Some programs are staffed by trained volunteers.

Investigate such programs in your school (through the health clinic or student services) or community (look in the yellow pages), and consider volunteering for one. The training and experience can help you understand both yourself and others.

3. Being assertive rather than passive or aggressive is a valuable skill that everyone can learn. To improve your ability to assert yourself appropriately, sign up for a workshop or class in assertiveness training on your campus or in your community.

Shyness is often the result of both high anxiety levels and lack of key social skills. To help overcome shyness, you need to learn to manage your fear of social situations and to develop social skills such as appropriate eye contact, initiating topics in conversations, and maintaining the flow of conversations by asking questions and making appropriate responses. As described in the chapter, repeated *exposure* to the source of one's fear—in this case, social situations—is the best method for reducing anxiety. When you practice new behaviors, they gradually become easier and you experience less anxiety. A counterproductive strategy is avoiding situations that make you anxious. Although this approach works in the short term—you eliminate your anxiety because you escape the situation—it keeps you from meeting new people and have new experiences. Another counterproductive strategy is self-medicating with alcohol or drugs. Being under their influence actually prevents you from learning new social skills and new ways to handle your anxiety.

To reduce your anxiety in social situations, try some of the following strategies:

- Remember that physical stress reactions are short-term responses to fear. Don't dwell on them—remind yourself that they will pass, and they will.

- Refocus your attention away from the stress reaction you're experiencing and toward the social task at hand. Your nervousness is much less visible than you think.

- Allow a warm-up period for new situations. Realize that you will feel more nervous at first, and take steps to relax and become more comfortable. Refer to the suggestions for deep breathing and other relaxation techniques in Chapter 2.

- If possible, take breaks during anxiety-producing situations. For example, if you're at a party, take a moment to visit the restroom or step outside. Alternate between speaking with good friends and striking up conversations with new acquaintances.

- Watch your interpretations; having a stress reaction doesn't mean that you don't belong in the group, that you're unattractive or unworthy, or that the situation is too much for you. Try thinking of yourself as excited or highly alert instead of anxious.

- Avoid cognitive distortions and practice realistic self-talk. Replace your self-critical thoughts with more supportive ones: "No one else is perfect, and I don't have to be either." "It would have been good if I had a funny story to tell, but the conversation was interesting anyway."

- Give yourself a reality check: Ask if you're really in a life-threatening situation (or just at a party); if the outcome you're imagining is really likely (or the worst thing that could possibly happen); or if you're the only one who feels nervous (or if many other people might feel the same way).

- Don't think of conversations as evaluations; remind yourself that you don't have to prove yourself with every social interaction. And remember that most people are thinking more about themselves than they are about you.

Starting and maintaining conversations can be difficult for shy people, who may feel overwhelmed by their physical stress reaction. If small talk is a problem for you, try the following strategies:

- Introduce yourself early in the conversation. If you tend to forget names, repeat your new acquaintance's name to help fix it in your mind ("Nice to meet you, Amelia.").

- Ask questions, and look for shared topics of interest. Simple, open-ended questions like "How's your presentation coming along?" or "How do you know our host?" encourage others to carry the conversation for a while and help bring forth a variety of subjects.

- Take turns talking, and elaborate on your answers. Simple "yes" and "no" answers don't move the conversation along. Try to relate something in your life—a course you're taking or a hobby you have—to something in the other person's life. Match self-disclosure with self-disclosure.

- Have something to say. Expand your mind and become knowledgeable about current events and local or campus news. If you have specialized knowledge about a topic, practice discussing it in ways that both beginners and experts can understand and appreciate.

- If you get stuck for something to say, try giving a compliment ("Great presentation!" or "I love your earrings.") or performing a social grace (pass the chips or get someone a drink).

- Be an active listener. Reward the other person with your full attention and with regular responses. Make frequent eye contact and maintain a relaxed but alert posture. (See Chapter 4 for more on being an active listener.)

At first, your new behaviors will likely make you anxious. Don't give up—things *will* get easier. Create lots of opportunities to practice your new behaviors; your goal is to make them routine activities. For example, striking up a conversation with someone in a registration or movie line can help you practice your small-talk skills in a nonthreatening setting. Once you are comfortable doing that, you might try initiating brief conversations with classmates about academic topics—the upcoming midterm, for example, or an assignment. Following that, you might try something more challenging, such as discussing a more personal topic or meeting new people in a social setting.

Regular practice and stress-management skills are critical. Using these techniques, you can increase your social skills and confidence level at the same time that you decrease your anxiety. Eventually, you'll be able to sustain social interactions with comfort and enjoyment. If you find that social anxiety is a major problem for you and self-help techniques don't seem to work, consider looking into a shyness clinic or treatment program on your campus.

SOURCES: Carducci, B. J. 1999. *Shyness: A Bold New Approach.* New York: Perennial. University of Texas at Dallas, Student Counseling Center. 2000. *Overcoming Social Anxiety* (http://www.utdallas.edu/student/slife/counseling/anxiety.html; retrieved August 31, 2000).

1. Do you remember incidents or moments from childhood that stand out as wonderful or horrible? Write a short essay about two such incidents, including what your feelings were and what you think you learned from them. Then describe what you would do now in the same situations and why.

2. *Critical Thinking* In the past, some political candidates have dropped out of a race or been defeated after it was revealed that they had undergone psychiatric treatment or some other form of therapy. Do you think a person who has been treated for a mental illness should be excluded from holding a public office or from any other profession? Why or why not? Does your position depend on the type of illness or the treatment the individual received? In your health journal, write a brief essay explaining your position.

3. Think about a person you respect. Describe him or her in writing, listing the qualities you admire. Do you have any of those qualities? What does your list say about the kind of person you want to be?

FOR MORE INFORMATION

Books

Carducci, B. J. 1999. *Shyness: A Bold New Approach.* New York: HarperCollins. *Explores the reasons for shyness and gives lots of useful advice for dealing with it in yourself and in your children.*

Casey, N. 2001. *Unholy Ghost: Writers on Depression.* New York: William Morrow. *An eloquent collection of essays about depression.*

Frances, A., and M. B. First. 1999. *Your Mental Health: A Layman's Guide to the Psychiatrist's Bible.* New York: Scribner. *A resource-packed reference with information on dozens of mental disorders; based on the APA's DSM-IV.*

Grohol, J. M., and E. L. Zuckerman. 2000. *An Insider's Guide to Mental Health Resources Online, 2000–2001 Edition.* New York: Guilford Press. *Explains and rates Internet search engines, newsgroups, and Web sites devoted to mental health.*

Hyman, B. M., and C. Pedrick. 1999. *The OCD Workbook: Your Guide to Breaking Free from Obsessive-Compulsive Disorder.* Oakland, Calif.: New Harbinger. *A self-directed program for blocking rituals, reducing fears, and changing unhealthy thought patterns.*

Mondimore, F. M. 1999. *Bipolar Disorder: A Guide for Patients.* Baltimore: Johns Hopkins University Press. *Covers the symptoms, diagnosis, and treatment of bipolar (or manic depressive) disorder.*

Schwartz, S. 2000. *Abnormal Psychology: A Discovery Approach.* Mountain View, Calif.: Mayfield. *Provides a comprehensive introduction to psychological disorders.*

Seligman, M. E. P. 1998. *Learned Optimism.* New York: Pocket Books. *A discussion of the effects of pessimism, optimism, and learned helplessness, with suggestions for change.*

Wolpert, L. 2000. *Malignant Sadness: The Anatomy of Depression.* New York: Free Press. A look at the nature of depression, with information for people with the disorder and their families.

Zuercher-White, E. 1998. *An End to Panic,* 2nd ed. Oakland, Calif.: New Harbinger. *Presents a variety of standard self-help techniques, including controlling breathing and developing more realistic self-talk.*

WW. Organizations, Hotlines, and Web Sites

American Association of Suicidology. Provides information about suicide and resources for people in crisis.
http://www.suicidology.org

American Psychiatric Association (APA). Provides public information by pamphlet or online about a variety of topics, including depression, anxiety, eating disorders, and psychiatric medications.

202-682-6000; 888-357-7924
http://www.psych.org

American Psychological Association Consumer HelpCenter. Provides information about common challenges to psychological health and about how to obtain professional help.
800-964-2000
http://helping.apa.org

Anxiety Disorders Association of America (ADAA). Provides information and resources related to anxiety disorders, including listings of support groups.
301-231-9350
http://www.adaa.org

Depression.com. A commercial site that presents information about drug treatment of depression.
http://www.depression.com

Internet Mental Health. An encyclopedia of mental health information, including medical diagnostic criteria.
http://www.mentalhealth.com

Mental Health Net. A comprehensive guide to mental health online, including background information and links for many topics.
http://www.cmhc.com

NAMI (National Alliance for the Mentally Ill). Provides information and support for people who are affected by mental illness.
800-950-NAMI (Help Line)
http://www.nami.org

National Depressive and Manic-Depressive Association (NDMDA). Provides educational materials and information about support groups and other resources.
800-82-NDMDA
http://www.ndmda.org

National Institute of Mental Health (NIMH). Provides helpful information about anxiety, depression, eating disorders, and other challenges to psychological health.
800-421-4211 (NIMH information line); 301-443-4513
http://www.nimh.nih.gov

National Mental Health Association. Provides consumer information on a variety of issues, including how to find help.
800-969-NMHA
http://www.nmha.org

National Mental Health Services Knowledge and Exchange Network (KEN). A one-stop source for information and resources relating to mental health.

800-789-CMHS

http://www.mentalhealth.org

Psych Central: Dr. John Grohol's Mental Health Page. A guide to psychology, support, and mental health issues, resources, and people on the Internet.

http://psychcentral.com

Student Counseling Virtual Pamphlet Collection. Provides links to more than 400 pamphlets produced by different student counseling centers; topics range from depression and anxiety to time management and assertiveness.

http://counseling.uchicago.edu/vpc

The following sites include interactive online assessments for various psychological problems:

Depression-screening.org: http://www.depression-screening.org

Freedom from Fear: http://www.freedomfromfear.com

New York University Department of Psychiatry:
    http://www.med.nyu.edu/Psych/public.html

SELECTED BIBLIOGRAPHY

Agency for Health Care Policy and Research (AHCPR). 1999. *Treatment of Depression—Newer Pharmacotherapies.* Rockville, Md.: AHCPR Pub. No. 99-E014.

American Psychiatric Association. 2000. *Diagnostic and Statistical Manual of Mental Disorders,* Fourth Edition, Text Revision *(DSM-IV-TR).* Washington, D.C.: American Psychiatric. Association Press.

Baare, W. F., et al. 2001. Volumes of brain structures in twins discordant for schizophrenia. *Archives of General Psychiatry* 58(1): 33–40.

Chang, E. C., and W. B. Bridewell. 1998. Irrational beliefs, optimism, pessimism, and psychological distress: A preliminary examination of differential effects in a college population. *Journal of Clinical Psychology* 54(2): 137–142.

Dodgson, P. G., and J. V. Wood. 1998. Self-esteem and the cognitive accessibility of strengths and weaknesses after failure. *Journal of Personality and Social Psychology* 75(1): 178–197.

Frances, A., and M. B. First. 1998. *Your Mental Health: A Layman's Guide to the Psychiatrist's Bible.* New York: Scribner.

Generalized anxiety disorder. 2000. *Journal of the American Medical Association Patient Page* 283(23): 3156.

Hinsie, L. E. 1999. The treatment of schizophrenia: A survey of the literature. *Psychiatric Quarterly* 70(1): 5–26.

Jackson, T. 1999. Differences in psychosocial experiences of employed, unemployed, and student samples of young adults. *Journal of Psychology* 133(1): 49–60.

Kender, K. S., and C. A. Prescott. 1999. A population-based twin study of lifetime major depression in men and women. *Archives of General Psychiatry* 56(1): 39–44.

Lam, R. W., et al. 2000. Effects of light therapy on suicidal ideation in patients with winter depression. *Journal of Clinical Psychiatry* 61(1): 30–32.

Maruta, T., et al. 2000. Optimists vs. pessimists: Survival rate among medical patients over a 30-year period. *Mayo Clinic Proceedings* 75(2): 140–143.

Nathan, P. E., and J. M. Gorman (eds.). 1998. *A Guide to Treatments That Work.* New York: Oxford University Press.

National Institutes of Health, National Center for Complementary and Alternative Medicine. 2000. *Factsheet: St. John's Wort* (http://nccam.nih.gov/nccam/fcp/factsheets/stjohnswort/stjohnswort.htm; retrieved May 9, 2000).

Nolen-Hoeksema, S., C. Grayson, and J. Larson. 1999. Explaining the gender difference in depressive symptoms. *Journal of Personality and Social Psychology* 77(5): 1061–1072.

Panic disorder. 2000. *Journal of the American Medical Association Patient Page* 283(19): 2612.

Perkonnigg, A., et al. 2000. Traumatic events and posttraumatic stress disorder in the community: Prevalence, risk factors, and comorbidity. *Acta Psychiatrica Scandinavica* 101: 46–59.

Pini, S., et al. 2001. Insight into illness in schizophrenia, schizo affective disorder, and mood disorders with psychotic features. *American Journal of Psychiatry* 158(1): 122–125.

Raikkonen, K., et al. 1999. Effects of optimism, pessimism, and trait anxiety on ambulatory blood pressure and mood during everyday life. *Journal of Personal and Social Psychology* 76(1): 104–113.

Reynolds, C. F., et al. 1999. Nortriptyline and interpersonal psychotherapy as maintenance therapies for recurrent major depression. *Journal of the American Medical Association* 281: 39–45.

Rothwell, J. D. 2000. *In the Company of Others: An Introduction to Communication.* Mountain View, Calif.: Mayfield.

Schwartz, S. 2000. *Abnormal Psychology: A Discovery Approach.* Mountain View, Calif.: Mayfield.

Sheldon, K. M., and L. Houser-Marko. 2001. Self-concordance, goal attainment, and the pursuit of happiness: Can there be an upward spiral? *Journal of Personality and Social Psychology* 80(1): 152–165.

Snow, V., S. Lascher, and C. Mottur-Pilson. 2000. Pharmacological treatment of acute major depression and dysthymia. *Annals of Internal Medicine* 132(9): 738–742.

Spicer, R. S., and T. R. Miller. 2000. Suicide acts in 8 states: incidence and case fatality rates by demographics and method. *American Journal of Public Health* 90(12): 1885–1891.

Stein, M. B., et al. 1998. Paroxetine treatment of generalized social phobia. *Journal of the American Medical Association* 280(8): 708–713.

Stein, M. B., K. L. Jang, and W. J. Livesley. 1999. Heritability of anxiety sensitivity: A twin study. *American Journal of Psychiatry* 156(2): 246–251.

Treating depression with electroconvulsive therapy. 2001. *Journal of the American Medical Association* 285(10): 1390.

U.S. Department of Health and Human Services. 1999. *Mental Health: A Report of the Surgeon General.* Rockville, Md.: DHHS.

Vaillant, G. E. 1977. *Adaptation to Life.* Boston: Little, Brown.

Van Ameringen, M., C. Mancini, and J. M. Oakman. 1998. The relationship of behavioral inhibition and shyness to anxiety disorder. *Journal of Nervous and Mental Disease* 186(7): 425–431.

Weissman, M. M. 1998. Cross-national epidemiology of obsessive-compulsive disorder. *CNS Spectrums* 3(5 Suppl 1): 6–9.

Williams, J. W., et al. 2000. A systematic review of newer pharmacotherapies for depression in adults: Evidence report summary. *Annals of Internal Medicine* 132(9): 743–756.

Wirz-Justice, A. 1998. Beginning to see the light. *Archives of General Psychiatry* 55: 861–862.

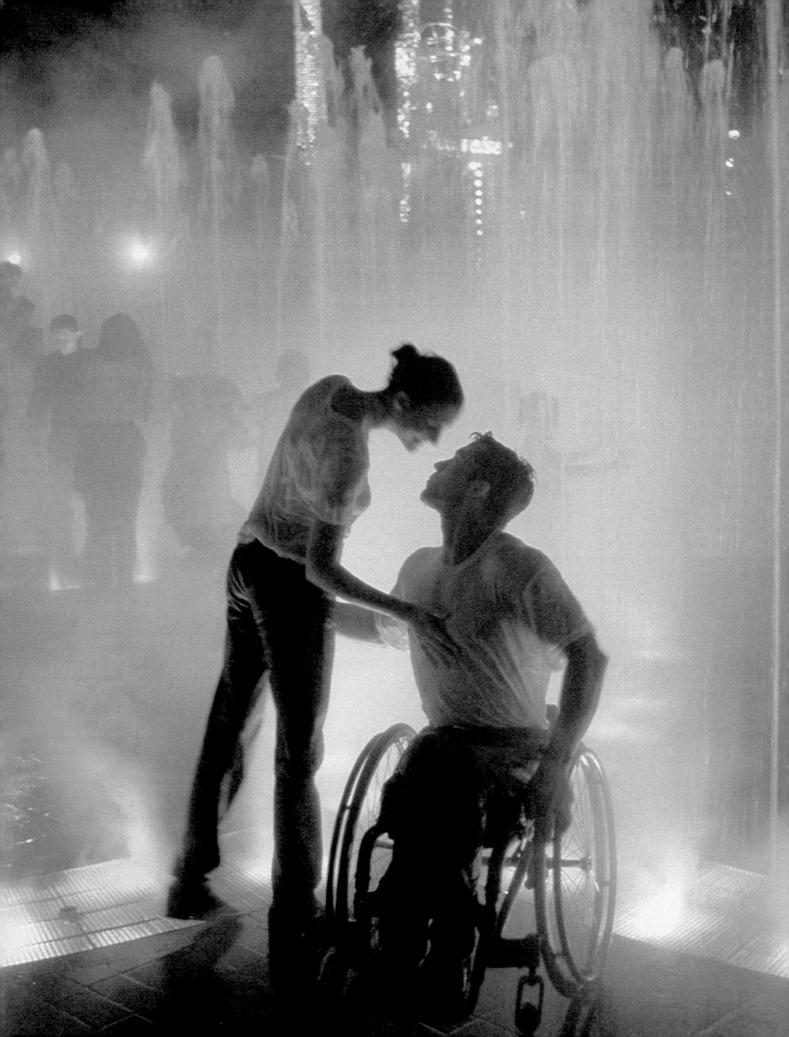

LOOKING AHEAD

After reading this chapter, you should be able to

- Explain the qualities that help people develop intimate relationships
- Describe different types of love relationships and the stages they often go through
- Describe common challenges of forming and maintaining intimate relationships
- Discuss relationship options available to adults today
- List some characteristics of successful families and some potential problems families face
- Explain some of the joys and challenges of being a parent

Intimate Relationships and Communication

4

TEST YOUR KNOWLEDGE

1. Couples who live together before marriage are less likely to get divorced than those who don't.
   True or false?

2. Conflict and fighting are usually signs of trouble in intimate relationships.
   True or false?

3. About what percentage of all U.S. married couples are interracial couples?
   a. 1%
   b. 5%
   c. 10%

4. Married people tend to be healthier and to live longer than unmarried people.
   True or false?

5. The love that lesbians and gay men experience is similar in quality to that experienced by heterosexuals.
   True or false?

6. What percentage of American households conform to the traditional model of wage-earning father, stay-at-home mother, and children?
   a. 5%
   b. 15%
   c. 30%

ANSWERS

1. FALSE. Studies have found that couples who cohabit before they get married are just as likely to divorce as those who don't cohabit.

2. FALSE. Conflict itself isn't a sign of trouble; it may mean a relationship is growing. What's important is how the partners handle the conflict.

3. B. When cohabitation is also considered, interracial intimate partnerships are more common. For example, among married Asian Americans, 25% of women and 16% of men have white spouses; among cohabiting Asian Americans, 45% of women and 37% of men have white partners.

4. TRUE. One explanation is that marriage encourages healthy behaviors, and surveys have found that married people are more likely to wear safety belts, be physically active, and not smoke.

5. TRUE. Like heterosexual relationships, gay and lesbian partnerships provide intimacy, passion, and security. Most gay men and lesbians experience at least one long-term relationship with a single partner.

6. B. Dual-career couples now represent almost half of the U.S. labor force.

Human beings need social relationships; we cannot thrive as solitary creatures. Nor could the human species survive if adults didn't cherish and support each other, if we didn't form strong mutual attachments with our infants, and if we didn't create families in which to raise children. Simply put, people need people.

Although people are held together in relationships by a variety of factors, the foundation of many relationships is love. Love in its many forms—romantic, passionate, platonic, parental—is the wellspring from which much of life's meaning and delight flows. In our culture, it binds us together as partners, parents, children, and friends. People devote tremendous energy to seeking mates, nurturing intimate relationships, keeping up friendships, maintaining marriages—all for the pleasure of loving and being loved.

Many human needs are satisfied in intimate relationships: the need for approval and affirmation, for companionship, for meaningful ties and a sense of belonging, for sexual satisfaction. Many of society's needs are fulfilled by relationships, too—most notably, the need to nurture and socialize children. Overall, healthy intimate relationships are an important contributor to the well-being of both individuals and society.

Ww. DEVELOPING INTIMATE RELATIONSHIPS

People who develop successful intimate relationships believe in themselves and in the people around them. They are willing to give of themselves—to share their ideas, feelings, time, needs—and to accept what others want to give them.

Self-Concept and Self-Esteem

The principal thing that we all bring to our relationships is our *selves*. To have successful relationships, we must first accept and feel good about ourselves. A positive self-concept and a healthy level of self-esteem help us love and respect others. How and where do we acquire a positive sense of self?

As discussed in Chapter 3, the roots of our identity and sense of self can be found in childhood, in the relationships we had with our parents and other family members. As adults, we probably have a sense that we're basically lovable, worthwhile people and that we can trust others if, as babies and children, we felt loved, valued, and respected; if adults responded to our needs in a reasonably appropriate way; and if they gave us the freedom to explore and develop a sense of being separate individuals.

Our personal identity isn't fixed or frozen. According to psychologist Erik Erikson, it continues to develop as we encounter and resolve various crises at each stage of life. The fundamental tasks of early childhood are the development of trust during infancy and of autonomy during toddlerhood. From these experiences and interactions we construct our first ideas about who we are. (For a more detailed discussion of Erikson's developmental theory, see Chapter 3.)

Another thing we learn in early childhood is **gender role**—the activities, abilities, and characteristics our culture deems appropriate for us based on whether we're male or female. In our society, men have traditionally been expected to work and provide for their families; to be aggressive, competitive, and power-oriented; and to use thinking and logic to solve problems. Women have been expected to take care of home and children; to be cooperative, supportive, and nurturing; and to approach life emotionally and intuitively. Although much more egalitarian gender roles are emerging in our society, the stereotypes we absorb in childhood tend to be deeply ingrained.

Our ways of relating to others may also be rooted in childhood. Some researchers have suggested that our adult styles of loving may be based on the style of **attachment** we established in infancy with our mother, father, or other primary caregiver. According to this view, people who are secure in their intimate relationships probably had a secure, trusting, mutually satisfying attachment to their mother, father, or other parenting figure. As adults, they find it relatively easy to get close to others. They don't worry about being abandoned or having someone get too close to them. They feel that other people like them and are generally well intentioned.

People who are clinging and dependent in their relationships may have had an "anxious/ambivalent" attachment, in which a parent's inconsistent responses made them unsure that their needs would be met. As adults, they worry about whether their partners really love them and will stay with them. They tend to feel that others don't want to get as close as they do. They want to merge completely with another person, which sometimes scares others away.

People who seem to run from relationships may have had an "anxious/avoidant" attachment, in which a parent's inappropriate responses made them want to escape from his or her sphere of influence. As adults, they feel uncomfortable being close to others. They're distrustful and fearful of becoming dependent. Their partners usually want more intimacy than they do.

Even if people's earliest experiences and relationships were less than ideal, however, they can still establish satisfying relationships in adulthood. People can be resilient and flexible. They have the capacity to change their ideas, beliefs, and behavior patterns. They can learn ways to

Terms

gender role A culturally expected pattern of behavior and attitudes determined by whether a person is male or female.

attachment The emotional tie between an infant and his or her caregiver or between two people in an intimate relationship.

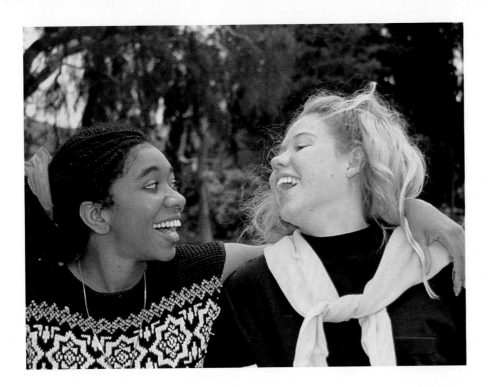

Close relationships without a sexual component are more common than those with sexual activity. Friendship satisfies our need for affection, affirmation, sharing, and companionship.

raise their self-esteem; they can become more trusting, accepting, and appreciative of others; and they can acquire the communication and conflict-resolution skills for maintaining successful relationships. Although it helps to have a good start in life, it may be even more important to begin again, right from where you are.

Friendship

The first relationships we form outside the family are friendships. With members of either the same or the other sex, friendships give people the opportunity to share themselves and discover others. The friendships we form in childhood are important in our development; through them we learn about tolerance, sharing, and trust.

Friendships usually include most or all of the following characteristics:

- *Companionship.* Friends are relaxed and happy in each other's company. They typically have common values and interests and make plans to spend time together.

- *Respect.* Friends have a basic respect for each other's humanity and individuality. Good friends respect each other's feelings and opinions and work to resolve their differences without demeaning or insulting each other. They also show their respect by being honest with one another (see the box "Being a Good Friend").

- *Acceptance.* Friends accept each other—"warts and all." They feel free to be themselves and express

their feelings spontaneously without fear of ridicule or criticism.

- *Help.* Sharing time, energy, and even material goods is important to friendship. Friends know they can rely on each other in times of need. They feel they can ask for help when the going gets tough.

- *Trust.* Friends are secure in the knowledge that they will not intentionally hurt each other. They feel safe confiding in one another.

- *Loyalty.* Friends can count on each other. They stand up for each other in both word and deed.

- *Mutuality.* Friends retain their individual identities, but close friendships are characterized by a sense of mutuality—"what affects you affects me." Friends share the ups and downs in each other's lives.

- *Reciprocity.* Friendships are reciprocal. There is give-and-take between friends and the feeling that both share joys and burdens more or less equally over time.

Intimate partnerships are like friendships in many ways, but they have additional characteristics. These relationships usually include sexual desire and expression, a greater demand for exclusiveness, and deeper levels of caring. Friendships are usually considered more stable and longer lasting than intimate partnerships. Friends are often more accepting and less critical than lovers, probably because their expectations are different. Like love relationships, friendships bind society together, providing people with emotional support and buffering them from stress.

How to Make Friends

- Find people with interests similar to your own. Join a club, participate in sports, do volunteer work, or join a discussion group to meet people with common interests.

- Be a good listener. Take a genuine interest in people. Solicit their opinions, and take time to listen to their problems and ideas.

- Take risks. If you meet someone interesting, ask him or her to join you for a meal or an event you would both enjoy.

How to Be a Good Friend

- Be trustworthy. Honor all confidences, and don't talk about your friend behind his or her back.

- Tell your friend about yourself. Self-disclosure—letting your friend know about your real concerns and joys—signals trust.

- Be supportive and kind. Be there when your friend is going through a rough time. Don't criticize your friend or offer unsolicited advice.

- Develop your capacity for intimacy. Intimate relationships are genuine, spontaneous, and caring.

- Don't expect perfection. Like any relationship, your friendship may go through difficult times. Talk through conflicts as they arise.

COMMUNICATE!   Intimate relationships are crucial for your overall well-being. You can help keep friendships strong by offering your friends support when they share feelings such as anger, disappointment, and frustration. The next time a friend shares a problem with you, listen closely and empathize with her or his feelings. Offer supportive statements and, if appropriate, your help. For example, "I understand your frustration; you've been working very hard on that project. Is there anything I can do to help?"

Love, Sex, and Intimacy

Love is one of the most basic and profound human emotions. It is a powerful force in all our intimate relationships. Love encompasses opposites: affection and anger, excitement and boredom, stability and change, bonds and freedom. Love does not give us perfect happiness, but it does give our lives meaning.

In many kinds of adult relationships, love is closely intertwined with sexuality. In the past, marriage was considered the only acceptable context for sexual activities, but for many people today, sex is legitimized by love. Many couples, both heterosexual and homosexual, live together in committed relationships. We now use personal standards rather than social norms to make decisions about sex. This trend toward personal responsibility results in even more of an emphasis on love than in the past.

For most people, love, sex, and commitment are closely linked ideals in intimate relationships. Love reflects the positive factors that draw people together and sustain them in a relationship. It includes trust, caring, respect, loyalty, interest in the other, and concern for the other's well-being. Sex brings excitement and passion to the relationship. It intensifies the relationship and adds fascination and pleasure. Commitment, the determination to continue, reflects the stable factors that help maintain the relationship. Responsibility, reliability, and faithfulness are characteristics of commitment. Although love, sex, and commitment are related, they are not necessarily connected. One can exist without the others. Despite the various "faces" of love, sex, and commitment, most of us long for a special relationship that contains them all.

Other elements can be identified as features of love, such as euphoria, preoccupation with the loved one, idealization of the loved one, and so on, but these tend to be temporary. These characteristics may include **infatuation**, which will fade or deepen into something more substantial. As relationships progress, the central aspects of love and commitment take on more importance.

Another way of looking at love has been proposed by psychologist Robert Sternberg. He sees love as being composed of intimacy, passion, and commitment (Figure 4-1). Intimacy refers to the feelings of warmth and closeness we have with someone we love. Passion refers to romance, attraction, and sexuality. Commitment refers to both the short-term decision that you love someone and the long-term commitment to be in the relationship.

According to Sternberg, these three elements can be enlarged, diminished, or combined in different ways. Each combination gives a different kind of love:

- *Liking* (intimacy only): Love between friends.

- *Infatuation* (passion only): An idealizing, obsessive, all-consuming love, characterized by a high degree of physical and emotional arousal; often unrequited; "love at first sight."

Terms   **infatuation** An idealizing, obsessive attraction, characterized by a high degree of physical arousal.

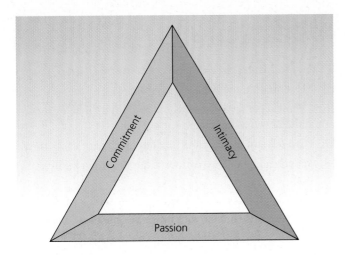

Figure 4-1   The love triangle.   SOURCE: Stemberg, R., and M. Barnes. 1988. *The Psychology of Love.* New Haven: Yale University Press, p. 37.

- *Romantic* (intimacy and passion): Love in which commitment may develop over time.

- *Fatuous* (passion and commitment): Deceptive love, the "whirlwind affair"; as passion fades, all that's left is commitment, but without time and intimacy, it's a poor foundation for an enduring relationship.

- *Empty* (commitment only): Dutiful love; also a poor foundation for a relationship.

- *Companionate* (intimacy and commitment): Essentially a committed friendship; often begins as romantic love, but as passion diminishes and intimacy increases, it is transformed into companionate love.

- *Consummate* (all three elements): The love that dreams are made of; difficult to sustain.

Men and women tend to have different views of the relationship between love (or intimacy) and sex (or passion). Numerous studies have found that men can separate love from sex rather easily, although many men find that their most erotic sexual experiences occur in the context of a love relationship. Women generally view sex from the point of view of a relationship. Some people believe you can have satisfying sex without love—with friends, acquaintances, or strangers. Although sex with love is an important norm in our culture, it is frequently disregarded in practice, as the high incidence of extrarelational affairs attests.

The Pleasure and Pain of Love   The experience of intense love has confused and tormented lovers throughout history. They live in a tumultuous state of excitement, subject to wildly fluctuating feelings of joy and despair. They lose their appetite, can't sleep, and can think of nothing but the loved one. Is this happiness? Misery? Or both?

The contradictory nature of passionate love can be understood by recognizing that human emotions have two components: physiological arousal and an emotional explanation for the arousal. (For a discussion of the biochemical and hormonal processes involved in arousal, see the description of the stress response in Chapter 2.) Love is just one of many emotions accompanied by physiological arousal; numerous unpleasant ones can also generate arousal, such as fear, rejection, frustration, and challenge. Although experiences like attraction and sexual desire are pleasant, extreme excitement is similar to fear and is unpleasant. For this reason, passionate love may be too intense to enjoy. Over time, the physical intensity and excitement tend to diminish. When this happens, pleasure may actually increase.

The Transformation of Love   All human relationships change over time, and love relationships are no exception. At first, love is likely to be characterized by high levels of passion and rapidly increasing intimacy. After a while, passion decreases as we become habituated to it and to the person. Generally, increasing the time spent together does not increase arousal.

Sometimes intimacy continues to grow at a deeper, less conscious level; at other times, the couple may drift apart. Commitment isn't necessarily diminished or altered by time. It grows more slowly and is maintained as long as we judge the relationship to be successful. If the relationship begins to deteriorate, the level of commitment usually decreases.

The disappearance of romance or passionate love is often experienced as a crisis in a relationship. If a more lasting love fails to emerge, the relationship will likely break up, and each person will search for another who will once again ignite his or her passion. Love does not necessarily have to be intensely passionate. When intensity diminishes, partners often discover a more enduring love. They can now move from absorption in each other to a relationship that includes external goals and projects, friends, and family. In this kind of intimate, more secure love, satisfaction comes not just from the relationship itself but also from achieving other creative goals, such as work or child rearing. The key to successful relationships is in transforming passion into an intimate love, based on closeness, caring, and the promise of a shared future. Only with the passage of time can love mature and deepen, allowing us to truly grow both psychologically and spiritually.

Challenges in Relationships

Although many people believe that love naturally makes an intimate relationship easy to begin and maintain, there are, in fact, often obstacles and challenges. Even in the best of circumstances, there are times when a loving relationship will be tested. Individuals bring to a relationship diverse needs and wants, some of which emerge only at times of change or stress. Common relationship challenges

Emotionally intelligent couples have richly detailed "love maps"—they know about each other's history, major goals and beliefs, and day-to-day struggles. To assess the quality of your current love maps, answer each of the following questions with "true" or "false."

1. I can name my partner's best friends.

2. I can tell you what stresses my partner is currently facing.

3. I know the names of some of the people who have been irritating my partner lately.

4. I can tell you some of my partner's life dreams.

5. I am very familiar with my partner's religious beliefs and ideas.

6. I can tell you about my partner's basic philosophy of life.

7. I can list the relatives my partner likes the least.

8. I know my partner's favorite music.

9. I can list my partner's three favorite movies.

10. My partner is familiar with my current stresses.

11. I know the three most special times in my partner's life.

12. I can tell you the most stressful thing that happened to my partner as a child.

13. I can list my partner's major aspirations and hopes in life.

14. I know my partner's major current worries.

15. My partner knows who my friends are.

16. I know what my partner would want to do if he or she suddenly won the lottery.

17. I can tell you in detail my first impressions of my partner.

18. Periodically, I ask my partner about his or her world right now.

19. I feel that my partner knows me pretty well.

20. My partner is familiar with my hopes and aspirations.

Scoring: Give yourself one point for each "true" answer.

10 or above: This is an area of strength in your relationship. You have a fairly detailed map of your partner's everyday life, hopes, fears, and dreams. If you maintain this level of knowledge and understanding of each other, you'll be well equipped to handle any problem areas that crop up in your relationship.

Below 10: Your relationship could stand some improvement in this area. By taking the time to learn more about your partner now, you'll find your relationship becomes stronger.

SOURCE: Gottman, J. M., and N. Silver. 1999. *The Seven Principles for Making Marriage Work.* New York: Three Rivers Press.

---

relate to self-disclosure, commitment, expectations, competitiveness, and jealousy.

Honesty and Openness
Everyone looks for honesty and openness in an intimate relationship. However, especially at the beginning of a relationship, partners tend to engage in a certain amount of pretense in an effort to present themselves in the best possible manner. It's usually best to be yourself from the start to give both you and your potential partner a chance to find out if you are comfortable with each other's beliefs, interests, and lifestyles.

Getting close to another person by sharing thoughts and feelings is emotionally risky, but it is necessary for a relationship to deepen. Take your time, and self-disclose at a slow but steady rate—one that doesn't make you feel too vulnerable or your partner too uncomfortable. Over time, you and your partner will learn more about each other and feel more comfortable sharing. In fact, intimate familiarity with your partner's life is a key characteristic of successful long-term relationships (see the box "Love Maps Questionnaire").

Unequal or Premature Commitment
Sometimes one person in an intimate partnership becomes more serious about the relationship than the other partner. In this situation, it can be very difficult to maintain a friendship without hurting the other person. Sometimes a couple makes a premature commitment, and then one of the partners has second thoughts and wants to break off the relationship. Sometimes both partners begin to realize that something is wrong, but each is afraid to tell the other. Most such problems can be dealt with only by honest and sensitive communication.

Unrealistic Expectations
Each partner brings hopes and expectations to a relationship, some of which may be unrealistic, unfair, and, ultimately, very damaging to the relationship. For example, if you believe that love will eliminate all of your problems, you may start to blame your partner for anything that goes wrong in your life. Other common expectations that can hurt a relationship include the following:

- *Expecting your partner to change.* There are probably some things about your partner that you like more than others. It's OK to discuss them with your partner; however, it's unfair to demand that your partner change to meet all of your expectations. Accept the differences you see between your ideal and the reality.

- *Assuming that your partner has all the same opinions, priorities, interests, and goals as you.* You may share many things with your partner, but don't assume that you think the same about everything—or that you have to in order for the relationship to succeed. Agreement on key issues is important, but differences can enhance a relationship as long as partners understand and respect each other's points of view.

- *Believing that a relationship will fulfill all of your personal, financial, intellectual, and social needs.* Expecting a relationship to fulfill all your needs places too much pressure on your partner and on your relationship, and it will inevitably lead to disappointment. For your own well-being, it's important to maintain some degree of autonomy and self-sufficiency.

Competitiveness   American social norms encourage a certain amount of healthy competition between intimate partners and friends. Games and competitive sports add flavor to the bonding process—as long as the focus is on fun. If one partner always feels the strong need to compete and win, it can detract from the sense of connectedness, interdependence, equality, and mutuality between partners. The same can be said for a perfectionistic need to be right in every instance—to "win" every argument.

Even if you're convinced you're right, a loving relationship won't work if you get everything your own way—it's just not fair. If competitiveness is a problem for you, ask yourself if your need to win is more important than your partner's feelings or the future of your relationship. Try engaging in noncompetitive activities or in an activity where you are a beginner and your partner excels. Accept that your partner may hold different views on issues than you do—and that those views may be just as valid and important to your partner as your own views are to you.

Balancing Time Spent Together and Apart   You may enjoy time together with your partner but you may also want to spend time alone or with other friends. If time apart is interpreted as rejection or lack of commitment, it can damage a relationship. It's important to talk with your partner about what time apart means and to share your feelings about what you expect from the relationship in terms of time together. Consider your partner's feelings carefully, and try to reach a compromise that satisfies both of you.

Differences in expectations about time spent together can mirror differences in ideas about emotional closeness. Any romantic relationship involves giving up some degree of autonomy in order to develop an identity as a couple. It's important to remember that every individual is unique and has different needs for distance and closeness in a relationship. As described earlier in the chapter, attachment styles developed early in life can affect people's level of comfort in close relationships. In addition, traditional gender roles tend to teach women to be caretakers of relationships and men to be independent and self-reliant.

Jealousy   Jealousy is the angry, painful response to a partner's real, imagined, or likely involvement with a third person. Some people think that the existence of jealousy proves the existence of love, but jealousy is actually a more accurate yardstick for measuring insecurity or possessiveness. In its irrational and extreme forms, jealousy can destroy a relationship by its insistent demands and attempts at control. Jealousy is a factor in precipitating violence in dating relationships among both high school and college students, and abusive spouses often use jealousy to justify their violence. (Problems with control and violence in relationships are discusssed in Chapter 23.) People with a healthy level of self-esteem are less likely to feel jealous. When jealousy occurs in a relationship, it's important for the partners to communicate clearly with each other about their feelings.

Successful Relationships

A true intimate relationship is characterized by a conscious sense of connectedness to another person. It emerges after a period of deep sharing, and it reflects a warm, caring, and trusting concern between partners. Successful relationships result in a heightened sense of self-worth for both partners.

What steps can you take to build a successful relationship? To meet the relationship challenges described in this section, good communication and conflict-resolution skills are critical. You need to be able to communicate your needs and wants clearly, listen to your partner, negotiate, and compromise. These skills are described in detail in the next section of the chapter.

Another key to successful relationships is the ability to ask for and give support. Partners need to know that they can count on each other during difficult times. If you are having trouble getting or giving the support that you or your partner needs, try some of the suggestions in the box "Strategies for Enhancing Support in Relationships."

Ending a Relationship

Even when a couple starts out with the best of intentions, an intimate relationship may not last. The couple may have been mismatched to begin with, or the relationship may have failed to thrive and the partners then turned elsewhere for satisfaction. Some breakups occur quickly following direct action by one or both partners, but many others occur over an extended period during which partners repeatedly consider both breaking up and reconciling.

Ending an intimate relationship is usually difficult and painful. Both partners may feel attacked and abandoned, but feelings of distress are likely to be more acute for the rejected partner. If you are involved in a breakup, following these guidelines may help make the ending easier:

- *Give the relationship a fair chance before breaking up.* If it's still not working, you'll know you did everything you could.

- *Be aware of the importance of support.* Time and energy spent on support will help both you and your partner deal with stress and create a positive atmosphere that will help when differences or conflicts do occur.

- *Learn to ask for help from your partner.* Try different ways of asking for help and support from your partner and make note of which approaches work best for your relationship.

- *Help your partner the way she or he would like to be helped.* Some people prefer empathy and emotional support, while others like more practical help with problems.

- *Avoid negativity, especially when being asked for help.* Asking for help puts a person in a vulnerable position. If your partner asks for your aid, be gracious and supportive; don't use phrases like "I told you so" or "You should have just . . ." Otherwise, your partner may learn not to ask for your help or support at all.

- *Make positive attributions.* If you're unsure about the reasons for your partner's behavior, give her or him the benefit of the doubt. For example, if your partner arrives for a date 30 minutes late and in a bad mood, assume it's because she or he had a bad day rather than attributing it to a character flaw or relationship problem. Offer appropriate support.

- *Help yourself.* Develop coping strategies for times your partner won't be available. These might include things you can do for yourself, such as going for a walk, or other people you can turn to for support.

- *Keep relationship problems separate.* Avoid bringing up relationship problems when you are offering or asking for help.

- *Avoid giving advice.* Immediately offering advice when asked for help implies that you are smarter or more capable than your partner at solving your partner's difficulty. Begin by providing emotional support and validating your partner's feelings. Then, if asked, help brainstorm solutions.

SOURCE: Plante, T., and K. Sullivan. 2000. *Getting Together and Staying Together: The Stanford Course on Intimate Relationships.* Bloomington, Ind.: 1stBooks Library.

- *Be fair and honest.* If you're the one initiating the breakup, don't try to make your partner feel responsible.

- *Be tactful and compassionate.* You can leave the relationship without deliberately damaging your partner's self-esteem. Emphasize your mutual incompatibility, and admit your own contributions to the problem.

- *If you are the rejected person, give yourself time to resolve your anger and pain.* Mobilize your coping resources, including social support and other stress-management techniques. You may go through a process of mourning the relationship, experiencing disbelief, anger, sadness, and finally acceptance. Remember that there are actually many people with whom you can potentially have an intimate relationship.

- *Recognize the value in the experience.* You honor the feelings that you shared with your partner by validating the relationship as a worthwhile experience. Ending a close relationship can teach you valuable lessons about your needs, preferences, strengths, and weaknesses. Use your insights to increase your chance of success in your next relationship.

Use the recovery period following a breakup for self-renewal. Redirect more of your attention to yourself, and reconnect with people and areas of your life that may have been neglected as a result of the relationship. Time will help heal the pain of the loss of the relationship.

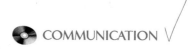

COMMUNICATION

The key to developing and maintaining any type of intimate relationship is good communication. Most of the time, we don't actually think about communicating; we simply talk and behave naturally. But when problems arise—when we feel others don't understand us or when someone accuses us of not listening—we become aware of our limitations or, more commonly, what we think are other people's limitations. Miscommunication creates frustration and distances us from our friends and partners.

Nonverbal Communication

As much as 65% of face-to-face communication is nonverbal. Even when we're silent, we're communicating. We send messages when we look at someone or look away, lean forward or sit back, smile or frown. Especially important forms of nonverbal communication are touch, eye contact, and proximity. If someone we're talking to touches our hand or arm, looks into our eyes, and leans toward us when we talk, we get the message that the person is interested in us and cares about what we're saying. If a person keeps looking around the room while we're talking or takes a step backward, we get the impression the person is uninterested or wants to end the conversation.

The ability to interpret nonverbal messages correctly is important to the success of relationships. It's also important, when sending messages, to make sure our body language agrees with our words. When our verbal and nonverbal messages don't correspond, we send a mixed message.

Communication Skills

Three keys to good communication in relationships are self-disclosure, listening, and feedback.

• *Self-disclosure* involves revealing personal information that we ordinarily wouldn't reveal because of the risk involved. It usually increases feelings of closeness and moves the relationship to a deeper level of intimacy. Friends often disclose the most to each other, sharing feelings, experiences, hopes, and disappointments; married couples sometimes share less because they think they already know everything there is to know about each other.

• *Listening,* the second component of good communication, is a rare skill. Good listening skills require that we spend more time and energy trying to fully understand another person's "story" and less time judging, evaluating, blaming, advising, analyzing, or trying to control. Empathy, warmth, respect, and genuineness are qualities of skillful listeners. Attentive listening encourages friends or partners to share more and, in turn, to be attentive listeners. To connect with other people and develop real emotional intimacy, listening is essential.

• *Feedback,* a constructive response to another's self-disclosure, is the third key to good communication. Giving positive feedback means acknowledging that the friend's or partner's feelings are valid—no matter how upsetting or troubling—and offering self-disclosure in response. If, for example, your partner discloses unhappiness about your relationship, it is more constructive to say that you're concerned or saddened by that and want to hear more about it than to get angry, to blame, to try to inflict pain, or to withdraw. Self-disclosure and feedback can open the door to change, whereas other responses block communication and change. (For tips on improving your skills, see the box "Guidelines for Effective Communication".)

Gender and Communication

Some of the difficulties people encounter in relationships can be traced to common gender differences in communication. Many authorities believe that, because of the way they've been raised, men and women generally approach conversation and communication differently. According to this view, men tend to use conversation in a competitive way, perhaps hoping to establish dominance in relationships. When male conversations are over, men often find themselves in a one-up or a one-down position. Women tend to use conversation in a more *affiliative* way, perhaps hoping to establish friendships. They negotiate various degrees of closeness, seeking to give and receive support. Men tend to talk more—though without disclosing more—and listen less. Women tend to use good listening skills like eye contact, frequent nodding, focused attention, and asking relevant questions.

Although these are generalized patterns, they can translate into problems in specific conversations. Even when a man and a woman are talking about the same subject, their unconscious goals may be very different. The woman may be looking for understanding and closeness, while the man may be trying to demonstrate his competence by giving advice and solving problems. Both styles are valid; the problem comes when differences in styles result in poor communication and misunderstanding.

Sometimes communication is not the problem in a relationship—the partners understand each other all too well. The problem is that they're unable or unwilling to change or compromise. Although good communication can't salvage a bad relationship, it does enable couples to see their differences and make more informed decisions.

Conflict and Conflict Resolution

Conflict is natural in intimate relationships. No matter how close two people become, they still remain separate individuals with their own needs, desires, past experiences, and ways of seeing the world. In fact, the closer the relationship, the more differences and the more opportunities for conflict there will be. Conflict itself isn't dangerous to a relationship; it may simply indicate that the relationship is growing. But if it isn't handled in a constructive way, it will damage—and ultimately destroy—the relationship.

Conflict is often accompanied by anger—a natural emotion, but one that can be difficult to handle. If we express anger, we run the risk of creating distrust, fear, and distance; if we act it out without thinking things through, we can cause the conflict to escalate; if we suppress it, it turns into resentment and hostility. The best way to handle anger in a relationship is to recognize it as a symptom of something that requires attention and needs to be changed. When angry, partners should back off until they calm down and then come back to the issue later and try to resolve it rationally. Negotiation will help dissipate the anger so the conflict can be resolved.

Although the sources of conflict for couples change over time, they primarily revolve around the basic tasks of living together: dividing the housework, handling money, spending time together, and so on. Sexual interaction is also a source of disagreement for many couples.

Although there are numerous theories on and approaches to conflict resolution, some basic strategies are generally useful in successfully negotiating with a partner:

1. *Clarify the issue.* Take responsibility for thinking through your feelings and discovering what's really bothering you. Agree that one partner will speak first and have the chance to speak fully while the other listens.

Getting Started

- When you want to have a serious discussion with your partner, find an appropriate time and place. Choose a block of time when you will not be interrupted or rushed and a place that is private.

- Face your partner and maintain eye contact. Use nonverbal feedback to show that you are interested and involved in the communication process.

Being an Effective Speaker

- State your concern or issue as clearly as you can.

- Use "I" statements—statements about how *you* feel—rather than statements beginning with "You," which tell another person how you think he or she feels. When you use "I" statements, you are taking responsibility for your feelings. "You" statements are often blaming or accusatory and will probably get a defensive or resentful response. The statement "I feel unloved," for example, sends a clearer, less blaming message than the statement "You don't love me."

- Focus on a specific behavior rather than on the whole person. Be specific about the behavior you like or don't like. Avoid generalizations beginning with "You always" or "You never." Such statements make people feel defensive.

- Make constructive requests. Opening your request with "I would like" keeps the focus on your needs rather than your partner's supposed deficiencies.

- Avoid blaming, accusing, and belittling. Even if you are right, you have little to gain by putting your partner down. Studies have shown that when people feel criticized or attacked, they are less able to think rationally or solve problems constructively.

- Ask for action ahead of time, not after the fact. Tell your partner what you would like to have happen in the future; don't wait for him or her to blow it and then express anger or disappointment.

Being an Effective Listener

- Provide appropriate nonverbal feedback (nodding, smiling, making eye contact, and so on).

- Don't interrupt.

- Develop the skill of reflective listening. Don't judge, evaluate, analyze, or offer solutions (unless asked to do so). Your partner may just need to have you there in order to sort out feelings. By jumping in right away to "fix" the problem, you may actually be cutting off communication.

- Don't give unsolicited advice. Giving advice implies that you know more about what a person needs to do than he or she does; therefore, it often evokes anger or resentment.

- Clarify your understanding of what your partner is saying by restating it in your own words and asking if your understanding is correct. "I think you're saying that you would feel uncomfortable having dinner with my parents and that you'd prefer to meet them in a more casual setting. Is that right?" This type of specific feedback prevents misunderstandings and helps validate the speaker's feelings and message.

- Be sure you are really listening, not off somewhere in your mind rehearsing your reply. Try to tune in to your partner's feelings as well as the words.

- Let your partner know that you value what he or she is saying and want to understand. Respect for the other person is the cornerstone of effective communication.

Then reverse the roles. Try to understand the other partner's position fully by repeating what you've heard and asking questions to clarify or elicit more information. Agree to talk only about the topic at hand and not get distracted by other issues. Sum up what your partner has said.

2. *Find out what each person wants.* Ask your partner to express his or her desires. Don't assume you know what your partner wants and speak for him or her. Clarify and summarize.

3. *Identify various alternatives for getting each person what he or she wants.* Practice brainstorming to generate a variety of options.

4. *Decide how to negotiate.* Work out some agreements or plans for change; for example, one partner will do one task and the other will do another task, or one partner will do a task in exchange for something he or she wants. Be willing to compromise, and avoid trying to "win." Find a solution that satisfies both partners.

5. *Solidify the agreements.* Go over the plan verbally and write it down, if necessary, to ensure that you both understand and agree to it.

6. *Review and renegotiate.* Decide on a time frame for trying out the new plan, and set a time to discuss how it's working. Make adjustments as needed.

To resolve conflicts, partners have to feel safe in voicing disagreements. They have to trust that the discussion won't get out of control, that they won't be abandoned by the other, and that the partner won't take advantage of their vulnerability. Partners should follow some basic ground rules when they argue, such as avoiding ultimatums, resisting the urge to give the silent treatment, refusing to "hit below the belt," and not using sex to smooth over disagreements.

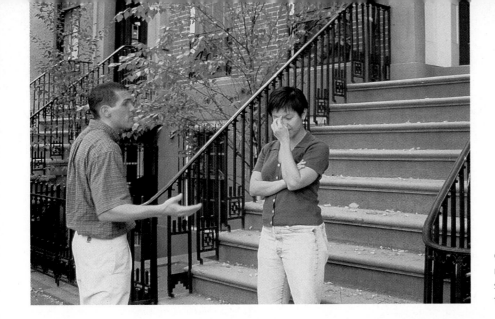

Conflict is an inevitable part of any intimate relationship. Couples need to develop constructive ways of resolving conflicts in order to maintain a healthy relationship.

When you do argue, maintain a spirit of good will and avoid being harshly critical or contemptuous. Remember—you care about your partner and want things to work out. See the disagreement as a difficulty that the two of you have together rather than as something your partner does to you. Finish any serious discussions on a positive note by expressing your respect and affection for your partner and your appreciation for having been listened to. If you and your partner find that you argue again and again over the same issue, it may be better to stop trying to resolve that problem and instead come to accept the differences between you.

> **COMMUNICATE!** A key strategy for effective communication is to use "I" statements that describe how you feel rather than "you" statements to describe how you think another person is acting or feeling. Try thinking of three "you" statements that you would like to make to someone you know, and then translate each one into an "I" statement. For example, "You never do anything to clean up the apartment" could be changed to "I get irritated when I realize that I've been doing most of the housework around the apartment. I'd like to talk about setting up a schedule for sharing the chores." Once you become familiar with "I" statements, try substituting them for "you" statements.

PAIRING AND SINGLEHOOD

Although most people eventually marry, everyone spends some time as a single person, and nearly all make some attempt, consciously or unconsciously, to find a partner. Intimate relationships are as important for singles as for couples.

Choosing a Partner

Most men and women select partners for long-term relationships through a fairly predictable process, although they may not be consciously aware of it. Most people pair with someone who lives in the same geographic area and who is similar in ethnic and socioeconomic background, educational level, lifestyle, physical attractiveness, and other traits. In simple terms, people select partners like themselves.

First attraction is based on easily observable characteristics: looks, dress, social status, and reciprocated interest. Once the euphoria of romantic love winds down, personality traits and behaviors become more significant factors in how the partners view each other. Through sharing and self-disclosure, they gradually gain a deeper knowledge of each other. The emphasis shifts to basic values, such as religious beliefs, political affiliation, sexual attitudes, and future aspirations regarding career, family, and children. At some point, they decide whether the relationship feels viable and is worthy of their continued commitment. If they are compatible, many people gradually discover deeper, more enduring forms of love.

Perhaps the most important question for potential mates is, How much do we have in common? Although differences add interest to a relationship, similarities increase the chances of a relationship's success. If there are major differences, partners should first ask, How accepting of differences are we? Then, How well do we communicate? Acceptance and communication skills go a long way toward making a relationship work, no matter how different the partners. Areas in which differences can affect the relationship include values, religion, ethnicity, attitudes toward sexuality and gender roles, socioeconomic status, familiarity with the other's culture, and interactions

Today more than ever we have opportunities to make friends with people from other ethnic groups and cultures. Yet how many of us are encouraged to reach out to those who are different from ourselves? Probably not many. Studies confirm that many families continue to instill negative attitudes toward people of other cultures and ethnicities. For this reason and others, friendships and intimate relationships with people different from ourselves can pose challenges. Yet once these challenges are overcome, these relationships can be mutually fulfilling.

What makes intercultural relationships more challenging? You and a friend from a different cultural background may find that you differ in how you communicate, what you value, and how you view the world. You may encounter disapproval about your relationship from friends and family. And because of these obstacles, you may experience more anxiety during the early stages of your relationship than you would with a friend from a similar cultural heritage.

Intimate partners with different cultural backgrounds may find that their relationship requires special effort to maintain. They bring two unique worlds to their partnership, and for their relationship to last, they must make room for both of these

worlds. Communication is particularly important—and challenging. Many interethnic couples say that they must explain themselves more frequently, both to each other and to their respective families and communities. If family response to the relationship is negative, an intercultural couple will need to develop their own social support network.

Despite these challenges, increasing numbers of people are establishing friendships and intimate relationships with people outside their own ethnic and cultural heritage. If you develop such a relationship, you and your friend or partner will probably find that it has many special benefits:

- You will get a chance to learn about each other's worlds and unique experiences. You may acquire new skills and information.

- You will build a strong relationship based not only on your similarities but also on your differences.

- You will learn respect, tolerance, and acceptance for people who are different from yourself—key steps in breaking down stereotypes of all kinds.

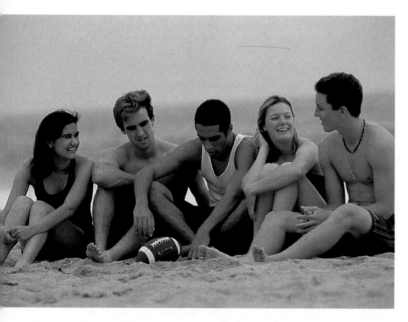

For many college students today, group activities have replaced dating as a way to meet and get to know potential partners.

with the extended family (see the box "Intercultural Friendships and Intimate Relationships").

Dating

Every culture has certain rituals for pairing and finding mates. Parent-arranged marriages, still the norm in many

cultures, are often very stable and permanent. Although the American cultural norm is personal choice in courtship and mate selection, the popularity of dating services (complete with personality tests and videotapes of prospects) and online matchmaking suggests that many people do want help finding a suitable partner (see the box "Online Relationships").

Most Americans—whether single, divorced, or widowed, heterosexual or gay, younger or older—find romantic partners through some form of dating. They narrow the field through a process of getting to know each other. Dating often revolves around a mutually enjoyable activity, such as seeing a movie or having dinner. In the traditional male-female dating pattern, the man takes the lead, initiating the date, while the woman waits to be called. In this pattern, casual dating might evolve into steady or exclusive dating, then engagement, and finally marriage.

For many young people today, traditional dating has given way to a more casual form of getting together in groups. Greater equality between the sexes is at the root of this change. Rather than strictly as couples, people go out in groups, and each person pays his or her way. A man and woman may begin to spend more time together, but often in the group context. If sexual involvement develops, it is more likely to be based on friendship, respect, and common interests than on expectations related to gender roles. In this model, mate selection may progress from getting together to living together to marriage.

More and more, people are looking to the Internet to find friends and partners. Communications with others in cyberspace can enable people to be themselves in a relaxed atmosphere, to try out other personas, and to confide in others in a private way. The Internet can also serve as "training wheels" for those who wish to develop their social skills.

The Internet is a good tool for locating people who share your hobbies and interests—whether that's Volkswagens, Sherlock Holmes mysteries, or baseball. You may or may not end up visiting a new contact in person, but if your goal is to communicate with someone about a common interest, e-mail, newsgroups, listservs, and chat rooms are all good options. (Refer to Appendix C for some basic guidelines about finding and using these Internet resources.)

People looking for intimate partners are also using the Internet. By getting to know someone online, you can make that "first impression" in the comfort of your living room. In online relationships, people will respond to you based on who you are rather than on your appearance. And with more than 100 million users of the World Wide Web in the United States alone, you have many more people to interact with than on your campus or in your neighborhood.

There are drawbacks to meeting partners online, however. People can misrepresent themselves, pretending to be very different—older or younger or even of a different sex—than they really are. Investing time and emotional resources in an unrealistic romance can be painful. There have also been a few in-

stances in which online romances have become dangerous or even deadly. (see Chapter 23 for information on cyberstalking). If you decide to meet someone in person whom you have previously met only online, here are some strategies that can help keep you safe:

- To increase your chances of meeting people interested in you as a person, avoid sexually oriented Internet sites.

- Until you know much more about a cyberfriend, don't give out personal information, including your real full name, school, or place of employment.

- Schedule a phone conversation or a series of phone conversations before deciding whether or not to meet an online friend in person.

- Don't agree to meet someone face to face unless you feel completely comfortable about it. Always meet initially in a very public place—a museum, a coffee shop, a restaurant. Bring along a friend to further increase your safety.

Finally, take care that your pursuit of online relationships does not interfere with your other interpersonal relationships and social activities. As described in Chapter 3, researchers have found that extensive use of the Internet is associated with greater loneliness, less communication with family members, and fewer social contacts. To maximize your emotional and interpersonal wellness, use the Internet to widen your circle of friends, not shrink it.

COMMUNICATE!   College offers many opportunities to expand your social network. If you're shy about meeting new people, work out in advance what you will say. The next time you want to strike up a conversation with a new acquaintance, try starting out by introducing yourself. Mention the physical context of the conversation, such as the location, weather, or ongoing event. Ask questions that will engage the other person, such as "Is this the first art history class you've taken?" or "Have you been to a lot of basketball games this season?"

Living Together

According to the U.S. Bureau of the Census, over 4 million heterosexual couples and an estimated 1.5 million gay and lesbian couples are currently living together. Living together, or **cohabitation,** is one of the most rapid and dramatic social changes that has ever occurred in our society. It seems to be gaining acceptance as part of the normal mate selection process. By age 30, about half of all men and women will have cohabited. The only thing separating those who cohabit from those who don't is reli-

gion. Several factors are involved in this change, including greater acceptance of premarital sex, increased availability of contraceptives, the tendency for people to wait longer before getting married, and a larger pool of single and divorced individuals.

Cohabitation is more popular among younger people than older, although a significant number of older couples live together without marrying to avoid losing a source of income, such as Social Security benefits, if they were to marry. Living together provides many of the benefits of marriage: companionship; a setting for an enjoyable and meaningful relationship; the opportunity to develop greater intimacy through learning, compromising, and sharing; a satisfying sex life; and a way to save on living costs.

Living together has certain advantages over marriage. For one thing, it can give the partners a greater sense of autonomy. Not bound by the social rules and expectations

---

cohabitation Living together in a sexual relationship without being married.

Terms

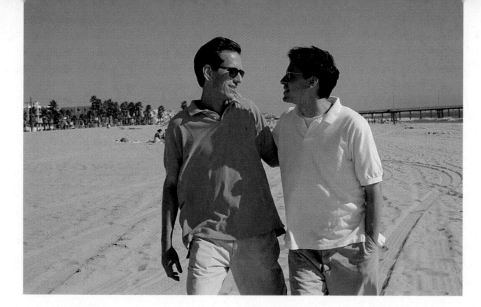

Greater openness has made gay men and lesbians more visible than they used to be, although they still constitute a minority of the population. Most gay men and lesbians have experienced at least one long-term relationship with a single partner.

that are part of the institution of marriage, partners may find it easier to keep their identity and more of their independence. Cohabitation doesn't incur the same obligations as marriage. If things don't work out, the partners may find it easier to leave a relationship that hasn't been legally sanctioned.

But living together has some liabilities, too. In most cases, the legal protections of marriage are absent, such as health insurance benefits and property and inheritance rights. These considerations can be particularly serious if the couple has children, from either former relationships or the current partnership. Since social acceptance of cohabitation is not universal, couples may feel family pressure to marry or otherwise change their living arrangements, especially if they have young children. The general trend, however, is toward legitimizing nonmarital partnerships; for example, some employers and communities now extend benefits to unmarried domestic partners.

Although many people choose cohabitation as a kind of trial marriage, unmarried partnerships tend to be less stable than marriages. In a survey of women age 15 to 44 who had cohabited, fewer than half were still living—married (37%) or unmarried (10%)—with their first live-in partner; 34% had dissolved the relationship prior to marriage, and 21% had married and then divorced their partner. There is little evidence that cohabitation before marriage leads to happier or longer-

lasting marriages; in fact, some studies have found slightly less marital satisfaction among couples who had previously cohabited. Researchers speculate that people who have cohabited might have higher expectations for marriage or might be less likely to adapt well to traditional marital roles.

Gay and Lesbian Partnerships

Regardless of **sexual orientation,** most people look for love in a close, satisfying, committed relationship. Gay and lesbian, or **homosexual,** couples have many similarities with **heterosexual** couples. According to one study, most gay men and lesbians have experienced at least one long-term relationship with a single partner. Like heterosexual relationships, gay and lesbian partnerships provide intimacy, passion, and security.

One difference between heterosexual and homosexual couples is that gay and lesbian couples tend to adopt "best friend" roles in their relationship rather than traditional gender roles. Domestic tasks are shared or split, and both partners usually support themselves financially. Another difference is that gay and lesbian couples often have to deal with societal hostility or ambivalence toward their relationships—in contrast to the social approval given to heterosexual couples (see the box "Same-Sex Marriage and Civil Unions). Consequently, community may be more important as a source of identity and social support than it is for heterosexuals.

Singlehood

Despite the prevalence and popularity of marriage, a significant proportion of adults in our society are unmarried—more than 90 million individuals. They are a diverse group, encompassing young people who have not married yet but plan to in the future, people who are living together (gay or heterosexual), divorced and widowed people, and those who would like to marry but haven't

Terms   **sexual orientation** A consistent pattern of emotional and sexual attraction based on biological sex; it exists along a continuum that ranges from exclusive heterosexuality (attraction to people of the other sex) through bisexuality (attraction to people of both sexes) to exclusive homosexuality (attraction to people of one's own sex).

homosexual Emotional and sexual attraction to people of one's own sex.

heterosexual Emotional and sexual attraction to people of the other sex.

On July 1, 2000, Vermont became the first state to offer the option of "civil union" to people for whom legal marriage is not an option. This was the date a law went into effect as a result of a Vermont Supreme Court ruling that same-sex couples were entitled to the same benefits and protections given to married couples, including rights relating to medical decisions and health care; parenting, child custody, and child support; inheritance; state income taxes; and other issues.

A civil union is a legal status parallel to civil marriage (the Vermont legislature decided not to use the word *marriage* for these unions), and for the purposes of Vermont law, civil union spouses are treated as legally married. Same-sex couples from other states may travel to Vermont to enter civil unions, but their status back in their home states is unclear. In fact, more than 30 states have enacted "defense of marriage acts" (DOMAs), which attempt to deny the validity of same-sex unions by defining marriage as a union between a man and a woman. There is also a federal DOMA, signed by President Clinton in 1996, which denies to same-sex couples the 1,049 federal benefits of marriage, including federal tax status, Social Security, survivor and pension benefits, and immigration rights. The federal DOMA also allows states to ignore same-sex marriages that may be legitimized by other states. Such action might otherwise be in violation of the U.S. Constitution's provision that each state will give "full faith and credit" to the laws of other states. (Currently the Netherlands is the only country to offer *marriage* and its associated legal benefits to same-sex partners; it began recognizing such unions in April 2001.)

What cases are made for and against civil union and same-sex marriage? Opponents put forth numerous arguments, including that the purpose of marriage is to procreate, that the Bible forbids same-sex unions, that homosexuals are seeking special rights, and that the majority of the population opposes such unions. The primary argument, however, is that same-sex marriage undermines the sanctity and validity of marriage as it is traditionally understood and thus undermines society. Rules and restrictions on who can marry preserve the value of the institution of marriage, according to this view. The underlying assumption of this position is that homosexual behavior is a choice and that people can change their orientation, though the process is difficult.

Proponents of civil union and same-sex marriage believe that homosexuality is outside the control of the individual and results from genetic and environmental factors that create an unchangeable orientation by adolescence or adulthood. The issue of same-sex union is then seen as one of basic civil rights, in which a group is being denied rights on the basis of something as unalterable as skin color. To the argument that marriage has a traditional meaning in our society, proponents respond that, on the contrary, marriage is an evolving institution that changes as society changes. Prior to 1967, marriage between whites and African Americans was prohibited in the United States; before the Civil War, African Americans were not allowed to marry at all. A generation ago, proponents go on, women's rights were restricted, gender roles were rigid, and divorce was rare. Today, most committed couples live together before getting married, many women have children outside of marriage, many families are headed by a single parent, and two-career couples who choose not to have children at all are increasingly common. These and other trends, according to this view, are leading people to broaden their definition of marriage and to see same-sex marriage as just another variation.

Both opponents and proponents point out that marriage is healthy for both men and women and is the main social institution promoting family values; both sides see this assertion as supportive of their position. What remains to be seen is how society in general is going to view same-sex marriage in the future—as a furthering of American values or as an attack on them.

found a mate. The category includes people who are single both by choice and by chance. The largest group of unmarried adults has never been married (Figure 4-2).

Several factors contribute to the growing number of single people. One is the changing view of singlehood, which is increasingly being viewed as a legitimate alternative to marriage. Education and career are delaying the age at which young people are marrying. The median age for marriage is now 26.8 years for men and 25.0 years for women. More young people are living with their parents as they complete their education, seek jobs, or strive for financial independence. Many other single people live together without being married. Gay people who would marry their partners if they were legally permitted to do so are counted among the single population. High divorce rates mean more singles, and people who have experienced divorce in their families may have more negative attitudes about marriage and more positive attitudes about singlehood.

Being single doesn't mean not having close relationships, however. Single people may date, enjoy active and fulfilling social lives, and have a variety of sexual experiences and relationships. Other advantages of being single include more opportunities for personal and career development without concern for family obligations and more freedom and control in making life choices. Disadvantages include loneliness and a lack of companionship, as well as economic hardships (mainly for single women). Single men and women both experience some discrimination and often are pressured to get married.

Nearly everyone has at least one episode of being single in adult life, whether prior to marriage, between marriages, following divorce or the death of a spouse, or for the entire adult life span. How enjoyable and valuable this single time is depends on several factors, including how deliberately the person has chosen it; how satisfied the person is with social relationships, standard of living, and

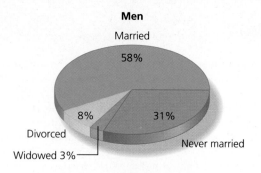

Men

Married
58%

Divorced
8%

Never married
31%

Widowed 3%

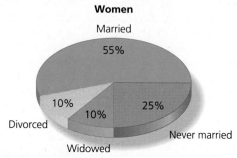

Women

Married
55%

Divorced
10%

Widowed
10%

Never married
25%

Figure 4-2   Marital status of the U.S. population age 15 years and older.   SOURCE: U.S. Bureau of the Census. 1999. *Marital Status of the Population 15 Years Old and Over, by Sex and Race: 1950 to Present* (http://www.census.gov/population/socdemo/ms-la/tabms-1.txt; retrieved January 24, 2001).

job; how comfortable the person feels when alone; and how resourceful and energetic the person is about creating an interesting and fulfilling life.

MARRIAGE

About 95% of all Americans marry at some time in their lives. Marriage continues to remain popular because it satisfies several basic needs. There are many important social, moral, economic, and political aspects of marriage, all of which have changed over the years. In the past, people married mainly for practical reasons, such as raising children or forming an economic unit. Today, people marry more for personal, emotional reasons. This shift places a greater burden on marriage to fulfill certain expectations that are sometimes unreasonably high. People may assume that all their emotional needs will be met by their partner; they may think that fascination and passion will always remain at high levels; they may simply expect to "live happily ever after." When people enter marriage with such preconceptions, it may be harder for them to appreciate the benefits that marriage really offers.

Benefits of Marriage

The primary functions and benefits of marriage are those of any intimate relationship: affection, personal affirma-

tion, companionship, sexual fulfillment, emotional growth. Marriage also provides a setting in which to raise children, although an increasing number of couples choose to remain childless, and people can also choose to raise children without being married. Marriage is also important for providing for the future. By committing themselves to the relationship, people establish themselves with lifelong companions as well as some insurance for their later years (see the box "Intimate Relationships Are Good for Your Health").

Issues in Marriage

Although we might like to believe otherwise, love is not enough to make a successful marriage. Couples have to be strong and successful in their relationship before getting married, because relationship problems will be magnified rather than solved by marriage. The following relationship characteristics appear to be the best predictors of a happy marriage:

- The partners have realistic expectations about their relationship.
- Each feels good about the personality of the other.
- They communicate well.
- They have effective ways of resolving conflicts.
- They agree on religious/ethical values.
- They have an egalitarian role relationship.
- They have a good balance of individual versus joint interests and leisure activities.

Once married, couples must face many adjustment tasks. In addition to providing each other with emotional support, they have to negotiate and establish marital roles, establish domestic and career priorities, manage their finances, make sexual adjustments, manage boundaries and relationships with their extended family, and participate in the larger community.

Marital roles and responsibilities have undergone profound changes in recent years. Many couples no longer accept traditional role assumptions, such as that the husband is solely responsible for supporting the family and the wife is solely responsible for domestic work. Today, many husbands share domestic tasks and many wives work outside the home. In fact, over 50% of married women are in the labor force, including women with babies under 1 year of age. Although women still take most of the responsibility for home and children even when they work and although men still suffer more job-related stress and health problems than women do, the trend is toward an equalization of responsibilities.

The Role of Commitment

Coping with all these challenges requires that couples be committed to remaining in the relationship through its inevitable ups and downs. They will need to be tolerant of

Research studies consistently underscore the importance of strengthening your family and social ties to help maintain emotional and physical wellness. Living alone, or simply feeling alone, can have a negative effect on both your state of mind and your physical health. Married people, on average, live longer than unmarried people—whether single, divorced, or widowed—and they score higher on measures of mental health. Findings suggest that there is something intrinsically beneficial about the long-term commitment that marriage represents.

People with strong social ties are less likely to become ill and tend to recover more quickly if they do. The benefits of intimate relationships have been demonstrated for a range of conditions: People with strong social support are less likely to catch colds. They recover better from heart attacks and live longer with heart disease. Among men with prostate cancer, those who are married live significantly longer than those who are single, divorced, or widowed; women with breast cancer live longer if they participate in a support group.

What is it about social relationships that supports wellness? Friends and partners may encourage and reinforce healthy habits, such as exercising, eating right, and seeing a physician when needed. In times of illness, a loving partner can provide both practical help and emotional support. Feeling loved, esteemed, and valued brings comfort at a time of vulnerability, reduces anxiety, and mitigates the damaging effects of stress.

Although good relationships may help the sick get better, bad relationships may have the opposite effect. The impact of relationship quality on the course of illness may be partly explained by effects on the immune system: A study of married couples whose fighting went beyond normal conflict and into criticism and name-calling found them to have weaker immune responses than couples whose arguments were more civil. (The immune effects were particularly strong among the wives, leading some researchers to postulate that women may be more aware of and affected by relationship problems.)

Marriage, of course, isn't the only support system available. Whether married or single, if you have supportive people in your life, you are likely to enjoy better physical and emotional health than if you feel isolated and alone. So when you start planning lifestyle changes to improve your health and well-being, don't forget to nurture your relationships with family and friends. Relationships are powerful medicine.

---

each other's imperfections and keep their perspective and sense of humor. Commitment is based on conscious choice rather than on feelings, which, by their very nature, are transitory. Commitment is a promise of a shared future, a promise to be together, come what may. Committed partners put effort and energy into the relationship, no matter how they feel. They take time to attend to their partner, give compliments, and face conflict when necessary.

Commitment has become an important concept in recent years. We talk about people who are afraid of commitment or of "making a commitment" to a person or a relationship. To many people, commitment is a more important goal than living together or marriage.

Separation and Divorce

People marrying today have a 50–55% chance of divorcing. The high rate of divorce in the United States reflects our extremely high expectations for emotional fulfillment and satisfaction in marriage. It also indicates that we no longer believe in the permanence of marriage.

The process of divorce usually begins with an emotional separation. Often one partner is unhappy and looks beyond the relationship for other forms of validation. Dissatisfaction increases until the unhappy partner decides he or she can no longer stay. Physical separation follows, although it may take some time for the relationship to be over emotionally.

Except for the death of a spouse or family member, divorce is the greatest stress-producing event in life. Both men and women experience turmoil, depression, and lowered self-esteem during and after divorce. People experience separation distress and loneliness for about a year and then begin a recovery period of 1–3 years. During this time they gradually construct a postdivorce identity, along with a new pattern of life. Most people are surprised by how long it takes to recover from divorce. Children are especially vulnerable to the trauma of divorce, and sometimes counseling is appropriate to help them adjust to the changes in their lives.

Despite the distress of separation and divorce, the negative effects are usually balanced sooner or later by the possibility of finding a more suitable partner, constructing a new life, and developing new aspects of the self. About 75% of all people who divorce remarry, often within 5 years. One result of the high divorce and remarriage rate is a growing number of stepfamilies (discussed in the next section).

WWW. FAMILY LIFE

American families are very different today than they were even a few decades ago. Currently, about half of all families are based on a first marriage; almost one-third are headed by a single parent; the remainder are remarriages or involve some other arrangement. Despite the tremendous variation apparent in American families, certain patterns can still be discerned.

For many young adults, the family life cycle begins with marriage. This first stage, when newlyweds are learning how to live together, ends abruptly when they have a baby. New parents have a new set of responsibilities, and their roles change profoundly and irreversibly: no more spontaneous outings to see a movie or leisurely Sunday mornings sipping coffee and browsing through the newspaper. The third member of the family, the new infant, demands around-the-clock attention.

Becoming a Parent

Few new parents have any preparation for the job of parenting, yet they have to assume that role literally overnight. They have to learn quickly how to hold a baby, how to change it, how to feed it, how to interpret its cries. No wonder the birth of the first child is one of the most stressful transitions for any couple.

Even couples with an egalitarian relationship before their first child is born find that their marital roles become more traditional with the arrival of the new baby. The father becomes the principal provider and protector, and the mother becomes the primary nurturer. Most research indicates that mothers have to make greater changes in their lives than fathers do. Although men today spend more time caring for their infants than ever before, women still take the ultimate responsibility for seeing that the baby is fed, clean, and comfortable. In addition, women are usually the ones who make job changes; they may quit working or reduce their hours in order to stay home with the baby for several months or more, or they may try to juggle the multiple roles of mother, homemaker, and employee and feel guilty that they never have enough time to do justice to any of these roles.

Not surprisingly, marital satisfaction often declines after the birth of the first child. The wife who has stopped working may feel she is cut off from the world; the wife who is trying to fulfill duties both at home and on the job may feel overburdened and resentful. The husband may have a hard time adjusting to having to share his wife's love and attention with the baby.

But marital dissatisfaction after the baby is born is not inevitable. Couples who successfully weather the stresses of a new baby seem to have these three characteristics in common:

1. They had developed a strong relationship before the baby was born.

2. They had planned to have the child and want it very much.

3. They communicate well about their feelings and expectations.

Parenting and the Family Life Cycle

Sometimes being a parent is a source of unparalleled pleasure and pride—the first smile (at you), the first word, the first home run. But at other times, parenting can seem like an overwhelming responsibility. How can you be sure you're not making some mistake that will stunt your child's physical, psychological, or emotional growth?

There is really no "right" way to raise children to ensure that they become healthy and happy. Of course, parents must provide for basic physical needs, such as food, shelter, clothing, and medical care. They must also help children develop a positive self-concept, as discussed earlier. But how do parents know how to best accomplish this? Does it mean they must give the child everything he or she wants and never say "No"? Of course not, but there is no set of hard-and-fast rules to guide parents in all situations.

Exactly what a parent does on any given occasion depends on a variety of factors, including values, beliefs, experience, and both the parent's and the child's personalities. Parents should try to remember that raising a child is an ongoing process. No single action is likely to either form or deform a child's personality forever. The important thing is to keep seeking ways to promote satisfaction for all family members—including the parents! It is also important for parents to develop and maintain confidence in their parenting skills, their common sense—and, above all, their love for their children.

At each stage of the family life cycle, the relationship between parents and children changes. And with those changes come new challenges. The parents' primary responsibility to a small, helpless baby is to ensure its physical well-being around the clock. As babies grow into toddlers and begin to crawl and walk and talk, they begin to be able to take care of some of their own physical needs. For parents, the challenge at this stage is to strike a balance between giving children the freedom to explore and setting limits that will keep the children safe and secure. As children grow toward adolescence, parents need to give them increasing independence and gradually be willing to let them risk success or failure on their own.

Marital satisfaction for most couples tends to decline somewhat while the children are in school. Reasons include the financial and emotional pressures of a growing family and the increased job and community responsibilities of parents in their thirties, forties, and fifties. Once the last child has left home, marital satisfaction usually increases because the couple have time to enjoy each other once more.

Single Parents

Chances are that you know a number of families who haven't followed the traditional family life cycle, or perhaps you're a member of such a family yourself. According to the U.S. Bureau of the Census, about 28% of all children under 18 live with only one parent (Figure 4-3). Today the family life cycle for many women is marriage, motherhood, divorce, single parenthood, remarriage, and widowhood.

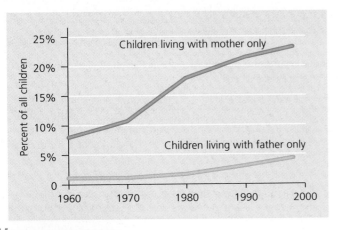

Figure 4-3 The growth of single-parent families in the United States.   Since 1960, the number of children living in single-parent families has risen from about 9% to nearly 28%. Although the majority of these children live with their mother, a growing number of single-parent households are headed by fathers.   SOURCE: U.S. Bureau of the Census. 1999. *Living Arrangement of Children Under 18 Years Old: 1960 to Present* (http://www.census.gov/population/socdemo/ms-la/tabch-1.txt; retrieved January 24, 2001).

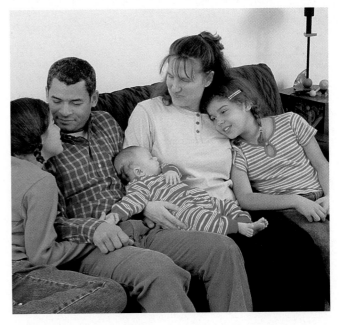

Almost one out of every five American families is a stepfamily, in which parents bring children from a previous marriage into a new family unit.

In some single-parent families, the traditional family life cycle is reversed and the baby comes before the marriage. In these families, the single parent is usually a teenage mother; she may very well be African American or Latina, and she may never get married or may not marry for several years. In 1998, about 60% of all African American children were living with single parents, as were 33% of Latino children. In single-parent families that are the result of divorce, the mother usually has custody of the children, but about 15% of single-parent families are headed by fathers. About 6% of children under 18 live with grandparents.

Economic difficulties are the primary problem for single mothers, especially for unmarried mothers who have not finished high school and have difficulty finding work. Divorced mothers usually experience a sharp drop in income the first few years on their own, but if they have job skills or education, they usually can eventually support themselves and their children adequately. Other problems for single mothers are the often-conflicting demands of playing both father and mother and the difficulty of satisfying their own needs for adult companionship and affection.

Financial pressures are also a complaint of single fathers, but they do not experience them to the extent that single mothers do. Because they are likely to have less practice than mothers in juggling parental and professional roles, they may worry that they do not spend enough time with their children. Because single father-hood is not as common as single motherhood, however, the men who choose it are likely to be stable, established, and strongly motivated to be with their children.

Research about the effect on children of growing up in a single-parent family is inconclusive. Evidence seems to indicate that these children tend to have less success in school and in their careers than children from two-parent families, but these effects may be associated more strongly with low educational attainment of the single parent rather than the absence of the second parent. Two-parent families are not necessarily better if one of the parents spends little time relating to the children or is physically or emotionally abusive.

Stepfamilies

Single parenthood is usually a transitional stage; about three out of four divorced women and about four out of five divorced men will ultimately remarry. Overall, almost half the marriages in the United States are remarriages for the husband, the wife, or both. If either brings children from a previous marriage into the new family unit, a stepfamily (or "blended family") is formed.

Stepfamilies are significantly different from primary families and should not be expected to duplicate the emotions and relationships of a primary family. Research has shown that healthy stepfamilies are less cohesive and more adaptable than healthy primary families; they have a greater capacity to allow for individual differences and

Life is full of challenges; the key to life in a strong family is to work together to meet those challenges. The following are strategies used by strong families for dealing with life's difficulties:

- *Look for something positive in difficult situations.* No matter how difficult, most problems teach us something about ourselves and others that we can draw on in future situations.

- *Pull together.* Think of the problem not as one family member's difficulty but as a challenge for the family as a whole.

- *Get help outside the family.* Call on extended family members, supportive friends, neighbors, colleagues, church or synagogue members, and community professionals.

- *Create open channels of communication.* Challenges cannot be met when communication shuts down.

- *Keep things in perspective.* "These things, too, shall pass."

- *Adopt new roles in a flexible manner.* Crises often demand that individuals learn new approaches to life and take on different responsibilities.

- *Focus to minimize fragmentation.* Look at the big picture. Focusing on the details rather than the essentials can make people edgy, even hysterical.

- *Give up on worry, or put it in a box.* Worrying itself usually causes more misery than the problem at hand. Sometimes it's best to stuff the worry down or to resolve to worry

10 minutes a day and then forget about it. The mind simply has to rest.

- *Eat well, exercise, love each other, and get adequate sleep.* We often forget that we are biological beings. Like kindergartners, we need a good lunch and time to play. We need to have our hair stroked, we need a good hug, and we need a good nap.

- *Create a life full of meaning and purpose.* We all face severe crises in life. These challenges are simply unavoidable. Sometimes it helps to focus on others, to offer service to the community. Giving of ourselves brings a richness and dignity to our lives, in spite of the troubles we endure.

- *Actively meet challenges head-on.* Life's disasters do not go away when we look in another direction.

- *Go with the flow to some degree.* Sometimes we are relatively powerless in the face of a crisis. Simply saying to ourselves that things will get better with time can be useful.

- *Be prepared in advance for life's challenges.* Healthy family relationships are like an ample bank balance: If our relational accounts are in order, we will be able to weather life's most difficult storms—together.

SOURCE: Olson, D. H., and J. DeFrain. 2000. *Marriage and the Family: Diversity and Strengths*, 3rd ed. Mountain View, Calif.: Mayfield.

accept that biologically related family members will have emotionally closer relationships. Stepfamilies gradually gain more of a sense of being a family as they build a history of shared daily experiences and major life events.

Successful Families

Family life can be extremely challenging. A strong family is not a family without problems; it's a family that copes successfully with stress and crisis (see the box "Strategies of Strong Families"). Many families move through life without a clear direction. Successful families are intentionally more connected—members share experiences and meanings. An excellent way to build strong family ties is to develop family rituals—organized, repeated activities that have meaning for family members. Family rituals may include everyday activities like family meals, shared household chores, and bedtime stories; celebration of wedding anniversaries, birthdays, Father's Day, Mother's Day, and other special anniversaries; and broader family or community activities such as weddings, reunions, and graduations.

Although there is tremendous variation in American families, researchers have proposed that six major qualities or themes appear in strong families.

1. *Commitment.* The family is very important to its members; sexual fidelity between partners is included in commitment.

2. *Appreciation.* Family members care about one another and express their appreciation. The home is a positive place for family members.

3. *Communication.* Family members spend time listening to one another and enjoying one another's company. They talk about disagreements and attempt to solve problems.

4. *Time together.* Family members do things together, often simple activities that don't cost money.

5. *Spiritual wellness.* The family promotes sharing, love, and compassion for other human beings.

6. *Coping with stress and crisis.* When faced with illness, death, marital conflict, or other crises, family members pull together, seek help, and use other coping strategies to meet the challenge.

It may surprise some people that members of strong families are often seen at counseling centers. They know that the smartest thing to do in some situations is to get help. Many resources are available for individuals and families seeking counseling; people can turn to physicians, clergy, marriage and family counselors, psychologists, or other trained professionals.

Families—and intimate relationships of all kinds—are essential to our overall wellness. A fulfilling life nearly always involves other people. Whether we're single or married, young or old, heterosexual or gay, we continue to need meaningful relationships throughout life.

SUMMARY

- Healthy intimate relationships are an important component of the well-being of both individuals and society. Many intimate relationships are held together by love.

- Successful relationships begin with a positive sense of self and reasonably high self-esteem. Personal identity, gender roles, and styles of attachment are all rooted in childhood experiences.

- The characteristics of friendship include companionship, respect, acceptance, help, trust, loyalty, and reciprocity.

- Love, sex, and commitment are closely linked ideals in intimate relationships. Love includes trust, caring, respect, and loyalty. Sex brings excitement, fascination, and passion to the relationship.

- Sternberg sees love as composed of intimacy, passion, and commitment. He defines seven types of love based on various combinations of these elements, ranging from friendship to consummate love.

- Common challenges in relationships relate to issues of self-disclosure, commitment, expectations, competitiveness, balancing time spent together and apart, and jealousy. Partners in successful relationships have strong communication skills and support each other in difficult times.

- The keys to good communication in relationships are self-disclosure, listening, and feedback.

- Cultural differences in how men and women have learned to communicate can create misunderstandings and frustration in relationships.

- Conflict is inevitable in intimate relationships; partners need to have constructive ways to negotiate their differences.

- People usually choose partners like themselves. If partners are very different, acceptance and good communication skills are necessary to maintain the relationship.

- Most Americans find partners through dating or getting together in groups. Cohabitation is a growing social pattern that allows partners to get to know each other intimately without being married.

- Gay and lesbian partnerships are similar to heterosexual relationships, with some differences. Partners often don't conform to traditional gender roles, and they may experience hostility or ambivalence rather than approval toward their partnerships from society.

- Singlehood is a growing option in our society. Advantages include greater variety in sex partners and more freedom in making life decisions; disadvantages include loneliness and possible economic hardship, especially for single women.

- Marriage fulfills many functions for individuals and society. It can provide people with affection, affirmation, and sexual fulfillment; a context for child rearing; and the promise of lifelong companionship.

- Love isn't enough to ensure a successful marriage. Partners have to be realistic, feel good about each other, have communication and conflict-resolution skills, share values, and have a balance of individual and joint interests.

- Commitment helps maintain a relationship over time and through difficult changes.

- When problems can't be worked out, people often separate and divorce. Divorce is traumatic for all involved, especially children, but the negative effects are usually balanced in time by positive ones.

- At each stage of the family life cycle, relationships change. Marital satisfaction may be lower during the child-rearing years and higher later.

- Many families today are single-parent families. Problems for single parents include economic difficulties, conflicting demands, and time pressures.
- Stepfamilies are formed when single or divorced people remarry and create new family units. Stepfamilies gradually gain more of a sense of being a family as they build a history of shared experiences.

- Important qualities of successful families include commitment to the family, appreciation of family members, communication, time spent together, spiritual wellness, and effective methods of dealing with stress.

TAKE ACTION

1. Take an informal survey among your friends of what they find attractive in a member of the other sex and what they look for in a romantic partner. Are there substantial differences between people? Do men and women look for different things?

2. Ask your parents what their experiences of dating and courtship were like. How are they different from your experiences? What do your parents think of current customs?

WWW. JOURNAL ENTRY

1. What are you looking for in an intimate relationship? In your health journal, make a list of the needs you would like to have met by a partner. Are they needs that you can realistically expect to have satisfied in a relationship?

2. **Critical Thinking** What approach do you take when it comes to communicating your feelings and needs to others? Think of a particular issue that has been bothering you, and write down the statements you would make if you were discussing it. Examine

your statements to see whether unrelated feelings or issues are coming through in them. Devise a strategy for dealing with the issue, using the guidelines given in this chapter on conflict resolution.

3. Make a list of your family's strengths and weaknesses. What do you like best about your family? What would you like to change? Choose one weakness, and develop strategies for dealing with it that you and your family can work on together.

FOR MORE INFORMATION

For resources in your area, check your campus directory for a counseling center or peer counseling program, or check the agencies listed in the Mental Health section of the phone book.

Books

Amatea, E., N. M. Brown, and E. S. Amatea. 2000. *Love and Intimate Relationships: Journeys of the Heart.* New York: Brunner/Mazel. *Provides a synthesis of theoretical perspectives as well as advice for enhancing relationships.*

Christensen, A., and N. Jacobson. 2000. *Reconcilable Differences.* New York: Guilford Press. *A guide to resolving conflicts and building intimacy in relationships.*

DeGenova, M. K., and F. P. Rice. 2002. *Intimate Relationships, Marriages, and Families.* 5th ed. Mountain View, Calif.: Mayfield. *A comprehensive look at intimate relationships.*

Gottman, J. M., and N. Silver. 1999. *Seven Principles for Making Marriage Work.* New York: Crown. *Research-based advice for keeping relationships on track.*

Ornish, D. 1998. *Love and Survival: The Scientific Basis for the Healing Power of Intimacy.* New York: HarperCollins. *A discussion of the positive health effects of intimate relationships.*

Plante, T., and K. Sullivan. 2000. *Getting Together and Staying Together: The Stanford Course on Intimate Relationships.* Bloomington, Ind.: 1stBooks Library. *Provides a concise and practical approach*

to intimate relationships based on both clinical practice and scientific research.

Sternberg, R. J. 1998. *Cupid's Arrow: The Course of Love Through Time.* New York: SIGS Books and Multimedia. *A review of Sternberg's triangular theory of love, with self-help advice.*

WWW. Organizations and Web Sites

American Association for Marriage and Family Therapy. Provides information on a variety of relationship issues and referrals to therapists.
202-452-0109
http://www.aamft.org

Association for Couples in Marriage Enrichment (ACME). An organization that promotes activities to strengthen marriage; a resource for books, tapes, and other materials.
800-634-8325
http://www.marriageenrichment.com

Family Education Network. Provides information about education, safety, health, and other family-related issues.
http://www.familyeducation.com

Go Ask Alice. Professional and peer educators provide answers to questions on many topics relating to interpersonal relationships and communication.
http://www.goaskalice.columbia.edu

Life Innovations. Provides materials for premarital counseling and marital enrichment.

800-331-1661

http://www.lifeinnovation.com

Parents Without Partners (PWP). Provides educational programs, literature, and support groups for single parents and their children. Call for a referral to a local chapter.

800-637-7974

http://www.parentswithoutpartners.org

Student Counseling Virtual Pamphlet Collection. Provides links to pamphlets produced by different student counseling centers; topics include relationships, sexual orientation, and assertiveness.

http://counseling.uchicago.edu/vpc

United States Census Bureau. Provides current statistics on births, marriages, and living arrangements.

http://www.census.gov

Whole Family Center. Provides information on all types of family relationships; the site includes an online magazine and examples of real-life dramas for teens, couples, and parents.

http://www.wholefamily.com

Yahoo/Lesbians, Gays, and Bisexuals. A Web site and search engine that contains many links to information and support for lesbians and gays.

http://dir.yahoo.com/society_and_culture/cultures_and_groups

See also the listings for Chapters 3 and 8.

SELECTED BIBLIOGRAPHY

Andrews, V. 1999. You've got mail: But you may want it stamped Return to Sender. *Health Scout,* February 12 (http://www.healthscout.com/cig-bin/WebObjects/af/hsaf.woa?ap=19&id=60996; retrieved February 18, 1999).

Baker, B., et al. 2000. The influence of marital adjustment on 3-year left ventricular mass and ambulatory blood pressure in mild hypertension. *Archives of Internal Medicine* 160(22): 3453–3458.

Battaglia, D. M., D. Datteri, and C. Lord. 1998. Breaking up is (relatively) easy to do: A script for the dissolutions of close relationships. *Journal of Social and Personal Relationships* 15(6): 829–845.

Bergner, R. M. 2000. Love and barriers to love. An analysis for psychotherapists and others. *American Journal of Psychotherapy* 54(1): 1–17.

Brown, S., and A. Booth. 1996. Cohabitation versus marriage: A comparison of relationship quality. *Journal of Marriage and the Family* 58: 668–678.

Christensen, A., and N. Jacobson. 2000. *Reconcilable Differences.* New York: Guilford Press.

Columbia University Health Education Program. 1997. *Go Ask Alice: Looking for Love on the Information Superhighway* (http://www.goaskalice.columbia.edu/1185.html; retrieved September 4, 1998).

DeGenova, M. K., and F. P. Rice. 2002. *Intimate Relationships, Marriages, and Families.* Mountain View, Calif.: Mayfield.

Feeney, J. 1999. Issues of closeness and distance in dating relationships: Effects of sex and attachment style. *Journal of Social and Personal Relationships* 16(5): 571–590.

Fletcher, G. J., et al. 1999. Ideals in intimate relationships. *Journal of Personality and Social Psychology* 76(1): 72–89.

Friends may be good for your heart. 1999. *Health News,* January.

Grote, N. K., and M. S. Clark. 2001. Perceiving unfairness in the family: Cause or consequence of marital distress? *Journal of Personality and Social Psychology* 80(2): 281–293.

Harvey, E. 1999. Short-term and long-term effects of early parental employment on children of the National Longitudinal Survey of Youth. *Developmental Psychology* 35(2): 445–459.

Heller, P. E., and B. Wood. 2000. The influence of religious and ethnic differences on marital intimacy: Intermarriage versus intramarriage. *Journal of Marital and Family Therapy* 26(2): 241–252.

Heller, P. E., et al. 1998. The process of intimacy: Similarity, understanding, and gender. *Journal of Family Therapy* 24(3): 273–288.

Hutson, T. L., et al. 2001. The connubial crucible: Newlywed years as predictors of marital delight, distress, and divorce. *Journal of Personality and Social Psychology* 80(2): 237–52.

Kiecolt-Glaser, J. K., et al. 1998. Marital stress: Immunologic, neuroendocrine, and autonomic correlates. *Annals of the New York Academy of Science* 840: 656–663.

Lewis, J. M. 1998. For better or worse: Interpersonal relationships and individual outcome. *American Journal of Psychiatry* 155(5): 582–589.

Marital status and survival in prostate cancer. 1998. *Harvard Men's Health Watch,* August.

Olson, D., and J. DeFrain. 2000. *Marriage and the Family,* 3rd ed. Mountain View, Calif.: Mayfield.

Orth-Gomér, K., et al. 2000. Marital stress worsens prognosis in women with coronary heart disease. *Journal of the American Medical Association* 284(23): 3008–3014.

Payne, M. 1998. "Waiting for lightning to strike": Social support for interracial couples. In *Readings in Cultural Contexts,* ed. J. N. Martin, T. K. Nakayama, and L. A. Flores. Mountain View, Calif.: Mayfield.

Plante, T., and K. Sullivan. 2000. *Getting Together and Staying Together: The Stanford Course on Intimate Relationships.* Bloomington, Ind.: 1stBooks Library.

Roy, R., et al. 2000. Beyond intimacy: Conceptualizing sex differences in same sex friendships. *Journal of Psychology* 134(1): 93–101.

Sprecher, S. 1999. "I love you more today than yesterday." Romantic partners' perceptions of changes in love and related affect over time. *Journal of Personality and Social Psychology* 76(1): 46–53.

Strong, B., et al. 2002. B., *Human Sexuality: Diversity in Contemporary America,* 4th ed. Mountain View, Calif.: Mayfield.

Suler, J. 1997. *The Final Showdown Between In-Person and Cyberspace Relationships* (http://www1.rider.edu/users/suler/psycyber/showdown.html; retrieved August 28, 2000).

University of Florida Counseling Center. 2000. *Handling Common Relationship Problems* (http://www.counsel.ufl.edu/CounselNet/cnetrelprob.htm; retrieved August 26, 2000).

University of Michigan Institute for Social Research. 2000. *Intimate Relationships Between Races More Common Than Thought* (http://www.umich.edu/~newsinfo/Releases/2000/Mar00/ro32300a.html; retrieved March 27, 2000).

University of Wisconsin—Eau Claire, Counseling Services. 2000. *Building Healthy Relationships* (http://www.UWEC.EDU/admin/counsel/pubs/bhr.htm; retrieved August 26, 2000).

Watson, D., B. Hubbard, and D. Wiese. 2000. General traits of personality and affectivity as predictors of satisfaction in intimate relationships: Evidence from self- and partner-ratings. *Journal of Personality* 68(3): 413–449.

White, L., and J. G. Gilbreth. 2001. When children have two fathers: Effects of relationships with stepfathers and noncustodial fathers on adolescent outcomes. *Journal of Marriage and Family* 63(1): 155–167.

Yeung, W. J., et al. 2001. Children's time with fathers in intact families. *Journal of Marriage and Family* 63(1): 136–154.

Zak, A. M., et al. 1998. Assessments of trust in intimate relationships and the self-perception process. *Journal of Social Psychology* 138(2): 217–228.

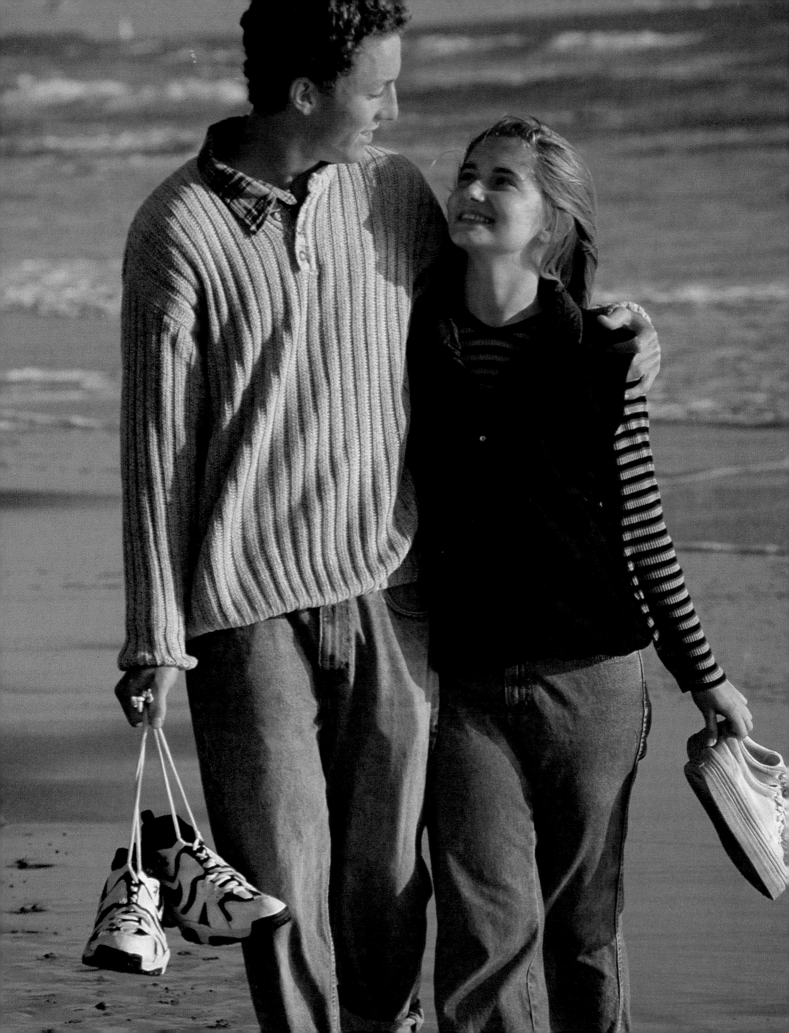

After reading this chapter, you should be able to

- Describe the structure and function of the female and male sex organs

- Explain the changes in sexual functioning that occur across the life span

- Describe how the sex organs function during sexual activity and list common causes of sexual problems

- Outline the factors that influence sexual behavior and the various ways human sexuality can be expressed

- Describe guidelines for safe, responsible sexual behavior

Sex and Your Body

5

TEST YOUR KNOWLEDGE

1. Early in development, all embryos begin as female.
   True or false?

2. Which of the following is a risk factor for erectile dysfunction ("impotence")?
   a. smoking
   b. overweight
   c. physical inactivity

3. Calcium supplements may reduce symptoms of premenstrual syndrome (PMS) in some women.
   True or false?

4. Alcohol consumption by young people is associated with unplanned, unprotected sexual activity and higher rates of sexually transmitted diseases (STDs).
   True or false?

5. Women's motivations for having sex are usually to express love, while men's motives are usually physical.
   True or false?

6. About how many sexual references, innuendoes, and jokes does a typical teenager view on television each year?
   a. 150
   b. 1500
   c. 15,000

ANSWERS

1. **TRUE.** Without the influence of sex hormones, all embryos would develop into females.

2. **ALL THREE.** 70–80% of cases of erectile dysfunction are thought to involve physical factors.

3. **TRUE.** Other self-help strategies for PMS include exercise, stress reduction, and a diet low in fat and rich in complex carbohydrates.

4. **TRUE.** Studies have shown that raising the drinking age and increasing the price of beer (through taxes) leads to a decrease in STD rates among young adults.

5. **FALSE.** While this statement is often true for men and women under 40, after age 40, physical gratification becomes the more common motivation for women, while emotional expression becomes more important for men.

6. **C.** Of these, fewer than 170 deal with abstinence, contraception, sexually transmitted diseases, or pregnancy.

Humans are sexual beings. Sexual activity is the source of our most intense physical pleasures, a central ingredient in many of our intimate emotional relationships, and, of course, the key to the reproduction of our species.

Sexuality is more than just sexual behavior. It includes biological sex (being biologically male or female), gender (masculine and feminine behaviors), sexual anatomy and physiology, sexual functioning and practices, and social and sexual interactions with others. Our individual sense of identity is powerfully influenced by our sexuality. We think of ourselves in very fundamental ways as male or female; as heterosexual or homosexual; as single, attached, married, or divorced. Sexuality is a complex, interacting group of inborn, biological characteristics and acquired behaviors people learn in the course of growing up in a particular family, community, and society.

Sexuality arouses intense feelings, and communicating about it is highly emotionally charged. Because of its basic role in human life, sexual expression is usually regulated with restrictions and taboos—written and unwritten laws specifying which functions and behaviors are acceptable and "normal" and which are unacceptable and "abnormal." Young people growing up in the United States are bombarded with conflicting messages about sex from television, movies, magazines, and popular music. The mass media suggest that the average person is a sexual athlete who continually jumps in and out of bed without using contraception, producing offspring, or contracting disease. Although parents, educators, and other responsible adults present a more balanced picture,

they may convey their own hidden messages as well. Ignorance, confusion, and fear are often the result.

Basic information about the body and about sexual functioning and behavior are vital to healthy adult life. Once we understand the facts, we have a better basis for evaluating the messages we get and for making informed, responsible choices about our sexual activities. If you have questions about aspects of your physical sexuality, this chapter will provide you with some answers.

Ww. SEXUAL ANATOMY

In spite of their different appearance, the sex organs of men and women arise from the same structures and fulfill similar functions. Each person has a pair of **gonads;** ovaries are the female gonads, and testes are the male gonads. The gonads produce **germ cells** and sex hormones. The germ cells are ova (eggs) in females and sperm in males. Ova and sperm are the basic units of reproduction; their union results in the creation of a new life.

Female Sex Organs

The external sex organs, or genitals, of the female are called the **vulva** (Figure 5-1a). The mons pubis, a rounded mass of fatty tissue over the pubic bone, becomes covered with hair during puberty (biological maturation). Below it are two paired folds of skin called the labia majora (major lips) and the labia minora (minor lips). Enclosed within are the clitoris, the opening of the urethra, and the opening of the vagina. The **clitoris** is highly sensitive to touch and plays an important role in female sexual arousal and orgasm. The clitoris, like the penis, consists of a shaft, glans, and spongy tissue that fills with blood during sexual excitement. The glans is the most sensitive part of the clitoris and is covered by the clitoral hood, or **prepuce,** which is formed from the upper portion of the labia minora.

The female urethra leads directly from the urinary bladder to its opening between the clitoris and the opening of the vagina; it conducts urine from the bladder to the outside of the body. Unlike the male urethra, it is independent of the genitals.

The vaginal opening is partially covered by the hymen. This membrane can be stretched or torn during athletic activity or when a woman has sexual intercourse for the first time. The idea that an intact hymen is the sign of a virgin is a myth. The **vagina** is the passage that leads to the internal reproductive organs (Figure 5-1b). It is the female structure for heterosexual sexual intercourse and also serves as the birth canal. Its soft, flexible walls are normally in contact with each other. A cylinder of muscles surrounds the vagina. During sexual excitement, the tension in these muscles increases and the walls of the vagina swell with blood.

Terms

sexuality A dimension of personality shaped by biological, psychosocial, and cultural forces and concerning all aspects of sexual behavior.

gonads The primary reproductive organs that produce germ cells and sex hormones; the ovaries and testes.

germ cells Sperm and ova (eggs).

vulva The external female genitals, or sex organs.

clitoris The highly sensitive female genital structure.

prepuce The foreskin of the clitoris or penis.

vagina The passage leading from the female genitals to the internal reproductive organs; the birth canal.

cervix The end of the uterus opening toward the vagina.

uterus The hollow, thick-walled, muscular organ in which the fertilized egg develops; the womb.

ovary One of two female reproductive glands that produce ova (eggs) and sex hormones; ovaries are the female gonads.

penis The male genital structure consisting of spongy tissue that becomes engorged with blood during sexual excitement.

scrotum The loose sac of skin and muscle fibers that contains the testes.

testis One of two male gonads, the site of sperm production; plural, *testes*. Also called *testicle*.

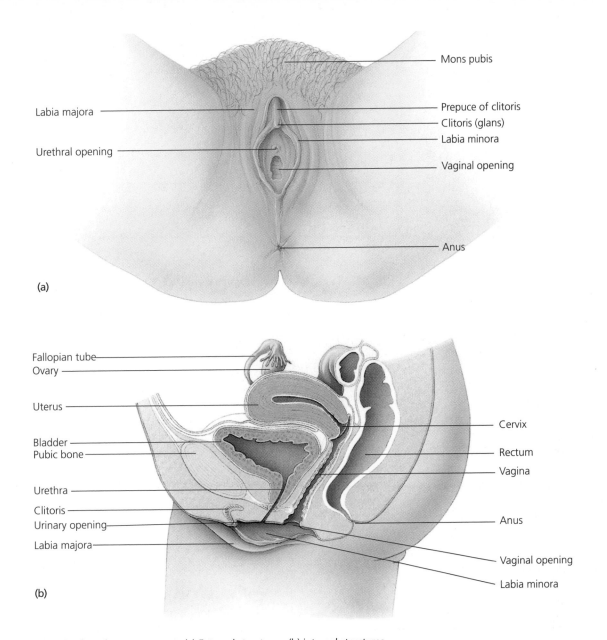

Labels (top figure, a):
Mons pubis
Labia majora
Prepuce of clitoris
Clitoris (glans)
Labia minora
Urethral opening
Vaginal opening
Anus
(a)

Labels (bottom figure, b):
Fallopian tube
Ovary
Uterus
Bladder
Pubic bone
Urethra
Clitoris
Urinary opening
Labia majora
Cervix
Rectum
Vagina
Anus
Vaginal opening
Labia minora
(b)

Figure 5-1   The female sex organs.   (a) External structures; (b) internal structures.

Projecting into the upper part of the vagina is the **cervix**, the neck of the uterus. Inside the pear-shaped **uterus**, which slants forward above the bladder, the fertilized egg is implanted and grows into a *fetus*. A pair of *fallopian tubes* (or *oviducts*) extend from the top of the uterus. The end of each oviduct surrounds an **ovary** and guides the mature ovum down into the uterus after the egg bursts from its follicle on the surface of the ovary.

Male Sex Organs

A man's external sex organs, or genitals, are the penis and the scrotum (Figure 5-2a). The **penis** consists of spongy tissue that becomes engorged with blood during sexual excitement, causing the organ to enlarge and become erect. The **scrotum** is a pouch that contains a pair of **testes**. The purpose of the scrotum is to maintain the testes at a temperature approximately 5°F below that of the rest of the body—that is, at about 93.6°F. The process of sperm production is extremely heat-sensitive. In hot temperatures the muscles in the scrotum relax, and the testes move away from the heat of the body. Conversely, in cold temperatures the muscles of the scrotum contract, and the testes move upward toward the body. This ability to regulate the temperature of the testes is important because elevated testicular temperature can interfere with normal sperm production.

Through the entire length of the penis runs the urethra, which can carry both urine and *semen*, the sperm-carrying fluid, to the opening at the tip of the glans (Figure 5-2b).

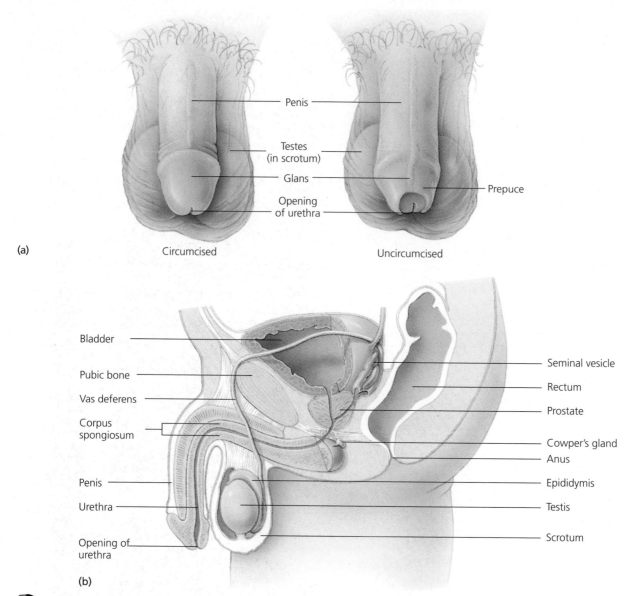

Figure 5-2   The male sex organs.   (a) External structures; (b) internal structures.

Although urine and semen share a common passage, they are prevented from mixing together by muscles that control their entry into the urethra.

The testes contain tightly packed seminiferous tubules within which sperm are produced. These tubules end in a maze of ducts that flow into a single storage tube called the *epididymis,* on the surface of each testis. This tube leads to the *vas deferens,* a tube that rises into the abdominal cavity. Inside the prostate gland, the two vasa deferentia join the ducts of the two *seminal vesicles,* whose secretions provide nutrients to semen. The *prostate gland* produces some of the fluid in semen that nourishes and transports sperm. The tubes of the seminal vesicle and the vas deferens on each side lead to the *ejaculatory duct,* which joins the urethra. The *Cowper's glands* (bulbourethral glands) are two small structures flanking the ure-

thra. During sexual arousal, these glands secrete a clear, mucuslike fluid that appears at the tip of the penis. The exact purpose of preejaculatory fluid is not known, but it may buffer sperm against any acidic urine in the urethra during ejaculation and help lubricate the urethra to facilitate the passage of sperm. In some men, preejaculatory fluid may contain sperm, so withdrawal of the penis before ejaculation is not a reliable form of contraception.

Circumcision   The smooth, rounded tip of the penis is the highly sensitive **glans,** an important component in sexual arousal. The glans is partially covered by the foreskin, or prepuce, a retractable fold of skin that is removed by **circumcision** in about 60–70% of newborn males in the United States. Circumcision is performed for cultural, religious, and hygienic reasons, and rates of circumcision vary widely among different groups. Worldwide, the rate is about 20%. Most Europeans, Asians, South and Central Americans, and Africans do not perform circumcision; Jews and Muslims are the major groups who circumcise for religious reasons.

The pros and cons of this simple procedure have been widely debated. Proponents argue that it promotes cleanliness and reduces the risk of urinary tract infections (UTIs) in newborns and penile cancer and sexually transmitted diseases (STDs) later in life. Research findings have been mixed; for example, a recent U.S. survey found no relationship between STD risk and circumcision, while international studies have shown a greater risk for STDs among uncircumcised males. Cultural as well as anatomical factors may explain these findings, and behavior is a far more important risk factor for STDs than circumcision status.

Opponents of circumcision state that it is an unnecessary surgical procedure that causes pain and puts a baby at risk for complications. Opponents also argue that by removing the foreskin, circumcision exposes the glans of the penis to constant irritation by clothing, thereby reducing its sensitivity; research into this issue has been inconclusive. In part because the overall risk of penile cancer and infant UTIs is low, the American Academy of Pediatrics (AAP) takes the position that although circumcision has potential medical benefits, the research is not sufficient to recommend the procedure routinely. When circumcision is performed, the AAP recommends that painkilling medication be provided.

While the debate focuses on medical concerns, most parents make their decision based on social or cultural factors. Fathers tend to want their sons to look like them and their peers. If a father is circumcised, he will most likely want his son to be circumcised, and vice versa. Whether or not to circumcise is a decision each family must make individually.

COMMUNICATE! Movies, magazines, and advertisements are filled with glamorous images of the human body, male and female. What messages are the media communicating about what's desirable and what isn't? How do they do so? What effect do these images have on your sense of your own body and your expectations for others?

HORMONES AND THE REPRODUCTIVE LIFE CYCLE

Many cultural and personal factors help shape the expression of your sexuality. But biology also plays an important role, particularly through the action of *hormones,* chemical messengers that are secreted directly into the bloodstream by the **endocrine glands.** The sex hormones produced by the ovaries or testes have a major influence on the development and function of the reproductive system throughout life. The sex hormones made by the testes are called **androgens,** the most important of which is *testosterone.* The female sex hormones, produced by the ovaries, belong to two groups: **estrogens** and **progestins,** the most important of which is *progesterone.* The cortex of the **adrenal glands** also produces androgens in both males and females.

The hormones produced by the testes, the ovaries, and the adrenal glands are regulated by the hormones of the **pituitary gland,** located at the base of the brain. This gland in turn is controlled by hormones produced by the **hypothalamus** in the brain. Sex hormones exert their primary developmental influences first in the embryo stage and later during adolescence.

Differentiation of the Embryo

The biological sex of an individual is determined by the fertilizing sperm at the time of conception. All human cells normally contain 23 pairs of chromosomes. In 22 of the pairs, the two partner chromosomes match. But in the twenty-third pair, the **sex chromosomes,** two configurations are possible. Individuals with two matching X chromosomes are female, and individuals with one X and one Y chromosome (a much shorter chromosome carrying specialized genes) are male. Thus, at the time of conception, the genetic sex is established: Females are XX and males are XY. The genetic sex will dictate whether the undifferentiated gonads will become ovaries or testes. If a Y chromosome is present, the gonads will become testes; the testes will produce the male hormone **testosterone.**

Terms

glans The rounded head of the penis or the clitoris.

circumcision Surgical removal of the foreskin of the penis.

endocrine glands Glands that produce hormones.

androgens Male sex hormones produced by the testes in males and by the adrenal glands in both sexes.

estrogens A class of female sex hormones, produced by the ovaries, that bring about sexual maturation at puberty and maintain reproductive functions.

progestins A class of female sex hormones, produced by the ovaries, that sustain reproductive functions.

adrenal glands Endocrine glands, located over the kidneys, that produce androgens (among other hormones).

pituitary gland An endocrine gland at the base of the brain that produces follicle-stimulating hormone (FSH) and luteinizing hormone (LH), among others.

hypothalamus A region of the brain above the pituitary gland whose hormones control the secretions of the pituitary; also involved in the nervous control of sexual functions.

sex chromosomes The X and Y chromosomes, which determine an individual's biological sex.

testosterone The most important androgen (male sex hormone); stimulates an embryo to develop into a male and induces the development of male secondary sex characteristics during puberty.

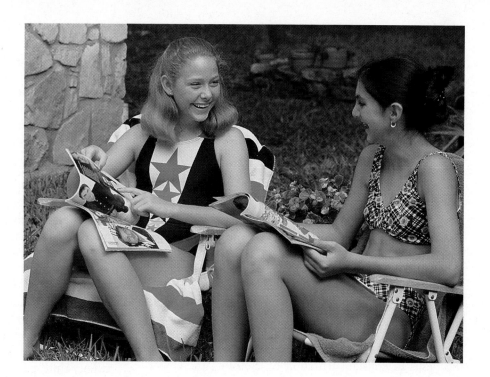

The physical changes of puberty usually begin between the ages of 8 and 13 for girls and 10 and 14 for boys. Once they reach puberty, these adolescents are biologically adults, but it will take another 5–10 years for them to become adults in social and psychological terms.

Testosterone circulates throughout the body and causes the undifferentiated reproductive structures to develop into male sex organs (penis, scrotum, and so on). If a Y chromosome is not present, the gonads become ovaries and the reproductive structures develop into female sex organs (clitoris, labia, and so on).

Each male and female reproductive structure develops from the same undifferentiated tissue, so that every structure in one sex has its developmental counterpart in the other. Therefore, the penis corresponds to the clitoris and the scrotum to the labia majora. It is the presence or absence of testosterone that determines which way the tissue will develop.

Female Sexual Maturation

Although humans are fully sexually differentiated at birth, the differences between males and females are accentu-

ated at **puberty,** the period during which the reproductive system matures, secondary sex characteristics develop, and the bodies of males and females come to appear more distinctive. The changes of puberty are induced by testosterone in the male and estrogen and **progesterone** in the female.

Physical Changes   The first sign of puberty in girls is breast development, followed by a rounding of the hips and buttocks. As the breasts develop, hair appears in the pubic region and later in the underarms. Shortly after the onset of breast development, girls show an increase in growth rate. Breast development usually begins between ages 8 and 13, and the time of rapid body growth occurs between ages 9 and 15. Estrogens and progestins from the ovaries, as well as androgens from the adrenal glands, are responsible for the female secondary sex characteristics, the physical changes that occur at puberty.

The Menstrual Cycle   A major landmark of puberty for young women is the onset of the **menstrual cycle,** the monthly ovarian cycle that leads to menstruation (loss of blood and tissue lining the uterus) in the absence of pregnancy. The first *menstrual period*, or menarche, occurs at the average age of 12.8 years in the United States, but it may also normally start several years earlier or later.

The menstrual cycle consists of four phases: (1) menses, (2) the estrogenic phase, (3) ovulation, and (4) the progestational phase (Figure 5-3). Day 1 of the cycle is considered to be the day of the onset of bleeding. For the purposes of our discussion, a cycle of 28 days will be used; however, normal cycles vary in length.

Terms

puberty The period of biological maturation during adolescence.

progesterone The most important progestin (female sex hormone); induces the development of female secondary sex characteristics during puberty, regulates the menstrual cycle, and sustains pregnancy.

menstrual cycle The monthly ovarian cycle, regulated by pituitary and ovarian hormones; in the absence of pregnancy, menstruation occurs.

corpus luteum The part of the ovarian follicle left after ovulation, which secretes estrogen and progesterone during the second half of the menstrual cycle.

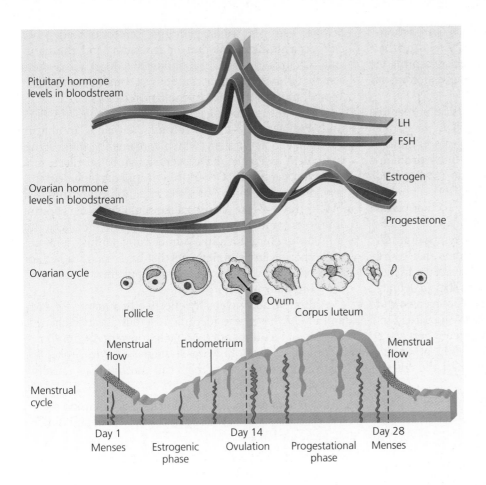

Pituitary hormone levels in bloodstream

LH

FSH

Ovarian hormone levels in bloodstream

Estrogen

Progesterone

Ovarian cycle

Ovum

Follicle

Corpus luteum

Menstrual flow

Endometrium

Menstrual flow

Menstrual cycle

Day 1
Menses

Day 14
Ovulation

Day 28
Menses

Estrogenic phase

Progestational phase

Figure 5-3   The menstrual cycle. The anterior pituitary releases FSH and LH, which stimulate the ovarian follicle to develop and release a mature egg. The ovarian follicle releases estrogen and progesterone, which stimulate the endometrium to continue to develop so that it will be ready to receive and nourish a fertilized egg. Unless pregnancy occurs, ovarian hormone levels fall and the endometrium sloughs off (menses).

During menses, characterized by the menstrual flow, hormones from the ovaries and anterior pituitary gland occur in relatively low amounts. This phase of the cycle usually lasts from day 1 to about day 5.

The estrogenic phase begins when the menstrual flow ceases, and the anterior pituitary begins to produce increasing amounts of follicle-stimulating hormone (FSH) and luteinizing hormone (LH). Under the influence of FSH, an egg-containing ovarian *follicle* begins to mature, producing increasingly higher amounts of estrogens. Stimulated by estrogen, the uterine lining, the *endometrium,* thickens with large numbers of blood vessels and uterine glands.

A surge of a potent estrogen called estradiol from the follicle causes the anterior pituitary to release a large burst of LH and a smaller amount of FSH. The high concentration of LH stimulates the developing follicle to release its ovum. This event is known as *ovulation.* After ovulation, the follicle is transformed into the **corpus luteum,** which produces progesterone and estrogen. Ovulation usually occurs about 14 days prior to the onset of menstrual flow, a fact that can be used to predict the most fertile time during the menstrual cycle, useful in both fertility treatment and natural family planning methods (see Chapter 6).

During the progestational phase of the cycle, the amount of progesterone secreted from the corpus luteum increases and remains high until the onset of the next menses. Under the influence of estrogen and progesterone, the endometrium continues to develop, readying itself to receive and nourish a fertilized ovum. When pregnancy occurs, the fertilized egg produces the hormone human chorionic gonadotropin (HCG), which maintains the corpus luteum. Thus, levels of ovarian hormones remain high and the uterine lining is preserved, preventing menses.

If pregnancy does not occur, the corpus luteum degenerates, and estrogen and progesterone levels gradually fall. Below certain hormonal levels, the endometrium can no longer be maintained, and it begins to slough off, initiating menses. As the levels of ovarian hormones fall, a slight rise in LH and FSH occurs, and a new menstrual cycle begins.

MENSTRUAL PROBLEMS   Menstruation is a normal biological process, but it may cause physical or psychological problems. *Dysmenorrhea* is characterized by cramps in the lower abdomen, backache, vomiting, nausea, a bloated feeling, diarrhea, and loss of appetite. Some of these symptoms can be attributed to uterine muscular contractions caused by chemicals called prostaglandins. Any drug that blocks the effects of prostaglandins, such as aspirin or ibuprofen, will usually alleviate some of the symptoms of dysmenorrhea.

Many women experience transient physical and emotional symptoms prior to the onset of their menstrual flow. Depending on their severity, these symptoms may be categorized as one of three related conditions: **premenstrual tension, premenstrual syndrome (PMS), and premenstrual dysphoric disorder (PMDD)**. Premenstrual tension symptoms are mild and may include negative mood changes and physical symptoms such as abdominal cramping and backache. More severe symptoms are classified as PMS; very severe symptoms that cause impairment in social functioning and work-related activities are classified as PMDD. All three conditions share a definite pattern: Symptoms appear prior to the onset of menses and disappear within a few days after the start of menstruation. It is estimated that as many as 75% of women report some discomfort prior to the onset of menses, 20–50% of women experience PMS symptoms, and 3–10% meet the criteria for PMDD.

Many symptoms are associated with PMS and PMDD, including physical changes such as breast tenderness, water retention (bloating), headache, and fatigue; insomnia or excessive sleep; appetite changes and food cravings; irritability, anger, and increased interpersonal conflict; mood swings; depression and sadness; anxiety and tearfulness; inability to concentrate; social withdrawal; and the sense that one is out of control or overwhelmed. The key to diagnosing PMS and PMDD is to keep a daily diary of symptoms over several menstrual cycles. PMDD is distinguished from PMS by the severity of symptoms, which in PMDD interfere significantly with work or school and with usual social activities and relationships.

Despite many research studies, the causes of PMS and PMDD are still unknown, and it is unclear why some women are more vulnerable than others. Research has focused on a variety of substances in the body that may fluctuate with the menstrual cycle, including progesterone, estrogen, prostaglandins, serotonin and other neurotransmitters, calcium, magnesium, and the naturally occurring opiate beta-endorphin. Most researchers feel that PMS is probably caused by a combination of hormonal, nutritional, and psychological factors.

There are no completely effective therapies for PMS and PMDD. Selective serotonin reuptake inhibitors (SSRIs) such as Sarafem, which contains the same active ingredient as Prozac, have been shown to be effective at reducing symptoms. Other drug treatments include estrogen, diuretics to minimize water retention, and drugs that block the effects of prostaglandins such as aspirin, ibuprofen, and more potent prescription prostaglandin inhibitors. There are also a number of vitamins, minerals, and other dietary supplements that have been studied for PMS relief; see the box "Dietary Supplements and PMS" for more information.

Although no universally effective treatments for PMS and PMDD have been identified, certain lifestyle changes are often recommended to help prevent or minimize symptoms. The following strategies provide relief for many women, and all of them can contribute to a healthy lifestyle at any time.

- *Limit salt intake.* Salt promotes water retention and bloating. Avoid adding salt to your food, and don't eat salty snacks.
- *Exercise.* Women who exercise experience fewer symptoms both before and after their menstrual periods.
- *Don't use alcohol or tobacco.* Alcohol and tobacco may aggravate certain symptoms of PMS and PMDD.
- *Eat a nutritious diet.* Choose a low-fat diet rich in complex carbohydrates from vegetables, fruits, and whole-grain breads, cereals, and pasta. Obtain an adequate calcium intake from calcium-rich foods and, if needed, supplements. Minimize your intake of sugar and caffeine, and avoid chocolate, which is rich in both.
- *Relax.* Stress reduction is always beneficial, and stressful events can trigger PMS symptoms. Try relaxation techniques during the premenstrual time.

If symptoms persist, keep a daily diary to track both the types of symptoms you experience and their severity. See your physician for an evaluation and to learn more about treatments that are available only with a prescription.

Male Sexual Maturation

Reproductive maturation of boys occurs about 2 years later than that of girls; it usually begins at about age 10 or 11. Physical changes include enlargement of the testes, development of pubic hair, growth of the penis, the onset of ejaculation (usually at about age 11 or 12), deepening of the voice, the appearance of facial hair, and a period of rapid growth.

Terms

premenstrual tension Mild physical and emotional changes associated with the time before the onset of menses; symptoms can include abdominal cramping and backache.

premenstrual syndrome (PMS) A disorder characterized by physical discomfort, psychological distress, and behavioral changes that begin after ovulation and cease when menstruation begins.

premenstrual dysphoric disorder (PMDD) Severe form of PMS, characterized by symptoms serious enough to interfere with work or school or with social activities and relationships.

menopause The cessation of menstruation, occurring gradually around age 50.

Many dietary supplements have been promoted for relief of the symptoms of PMS; those described below are among the most commonly advocated compounds. Only one supplement, calcium, has been shown to provide relief in rigorous clinical studies; several others show promise, but more research is needed.

- *Calcium.* Blood calcium levels are lower during the premenstrual period, and careful research studies have shown calcium supplements to be effective at relieving symptoms of PMS. The amount of calcium taken by women in these studies, 1000–1200 mg per day, is within accepted safety limits for calcium intake and may also be beneficial for building and maintaining bone density (see Chapter 12 for more on recommended intakes of vitamins and minerals).

- *Magnesium.* Levels of magnesium in certain body cells are lower in women with PMS, and magnesium is involved in neurotransmitter activity. Results of small studies of the effects of magnesium have been promising, but larger trials are needed. Magnesium supplements can cause side effects, including diarrhea, in some people and so should be used with caution.

- *Vitamin B-6.* Vitamin B-6 plays an important role in the synthesis of neurotransmitters, so researchers have proposed that taking supplements of vitamin B-6 may help reduce mood-related symptoms of PMS. Research into the effects of vitamin B-6 has yielded mixed results, however. In addition, long-term use of high doses of vitamin B-6 can cause permanent nerve damage.

- *Vitamin E.* Although the mechanism is unclear, one study found that vitamin E supplements may improve PMS symptoms. Further research is needed.

- *Carbohydrates.* Some women with PMS report craving carbohydrate-rich foods, a change in diet that may actually improve the mood-related symptoms of PMS. Increased intake of carbohydrates may increase blood levels of tryptophan, an amino acid the body uses to produce the neurotransmitter serotonin. Although some dietary supplements containing mixtures of carbohydrates have been marketed for PMS symptoms, it is unclear whether these are any more effective than changing the diet to include more carbohydrate-rich fruits, vegetables, and grains.

Other compounds under study include evening primrose oil, black cohash, and chaste tree fruit (*vitex agnus-castus*). If you decide to try any of these or other dietary supplements for PMS, you should discuss your use of supplements with a qualified health professional. Some herbal products interact with prescription and over-the-counter drugs as well as other herbs; in addition, some may be toxic at high doses or dangerous during pregnancy. Refer to Chapters 12 and 21 for more information on dietary supplements.

SOURCE: Bendich, A. 2000. Review: The potential for dietary supplements to reduce premenstrual syndrome (PMS) symptoms. *Journal of the American College of Nutrition* 19(1): 3–12.

Aging and Human Sexuality

Changes in hormone production and sexual functioning occur as we age. As a woman approaches age 50, her ovaries gradually cease to function and she enters **menopause,** the cessation of menstruation. For some women, the associated drop in hormone production causes symptoms that are troublesome. The most common physical symptoms of menopause are hot flashes, sensations of warmth rising to the face from the upper chest, with or without perspiration and chills. Other symptoms include headaches, dizziness, palpitations, and joint pains. Osteoporosis—decreasing bone density—can develop, making older women more vulnerable to fractures. Some menopausal women become moody, even markedly depressed, and they may also experience fatigue, irritability, and forgetfulness. Hormone replacement therapy can significantly relieve most of these symptoms, but it may increase some women's risk of certain types of cancer.

As a result of decreased estrogen production, the vaginal walls become thin, and lubrication in response to sexual arousal diminishes; sexual intercourse may become painful. Hormonal treatment or the use of lubricants during intercourse can minimize these problems. See Chapter 19 for more on the physical changes associated with menopause and aging.

Some women have a difficult time making the psychological adjustment to this stage of life, associating it with a loss of youth and sexual attractiveness. Others welcome it as a time of increased personal freedom, when the responsibilities of child rearing are over, and sex can be enjoyed without the fear of pregnancy. For many, menopause is seen as signaling the end of one phase of life and the beginning of another, equally meaningful, one. A recent poll of menopausal women found that more than half reported being happier now than in their younger years.

In men, testosterone production gradually decreases with age. As they get older, men depend more on direct physical stimulation for sexual arousal. They take longer to get an erection and find it more difficult to maintain; orgasmic contractions are less intense.

Many men go through a period of reassessment and readjustment in middle age, which may have repercussions for their sexuality. However, a study that followed more than 3000 people for 10 years found that far from being a time of dissatisfaction and "midlife crisis," the middle

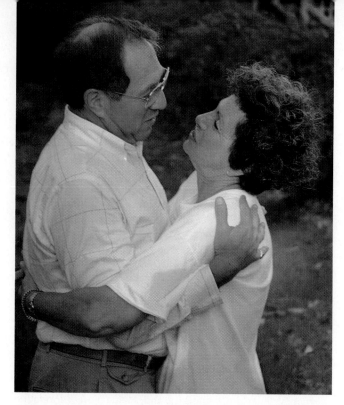

Although sexual physiology changes as people get older, many men and women readily adjust to these alterations. Sexual activity can continue throughout life for people like this healthy and vigorous older couple.

years are a fulfilling time of life characterized by satisfying relationships. As with women, sexual activity can continue to be a source of pleasure and satisfaction for men as they grow older. A recent survey found that nearly half of all Americans age 60 or older engage in sexual activity at least once a month.

SEXUAL FUNCTIONING

In this section, we discuss sexual physiology—how the sex organs function during sexual activity—and problems that can occur with sexual functioning. Sexual activity is based on stimulus and response. Erotic stimulation leads to sexual arousal (excitement), which may culminate in the intensely pleasurable experience of orgasm. But sexual activity should not be thought of only in terms of the sex organs. Responses to sexual stimulation involve not just the genitals but the entire body—and the mind as well.

Sexual Stimulation

Sexual excitement can come from many sources, both physical and psychological. Although physical stimuli have an obvious and direct effect, some people believe psychological stimuli—thoughts, fantasies, desires, per-

ceptions—are even more powerfully erotic. Regardless of the source of erotic stimuli, all stimulation has a physical basis, which is given meaning by the brain.

Physical Stimulation Physical stimulation comes through the senses: We are aroused by things we see, hear, taste, smell, and feel. It has even been suggested that we may be attracted and aroused by molecules of specific chemicals, called *pheromones,* that are produced by other people's bodies to create sexual excitement. Most often, sexual stimuli come from other people, but they may also come from books, photographs, paintings, songs, films, or other sources.

The most obvious and effective physical stimulation is touching. Even though culturally defined practices vary and individual people have different preferences, most sexual encounters eventually involve some form of touching with hands, lips, and body surfaces. Kissing, caressing, fondling, and hugging are as much a part of sexual encounters as they are of expressing affection.

The most intense form of stimulation by touching involves the genitals. The clitoris and the glans of the penis are particularly sensitive to such stimulation. Other highly responsive areas include the vaginal opening, the nipples, the breasts, the insides of the thighs, the buttocks, the anal region, the scrotum, the lips, and the earlobes. Such sexually sensitive areas, or **erogenous zones,** are especially susceptible to sexual arousal for most people, most of the time. Often, though, it's not *what* is touched but how, for how long, and by whom that determine the response. Under the right circumstances, touching any part of the body can cause sexual arousal.

Psychological Stimulation Sexual arousal also has an important psychological component, regardless of the nature of the physical stimulation. Fantasies, ideas, memories of past experiences, and mood can all generate sexual excitement. Erotic thoughts may be linked to an imagined person or situation or to a sexual experience from the past. Fantasies may involve activities a person doesn't actually wish to experience in reality, usually because they're dangerous, frightening, or forbidden.

Arousal is also powerfully influenced by emotions. How you feel about a person and how the person feels about you matter tremendously in how sexually responsive you are likely to be. Even the most direct forms of physical stimulation carry emotional overtones. Kissing, caressing, and fondling express affection and caring. The emotional charge they give to a sexual interaction is at least as significant to sexual arousal as the purely physical stimulation achieved by touching.

The Sexual Response Cycle

Noted sex researchers William Masters and Virginia Johnson were the first to describe in detail the human sexual response cycle. Men and women respond physiologically with a predictable set of reactions, regardless of the nature of the stimulation (Figure 5-4).

Two physiological mechanisms explain most genital and bodily reactions during sexual arousal and orgasm. These mechanisms are vasocongestion and myotonia. **Vasocongestion** is the engorgement of tissues that results when more blood flows into an organ than is flowing out. Thus, the penis becomes erect on the same principle that makes a garden hose become stiff when the water is turned on. **Myotonia** is increased muscular tension, which culminates in rhythmical muscular contractions during orgasm.

Four phases characterize the sexual response cycle:

1. In the *excitement phase,* the penis becomes erect as its tissues become engorged with blood. The testes expand and are pulled upward within the scrotum. In women, the clitoris and the labia are similarly engorged with blood, and the vaginal walls become moist with lubricating fluid.

2. The *plateau phase* is an extension of the excitement phase. Reactions become more marked: In men, the penis becomes harder, and the testes larger. In women, the lower part of the vagina swells, while its upper end expands and vaginal lubrication increases.

3. In the *orgasmic phase,* or **orgasm,** rhythmic contractions occur along the man's penis, urethra, prostate gland, seminal vesicles, and muscles in the pelvic and anal regions. These involuntary muscular contractions lead to the ejaculation of **semen,** which consists of sperm cells from the testes and secretions from the prostate gland and seminal vesicles. In women, contractions occur in the lower part of the vagina and in the uterus, as well as in the pelvic region and the anus.

4. In the *resolution phase,* all the changes initiated during the excitement phase are reversed. Excess blood drains from tissues, the muscles in the region relax, and the genital structures return to their unstimulated state.

More general physical reactions accompany the genital changes in both men and women. Beginning with the excitement phase, nipples become erect, the woman's breasts begin to swell, and in both sexes the skin of the chest becomes flushed; these changes are more marked in women. The heart rate doubles by the plateau phase, and respiration becomes faster. During orgasm, breathing becomes irregular and the person may moan or cry out. A feeling of warmth leads to increased sweating during the resolution phase. Deep relaxation and a sense of well-being pervade the body and the mind.

Male and female reactions during the sexual response cycle differ somewhat. Generally, the male pattern is more uniform, whereas the female pattern is more varied. For instance, the female excitement phase may lead directly to orgasm, or orgasmic and plateau phases may be fused.

Male orgasm is marked by the ejaculation of semen. After ejaculation, men enter a *refractory period,* during which they cannot be restimulated to orgasm. Women do not have a refractory period, and immediate restimulation to orgasm is possible.

WWW. Sexual Problems

Both physical and psychological factors can interfere with sexual functioning. If you are in poor physical health or experiencing high levels of stress or anxiety, sexual functioning may be negatively affected. Difficulties may be caused by infection and other sexual health problems. Disturbances in sexual desire, performance, or satisfaction are referred to as **sexual dysfunctions.**

Common Sexual Health Problems Some problems with sexual functioning are due to treatable or preventable infections or other sexual health problems. Conditions that affect women include the following:

- *Vaginitis,* inflammation of the vagina, is caused by a variety of organisms: *Candida* (yeast infection), *Trichomonas* (trichomoniasis), and the overgrowth of a variety of bacteria (bacterial vaginosis). Symptoms include vaginal discharge, vaginal irritation, and pain during intercourse. (See Chapters 17 and 18 for more on yeast infection, trichomoniasis, and bacterial vaginosis.)

- *Endometriosis* is the growth of endometrial tissue (tissue normally found lining the uterus) outside of the uterus. It occurs most often in women of childbearing age, and pain in the lower abdomen and pelvis is the most common symptom. Painful premenstrual intercourse may occur. Endometriosis can cause serious problems if left untreated because the endometrial tissue can scar and partially or completely block the oviducts, causing infertility (difficulty conceiving) or sterility (the inability to conceive). Endometriosis is treated with hormone therapy and/or surgery.

- *Pelvic inflammatory disease (PID)* is an infection of the uterus, oviducts, or ovaries, caused when microorganisms spread to these areas from the vagina.

erogenous zone Any region of the body highly responsive to sexual stimulation.

vasocongestion The accumulation of blood in tissues and organs.

myotonia Increased muscular tension.

orgasm The discharge of accumulated sexual tension with characteristic genital and bodily manifestations and a subjective sensation of intense pleasure.

semen Seminal fluid, consisting of sperm cells and secretions from the prostate gland and seminal vesicles.

sexual dysfunction A disturbance in sexual desire, performance, or satisfaction.

Terms

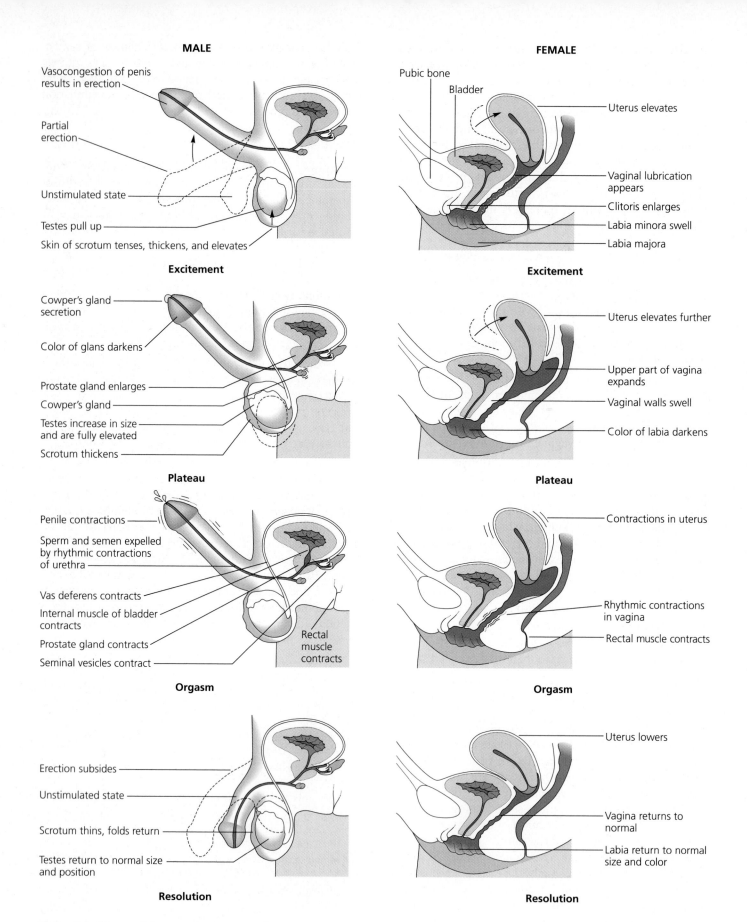

MALE

Vasocongestion of penis results in erection

Partial erection

Unstimulated state

Testes pull up

Skin of scrotum tenses, thickens, and elevates

Excitement

Cowper's gland secretion

Color of glans darkens

Prostate gland enlarges

Cowper's gland

Testes increase in size and are fully elevated

Scrotum thickens

Plateau

Penile contractions

Sperm and semen expelled by rhythmic contractions of urethra

Vas deferens contracts

Internal muscle of bladder contracts

Prostate gland contracts

Seminal vesicles contract

Rectal muscle contracts

Orgasm

Erection subsides

Unstimulated state

Scrotum thins, folds return

Testes return to normal size and position

Resolution

FEMALE

Pubic bone

Bladder

Uterus elevates

Vaginal lubrication appears

Clitoris enlarges

Labia minora swell

Labia majora

Excitement

Uterus elevates further

Upper part of vagina expands

Vaginal walls swell

Color of labia darkens

Plateau

Contractions in uterus

Rhythmic contractions in vagina

Rectal muscle contracts

Orgasm

Uterus lowers

Vagina returns to normal

Labia return to normal size and color

Resolution

Figure 5-4   Stages of the sexual response cycle.

Approximately 50–75% of PID cases are caused by sexually transmitted organisms associated with diseases such as gonorrhea and chlamydia. PID can cause scarring of the oviducts, resulting in infertility or sterility. Symptoms include pain in the abdomen and pelvis, fever, and possibly pain during intercourse. (Sexually transmitted diseases are discussed in detail in Chapter 18.)

Sexual health problems that affect men include the following:

- *Prostatitis* is inflammation or infection of the prostate gland. Symptoms are fever, chills, pain in the genital region, frequent urination, and, in some cases, painful ejaculation. More common in men over 40, prostatitis is treated with antibiotics.

- *Testicular cancer* occurs most commonly in men in their twenties and thirties. A rare cancer, it has a very high cure rate if detected early. A testicular self-exam should be performed regularly (see Chapter 16).

Sexual Dysfunctions The term *sexual dysfunction* encompasses disturbances in sexual desire, performance, or satisfaction. A wide variety of physical conditions and drugs may interfere with sexual functioning; psychological causes and problems in intimate relationships can be important factors in some cases. The same two mechanisms—vasocongestion and myotonia—that are the basis of the sexual response cycle are also at the root of the main forms of sexual disturbance: an inability to become aroused and problems experiencing orgasm.

COMMON SEXUAL DYSFUNCTIONS Common sexual dysfunctions in men include **erectile dysfunction** (previously called impotence), the inability to have or maintain an erection sufficient for sexual intercourse; **premature ejaculation**, ejaculation before or just on penetration of the vagina or anus; and **retarded ejaculation,** the inability to ejaculate once an erection is achieved. Many men experience occasional difficulty achieving an erection or ejaculating because of excessive alcohol consumption, fatigue, or stress. In fact, it is estimated that 50% of all American men experience occasional bouts of erectile dysfunction and retarded ejaculation.

Two sexual dysfunctions in women are **vaginismus,** in which the woman experiences painful involuntary muscular spasms when sexual intercourse is attempted, and **orgasmic dysfunction,** the inability to experience orgasm. Vaginismus is a conditioned reflex probably related to fear of intercourse. Orgasmic dysfunction has been the subject of a great deal of discussion over the years, as people debated the nature of the female orgasm and what constitutes dysfunction in women. Many women experience orgasm but not during intercourse, or they experience orgasm during intercourse only if the clitoris is directly stimulated at the same time. In general, the inability to experience orgasm under certain circumstances is a problem only if the woman considers it so.

TREATING SEXUAL DYSFUNCTION Most forms of sexual dysfunction are treatable. The first step is to have a thorough physical examination to identify any underlying medical condition that may be responsible for the problem. Heart disease and diabetes, for example, may cause erectile dysfunction; in fact, up to 80% of all erectile problems are thought to be due to physical factors, particularly vascular problems involving restriction of blood flow. Smoking affects blood vessels and blood flow in the penis and is an independent risk factor for erectile dysfunction. Drugs and medications, especially alcohol and medications used to treat high blood pressure, may also inhibit sexual responses.

If physical problems continue to interfere with sexual response, many treatments are available, particularly for erectile dysfunction. Older treatments include a variety of methods that induce blood flow into the penis—vacuum pumps or drugs that are injected directly into the penis or inserted into the urethra in pellet form—and rigid or inflatable implants. In 1998, Viagra (sildenafil citrate), the first-ever prescription pill for erectile dysfunction, was introduced; it quickly became the most successful new prescription drug in history. Viagra doesn't cause an erection, but it enhances blood flow into the penis, thereby allowing an erection when sexual stimulation occurs. It has been shown to be effective in as many as 70% of men with erectile dysfunction, allowing them to achieve erections comparable for their age group. It does not enhance sex drive or sexual response in men who can already achieve an erection.

If no physical problem is found, a sexual dysfunction may be psychosocial in origin. Psychosocial causes of dysfunction include troubled relationships, a lack of sexual skills, irrational attitudes and beliefs, anxiety, and psychosexual trauma, such as sexual abuse or rape. Many of these problems can be addressed by sex therapy methods that seek to modify the beliefs and behavior patterns that are interfering with satisfactory sexual relationships. A therapist may recommend books or films to help counter sexual myths and teach sexual skills. A therapist can also promote open discussion between partners and suggest specific activities or techniques. For example, premature ejaculation is often treated by the squeeze technique, in which the tip of the penis is squeezed when the man feels he is about to ejaculate.

erectile dysfunction The inability to have or maintain an erection.

premature ejaculation Involuntary orgasm before or shortly after the penis enters the vagina or anus; ejaculation that takes place sooner than desired.

retarded ejaculation The inability to ejaculate when one wishes to during intercourse.

vaginismus Painful, involuntary muscular contractions in the vagina that occur when sexual intercourse is attempted.

orgasmic dysfunction The inability to experience orgasm.

Terms

Women who seek treatment for orgasmic dysfunction often have not had the chance to learn through trial and error what types of stimulation will excite them and bring them to orgasm. Most sex therapists prefer to treat this problem with **masturbation** (genital self-stimulation). Women are taught about their own anatomy and sexual responses and then are encouraged to experiment with masturbation until they experience orgasm. Once they can masturbate to orgasm, they can transfer this learning to sexual intercourse with a partner. The use of Viagra has been studied in women, but it was not found to be more effective than a placebo; other substances being tested for the treatment of female sexual dysfunction include prostaglandin creams and testosterone patches. Another option is a device recently approved by the FDA that creates suction over the clitoris in order to increase blood flow and sensation.

Sexual problems are closely tied to emotional and psychological concerns and with a person's perceptions, thoughts, beliefs, values, and relationships with others.

COMMUNICATE! Many people have difficulty asking their physician questions about sexual matters, especially sexual functioning, yet physicians are usually an excellent resource for information and help. If you have questions you'd like answered, try writing them down as they occur to you. A week or two before you see your physician, read them out loud at home to get used to the idea of talking about them. Bring the list with you to your appointment. Try beginning with something that's easy to say, such as, "Doctor, I have a couple of questions I'd like to ask you."

WW. SEXUAL BEHAVIOR

Many behaviors stem from sexual impulses, and sexual expression takes a variety of forms. Probably the most basic aspect of sexuality is reproduction, the process of producing offspring. As important as reproduction is, the intention of creating a child accounts for only a small measure of sexual activity; most people have sex for other reasons as well.

Sexual excitement and satisfaction are aspects of sexual behavior separate from reproduction. The intensely pleasurable sensations of arousal and orgasm are probably the strongest motivators for human sexual behavior. People are infinitely varied in the ways they seek to experience erotic pleasure. In this section, we examine how sexual behavior develops and take a closer look at different sexual behaviors.

The Development of Sexual Behavior

Sexual behavior is a product of many factors, including genetics, physiology, psychology, and social and cultural influences. Our behavior is shaped by the interplay of our biological predispositions and our learning experiences throughout life.

Gender Roles and Gender Identity   The term *gender* is usually used to refer to the state of being male or female; people often use the word *sex* to mean the same thing. Strictly speaking, *sex* refers only to being biologically male or female, while *gender* encompasses both your biological sex and your masculine or feminine behaviors. As mentioned in Chapter 4, your gender role is everything you do in your daily life that expresses your maleness or femaleness to others, including dress, speech patterns, and mannerisms. Your **gender identity** is your personal, inner sense of being male or female.

Biological sex, gender role, and gender identity are usually in agreement, but some people experience conflict among them. For example, a male who feels trapped in the body of a male and who wants to be a female may exhibit the gender role of a male, but his gender identity is that of a female. The umbrella term *transgender* is often used to describe any individual whose appearance, personal characteristics, or behavior differ from the social and cultural norms for males and females. Transgendered individuals include the following:

- Transsexual men and women, who feel their biological sex does not match their gender identity. Transsexuals may seek sex reassignment, which involves surgery to change the appearance of the genitals and hormonal treatments to induce secondary sex characteristics such as breasts or facial hair.

- Cross-dressers ("transvestites"), who enjoy wearing clothing identified with the other gender. Cross-dressing covers a broad range of behaviors, from wearing one article of clothing of the other sex in a private location to wearing an entire outfit in public.

- Intersexed individuals, who were born with ambiguous genitals—neither fully female nor fully male—due to genetic or hormonal abnormalities. Intersexed individuals may or may not have undergone surgery as infants to assign them to a particular sex.

- Men or women, regardless of sexual orientation, whose appearance, characteristics, or behavior is perceived as gender atypical in their society or culture.

Terms
masturbation Self-stimulation for the purpose of sexual arousal and orgasm.

gender identity A person's personal, internal sense of maleness or femaleness.

BIOLOGICAL AND CULTURAL INFLUENCES   Some gender characteristics are determined biologically, such as the genitals a person is born with and the secondary sex characteristics that develop at puberty. Others are defined by society and learned in the course of growing up. From birth, children are encouraged to behave in ways their culture deems appropriate for one sex or the other. In our society, parents usually give children gender-specific names, clothes, and toys, and children may model their own behavior after their same-sex parent. People are far more likely to tell a boy why the car is accelerating and a girl why the cookies aren't chewy. Family and friends create an environment that teaches the child how to act appropriately as a girl or a boy. Teachers, television, books, and even strangers model these gender roles.

Gender roles vary from one society to another and from one time to another. In the United States today, for example, many women shave their legs and wear makeup; in Muslim countries, women wear robes and veils that conceal their face and body. Each set of behaviors expresses some learned aspect of the female gender role in that society, and each set would be inappropriate in the other society. Standards of sexual attractiveness also vary from one culture to another; see the box "Attracting a Partner in Different Cultures."

An extreme example of how cultural traditions can affect gender roles and sexual activity is female genital mutilation, a procedure often called "female circumcision." In over 20 African countries, some parts of Asia and the Middle East, and immigrant communities elsewhere, female infants, children, or young women may undergo a procedure in which parts of the clitoris and labia are removed. In some procedures, only the hood of the clitoris is removed. In others, the entire clitoris, labia minora, and parts of the labia majora are removed. The sides of the labia majora may be sewn together, leaving only a small opening for the passage of urine and menstrual blood. The effects of these painful procedures can include bleeding, infection, the inability to enjoy sex, and infertility.

The practice probably developed as a way of controlling women's sexuality and ensuring that a woman would be a virgin at the time of marriage. Upon marriage, the husband reopens the labia to allow intercourse and childbirth. It is interesting to note that surgery to remove all or part of the clitoris was practiced by physicians in the nineteenth century in both England and the United States, primarily as a "cure" for masturbation.

Many countries, including the United Kingdom, Sweden, and Belgium, now have laws against female genital mutilation, and the World Health Organization and other groups are trying to educate people about the negative medical consequences of the procedures.

GENDER-ROLE FLEXIBILITY   Historically, gender roles have tended to highlight and emphasize the differences between males and females, but new gender roles are

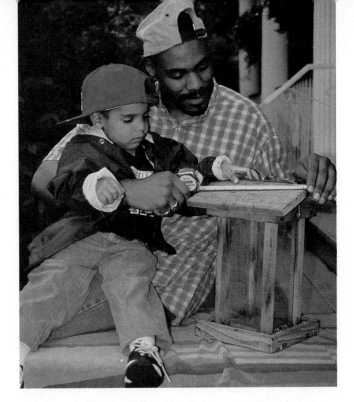

Our sense of gender identity and many of our gender-role behaviors are overwhelmingly influenced by cultural factors. This young boy is learning gender-specific behaviors by imitating his father.

emerging in our society that reflect more of a mix of male and female characteristics and behaviors. This tendency toward *androgyny* greatly broadens the range of experiences available to both males and females. Androgynous adults are less stereotyped in their thinking; in how they look, dress, and act; in how they divide work in the home; in how they think about jobs and careers; and in how they express themselves sexually. Women today are able, and even expected, to be much more assertive, competitive, ambitious, and powerful than they were allowed to be in the past; likewise, men can be more sensitive, articulate, nurturing, and emotionally expressive.

Gender, Sexuality, and the Mass Media   Many of our ideas about sexuality and gender roles are shaped by the mass media. Television, movies, music, magazines, and advertisements are awash with sexual images. These images are usually of young, sexy people promising passionately fulfilling relationships. Women and men are often portrayed in traditional gender roles, with provocatively dressed women in need of protection interacting with aggressive and muscular men.

Media images of sexuality are often more influential than the family in shaping the sexual attitudes and behavior of adolescents and college students. Yet these images are usually unrealistic and help perpetuate stereotypes of women and men in our society. The mass media rarely portray people negotiating safer sex or communicating seriously about other sexual issues.

While each of us has our own standard of what physical characteristics we consider to be beautiful or handsome, most of us could agree on what is attractive in our culture today. Standards of beauty change over time within a given culture, and standards of attractiveness vary across different cultures. Here's how partners are attracted in two cultures.

A man in the southeastern United States is getting ready for a date. He really wants to impress her tonight, so he puts on his best slacks and new shirt. He dabs on extra after-shave lotion, brushes his teeth for the second time, rinses with mouthwash, and makes sure his well-washed hair is held in place with a bit of hair spray. He's ready.

Thousands of miles away on a remote island in Southeast Asia, another man is getting ready to court a potential mate. He lives on one of the Sulu Islands in the southern Philippines. He has put heavily scented wax on his hair and put white powder on his face. He checks his pinky fingernail and is satisfied that it has grown very long in the past few weeks. He is pleased with the color of nail polish on it. He is dressed in very loose-fitting clothes that reveal his genitals. He's ready.

Back in the United States, a woman is using a multitude of cosmetics—powders, lipstick, hair spray, perfume, eyeliner, and eye shadow—in preparation for her date. She has purchased a nice dress with matching shoes especially for tonight, and her hair is in a new and different style. She's ready.

The potential mate of the man in the Philippines is very excited about meeting him tonight. She will go with other young women and men to the local beach for conversation and the playing of music. Like other women in her culture, she does not wash her hair often, but frequently combs coconut oil through it. Men find this very sexy, and she is happy with the amount of oil in her hair. She puts on some white face powder and perfume, touches up her nail polish, and then puts on lipstick. She is pleased with her appearance and decides to put a spot of lipstick on each cheek. She's ready.

Obviously, each of the cultures described above has its own standard of attractiveness, but it's also clear that there are similarities. In both cases the women use perfume and pay particular attention to their hair. The men also use scent in an attempt to attract a mate. Although cultural standards differ in some ways, we are all intent on securing the most attractive mate, in our own eyes, that we can.

SOURCE: Nimmo, H. A. 1991. Bajau sex and reproduction. In *Human Sexuality: Cross-Cultural Readings*, ed. B. du Toit. New York: McGraw-Hill.

Childhood Sexual Behavior   The capacity to respond sexually is present at birth. Ultrasound studies suggest that boys experience erections in the uterus. After birth, both sexes have the capacity for orgasm, though many babies may not experience it. As people grow, many discover this capacity through self-exploration. Sexual behaviors gradually emerge in childhood; self-exploration and touching the genitals are common forms of play, observed among infants as young as 6 months. They gradually lead to more deliberate forms of masturbation, with or without orgasm.

Children often engage in sexual play with playmates by exploring each other's genitals. These activities are often part of games like "playing house" or "playing doctor." By age 12, 40% of boys have engaged in sex play; the peak exploration age for girls is 9, by which time 14% have had such experiences.

COMMUNICATE!   Parents are often embarrassed to talk about sex with their children and adolescents, yet honest and factual discussions of sexuality are among the most important conversations to have with children. Many experts advise giving the very youngest children short and simple answers that respond only to their immediate concerns and adding details as they mature. Choose one topic, like intercourse or homosexuality, and practice what you would say to open a conversation with your own child about it.

Adolescent Sexuality   A person who has experienced puberty is biologically an adult. But in psychological and social terms, people take 5–10 more years to attain full adult status. This discrepancy between biological and social maturity creates considerable confusion over what constitutes appropriate sexual behavior during adolescence.

Sexual fantasies and dreams become more common and explicit in adolescence than at earlier ages, often as an accompaniment to masturbation. Research has shown that about 80% of teenage boys and 55% of teenage girls masturbate more or less regularly. Once puberty is reached, orgasm in boys is accompanied by ejaculation. Teenage boys also experience **nocturnal emissions** ("wet dreams"). Some girls also have orgasmic dreams. In general, masturbation does not carry the social stigma and imagined perils of former times, but adolescents—and many adults as well—are often still embarrassed by it.

Sexual interaction during adolescence usually takes place between peers in the context of dating. Sexual intimacy is usually expressed in such relationships through petting and necking, which may involve kissing, caressing, and stimulating the breasts and genitals. These activities lead to arousal but may not culminate in orgasm.

Many American teenagers also engage in premarital sexual relations. Recent surveys indicate that the average age of first sexual intercourse is about 17.2 years for girls and 16.6 years for boys; among high school students,

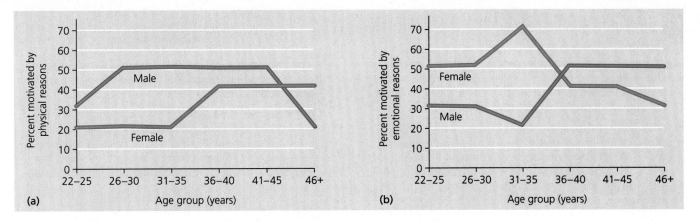

Figure 5-5 Motivations for engaging in sex by age and gender. (a) The physical motive.
(b) The emotional motive.   SOURCES: Data from Laumann, E., et al. 1994. *The Social Organization of Sexual-ity: Sexual Practices in the United States*. Chicago: University of Chicago Press. Sprague, J., and D. Quadagno. 1989. Gender and sexual motivation. *Journal of Psychology and Human Sexuality* 2: 57–76.

48.8% of males and 47.7% of females report that they have had sexual intercourse. Rates for premarital sex vary considerably from one group to another, however, based on ethnic, educational, socioeconomic, religious, geographic, and other factors. Engaging in sexual intercourse for the first time is affected by these same factors, plus psychological readiness, fear of consequences, being in love, going steady, peer pressure, and the need to act like an adult, gain popularity, or rebel. Some people thoughtfully weigh decisions and others plunge recklessly.

Adolescent sexual behaviors are not confined to heterosexual relationships. Beginning in childhood, sex play involves members of one's own sex as well as of the other sex. Homosexual attractions, with or without sexual encounters, are likewise common in adolescence. For many these are youthful experiments and don't mean that participants will ultimately be homosexual. For a minority they may be a factor in adult sexual orientation. Most adult gay men and women trace their preferences to their early years.

Adult Sexuality   Early adulthood is a time when people make important life choices—a time of increasing responsibility in terms of interpersonal relationships and family life (see the box "Sexual Decision Making"). In recent years, both in the United States and abroad, there has been a definite trend toward marriage at a later age than in past decades. And before marriage, more young adults are driven by an internal need to become sexually knowledgeable. Today, more people in their twenties believe that becoming sexually experienced rather than preserving virginity is an important prelude to selecting a mate. Take the quiz in the box "Your Sexual Attitudes" to explore your own beliefs and opinions about sex.

A survey investigating women's and men's motivations for engaging in sexual activities found that motivations

change with age (Figure 5-5). Younger men state that they engage in sex for physical reasons, while women of the same age state that they engage in sex for emotional reasons. As men and women get older, their motives change; men more often engage in sex for emotional reasons, and women more often for physical reasons. In the oldest age groups, women and men actually switch their motives for sex from those of the earliest age groups.

Adult sexuality can include any of the sexual behaviors and practices described in this chapter. In mature love relationships, people ideally can integrate all the aspects of intimacy—physical, sexual, emotional—so that sexuality is a deeply meaningful part of how they express love.

Sexuality in Illness and Disability   Any disease or disability that affects mobility, well-being, self-esteem, or body image has the potential to affect sexual expression. People with chronic diseases or disabilities often have special needs regarding their sexual behavior. They must also confront widespread myths that they are asexual. In our culture, only people conforming to a narrow standard of youth, attractiveness, and ability are seen as sexual beings. But sexuality is integral to all of us, regardless of our physical status.

The diagnosis of a chronic illness or the onset of a disability usually requires major adjustments in many areas of life, including sexuality. At first, sexual activity may take a low priority because of fear and the loss of self-esteem. Individuals and couples can learn to become creative about sexual expression and develop new approaches based on the limitations of the disability.

nocturnal emissions Orgasm and ejaculation (wet dream) during sleep.

Terms

Choosing to have sex can change a relationship and an individual's life. In making decisions about sexual activity, you owe it to yourself and your partner to honestly think and talk about your choices. Consider the following issues:

- *Your background, beliefs, and goals.* What are your religious, moral, and/or personal values regarding relationships and sex? What are your priorities at this time, and how will a sexual relationship fit into your goals and plans for the future? Are you physically, emotionally, and financially ready to accept the potential consequences of the choices you make? How will you feel if you act in ways that are not consistent with your values and goals?

- *Your relationship with your partner.* How do you feel about your partner and your relationship? Do you respect and trust one another? Do you feel comfortable talking about sexual issues, and have you discussed contraception, preg-

nancy, and safer sex? How do you think having sex will affect your relationship and how you feel about yourself and your partner? What does having sex mean to each of you?

- *Your reasons for having sex.* Are you feeling pressured to have sex? Are you afraid of losing your partner if you say no? Are you too embarrassed, shy, or insecure to say no or discuss waiting? Are you being honest with yourself and your partner about your reasons for moving into a sexual relationship?

Personal decisions about sex should always be respected. You have the right to make your own choices and to do only what you feel comfortable with. When you make choices about sex based on self-respect, along with physical, emotional, and spiritual considerations, you'll be more likely to feel good about your decisions—now and in the future—and to enhance your health and well-being.

Developing a positive body image is often a particularly important, and difficult, adjustment for people with physical illness or limitations.

Sexual Orientation

As discussed in Chapter 4, sexual orientation is a consistent pattern of emotional and sexual attraction based on biological sex. It exists along a continuum that ranges from exclusive heterosexuality (attraction to people of the other sex) through bisexuality (attraction to people of both sexes) to exclusive homosexuality (attraction to people of one's own sex). The terms *straight* and *gay* are often used to refer to heterosexuals and homosexuals, respectively, and female homosexuals are also referred to as lesbians. Sexual orientation involves feelings and self-concept, and individuals may or may not express their sexual orientation in their behavior.

In a national survey, 2–5% of men had engaged in homosexual sex at some point in their lives, and 1–3% identified themselves as homosexuals. Of the women surveyed, 4% stated that they had engaged in homosexual sex at some point in their lives, and 1.5% identified themselves as homosexuals. These numbers are lower than in past surveys. But do people tell the truth in surveys that probe very sensitive and private aspects of their lives? This question is always an issue.

Heterosexuality   The great majority of people are heterosexual. The heterosexual lifestyle usually includes all the behavior and relationship patterns described in Chapter 4: dating, engagement and/or living together, and marriage.

Homosexuality   Homosexuality exists in almost all cultures. Many homosexual couples form long-lasting close and stable ties (refer to Chapter 4 for information on same-sex marriage and civil unions). The lifestyle of homosexual people depends largely on whether they are open about their sexual orientation. Those who feel forced to be secretive may lead a double life, one public and one private. Those who have "come out" participate more actively in gay activities and organizations.

Some people are threatened or upset by homosexuality, perhaps because homosexuals are viewed as different or because no one is sure how sexual orientation develops. The "gay liberation" movement of the 1970s and 1980s helped dispel some of the historical prejudice against gays and lesbians, but homosexuality still has not received widespread societal approval. In extreme cases, irrational fear or hatred of homosexuals—known as **homophobia**—causes people to discriminate against or even attack homosexuals.

The major difference between heterosexuals and homosexuals is in their choice of sex partners. Homosexual individuals are as different and varied from each other as are heterosexuals. Just like heterosexuals, lesbians and gay men may be in long-term, committed relationships or they may date different people. They have the same responsibilities and concerns as anyone else. They have job commitments, they raise children, and they seek to fulfill their potential in all areas of their lives. For homosexuals,

For each statement, circle the response that most closely reflects your position.

	Agree	Not Sure	Disagree
1. Sex education encourages young people to have sex.	1	2	3
2. Homosexuality is a healthy, normal expression of sexuality.	3	2	1
3. Members of the other sex will think more highly of you if you remain mysterious.	1	2	3
4. It's better to wait until marriage to have sex.	1	2	3
5. Abortion should be a personal, private choice for a woman.	3	2	1
6. It's natural for men to have more sexual freedom than women.	1	2	3
7. Condoms should not be made available to teenagers.	1	2	3
8. Access to pornography should not be restricted for adults.	3	2	1
9. A woman who is raped usually does something to provoke it.	1	2	3
10. Contraception is the woman's responsibility.	1	2	3
11. Feminism has had a positive influence on society.	3	2	1
12. Masturbation is a healthy expression of sexuality.	3	2	1
13. I have many friends of the other sex.	3	2	1
14. Prostitution should be legalized.	3	2	1
15. Women use sex for love; men use love for sex.	1	2	3
16. Our society is too sexually permissive.	1	2	3
17. The man should be the undisputed head of the household.	1	2	3
18. Having sex just for pleasure is OK.	3	2	1

Scoring

Add up the numbers you circled to obtain your overall score.

1–18   Traditional attitude about sexuality

19–36   Ambivalent or mixed attitude about sexuality

37–54   Open, progressive attitude about sexuality

---

bisexuals, and heterosexuals, sexual expression is but one facet of human experience.

Bisexuality   Some bisexual individuals are involved with partners of both sexes at the same time, while others may alternate between same-sex partners and partners of the other sex ("serial bisexuality"). HIV infection is a risk associated with bisexuality, particularly in cases where bisexual men don't disclose their sexual orientation to their female partners. The largest group of bisexuals are married men who have secret sexual involvements with men but who rarely have female sexual contacts outside marriage.

The Origins of Sexual Orientation   Many theories have been proposed to account for the development of sexual orientation. Biological theories have focused on genetic and hormonal influences. One study found structural differences between homosexual and heterosexual men in the brain region that controls sexual behavior. It remains unclear, however, whether this anatomical variation represents a cause or a result of sexual orientation. Another possible influence is differing levels of prenatal hormones, which may affect fetal brain development.

Evidence for a genetic basis for sexual orientation was provided by a recent study of 108 sets of female twins in which at least one twin was a lesbian. Researchers found that among the identical twins, both twins were lesbians in 48% of the cases; for the nonidentical twins, both twins were lesbians in 16% of the cases. Among adopted girls with a lesbian sister, only 6% of the adoptive siblings were homosexual. Although these results may suggest a genetic component to sexual orientation, other influences must also operate because identical twins do not all share the same orientation. There is no evidence that sexual orientation is determined solely by biological or genetic factors.

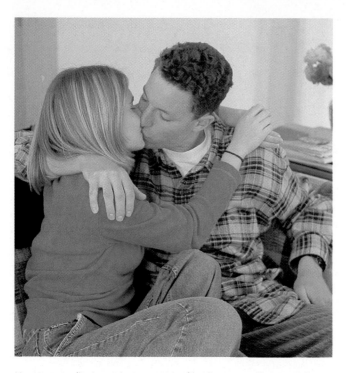

Human sexuality is not just a matter of bodies responding to each other. This couple's physical experiences together will be powerfully affected by their emotions, ideas, and values and by the quality of their relationship.

Many psychological theories have also been proposed. Researchers have looked at how much contact children have with members of the two sexes, at the types of relationships children have with their parents, and at family dynamics. Early negative experiences with heterosexuality or positive experiences with homosexuality have also been proposed as possible influences. The significant growth of single-parent families over the past 40 years has not been accompanied by large shifts in sexual orientation among Americans, so it is unlikely that family dynamics or early learning experiences are strong factors in determining sexual orientation.

Most scientists today agree that sexual orientation is most likely the result of the complex interaction of biological, psychological, and social factors, possibly different in the case of each individual.

Varieties of Human Sexual Behavior

Most people express their sexuality in a variety of ways. Some sexual behaviors are aimed at self-stimulation only, such as masturbation, while other practices involve interaction with others in behaviors such as kissing and intercourse. Some people choose not to express their sexuality and practice celibacy instead.

Celibacy   Continuous abstention from sexual activities, termed **celibacy,** can be a conscious and deliberate choice, or it can be necessitated by circumstances. Health

considerations and religious and moral beliefs may lead some people to celibacy, particularly until marriage or until an acceptable partner appears. A disadvantage of the celibate life is that it may lack physical contact and affection.

Many people use the related term *abstinence* to refer to avoidance of just one sexual activity—intercourse. The use of abstinence to prevent pregnancy and sexually transmitted diseases is discussed in Chapters 6 and 18.

Autoeroticism and Masturbation   The most common form of **autoeroticism** is **erotic fantasy,** creating imaginary experiences that range from fleeting thoughts to elaborate scenarios. Fantasies may be replays of past sexual experiences or fabrications based on unfulfilled wishes or taken from books, drawings, or photographs.

Masturbation involves manually stimulating the genitals, rubbing them against objects (such as a pillow), or using stimulating devices such as vibrators. Although commonly associated with adolescence, masturbation is practiced by many throughout adult life. It may be used as a substitute for sexual intercourse or as part of sexual activity with a partner. Masturbation gives a person control over the pace, time, and method of sexual release and pleasure. On average, two out of three college students masturbate a few times a week, others do it more or less frequently, and some don't do it at all.

Touching and Foreplay   Tactile stimulation, or touching, is integral to sexual experiences, whether in the form of massage, kissing, fondling, or holding. Our entire body surface is a sensory organ, and touching almost anywhere can enhance intimacy and sexual arousal. As mentioned earlier, some body areas, the erogenous zones, are much more sensitive to touch as a sexual stimulus than others. Touching can convey a variety of messages, including affection, comfort, and a desire for further sexual contact.

During arousal, many men and women manually and orally stimulate each other by touching, stroking, and caressing their partner's genitals. Men and women vary greatly in their preferences for the type, pacing, and vigor of such **foreplay.** Working out the details to accommodate each other's pleasure is a key to enjoying these activities. Direct communication about preferences can enhance sexual pleasure and protect both partners from physical and psychological discomfort.

Oral-Genital Stimulation   **Cunnilingus** (the stimulation of the female genitals with the lips and tongue) and **fellatio** (the stimulation of the penis with the mouth) are quite common practices. Although prevalence varies in different populations, 70–90% of men and women report that they have engaged in oral sex. Oral sex may be practiced either as part of foreplay or as a sex act culminating in orgasm. Like all acts of sexual expression between two people, oral sex requires the cooperation and consent of both partners. If they disagree about its acceptability, they need to discuss their feelings and try to reach a mutually pleasing solution.

Anal Intercourse   About 10% of heterosexuals and 50% of homosexual males regularly practice anal stimulation and penetration by the penis or a finger. The receiver does not usually reach orgasm from anal intercourse, though men usually experience orgasm while penetrating. Many people have strongly negative attitudes toward anal sex because they consider it unclean, unnatural, or unappealing. Because the anus is composed of delicate tissues that tear easily under such pressure, anal intercourse is one of the riskiest of sexual behaviors associated with the transmission of HIV and the bacteria that cause gonorrhea and syphilis. The use of condoms is highly recommended for anyone engaging in anal sex. Special care and precaution should be exercised if anal sex is practiced—cleanliness, lubrication, and gentle entry at the very least. Anything that is inserted into the anus should not subsequently be put into the vagina unless it has been thoroughly washed. Bacteria normally present in the anus can cause vaginal infections.

Sexual Intercourse   For most adults, most of the time, **sexual intercourse** is the ultimate sexual experience. Men and women engage in coitus—make love—to fulfill both sexual and psychological needs. The most common heterosexual practice is the man inserting his erect penis into the woman's dilated and lubricated vagina after sufficient arousal.

Much has been written on how to enhance pleasure through various coital techniques, positions, and practices. For a woman, the key factor in physical readiness for coitus is adequate vaginal lubrication, and in psychological readiness, being aroused and receptive. For a man, the setting and the partner must arouse him to attain and maintain an erection. Personal preferences vary, but most people prefer a safe, private setting. Candlelight and music, for example, can enhance the mood of the occasion. Psychological factors and the quality of the relationship are more important to overall sexual satisfaction than sophisticated or exotic sexual techniques.

Atypical and Problematic Sexual Behaviors

In American culture, many kinds of sexual behavior are accepted. However, some types of sexual expression are considered harmful; they may be against the law or classified as mental disorders, or both. Because sexual behavior occurs on a continuum, it is sometimes difficult to differentiate a behavior that is simply atypical from one that is harmful. When attempting to evaluate an unusual sexual behavior, experts consider the issues of consent between partners and whether physical or psychological harm is done to the individual or to others.

Sexual fantasies and behaviors that are consensual—agreed on by adult partners—but that are not statistically typical of American sexual behaviors are known as **atypical sexual behaviors.** An example of an atypical sexual behavior is the consensual use of sex toys. Those behaviors that are classified as mental disorders, or **paraphilias,** are characterized by recurring, intense sexual fantasies and urges that involve nonhuman objects, the suffering or humiliation of oneself or one's partner, or children or other nonconsenting individuals. Examples are peeping into strangers' homes, making obscene phone calls, and having sexual contact with children. The effects of paraphilic behavior on others range from minor upset to serious physical and long-term psychological harm.

The use of force and coercion in sexual relationships is one of the most serious problems in human interactions. The most extreme manifestation of **sexual coercion**—forcing a person to submit to another's sexual desires—is rape, but sexual coercion occurs in many more subtle forms, such as sexual harassment. Sexual coercion—including rape, the sexual abuse of children, and sexual harassment—is discussed in detail in Chapter 23.

Commercial Sex

Conflicting feelings about sexuality are apparent in the attitudes of Americans toward commercial sex: prostitution and sexually oriented materials such as videos, magazines, and books. Our society condemns sexually explicit material and prostitution, but it also provides their customers.

Pornography   Derived from the Greek word meaning "the writing of prostitutes," **pornography** is now often defined as obscene literature, art, or movies. A major problem in identifying pornographic material is that different

Terms

celibacy Continuous abstention from sexual activity.

autoeroticism Behavior aimed at sexual self-stimulation.

erotic fantasy Sexually arousing thoughts and daydreams.

foreplay Kissing, touching, and any form of oral or genital contact that stimulates people toward intercourse.

cunnilingus Oral stimulation of the female genitals.

fellatio Oral stimulation of the penis.

sexual intercourse Sexual relations involving genital union; also called *coitus,* and also known as making love.

atypical sexual behavior Consensual sexual behavior that is not statistically typical within a population.

paraphilia A mental disorder characterized by recurring, intense sexual fantasies and urges that involve nonhuman objects, the suffering or humiliation of oneself or one's partner, or children or other nonconsenting individuals.

sexual coercion The use of physical or psychological force or intimidation to make a person submit to sexual demands.

pornography The explicit or obscene depiction of sexual activities in pictures, writing, or other material.

About 15% of all Internet users report visiting sexual Internet sites. Most of these sites feature pornographic images and/or sexually oriented chat rooms. A survey of nearly 10,000 users of sexual Internet sites found that about the same number of men and women visit sexual sites; men are more likely to visit sites with visual images, while women are more likely to visit chat rooms. People in chat rooms may engage in a range of behaviors, from mild flirtation with a group of chat room visitors to private, real-time discussions of explicit sexual activities with another Internet user. Many cybersex participants report feeling some degree of sexual excitement; some masturbate while viewing erotic images online or engaging in sexual chat.

Research into cybersex has identified some potential benefits of easily available online sexual material. The anonymous nature of the Internet gives people a sense of freedom and allows them to try out different identities and to seek sexual fulfillment in ways that they would not feel comfortable doing in real life. They may feel freer to talk openly about their sexual concerns or fantasies. A great deal of factual information about sexual behavior, contraception, and STDs is available for people who might not otherwise access such information; sexually oriented products such as condoms are also easily obtainable. Online sexual information may facilitate candid discussions between partners. In addition, the Internet provides opportunities for social contact and support among people with special concerns who might otherwise feel isolated; for example, rape survivors, people with herpes, or people with disabilities can meet online to share experiences and discuss sexual issues with their peers.

However, cybersex can cause problems for some people. Surveys indicate that about 5–8% of people who use the Internet for sex spend more than 11 hours per week online, with some people spending more than 50 hours per week online for sexual pursuits. This group is much more likely to report problems with work or interpersonal relationships than are people who spend lesser amounts of time online (see Chapter 9 for more on compulsive and addictive behaviors). For people who already feel isolated and lonely, cybersex may increase their social isolation as they spend more time online and less time reaching out to others in person. Online sexual encounters may offer the illusion of intimacy, but they do not have all the complexities or all the benefits of long-term, real-world intimate relationships.

For people involved in committed relationships, cybersex may be viewed as emotional infidelity and a threat to the relationship. People are likely to feel betrayed if they discover their partner has secretly been investing time and energy in online sexual interaction with others. In addition, the availability of certain types of sexual materials may reinforce abusive or problematic behaviors. For example, people have used the Internet to obtain child pornography and to contact young people and solicit meetings.

As described in Chapter 4, some people use the Internet to look for intimate partners whom they can meet face to face. Although online interaction has some special advantages for meeting people, including the opportunity to focus on interests and values before physical appearance, there are also potential dangers. Refer to Chapter 4 for more on the potential benefits and costs of looking for intimate partnerships online.

SOURCES: Cooper, A., et al. 1999. Sexuality on the Internet: From sexual exploration to pathological expression. *Professional Psychology Research and Practice* 30(2). McClam, E. 2000. Cyber-sex addiction mushrooms in Internet climate of anonymity. *San Francisco Examiner*, May 6. Thompson, N. 2000. Sex in the digital city. *Washington Monthly*, July/August.

---

people and communities have different opinions about what is obscene. Differing definitions of obscenity have led to many legal battles over potentially pornographic materials. Currently, the sale and rental of pornographic materials is restricted so that only adults can legally obtain them; materials depicting children in sexual contexts are illegal in any format or setting.

The appearance of thousands of sexually oriented Web sites has expanded the number of people with access to pornographic materials and has made enforcing pornography laws more difficult. People who might have hesitated to buy magazines or rent videos in person can now access sexually explicit material privately and anonymously (see the box "Cybersex"). Of special concern is the increased availability of illegal materials such as child pornography that previously could be acquired only with great difficulty and at great legal risk. Web sites that sell pornography take in more than $1 billion each year, and there are many online newsgroups where visitors exchange materials for free. Adult Web sites typically have the warning "You must be 18 to enter," but these warnings are not effective if users can simply click a button to verify their age. More effective are screening software programs that can be installed on individual computers; these programs block access to adults-only Web sites and newsgroups. Other strategies to keep minors from accessing pornography online include subscription-based adult verification services and credit card requirements.

Many people distinguish between "soft porn" and "hard porn" materials. Soft porn, often marketed for couples, typically includes an apparently loving couple having sex in a relaxed setting. There is mutual kissing and touching, and both partners are shown as having a positive experience. In hard porn, there is usually little mu-

Terms   **prostitution** The exchange of sexual services for money.

To talk with your partner about sexuality, follow the general suggestions for effective communication given in Chapter 4. Getting started may be the most difficult part. Some people feel more comfortable if they begin by talking about talking—that is, initiating a discussion about why people are so uncomfortable talking about sexuality. Talking about sexual histories—how partners first learned about sex or how family and cultural background influenced sexual values and attitudes—is another way to get started. Reading about sex can also be a good beginning: Partners can read an article or book and then discuss their reactions.

Be honest about what you feel and what you want from your partner. Cultural and personal obstacles to discussing sexual subjects can be difficult to overcome, but self-disclosure is important for successful relationships. Research indicates that when one partner openly discusses attitudes and feelings, the other partner is more likely to do the same. If your partner seems hesitant to open up, try asking open-ended or either/or questions: "Where do you like to be touched?" or "Would you like to talk about this now or wait until later?"

If something is bothering you about your sexual relationship, choose a good time to initiate a discussion with your partner. Be specific and direct but also tactful. Focus on what you actually observe, rather than on what you think the behavior means. "You didn't touch or hug me when your friends were around" is an observation. "You're ashamed of me around your friends" is an inference about your partner's feelings. Try focusing on a specific behavior that concerns you rather than on the person as a whole—your partner can change behaviors but not his or her entire personality. For example, you could say, "I'd like you to take a few minutes away from studying to kiss me," instead of "You're so caught up in your work, you never have time for me."

If you are going to make a statement that your partner may interpret as criticism, try mixing it with something positive ("I love spending time with you, but I feel annoyed when you . . ."). On the other hand, if your partner says something that upsets you, don't lash back. An aggressive response may make you feel better in the short run, but it will not help the communication process or the quality of the relationship.

If you want to say no to some sexual activity, say no unequivocally. Don't send mixed messages. If you are afraid of hurting your partner's feelings, offer an alternative if it's appropriate—"I am uncomfortable with that. How about. . . ."

If you're in love, you may think that the sexual aspects of a relationship will work out magically without discussion. But partners who never talk about sex deny themselves the opportunity to increase their closeness and improve their relationship.

---

tual touching, and only the male appears to enjoy the experience. Hard porn sometimes explicitly depicts sexual violence and exploitation. Hard porn materials tend to be the focus of more criticism than soft porn materials.

Much of the debate about pornography focuses on whether it is harmful. Some people argue that adults who want to view pornographic materials in the privacy of their own homes should be allowed to do so. Others feel that the exposure to explicit sexual material can lead to delinquent or criminal behavior, such as rape or the sexual abuse of children. Currently, there is no reliable evidence that pornography by itself leads to violence or paraphilic behavior, and debate is likely to continue.

Prostitution   The exchange of sexual services for money is **prostitution**. Prostitutes may be men, women, or children, and the buyer of a prostitute's services is nearly always a man. Except in parts of Nevada, prostitution is illegal in the United States.

Sex with a prostitute provides the customer with sexual release without commitment, the expectation of intimacy, or the fear of rejection. Some men patronize prostitutes to have sex with a different type of partner than usual or to engage in a type of sex their usual partner will not permit. Most customers are white, middle-class, middle-aged, and married. Although they come from a wide variety of backgrounds, prostitutes are usually motivated to join the profession because of money.

AIDS is a major concern for prostitutes and their customers. Many prostitutes are injecting drug users or are involved with men who are. The rate of HIV infection among prostitutes varies widely, but in some parts of the country it is as high as 25–50%.

Responsible Sexual Behavior

Healthy sexuality is an important part of adult life. It can be a source of pleasurable experiences and emotions and an important part of intimate partnerships. But sexual behavior also carries many responsibilities, and you need to make choices about your sexuality that contribute to your well-being and that of your partner.

Open, Honest Communication   Each partner needs to clearly indicate what sexual involvement means to him or her. Does it mean love, fun, a permanent commitment, or something else? The intentions of both partners should be clear. For strategies on how to talk about sexual issues with your partner, refer to the box "Communicating About Sexuality."

Agreed-On Sexual Activities   No one should pressure or coerce a partner. Sexual behaviors should be consistent

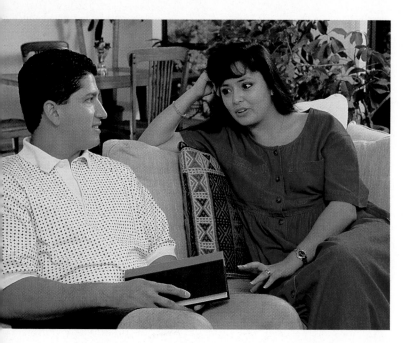

Sexual activity has many potential consequences, including pregnancy, disease, and emotional changes in the relationship. Responsible sexual behavior includes discussing these consequences openly and honestly.

with the sexual values, preferences, and comfort level of both partners. Everyone has the right to refuse sexual activity at any time.

Sexual Privacy   Intimate relationships involving sexual activity are based on trust, and that trust can be violated if partners reveal private information about the relationship to others. Sexual privacy also involves respecting other people—not engaging in activities in the presence of others that would make them uncomfortable. The question of how to handle bringing a partner back to a shared dorm room is something that many college students must address. Roommates should be respectful of one another and discuss the situation in advance to avoid embarrassing encounters.

Using Contraception   If pregnancy is not desired, contraception should be used during sexual intercourse. Both partners need to take responsibility for protecting against unwanted pregnancy. Partners should discuss contraception before sexual involvement begins. (See Chapter 6 for more information on contraception.)

Safer Sex   Both partners should be aware of and practice safer sex to guard against sexually transmitted diseases (STDs). Many sexual behaviors carry the risk of STDs, including HIV infection. Partners should be honest about their health and any medical conditions and work out a plan for protection. Behaviors that carry no risk of HIV infection are those that don't involve the exchange of

body fluids (blood, semen, and vaginal secretions). Anyone who is not in a mutually monogamous relationship with an uninfected partner and who wishes to have sex should always use a condom. (For more information on STDs and safer sex practices, see Chapter 18.)

Sober Sex   The use of alcohol or drugs in sexual situations increases the risk of unplanned, unprotected sexual activity. This is particularly true of young adults, many of whom engage in episodes of binge drinking during social events. The link between intoxication and unsafe sex is illustrated by a recent CDC study that found that states with higher drinking ages and higher beer taxes have lower rates of STDs. Alcohol and drugs impair judgment and should not be used in association with sexual activity.

Taking Responsibility for Consequences   Individuals should be aware of the physical and emotional consequences of their sexual behavior and accept responsibility for them. Consequences include pregnancy, STDs, and emotional changes in the relationship between partners.

Tips for Today

Wellness includes understanding and enjoying your own sexuality. This means understanding your sexual anatomy, physiology, and functioning; your sexual orientation; and the various ways of expressing your sexuality and of interacting sexually with others. A healthy sexual life is built on acceptance of yourself and good communication with your partner.

Right now you can

- Make a decision to deal with any sexual question or problem that you've been avoiding. Unless you're sure it's not a physical problem, begin by making an appointment with your physician.

- Take a few moments to reflect on and articulate to yourself exactly what your beliefs are about sexual relationships at this point in your life. Consider your values, emotions, plans, and resources; also consider whether you are acting in accordance with your beliefs.

- If you are in a sexual relationship, think about how you and your partner communicate about sex. If there's something you want to discuss, plan how you will broach the subject. Refer to the box "Communicating About Sexuality" for ideas on how to begin.

- If you are in a sexual relationship, ask yourself whether you are acting responsibly and in the best interest of yourself and your partner 100% of the time. For example, do you always respect each other's wishes and limits when it comes to sexual activity? Do you always avoid mixing sex and alcohol or drugs? If the answer to these or any similar questions is no, resolve to change that behavior.

SUMMARY

- The female external sex organs are called the vulva; the clitoris plays an important role in sexual arousal and orgasm. The vagina leads to the internal sex organs, including the uterus, oviducts, and ovaries.

- The male external sex organs are the penis and the scrotum; the glans of the penis is an important site of sexual arousal. Internal sexual structures include the testes, vasa deferentia, seminal vesicles, and prostate gland.

- The fertilizing sperm determines the sex of the individual. Specialized genes on the Y chromosome initiate the process of male sexual differentiation in the embryo.

- Hormones initiate the changes that occur during puberty: The reproductive system matures, secondary sex characteristics develop, and the bodies of males and females become more distinctive.

- The menstrual cycle consists of four phases: menses, the estrogenic phase, ovulation, and the progestational phase.

- The ovaries gradually cease to function as women approach age 50 and enter menopause. The pattern of male sexual responses changes with age, and testosterone production gradually decreases.

- Sexual activity is based on stimulus and response. Stimulation may be physical or psychological.

- Vasocongestion and myotonia are the primary physiological mechanisms of sexual arousal.

- The sexual response cycle has four stages: excitement, plateau, orgasm, and resolution.

- Physical and psychological problems can both interfere with sexual functioning. A treatment for sexual dysfunction first addresses any underlying medical conditions and then looks at psychosocial problems.

- Some gender characteristics are determined biologically, and others are defined by society. Children learn traits and behaviors traditionally deemed appropriate for one sex or the other.

- The ability to respond sexually is present at birth. Sexual behaviors emerging in childhood include self-exploration, perhaps leading to masturbation.

- Although puberty defines biological adulthood, people take 5–10 more years to reach social maturity. Sexual fantasies and dreams and nocturnal emissions characterize adolescent sexuality.

- A person's sexual orientation can be heterosexual, homosexual, or bisexual. Possible influences include genetics, hormonal factors, and early childhood experiences.

- Human sexual behaviors include celibacy, erotic fantasy, masturbation, touching, cunnilingus, fellatio, anal intercourse, and coitus.

- To evaluate whether an atypical sexual behavior is problematic, experts consider the issues of consent between partners and whether the behavior results in physical or psychological harm.

- Pornography and prostitution are examples of the commercialization of sex; sexual stimulation is exchanged for money.

- Responsible sexuality includes open, honest communication; agreed-on sexual activities; sexual privacy; using contraception; safer sex practices; sober sex; and taking responsibility for consequences.

TAKE ACTION

1. Many reputable self-help books about sexual functioning are available in libraries and bookstores. If you're not satisfied with your level of knowledge and understanding, consider consulting some other sources.

2. If you have an intimate sexual relationship with a regular partner, think honestly about what is satisfying about it and what you would like to change. Is there anything you want to discuss with your partner but have been afraid to bring up? Take a chance, and talk with your partner about it.

JOURNAL ENTRY

1. Sexual myths and misconceptions are common in our culture. In your health journal, make a list of statements about sexuality that you've heard but are not sure are accurate. Find out the facts by consulting books and pamphlets mentioned here or available through your school health center or library.

2. *Critical Thinking* Many states have laws prohibiting certain sexual behaviors. How much control do you think society should have over an individual's sexual practices? What types of behaviors do you think should be regulated and why? What behaviors should be left up to the discretion of the individual? Write an essay outlining your position; be sure to explain your reasoning.

3. If you think you may have PMS or PMDD, keep a diary of any physical, emotional, or behavioral symptoms that seem to fluctuate monthly; also keep track of when your period occurs. If you notice a definite cyclical character to your symptoms, consider the tips listed in this chapter.

4. *Critical Thinking* Consider one or two of your favorite television shows or movies. How are sexuality and sexual behavior presented? How many sexual references occur? What types of sexual behaviors are shown or alluded to? What impression would a viewer have about the typical sexual behaviors of the characters? Are any of the potential emotional or physical consequences of sexual behavior shown? Write a short essay outlining your findings, and state whether you think the depiction of sexuality is accurate. In your opinion, can the presentation of sexuality in the programs or movies you chose influence the behavior of viewers? Explain your reasoning.

FOR MORE INFORMATION

Books

Ammer, C. 2000. *The New A to Z of Women's Health: A Concise Encyclopedia.* New York: Facts on File. *Topics include the reproductive system, sexuality, STDs, and contraception.*

Boston Women's Health Book Collective. 1998. *Our Bodies, Ourselves for the New Century.* New York: Simon & Schuster. *Broad coverage of many women's health concerns, with an emphasis on psychological as well as physical factors. A favorite for many years; periodically updated.*

Colapinto, J. 2000. *As Nature Made Him: The Boy Who Was Raised as a Girl.* New York: HarperCollins. *Tells the fascinating story of a boy who, following a botched circumcision, is raised as a girl until the age of 14, at which time he chooses to live life as a male; offers interesting perspectives on the nature vs. nurture controversy surrounding gender identity.*

Dalton, K., and W. Holton. 2000. *Once a Month: Understanding and Treating PMS,* 6th ed. Alameda, Calif.: Hunter House. *An up-to-date discussion of symptoms and self-help strategies for PMS.*

Men's Health Books. 2000. *The Complete Book of Men's Health.* Emmaus, Penn.: Rodale. *A comprehensive guide to a healthy lifestyle, including information on communication and sexuality.*

Reuben, David. 2000. *Everything You Ever Wanted to Know About Sex.* New York: St. Martin's Press. *A frank and humorous look at sexuality in an accessible question-and-answer format.*

Signorile, M. 1996. *Outing Yourself: How to Come Out as Lesbian or Gay to Your Family, Friends, and Coworkers.* Hamden, Conn.: Fireside. *Offers advice for lesbians and gays who are working toward telling others about their sexual orientation.*

Strong, B., et al. 2002. *Human Sexuality: Diversity in Contemporary America,* 4th ed. Mountain View, Calif.: Mayfield. *A comprehensive introduction to human sexuality.*

W. Organizations and Web Sites

American Association of Sex Educators, Counselors, and Therapists (AASECT). Certifies sex educators, counselors, and therapists and provides listings of local therapists dealing with sexual problems.
http://www.aasect.org

Dr. Drew. Provides answers to frequently asked questions about sexuality and relationships, geared toward young adults.
http://www.drDrew.com

Facts of Life Netline. Provides answers to many commonly asked questions about sexuality.
http://www.netidea.com/sexologynetline/facts

Go Ask Alice. Professional and peer educators provide answers to questions on many topics relating to sexuality.
http://www.goaskalice.columbia.edu

The Kinsey Institute for Research in Sex, Gender, and Reproduction. One of the oldest and most respected institutions doing research on sexuality.
812-855-7686
http://www.indiana.edu/~kinsey

Male Health Center. A commercial site that provides a variety of information on male sexual health topics.
http://www.malehealthcenter.com

New York University Sexual Disorders Screening. Provides interactive online screening tests for common sexual disorders.
http://www.med.nyu.edu/Psych/screens/sdsm.html (men)
http://www.med.nyu.edu/Psych/screens/sdsf.html (women)

North American Menopause Society (NAMS). Provides general information about menopause and lists of local support groups and menopause clinicians; Web site includes a helpful section with answers to frequently asked questions.
440-442-7550
http://www.menopause.org

PMS Access/Women's Health America Group. Provides information about PMS and links to other sites dealing with PMS and women's health issues.
800-222-4767; 800-558-7046
http://www.womenshealth.com

San Jose Marital and Sexuality Centre. Provides articles on issues relating to cybersex and an online sexual compulsion assessment.
http://www.sex-centre.com

Sexuality Information and Education Council of the United States (SIECUS). Provides information on many aspects of sexuality and has an extensive library and numerous publications.
http://www.siecus.org

Talking with Kids. Provides advice for parents about talking with children about difficult issues, including sex, relationships, and STDs.

http://www.talkingwithkids.org

U.S. Food and Drug Administration/Viagra. Provides information and cautions about the use of sildenafil citrate (Viagra) to treat sexual dysfunction in men.

http://www.fda.gov/cder/consumerinfo/viagra

See also the listings for Chapters 4, 6–8, and 18.

SELECTED BIBLIOGRAPHY

Adler, R., M. S. Ottaway, and S. Gould. 2001. Circumcision: We have heard from the experts; now let's hear from the parents. *Pediatrics* 107(2): E20.

American Academy of Pediatrics. 2000. *Circumcision: Information for Parents* (http://www.aap.org/family/circ.htm; retrieved September 5, 2000).

American Academy of Pediatrics Task Force on Circumcision. 1999. Circumcision Policy Statement. *Pediatrics* 103(3): 686–693.

American College of Obstetricians and Gynecologists. 2000. *Premenstrual Syndrome.* Washington, D.C.: American College of Obstetricians and Gynecologists.

American Psychological Association. 1998. *Answers to Your Questions About Sexual Orientation and Homosexuality* (http://www.apa.org/publinfo/answers.html; retrieved May 22, 2000).

Barnard, N. D., et al. 2000. Diet and sex-hormone binding globulin, dysmenorrhea, and premenstrual symptoms. *Obstetrics and Gynecology* 95(2): 245–250.

Basson, R., et al. 2000. Efficacy and safety of sildenafil in estrogenized women with sexual dysfunction associated with female sexual arousal disorder. *Obstetrics and Gynecology* 95(4 Suppl 1): S54.

Burack, R. 1999. Teenage sexual behavior: Attitudes towards and declared sexual activity. *British Journal of Family Planning* 24(4): 145–148.

Centers for Disease Control and Prevention. 2000. Alcohol policy and sexually transmitted disease rates—United States, 1981–1995. *Morbidity and Mortality Weekly Report* 49(16): 346–349.

Christakis, D. A., et al. 2000. A trade-off analysis of routine newborn circumcision. *Pediatrics* 105(1 Pt 3): 246–249.

Cohen-Kettenis, P., and L. Gooren. 1999. Transsexualism: A review of etiology, diagnosis, and treatment. *Journal of Psychosomatic Research* 46: 315–333.

Currah, P., and S. Minter. 2000. *Transgender Equality: A Handbook for Activists and Policymakers.* Washington, D.C.: National Gay and Lesbian Task Force.

Food and Drug Administration. 2000. *FDA Approves Fluoxetine to Treat Premenstrual Dysphoric Disorder* (http://www.fda.gov/bbs/topics/ANSWERS/ANS01024.html; retrieved September 9, 2000).

Food and Drug Administration. 2000. *FDA Clears New Female Sexual Therapy Device* (http://www.fda.gov/bbs/topics/ANSWERS/ANS01012.html; retrieved September 6, 2000).

Goldstein, I. 2000. Male sexual circuitry. *Scientific American* 283(2): 70–75.

Joint United Nations Programme on HIV/AIDS (UNAIDS). 2000. Male circumcision and HIV infection. *Report on the Global HIV/AIDS Epidemic—June 2000* (http://www.unaids.org/epidemic_update/report/Epi_report_chap_prevention.htm; retrieved September 5, 2000).

Kraemer, G. R., and R. R. Kraemer. 1998. Premenstrual syndrome: Diagnosis and treatment experiences. *Journal of Women's Health* 7(7): 893–907.

Laumann, E. O., A. Paik, and R. C. Rosen. 1999. Sexual dysfunction in the United States: Prevalence and predictors. *Journal of the American Medical Association* 281: 537–544.

Leiblum, S. R. 2001. Critical overview of the new consensus-based definitions and classification of female sexual dysfunction. *Journal of Sex and Marital Therapy* 27(2): 159–67.

Moneyyirci-Delale, O., et al. 1998. Sex steroid hormones modulate serum ionized magnesium and calcium levels throughout the menstrual cycle. *Fertility and Sterility* 69: 958–962.

National Council on Aging. 1998. *Half of Older Americans Report They Are Sexually Active; 4 in 10 Want More Sex, Says New Survey* (http://www.ncoa.org/press/sexsurvey.htm; retrieved September 28, 1998).

North American Menopause Society. 1998. *Menopause Is the Beginning of a New, Fulfilling Stage of Life* (http://www.menopause.org/news.htm#anchor10312017; retrieved October 26, 1998).

Paz Galupo, M., and S. St. John. 2001. Benefits of cross-sexual orientation friendships among adolescent females. *Journal of Adolescence* 24(1): 83–93.

Schoen, E. J., C. J. Colby, and G. T. Ray. 2000. Newborn circumcision decreases incidence and costs of urinary tract infections during the first year of life. *Pediatrics* 105(4): 789–793.

Shakir, S. A., et al. 2001. Cardiovascular events in users of sildenafil: Results from first phase of prescription event monitoring in England. *British Medical Journal* 22(7287): 651–652.

Silence about sexual problems can hurt relationships. 1999. *Journal of the American Medical Association* 281: 210.

Steinberg, S., et al. 1999. A placebo-controlled clinical trial of L-tryptophan in premenstrual dysphoria. *Biological Psychiatry* 45(3): 313–320.

Strasburger, V. C., and E. Donnerstein. 1999. Children, adolescents, and the media: Issues and solutions. *Pediatrics* 103(1): 129–139.

Strong, B., et al. 2002. *Human Sexuality: Diversity in Contemporary America,* 4th ed. Mountain View, Calif.: Mayfield.

Thys-Jacobs, S., et al. 1998. Calcium carbonate and the premenstrual syndrome: Effects on premenstrual and menstrual symptoms. Premenstrual Syndrome Study Group. *American Journal of Obstetrics and Gynecology* 179(2): 444–452.

Upchurch, D. M., et al. 1998. Gender and ethnic differences in the timing of first sexual intercourse. *Family Planning Perspectives* 30(3): 121–127.

Waldo, C. R. 1998. Out on campus: Sexual orientation and academic climate in a university context. *American Journal of Community Psychology* 26(5): 745–774.

World Health Organization. 2000. *Fact Sheet: Female Genital Mutilation* (http://www.who.int/inf-fs/en/fact241.html; retrieved June 14, 2000).

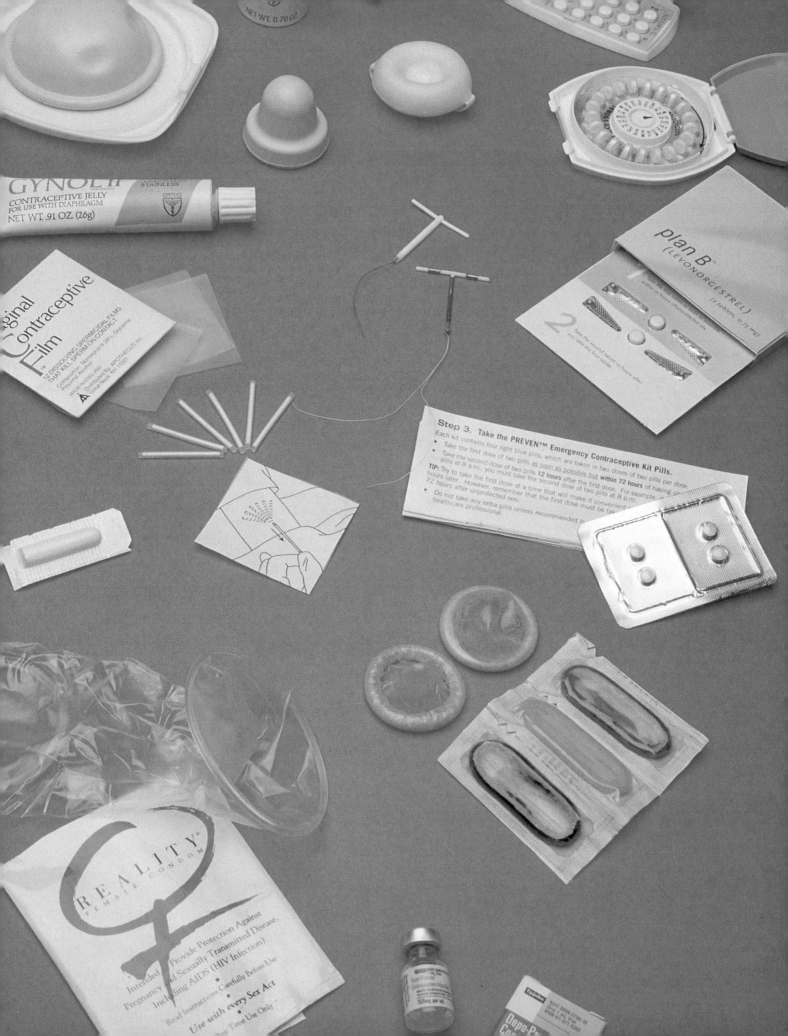

After reading this chapter, you should be able to

- Explain how contraceptives work and how to interpret information about a contraceptive method's effectiveness, risks, and benefits

- List the most popular contraceptives, and discuss their advantages, disadvantages, and effectiveness

- Discuss issues related to contraception, including nonmarital sexual relationships, gender differences, sex education for teenagers, and communication between partners

- Choose a method of contraception based on the needs of the user and the safety and effectiveness of the method

Contraception

TEST YOUR KNOWLEDGE

1. Which of the following contraceptive methods offers the best protection against pregnancy? Which offers the best protection against sexually transmitted diseases?
   a. oral contraceptives
   b. Norplant implants
   c. male condoms
   d. diaphragm with spermicidal foam

2. Emergency contraceptive pills should be taken within 72 hours of unprotected sex.
   True or false?

3. Hand lotion, Vaseline (petroleum jelly), and baby oil are good choices for condom lubricants.
   True or false?

4. About 90% of users of barrier contraceptive methods (male condom, diaphragm, and so on) use the method with each act of intercourse.
   True or false?

5. What percentage of women say they can't trust men to be responsible for contraception?
   a. 25%
   b. 50%
   c. 75%

In her lifetime, the ovaries of an average woman release over 400 eggs, one a month for about 35 years. Each egg is capable of developing into a human embryo if fertilized by one of the millions of sperm a man produces in every ejaculate. Furthermore, unlike most other mammals, humans are capable of sexual activity at any time of the month or year. These facts help explain why people have always had a compelling interest in controlling fertility and in preventing unwanted pregnancies. Historical writings dating back to the fourth century B.C. mention the use of douches, sponges, and crude methods of abortion. Other materials mentioned as potential contraceptives include lemon juice, parsley, seaweed, olive oil, camphor, and opium. Although not fully understood at the time, the underlying principle of these trial-and-error methods was the same as that of today's **contraceptives:** preventing **conception** by blocking the female's egg from uniting with the male's sperm, thereby preventing pregnancy.

Modern contraceptive methods are much more predictable and effective than in the past, and people today have many options when it comes to making decisions about their sexual and contraceptive behavior. (The statistical consequences of these decisions are shown in Table 6-1.) In addition to the primary purpose of preventing pregnancy, many types of contraception play an important role in protecting against **sexually transmitted diseases (STDs)**. Being informed about the realities and risks and making responsible decisions about sexual and contraceptive behavior are crucial components of lifelong wellness. But because such decisions are emotional, complex, and difficult, people tend to avoid them or deal with them ineffectively.

While biological, social, and media pressures often encourage sexual activity at ever-younger ages, few forces in the United States support a factual, realistic discussion of

VITAL STATISTICS

Table 6-1 **Worldwide Sexual Behavior and Its Consequences**

	Estimated Daily Occurrence
Cases of curable STDs	910,000
Pregnancies	550,000
Births	360,000
Abortions	140,000
Cases of HIV infection	15,000
Deaths—from AIDS	7,700
—from childbirth complications	1,600
—from STDs (excluding AIDS)	500
—from unsafe abortions	200

SOURCES: United Nations Population Fund. 2000. *Rights for Sexual and Reproductive Health* (http://www.unfpa.org/modules/intercenter/reprights/sexual.htm; retrieved September 12, 2000). Joint United Nations Programme on HIV/AIDS. 2000. *Report on the Global HIV/AIDS Epidemic: Global Summary* (http://www.unaids.org/epidemic_update/report/Epi_report_chap_glo_estim.htm). World Health Organization. 2000.*The World Health Report 2000*. Geneva: World Health Organization. United Nations Population Division. 1999. The world at six billion. *Population Newsletter*, December. Safe Motherhood. 1998. *Unwanted Pregnancy* (http://www.safemotherhood.org/facts_and_figures/unwanted_pregnancy.htm; retrieved September 12, 2000).

the importance of either postponing sexual intercourse or using contraception when intercourse is chosen. Our present superficial approaches to education are clearly ineffective: The United States has one of the highest teen pregnancy rates of all developed nations. Because many of the changing roles of women are severely compromised by unplanned child rearing and because the option of abortion is becoming more restricted, the problem is even worse than the numbers show.

This chapter provides basic information on the various contraceptive methods, including their advantages and disadvantages. The issues raised should encourage you to think about your own beliefs and attitudes about sexual behavior and contraception and to discuss them with others. Among the most important choices of your life will be deciding what type of sexual involvement is best for you and when you are ready for a sexual relationship; equally critical is the commitment to always protect yourself against unwanted pregnancy and STDs.

PRINCIPLES OF CONTRACEPTION

A variety of effective approaches in preventing conception are based on different principles of birth control. **Barrier methods** work by physically blocking the sperm from

Terms

contraceptive Any agent that can prevent conception; condoms, diaphragms, intrauterine devices, and oral contraceptives are examples.

conception The fusion of ovum and sperm, resulting in a fertilized egg, or zygote.

sexually transmitted disease (STD) Any of several contagious diseases contracted through intimate sexual contact.

barrier method A contraceptive that acts as a physical barrier, blocking the sperm from uniting with the egg.

ovulation The release of the egg (ovum) from the ovaries.

contraceptive failure rate The percentage of women using a particular contraceptive method who experience an unintended pregnancy in the first year of use.

continuation rate The percentage of women who continue to use a particular contraceptive after a specified period of time.

oral contraceptive (OC) Any of various hormone compounds (estrogen and progestins) in pill form that prevent conception by preventing ovulation.

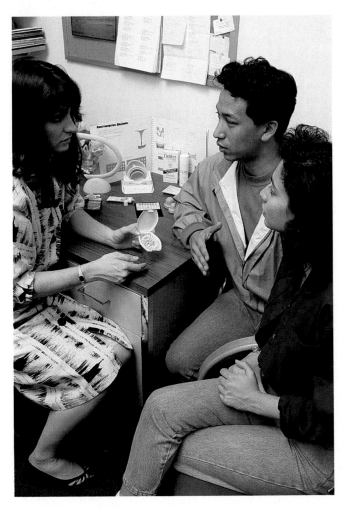
To be effective, contraceptives should be chosen thoughtfully and used correctly. A careful explanation by a health care professional will help this couple choose a method that is right for them.

basing your current choices on common misinformation.)

Effectiveness, one of the factors listed above, requires further explanation. Contraceptive effectiveness is partly determined by the reliability of the method itself—the failure rate if it were always used exactly as directed ("perfect use"). Effectiveness is also determined by characteristics of the user, including fertility of the individual, frequency of intercourse, and, more important, how consistently and correctly the method is used. This "typical use" **contraceptive failure rate** is based on studies that directly measure the percentage of women experiencing an unintended pregnancy in the first year of contraceptive use. For example, the 5% failure rate of oral contraceptives means 5 out of 100 typical users will become pregnant in the first year. This failure rate is likely to be lower for women who are consistently careful in following instructions and higher for those who are frequently careless. Similarly, the 20% failure rate of typical diaphragm use can be decreased or increased significantly by how correct and consistent the woman is in using the device.

Another measure of effectiveness is the **continuation rate**—the percentage of people who continue to use the method after a specified period of time. This measure is important because many unintended pregnancies occur when a method is stopped and not immediately replaced with another. Thus, a contraceptive with a high continuation rate would be more effective at preventing pregnancy than one with a low continuation rate.

We turn now to a description of the various contraceptive methods, discussing first those that are reversible and then those that are permanent.

reaching the egg. Diaphragms, condoms, and several other methods are based on this principle. *Hormonal methods,* such as oral contraceptives (birth control pills), alter the biochemistry of the woman's body, preventing **ovulation** (the release of the egg) and producing changes that make it more difficult for the sperm to reach the egg if ovulation does occur. So-called *natural methods* of contraception are based on the fact that egg and sperm have to be present at the same time if fertilization is to occur. Finally, *surgical methods*—female and male sterilization—more or less permanently prevent transport of the sperm or eggs to the site of conception.

All contraceptive methods have advantages and disadvantages that make them appropriate for some people but not for others or the best choice at one period of life but not at another. Factors that affect the choice of method include effectiveness, convenience, cost, reversibility, side effects and risks, and protection against STDs. Later in this chapter, we help you sort through these factors to decide on the method that's best for you. (See the box "Myths About Contraception" to make sure you're not

REVERSIBLE CONTRACEPTIVES

Reversibility is an extremely important consideration for young adults when they choose a contraceptive method, because most people either plan to have children or at least want to keep their options open until they're older. In this section we discuss the reversible contraceptives, beginning with the hormonal methods, then moving to the barrier methods, and finally covering the natural methods.

Oral Contraceptives: The Pill

A century ago or more, a researcher made a key observation: Ovulation does not occur during pregnancy. Further research brought to light the hormonal mechanism: During pregnancy, the corpus luteum secretes progesterone and estrogen in amounts high enough to suppress ovulation. (Refer to Chapter 5 for a complete discussion of the hormonal control of the menstrual cycle.) **Oral contraceptives (OCs),** or birth control pills, prevent ovulation

Myth   Taking borrowed birth control pills for a few days before having sexual relations gives reliable protection against pregnancy.

Fact   Instructions for taking birth control pills must be followed carefully to provide effective contraception. With most pills, this means starting them with a menstrual period and then taking one every day.

Myth   Pregnancy never occurs when unprotected intercourse takes place just before or just after a menstrual period.

Fact   Menstrual cycles may be irregular, and ovulation may occur at unpredictable times.

Myth   During sexual relations, sperm enter the vagina only during ejaculation and never before.

Fact   The small amounts of fluid secreted before ejaculation may contain sperm. This is why withdrawing the penis from the vagina just prior to ejaculation is not an effective method of contraception.

Myth   If semen is deposited just outside the vaginal entrance, pregnancy cannot occur.

Fact   Although sperm usually live about 72 hours within the woman's body, they can live up to 6 or 7 days and are capable of traveling through the vagina and up into the uterus and oviducts.

Myth   Douching immediately after sexual relations can prevent sperm from reaching and fertilizing an egg.

Fact   During ejaculation (within the vagina), some sperm begin to enter the cervix and uterus. Since they are no longer in the vagina, it is impossible to remove them by douching after sexual relations. Douching may actually push the sperm up farther.

Myth   A woman who is breastfeeding does not have to use any contraceptive method to prevent pregnancy.

Fact   Frequent and regular breastfeeding may at times prevent ovulation, but not consistently and reliably. Ovulation and pregnancy may occur before the first period after delivering a baby.

Myth   Women can't become pregnant the first time they have intercourse.

Fact   *Any time* intercourse without protection takes place, sperm may unite with an egg to begin a pregnancy. There is nothing unique about first intercourse to prevent this.

Myth   Taking a "rest" from the pill periodically is necessary for safety.

Fact   There are no known medical benefits from taking a prolonged break from OC use; the risks and benefits of ongoing pill use should be evaluated for each individual. Pregnancy commonly occurs when one contraceptive method is stopped and not effectively replaced by another method.

Myth   Pregnancy is impossible if partners have sex while standing up.

Fact   Sperm can travel and reach the ovum regardless of body position.

---

by mimicking the hormonal activity of the corpus luteum. The active ingredients in OCs are estrogen and progestins, laboratory-made compounds that are closely related to progesterone.

In addition to preventing ovulation, the birth control pill has other backup contraceptive effects. It inhibits the movement of sperm by thickening the cervical mucus, alters the rate of ovum transport by means of its hormonal effects on the oviducts, and may prevent implantation by changing the lining of the uterus, in the unlikely event that a fertilized ovum reaches that area.

The most common type of OC is the combination pill. Each 1-month packet contains 3 weeks of pills that combine varying types and amounts of estrogen and progestin. Most packets also include a 1-week supply of inactive pills to be taken following the hormone pills; others instruct the woman to simply take no pills at all for 1 week before starting the next cycle. During the week in which no hormones are taken, a light menstrual period occurs. Many different types of combination pills are available today, and if minor problems occur with one brand, women can switch to another.

A second, much less common, type of OC is the minipill, a small dose of a synthetic progesterone taken every day of the month. Because the minipill contains no estrogen, it has fewer side effects and health risks, but it also carries a higher risk of pregnancy and irregular bleeding.

A woman is usually advised to start the first cycle of pills with a menstrual period to increase effectiveness and eliminate the possibility of unsuspected pregnancy. She must take each month's pills completely and according to instructions. Taking a few pills just prior to having sexual intercourse will not provide effective contraception.

Hormonal adjustments that occur during the first cycle or two may cause slight bleeding between periods. This spotting is considered normal. Full effectiveness cannot be guaranteed during the first week because maximal levels of hormones haven't yet been reached. A backup method is recommended during the first week and any subsequent cycle in which the woman forgets to take any pills.

Terms   **fertility** The ability to reproduce.

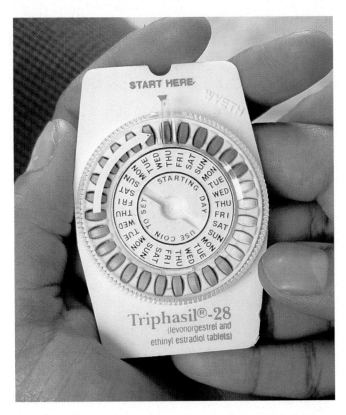

Oral contraceptives are the most popular reversible method of contraception among American women. When used correctly, oral contraceptives are highly effective.

Since its approval by the FDA in 1960, the pill has remained a popular contraceptive in the United States. OC use declined temporarily in the late 1970s following publicity regarding possible increased risks of heart attack and stroke. However, these risks have been substantially reduced by the use of lower-dosage pills (those with 50 micrograms or less of estrogen) and the identification of women at higher risk for complications. Today, OCs are the most widely used form of contraception among unmarried women and are second only to sterilization among married women.

Advantages   The main advantage of the oral contraceptive is its high degree of effectiveness in preventing pregnancy. Nearly all unplanned pregnancies result because the pills were not taken as directed. The pill is relatively simple to use and does not require any interruptions that could hinder sexual spontaneity. Most women also enjoy the predictable regularity of periods, as well as the decrease in cramps and blood loss. For young women, the reversibility of the pill is especially important; **fertility**—the ability to reproduce—returns after the pill is discontinued (although not always immediately).

Medical advantages include a decreased incidence of benign breast disease, iron-deficiency anemia, pelvic in-

flammatory disease (PID), ectopic pregnancy, endometrial cancer (of the lining of the uterus), and ovarian cancer. Women who have never used the pill are twice as likely to develop endometrial or ovarian cancer as those who have taken it for at least 12 months.

Disadvantages   Although oral contraceptives do lower the risk of PID, they do not protect against HIV infection or other STDs in the lower reproductive tract. OCs have been associated with increased cervical chlamydia. Regular condom use is recommended for an OC user, unless she is in a long-term, mutually monogamous relationship with an uninfected partner.

The hormones in birth control pills influence all tissues of the body, and they can lead to a variety of minor disturbances. Symptoms of early pregnancy—morning nausea, weight gain, and swollen breasts, for example—may appear during the first few months of OC use. They usually disappear by the fourth cycle. Other side effects include depression, nervousness, changes in sex drive, dizziness, generalized headaches, migraine, bleeding between periods, and changes in the lining of the walls of the vagina, with an increase in clear or white vaginal discharge. Chloasma, or "mask of pregnancy," sometimes occurs, causing brown "giant freckles" to appear on the face. Acne may develop or worsen, but in most women, using the pill causes acne to clear up, and it is sometimes prescribed for that purpose.

Serious side effects have been reported in a small number of women. These include blood clots, stroke, and heart attack, concentrated mostly in older women who smoke or have a history of circulatory disease. Recent studies have shown very little, if any, increased risk of heart attack for healthy young nonsmoking women on lower-dosage pills. OC users may be slightly more prone to stroke, high blood pressure, blood clots in the legs and arms, and benign liver tumors that may rupture and bleed. OC use is also associated with a slight increase in the diagnosis of breast and cervical cancer; however, earlier detection and other variables such as number of sexual partners may account for much of this increase. Most adverse effects of OCs disappear after pill use is discontinued, and studies show no long-term effect on mortality.

Birth control pills are not recommended for women with a history of blood clots, heart disease or stroke, any form of cancer or liver tumor, or impaired liver function. Women with certain other health conditions or behaviors, including migraines, high blood pressure, cigarette smoking, and sickle-cell disease, require close monitoring.

In trying to decide whether to use oral contraceptives, each woman needs to weigh the benefits against the risks. To make an informed decision, she should seek the help of a health care professional in evaluating the known risk variables that apply to her (see the box "Obtaining a Contraceptive from a Health Clinic or Physician"). A woman can take several steps to decrease her risk from OC use:

If you are a woman who is considering a method of contraception that requires a prescription or professional fitting or insertion, you'll need to go to a health clinic or a physician to get it. Many of the female methods—including the hormonal methods, IUDs, and the diaphragm and cervical cap—require at least an initial professional visit. The thought of visiting a physician's office or health clinic to discuss and obtain contraception makes many people nervous. Keep in mind that the people in the office are health care professionals who will not pass moral judgment on you. They are dedicated to meeting your health care needs. Knowing what to expect can help you get more from your visit.

Before Your Visit

You can prepare for a more successful visit by doing the following:

1. Pull together your personal and family medical history. Make sure it's accurate and up-to-date.

2. Review the section in this chapter entitled "Which Contraceptive Method Is Right for You?" Carefully consider each topic, and discuss it with your partner if that would be helpful.

3. Write down any questions you have. Clarify in your own mind what you need to find out about your contraceptive options.

4. If you have questions about sexually transmitted diseases or other aspects of sexuality, write those down too.

5. If you like, plan to have your partner, a friend, or a family member accompany you to your appointment.

During Your Visit

When you arrive, you'll probably be asked to fill out forms covering your background and medical history. A physician or staff member will then review the various contraceptive methods with you and answer your questions. She or he can help you evaluate the key factors affecting your choice of method, including health risks, lifestyle factors, cost, and protection against STDs. You may have blood and urine samples taken for lab tests.

The Physical Exam

Your physical exam will probably include a check of your breasts, external genitals, and abdomen, plus a Pap test and possible screening for certain STDs. The exam will help ensure that you can safely use the method you have chosen, as well as protect your overall health. If this is your first pelvic exam and/or you feel nervous or uncomfortable, tell the clinician, and ask her or him to explain each step of the examination.

For the pelvic exam, you will be asked to lie on your back on an examination table, with your feet in metal stirrups and your knees bent. The exam doesn't usually hurt. An instrument called a speculum will be inserted into the vagina to hold it open so the clinician can look at the cervix and vaginal walls. For the Pap test, the clinician will scrape some cells from the cervix and place them on a glass slide. These cells will be analyzed for any signs of cancer. You may feel a slight pressure while the cells are collected. The clinician will also check your internal organs by placing two gloved fingers into the vagina and the other hand on the lower abdomen. He or she will palpate (examine by touching) the uterus and ovaries to check for any abnormalities.

If you're getting a diaphragm or a cervical cap, you will be fitted for it at this time. The clinician will probably try different sizes to find the best fit and then will show you how to insert and remove it.

Following Your Exam

After your exam, a health care worker will either provide you with your contraceptive, arrange for a further appointment (if necessary), or give you a prescription. Make sure you know exactly how to use the method you've chosen. Written instructions and information may be available. Be sure you have a phone number you can call if you have questions later.

1. Request a low-dosage pill.

2. Stop smoking.

3. Follow the dosage carefully and consistently.

4. Be alert to preliminary danger signals, which can be remembered with the word ACHES:

    Abdominal pain (severe)

    Chest pain (severe), cough, shortness of breath or sharp pain on breathing in

    Headaches (severe), dizziness, weakness, or numbness, especially if one-sided

    Eye problems (vision loss or blurring) and/or speech problems

    Severe leg pain (calf or thigh)

5. Have regular checkups to monitor blood pressure, weight, and urine, and have an annual examination of the thyroid, breasts, abdomen, and pelvis.

6. Have regular **Pap tests** to check for early cervical changes. Because OC use may temporarily increase some women's susceptibility to the STDs chlamydia and gonorrhea, regular screening for those diseases is also recommended, especially when condoms aren't being used.

Terms   **Pap test** A scraping of cells from the cervix for examination under a microscope to detect cancer.

Table 6-2	Contraceptive Risks
Contraceptive Method	**Risk of Death in Any Given Year**
Oral contraceptives	
Nonsmoker	1 in 66,700
Age less than 35	1 in 200,000
Age 35–44	1 in 28,600
Heavy smoker (25 or more cigarettes/day)	1 in 1,700
Age less than 35	1 in 5,300
Age 35–44	1 in 700
IUDs	1 in 10,000,000
Barrier methods, spermicides	none
Fertility awareness methods, withdrawal	none
Sterilization	
Laparoscopic tubal ligation	1 in 38,500
Hysterectomy	1 in 1,600
Vasectomy	1 in 1,000,000
Pregnancy and childbirth	1 in 10,000

SOURCE: Hatcher, R. A., et al. 1998. *Contraceptive Technology,* 17th rev. ed. New York: Ardent Media. Reprinted by permission of Irvington Publishing.

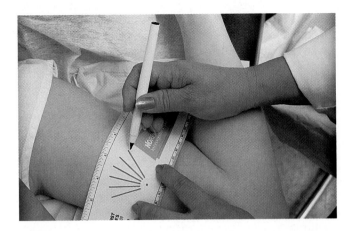

Contraceptive implants, filled with synthetic hormones and inserted under the skin on the arm or leg, can provide 5 years of protection against pregnancy.

For most women, the known, directly associated risk of death from taking birth control pills is much lower than the risk of death from pregnancy (Table 6-2).

Effectiveness Oral contraceptive effectiveness varies substantially because it depends so much on individual factors. If taken exactly as directed, the failure rate is extremely low (0.1%). However, among average users, lapses such as forgetting to take a pill do occur, and a typical first-year failure rate is 5%. The continuation rate for OCs also varies; the average rate is 71% after 1 year.

Contraceptive Implants

Contraceptive implants are placed under the skin and deliver a small but steady dose of hormones over a period of several years. Implants have been used for more than 25 years in various countries, including several in Europe, South America, Asia, and Scandinavia. In 1990, the Norplant contraceptive implant became available in the United States. Norplant consists of six flexible, matchstick-sized capsules that contain progestin, a synthetic progesterone. The capsules are placed under the skin, usually on the inside of a woman's upper arm in a fan-

shaped configuration. The procedure can be done in less than 15 minutes, with a local anesthetic and only one very small incision; no stitches are required. The progestin in Norplant has several contraceptive effects: Hormonal shifts may inhibit ovulation and affect development of the uterine lining, thickening of cervical mucus inhibits the movement of sperm, and transport of the egg through the fallopian tubes may be slowed.

The use of Norplant by American women dropped substantially after its first few years of availability because of ongoing lawsuits and related complaints (see "Disadvantages," which follows). Other types of contraceptive implants are available in other countries and may soon be available in the United States; these include a single capsule device, Implanon, and the two-capsule Norplant 2. In studies, these implants have been easier to insert and remove than the six-capsule Norplant; Implanon comes preloaded in a disposable applicator. Contraceptive implants are best suited for women who wish to have continuous and long-term protection against pregnancy.

Advantages Norplant implants are the most effective reversible method of contraception now available. After insertion of the implants, no further action is required for up to 5 years of protection; at the same time, contraceptive effects are quickly reversed upon removal. Because Norplant, unlike the combination pill, contains no estrogen, it carries a lower risk of certain side effects, such as blood clots and other cardiovascular complications. In addition, the progestin is released at a steady rate, in smaller quantities than are found in oral contraceptives. The thickened cervical mucus resulting from Norplant use has a protective effect against PID.

Disadvantages As with the pill, Norplant gives no protection against HIV infection and STDs in the lower reproductive tract. Although the implants are barely visible, their appearance may bother some women. The initial cost can be substantial (but protection is provided for 5 years). Only specially trained practitioners can insert or remove the implants, and removal is sometimes difficult. Lawsuits filed against the manufacturer of Norplant have focused on removal difficulties and inadequate warnings about side effects. A further problem with Norplant has been the discovery of certain product lots with low hormone levels and reduced effectiveness. To help address some of the problems with Norplant, the manufacturer offers a consumer information hotline (800-934-5556).

The most common side effects of contraceptive implants are menstrual irregularities, including longer menstrual periods, spotting between periods, or having no bleeding at all. The menstrual cycle usually becomes more regular after 1 year of use. Less common side effects include headaches, weight gain, breast tenderness, nausea, acne, and mood swings. Cautions and more serious health concerns are similar to those associated with oral contraceptives but are less common.

Effectiveness   Typical failure rates are very low (0.05%) in the first year, increasing slowly with each additional year of use. The cumulative failure rate of Norplant at the end of 5 years is about 3.7%; the continuation rate is about 88%.

Injectable Contraceptives

Hormonal contraceptive injections were developed in the 1960s and are currently being used in at least 80 countries throughout the world. The first injectable contraceptive approved for use in the United States was Depo-Provera, which uses long-acting progestins. Injected in the arm or buttocks, Depo-Provera is usually given every 12 weeks, although it actually provides effective contraception for a few weeks beyond that. As another progestin-only contraceptive, it prevents pregnancy in the same ways as Norplant.

Lunelle, an injectable containing both estrogen and progestin, was approved for use in the United States in 2000. Lunelle injections are given every month rather than every 3 months as with Depo-Provera. Lunelle prevents pregnancy in the same way as OCs.

Advantages   Injectable contraceptives are highly effective and require little action on the part of the user. Because the injections leave no trace and involve no ongoing supplies, injectables allow women almost total privacy in their decision to use contraception. Like Norplant, Depo-Provera has no estrogen-related side effects; it requires only periodic injections rather than the minor surgical

procedures of implant insertion and removal. Lunelle, which does contain estrogen, has many of the same benefits as oral contraceptives and may be preferred by women who do not want to take a pill every day.

Disadvantages   Injectable contraceptives provide no protection against HIV infection and STDs in the lower reproductive tract. A woman must visit a health care facility every month (Lunelle) or every three months (Depo-Provera) to receive the injections. The side effects of Depo-Provera are similar to those of Norplant; menstrual irregularities are the most common, and after 1 year of using Depo-Provera, many women have no menstrual bleeding at all. Lunelle causes less menstrual irregularity than Depo-Provera. Weight gain is a common side effect of both Depo-Provera and Lunelle. After discontinuing the use of Depo-Provera, women may experience temporary infertility for up to 12 months; with Lunelle, fertility usually returns within 2–3 months of the last injection.

Reasons for not using Depo-Provera are similar to those for not using Norplant; contraindications for Lunelle are similar to those for OCs. Although early animal studies indicated that Depo-Provera increases the risk of breast and other cancers, the FDA has concluded that worldwide studies and years of human use have shown the risk of cancer in humans to be minimal or nonexistent. Recent research suggests that extended use of Depo-Provera or Lunelle may be associated with decreased bone density, a risk factor for osteoporosis (see Chapter 12). In studies, bone density returned to normal when Depo-Provera was discontinued; more research is needed to clarify the effects of injectable contraceptives on bone density. The long-term effects of Lunelle have not yet been firmly established but are expected to be similar to those for OCs.

Effectiveness   Typical failure rates with Depo-Provera are 0.3%; those reported for Lunelle are 0.2–0.4%. The 1-year continuation rate for Depo-Provera is about 42%.

Emergency Contraception

Emergency contraception refers to postcoital methods—those used after unprotected sexual intercourse. An emergency contraceptive may be appropriate if a regularly used method has failed (for example, if a condom breaks) or if unprotected sex has occurred. Emergency contraceptives are designed only for emergency use and should not be relied on as a regular method.

The most frequently used emergency contraceptive is a two-dose regimen of certain combination oral contraceptives. These pills have been packaged as emergency contraceptives for more than a decade in Great Britain, Germany, and other countries. Although long approved by the FDA as contraceptives and prescribed by some physicians for emergency use, these OCs have only re-

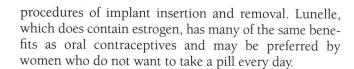

Terms   **abortifacient** An agent or substance that induces abortion.

intrauterine device (IUD) A plastic device inserted into the uterus as a contraceptive.

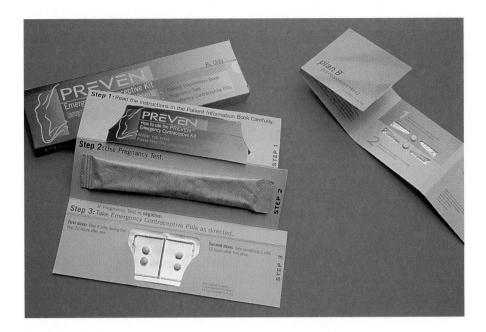

Emergency hormonal contraceptives reduce the risk of pregnancy by about 75% if taken within 72 hours of unprotected intercourse. The most commonly used regimens for emergency contraception involve taking two doses of hormones about 12 hours apart.

cently been approved specifically for postcoital purposes in the United States. In 1996, an FDA advisory panel concluded that six brands of OCs already available in the United States are safe and effective for emergency contraception, reducing the risk of pregnancy by 75%.

Researchers are still uncertain precisely how OCs work as emergency contraceptives. Opponents of their use argue that if they act by preventing implantation of a fertilized egg, they may actually be **abortifacients;** however, recent evidence indicates that prevention of implantation may not be their primary mode of action. Postcoital pills also appear to inhibit or delay ovulation and to alter the transport of sperm and/or eggs.

By 2000, two FDA-approved products specifically designed for emergency contraception were available in the United States—Preven, which contains both estrogen and progestin, and Plan B, which contains only progestin. These and other regimens for emergency contraception involve taking two doses of hormones 12 hours apart. The first dose must be taken within 72 hours after intercourse (the sooner, the better). The most common side effects are nausea, vomiting, and breast tenderness. Early indications are that Plan B may be more effective than Preven and cause less nausea and vomiting; if taken within 24 hours after intercourse, Plan B may prevent as many as 95% of expected pregnancies.

Intrauterine devices, discussed in the next section, can also be used for emergency contraception: If inserted within 5 days of unprotected intercourse, they are even more effective than OCs. However, because their use is more complicated, they are not used nearly as frequently. In addition, mifepristone, the "abortion pill," is being studied as another possible option (see Chapter 7 for more on mifepristone).

For more on options for emergency contraception, refer to the resources in the For More Information section at the end of the chapter.

The Intrauterine Device (IUD)

The **intrauterine device (IUD)** is a small plastic device placed in the uterus as a contraceptive. At the height of its popularity in the early 1970s, about 10% of all women using contraceptives in the United States had an IUD. But in the late 1970s, IUD use began to decline, mostly as a result of publicity about the increased risk of serious infections associated with the popular Dalkon Shield and its withdrawal from the market. Three IUDs are now available in the U.S.: the hormone-releasing Progestasert, which requires replacement every year; the Copper T-380A (also known as the Para-Gard), which gives protection for up to 10 years; and the Levonorgestral IUD (Mirena), approved in 2000, which releases small amounts of progestin and is effective for up to 5–10 years. By 2000, fewer than 1% of all American women who used contraception had IUDs.

Researchers do not know exactly how IUDs prevent pregnancy. Current evidence suggests that they work primarily by preventing fertilization. IUDs may cause biochemical changes in the uterus and affect the movement of sperm and eggs; although less likely, they may also interfere with implantation of fertilized eggs. Progestasert and Mirena slowly release very small amounts of hormones, which impedes fertilization or implantation.

An IUD must be inserted and removed by a trained professional. It can be inserted at any time during the menstrual cycle, as long as the woman is not pregnant. The device is threaded into a sterile inserter, which is introduced

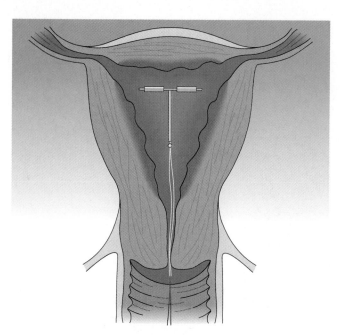

Figure 6-1   An IUD (Copper T-380A) properly positioned in the uterus.   The attached threads that protrude from the cervix into the upper vagina allow the woman to check to make sure that the IUD is in place.

through the cervix; a plunger pushes the IUD into the uterus. The threads protruding from the cervix are trimmed so that only 1–1.5 inches remain in the upper vagina (Figure 6-1).

Advantages   Intrauterine devices are highly reliable and are simple and convenient to use, requiring no attention except for a periodic check of the string position. They do not require the woman to anticipate or interrupt sexual activity. Usually IUDs have only localized side effects, and in the absence of complications, they are considered a fully reversible contraceptive. In most cases, fertility is restored as soon as the IUD is removed. The long-term expense of using an IUD is low.

Disadvantages   Most side effects of IUD use are limited to the genital tract. Heavy menstrual flow and bleeding and spotting between periods may occur, although with Mirena, menstrual periods tend to become shorter and lighter over time. Another side effect is pain, particularly

uterine cramps and backache, which seem to occur most often in women who have never been pregnant. Spontaneous expulsion of the IUD happens to 5–6% of women within the first year, most commonly during the first months after insertion. The older the woman is and the more children she has had, the less likely she is to expel the device. In about 1 of 1000 insertions, the IUD punctures the wall of the uterus and may migrate into the abdominal cavity.

A serious but rare complication of IUD use is pelvic inflammatory disease (PID). Most pelvic infections among IUD users are relatively mild and can be treated successfully with antibiotics. However, early and adequate treatment is critical, for a lingering infection can lead to tubal scarring and subsequent infertility.

Some physicians advise against the use of IUDs by young women who have never been pregnant because of the increased incidence of side effects in this group and the risk of infection with the possibility of subsequent infertility. IUDs are not recommended for women of any age who have a history of pelvic infection or who are at high risk for STDs. They are also unsuitable for women with suspected pregnancy, large tumors of the uterus or other anatomical abnormalities, irregular or unexplained bleeding, a history of ectopic pregnancy, or rheumatic heart disease. No evidence has been found linking IUD use to cancer, but the long-term effects are not well known. IUDs offer no protection against STDs.

Early IUD danger signals are abdominal pain, fever, chills, foul-smelling vaginal discharge, irregular menstrual periods, and other unusual vaginal bleeding. A change in string length should also be noted. An annual checkup is important and should include a Pap test and a blood check for anemia if menstrual flow has increased. (And in the case of Progestasert use, the IUD must be replaced every 12 months.)

Effectiveness   The typical failure rate of IUDs during the first year of use is 1–2%. Effectiveness can be increased by periodically checking to see that the device is in place and by using a backup method for the first few months after IUD insertion. If pregnancy occurs, the IUD should be removed to safeguard the health of the woman and to maintain the pregnancy. The continuation rate of IUDs is about 80% after 1 year of use.

Male Condoms

The **male condom** is a thin sheath designed to cover the penis during sexual intercourse. Most brands available in the United States are made of latex, although condoms made of polyurethane are also now available. Condoms prevent sperm from entering the vagina and provide protection against disease. Condoms are the most widely used barrier method and the third most popular of all

Terms

male condom A sheath, usually made of thin latex (synthetic rubber), that covers the penis during sexual intercourse; used for contraception and to prevent STDs.

ejaculation An abrupt discharge of semen from the penis after sexual stimulation.

spermicide A chemical agent that kills sperm.

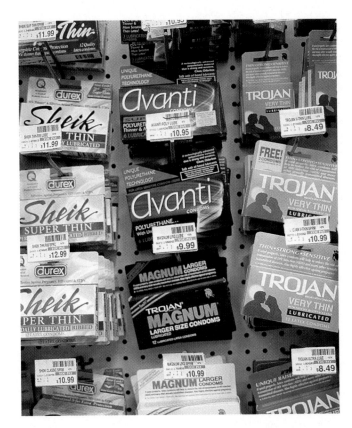

Condoms come in a variety of sizes, textures, and colors; some brands have a reservoir tip designed to collect semen. Used consistently and correctly, condoms provide the most reliable protection available against HIV infection for sexually active people.

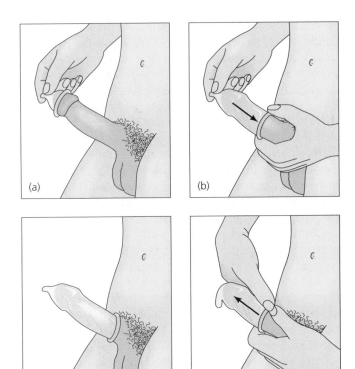

Figure 6-2 Use of the male condom. (a) Place the rolled-up condom over the head of the erect penis. Hold the top half-inch of the condom (with air squeezed out) to leave room for semen. (b) While holding the tip, unroll the condom onto the penis. Gently smooth out any air bubbles. (c) Unroll the condom down to the base of the penis. (d) To avoid spilling semen after ejaculation, hold the condom around the base of the penis as the penis is withdrawn. Remove the condom away from your partner, taking care not to spill any semen.

contraceptive methods used in the United States, after the pill and female sterilization.

Condom sales have increased dramatically in recent years, primarily because they provide some protection against all STDs and are the only method that provides substantial protection against HIV infection. At least one-third of all male condoms are bought by women. This figure will probably increase as more women become aware of the serious risks associated with STDs and assume the right to insist on condom use. Women are more likely to contract an STD from an infected partner than men are. Women also face additional health risks from STDs, including cervical cancer, PID, ectopic pregnancy (which is potentially life-threatening), and infertility. (See Chapter 18 for more information on STDs.)

The man or his partner must put the condom on the penis before it is inserted into the vagina, because the small amounts of fluid that may be secreted unnoticed prior to **ejaculation** often contain sperm capable of causing pregnancy. The rolled-up condom is placed over the head of the erect penis and unrolled down to the base of the penis, leaving a half-inch space (without air) at the tip to collect semen (Figure 6-2). Some brands of condoms have a reservoir tip designed for this purpose. Uncircum-

cised men must first pull back the foreskin of the penis. Partners must be careful not to damage the condom with fingernails, rings, or other rough objects.

Prelubricated condoms are available containing the **spermicide** nonoxynol-9, the same agent found in many of the contraceptive creams that women use. Spermicide condoms may decrease the risk of pregnancy, but the extent of decreased risk has not been established. Furthermore, these condoms have been associated with urinary tract infections in women.

If desired, users can lubricate their own condoms with contraceptive foam, creams, or jelly or with water-based preparations such as K-Y Jelly. Any product that contains mineral or vegetable oil—including baby oil, many lotions, regular Vaseline petroleum jelly, cooking oils (corn oil, Crisco, butter, and so on), and some vaginal lubricants and anti-fungal or anti-itch creams—should never be used with latex condoms; they can cause latex to begin to disintegrate within 60 seconds, thus greatly increasing the chance of condom breakage. (Polyurethane is not affected by oil-based products.)

When the man loses his erection after ejaculating, the condom loses its tight fit. To avoid spilling semen, the condom must be held around the base of the penis as the penis is withdrawn. If any semen is spilled on the vulva, sperm may find their way to the uterus.

Advantages Condoms are easy to purchase and are available without prescription or medical supervision (see the box "Buying and Using Over-the-Counter Contraceptives"). Simple to use, they provide for greater male participation in contraception. Their effects are immediately and completely reversible. In addition to being free of medical side effects (other than occasional allergic reactions), latex condoms help protect against STDs. Condoms made of polyurethane are appropriate for people who are allergic to latex; they also provide STD protection, but they are not as well studied as latex condoms, so their exact effectiveness is unknown. (Lambskin condoms permit the passage of HIV and other disease-causing organisms, so they can be used only for pregnancy prevention, not the prevention of STDs.) Except for abstinence, correct and consistent use of latex male condoms offers the most reliable available protection against the transmission of HIV.

Disadvantages The two most common complaints about condoms are that they diminish sensation and interfere with spontaneity. Although some people find these drawbacks serious, others consider them only minor disadvantages. Many couples learn to creatively integrate condom use into their sexual practices. Indeed, it can be a way to improve communication and share responsibility in a relationship.

Effectiveness In actual use, the failure rate of condoms varies considerably. First-year rates among typical users average about 14%. At least some pregnancies happen because the condom is carelessly removed after ejaculation. Some may also occur because of a break or a tear, which may happen 1–2 times in every 100 instances of use for latex condoms; some studies have found higher breakage and slippage rates for polyurethane condoms. Breakage is more common among inexperienced users. Other contributing factors include poorly fitting condoms, insufficient lubrication, excessively vigorous sex, and improper storage (because heat destroys rubber, latex condoms should not be stored for long periods in a wallet or a car's glove compartment). To help ensure quality, condoms should not be used past their expiration date or more than 5 years past their date of manufacture (2 years for those with spermicide). It is important to note, however, that most condom failures are due to inconsistent or improper use, not problems with condom quality.

If a condom breaks or is carelessly removed, the risk of pregnancy can be reduced somewhat by the immediate use of a vaginal spermicide. If postcoital (emergency) contraception is an appropriate option, a health care provider should be consulted as soon as possible. The effectiveness of the condom can be greatly improved and approaches that of oral contraceptives if a spermicidal foam is also inserted just *before* intercourse. The most common cause of pregnancy with condom users is "taking a chance"—that is, occasionally not using a condom at all—or waiting to use it until after preejaculate fluid (which may contain some sperm) has already entered the vagina.

> **COMMUNICATE!** Couples sometimes fail to use condoms or other contraceptive methods because they feel it reduces the spontaneity of sex or destroys a romantic atmosphere. If you are in a relationship and find yourself facing this problem, think about what you will do and practice what you will say. Talk with your partner ahead of time, and be confident about your right to control your own fertility. You might begin by saying something like, "I know you think using a condom is unromantic, but not using one means taking a chance on getting pregnant—and I'm not ready for that right now. Being worried doesn't make me feel very romantic. Let's talk about how we can use condoms and still stay in the mood."

Female Condoms

A female condom is a latex or polyurethane pouch that a woman or her partner inserts into her vagina. One brand, Reality, was approved in May 1993 for use in the United States. Although the female condom is preferred in certain situations because it requires less participation on the part of the male partner, its overall popularity remains far below that of the male condom.

The female condom currently available is a disposable device that comes in one size and consists of a soft, loose-fitting polyurethane sheath with two flexible rings (Figure 6-3). The ring at the closed end is inserted into the vagina and placed at the cervix much like a diaphragm. The ring at the open end remains outside the vagina. The walls of the condom protect the inside of the vagina.

The directions that accompany the condom should be followed closely. It can be inserted up to 8 hours before intercourse and should be used with the supplied lubricant or a spermicide to prevent penile irritation. As with male condoms, users need to take care not to tear the condom during insertion or removal. Following intercourse, the woman should remove the condom immediately, before standing up. By twisting and squeezing the outer ring, she can prevent the spilling of semen. A new condom should be used for each act of sexual intercourse. A female condom should not be used with a male condom because when the two are used together, slippage is more likely to occur.

You can buy several types of contraceptives without a prescription. These have several advantages—they are readily accessible and relatively inexpensive, they are moderately effective at preventing pregnancy, and some offer some protection against HIV infection and other STDs. But like all methods, over-the-counter contraceptives work only if they are used correctly. The following guidelines can help you maximize the effectiveness of your method of choice.

Male Condoms

- *Buy latex condoms.* If you're allergic to latex, use a polyurethane condom or wear a lambskin condom under a latex one. Lambskin condoms provide no STD protection; polyurethane condoms may provide protection against pregnancy and STDs comparable to latex condoms, but more studies are needed.

- *Buy and use condoms while they are fresh.* Packages have an expiration date or a manufacturing date. Don't use a condom after the expiration date or more than 5 years after the manufacturing date (2 years if it contains spermicide).

- *Try different styles and sizes.* Male condoms come in a variety of textures, colors, shapes, lubricants, and sizes. Shop around until you find a brand that's right for you. Condom widths and lengths vary by about 10–20%. A condom that is too tight may be uncomfortable and more likely to break; one that is too loose may slip off.

- *Use "thinner" condoms with caution.* Condoms advertised as "thinner" are often no thinner than others, and those that really are the thinnest tend to break more easily.

- *Don't remove the condom from an individual sealed wrapper until you're ready to use it.* Open the packet carefully. Don't use a condom if it's gummy, dried out, or discolored. Keep extra condoms on hand.

- *Store condoms correctly.* Don't leave condoms in extreme heat or cold, and don't carry them in a pocket wallet.

- *Use only water-based lubricants.* Never use oil-based lubricants like Vaseline or hand lotion, as they may cause a latex condom to break. Avoid oil-based vaginal products.

- *Use male condoms correctly* (see Figure 6-2). Use a new condom every time you have intercourse. Misuse is by far the leading reason that condoms fail.

Female Condoms

- *Make sure your condom comes with the necessary supplies and information.* The Reality female condom comes individually wrapped. With your condom, you should receive a leaflet containing instructions and a small bottle of additional lubricant.

- *Buy and use female condoms while they are fresh.* Check the expiration dates on the condom packet and the lubricant bottle.

- *Buy several condoms.* Buy one or more for practice before using one during sex. Have a backup in case you have a problem with insertion or use.

- *Read the leaflet instructions carefully.* Practice inserting the condom and checking that it's in the proper position.

- *Use the female condom correctly.* Make sure the penis is inserted into the pouch and that the outer ring is not pushed into the vagina. Add lubricant around the outer ring if needed.

Contraceptive Sponges

- *Buy and use contraceptive sponges when they are fresh.* Check the expiration date on each package.

- *Read and follow the package instructions carefully.* Moisten the sponge with water and place high in the vagina.

- *Use each sponge only once.* The sponge may be left in place for up to 24 hours without the addition of spermicide for repeated intercourse.

Spermicides

- *Try different types of spermicides.* You may find one type easier or more convenient to use. Foams come in aerosol cans and are similar to shaving cream in consistency. Foams are thicker than creams, which are thicker than jellies. Foams, creams, and jellies usually require applicators; spermicidal suppositories and films do not.

- *Read and follow the package directions carefully.* Cans of foam must be shaken before use. Jellies and creams are often inserted with an applicator just outside the entrance to the cervix. Suppositories and film must be placed with the finger.

- *Pay close attention to the timing of use.* Follow the package instructions for inserting the spermicide at the appropriate time before intercourse actually occurs. Spermicides have a fairly narrow window of effectiveness. Be sure to also allow the recommended amount of time for suppositories and films to dissolve.

- *Use an additional full dose for each additional act of intercourse.*

- *Leave the spermicide in place for 8 hours after the last act of intercourse.*

- *Consider using spermicides with another form of birth control.* These include a condom, diaphragm, or cervical cap. Combined use provides greater protection against pregnancy.

More than 60 medical, public health, and women's groups have filed petitions with the FDA urging the agency to change the status of emergency contraceptive pills from prescription to over the counter; several state legislatures are considering measures that would allow women to obtain the pills from a pharmacist without a prescription. If emergency contraceptive pills do become available over the counter, it will be important for users to follow the instructions carefully.

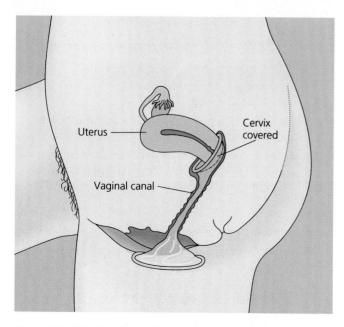

Figure 6-3　The female condom properly positioned.

Labels in figure: Uterus, Cervix covered, Vaginal canal

Advantages　For many women, the greatest advantage of the female condom is the control it gives them over contraception and STD prevention. Female condoms can be inserted before sexual activity and are thus less disruptive than male condoms. Because the outer part of the condom covers the area around the vaginal opening as well as the base of the penis during intercourse, it offers potentially better protection against genital warts or herpes. The polyurethane pouch can be used by people who are allergic to latex. And because polyurethane is thin and pliable, there is little loss of sensation. When used correctly, the female condom should theoretically provide protection against HIV transmission and STDs comparable to that of the latex male condom. However, in research involving typical users, the female condom was less effective in preventing both pregnancy and STDs.

Disadvantages　As with the traditional condom, interference with spontaneity is likely to be a common complaint. The outer ring, which hangs visibly outside the vagina, may be bothersome during foreplay; if so, couples may choose to put the device in just before intercourse. During coitus, both partners must take care that the penis is inserted into the pouch, not outside it, and that the de-

vice does not slip inside the vagina. For many couples, initial awkwardness and difficulty are largely eliminated after a few weeks' use. Female condoms, like male condoms, are made for one-time use. A single female condom costs about four times as much as a single male condom.

Effectiveness　The typical first-year failure rate of the female condom is 21%. For women who follow instructions carefully and consistently, the failure rate is considerably lower. The effectiveness of the female condom, like that of other barrier contraceptive methods, depends primarily on how it is used.

The Diaphragm with Spermicide

Before oral contraceptives were introduced, about 25% of all American couples who used any form of contraception relied on the **diaphragm.** Many former diaphragm users have been won over to the pill or to IUDs, but the diaphragm continues to offer advantages that are important to some couples. About 1.2% of all women who use contraception use a diaphragm.

The diaphragm is a dome-shaped cup of thin rubber stretched over a collapsible metal ring. When correctly used with spermicidal cream or jelly, the diaphragm covers the cervix, blocking sperm from entering the uterus.

A diaphragm can be obtained only by prescription. Because of individual anatomical differences, a diaphragm must be carefully fitted by a trained clinician to ensure both comfort and effectiveness. The fitting should be checked with each routine annual medical examination, as well as after childbirth, abortion, or a weight change of more than 10 pounds.

The woman spreads spermicidal jelly or cream on the diaphragm before inserting it and checking its placement (Figure 6-4). If more than 6 hours elapse between the time of insertion and the time of intercourse, additional spermicide must be applied. The diaphragm must be left in place for at least 6 hours after the last act of coitus to give the spermicide enough time to kill all the sperm.

To remove the diaphragm, the woman simply hooks the front rim down from the pubic bone with one finger and pulls it out. She should wash it with mild soap and water, rinse it, pat it dry, and then examine it for holes or cracks. Defects would most likely develop near the rim and can be spotted by looking at the diaphragm in front of a bright light. After inspecting the diaphragm, she should dust it with cornstarch (*not* talcum powder, which may damage it and irritate the vagina) and store it in its case.

Advantages　Diaphragm use is less intrusive than condom use because a diaphragm can be inserted up to 6 hours before intercourse. Its use can be limited to times of sexual activity only, and it allows for immediate and total reversibility. The diaphragm is free of medical side ef-

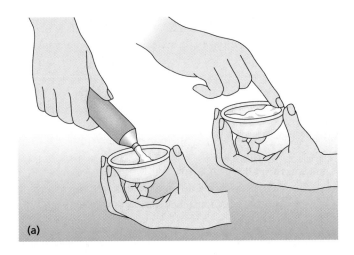

(a)

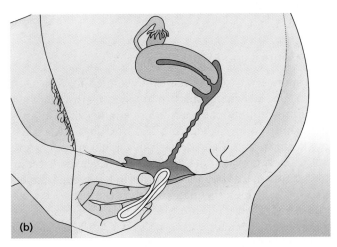

(b)

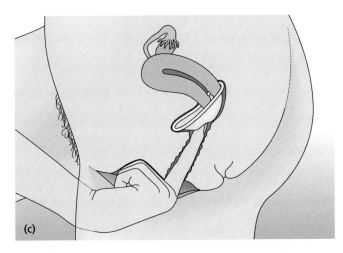

(c)

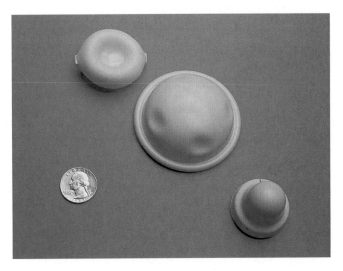

The diaphragm and cervical cap work by covering the mouth of the cervix, blocking sperm from entering the cervix; both require professional fitting. The sponge, which is available without a prescription, acts as a barrier, a spermicide, and a seminal fluid absorbent.

Figure 6-4   Use of the diaphragm.   Wash your hands with soap and water before inserting the diaphragm. It can be inserted while squatting, lying down, or standing with one foot raised. (a) Place about a tablespoon of spermicidal jelly or cream in the concave side of the diaphragm, and spread it around the inside of the diaphragm and around the rim. (b) Squeeze the diaphragm into a long narrow shape between the thumb and forefinger. Insert it into the vagina, and push it up along the back wall of the vagina as far as it will go. (c) Check its position to make sure the cervix is completely covered and that the front rim of the diaphragm is tucked behind the pubic bone.

fects (other than rare allergic reactions). When used along with spermicidal jelly or cream, it offers significant protection against gonorrhea and possibly chlamydia, STDs that are transmitted only by semen and for which the cervix is the sole site of entry. Diaphragm use can also protect the cervix from semen infected with the human papillomavirus, which has been implicated as an important factor in cellular changes in the cervix that can lead to cancer. However, the diaphragm is unlikely to protect against STDs that can be transmitted through vaginal or vulvar surfaces (in addition to the cervix), including HIV infection, genital herpes, and syphilis.

Disadvantages   Diaphragms must always be used with a spermicide, so a woman must keep both of these somewhat bulky supplies with her whenever she anticipates sexual activity. Diaphragms require extra attention, since they must be cleaned and stored with care to preserve their effectiveness. Some women cannot wear a diaphragm because of their vaginal or uterine anatomy. In other women, diaphragm use can cause an increase in bladder infections and may need to be discontinued if repeated infections occur. It has also been associated with a slightly increased risk of **toxic shock syndrome (TSS)**, an occasionally fatal bacterial infection. To diminish the risk of TSS, a woman should wash her hands carefully with soap and water before inserting or removing the diaphragm, should not use the diaphragm during menstruation or in the presence of an abnormal vaginal discharge, and should never leave the device in place for more than 24 hours.

Effectiveness   The effectiveness of the diaphragm mainly depends on whether it is used properly. In actual practice, women rarely use it correctly every time they have intercourse. Typical failure rates are 20% during the first year of use. The main causes of failure are incorrect insertion, inconsistent use, and inaccurate fitting. Sometimes, too, the vaginal walls expand during sexual stimulation, causing the diaphragm to be dislodged. If a diaphragm slips during intercourse, a woman may choose to contact her physician to discuss use of emergency contraception.

The Cervical Cap

The **cervical cap,** another barrier device, is a thimble-shaped rubber or plastic cup that fits snugly over the cervix and is held in place by suction. The cap comes in various sizes and must be fitted by a trained clinician. It is used in a manner similar to that of the diaphragm, a small amount of spermicide being placed in the cup before each insertion.

Advantages   Advantages of the cervical cap are similar to those associated with diaphragm use and include partial STD protection. It is an alternative for women who cannot use a diaphragm because of anatomical reasons or recurrent urinary tract infections. Because the cap fits tightly, it does not require a fresh dose of spermicide with repeated intercourse. It may be left in place for up to 48 hours (compared with 24 hours for the diaphragm).

Disadvantages   Along with most of the disadvantages associated with the diaphragm, difficulty with insertion and removal is more common for cervical cap users. In addition, some studies have indicated that women who use the cap rather than the diaphragm initially have a higher rate of abnormal Pap test results. In most cases, these are due to inflammation or infections of the cervix, conditions that are easily treatable. As a safety precaution, the FDA requires that the cap be prescribed only for women with normal Pap tests and that a repeat Pap test be done after 3 months of use to confirm that no changes have occurred. Because there may be a slightly increased risk of TSS with prolonged use, the cap should not be left in place for more than 48 hours.

Effectiveness   Studies indicate that for women who have never had children, cervical cap failure rate is about 20%, similar to that of the diaphragm. For women who have given birth, the failure rate goes up to about 40%.

Terms
> **cervical cap** A thimble-shaped cup that fits over the cervix, to be used with spermicide.
>
> **sponge** A contraceptive device about 2 inches in diameter that fits over the cervix and acts as a barrier, spermicide, and seminal fluid absorbent.
>
> **douche** To apply a stream of water or other solutions to a body part or cavity such as the vagina; not a contraceptive technique.

COMMUNICATE!   Many types of contraception have to be prescribed and/or fitted by a physician. If you are planning a visit with your physician to obtain a contraceptive, be sure you understand all the implications of the method you choose. Make a list of your questions ahead of time so you don't forget any of them when you're in the office or exam room. Some questions to ask are "How does this contraceptive work?" "How often do I have to use/take/replace it?" "Does it have any side effects?" "What is its effectiveness, and what can I do to make sure it is as effective for me as possible?" "What should I do if I want to stop using/taking it?" "Will it have any permanent effect on my fertility?" "How much is it going to cost?" Think about any other issues that are important to you, and practice wording the questions you need to ask.

The Contraceptive Sponge

The **sponge** was sold in the United States between 1983 and 1995, at which time the original manufacturer decided to withdraw the contraceptive rather than to bring its manufacturing plant up to FDA standards. The safety or effectiveness of the sponge itself was never in question, and FDA approval of the product was never rescinded. A new company has bought the rights to the sponge and expects to have it on the market in the near future.

The sponge is a round, absorbent device about 2 inches in diameter with a polyester loop on one side (for removal) and a concave dimple on the other side, which helps it fit snugly over the cervix. The sponge is made of polyurethane and is presaturated with the same spermicide that is used in contraceptive creams and foams. The spermicide is activated when moistened with a small amount of water just before insertion. The sponge, which can be used only once, acts as a barrier, as a spermicide, and as a seminal fluid absorbent.

Advantages   The sponge offers advantages similar to those of the diaphragm and cervical cap, including partial STD protection. In addition, sponges can be obtained without a professional fitting, and they may be safely left in place for 24 hours without the addition of spermicide for repeated intercourse.

Disadvantages   Reported disadvantages include difficulty with removal and an unpleasant odor if left in place for more than 18 hours. Allergic reactions, such as irritation of the labia, are more common with the sponge than with other spermicide products, probably because the overall dose contained in each sponge is significantly higher than that used with other methods. (It contains 1 gram of spermicide compared with the 60–100 mg present in one application of other spermicidal products.) Because the sponge has also been associated with toxic

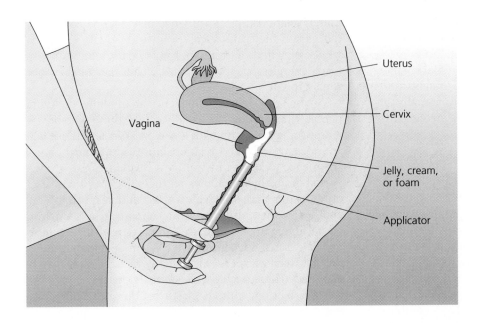

Figure 6-5 The application of spermicide.

shock syndrome, the same precautions must be taken as described for diaphragm use. A sponge user should be especially alert for symptoms of TSS when the sponge has been difficult to remove or was not removed intact. It is not known how much spermicide is absorbed through the vaginal walls with this device or what possible effects are caused by recurring, extended exposure.

Effectiveness   The typical effectiveness of the sponge is similar to that of the diaphragm (20% failure rate during the first year of use) for women who have never experienced childbirth. For women who have had a child, however, sponge effectiveness is significantly lower than diaphragm effectiveness. One possible explanation is that the one size now marketed may be insufficient to adequately cover the cervix after childbirth. To ensure effectiveness, the user should carefully check the expiration date on each sponge, as shelf life is limited.

Vaginal Spermicides

Spermicidal compounds developed for use with a diaphragm have been adapted for use without a diaphragm by combining them with a bulky base. Foams, creams, jellies, suppositories, and films are all available. Foam is sold in an aerosol bottle or a metal container with an applicator that fits on the nozzle. Creams and jellies are sold in tubes with an applicator that can be screwed onto the opening of the tube (Figure 6-5).

Foams, creams, and jellies must be placed deep in the vagina near the cervical entrance and must be inserted no more than 30 minutes before intercourse. After an hour, their effectiveness is drastically reduced, and a new dose must be inserted. Another application is also required before each repeated act of coitus. If the woman wants to **douche**, she should wait for at least 6 hours after the last

intercourse to make sure that there has been time for the spermicide to kill all the sperm; douching is not recommended, however, because it can irritate vaginal tissue and increase the risk of various infections.

The spermicidal suppository is small and easily inserted like a tampon. Because body heat is needed to dissolve and activate the suppository, it is important to wait at least 15 minutes after insertion before having intercourse. The suppository's spermicidal effects are limited in time, and coitus should take place within 1 hour of insertion. A new suppository is required for every act of intercourse.

The vaginal contraceptive film (VCF) is a paper-thin 2-inch square of film that contains spermicide. It is folded over one or two fingers and placed high in the vagina, as close to the cervix as possible. In about 15 minutes the film dissolves into a spermicidal gel that is effective for about 1 hour. A new film must be inserted for each act of intercourse.

Advantages   The use of vaginal spermicides is relatively simple and can be limited to times of sexual activity. They are readily available in most drugstores and do not require a prescription or a pelvic examination. Spermicides allow for complete and immediate reversibility, and the only medical side effects are occasional allergic reactions. Vaginal spermicides may provide limited protection against some STDs but should never be used instead of condoms for reliable protection, especially when there is any risk of HIV infection.

Disadvantages   When used alone, vaginal spermicides must be inserted shortly before intercourse, so their use may be seen as an annoying disruption. Some women find the slight increase in vaginal fluids after spermicide use unpleasant. Spermicides can alter the balance of bacteria in the vagina. Because this may increase the risk of urinary tract infections, women who are especially prone to these infections may want to avoid spermicides. Overuse of spermicides can irritate vaginal tissues; if this occurs, the risk of HIV transmission may actually increase. The potential risks of long-term use are currently being studied.

Effectiveness   The reported effectiveness rates of vaginal spermicides vary widely, depending partly on how consistently and carefully instructions are followed. The typical failure rate is about 26% during the first year of use. Of the various types of spermicides, foam is probably the most effective, because its effervescent mass forms a more dense and evenly distributed barrier to the cervical opening. Creams and jellies provide only minimal protection unless used with a diaphragm or cervical cap. Spermicide use is generally recommended only in combination with other barrier methods or as a backup with other contraceptives.

Abstinence, Fertility Awareness, and Withdrawal

Millions of people throughout the world do not use any of the contraceptive methods we have described, because of religious conviction or cultural prohibitions or because of poverty or lack of information and supplies. If they use any method at all, they are likely to use one of the following relatively "natural" methods of attempting to prevent conception.

Abstinence   The decision not to engage in sexual intercourse for a chosen period of time, or **abstinence,** has been practiced throughout history for a variety of reasons. Until relatively recently, many people abstained because they had no other contraceptive measures. Today, with other methods available, about 1.5% of all American women rely on periodic abstinence as a contraceptive method. To some, other methods simply seem unsuitable. Concern about possible side effects, STDs, and unwanted pregnancy may be factors. For others, the most important reason for choosing abstinence is a moral one, based on cultural or religious beliefs or strongly held personal values (see the box "Sexual Decision Making" on p. 130). Individuals may feel that sexual intercourse is appropriate only for married couples or for people in serious, committed relationships. Abstinence may also be considered the wisest choice in terms of an individual's emotional needs. A period of abstinence may be useful as a time to focus energies on other aspects of interpersonal or personal growth.

Anyone can practice abstinence at any time, including people who are not yet sexually active, those who are beginning a relationship with a new partner, and those who are not currently in a relationship. Couples may choose abstinence to allow time for their relationship to grow. A period of abstinence allows partners to get to know each other better and to develop trust and respect for one another. Many couples who do choose to abstain from sexual intercourse in the traditional sense turn to other mutually satisfying alternatives. When open communication between partners exists, many new avenues may be explored. These may include dancing, massage, hugging, kissing, petting, mutual masturbation, and oral-genital sex. Sexual feelings and intimacy may be expressed and satisfied through a wide range of activities.

The Fertility Awareness Method   The basis for the **fertility awareness method (FAM)** is abstinence from coitus during the fertile phase of a woman's menstrual cycle. Ordinarily only one egg is released by the ovaries each month, and it lives about 24 hours unless it is fertilized. Sperm deposited in the vagina are on average capable of fertilizing an egg for about 6–7 days, so conception can theoretically occur only during 8 days of any cycle. Predicting which 8 days is difficult. It is done by either the calendar method or the temperature method. Information on cyclical changes of the cervical mucus can also help determine the time of ovulation.

The *calendar method* is based on the knowledge that the average woman releases an egg 14–16 days before her next period begins. Few women menstruate with complete regularity, so a record of the menstrual cycle must be kept for 12 months, during which time some other method of contraception must be used. The first day of each period is counted as day 1. To determine the first fertile, or "unsafe," day of the cycle, subtract 18 from the number of days in the shortest cycle (Figure 6-6). To determine the last unsafe day of the cycle, subtract 11 from the number of days in the longest cycle.

The *temperature method* is based on the knowledge that a woman's body temperature drops slightly just before ovulation and rises slightly after ovulation. A woman using the temperature method records her basal (resting) body temperature (BBT) every morning before getting out of bed and before eating or drinking anything. Once the temperature pattern is apparent (usually after about 3 months), the unsafe period for intercourse can be calculated as the interval from day 5 (day 1 is the first day of the period) until 3 days after the rise in BBT. To arrive at a shorter unsafe period, some women combine the calendar and temperature methods, calculating the first unsafe

Terms   **abstinence** Avoidance of sexual intercourse; a method of contraception.

fertility awareness method (FAM) A method of preventing conception based on avoiding intercourse during the fertile phase of a woman's cycle.

sterilization Surgically altering the reproductive system to prevent pregnancy. Vasectomy is the procedure in males; tubal sterilization or hysterectomy is the procedure in females.

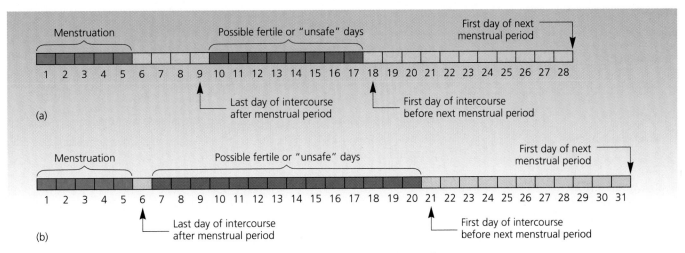

Figure 6-6 The fertility awareness method of contraception. This chart shows the safe and unsafe days for (a) a woman with a regular 28-day cycle and (b) a woman with an irregular cycle, ranging from 25 to 31 days.

day from the shortest cycle of the calendar chart and the last unsafe day as the third day after a rise in BBT.

The *mucus method* (or Billings method) is based on changes in the cervical secretions throughout the menstrual cycle. During the estrogenic phase, cervical mucus increases and is clear and slippery. At the time of ovulation, some women can detect a slight change in the texture of the mucus and find that it is more likely to form an elastic thread when stretched between thumb and finger. After ovulation, these secretions become cloudy and sticky and decrease in quantity. Infertile, safe days are likely to occur during the relatively dry days just before and after menstruation. These additional clues have been found to be helpful by some couples who rely on the fertility awareness method. One problem that may interfere with this method is that vaginal infections or vaginal products or medication can also alter the cervical mucus.

FAM is not recommended for women who have very irregular cycles—about 15% of all menstruating women. Any woman for whom pregnancy would be a serious problem should not rely on FAM alone, because the failure rate is high—approximately 25% during the first year of use. FAM offers no protection against STDs.

Withdrawal In withdrawal, or coitus interruptus, the male removes his penis from the vagina just before he ejaculates. Withdrawal has a relatively high failure rate because the male has to overcome a powerful biological urge. In addition, because preejaculatory fluid may contain viable sperm, pregnancy can occur even if the man withdraws prior to ejaculation. Sexual pleasure is often affected because the man must remain in control and the sexual experience of both partners is interrupted.

Withdrawal is probably about as effective as the di-

aphragm and cervical cap. Men who are less experienced with sexual intercourse and withdrawal or who have difficulty in foretelling when ejaculation will occur have higher failure rates. Withdrawal does not protect against STDs.

Combining Methods

Couples can choose to combine the preceding methods in a variety of ways, both to add STD protection and/or to increase contraceptive effectiveness. For example, condoms are strongly recommended along with OCs whenever there is a risk of STDs (Table 6-3). Foam may be added to condom use to increase protection against both STDs and pregnancy. For many couples, and especially for women, the added benefits will far outweigh the extra effort and expense.

Table 6-4 summarizes the effectiveness and cost of available contraceptive methods.

PERMANENT CONTRACEPTION: STERILIZATION

Sterilization is permanent, and it is highly effective at preventing pregnancy. For these reasons, it is becoming an increasingly popular method of contraception. At present it is the most commonly used method in the United States and in the world. It is especially popular among couples who have been married 10 or more years, as well as couples who have had all the children they intend. Sterilization provides no protection against STDs.

An important consideration in choosing sterilization is that, in most cases, it cannot be reversed and should be considered permanent. Although the chances of restoring

Table 6-3 Contraceptive Methods and STD Protection

Method	Level of Protection
Hormonal methods	Do not protect against HIV or STDs in lower reproductive tract; increase risk of cervical chlamydia; provide some protection against PID.
IUD	Does not protect against STDs; associated with PID in first month after insertion.
Latex male condom	Best method for protection against STDs (if used correctly); does not protect against infections from lesions that are not covered by the condom. (Polyurethane condoms should provide protection, but definitive findings are not yet available; lambskin condoms do not protect against STDs.)
Female condom	Theoretically should reduce the risk of STDs, but research results are not yet available.
Diaphragm, sponge, or cervical cap	Protects against cervical infections and PID. Research results regarding HIV protection are contradictory, but diaphragms, sponges, and cervical caps are not as effective as male condoms.
Spermicide	Modestly reduces the risk of cervical gonorrhea, chlamydia, and PID; effectiveness against other STDs is uncertain. If vaginal irritation occurs, infection risk may increase.
FAM	Does not protect against STDs.
Sterilization	Does not protect against STDs.
Abstinence	Complete protection against STDs (as long as all activities that involve the exchange of body fluids are avoided).

Abstinence or sex with a mutually monogamous, uninfected partner is the surest way to protect yourself against HIV and other STDs. Barring this, correct and consistent use of latex male condoms provides the best protection against STDs.

fertility are being increased by modern surgical techniques, such operations are costly, and pregnancy can never be guaranteed. Some couples choosing male sterilization store sperm as a way of extending the option of childbearing.

Some studies indicate that male sterilization is preferable to female sterilization in a variety of ways. The overall cost of a female procedure is about four times that of a male procedure, and women are much more likely than men to experience both minor and major complications following the operation. Furthermore, feelings of regret seem to be somewhat more prevalent in women than in men after sterilization.

Although some physicians will perform surgery for sterilization on request, most require a thorough discussion with both partners before the operation. Most physicians also recommend that people who have religious conflicts, psychological problems related to sex, or unstable marriages not be sterilized. Young couples who might later change their minds are also frequently advised not to undergo sterilization.

Male Sterilization: Vasectomy

The procedure for male sterilization, **vasectomy,** involves severing the **vasa deferentia,** two tiny ducts that transport sperm from the testes to the seminal vesicles (see Figure 5-2). The testes continue to produce sperm, but the sperm are absorbed into the body. Because the testes contribute only about 10% of the total seminal fluid, the actual quantity of ejaculate is only slightly reduced. Hormone production from the testes continues with very little change, and secondary sex characteristics are not altered.

Vasectomy is ordinarily performed in a physician's office and takes about 30 minutes. A local anesthetic is injected into the skin of the scrotum near the vasa. Small incisions are made at the upper end of the scrotum where it joins the body, and the vas deferens on each side is exposed, severed, and tied off or sealed by electrocautery. The incisions are then closed with sutures, and a small dressing is applied (Figure 6-7). Pain and swelling are usually slight and can be relieved with ice compresses, aspirin, and the use of a scrotal support. Bleeding and infection occasionally develop but are usually easily treated.

Terms

vasectomy The surgical severing of the ducts that carry sperm to the ejaculatory duct.

vasa deferentia The two ducts that carry sperm to the ejaculatory duct, singular, vas deferens.

Table 6-4 Contraceptive Effectiveness and Costs

| Method | Percentage of Women Experiencing an Unintended Pregnancy in the First Year of Use | | Approximate Annual Cost[a] |
	Typical Use	Perfect Use	
Norplant	0.05%	0.05%	$160 if left in for 5 years
Male sterilization (vasectomy)	0.15	0.10	$750 (one-time cost)
Depo-Provera	0.30	0.30	$280
Female sterilization	0.50	0.50	$2500 (one-time cost)
Copper T IUD	0.8	0.6	$50 if left in for 10 years
Progestasert IUD	2.0	1.5	$360
Oral contraceptives	5		$300
Combination		0.1	
Progestin only		0.5	
Male condom (latex)	14	3	$40
Withdrawal	19	4	none
Diaphragm with spermicide	20	6	$130
Sponge[b]	20	9	$125
Cervical cap[b]	20	9	$130
Female condom	21	5	$200
Fertility awareness method	25		none
Calendar alone		9	
Combination of FAM methods		2	
Spermicides	26	6	$80
Chance	85	85	none

[a] Based on costs in a managed-care setting; costs will vary, as will insurance coverage.
[b] For women who have given birth, the rates of unintended pregnancy increase to 40% for typical use and 26% (cervical cap) and 20% (sponge) for perfect use.

SOURCE: Hatcher, R. A., et al. 1998. *Contraceptive Technology*, 17th rev. ed. New York: Ardent Media. Reprinted by permission of Irvington Publishing.

Fewer complications occur with an alternative procedure involving a midline puncture rather than incisions; this "no-scalpel" technique is used in about 30% of vasectomies performed in the United States. After either procedure, most men are ready to return to work in 2 days.

Men can have sex again as soon as they feel no further discomfort, usually after about a week. Another method of contraception must be used for the next 20 ejaculations or 3 months after vasectomy, however, because sperm produced before the operation may still be present in the semen. Microscopic examination of a semen sample can confirm that sperm are no longer present in the ejaculate.

No strong links have been found between vasectomy and chronic diseases, and the bulk of the evidence now indicates that men with vasectomies are not at increased risk for heart disease, prostate cancer, or testicular cancer. However, research into the long-term health effects of vasectomy is ongoing.

Vasectomy is highly effective. In a small number of cases, a severed vas rejoins itself, so some physicians advise yearly examination of a semen sample. The overall failure rate for vasectomy is 0.15%.

Although some surgeons report pregnancy rates of about 80% for partners of men who have their vasectomies reversed within 10 years of the original procedure, most studies report figures in the 50% range. In at least half of all men who have had vasectomies, the process of absorbing sperm (instead of ejaculating it) results in antisperm antibodies that may interfere with later fertility.

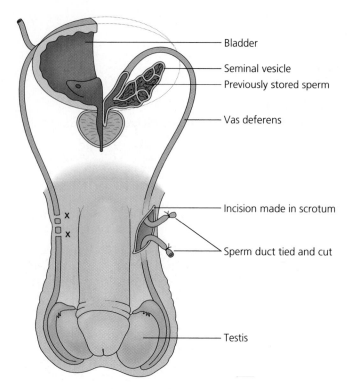

— Bladder

— Seminal vesicle
— Previously stored sperm

— Vas deferens

— Incision made in scrotum

— Sperm duct tied and cut

— Testis

Figure 6-7 Vasectomy. This surgical procedure involves severing the vasa deferentia, thereby preventing sperm from being transported and ejaculated.

Other factors, such as length of time between the vasectomy and the reversal surgery, may also be important predictors of reversal success.

Female Sterilization

The most common method of female sterilization involves severing, or in some manner blocking, the oviducts, thereby preventing the egg from reaching the uterus and the sperm from entering the fallopian tubes (see Figure 5-1). Ovulation and menstruation continue, but the unfertilized eggs are released into the abdominal cavity and absorbed. Although progesterone levels in the blood may decline slightly, hormone production by the ovaries and secondary sex characteristics are generally not affected.

Tubal sterilization is most commonly performed by a method called **laparoscopy.** A laparoscope, a tube containing a small light, is inserted through a small abdominal incision, and the surgeon looks through it to locate the fallopian tubes. Instruments are passed either through the laparoscope or through a second small incision, and the two fallopian tubes are sealed off with ties or staples or by

Terms

tubal sterilization Severing or in some manner blocking the oviducts, preventing eggs from reaching the uterus.

laparoscopy Examining the internal organs by inserting a tube containing a small light through an abdominal incision.

hysterectomy Total or partial surgical removal of the uterus.

electrocautery (Figure 6-8). Either a local or a general anesthetic can be used. The operation takes about 15 minutes, and women can usually leave the hospital 2–4 hours after surgery. Tubal sterilization can also be performed shortly after a vaginal delivery, or in the case of cesarean section immediately after the uterine incision is repaired.

Although female sterilization is somewhat riskier than male sterilization, with a complication rate of about 0.1–7%, it is the more common procedure (see the box "Contraceptive Use Among American Women"). Potential problems include bowel injury, wound infection, and bleeding. Serious complications are rare, and the death rate is low.

The failure rate for tubal sterilization is about 0.5%. When pregnancies do occur, an increased percentage of them are ectopic. Some complaints of long-term abdominal discomfort and menstrual irregularity following tubal sterilization have been reported. Reversibility rates of current methods are about 50–70%. A new method currently being considered for use involves a clip that can be clamped around the fallopian tube; this method may provide a better chance of later reversal. However, it is also associated with a higher failure rate.

Hysterectomy, removal of the uterus, is the preferred method of sterilization for only a small number of women, usually those with preexisting menstrual problems. Because of the risks involved, hysterectomy is not recommended unless the woman has disease or damage of the uterus and future surgery appears inevitable.

ISSUES IN CONTRACEPTION

The subject of contraception is closely tied to several issues that are currently receiving much attention in the United States—issues like premarital sexual relations, gender differences, and sexuality education for teens.

When Is It OK to Begin Having Sexual Relations?

One issue that strongly affects a society's approach to contraception is the question of at what age it's acceptable to begin having sex. Opinions on this issue often determine one's views on sexuality education and contraception accessibility. Americans have a wide range of opinions: only after marriage; when 18 years or older; when in a loving, stable relationship; when the partners have completed their education and/or could support a child; whenever both partners feel ready and are using protection against pregnancy and STDs.

Opinions about appropriate sexual behavior shift from one decade to another. Although attitudes became more liberal during the 1960s and 1970s, people started having more restrictive views in the 1980s and 1990s. Today, the most common reasons for disapproving of sex are the risk

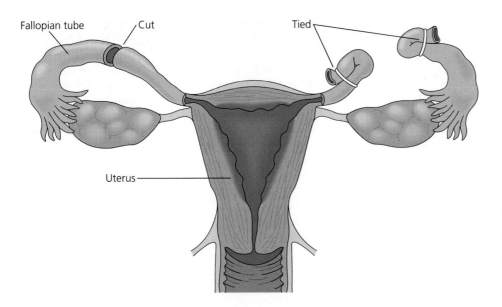

Fallopian tube | Cut | Tied

Uterus

Figure 6-8 Tubal sterilization. This procedure involves severing or blocking the fallopian tubes, thereby preventing eggs from traveling from the ovaries to the uterus. It is a more complex procedure than vasectomy.

of exposure to STDs, the risk of pregnancy, and moral or religious beliefs. According to recent data, most of today's young Americans are somewhat permissive regarding premarital sex. While many approve of sexual relations for couples who are seriously dating or engaged to be married, they are less accepting of sexual intercourse on a first date or at the casual dating stage.

Closely related to the issue of beginning sexual relations is a more personal question: What would you consider the ideal amount of previous sexual experience for you and your partner? Again, opinions vary, especially in terms of what is desirable for men and for women. While limited experience is still more commonly deemed desirable for women, being "sexually experienced" is often valued more highly for men.

As more women consider careers for themselves and therefore often delay childbearing and even marriage, the likelihood of sexual activity and the critical need for pregnancy and STD prevention only increase. As a result, making decisions about sexual activity and contraception becomes even more important to those starting college or a career. Unfortunately, however, many individuals in this age group—even those who protect their health in all other areas of their life—end up taking high risks in their sexual behavior. Ambivalence and a lack of communication about who will "take charge" are common and are partly due to the denial of, and hypocrisy about, sexual behavior that exists in our society. (For guidelines on improving your own communication, see the box "Talking with a Partner About Contraception.")

Contraception and Gender Differences

A second issue, one all couples must confront, is the differing significance of contraception to women and men. The consequences of not using contraception are markedly different for men and women. In past years, women have accepted the primary responsibility of contraception, along with related side effects and health risks, partly because of the wider spectrum of methods available to them and partly because women have greater personal investment in preventing pregnancy and childbearing. Men still have very few contraceptive options, with condoms being the only reversible method currently available (see the box "Future Methods of Contraception"). Recently, however, their participation has become critical, since condom use is central to safer sex, even when OCs or other female methods are being used.

Although dependent primarily on the cooperation of the man, condom use and the prevention of STDs has potentially greater consequences for the woman. While men may suffer only local and short-term effects from the most common diseases (not including HIV infection), women face an increased risk of serious long-term effects, such as cervical cancer and/or pelvic infection with associated infertility, from these same prevalent STDs. In addition, women are more likely to contract HIV from an infected partner than men are. In other words, although dependent on the male, condom use is clearly a more important issue for women. The female condom may offer a helpful alternative, but cooperation of the male partner is still needed to ensure correct use.

The experience of an unintended pregnancy is very different for the two involved partners. While men do suffer emotional stress from such an unexpected occurrence (and sometimes share financial and/or custodial responsibilities), women are much more intimately affected, obviously by the biological process of pregnancy itself, as well as the outcome: abortion, adoption, or parenting. In addition, our societal attitudes are more severely punitive toward the woman and place much greater responsibility and blame on her when an unintended pregnancy occurs;

About 60 million women in the United States are in their child-bearing years (15–44) and thus face decisions about contraception. Overall, about 64% of American women use some form of contraception, and most of the remaining 36% are either sterile, pregnant or trying to become pregnant, or not sexually active. Only 5% of American women are fertile, sexually active, and not seeking pregnancy; this small group accounts for almost half of the 3 million unintended pregnancies that occur each year. The unintended pregnancies that occur among contraceptive users are usually the result of inconsistent or incorrect use of methods. For example, in a large-scale survey asking women about their use of contraception in the previous 3 months, 13% of pill users reported missing two or more pills, and 20% of barrier method users reported that they actually used their method of choice only half the time—or less.

Female sterilization and oral contraceptives are the two most popular methods among American women (see figure). However, choice of contraceptive method and consistency of use vary with age, marital status, and other factors:

- *Age:* Sterilization is much more common among older women, particularly those who are over 35 years of age and/or who have had children. Older women are also much more likely to use reversible methods consistently—they are least likely to miss pills and most likely to use barrier methods during every act of intercourse. Young women between the ages of 15 and 17 years who use OCs are more likely by far to miss pills than women in any other age group.

- *Marital status:* Women who are or have been married have much higher rates of sterilization than women who have never been married. Those who have never been married have high rates of OC and condom usage.

- *Ethnicity:* Overall rates of contraceptive use and use of female sterilization and OCs are highest among white women. Implants and injectables are more often used by African American women and Latinas, and IUD use is highest among Latinas. Condom use is highest among Asian American women and similar across other ethnic groups. Male sterilization is much more common among white men than among men of other ethnic groups.

- *Socioeconomic status and educational attainment:* Low socioeconomic status and low educational attainment are associated with high rates of female sterilization and low rates of pill and condom use. However, women who are poor or have low educational attainment and who do use OCs have higher rates of consistent use than women who are wealthier or have more education.

Some trends in contraceptive use may also reflect the differing priorities and experiences of women and men. For example, female sterilization is more expensive and carries greater health risks than male sterilization—yet it is more than twice as common. (Worldwide, female sterilization is more than four times as common as male sterilization.) This pattern may reflect culturally defined gender roles and the fact that women are more directly affected by unintended pregnancy. In surveys, women rate pregnancy prevention as the single most important factor when choosing a contraceptive method; in contrast, men rate STD prevention as equally important.

SOURCES: Alan Guttmacher Institute. 2000. *Facts in Brief: Contraceptive Use* (http://www.agi-usa.org/ pubs/fb_contr_use.html; retrieved March 24, 2001). Grady, W. R., D. H. Klepinger, and A. Nelson-Wally. 1999. Contraceptive characteristics: The perceptions and priorities of men and women. *Family Planning Perspectives* 31(4): 168–175. National Center for Health Statistics. 1997. Fertility, family planning, and women's health: New data from the 1995 survey of family growth. *Vital and Health Statistics* 23(19).

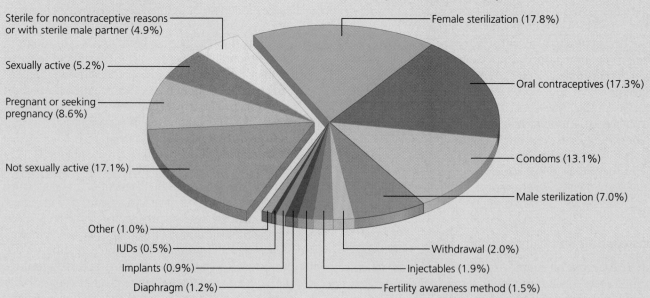

Women not using contraception (35.8% of U.S. women)

- Sterile for noncontraceptive reasons or with sterile male partner (4.9%)
- Sexually active (5.2%)
- Pregnant or seeking pregnancy (8.6%)
- Not sexually active (17.1%)
- Other (1.0%)
- IUDs (0.5%)
- Implants (0.9%)
- Diaphragm (1.2%)

Method reported by women using contraception (64.2% of U.S. women)

- Female sterilization (17.8%)
- Oral contraceptives (17.3%)
- Condoms (13.1%)
- Male sterilization (7.0%)
- Withdrawal (2.0%)
- Injectables (1.9%)
- Fertility awareness method (1.5%)

Contraceptive use among American women age 15–44 years.

Many people have a difficult time talking about contraception with a potential sex partner. How should you bring it up? And whose responsibility is it, anyway? Talking about the subject may be embarrassing at first, but imagine the possible consequences of *not* talking about it. An unintended pregnancy or a sexually transmitted disease could profoundly affect you for the rest of your life. Talking about contraception is one way of showing that you care about yourself, your partner, and your future.

Before you talk with your partner, explore your own thoughts and feelings. Find out the facts about different methods of contraception, and decide which one you think would be most appropriate for you. If you're nervous about having this discussion with your partner, it may help to practice with a friend.

Pick a good time to bring up the subject. Don't wait until you've started to have sex. A time when you're both feeling comfortable and relaxed will maximize your chances of having a good discussion. Tell your partner what you know about contraception and how you feel about using it, and talk about what steps you both need to take to get and use a method you can live with. Listen to what your partner has to say, and try to understand his or her point of view. You may need to have more than one discussion, and it may take some time for both of you to feel comfortable with the subject. *But don't have sex until this issue is resolved.*

If you want your partner to be involved but he or she isn't interested in talking about contraception, or if he or she leaves all the responsibility for it up to you, consider whether this is really a person you want to be sexually involved with. If you decide to go ahead with the involvement, you may want to enlist the support of a friend, family member, or health care worker to help you make and implement decisions about the essential issue of contraception.

---

the focus is almost entirely on the "girl who got into trouble" or the "unwed mother," with no mention of the "unwed father." The current trend of cutting welfare support for single mothers means that this increasing number of young women and their children will live with even greater disadvantages.

Fortunately, there is growing interest in the roles and responsibilities of men in family planning. More leaders in the health care field are recognizing that few educational materials and clinical programs focus on male contraception and reproductive health. Men can increase their participation in contraception by initiating and supporting communication regarding contraception and STD protection, buying and using condoms whenever appropriate, helping pay contraceptive costs, and being available for shared responsibility in the resolution of an unintended pregnancy, should one occur.

Sexuality and Contraceptive Education for Teenagers

A third controversial issue is sexuality education and pregnancy prevention programs for teenagers. Again, opinion in the United States is sharply divided. Certain religious groups are concerned that more sexuality education and especially the availability of contraceptives will lead to more sexual activity and promiscuity. They maintain that greater access to improved contraception was a key factor contributing to the sexual revolution in the 1960s and that the ensuing liberal sexual attitudes have been generally more destructive than helpful. They point to an increase in divorce, a rise in STDs, and a general relaxing of standards of morality as related negative effects.

Many in this group urge that sexuality education be

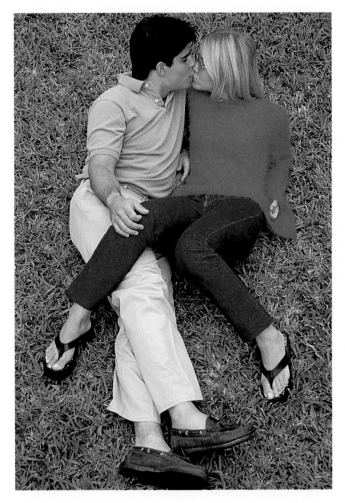

How old should people be when they become sexually active? The answer depends on the personal values, beliefs, and experiences of the individuals involved.

Even the best of the present methods of contraception have drawbacks, and the search continues for the ideal method—more effective, safer, cheaper, easier to use, more readily available, easily reversible, and acceptable to more people. Many new methods are widely used in other countries long before they become available in the United States. This delay is partly due to higher costs of safety testing in the United States, greater liability risks for manufacturers, and lower levels of government funding for contraceptive research.

Despite delays, the past decade has seen several new methods approved and marketed in the United States, a trend that is likely to continue. The options expected to become available in the near future are variations of current methods: new combinations of hormones in OCs, implants, injectables, and emergency contraceptives; new designs for IUDs and condoms; and new spermicides and microbicides that are effective in destroying viruses and bacteria as well as sperm. Some of the other methods being studied are described below.

New Ways of Delivering Hormones

Several new techniques for delivering hormones are currently being developed. The *contraceptive patch,* which releases estrogen and progestin, is similar to the patches used in nicotine replacement therapy. About the size of a half-dollar, the patch can be worn on an arm, the abdomen, or the buttocks. It works like OCs and is highly effective in preventing pregnancy.

The *vaginal ring* resembles the rim of a diaphragm and is molded with a mixture of progestin and estrogen. A woman inserts the ring herself and wears it for 3 weeks, during which time the hormones are absorbed into her bloodstream, preventing ovulation. Menstruation follows removal, and then a new ring is inserted.

Similar to Norplant, *biodegradable implants* are placed under the skin and deliver small doses of hormones over a long period of time. Unlike Norplant, the capsules dissolve over time, eliminating the need for surgical removal. *Injectable microspheres,* tiny clusters of molecules filled with hormones, also dissolve as they deliver a steady dose of hormones over many months.

New Barrier Methods

Lea's Shield is a one-size-fits-all diaphragm-like device that does not require fitting by a clinician. Made of silicone, it can be used by those allergic to latex and is not damaged by petroleum-based products. Lea's Shield is already available in Canada and parts of Europe. FemCap, also made of silicone, is a prescription barrier contraceptive shaped like a sailor's hat with a dome that covers the cervix. It is designed to fit more comfortably and to dislodge less frequently than conventional cervical caps.

Home Tests to Increase the Effectiveness of FAM

A computerized aid for FAM that uses the results of home urine tests is currently available in England, Germany, the Netherlands, and several other countries. The handheld Persona device tracks levels of two hormones and tells a woman when she is fertile. On fertile days, a couple must abstain from intercourse or use another method. If used correctly, Persona decreases the failure rate of FAM to about 6%.

Hormonal Contraceptives for Men

Male and female hormones can interfere with sperm development in the male, just as they suppress ovulation in the female. One promising contraceptive under study combines a daily pill containing a progestin with a testosterone pellet implanted under the skin and replaced every 12 weeks. This combination has been shown to reduce sperm production to zero, although some men report side effects similar to those women may experience when taking OCs: headaches, acne, and increased appetite.

Contraceptive Immunization

Immunity to fertility has occasionally (though rarely) occurred as a result of a man's being unintentionally sensitized to his own sperm cells. He then produces antibodies that inactivate sperm as if they were disease organisms. In theory, a woman could be purposely sensitized against her own egg cells or against her partner's sperm cells. Another immunocontraceptive under study targets just the zona pellucida (ZP), the protein covering of the egg cell. Immunization against ZP would temporarily block sperm from penetrating the egg without affecting normal egg development.

Reversible Sterilization

Present methods of sterilization in both men and women are reversible 50–70% of the time. Several new techniques are being studied in the hope that restoring fertility can be made easier and more predictable. These techniques include injecting liquid silicone into the fallopian tubes, where it solidifies and forms a plug, and placing various types of clips and plugs on the vasa to totally block sperm flow. These plugs or clips could then be removed if an individual wanted to restore fertility.

handled in the home, where parents can instill moral values, including premarital abstinence. According to some in this group, young people should primarily be taught to "just say no." They see most public education about contraception, especially facilities that make supplies available, as only increasing the problem.

Other groups argue that encouraging the public availability of contraceptive information and supplies does not necessarily result in an increase in promiscuous sexual behavior, pointing to the fact that many young teenagers are already pregnant when they first visit a health care facility. These groups assert that parents are not effectively dealing with the issues and that a broader, coordinated approach involving public institutions, including schools, is needed, along with parental input. Many current programs focus on postponing sexual involvement but also emphasize contraceptive use for individuals who are sexually active. Increased availability of contraceptive information and methods is considered a necessary and realistic part of this approach.

Proponents of sexuality and contraceptive education for teenagers point to countries, such as the Netherlands, that have a far lower incidence of teenage pregnancy than the United States (1.8% and 12.8%, respectively). While Dutch teens are just as likely as American teens to engage in intercourse, they are far more likely to use contraception. In the Netherlands, sexuality and contraceptive education are extensive and quite explicit in radio and television programming, and national health insurance and state-financed clinics provide and fund contraception.

Recent studies have revealed an encouraging new trend toward safer sexual practices among American high school students. In a large-scale survey conducted in 1999, 50% of students surveyed said that they had never had intercourse, and more than 60% had abstained from intercourse during the previous 3 months. Among sexually active high school students, nearly 60% reported that they or their partner had used a condom the last time they had intercourse. These statistics help explain recent declines in the birth rate for teenagers, which hit an all-time low in 1999.

While sexuality and contraceptive education in public facilities remains a volatile issue, there is overall growing support for such programs. Studies show that sexually active students who receive sexuality education are more likely to use contraceptives and that those who are not sexually active are not encouraged to initiate having sex. However, these programs are receiving increasing support mainly because of the prevalent fear of HIV infection and other STDs. In fact, in some cases the focus of "sex ed" is almost exclusively on disease prevention. Although not as deadly as the AIDS epidemic, the nearly 1 million teenage pregnancies that occur each year in the United States are a serious public health problem and warrant much greater national attention than they have received thus far.

> **COMMUNICATE!** Did your parents tell you anything about contraception? If so, was it what you needed or wanted to know? Think about what you would ideally have wanted someone to tell you. Then imagine saying something similar to your own adolescents (or young people you care about). You might begin by saying something like, "I want you to know I respect your privacy and your right to make decisions. I also love you and want to be sure you're able to protect yourself if you choose to have sex."

WWW. WHICH CONTRACEPTIVE METHOD IS RIGHT FOR YOU?

The process of choosing and using a contraceptive method can be complex and varies greatly from one cou-

ple to another. Each person must consider many variables in deciding which method is most acceptable and appropriate for her or him. Important considerations include those listed here:

1. *Health risks.* Is there anything in your personal or family medical history that would affect your choice of method? For each method you consider, what are the potential health risks that apply to you? For example, IUDs are not recommended for young women without children because of an increased risk of pelvic infection and subsequent infertility. Hormonal methods should be used only after a clinical evaluation of your medical history. Other methods have only minor and local side effects. If necessary, talk with your physician about the potential health effects of different methods for you.

2. *The implications of an unplanned pregnancy.* How would an unplanned pregnancy affect you and your future? What are your feelings regarding the options—abortion, adoption, or raising a child? If effectiveness is of critical importance to you, carefully consider the ways the effectiveness of each method can be improved. Abstinence is 100% effective, if maintained. If used correctly, hormonal methods offer very good protection against pregnancy. Barrier methods can be combined with spermicides to improve their effectiveness.

3. *STD risk.* How likely are you to be exposed to any sexually transmitted diseases? Have you and your partner been screened for STDs recently? Have you openly and honestly discussed your past sexual behavior? Condom use is of critical importance whenever any risk of STDs is present. This is especially true when you are not in an exclusive, long-term relationship or when you are taking the pill, because cervical changes that occur during hormone use may increase vulnerability to certain diseases. Abstinence or activities that don't involve intercourse or any other exchange of body fluids can be a satisfactory alternative for some people.

4. *Convenience and comfort level.* How do your partner and you view each of the methods? Which would you most likely use consistently? The hormonal methods are generally ranked high in this category, unless there are negative side effects and health risks or forgetting to take pills is a problem for you. Some people think condom use disrupts spontaneity and lowers penile sensitivity. (Creative approaches to condom use and improved quality can decrease these concerns.) The diaphragm, cervical cap, contraceptive sponge, female condom, and spermicides can be inserted before intercourse begins but are still considered a significant inconvenience by some.

5. *Type of relationship.* How easy is it for you to talk with your partner about contraception? How willing is he or she to be involved? Barrier methods require more motivation and a sense of responsibility from *each*

ASSESS YOURSELF · Which Contraceptive Method Is Right for You and Your Partner?

If you are sexually active, you need to use the contraceptive method that will work best for you. A number of factors may be involved in your decision. The following questions will help you sort out these factors and choose an appropriate method. Answer yes (Y) or no (N) for each statement as it applies to you and, if appropriate, your partner.

_____ 1. I like sexual spontaneity and don't want to be bothered with contraception at the time of sexual intercourse.

_____ 2. I need a contraceptive immediately.

_____ 3. It is very important that I do not become pregnant now.

_____ 4. I want a contraceptive method that will protect me and my partner against sexually transmitted diseases.

_____ 5. I prefer a contraceptive method that requires the cooperation and involvement of both partners.

_____ 6. I have sexual intercourse frequently.

_____ 7. I have sexual intercourse infrequently.

_____ 8. I am forgetful or have a variable daily routine.

_____ 9. I have more than one sex partner.

_____ 10. I have heavy periods with cramps.

_____ 11. I prefer a method that requires little or no action or bother on my part.

_____ 12. I am a nursing mother.

_____ 13. I want the option of conceiving immediately after discontinuing contraception.

_____ 14. I want a contraceptive method with few or no side effects.

If you answered "yes" to the statements whose numbers are listed in the left columns below, the method in the right columns might be a good choice for you.

1, 3, 6, 10, 11	Oral contraceptives	5, 7, 12, 13, 14	Diaphragm and spermicide, cervical cap
1, 3, 6, 8, 10, 11	Contraceptive implants	2, 5, 7, 8, 12, 13, 14	Vaginal spermicides and sponge
1, 3, 6, 8, 10, 11, 12	Contraceptive injectables	5, 7, 13, 14	FAM and withdrawal
1, 3, 6, 8, 11, 12, 13	IUD		
2, 4, 5, 7, 8, 9, 12, 13, 14	Condoms (male and female)		

Your answers may indicate that more than one method would be appropriate for you. To help narrow your choices, circle the numbers of the statements that are *most* important for you. Before you make a final choice, talk with your partner(s) and your physician. Consider your own lifestyle and preferences, as well as the features of each method (effectiveness, side effects, costs, and so on). For maximum protection against pregnancy and STDs, you might want to consider combining two methods. It's also a good idea to be prepared for change; the method that seems right for you now may be inappropriate if your circumstances become different.

partner than hormonal methods do. When the method depends on the cooperation of one's partner, assertiveness is necessary, no matter how difficult. This is especially true in new relationships, when condom use is most important. When sexual activity is infrequent, a barrier method may make more sense than an IUD or one of the hormonal methods.

6. *Ease and cost of obtaining and maintaining each method.* If a physical exam and clinic follow-up is required, how readily accessible is this to you? Can you and your partner afford the associated expenses of the method? Investigate the costs of different methods (see Table 6-4). Find out if your insurance covers any of the costs.

7. *Religious or philosophical beliefs.* Are any of the methods unacceptable to you because of your personal beliefs? For some, abstinence and/or FAM may be the only permissible contraceptive methods.

Whatever your needs, circumstances, or beliefs, *do* make a choice about contraception. Not choosing anything is the one method known *not* to work. (To help make a choice that's right for you, take the quiz in the box "Which Contraceptive Method Is Right for You and Your Partner?") This is an area in which taking charge of your health has immediate and profound implications for your future. The method you choose today won't necessarily be the one you'll want to use your whole life or even next year. But it should be one that works for you right now.

Your decisions about contraception are among the most important you will make in your life. They affect your physical and emotional health, your relationship and family choices, and your career and life plans. Decisions about contraception are far too important to leave to chance!

Right now you can

- Close your eyes and visualize the life you hope to have in 5 years, 10 years, and 15 years. Does it include a relationship, a family, children? Are you doing anything right now—such as taking a chance on an unintended pregnancy—that could prevent you from realizing your dreams?

- If you are sexually active or considering becoming so, make an appointment with a physician or health care practitioner to discuss which contraceptive method is right for you.

- If you are sexually active, consider whether your sexual health or the nature of your relationship with your partner has changed since you made your current contraceptive choices. If you want to make changes, think about how to do so and how to discuss such changes with your partner.

SUMMARY

- Barrier methods of contraception physically prevent sperm from reaching the egg; hormonal methods are designed to prevent ovulation, fertilization, and/or implantation; and surgical methods permanently block the movement of sperm or eggs to the site of conception.

- The choice of contraceptive method depends on effectiveness, convenience, cost, reversibility, side effects and risk factors, and protection against STDs. The concept of effectiveness includes failure rate and continuation rate.

- In oral contraceptives (OCs), a combination of estrogen and progestins prevents ovulation, inhibits the movement of sperm, and affects the uterine lining so that implantation is prevented.

- Contraceptive implants consist of hormone-filled capsules inserted under the skin that release steady doses of synthetic progesterone, providing effective, reversible protection for up to 5 years.

- Depo-Provera injections contain a long-acting progestin that protects against pregnancy for a period of 3 months. Lunelle injections contain both estrogen and progestin and must be repeated every month.

- The most commonly used emergency contraceptives are two-dose regimens of combined or progesterone-only oral contraceptives.

- How IUDs work is not clearly understood; they may cause biochemical changes in the uterus, affect movement of sperm and eggs, or interfere with the implantation of the egg in the uterus.

- Advantages of male condoms include availability and ease of purchase, simplicity of use, immediate reversibility, STD protection, and freedom from side effects.

- Female condoms consist of a polyurethane or latex sheath that can be inserted well before intercourse. They may be less reliable than male condoms in preventing pregnancy and the transmission of STDs.

- When used correctly, with spermicidal cream or jelly, a diaphragm or cervical cap covers the cervix and blocks sperm from entering.

- The contraceptive sponge is a round device that is saturated with spermicide. Sponges act as barriers, spermicides, and absorbers of seminal fluid.

- Vaginal spermicides come in the form of foams, creams, jellies, suppositories, and film.

- Abstinence may be chosen out of fear of STDs or because of personal needs.

- The fertility awareness method (FAM) is based on avoiding coitus during the fertile phase of a woman's menstrual cycle. The calendar method, basal body temperature method, or mucus method may be used to determine the fertile period.

- In withdrawal, the male must remove his penis from the vagina before he ejaculates.

- Combining methods can increase contraceptive effectiveness and help protect against STDs.

- Sterilization is considered permanent; reversibility can never be guaranteed. Male sterilization may be preferable to female sterilization because it is less expensive, has fewer complications, and causes fewer feelings of regret.

- Vasectomy—male sterilization—involves severing the vasa deferentia. Female sterilization involves severing or blocking the oviducts so that the egg cannot reach the uterus.

- Opinions on when to begin having sexual relations are tied to views on sexuality education and contraception accessibility. Because women today frequently delay childbearing, decisions about sexual activity and contraception are essential for optimal health.

- Although using condoms depends on male cooperation, the implications of not using them are greater for women, in terms of both pregnancy and the consequences of STDs.

- Opinion in the United States is divided on the issues of sexuality education and availability of contraceptives for teenagers.

- Issues to be considered in choosing a contraceptive include the individual health risks of each method, the implications of an unplanned pregnancy, STD risk, convenience and comfort level, type of relationship, the cost and ease of obtaining and maintaining each method, and religious or philosophical beliefs.

TAKE ACTION

1. Make an appointment with a physician or other health care provider to review the health risks of different contraceptive methods as they apply to you. For each method, determine whether any risk factors associated with its use apply to you or your partner.

2. Visit a local drugstore and make a list of the contraceptives they sell, along with their prices. Next, investigate the costs of prescription contraceptive methods by contacting your physician, medical clinic, and/or pharmacy. Estimate the annual cost of regular use for each method, and rank the methods from most to least expensive.

3. Devise a public service campaign that will encourage men to become more involved in contraception. Your campaign might use techniques such as TV and print advertisements, radio announcements, and posters. Look at other public service campaigns and advertisements for ideas. What sorts of images do you think would be motivational? What sort of tone and message do you think would be most effective?

W. JOURNAL ENTRY

1. Consider the different methods of contraception described in this chapter. In your health journal, rank the methods according to how they suit your particular lifestyle. Take into account such considerations as convenience, cost, and how often you have sexual intercourse.

2. In your health journal, list the positive behaviors and attitudes that help you adhere to your beliefs about contraception. (For example, not getting drunk would probably help prevent you from making an unwise choice.) Are there ways you can strengthen these behaviors? Then list behaviors and attitudes that might interfere with your effective use of contraception. Can you do anything to change or improve any of these?

3. *Critical Thinking* What are your feelings about sexuality education for children and teenagers? Write a brief essay that presents the main arguments, both pro and con. Conclude with a description of the sexuality education you received and a statement of your own opinion on whether sexuality education is valuable. Are you satisfied with what you were taught? What effect did it have on your sexual behavior? In general, do you think sexuality education promotes responsibility or promiscuity? Or neither?

FOR MORE INFORMATION

Books

Boston Women's Health Book Collective. 1998. *Our Bodies, Ourselves for the New Century.* New York: Simon & Schuster. *Broad coverage of many women's health concerns, with extensive coverage of contraception.*

Glasier, A., and B. Winikoff. 2000. *Fast Facts: Contraception.* Oxford: Health Press. *Basic facts and figures related to contraceptive methods, including future trends. Succinct and easy to read.*

Hatcher, R. A., et al. 1998. *Contraceptive Technology,* 17th rev. ed. New York: Ardent Media. *A reliable source of up-to-date information on contraception.*

Hatcher, R. A., et al. 2000. *Safely Sexual.* New York: Ardent Media. *Realistic recommendations on the prevention of unplanned pregnancy, as well as HIV infection and other STDs.*

Knowles, J., and M. Ringel. 1998. *All About Birth Control: A Personal Guide.* New York: Three Rivers Press. *Provides detailed descriptions of each contraceptive method.*

Tone, A. 2001. *Devices and Desires: Men, Women, and the Commercialization of Contraception in the United States.* New York: Hill and Wang. *An engaging history of contraception in America.*

W. Organizations, Hotlines, and Web Sites

The Alan Guttmacher Institute. A nonprofit institute for reproductive health research, policy analysis, and public education.
212-248-1111
http://www.agi-usa.org

Ann Rose's Ultimate Birth Control Links Page. A Web site with information on methods of birth control and decision-making strategies.
http://gynpages.com/ultimate

Association of Reproductive Health Professionals. Offers educational materials about family planning, contraception, and other reproductive health issues; the Web site includes an interactive questionnaire to help people choose contraceptive methods.

202-466-3825

http://www.arhp.org

Emergency Contraception Hotline. Provides information and referrals.

888-NOT-2-LATE

Emergency Contraception Web Site. Provides extensive information about emergency contraception; sponsored by the Office of Population Research at Princeton University.

http://ec.princeton.edu

It's Your Sex Life. Provides information about sexuality, relationships, contraceptives, and STDs; geared toward teenagers and young adults.

http://www.itsyoursexlife.com

Managing Contraception. Provides brief descriptions and tips for using many forms of contraception.

http://www.managingcontraception.com

Planned Parenthood Federation of America. Provides information on family planning, contraception, and abortion and provides counseling services.

800-669-0156 (to order publications)

800-230-PLAN (for a list of health centers)

http://www.plannedparenthood.org

Reproductive Health Online (Reproline). Presents information on contraceptive methods currently available and those under study for future use.

http://www.reproline.jhu.edu

The following are some of the many organizations focusing on family planning and reproductive health issues worldwide:

Family Health International

http://www.fhi.org

Global Reproductive Health Forum at Harvard

http://www.hsph.harvard.edu/Organizations/healthnet

International Planned Parenthood Federation

http://www.ippf.org

Safe Motherhood

http://www.safemotherhood.org

United Nations Population Fund

http://www.unfpa.org

See also the listings for Chapters 5, 7, 8, and 18.

SELECTED BIBLIOGRAPHY

Beral, V., et al. 1999. Mortality association with oral contraceptive use: 25 year follow up of cohort of 46,000 women from Royal College of General Practitioners' oral contraception study. *British Medical Journal* 318: 96–100.

Berenson, A. B., et al. 2000. A prospective study of the effects of oral and injectable contraception on bone mineral density. *Obstetrics and Gynecology* 95(4) (Suppl 1): S6.

Burke, W. 2000. Oral contraceptives and breast cancer: A note of caution for high-risk women. *Journal of the American Medical Association* 284(14): 1837–1838.

Burkman, R. T. 2001. Oral contraceptives: Current status. *Clinical Obstetrics and Gynecology* 44(1): 62–72.

Centers for Disease Control and Prevention. 2000. National and state-specific pregnancy rates among adolescents—United States, 1995–1997. *Morbidity and Mortality Weekly Report* 49(27): 605–611.

Centers for Disease Control and Prevention. 2000. Youth risk behavior surveillance—United States, 1999. *MMWR Surveillance Summaries* 49(SS05): 1–96.

Croxatto, H. B. 2000. Progestagen implants. *International Planned Parenthood Federation Medical Bulletin* 34(1): 1–3.

Davis, K. R., and S. C. Weller. 1999. The effectiveness of condoms in reducing heterosexual transmission of HIV. *Family Planning Perspectives* 31(6): 272–279.

Diaz, S. 1999. Contraceptive vaginal rings. *International Planned Parenthood Federation Medical Bulletin* 33(1): 3–4.

Dunn, N., et al. 2000. Oral contraceptives and myocardial infarction: A meta-analysis. *Journal of the American Medical Association* 284(1): 72–78.

Innovations in other barrier methods. 1999. *Population Reports*, Series H, Number 9, 27(1): 19.

International Medical Advisory Panel (IMAP). 2000. IMAP statement on the non-latex condom. 2000. *International Planned Parenthood Federation Medical Bulletin* 34(1): 3.

Kirby, D., et al. 1999. The impact of condom distribution in Seattle schools on sexual behavior and condom use. *American Journal of Public Health* 89(2): 182–187.

Le, J., and C. Tsourounis. 2001. Implanon: A critical review. *Annals of Pharmacotherapy* 35(3): 329–36.

McClanahan, P., et al. 2000. Characteristics of Norplant users. *Journal of Obstetric, Gynecologic, and Neonatal Nursing* 29(3): 275–281.

Microbicides, vaccines will cut unintended pregnancies and STDs. 2000. *Contraceptive Technology Update* 21(1): 1.

National Center for Health Statistics. 2000. Births: Preliminary data for 1999. *National Vital Statistics Reports* 48(14).

Perlman, S. E., et al. 2001. Contraception. Myths, facts and methods. *Journal of Reproductive Medicine* 46(2 Suppl): 169–77.

Petitti, D. B., et al. 2000. Steroid hormone contraception and bone mineral density: A cross-sectional study in an international population. *Obstetrics and Gynecology* 95(5): 736–744.

Princeton University Office of Population Research: Emergency Contraception World Wide Web Site. 2000. *Emergency Contraception* (http://ec.princeton.edu/info/ecp.html; retrieved July 19, 2000).

Rodrigues, I., F. Grou, and J. Joly. 2001. Effectiveness of emergency contraceptive pills between 72 and 120 hours after unprotected sexual intercourse. *American Journal of Obstetrics and Gynecology* 184(4): 531–537.

Rosen, A. D., and T. Rosen. 1999. Study of condom integrity after brief exposure to over-the-counter vaginal preparations. *Southern Medical Journal* 92(3): 305–307.

Santelli, J. S., et al. 2000. Adolescent sexual behavior: Estimates and trends from four nationally representative surveys. *Family Planning Perspectives* 32(4): 156–165.

Schwingl, P. J., and H. A. Guess. 2000. Safety and effectiveness of vasectomy. *Fertility and Sterility* 73(5): 923–936.

Shelton, J. D. 2001. Risk of clinical pelvic inflammatory disease attributable to an intrauterine device. *Lancet* 357(9254): 443.

Shulman, L. P., et al. 1999. Patient acceptability and satisfaction with Lunelle monthly contraceptive injection. *Contraception* 60(4): 215–222.

Skegg, D. C. G. 1999. Oral contraception and health: Long term study of mortality shows no overall effect in a developed country. *British Medical Journal* 318: 69–70.

Stephenson, J. 2000. Widely used spermicide may increase, not decrease, risk of HIV transmission. *Journal of the American Medical Association* 284(8): 949.

Tan, J. K., and H. Degreef. 2001. Oral contraceptives in the treatment of acne. *Skin Therapy Letter* 6(5): 1–3.

Trussel, J., et al. 2000. Access to emergency contraception. *Obstetrics and Gynecology* 95(2): 267–270.

Westhoff, C., and A. Davis. 2000. Tubal sterilization: Focus on the U.S. experience. *Fertility and Sterility* 73(5): 913–922.

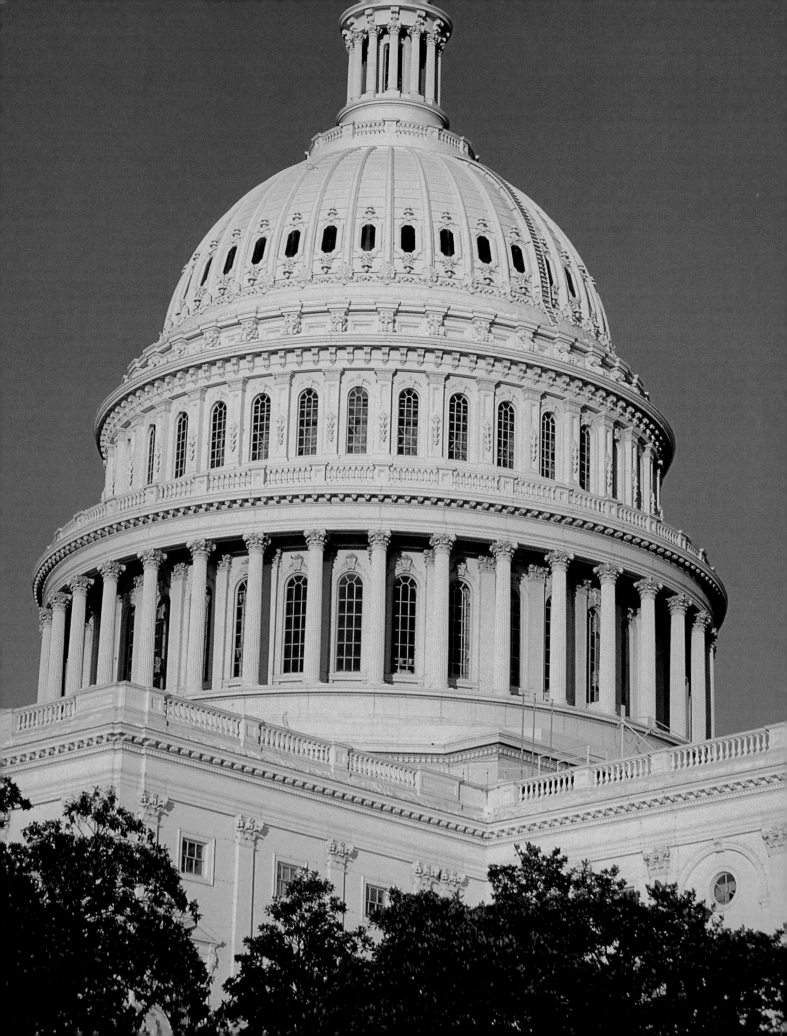

LOOKING AHEAD

After reading this chapter, you should be able to

- Describe the history and current legal status of abortion in the United States

- Explain the current debate over abortion, including the main points of the pro-choice and pro-life points of view

- Describe the methods of abortion available in the United States

- List possible physical and psychological effects of abortion

- Discuss the decision-making process a woman and her partner may go through when facing an unintended pregnancy

Abortion

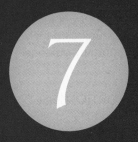

TEST YOUR KNOWLEDGE

1. The rate of abortion in the United States is going up.
   True or false?

2. About what percentage of abortions in the United States take place in the first 12 weeks of pregnancy?
   a. 60%
   b. 70%
   c. 80%
   d. 90%

3. A majority of Americans are in favor of the right to a legal abortion in some circumstances.
   True or false?

4. About how many American women have an abortion in any given year?
   a. 1 in 1000
   b. 1 in 100
   c. 1 in 50

5. About 25% of all pregnancies in the United States are unintended and about 25% of unintended pregnancies are terminated by abortion.
   True or false?

ANSWERS

1. **FALSE.** The rate of abortion rose during the 1970s, remained stable during the 1980s, and declined in the 1990s. The abortion rate in 1997 was the lowest recorded since 1975.

2. **D.** About 90% of all abortions take place in the first 12 weeks of pregnancy; more than 55% take place in the first 8 weeks.

3. **TRUE.** Current polls indicate that about 28% of Americans favor the right to legal abortion in all circumstances, and an additional 51% favor the right in some circumstances. About 19% of Americans think that abortion should be illegal in all circumstances.

4. **C.** At current rates, about 43% of American women will have had at least one abortion by the time they are 45 years old.

5. **FALSE.** About half of all pregnancies in the United States are unintended, and about half of these are terminated by abortion.

In the United States today, few issues are as complex and emotion filled as abortion. While most public attention has focused on legal definitions and restrictions, the most difficult aspects of abortion actually take place at a much more personal level. Because the majority of women having abortions are young, many college students have had some type of direct exposure to these more personal experiences of abortion. They are in a key position to understand and address the contributing factors as well as the broad effects of unintended pregnancies and abortion. Instead of simply attempting to legislate certain behaviors, they can choose to grapple with the complex human factors that go into the prevention as well as the "treatment" of unintended pregnancy. This chapter will provide basic information on abortion, including the current focuses of controversy. We hope it will act as a springboard for you to form your own views and, more important, personal plans for constructive action.

THE ABORTION ISSUE

The discussion that follows presents various perspectives on abortion. The word **abortion,** by strict definition, means the expulsion of an embryo or fetus from the uterus before it is sufficiently developed to survive. As commonly used, however, *abortion* refers only to those expulsions that are artificially induced by mechanical means or drugs, and *miscarriage* is generally used for a spontaneous abortion, one that occurs naturally with no causal intervention. In this chapter, *abortion* will mean a deliberately induced expulsion.

The History of Abortion in the United States

For more than two centuries, abortion policy in the United States followed English common law, which made the practice a crime only when performed after "quickening" (fetal movement that begins at about 20 weeks). There was little public objection to this policy until the early 1800s, when an anti-abortion movement began, led primarily by physicians who questioned the doctrine of quickening and who objected to the growing practice of abortion by untrained persons (in part because it weakened their control of medical services).

This anti-abortion drive gained minimal attention until the mid-1800s, when newspaper advertisements for abortion preparations became common and concern grew that women were using abortion as a means of birth control (and perhaps to cover up extramarital activity). There was much discussion about the corruption of

morality among women in the United States, and by the 1900s, abortion was illegal in every state. These anti-abortion laws stayed in effect until the 1960s, when courts began to invalidate them on the grounds of constitutional vagueness and violation of the right to privacy.

Current Legal Status

In 1973, the U.S. Supreme Court made abortion legal in the landmark case of *Roe v. Wade*. To replace the restrictions most states still imposed at that time, the justices devised new standards to govern abortion decisions. They divided pregnancy into three parts, or trimesters, giving a pregnant woman less choice about abortion as she advances toward full term. In the first trimester, the abortion decision must be left to the judgment of the pregnant woman and her physician. During the second trimester, similar rights remain but a state may regulate factors that protect the health of the woman, such as type of facility where an abortion may be performed. In the third trimester, when the fetus is viable (capable of survival outside of the uterus), a state may regulate and even bar all abortions except those considered necessary to preserve the mother's life or health.

Since 1973, repeated campaigns have been waged to overturn the *Roe v. Wade* decision and to ban abortion altogether. Although abortion remains legal throughout the United States, rulings by the Supreme Court in 1989 (*Webster v. Reproductive Health Services*) and 1992 (*Planned Parenthood of Southeastern Pennsylvania v. Casey*) allow states to regulate abortion throughout pregnancy as long as an "undue burden" is not imposed on women seeking the procedure. As a result, states have passed a variety of laws that have had the effect of reducing women's access to abortion. These laws include bans on the use of public funding, employees, and facilities for abortion services; mandatory counseling and waiting periods; insurance prohibitions; and requirements for parental consent for minors.

In addition to state abortion restrictions, the U.S. Congress has barred the use of federal Medicaid funds to pay for abortions, except when a woman's life is in danger or in cases of rape or incest. Currently, only 18 states provide nonfederal public money to assist poor women seeking abortions. Concerns have been raised that a two-tiered system has been created—one for women with means and another for those without.

Opponents of abortion, unsuccessful so far in their efforts to see *Roe v. Wade* overturned or a constitutional amendment passed to outlaw abortion, have recently focused on specific methods of abortion. For example, many states have passed legislation outlawing a particular method of late-term abortion referred to by abortion opponents as "partial birth abortion." (*Partial birth abortion* is a nonmedical term for a rarely used late abortion method discussed later in this chapter.) However, a Ne-

Terms   **abortion** The expulsion or removal of an embryo or fetus from the uterus.

braska ban on "partial birth abortion" was struck down in a 5 to 4 decision by the Supreme Court in June 2000 (*Stenberg v. Carhart*); the judges in the majority view found that the ban placed an undue burden on women seeking abortion and that it failed to take into consideration the need to protect women's health. Similar laws in other states are also likely to be ruled unconstitutional.

Legal and legislative efforts have also targeted medications that can be used to induce abortion. The drug mifepristone (RU-486) was used extensively in other countries to perform nonsurgical early abortions for years before being approved for use in the United States. Mifepristone is discussed in greater detail later in the chapter.

Both pro-choice and pro-life groups are likely to remain active, seeking to advance their positions both by promoting legislation and by supporting political candidates who share their views.

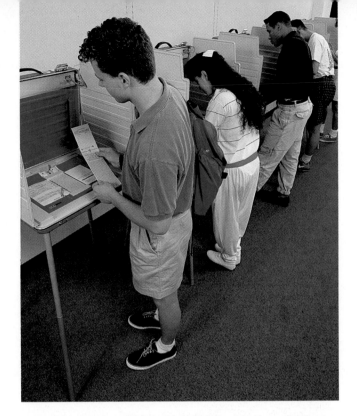

Voting for political candidates with well-defined views on abortion is one way individuals can influence the legal status of abortion in the United States.

COMMUNICATE! What are your government representatives' views on abortion? Contact their offices or go to their Web pages to find out their positions. Do they present clearly thought-out and articulated views? Do you see any fallacies in their thinking, such as false dilemma (presenting only two options when more are available), ad hominem (attacking the person making a claim rather than the claim itself), slippery slope (arguing that one action or event leads inevitably to a progression of additional actions or events), or false analogy (claiming that two things that are alike in one way are also alike in other ways)? If you see these or other flaws in logic, consider communicating with the representatives to seek clarification. If their views are not in line with your own, also consider letting them know where you stand.

Moral Considerations

Along with the legal debates are ongoing arguments between pro-life and pro-choice groups regarding the ethics of abortion (see the two "Opposing Views" boxes). Central to the pro-life position is the belief that the fertilized egg must be valued as a human being from the moment of conception and that abortion at any time is equivalent to murder. This group holds that any woman who has sexual intercourse knows that pregnancy is a possibility, and should she willingly have intercourse and get pregnant, she is morally obligated to carry the pregnancy through. Pro-life followers encourage adoption for women who feel they are unable to raise the child and point out how many couples are seeking babies for adoption. Pro-life individuals do not consider the availability of legal abortion essential to women's well-being but view it instead as having an overall destructive effect on our traditional morals and values.

By contrast, the pro-choice viewpoint holds that distinctions must be made between the stages of fetal development and that preserving the fetus early in pregnancy (or *gestation*) is not always the ultimate moral concern. Members of this group maintain that women must have the freedom to decide whether and when to have children; they argue that pregnancy can result from contraceptive failure or other factors out of a woman's control. When pregnancy does occur, pro-choice individuals believe that the most moral decision possible must be determined according to each situation and that, in some cases, greater injustice would result if abortion were not an option. If legal abortions were not available, pro-choice supporters say, "back-alley shops" and do-it-yourself techniques, with their many health risks, as well as the births of unplanned children, would again grow in number. Others argue that discrimination in health care would result, since wealthy women could more easily make the travel arrangements necessary for a legal abortion elsewhere.

Some people strongly identify exclusively with either the pro-life or the pro-choice stance, but many have moral beliefs that are blurred, less defined, and in some cases a mixture of the two. Many people instinctively feel that the fetus gains increasing human value as a pregnancy advances. In this view, early abortion, especially before the 8th week, is acceptable, whereas later abortion,

Kate Michelman

Pro-choice is not pro-abortion. Pro-choice is pro-freedom, pro-family, and pro-children. Pro-choice is about the lives, health, and security of women, their children, and their families. It's about freedom—freedom of religion, freedom of conscience, freedom of speech, and the right to privacy. It's about the freedom to choose whether or not to bear a child. No other choice has more impact on our community and our nation.

Reducing the *need* for abortion should be our nation's goal. No one wants an abortion. We all wish we could sail through life without difficult, painful choices. But we live in a complex and uncertain world filled with risk, temptation, illusion, and sometimes terror. No matter how strong the outer protection of love, marriage, income, and stability, each pregnancy comes down to a separate judgment, a different choice.

Women should have the freedom to make that choice.

For most women, the choice of abortion is the hardest choice of all. Abortion is not a choice of convenience. It's a choice wrapped in questions of morality, religion, and ethics. Abortion is filled with wrenching ambivalence and deep matters of the heart. Abortion or not, a woman's right to make this decision should be guaranteed.

In 1973 the question before the Supreme Court in *Roe v. Wade* was: Who should make the deeply personal and profound decision about pregnancy and childbirth? Answer: The woman.

Roe is a compromise that balances the woman and the unborn. It favors one at first and then the other as the pregnancy advances. It chooses the middle ground, the essence of pro-choice. *Roe* is neither libertine nor Draconian. It is neither pro-abortion nor anti-abortion. *Roe* strikes a delicate balance between freedom and responsibility.

For years women have considered the right to choose an abortion to be a basic freedom, no less than freedom of speech or freedom of worship. However, in June 1992 the *Casey* decision imposed restrictions that pushed *Roe* to the very precipice. The Court took the most fundamental American freedom and shattered it into jagged parts.

People once said we shouldn't make choice a political issue. I wish we didn't have to. I wish we could count on the fundamental American right to privacy and dignity. But we've learned the hard way that we can't.

The pro-choice agenda goes beyond the right to choose abortion. It is aimed at creating an America that respects the lives of women, protects the lives of children, and makes whole and happy families.

In a nation with one of the highest rates of unintended pregnancy, we must address the social conditions that force millions of women each year to face the abortion question. Contraception is still hidden behind counters. Expectant mothers still give birth without prenatal care. When it comes to birth control, America is an underdeveloped nation.

America's national policy is fragmented and incoherent. We strongly believe that government has the obligation to pull the pieces together and form a comprehensive reproductive health policy. The central goal of the pro-choice agenda is to reduce abortions. The pro-choice plan seeks to ensure that women who choose to have children can do so in a supportive and healthy environment. We need fundamental and widespread education in human development and sexuality. Our children must understand not just the mechanics of sex and contraception but also the tremendous consequences of pregnancy and birth. It is not enough to counsel abstinence. We've got to foster joint parent/school programs to educate our children about the realities of sex, contraception, and choice. We need to clarify the options and consequences of having children—not just the joys, but the responsibilities; not just the gifts, but the costs.

Federal grants to nonprofit organizations for family planning services have been drastically cut. This trend must be reversed. We also urge the federal government to get behind school-linked health clinics. To effectively promote child and teen health, a comprehensive plan must include counseling on pregnancy prevention, drugs, and jobs. Any national reproductive health care plan must guarantee access to prenatal care, treatment for drug-dependent pregnant women, child care, and family and medical leave.

This is not an insurmountable agenda. These are not demands from the political extremes or appeals to break the bank. These are the simple, minimum steps toward a civilized, humane, durable reproductive policy—a policy Americans support.

Kate Michelman is president of the National Abortion and Reproductive Rights Action League. Reprinted by permission of HealthLine.

when the fetus appears more like an infant, is unacceptable. Although the most vocal groups in the abortion debate tend to paint a black-and-white picture, the majority of Americans view abortion as a complex issue without any easy answers.

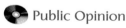 Public Opinion

In general, U.S. public opinion on abortion seems to change, depending on the specific situation. Many individuals approve of legal abortion as an option when destructive health or welfare consequences could result from continuing pregnancy, but they do not advocate abortion as a simple way out of an inconvenient situation. Overall, most adults in the United States continue to approve of legal abortion and are opposed to overturning the basic right to abortion established in *Roe v. Wade* (Figure 7-1). But the amount of public support varies considerably, depending on the circumstances surrounding the abortion request (Table 7-1).

J. C. Willke, M.D.

In considering abortion, the first question to ask is: What is this that grows within the woman? Is this human life? Or when will it be? If it's not human life, then a case can be made to permit abortion. If, however, this being is fully human, sexed, alive, complete, and intact from the first-cell stage, then a second human life exists and we have a collision of the rights of two humans.

So, first, let's ask: Is this human life? The answer lies in books on biology, embryology, and fetology. In these sciences there is no disagreement on the facts of when human life begins. At the union of sperm and ovum there exists a living, single-celled, complete human organism. It is already male or female, is alive and growing, and is human, as the 46 human chromosomes in the cell's nucleus mark this microscopic being as a member of the human family. This is arguably the most complicated cell in the entire world; it contains more information than could be contained in all of NASA's computers. As this single-celled human organism divides and subdivides, each cell in turn contains progressively less information, is more specialized.

At 1 week of life, this embryonic human attaches to the nutrient lining of the woman's womb and soon sends into her body a hormonal message that stops her period. About 4 days after the time when the woman's period would have begun, the embryo's heart begins to beat. At 40 days, brain waves can be recorded. By 10 weeks, the structure of the body is completely formed. By 3 months, all organ systems are functioning. To deny that fully human life begins at fertilization is to deny the known facts of fetal development and biological science.

Some argue that life existed in the sperm and ovum and will exist in the future. True, but we are not asking about generic life, but rather about this one unique individual's human life, which begins at fertilization and ends at death.

Some would measure the beginning of human life with a theologic yardstick, speaking of soul, God, and creation. In a secular state, however, we cannot use a theologic belief to define when human life begins for the purpose of making laws that either protect or allow the destruction of that life.

Others use various philosophical definitions of when the fullness of humanness exists, such as when cognition and self-consciousness are possible, when love is exchanged, when a being is declared to be "humanized" or "socialized," or when certain biological mileposts are reached. Though these definitions are arrived at by intellectual processes, they cannot be scientifically proven. Open to disagreement among people of good will, these definitions are also beliefs. We should not impose either religious or philosophical beliefs upon others in our culture. If one defines human life from the facts of natural science, then human life, complete and intact, begins at fertilization. That is a fact that we must face and work with.

Because this is human life from the very moment of conception, the issues touching that life are those of civil rights and human rights and the laws protecting those rights.

Let's ask a second question: Should there be equal protection under the law for all living humans? Or should the law discriminate fatally against entire classes of humans, in this case against those still living in the womb?

Interestingly enough, our nation faced a similar situation once before—slavery. In 1857, the Supreme Court ruled in the Dred Scott case that black people were not legal persons before the law. They were the property of the slave owner, who could buy, sell, or even kill them. Abolitionists' protests were countered: "Now look, you find slavery morally offensive? Well, you don't have to own a slave. But don't force your morality on the owner, for he has the constitutional right to choose to own a slave." In 1973, the Court did it again. In *Roe v. Wade*, also by a 7 to 2 margin, it ruled that unborn people were not legal persons. They were the property of the owner (the mother), who could keep or kill. Pro-lifers objected, to hear the same response. "Look, you find abortion morally offensive. Well, you don't have to have one. But don't force your morality on the owner (the woman), for she now has the constitutional right to choose, to kill."

The *Dred Scott* decision discriminated by skin color; *Roe v. Wade* discriminates by place of residence: still living in the womb. Each is a civil rights outrage.

A woman has a right to her own body, but to say that the little passenger residing within her is a part of her body is to utter a biological absurdity.

But she does not want this child? Since when does anyone's right to live depend upon someone else wanting them? Killing the unwanted is a monstrous evil.

A woman's issue? Women make up the overwhelming majority in the pro-life movement, and opinion polls consistently show more opposition to abortion from females than from males.

So, should a woman have the right to choose? I have a right to free speech, but not to shout "fire" in a theater. A person's right to anything stops when it injures or kills another living human.

No one should minimize the problems of pregnant women. With adequate counseling, informed consent, and the involvement of parents, husbands, and friends, we can help solve most of their problems—but sadly, never all of them. The pivotal question is: Should any civilized nation give to one citizen the absolute legal right to kill another to solve that first person's personal problem? I think not. We must give women far more help, both privately and publicly, than is available today. But we simply cannot continue to solve their personal problems by allowing the ghastly violence of killing tiny, innocent humans.

J. C. Willke is president of the Life Issues Institute and The International Right to Life Federation. Reprinted by permission of HealthLine.

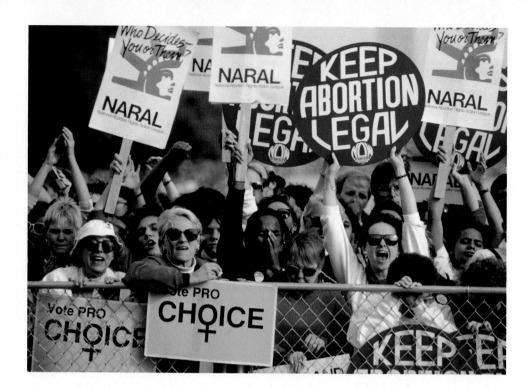

Pro-choice groups believe that the decision to end or continue a pregnancy is a personal matter that should be left up to the individual.

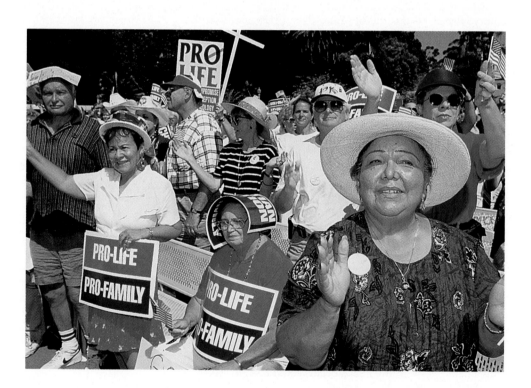

Pro-life groups oppose abortion on the basis of their belief that life begins at the moment of conception.

For example, people who feel that abortion should be available in early pregnancy often question at which stage in later pregnancy the fetus's rights should take precedence over the woman's rights. The 1973 U.S. Supreme Court decision considered viability the key criterion in establishing the point beyond which a woman's right to choose abortion becomes markedly restricted. In 1973, viability was generally considered to be about 26–28 weeks. Today it is about 24 weeks, with isolated cases of survival at 23 weeks. Although neonatal intensive care units continue to advance technologically, most experts feel that viability cannot be expected beyond this limit.

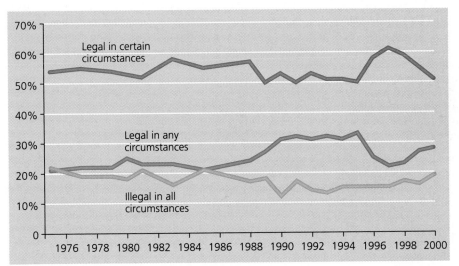

Ww. VITAL STATISTICS

Figure 7-1 Public opinion about abortion. This graph represents responses to the question: Do you think abortions should be legal under any circumstances, legal only under certain circumstances, or illegal in all circumstances? SOURCE: Gallup Organization. 2001. *Majority of Americans Say* Roe v. Wade *Decision Should Stand* (http://www.gallup.com/poll/releases/pr010122.asp; retrieved January 24, 2001).

Ww. VITAL STATISTICS

Table 7-1 **Views on Abortion**

1. Should a pregnant woman be able to obtain an abortion in the following circumstances?

	Yes
Her life is endangered.	84%
Her physical health is endangered.	81%
The pregnancy was caused by rape or incest.	78%
Her mental health is endangered.	64%
The baby is physically or mentally impaired.	53%
The woman or family cannot afford to raise the child.	34%

2. Should a woman be permitted to have an abortion during the following stages of pregnancy?

	Yes
In the first 3 months	65%
In the second 3 months	24%
In the last 3 months	8%

SOURCE: Gallup Organization. 2000. *Abortion Issues* (http://www.gallup.com/poll/Indicators/indabortion.asp; retrieved September 22, 2000).

Other individuals associate fetal rights not with viability but with earlier developmental characteristics such as the onset of heartbeat, brain size, and nervous system maturity. Still others argue that the embryo becomes a human being at the point of individuation or twinning, which occurs about 2 weeks after conception. (Before that time, the embryo has not yet differentiated into either a single or an identical twin pregnancy.) Others believe that the moment of conception is the only critical point to consider. For them, all other developmental stages are irrelevant to the abortion debate. As can be seen from such wide variation of opinion, objective measures of humanness and clear-cut guidelines regarding fetal rights are elusive, and decisions ambiguous.

Although opinions vary as to whether, or when, abortion rights should be tightly regulated by law, most people agree that abortions done later in pregnancy present more difficulties in personal, medical, philosophical, and social terms. Of all abortions done after the 12th week of gestation, more than 35% are performed on teenagers. Possible explanations include teenagers' ignorance, denial, fear, and lack of supportive family or friends, as well as state regulatory hurdles faced by teenagers. Other typical recipients of late abortions include low-income women, who may have more difficulty finding suitable facilities as well as necessary funds, and premenopausal women who fail to recognize a delayed period as pregnancy. Another small group of women who may seek late abortion are those who have learned through genetic tests that the fetus has a specific abnormality.

Personal Considerations

For the pregnant woman who is considering abortion, the usual legal and moral arguments may sound meaningless as she attempts to weigh the many short- and long-term ramifications for all lives directly concerned. If she chooses abortion, can she accept that decision in terms of her own religious and moral beliefs? What are her long-range feelings likely to be regarding this decision? What are her partner's feelings regarding abortion, and how will she deal with his responses? Does she have a supportive

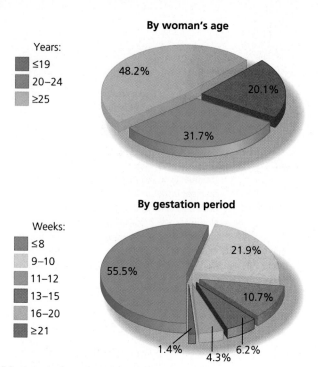

By woman's age

Years:
- ≤19
- 20–24
- ≥25

48.2%
20.1%
31.7%

By gestation period

Weeks:
- ≤8
- 9–10
- 11–12
- 13–15
- 16–20
- ≥21

21.9%
55.5%
10.7%
1.4%
4.3%
6.2%

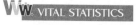

Figure 7-2 Distribution of abortions by the woman's age and by the weeks of gestation. SOURCE: Centers for Disease Control and Prevention. 2000. Abortion surveillance—United States, 1997. *Morbidity and Mortality Weekly Report* 49(SS–11).

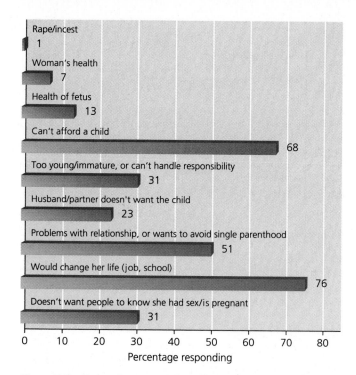

Reason	Percentage responding
Rape/incest	1
Woman's health	7
Health of fetus	13
Can't afford a child	68
Too young/immature, or can't handle responsibility	31
Husband/partner doesn't want the child	23
Problems with relationship, or wants to avoid single parenthood	51
Would change her life (job, school)	76
Doesn't want people to know she had sex/is pregnant	31

Percentage responding

Figure 7-3 The reasons women choose abortions. The respondents in this study were allowed to give more than one answer. SOURCE: Data from the Alan Guttmacher Institute.

relative or friend who will help her through this time of emotional adjustment? Which medical facility offering abortions would be most suitable for her? What about transportation and costs? (Figures 7-2 and 7-3 present statistical information about women who choose abortion.)

For the woman who decides against abortion and chooses instead to continue the pregnancy, there are other questions. If she decides to raise the child herself, will she have the resources to do it well? Is a supportive, lasting relationship with her partner likely? If not, how does she feel about being a single parent? Are family members available to help with the many demands of child rearing? If she is young, what will be the effects on her own growth? Will she be able to continue with her educational and personal goals? What about the ongoing financial responsibilities?

If the pregnant woman considers adoption, she will have to try to predict what her emotional responses will be throughout the full-term pregnancy and the adoption process. What are her long-range feelings likely to be? What is the best setting for her during her pregnancy? How can she best maintain continuity with the rest of her life and her long-term goals? What type of adoption would be most appropriate? (The box "The Adoption Option" addresses some of these questions.)

Current Trends

Clearly, all responses to unintended pregnancy can be difficult, including abortion and especially late abortion. Fortunately, with the increased accessibility to legalized abortion following the mid-1970s, the rate of late abortions dropped steadily, until fewer than 1% of all abortions were performed at more than 20 weeks and fewer than 12% at more than 12 weeks by the 1990s. The overall abortion *rate* rose during most of the 1970s, leveled off around 1980, and decreased in the 1990s (Figure 7-4). Possible future influences on the number, rate, and timing of abortions in the United States include legal decisions, more widespread availability of emergency contraceptives, and the increasing use of medical abortion. (See Chapter 6 for more on emergency contraception; medical abortion is discussed later in this chapter.)

Since the 1989 *Webster* and 1992 *Casey* decisions, many states have imposed additional restrictions on abortion. By 2001, 30 states required mandatory counseling, followed in 19 states by a waiting period; 42 states required parental consent or notification for minors; more than half of the states banned certain abortion procedures; and 32 states restricted the use of public funds for abortion. Overall, the number of laws restricting abortion in the states has more than quadrupled since 1995. Research into the effects of these restrictions has been mixed. Some studies indicate that parental consent and notification laws may result in minors traveling out of

One of the options available to a woman facing an unplanned pregnancy is adoption. Between 1952 and 1972, nearly 9% of unmarried pregnant women gave their children up for adoption; currently, however, only about 2% of women choose to place a child for adoption. This decline is probably due to a variety of factors, including increased rates of contraceptive use and an easing of the social stigma of single parenthood. The drop in adoption rates in the 1970s probably reflected an increase in the abortion rate following the 1973 legalization of abortion; however, since 1990 adoption rates have remained steady, while the abortion rate has declined, indicating that women are not choosing abortion over adoption. Women who place their children for adoption tend to come from higher socioeconomic backgrounds and to have higher levels of educational attainment than those who choose to keep their babies or have an abortion. They are also likely to have greater educational and vocational goals for themselves than those who keep their children. Often, women who choose adoption come from supportive families who assist them throughout the experience.

If you are pregnant and considering adoption, make sure you explore all possibilities before you make a final choice. The decision to go through an unwanted pregnancy and then give the baby to another family is difficult and takes tremendous love, maturity, and courage. Adoption is permanent: The adoptive parents will raise your child and have legal authority for his or her welfare. Think about your life now and in the future as you weigh alternatives. There are many people who can help you consider your options, including your partner, friends, family members, or a professional counselor at a crisis pregnancy center, family planning clinic, or family services, social services, or adoption agency. A counselor should always treat you with respect and be willing to discuss all your options with you—keeping the baby, having an abortion, or arranging an adoption. If you aren't comfortable with a particular counselor, find a different one.

There are two types of adoptions, confidential and open. In confidential adoption, the birth parents and the adoptive parents never know each other. Adoptive parents will be given any information, such as medical information, that they would need to help take care of the child. A later meeting between the child and birth parents is possible in confidential adoption, however, if the birth parents leave information with the agency or lawyer who handled the adoption and/or in a national adoption registry.

In an open adoption, the birth parents and adoptive parents know something about each other. There are different levels of openness, ranging from reading a brief description of prospective adoptive parents to meeting them and sharing full informa-

tion. Birth parents may also be able to arrange to stay in touch with the family over the years, by visiting, calling, or writing. Some women feel that an open adoption enables them to keep in touch with a baby they will always love; others feel that this would be too difficult and decide against contact with the adoptive family.

In all states, you can work with a licensed child-placing (adoption) agency. In most, you can also work directly with an adopting couple or their attorney; this is called a private or independent adoption. Prospective adoptive parents can be located through personal ads, a physician, adoptive parent support groups, national matching services, and family members and friends. To find an agency or lawyer who will arrange the type of adoption you want, ask about their rules and procedures. For example, will you receive financial help and counseling? Will you be able to have the amount of information about the adoptive parents and the amount of contact with the baby that you want? If your baby is a child of color and it is important to you that the adoptive parents are of the same ethnic or racial background, ask if the agency or attorney has such families approved and waiting for placement. Some agencies specialize in finding families for children of color.

You will also need to consider the reaction and rights of the birth father. A woman can choose to have an abortion without the consent or knowledge of the father, but once the baby is born, the father has certain rights. These rights vary from state to state, but, at a minimum, most states require that the birth father be notified of the adoption. In some states, the birth father may be able to take the child even if the mother prefers that the child go to an adoptive family. In the past, few birth fathers took part in the adoption process, but some agencies now report that as many as one-quarter of fathers have some involvement in their child's placement. If you are considering placing a child for adoption, it is important to find out about birth fathers' rights in your state and to make appropriate arrangements.

As with abortion, there are emotional and physical risks associated with pregnancy, childbirth, and adoption. Throughout the adoption process, make sure that you have the help you need and that you carefully consider all your options. Deciding how to handle an unplanned pregnancy is important, and you have the power to make your own decisions.

SOURCES: National Adoption Information Clearinghouse. 2000. *Are You Pregnant and Thinking About Adoption?* (http://www.calib.com/naic/pubs/f_pregna.htm; retrieved September 21, 2000). National Adoption Information Clearinghouse. 2000. *Placing Children for Adoption* (http://www.calib.com/naic/pubs/s_place.htm; retrieved September 21, 2000).

state to obtain abortions. Mandatory delay laws have been found to influence the number and timing of abortions. Further research is needed to establish whether these types of restrictions constitute an "undue burden" for women seeking abortions.

Adding to the legal restrictions is the growing scarcity of physicians willing to provide abortion services. Currently, 86% of all U.S. counties, 90% of rural counties, and about 30% of metropolitan areas have no abortion providers. It is unclear whether the approval of mifepristone

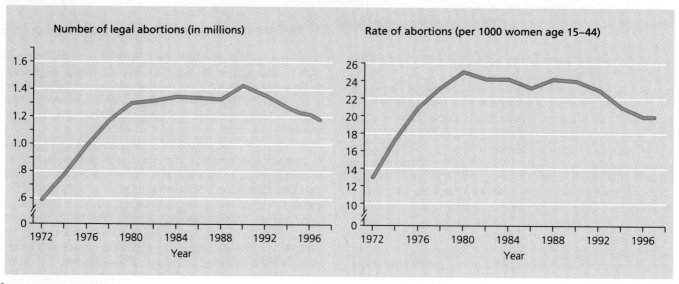

Figure 7-4 Abortion rates in the United States. SOURCE: Centers for Disease Control and Prevention. 2000. Abortion surveillance—United States, 1997. *Morbidity and Mortality Weekly Report* 49(SS–11).

for medical abortion will significantly affect these numbers. The diminishing number of providers is due in part to increased anti-abortion protests and violence, including arson, bombings, and the murders of several physicians and clinic workers. Women living in areas that have restrictive laws and few abortion providers may continue to obtain abortions, but they are likely to face significant increases in expense and time delays. If the constitutional right to abortion is to be maintained, these obstacles need to be carefully considered.

Unless accompanied by a greater effort at preventing unwanted pregnancy, especially among the young single women who make up the majority of those seeking abortions, legal changes alone will probably not dramatically reduce the number of abortions. At current rates, about 43% of American women will have at least one abortion by the time they are 45 years old. For a broader perspective, see the box "Abortion Around the World."

We hope the recent surge of public interest in sexual behavior, largely due to the fear of STDs, will lead to more open discussions of sexuality and contraception for individuals who choose to be sexually active. With more communication and a better understanding of one's personal need for intimacy and closeness, individuals and couples can perhaps make informed, responsible decisions about the best way to meet those needs. For those who choose to include sexual intercourse as part of their relationships, contraception should be made readily available and correctly used (see Chapter 6). Other measures that might help decrease the demand for abortion include the fol-

lowing economic and social reforms: increased options for working women, more dual parenting, maternal/paternal leaves, improved child care facilities, and quality prenatal and postnatal care available for all people regardless of socioeconomic status.

> **COMMUNICATE!** If you and your partner must discuss whether to obtain an abortion, try first to agree about whose choice it is. Once you have established how much input each of you will have in the decision, you can address the many questions surrounding the decision itself. It will be easier to think things through if your respective roles are clear.

METHODS OF ABORTION

Abortion methods can be divided into two categories: surgical and medical. Surgical abortion is by far the most common, accounting for about 98% of all abortions performed in the United States. Medical abortion, in which medications are used to induce abortion, may become more common following the approval in 2000 of mifepristone (Mifeprex). Emergency contraception—pills taken or IUDs inserted immediately after unprotected sexual intercourse—are generally not considered abortifacients (agents that produce abortion) from a medical viewpoint, because they act before implantation of the fertilized egg, if one is present (see Chapter 6). Therefore, these topics are not discussed here.

As one would expect, the legal status, availability, and safety of abortion varies widely around the world. Of the 46 million abortions performed each year worldwide, about 26 million are legal and 20 million illegal (see the figure).

- 25% of the world's people live in countries where laws ban abortion entirely or permit it only to save the life of a pregnant woman.

- 14% of the world's people live in countries with somewhat less restrictive laws that permit abortion to protect a pregnant woman's physical or mental health.

- 61% of the world's people live in countries where abortion is permitted either for a wide range of reasons or without restriction as to reason. Many of these countries do have regulations or restrictions such as third-party authorizations, waiting periods, or mandatory counseling, and many place limits on gestational age and the types of facilities where abortions can be performed.

Even in countries where abortion is illegal, women still undergo abortions. In fact, many countries with strict anti-abortion laws have high rates of abortion and, because most procedures are carried out secretly in unsafe conditions, high rates of serious complications. Nearly all of the 80,000 abortion-related deaths each year occur in countries with strict abortion laws. In countries where abortion is legal, widely available at low cost, and performed under safe conditions, abortion rates are relatively low and serious complications rare. (Widespread availability of contraception is another factor associated with low rates of abortion.)

Legal status is not the sole determinant of the availability of safe abortion services, however. How the laws are interpreted and enforced can be just as critical. For example, in some countries that allow abortion for mental health reasons, the law is interpreted to allow the majority of women seeking abortions to obtain them; in other countries with comparable laws, few abortions are allowed. Enforcement also varies. For example, in Mozambique, where abortion is officially banned, women can obtain abortions on request at many hospitals, and abortion-related legal charges are rarely filed. In other countries, laws are strictly enforced, and both women who have abortions and abortion providers are prosecuted. It is estimated that two-thirds of women currently in prison in Nepal have been convicted of undergoing illegal abortions. Strict enforcement of anti-abortion laws tends to disproportionately affect poor women because wealthier women can pay to obtain discreet, safe abortions from private physicians, thus avoiding the more tightly regulated public hospitals.

The attitudes and beliefs of the medical community also influence the availability of abortion services. For example, in Nigeria, many physicians will perform abortions in spite of legal bans because the medical community believes in the need for safe abortion services. On the flip side, major medical associations in Poland and the Republic of Ireland have adopted guidelines that are stricter than their country's laws.

The number and location of abortion providers and the cost of abortion services also influence the true availability of abortion in a particular country, regardless of its actual legal status. Community and physician opposition to abortion has left parts of the United States, Austria, and Germany without abortion providers, despite the fact that abortion is legal in all three countries. In contrast, policies in Denmark go beyond just permitting safe abortion to ensuring that services are widely available: There, each county must have at least one hospital that has the capacity to perform abortions, and services are free.

SOURCES: Berer, M. 2000. Making abortions safe: A matter of good public health policy and practice. *Bulletin of the World Health Organization* 78(5): 580–592. Henshaw, S. K., S. Singh, and T. Hass. 1999. The incidence of abortion worldwide. *International Family Planning Perspectives* 25: S30–S38. Rahman, A., L. Katzive, and S. K. Henshaw. 1998. A global review of laws on induced abortion, 1985–1997. *International Family Planning Perspectives* 24(2): 56–64.

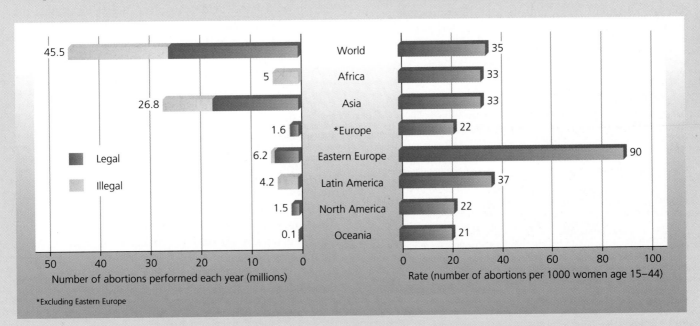

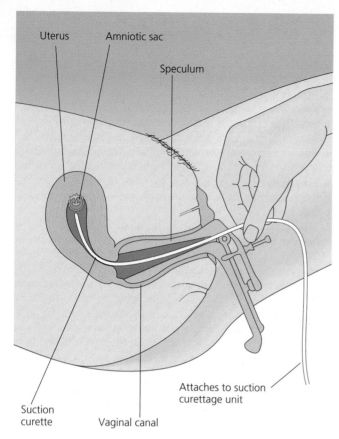

Uterus Amniotic sac

Speculum

Attaches to suction
curettage unit

Suction
curette   Vaginal canal

Figure 7-5   Suction curettage.   This procedure takes 5–10 minutes and can be performed up to the 12th week of pregnancy.

Suction Curettage

First developed in China in 1958, **suction curettage** (also called *vacuum aspiration*) is the most common method for abortions from the 6th to the 12th week of pregnancy. It is used in about 90% of all abortions performed in the United States. The procedure can be done quickly, usually on an outpatient basis, and the risk of complications is small.

Terms
- **suction curettage** Removal of the embryo or fetus by means of suction; also called *vacuum aspiration*.
- **local anesthetic** A drug that blocks the nerves carrying pain sensations to the brain; in abortion and childbirth, the nerves running from the pelvic area to the brain are affected while the woman is left awake and alert.
- **manual vacuum aspiration (MVA)** The vacuum aspiration of uterine contents shortly after a missed period using a handheld syringe.
- **ectopic pregnancy** An abnormal pregnancy that develops outside of the uterus, usually in a fallopian tube (oviduct).
- **dilation and evacuation (D & E)** The method of abortion most commonly used between 13 and 15 weeks of pregnancy. Following dilation of the cervix, both vacuum aspiration and curettage instruments are used as needed.

A sedative may be given, along with a **local anesthetic**. A speculum is inserted into the vagina, and the cervix is cleansed with a surgical solution. The cervix is dilated and a suction curette, a specially designed hollow tube, is then inserted into the uterus (Figure 7-5). The curette is attached to the rubber tubing of an electric pump, and suction is applied. In 20–30 seconds, the uterus is emptied. Moderate cramping is common during evacuation. To ensure that no fragments of tissue are left in the uterus, the doctor usually scrapes the uterine lining with a metal curette, an instrument with a spoonlike tip. The entire suction curettage procedure takes only 5–10 minutes.

After a few hours in a recovering area, the woman can return home. She is usually instructed not to have intercourse or use tampons for several weeks after the abortion and to return for a 2-week postabortion examination. This follow-up exam is important to verify that the abortion was complete and that no signs of infection are present.

Manual Vacuum Aspiration

Accurate and easy-to-use home pregnancy tests have made it increasingly common for women to know they are pregnant at very early stages of gestation, just at the time of a missed period. If a pregnant woman seeking an abortion is only 4 or 5 weeks past the time of her last period, she is sometimes told to wait several weeks before having the procedure. This is because suction curettage is believed to be safer and more effective when performed at least 6 or 7 weeks after the last menstrual period. A relatively new option for women at the very earliest stages of pregnancy is a surgical procedure called **manual vacuum aspiration (MVA)**. This method is not available in all clinics, but as more experience is gained with this procedure, MVA may become increasingly available to women who desire very early surgical abortion.

In MVA, the cervix is dilated and a plastic tube attached to a hand-held syringe is inserted through the cervix. The uterus is emptied with gentle suction provided by the syringe. Careful inspection of the aspirated material is critical to ensure that the gestational sac has been removed. Utrasonography and follow-up pregnancy testing are also used to make sure that the abortion is complete and that there is no **ectopic pregnancy** (a pregnancy that develops outside of the uterus, usually in the fallopian tubes).

Abortion After the First Trimester

Only about 1 in 10 abortions is performed after the 12th week of pregnancy. The method most commonly used for abortion from 13 to 24 weeks of pregnancy is **dilation and evacuation (D & E)**. The cervix is opened using dilators, which gradually expand the cervix overnight while the woman is at home. The next day, the uterus is emptied using surgical instruments and the aspirating

In September 2000, the FDA approved the use of mifepristone (trade name Mifeprex) in the United States for the termination of early pregnancy. Mifepristone, also known as RU-486 or the "abortion pill," has been mired in controversy for the past two decades. It was first approved for use for medical abortion in France in 1988. Protests in the United States, France, and Germany led the manufacturer to temporarily take the drug off the market, but distribution was resumed by the order of the French minister of health in the interests of public health. Since then, more than 600,000 women in Europe have had medical abortions using mifepristone. The drug has also been approved for use in the United Kingdom, China, Russia, Israel, and much of Europe.

Despite political opposition, clinical trials of the drug were allowed in the United States during the mid-1990s. In 1996, the FDA stated that mifepristone is safe and effective for abortion in early pregnancy and that it could be approved for use if concerns regarding manufacturing and labeling were resolved. However, political and manufacturing issues delayed final approval until 2000.

Pro-life groups in the United States have strongly opposed the approval of mifepristone, at least in part because of concerns that it would make abortion easier to obtain and more common. Groups that target abortion clinics and providers would have a more difficult time organizing protests if medical abortion were widely available in the privacy of a physician's office. Opponents of mifepristone also point to the drug's side effects and potential health risks.

Those in favor of the drug's approval argue that ready access to very early medical abortion would help decrease the need for riskier late abortions. Widespread availability of mifepristone could also help ensure access to abortion services for poor women and women who live in areas with no providers of surgical abortion. Surveys indicate that some physicians who do not currently provide surgical abortions would be willing to prescribe mifepristone. There are some special requirements, however: Physicians who distribute mifepristone must be able to accurately determine the duration of a pregnancy and to detect an ectopic pregnancy; they must also be able to either provide surgical intervention in cases of incomplete abortion or severe bleeding or arrange in advance to provide such care through others.

The FDA approval of mifepristone is unlikely to end the controversy. Individuals and groups opposed to abortion have promised to work through legislative and legal channels in an effort to have the drug removed from the market or its use restricted. Changes in the makeup of the U.S. Supreme Court or Cabinet could also affect the status of mifepristone. It is also unclear how the use of mifepristone will fit into current legal requirements in some states for such things as waiting periods and parental notification; states may also pass additional laws specifically related to mifepristone.

On the national level, legislation has been introduced to ban all drugs that can be used to induce abortion. If passed, such a law could have effects far beyond a ban on mifepristone, because some medications used to treat serious illnesses also induce abortion. For example, methotrexate is widely used to treat both cancer and rheumatoid arthritis. Mifepristone itself may have potential medical uses besides pregnancy termination, including treatment of breast cancer, endometriosis, and glaucoma. Banning all drugs that can be used to induce abortion could limit the development of new therapies for a variety of diseases. Other proposed legislation would require formal training and certification for any physician who plans to prescribe mifepristone.

Even if the drug remains available and is offered by a significant number of physicians, it is unclear what effect it will have on patterns and rates of abortion in the United States. In France, where the drug has been used extensively, the abortion rate has actually declined since the drug was introduced. Mifepristone is used in about 20–30% of all abortions performed in France; as in the United States, surgical abortion is still used in the majority of cases.

machine. The more advanced the pregnancy, the higher the incidence of complications.

Partial birth abortion is a nonmedical term for a particular type of D & E. In this procedure, the fetal limbs and body are delivered first and then the skull is collapsed to allow it to pass more easily through the cervix. This procedure is performed only rarely, but it can be useful in the presence of particular fetal anomalies such as severe hydrocephalus (a condition is which fluid collects around the brain, causing brain damage and an enlarged head). This procedure has been the target of abortion opponents.

Labor induction is another infrequently used method of late abortion. Prostaglandins, chemicals that cause uterine contractions, are used to induce labor, sometimes in conjunction with injections of salt or urea into the uterus. The delivery of the fetus usually occurs in 6 to 24 hours. The woman is hospitalized during this process. Fewer than 1% of abortions performed in the United States use the induction method.

Medical Abortion

Ending a pregnancy with medications rather than surgery is an option for women who are in the early phase of pregnancy. Medical abortion is commonly used in other parts of the world, but its use in the United States has been very limited, mainly for political reasons (see the box "Mifepristone: A Tangled Web of Medicine and Politics"). Medical abortion is generally used in very early pregnancy, within 49 days of the last menstrual period. The combination of drugs that is given causes the embryo and products of conception to be passed out through the vagina, as in a natural miscarriage. An ultrasound may be performed before giving the medication to make sure that the pregnancy dates are accurate because complication rates for medical abortion are higher if the pregnancy is more advanced.

Advantages and Disadvantages of Medical Abortion
Medical abortion is generally safer than surgical abortion because it involves no anesthesia or surgical risks. Some women feel that medical abortion allows them to take more control of the procedure and gives them more privacy than a surgical abortion would. Medical abortion can also be done very early in pregnancy.

The major disadvantages of medical abortion are that the process takes days or even weeks to complete (early surgical abortion generally takes less than an hour and can be done under sedation) and that bleeding after the procedure often lasts longer than with surgical abortion. Medical abortion also generally requires more clinic visits (three) than surgical abortion. The cost to the patient of medical and surgical abortion is generally about the same.

Drugs Used for Medical Abortion
Mifepristone, misoprostol, and methotrexate are three widely used drugs for medical abortion. Mifepristone blocks the uterine absorption of progesterone, thereby causing the uterine lining and any fertilized egg to shed. Mifepristone can be administered under medical supervision up to 49 days following the last menstrual period. A woman takes a dose of mifepristone and follows it up two days later with a second drug, the prostaglandin analog misoprostol, which induces contractions. The two-drug regimen has a rate of completed abortion of about 92–95%; the success rate is highest early in pregnancy. Side effects include nausea, vomiting, diarrhea, and abdominal pain. Vaginal bleeding is often more prolonged than with surgical abortion (9–16 days), but total blood loss is similar. In a few cases, bleeding is heavy, and a follow-up suction curettage is necessary. With mifepristone and misoprostol, abortion can take anywhere from a few hours to several weeks; about 50% of abortions occur within 4 hours and 75% within 24 hours. Two weeks after taking mifepristone, a woman must return to her health care provider for a follow-up visit to ensure that the abortion is complete.

A second drug, methotrexate, can also be used with prostaglandin for early medical abortion. Methotrexate has been approved by the FDA for cancer treatment since 1953 and is also commonly used to treat rheumatoid arthritis. Although not approved specifically for early abortion, it has been used for that purpose. Methotrexate stops the embryonic or fetal cells from dividing; it is followed by a dose of prostaglandin in a regimen similar to

that for mifepristone. With this combination of drugs, 80–85% of women will abort within 2 weeks; up to 95% will abort within 30 days. Because mifepristone acts more quickly than methotrexate and is slightly more effective, it is likely that mifepristone will become the preferred medication for medical abortion.

COMPLICATIONS OF ABORTION

Along with questions regarding the actual procedure of abortion, many people have concerns about possible aftereffects. More information is gradually being gathered on this important subject.

Possible Physical Effects

The incidence of immediate problems following an abortion (infection, bleeding, trauma to the cervix or uterus, and incomplete abortion requiring repeat curettage) varies widely. The potential for problems is significantly reduced by a woman's good health, early timing of the abortion, use of the suction method and local anesthetic, performance by a well-trained clinician, and the availability and use of prompt follow-up care.

Problems related specifically to infection can be minimized through preabortion testing and treatment for gonorrhea, chlamydia, and other infections. Some clinicians routinely give antibiotics after an abortion, while others treat only those women who have a history or current symptoms of pelvic infection. Postabortion danger signs are

- Fever above 100°F
- Abdominal pain or swelling, cramping, or backache
- Abdominal tenderness (to pressure)
- Prolonged or heavy bleeding
- Foul-smelling vaginal discharge
- Vomiting or fainting
- Delay in resuming menstrual periods (6 weeks or more)

Some bleeding occurs during and after most abortions. However, excessive bleeding during or after the procedure is rare with early suction curettage. In later pregnancies, the use of uterus-contracting medications reduces the risk significantly. Because aspirin, ibuprofen, and other nonsteroidal anti-inflammatory drugs can increase bleeding, they should be avoided. For pain relief, acetaminophen and a heating pad are safe substitutes.

Cervical trauma or laceration and perforation of the uterus are also uncommon in early abortion performed by a well-trained clinician. In more advanced pregnancies, slow and careful dilation of the cervix before an abortion can diminish these risks. The use of a local or regional, instead of general, anesthetic also minimizes the risk of uterine perforation, because less relaxation of the uterus occurs.

Incomplete abortion means that some pregnancy tissue has remained in the uterus. With this condition, or when blood clots form in the uterus shortly after an abortion, severe cramping and signs of infection can occur, and a repeat suction curettage is usually needed. On rare occasions, a pregnancy may continue after an incomplete abortion. The recommended follow-up exam is important to establish that the abortion was complete.

Missed ectopic pregnancy is another potentially serious problem that can surface after an abortion. Surgical abortion techniques remove tissue from the uterus but will miss an ectopic pregnancy developing outside of the uterus. If an ectopic pregnancy goes untreated, the embryo can eventually become large enough to rupture the fallopian tube, causing potentially catastrophic bleeding. Tissue removed during an abortion is normally examined for evidence that the gestational sac or embryo has been removed. If there is any doubt, ultrasound and follow-up pregnancy testing can reveal whether an ectopic pregnancy is present.

Studies on long-term complications—subsequent infertility, spontaneous second abortions, premature delivery, and babies of low birth weight—have not revealed any major risks with the most common abortion methods. The risk of postabortion infertility seems to be very low, especially when any signs of infection are reported and treated promptly. There is also apparently no effect on the outcome of future pregnancies when an early suction curettage is performed with minimal cervical dilation; with later abortions and with repeated or multiple abortions, there is only a slight risk, if any. For Rh-negative women, dangerous sensitization (the buildup of antibodies) can be minimized by an injection of Rh-immune globulin given within 72 hours of the procedure.

A few studies have reported that women who have abortions have an increased risk of breast cancer. However, a well-designed 1997 study of 1.5 million Danish women found no connection between a woman's abortion history and her risk of breast cancer.

The overall risk of death is low. Mortality rates have decreased substantially since abortion was legalized in 1973 (Table 7-2).

Possible Psychological Effects

After an exhaustive review completed in 1988, the then surgeon general, C. Everett Koop, concluded that the available evidence failed to demonstrate either a negative or a positive long-term impact of abortion on mental health. More recent research has resulted in the same general conclusion. The psychological side effects of abortion are less clearly defined than the physical ones. Responses vary and depend on the individual woman's psychologi-

Table 7-2	Abortion Risks
	Risk of Death in Any Given Year
Legal abortion	
Before 9 weeks	1 in 262,800
9–12 weeks	1 in 100,100
13–15 weeks	1 in 34,400
After 15 weeks	1 in 10,200
Illegal abortion	1 in 3,000
Pregnancy and childbirth	1 in 10,000

SOURCES: Hatcher, R. A., et al. 1998. *Contraceptive Technology*, 17th rev. ed. New York: Ardent Media. Carlson, K. J., S. A. Eisenstat, and T. Ziporyn. 1996. *The Harvard Guide to Women's Health.* Cambridge, Mass.: Harvard University Press.

cal makeup, family background, current personal and social relationships, cultural attitudes, and many other factors. A woman who has specific goals with a somewhat structured life pattern may be able to incorporate her decision to have an abortion as the unequivocally "best" and acceptable course more easily than a woman who feels uncertain about her future.

Although many women experience great relief after an abortion and virtually no negative feelings, some go through a period of ambivalence. Along with relief, they often feel a mixture of other responses, such as guilt, regret, loss, sadness, and/or anger. When a woman feels she was pressured into sexual intercourse or into the abortion, she may feel bitter. If she had strongly believed abortion to be immoral, she may wonder if she is still a good person. Many of these feelings are strongest immediately after the abortion, when hormonal shifts are occurring; such feelings often pass quite rapidly. Others take time and fade only slowly. It is important for a woman to realize that such a mixture of feelings is natural.

For a woman who does experience psychological or emotional effects after an abortion, talking with a close friend or family member can be very helpful. Supportive people can help her feel positive about herself and her decision. Although a legal and common procedure in the United States, abortion is still treated very secretively in most of our society, so it is easy for a woman to feel unique, isolated, and alone. Some women may specifically seek out other women who have had an abortion. Many clinical centers that offer abortions make such peer counseling available. Other women find they can identify with case histories in books written on abortion, which can help them deal with their own reactions. In a few cases, unresolved emotions may persist, and a woman should seek professional counseling.

Susan

Susan was a first-year college student who was caught up in her new academic and social activities. Bill (another student) and she had been dating for about 3 months, when one evening she decided to "take a chance" and not use contraception because she had just finished her menstrual period. When her next period was 2 weeks overdue, she had a pregnancy test. It was positive.

From the moment she found out, Susan considered only one option: abortion. "I couldn't have raised a child," she said. "And I wouldn't bring a child into the world unless I could take the responsibility for it. I think it would be worse to ruin my future and a baby's life because of a mistake." When Bill first learned of the pregnancy, he became distant, but he did agree to help pay for the abortion. Soon, however, he withdrew completely and had no further contact with Susan.

The hardest time for Susan was before the abortion, when she found herself crying frequently. She talked a lot with a close girlfriend, who went with her to the clinic and stayed with her after the abortion. Like all women who have abortions, Susan needed comforting.

After the abortion, Susan felt very strongly that she had made the best decision, but she did occasionally wonder how she would feel in future years. After meeting a new boyfriend with whom she could talk openly, Susan felt more certain than ever that she had made the right choice.

Helen

Helen was attending a junior college and working part-time when she found out she was pregnant. She and Mike had met just a couple of months before the pregnancy. They both planned to become parents at some point in their lives, but this was earlier than either of them had expected. They discussed all the options, and they agreed that getting married and keeping their child was the only acceptable solution.

Helen gave up school for the time being, and Mike took on more hours at work to help pay for the additional expense of a child. Six months after they were married, their daughter was born. Helen and Mike say that it was at this period of their life that they really got to know each other. "Our apartment was so small, we couldn't help but learn everything about each other."

It's now eight years later, and Helen and Mike have two children. Mike works full-time but hopes to return to school and complete his degree in the future. Helen works part-time and attends evening classes twice a week. They'd like to move to a larger apartment and to travel more, but they can't afford to. "We've given up a lot, and it's still a struggle. But we're a happy family, and we know that we made the right choice for us."

Anna

Anna was shocked when she found out she was pregnant. She was sure she wasn't ready to be a parent herself; she was too young and still hadn't sorted out what she wanted from life. But Anna also felt that having an abortion would be wrong. So she decided to have the baby and put it up for adoption. "I myself am adopted, so adoption seemed a natural choice, and the best one available to me."

Her boyfriend broke up with her when she told him. But her parents were supportive and helped arrange for her baby's placement in a good home. Anna knew she would have to give her baby up as soon as it was born, but during her pregnancy she developed a powerful bond with her child. Anna delivered her son and left the hospital three days later. "I had to just give the baby to the nurse and walk out. My parents and I cried. I spent nine months preparing for that moment, but it was still so painful."

After a year Anna still hurts, but she doesn't regret her decision. "Keeping him would have changed my life completely, and I knew I wasn't ready to be a mother. I couldn't have given my son the kind of life I want him to have." She's proud that she went through her pregnancy. As an adopted child herself, Anna felt she owed her son the same chance that her biological mother gave her.

COMMUNICATE!   The decision to have an abortion is a difficult one, and the experience is emotional and often lonely. If a friend confides in you that she has recently had an abortion, she is most likely experiencing many conflicting feelings, including relief that an unwanted pregnancy is over; regret, grief, or mourning; shame or embarrassment; or perhaps anger toward her sexual partner. More than anything else, she may need to share her feelings with a caring friend. Whether or not you agree with the choice she has made, don't judge or blame her or try to make her see your point of view. Sometimes sympathetic listening—for example, "You sound really sad; I'm so sorry"—is the best communication.

DECISION MAKING AND UNINTENDED PREGNANCY

When faced with an unintended pregnancy, women differ greatly in their approach to decision making (see the box "Personal Decisions About Abortion"). Unprotected sexual intercourse may be followed immediately by a vague sense of anxiety. When symptoms of pregnancy appear, some women—especially young women—respond with denial, ascribing the delayed menstruation and other signs to other causes. Several days or weeks may elapse before the woman finally has the pregnancy confirmed (a major cause of late abortions). After a positive test, women often feel a mixture of anxiety, depression, guilt,

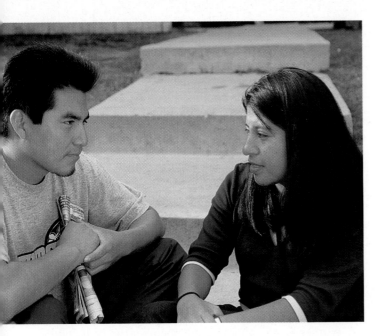

When an unintended pregnancy occurs, both partners can weigh important considerations and help choose an appropriate course of action.

and anger, sometimes tinged with some anticipation and delight. The actual decision making can vary widely. Some women calmly and resolutely make a choice within a very short time, while others, feeling panic and chaos, wrestle with the decision for several weeks. For some women, it is the first time in their lives that they feel unable to find a "right" answer and instead must settle for a "best" but difficult solution.

The response of a woman's partner can have a significant influence on how she experiences an unintended pregnancy. Men's emotional reactions can vary considerably. Some withdraw and choose to remain completely detached; others simply press for the most expedient solution (usually abortion). Still others feel very emotionally involved and wish to play an active role in decision making. Partners can be very helpful, both in weighing important considerations and in actually helping with the chosen course of action. Some couples find that an abortion experience draws them closer together; for others, it's the last straw in an already unstable relationship.

Parents can also be helpful. However, if there are serious disagreements, a stressful situation can become even more difficult. Over half of the states have parental consent or notification requirements, although there are "judicial bypass" procedures in which a judge can decide either that a minor is mature and can give informed consent or that an abortion would be in her best interest.

No matter which of the available options to unintended pregnancy is chosen, a series of questions is likely to arise that must be addressed (see the "Personal Considerations" section earlier in the chapter). Although a

prompt decision has critical advantages, careful deliberation is important. If there are strong feelings of uncertainty or ambivalence, hasty action should be avoided.

Having a supportive confidant, such as a partner, other close friend, or family member, can be very important in sorting out complex feelings. Along with listening and offering understanding and perspective, supportive people can help find suitable medical personnel and plan financial arrangements. Once a course of action has been chosen, a sense of moving ahead usually follows, and the next step toward resolution can occur.

Tips for Today

Abortion is a controversial and volatile issue in our society and a difficult choice for individuals. Legal, moral, personal, and medical considerations all enter into views and decisions about abortion. You may never have to face an unintended pregnancy, but you should know what choices you would have—abortion, adoption, parenthood—as well as where you stand on the issue.

Right now you can

- Take some time to examine your feelings about becoming a parent unexpectedly.

- Take time to consider your views on the morality of abortion. Refer to the boxes in this chapter for some thoughtful ideas about the subject.

- If you are sexually active, talk to your partner about abortion—do you have similar views and feelings, or are they different? How would you resolve a conflict?

- If you are sexually active, reexamine your contraceptive method and make sure you have made the right choice.

SUMMARY

- The common use of the word *abortion* refers only to artificially induced expulsion of the fetus.

- Until the mid-1800s, abortion in the United States was legal if it took place before the 20th week of pregnancy; more restrictive laws passed by the various states remained in effect until they began to be invalidated by courts in the 1960s.

- The 1973 *Roe v. Wade* Supreme Court case devised new standards to govern abortion decisions; based on the trimesters of pregnancy, it limited a woman's choices as her pregnancy advanced.

- Although the Supreme Court continued to uphold its 1973 decision, it gave states further power to regulate abortion in *Webster v. Reproductive Health Services* and *Planned Parenthood of Southeastern Pennsylvania v. Casey*

- The controversy between pro-life and pro-choice viewpoints focuses on the issue of when life begins. Pro-life groups believe that a fertilized egg is a human life from the moment of conception and that any abortion is a murder. Pro-choice groups distinguish between stages of fetal development and argue that a woman should make the final decision regarding her pregnancy.

- Overall public opinion in the United States supports legal abortion in at least some circumstances and opposes overturning *Roe v. Wade*. Opinion changes according to individual situations.

- Most people agree that abortions performed late in pregnancy present personal, medical, philosophical, and social problems.

- The woman considering abortion must think about her own religious and moral beliefs, her long-range reactions, support from others, and the cost and availability of the procedure.

- Suction curettage, the preferred method of abortion from the 6th to the 12th week of pregnancy, uses an electric pump to remove the uterine contents; the physician also scrapes the uterine lining with a metal curette.

- Manual vacuum aspiration is the aspiration of the uterine contents using suction provided by a hand-held syringe.

- The most common abortion method after the first trimester is dilation and evacuation (D & E), in which the uterus is emptied using aspiration and surgical instruments. Labor induction is used much less frequently.

- Medical abortion is performed with a combination of drugs very early in pregnancy; drugs used include mifepristone, misoprostol, and methotrexate.

- Physical complications following abortion can be minimized by overall good patient health, early timing, use of the suction method and a local anesthetic, a well-trained physician, and follow-up care.

- Psychological aftereffects of abortion vary with the individual. Many women go through a period of ambivalence; the strongest feelings usually occur immediately after the abortion. Having a supportive partner, friend, and/or family member can be helpful.

- Women who face unintended pregnancy differ in the way they make decisions; some make their choice calmly and quickly, while others struggle for weeks. It is often a matter of finding the "best," not necessarily the "right," solution.

TAKE ACTION

1. Survey your classmates about their position on the abortion issue. How many people consider themselves pro-choice and how many pro-life? How strong are their opinions? What, if anything, might cause them to change their minds? Do opinions seem to depend on age, gender, or any other factor?

2. Now that you have information about abortion, reevaluate your contraceptive practices. If they aren't adequate to prevent unintended pregnancy, make any changes you consider necessary to protect yourself and your partner.

W. JOURNAL ENTRY

1. *Critical Thinking* Write a one-page essay presenting your personal opinion on the abortion issue. Include arguments to refute the points typically made by the opposing side. Then write an essay presenting a convincing case for the opposite position. Make sure your arguments are clearly stated and that you can defend them, where appropriate, with facts.

2. Describe in writing the feelings you would have if you were faced with a decision about abortion right now. Decide on a course of action, and then project the consequences of your decision into the future. Describe how your decision might affect the course of your life and how you might feel about it a month from now, a year from now, 10 years from now, and 20 years from now.

FOR MORE INFORMATION

Books

Kaufmann, K. 1997. *The Abortion Resource Handbook*. New York: Simon & Schuster. *A resource for women seeking abortion, with information on legal, medical, and emotional aspects of abortion.*

National Abortion and Reproductive Rights Action League Foundation. 2001. *Who Decides? A State-by-State Review of Abortion and Reproductive Rights*. Washington, D.C.: NARAL Foundation. *An in-depth annual review of the legal status of reproductive rights in the United States.*

Pojman, L., and F. Beckwith, eds. 1998. *Abortion Controversy: 25 Years After Roe vs. Wade, a Reader,* 2nd ed. Belmont, Calif.: Wadsworth. *Includes academic articles from all perspectives of the abortion debate and abridged versions of key court decisions.*

Rein, M. L., et al., eds. 2000. *Abortion 2000: An Eternal Social and Moral Issue.* Wylie, Tex.: Information Plus. *A brief reference outlining the legal, political, and ethical issues relating to abortion.*

WWW. Organizations and Web Sites

Abortion Law Homepage. Includes an overview of the background and state of U.S abortion law, including the text of major legal decisions.

> http://hometown.aol.com/abtrbng

The Alan Guttmacher Institute. Publishes books and fact sheets on reproductive health issues; its journal, *The Guttmacher Report on Public Policy,* provides timely analysis of national reproductive health policy debates.

> 212-248-1111
> http://www.agi-usa.org

National Abortion and Reproductive Rights Action League. Provides information on the politics of the pro-choice movement.

> 202-973-3000
> http://www.naral.org

National Adoption Information Clearinghouse. Provides resources on all aspects of adoption.

> 888-251-0075
> http://www.calib.com/naic

National Right to Life Committee. Provides information on alternatives to abortion and the politics of the pro-life movement.

> 202-626-8800
> http://www.nrlc.org

Planned Parenthood Federation of America. Provides information on family planning, contraception, and abortion and provides counseling services.

> 800-669-0156 (to order publications)
> 800-230-PLAN (for a list of health centers)
> http://www.plannedparenthood.org.

Population Council: Abortion. Information on the development and testing of mifepristone from the holder of U.S. rights to the drug.

> http://www.popcouncil.org/rhfp/abortion.html

U.S. Food and Drug Administration: Mifepristone. Provides information on the testing, labeling, and use of mifepristone.

> http://www.fda.gov/cder/drug/infopage/mifepristone

See also the listings for Chapters 5, 6, and 8.

SELECTED BIBLIOGRAPHY

Alan Guttmacher Institute. 1999. *Facts in Brief: Induced Abortion Worldwide* (http://www.agi-usa.org/pubs/fb_0599.html; retrieved September 22, 2000).

Alan Guttmacher Institute. 2000. *Facts in Brief: Induced Abortion* (http://www.agi-usa.org/pubs/fb_induced_abortion.html; retrieved September 22, 2000).

American College of Obstetricians and Gynecologists. 2000. *Statement of the American College of Obstetricians and Gynecologists on the U.S. Supreme Court Abortion Case* Stenberg v. Carhart, *April 21, 2000* (http://www.acog.com/from_home/publications/press-releases/nr04-21-00.htm; retrieved July 5, 2000).

Annas G. J. 2001. Partial-birth abortion and the Supreme Court. *New England Journal of Medicine* 344(2): 152–156.

Blendon, R. J., et al. 2001. The implications of the 2000 election. *New England Journal of Medicine* 344(9): 679–684.

Carlson, M. 1998. The passive majority: What good is the right to an abortion if extremists can make it unavailable? *Time* 152(1): 60.

Centers for Disease Control and Prevention. 2000. Abortion surveillance— United States, 1997. *Morbidity and Mortality Weekly Report* 49(SS–11).

Christin-Maitre, S., P. Bouchar, and I. Spitz. 2000. Drug therapy: Medical termination of pregnancy: *New England Journal of Medicine* 342(13): 946–956.

Ellertson, C. 1997. Mandatory parental involvement in minors' abortions: Effects of the laws in Minnesota, Missouri, and Indiana. *American Journal of Public Health* 87(8): 1367–1374.

Gallup Organization. 2000. *Poll Releases: Approval of Controversial Abortion Drug RU-486 Proposed* (http://www.gallup.com/poll/releases/pr000607b.asp; retrieved June 12, 2000).

Grimes, D. 2000. Conferences with patients and doctors: A 26-year-old woman seeking an abortion. *Journal of the American Medical Association* 282(12): 1169–1175.

Henshaw, S. K. 1998. Abortion incidence and services in the United States, 1995–1996. *Family Planning Perspectives* 30(6): 263–270, 287.

Joyce, T., et al. 1997. The impact of Mississippi's mandatory delay law on abortions and births. *Journal of the American Medical Association* 278(8): 653–658.

Major, B., et al. 2000. Psychological responses of women after first-trimester abortion. *Archives of General Psychiatry* 57(8): 777–784.

Melbye, M., et al. 1997. Induced abortion and the risk of breast cancer. *New England Journal of Medicine* 336(2): 81–85.

National Abortion and Reproductive Rights Action League. 2001. *Who Decides: A State-by-State Review of Abortion and Reproductive Rights* (http://www.naral.org; retrieved February 12, 2001).

Parazzini, F., et al. 1998. Induced abortion in the first trimester of pregnancy and risk of miscarriage. *British Journal of Obstetrics and Gynaecology* 105(4): 418–421.

Planned Parenthood Federation of America. 1999. *Fact Sheet: How Abortion Is Provided* (http://www.plannedparenthood.org/library/ABORTION/howabort_fact.html; retrieved July 5, 2000).

Planned Parenthood Federation of America. 1999. *Mifepristone: A Brief History* (http://www.plannedparenthood.org/library/ABORTION/Mifepristone.html; retrieved June 12, 2000).

Population Council. 1998. *U.S Mifepristone Clinical Trial: Summary of Findings* (http://www.popcouncil.org/rhdev/mifepristone_ustrial.html; retrieved November 13, 1998).

Supreme Court of the United States. 2000. *Stenberg, Attorney General of Nebraska, et al. v. Carhart* (http://www.supremecourtus.gov/opinions/99pdf/99-830.pdf; retrieved September 22, 2000).

U.S. Food and Drug Administration, Center for Drug Evaluation and Research. 2000. *Mifepristone Questions and Answers* (http://www.fda.gov/cder/drug/infopage/mifepristone/mifepristone-qa.htm; retrieved September 28, 2000).

Wiebe, E. R. 2001. Misoprostol administration in medical abortion. A comparison of three regimens. *Journal of Reproductive Medicine* 46(2): 125–129.

Winikoff, B., et al. 1998. Acceptability and feasibility of early pregnancy termination by mifepristone-misoprostol. Results of a large multicenter trial in the United States. *Archives of Family Medicine* 7(4): 360–366.

Zapka, J. G., et al. 2001. The silent consumer: Women's reports and ratings of abortion services. *Medical Care* 39(1): 50–60.

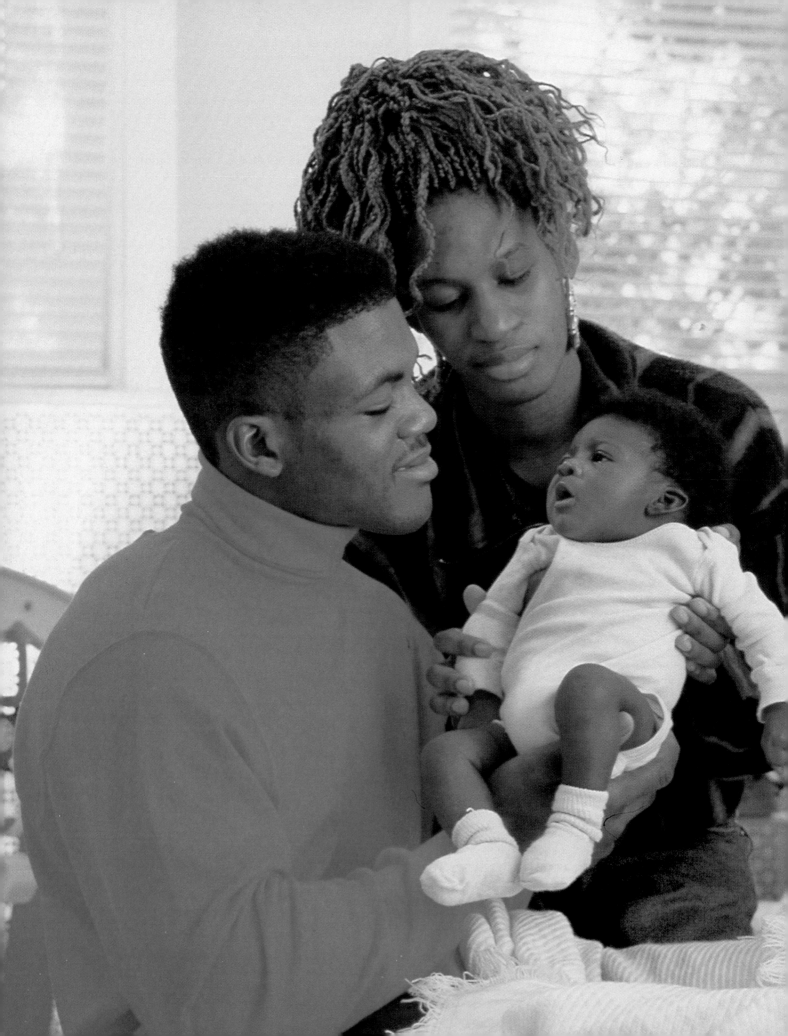

After reading this chapter, you should be able to

- List key issues to consider when deciding about parenthood

- Explain the process of conception, and describe the most common causes and treatments for infertility

- Describe the physical and emotional changes a pregnant woman typically experiences

- Discuss the stages of fetal development

- List the important components of good prenatal care

- Describe the process of labor and delivery

Pregnancy and Childbirth

8

TEST YOUR KNOWLEDGE

1. What is the approximate annual cost of raising a child?
   a. $3,900
   b. $8,900
   c. $15,900

2. What is the leading cause of female infertility?
   a. growths in the uterus
   b. exposure to radiation
   c. blocked fallopian tubes caused by STDs

3. Before conception and in the early weeks of pregnancy, adequate intake of which of the following nutrients can reduce the risk of spina bifida and other neural tube defects?
   a. iron
   b. folic acid
   c. calcium

4. High levels of stress during pregnancy can increase the risk of certain types of birth defects.
   True or false?

5. The position in which babies sleep has a significant impact on their risk of dying from sudden infant death syndrome (SIDS).
   True or false?

ANSWERS

1. **B.** On average, it costs about $8,900 per year to raise a child, for a total of about $160,000 to age 18.

2. **C.** If left untreated, the STDs gonorrhea and chlamydia can lead to tubal scarring and blockage. Leading causes of male infertility include low sperm count and poor sperm motility.

3. **B.** It is recommended that all reproductive-age women consume 400 μg of folic acid from fortified foods and/or supplements each day to reduce the risk of spina bifida and other neural tube defects.

4. **TRUE.** Although the overall risk is very low, women who experience severe emotional trauma around the time of conception or during the first trimester are more likely to have an infant with defects of the skull, spine, palate, or limbs; they are also at greater risk for preterm labor.

5. **TRUE.** The rate of SIDS in the United States has dropped over 40% since 1992, when an education campaign called "Back to Sleep" was implemented to teach parents and caregivers to put babies to bed on their backs instead of their stomachs.

Deciding whether to become a parent is one of the most important decisions you will ever make. Having a child changes your life forever, and deciding not to have children has equally far-reaching implications. Yet many people approach this momentous decision with only the vaguest notion of what is involved in pregnancy and childbirth. An estimated half of the approximately 4 million babies born every year in the United States are from unintentional pregnancies.

Today, with changing cultural expectations and increasingly sophisticated contraceptive technology, you have more choice about becoming a parent than people have ever had before. Until recently it was expected that virtually every married couple would have children. Now you can choose whether, when, and how you want to have a child. And you don't have to be part of a couple to have a child; the number of women choosing to have children on their own has risen dramatically. About one-third of all U.S. births are to unmarried women.

Pregnancy is a relatively comfortable experience for most women and the outcome predictably happy. Yet for some, problems occur. Some couples who have always planned for children may find that they are unable to conceive; others may face complications during pregnancy. Some problems are impossible to prevent, but you can make choices that minimize the risks and maximize the benefits for yourself, your partner, and your children.

Having a child is one of the most arduous, important, and rewarding enterprises that human beings undertake. The more you know about it—about conception and pregnancy, fetal development and prenatal care, childbirth and parenting—the more capable you will be of making intelligent, informed decisions about it. This chapter presents information you can use both now and later in your life to make the choices about pregnancy and childbirth that are right for you.

PREPARATION FOR PARENTHOOD

Before you decide whether or when to become a parent, you'll want to consider your suitability and readiness. If you make the decision to have a child, there are actions you can take before the pregnancy begins to help ensure a healthy outcome for all.

Deciding to Become a Parent

Many factors have to be taken into account when you are considering parenthood. Following are some questions you should ask yourself and some issues you should consider when making this decision. Some issues are relevant to both men and women; others apply only to women.

• *Your physical health and your age.* Are you in reasonably good health? If not, can you improve your health by changing your lifestyle, perhaps by modifying your diet or giving up cigarettes, alcohol, or drugs? Are you overweight? Do you have physical conditions, such as diabetes or high blood pressure, that will require extra care and medical attention during pregnancy? Do you or your partner have a family history of genetic problems that a baby might inherit? Does your age place you or your baby at risk? (Teenagers and women over 35 have a higher incidence of some problems.) Improving your health before pregnancy (discussed in the next section) can help ensure a trouble-free pregnancy and a healthy baby.

• *Your financial circumstances.* Can you afford a child? Will your health insurance cover the costs of pregnancy, delivery, and medical attention for mother and baby before and after the birth, including physicians' fees and hospital costs? Supplies for the baby are expensive, too—diapers, bedding, cribs, strollers, car seats, clothing, food and medical supplies, and child care. Depending on a variety of factors, including age of child, number of children, family income, and region of residence, the annual cost of raising a child averages about $8,900. The cost of raising a child to age 18 averages about $160,000 per child for a middle-class family with two children. If one parent has quit his or her job to care for the child or is on parental leave, the family must live on one income.

• *Your relationship with your partner.* Are you in a stable relationship, and do both of you want a child? Are your views compatible on such issues as child-rearing goals, the distribution of responsibility for the child, and work and housework obligations?

• *Your educational, career, and child care plans.* Have you completed as much of your education as you want right now? Have you established yourself in a career, if that is something you want to do? Have you investigated parental leave and company-sponsored child care? Do you and your partner agree on child care arrangements, and does such child care exist in your community? Some experts advise against full-time child care for babies under 1 year of age, but studies have found no permanent adverse effects of early child care on child development. Some people consider the child care issue the most difficult in parenting.

• *Your emotional readiness for parenthood.* Do you have the emotional discipline and stamina to care for and nurture an infant? Are you prepared to have a helpless baby completely dependent on you all day and all night? Are you willing to change your lifestyle to provide the best conditions for a baby's development, both before and after birth?

• *Your social support system.* Do you have a network of family and friends who will help you with the baby? Are there community resources you can call on for additional assistance? A family's social support system is one of the most important factors affecting its ability to adjust to a baby and cope with new responsibilities.

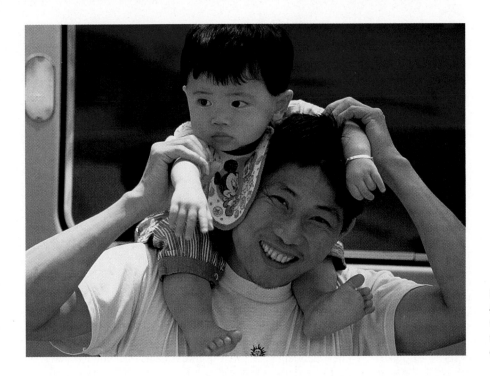

Having a child is one of the most important and rewarding experiences a person can undertake. Careful preparation can help maximize the benefits for both parents and children.

• *Your personal qualities, attitudes toward children, and aptitude for parenting.* Do you like infants, young children, and adolescents? Do you think time with children is time well spent? Do you feel good enough about yourself to love and respect others? Do you have safe ways of handling anger, frustration, and impatience?

• *Your philosophical or religious beliefs.* Some people question the value of bringing more people into an already overcrowded world. They feel that human beings have already fulfilled the biblical directive to be fruitful and multiply, and they choose not to have children.

COMMUNICATE! The media present images of many different kinds of families. Do you think any of these reflect a realistic view of parenthood? Which aspects strike you as positive, and which as negative? Are mothers presented differently from fathers? How has the media image of families influenced your feelings about being a parent? Consider what is being communicated to you by the media and what your response to it is.

Preconception Care

The birth of a healthy baby depends in part on the mother's overall wellness *before* conception. The U.S. Public Health Service recommends that all women receive health care to help them prepare for pregnancy. **Preconception care** should include an assessment of health risks, the promotion of healthy lifestyle behaviors, and any treatments necessary to reduce risk. Following are

some of the questions, tests, and treatments you and your partner may encounter during preconception care:

1. Do you have any preexisting medical conditions, such as diabetes, epilepsy, asthma, high blood pressure, or anemia? There may be things you can do to improve the chances of a trouble-free pregnancy and a positive outcome.

2. Are you taking any prescription or over-the-counter medications or dietary supplements? Some medications can harm the **fetus,** so you may need to change or discontinue their use to help ensure a healthy pregnancy.

3. Have you had any prior problems with pregnancy and delivery, including miscarriage, premature birth, ectopic pregnancy, or delivery complications? Some problems are due to physical or hormonal difficulties that can be treated.

4. Does your age place you at risk for infertility or health problems during pregnancy, or does it increase the likelihood that your baby may have a genetic or chromosomal disorder? Pregnant teenagers may need special nutritional counseling during pregnancy to meet the needs of their own growing body as well as the baby's. The incidence of Down syndrome increases with maternal age; genetic testing and counseling is often rec-

preconception care Health care in preparation for pregnancy.

fetus The developmental stage of a human from the 9th week after conception to the moment of birth.

Terms

Genes carry the chemical instructions that determine the development of hundreds of individual traits, including disease risks, in every human being. Many traits and conditions involve multiple genes and environmental influences. However, some diseases can be traced to a mutation in a single gene.

Children inherit one set of genes from each parent. If only one copy of an abnormal gene is necessary to produce a disease, then it is termed a *dominant* gene. Diseases that are carried by dominant genes seldom skip a generation: Anyone who carries the gene will probably get the disease. If two copies of an abnormal gene (one from each parent) are necessary for a disease to occur, then the gene is called *recessive*. Many common diseases caused by recessive genes occur disproportionately in certain ethnic groups. Prospective parents who come from the same ethnic group can be tested for any recessive diseases found in that group. If both are carriers, each of their children will have about a 25% chance of developing the disease.

Learning all you can about diseases that affect members of your ethnic group can be a lifesaver. Not only can you learn about the risk to your children, but you may also discover there are things you can do to manage the disease and reduce its impact.

• *Sickle-cell disease* affects about 1 out of every 500 African Americans and 1 out of every 1200 Latinos. In this disease, the red blood cells, which carry oxygen to the body's tissues, change shape; the normal doughnut-shaped cells become sickle-shaped. These altered cells carry less oxygen and clog small blood vessels.

People who inherit one gene for sickle-cell disease (about 1 in 12 African Americans) experience only mild symptoms; those with two genes become severely, often fatally, ill. Interestingly, people who inherit one sickle-cell gene are far more resistant to malaria than are those without the gene, leading geneticists to conclude that the sickle-cell trait might

have developed in tropical regions as an adaptation to the widespread presence of malaria.

If you are at risk for sickle-cell disease, you can

1. Get genetic counseling to help determine your family's genetic pattern and the degree of risk to you and your potential offspring

2. Take particular care to reduce stress and respond to minor infections, since red blood cells become sickle-shaped during periods of stress on the body

3. Get regular checkups and appropriate treatment

• *Hemochromatosis* ("iron overload") affects about 1 in 250 Americans; most at risk are people of Northern European (especially Irish), Mediterranean, and Hispanic descent. In people with hemochromatosis, the body absorbs and stores up to 10 times the normal amount of iron. Over time, iron deposits form in the joints, liver, heart, and pancreas. If untreated, hemochromatosis can cause organ failure and death.

Early symptoms are often vague, but early detection and treatment are necessary to prevent damage. If you have any family members with the disorder, get tested, routine testing may soon be recommended for all Americans. Treatment involves reducing iron stores by removing blood from the body (a process also known as phlebotomy or "bloodletting").

• *Tay-Sachs disease,* another recessive disorder, occurs annually in approximately 1 out of every 1000 Jews of Eastern European ancestry. People with Tay-Sachs disease are unable to metabolize fat properly; as a result, the brain and other nerve tissues deteriorate. Affected children begin by showing weaknesses in their movements and eventually develop blindness and seizures. This disease is fatal, and death usually occurs by age 3 or 4.

If you are of Eastern European Jewish ancestry and are planning to have children, genetic counseling will help you as-

ommended for women age 35 and older. Older women may also find that it is harder to become pregnant.

5.   Do you smoke, drink, or take other drugs? These habits are dangerous for the baby, and a health care professional can recommend treatment programs. If you are a heavy consumer of caffeine, cutting back before and during pregnancy is recommended.

6.   Do you currently have any infections, or do you need any additional vaccinations? Women at risk for hepatitis B or not immunized against rubella (German measles) should be vaccinated. Women not immune to parvovirus B19, which causes "fifth disease," or toxoplasmosis, a disease transmitted in contaminated food or by animals, especially cats, can find out how to prevent infection during pregnancy (both these diseases can cause miscarriage or complications in pregnancy and/or

for the developing fetus). Testing for tuberculosis and certain STDs can ensure treatment prior to pregnancy. (See Chapters 17 and 18 for more information about STDs and other infectious diseases.)

7.   Are you at risk for HIV infection (see Chapter 18)? If so, you should be tested before you or your partner becomes pregnant. Babies born to HIV-infected mothers can become infected.

8.   Do you eat a balanced diet? Are you particularly underweight or overweight? Do you suffer from an eating disorder? Do you have special dietary habits, such as being a vegetarian? Nutritional counseling can help you create a plan for healthy eating, before and during pregnancy. Your physician may also prescribe multivitamins, particularly folic acid. The U.S. Public Health Service recommends that all women of childbearing age take ex-

sess the chances that you and your mate will produce a child with Tay-Sachs disease.

• *Cystic fibrosis* occurs in 1 in every 2000 Caucasians per year; about 1 in 20 carries one copy of the cystic fibrosis gene. Because essential enzymes of the pancreas are deficient, thick mucus impairs functioning in the lungs and intestinal tracts of people with this disease. The disease is often fatal in early childhood, but medical treatments are increasingly effective in reducing symptoms and prolonging life. In some cases, symptoms do not appear until early adulthood.

If there is a history of cystic fibrosis in your family and you plan to have children, genetic tests and counseling can help in assessing the risk to your prospective offspring.

• *Thalassemia* is a blood disease found most often among Italians, Greeks, and, to a lesser extent, African Americans and Asians. When inherited from one parent, this form of anemia is mild; when two genes are present, the disease is severe and can cause fetal death or, after birth, a condition called Cooley's anemia. Children with this condition require repeated blood transfusions, eventually resulting in a damaging iron buildup. New medical interventions, such as genetic engineering, bone marrow transplants, and chemicals that bind with excess iron and remove it from the body, offer promise.

If you are at risk of carrying thalassemia, you can

1. Get regular checkups and monitor your health for symptoms

2. Learn symptom management

3. Get genetic counseling to assess the risk to your offspring

• *Lactose intolerance* is a condition affecting about 30–50 million Americans, including a majority of Asian Americans, Native Americans, and African Americans. Although all humans are dependent on milk in the early years, by about age 4 many lose the ability to absorb lactose, the chief nutrient in milk. This lactose intolerance results from an absence of lactase, an enzyme that permits the efficient digestion of milk. When lactose-intolerant people ingest more than 1–2 servings of milk or dairy products, they suffer from gas pains and diarrhea. Studies show that lactose intolerance is especially prevalent in cultures where milk is relatively unimportant after weaning, suggesting that evolutionary adaptation has played a role in its development.

If you suspect latcose intolerance, see your physician for a test. If you are lactose intolerant, use trial and error to determine how many servings of dairy products you can consume without symptoms. If you react to very small amounts of lactose, try lactose-reduced products or lactase drops or tablets.

• *Diabetes* is 55% more common among African Americans than white Americans; Native Americans and Latinos are also at increased risk. Asians have a predisosition for diabetes that may surface with American diets. See Chapter 14 for more on the many steps you can take if you are at risk for diabetes.

• *Osteoporosis* is more likely to develop in light-skinned people of Northern European ancestry than in dark-skinned people. This condition is a gradual loss of bone mass that can result in multiple fractures, crippling, deformity, and constant pain. See Chapter 19 for a detailed discussion of how to reduce your risk of osteoporosis.

Other health problems that have a hereditary component and that disproportionately affect certain ethnic groups include high blood pressure, alcoholism, and certain types of cancer.

tra folic acid because during the first few weeks of pregnancy it reduces the risk of neural tube defects such as spina bifida (see p. 210).

9. Were you a diethylstilbestrol (DES) baby? Daughters born to women who were given DES during pregnancy to prevent miscarriage—a common practice from the 1940s to the early 1970s—are at risk for a variety of problems with conception and pregnancy. DES daughters may need special monitoring and care to identify and treat problems as soon as they develop. (For more on DES, see Chapter 16.)

10. Do twins or multiple births run in either your or your partner's family? If so, this tendency may increase the likelihood of a multiple birth.

11. Do either you or your partner have a family history of any genetic disease? Have you or any family member had a child with a birth defect or mental impairment? Genetic testing and counseling can determine whether you are a carrier for a specific disease, what the effects of the disease would be, and whether a baby you conceive can be tested prenatally. Members of certain ethnic groups are at higher risk for genetic disorders that are more prevalent within their groups than in the general population. For more information on these disorders, refer to the box "Ethnicity and Genetic Diseases."

Additional tests or changes in behavior may be recommended if you have recently traveled outside the United States; if you work with chemicals, radiation, or toxic substances; if you participate in physically demanding or hazardous activities or occupations; or if you face significant psychosocial risks, including homelessness, an unsafe home environment, or mental illness.

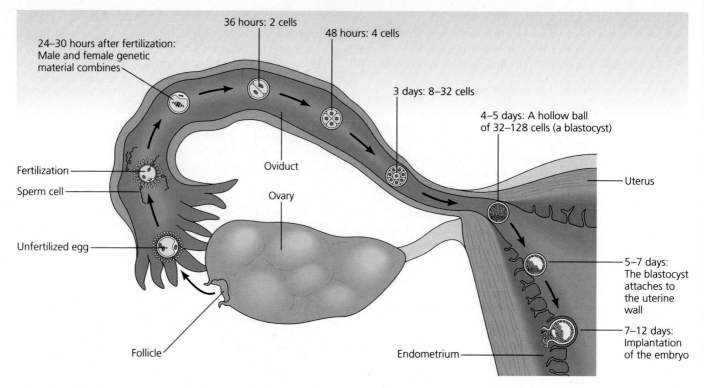

Figure 8-1 Fertilization and early development of the embryo. The unfertilized egg is released from an ovarian follicle into the oviduct, where it is fertilized by a sperm cell. As the fertilized egg moves through the oviduct toward the uterus, the genetic material from the egg and sperm combine, and the egg begins to divide. When the egg reaches the uterus, it is in the form of a hollow ball of cells called a blastocyst, which becomes implanted in the endometrium.

Labels in figure:
- 24–30 hours after fertilization: Male and female genetic material combines
- 36 hours: 2 cells
- 48 hours: 4 cells
- 3 days: 8–32 cells
- 4–5 days: A hollow ball of 32–128 cells (a blastocyst)
- Uterus
- 5–7 days: The blastocyst attaches to the uterine wall
- 7–12 days: Implantation of the embryo
- Endometrium
- Ovary
- Oviduct
- Fertilization
- Sperm cell
- Unfertilized egg
- Follicle

UNDERSTANDING FERTILITY

Conceiving a child is a highly complex process. Although many couples conceive readily, others can testify to the difficulties that can be encountered.

Www. Conception

The process of **conception** involves the **fertilization** of an egg (ovum) from a woman by a sperm from a man (Figure 8-1). Every month during a woman's fertile years, her body prepares itself for conception and pregnancy. In one of her **ovaries** an egg ripens and is released from its **follicle.** The egg, about the size of a pinpoint, travels through an **oviduct,** or **fallopian tube,** to the **uterus,** in 3–4 days. The lining of the uterus, or **endometrium,** has already thickened for the implantation of a **fertilized egg,** or zygote. If the egg is not fertilized, it lasts about 24 hours and then disintegrates. It is expelled along with the uterine lining during menstruation.

Sperm cells are produced in the man's **testes** and ejaculated from his penis into the woman's vagina during sexual intercourse (except in cases of artificial insemination or assisted reproduction; see p. 202). Sperm cells are much smaller than eggs. The typical ejaculate contains millions of sperm, but only a few complete the journey through the uterus and up the fallopian tube to the egg. Many sperm cells do not survive the acidic environment of the vagina. Once through the cervix and into the uterus, many sperm cells are diverted to the wrong oviduct or get stuck along the way. Of those that reach the egg, only one will penetrate its hard outer layer. As sperm approach the egg, they release enzymes that soften this outer layer. Enzymes from hundreds of sperm must be released in order for the egg's outer layer to soften enough to allow one sperm cell to penetrate. The first sperm cell that bumps into a spot that is soft enough can swim into the egg cell. It then merges with the nucleus of the egg, and fertilization occurs. The sperm's tail, its means of locomotion, gets stuck in the outer membrane and drops off, leaving the sperm head inside the egg. The egg then releases a chemical that makes it impenetrable by other sperm.

The ovum carries the hereditary characteristics of the mother and her ancestors; sperm cells carry the hereditary characteristics of the father and his ancestors. Each parent cell—egg or sperm—contains 23 chromosomes, each of which contains **genes,** packages of chemical instructions for the developing baby. Genes provide the blueprint for a unique individual (see the box "Creating a Family Health Tree").

As soon as fertilization occurs, the zygote starts to undergo the cell division that begins the growth process. It continues to divide as it travels through the oviduct to the uterus. Upon reaching the uterus, the cluster of cells, now called a blastocyst, becomes implanted in the endometrium.

The usual course of events is that one egg and one sperm unite to produce one fertilized egg and one baby. But if the ovaries release two (or more) eggs during ovulation, and if both eggs are fertilized, twins will develop. These twins will be no more alike than siblings from different pregnancies, because each will have come from a different fertilized egg. Twins who develop this way are referred to as **fraternal twins;** they may be the same sex or different sexes. Twins can also develop from the division of a single fertilized egg into two cells that develop separately. Because these babies share all genetic material, they will be **identical twins.**

Infertility

Although the main concern for many women and men, especially if they are young and single, is how *not* to get pregnant, the reverse is true for millions of couples who have difficulty conceiving. **Infertility** is usually defined as the inability to conceive after trying for a year or more. It affects about 6 million couples—10% of the reproductive-age population of the United States. Over a million couples seek treatment for infertility each year. Although the focus is often on women, up to 40% of the factors contributing to infertility are male, and in about 15% of infertile couples, both partners have problems. Therefore, it is important that each individual be evaluated.

Female Infertility   Female infertility usually results from one of two key causes—tubal blockage (40%) or failure to ovulate (40%). An additional 10% of cases of infertility are due to anatomical abnormalities, benign growths in the uterus, thyroid disease, and other uncommon conditions; the remaining 10% of cases are unexplained.

Blocked fallopian tubes are most commonly the result of *pelvic inflammatory disease (PID)*, a serious complication of several sexually transmitted diseases. Most cases of PID are associated with untreated cases of chlamydia or gonorrhea. More than 1.5 million cases of PID are treated each year, but physicians estimate that half may go untreated because of an absence of symptoms. Other causes of PID include unsterile abortions and certain types of older IUDs. Tubal blockages can also be caused by prior surgery or by *endometriosis,* a condition in which endometrial (uterine) tissue grows outside of the uterus. This tissue responds to hormones and can cause pain, bleeding, scarring, and adhesions. Endometriosis is typically treated with hormonal therapy and surgery.

Age impacts fertility; beginning at around age 30, a woman's fertility naturally begins to decline. Age is probably the main factor in ovulation failure. Exposure to toxic chemicals or radiation also appears to reduce fertility, as does cigarette smoking.

Male Infertility   The leading causes of infertility among men are low sperm count, lack of sperm motility (the ability to move spontaneously), misshapen sperm, and blocked passageways between the testes and the urethra. Smoking may cause reduced sperm counts and abnormal sperm. The sons of mothers who took DES may have increased sperm abnormalities and fertility problems. Certain prescription and illegal drugs also affect the number of sperm. Large doses of marijuana, for example, cause lower sperm counts and suppress certain reproductive hormones. Other causes of sperm problems include injury to the testicles, infection (especially from mumps during adulthood), birth defects, or subjecting the testes to high temperatures.

Some studies indicate that sperm counts worldwide have dropped by as much as 50% over the past 30 years. Evidence suggests that toxic substances such as lead, chemical pollutants, and radiation are responsible for this decrease. Recent research has also focused on a class of chemicals known as *endocrine disrupters*—substances found widely in the environment that mimic or interfere with the body's hormones, thereby causing problems with

Terms

conception The fusion of ovum and sperm, resulting in a fertilized egg.

fertilization The initiation of biological reproduction: the union of the nucleus of an egg cell with the nucleus of a sperm cell.

ovary One of the two female reproductive organs that produce ova (eggs) and sex hormones.

follicle One of many saclike structures within the ovary in which eggs mature.

oviduct (fallopian tube) One of two passages through which eggs travel from the ovaries to the uterus; the site of fertilization.

uterus The hollow, thick-walled, muscular organ in which the fertilized egg develops; the womb.

endometrium The mucous membrane that forms the inner lining of the cavity of the uterus.

fertilized egg The egg after penetration by a sperm; a zygote.

testis One of two male reproductive organs; the testes are the site of sperm production.

gene A package of chemical instructions, or hereditary material, that defines an individual's unique traits.

fraternal twins Twins who develop from separate fertilized eggs; not genetically identical.

identical twins Twins who develop from the division of a single zygote; genetically identical.

infertility The inability to conceive after trying for a year or more.

The genetic inheritance that each of us receives from our parents—and that our children receive from us—contains more than just physical characteristics, such as eye and hair color. Heredity also contributes to our risk of developing certain diseases and disorders. For certain uncommon illnesses such as hemophilia and sickle-cell disease, heredity is the primary cause; if your parents pass on the necessary genes, you'll get the disease. But heredity plays a subtler role in many other diseases, which are caused at least in part by environmental influences such as infection, cancer-causing chemicals, and physical inactivity. While your genes alone will not produce those diseases, they can determine how susceptible you are. Researchers have found a genetic influence in many common disorders, including heart disease, diabetes, depression, asthma, alcoholism, and certain forms of cancer.

Knowing that a specific disease runs in your family can save your life. It allows you to watch for early warning signs and get screening tests more often than you otherwise would. Changing health habits, too, can be valuable for people with a family history of certain diseases. An individual with a family history of high cholesterol and early heart disease can increase physical activity and pay special attention to diet.

In general, the more relatives with a genetically transmitted disease and the closer they are to you, the greater your risk. However, nongenetic factors—such as health habits—can also play a role. Signs of strong hereditary influence include early onset of the disease, appearance of the disease largely or exclusively on one side of the family, onset of the same disease at the same age in more than one relative, and developing the disease despite good health habits.

You can put together a simple family health tree by compiling a few key facts on your primary relatives: siblings, parents, aunts and uncles, and grandparents. Those facts include the date of birth, major diseases, health-related conditions and habits, and, for deceased relatives, the age at death as well as the cause. Because certain diseases are more common in particular ethnic groups, also record the ethnic background of each grandparent. Next, create a tree, using the example here as a guide.

Then show your tree to a physician or genetic counselor, who can help you target the health behaviors and screening tests that are most important for you and help determine whether genetic testing might be appropriate.

A Sample Family Health Tree and What It Means

The 55-year-old woman who prepared this family tree has a strong family history of osteoporosis on her mother's side. Based on this, her physician may suggest a bone density test to help gauge her risk and recommend bone-healthy lifestyle changes. She also has several close relatives on her father's side of the family who had high cholesterol levels and had heart attacks at an early age. These risk factors significantly increase her chance of having a heart attack.

The woman has two aunts who died of breast cancer, but there are several reasons not to be overly concerned. Aunts are second-degree relatives, more distantly related to her than her mother or sister (first-degree relatives). In addition, they came from different sides of the family, and they developed the disease quite late in life. Given these factors, it is likely that these cases of breast cancer did not have a significant genetic origin.

Looking at her family history can help this woman make important decisions about treatments and behaviors such as hormone replacement therapy (HRT) and moderate alcohol consumption, which may lower the risk of heart attack but which may also slightly increase the risk of breast cancer. Based on her family history, her physician may recommend HRT because she appears to be at much greater risk for heart problems than for breast cancer; in addition, HRT helps combat bone loss and may reduce her risk of osteoporosis-related fractures.

SOURCES: From "Prepare for the Future: Know Your Ancestors" and "Creating a Family Health Tree" © 1999 by Consumers Union of U.S., Inc. Yonkers, NY 10703-1057, a nonprofit organization. Excerpted with permission from the September 1999 issue of Consumer Reports on Health® for educational purposes only. No commercial use or photocopying permitted. Log on to www.ConsumerReports.org, or call 800-234-2188.

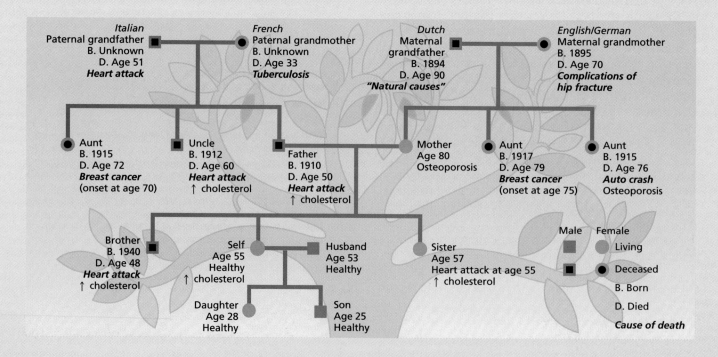

reproduction and development. Examples of hormone mimics include dioxin, PCBs, DDT, and compounds used in some plastics. Animal studies have linked prenatal exposure to endocrine disrupters with feminized genitalia and other reproductive problems in male offspring. Scientists do not yet know, however, what effects endocrine disrupters may have on human health and fertility.

Treating Infertility About 90% of infertile couples receive a physical diagnosis for their condition; for the remaining 10%, the cause of the infertility remains unexplained. Most cases of infertility are treated with conventional medical therapies: Surgery can repair oviducts, clear up endometriosis, and correct anatomical problems in both men and women. Fertility drugs can help women ovulate, although they carry the risk of causing multiple births. If these conventional treatments don't work, couples can turn to more advanced techniques (see the box "Infertility and Reproductive Technology"). However, most infertility treatments are expensive and emotionally draining, and their success is uncertain. Some infertile couples choose not to try to have children, while others turn to adoption. One measure you can take now to avoid infertility is to protect yourself against STDs and to treat promptly and completely any disease you do contract.

Emotional Responses to Infertility Couples who seek treatment for infertility have often already confronted the possibility of not being able to become biological parents. Many infertile couples feel they have lost control over a major area of their lives. They may lose perspective on the rest of their lives as they focus more and more on the reasons for their infertility and on treatment. Infertile couples may need to set their own limits on how much treatment they are willing to undergo. Support groups for infertile couples can provide help in this difficult situation, but there are few easy answers to infertility. If treatment is unsuccessful, couples must mourn the loss of the children they will never bear. They must make some kind of decision about their future, whether to pursue plans for adoption or another treatment or to adjust to childlessness and go on with their lives.

> **COMMUNICATE!** Some fertility problems may be at least partly inherited, so it can be useful to know your parents' fertility history. If you don't want to approach the issue directly, you can ask such questions as, "Was there a reason that you waited so long after you got married to have children?" or "Did you plan to have me when you did?" You may learn things you didn't know about other aspects of your parents' lives as well, such as their career aspirations or their socioeconomic status when they were younger.

PREGNANCY

Pregnancy is usually discussed in terms of **trimesters**—three periods of about 3 months (or 13 weeks) each. During the first trimester, the mother experiences a few physical changes and some fairly common symptoms. During the second trimester, often the most peaceful time of pregnancy, the mother gains weight, looks noticeably pregnant, and may experience a general sense of well-being if she is happy about having a child. The third trimester is the hardest for the mother because she must breathe, digest, excrete, and circulate blood for herself and the growing fetus. The weight of the fetus, the pressure of its body on her organs, and its increased demands on her system cause discomfort and fatigue and may make the mother increasingly impatient to give birth.

Pregnancy Tests

The earliest tests for pregnancy are chemical tests designed to detect the presence of **human chorionic gonadotropin (HCG),** a hormone produced by the implanted fertilized egg. These tests may be performed as early as 2 weeks after fertilization. Home pregnancy test kits, which are sold without a prescription in drugstores, come equipped with a small sample of red blood cells coated with HCG antibodies, to which the woman can add a small amount of her own urine. If the concentration of HCG is great enough, it will clump together with the HCG antibodies, indicating that the woman is pregnant. Home pregnancy tests can be very reliable, but the instructions must be followed carefully.

Changes in the Woman's Body

Hormonal changes begin as soon as the egg is fertilized, and for the next 9 months, the woman's body nourishes the fetus and adjusts to its growth. Let's take a closer look at the changes of early, middle, and late pregnancy (Figure 8-2).

Early Signs and Symptoms Early recognition of pregnancy is important, especially for women with physical problems and nutritional deficiencies. The following symptoms are not absolute indications of pregnancy, but they are reasons to visit a gynecologist:

- *A missed menstrual period.* If an egg has been fertilized and implanted in the uterine wall, the endometrium is retained to nourish the embryo. A woman

> **trimester** One of the three 3-month periods of pregnancy.
>
> **human chorionic gonadotropin (HCG)** A hormone produced by the fertilized egg that can be detected in the urine or blood of the mother within a few weeks of conception.

Terms

Assisted reproductive technology (ART) has come a long way since the first "test-tube baby" was born in 1978. Many new techniques have already been developed, and research in the areas of genetics and cloning promise even more breakthroughs. With these advances, however, come many medical and ethical questions.

Intrauterine Insemination

Male infertility can sometimes be overcome by collecting and concentrating the man's sperm and introducing it by syringe into a woman's vagina or uterus, a procedure known as **artificial (intrauterine) insemination.** The woman is often given fertility drugs to induce ovulation prior to the insemination procedure. The sperm can be provided by the woman's partner or, if there are severe problems with his sperm or he carries a serious genetic disorder, by a donor. Donor sperm are also used by single women and lesbian couples who wish to conceive using artificial insemination. The success rate is about 60%. There are about 30,000 births each year from intrauterine insemination.

In a new technique under development, sperm are sorted by the sex chromosome they carry prior to artificial insemination, thereby enabling couples to select the sex of their infant.

IVF, GIFT, and ZIFT

Three related techniques for overcoming infertility involve removing mature eggs from a woman's ovary. Fewer than 5% of infertile American couples who seek treatment try these techniques. In **in vitro fertilization (IVF),** the harvested eggs are mixed with sperm in a laboratory dish. If eggs are successfully fertilized, one or more of the resulting embryos is inserted into the woman's uterus. IVF is often used by women with blocked oviducts. In **gamete intrafallopian transfer (GIFT),** eggs and sperm are surgically placed into the fallopian tubes prior to fertilization. In **zygote intrafallopian transfer (ZIFT),** eggs are fertilized outside the woman's body and surgically introduced into the oviducts after they begin to divide. GIFT and ZIFT can be used by women who have at least one open fallopian tube.

Variations on these three techniques are also becoming available. Donor sperm, donor eggs, and even donor embryos can be used. Extra eggs can be harvested and fertilized and the resulting embryos frozen for later use. In cases of severe male infertility, intracytoplasmic sperm injection (ICSI), in which a single sperm is injected into a mature egg, may be used. Concerns have been raised about ICSI, however, because some studies have linked it to an increase in genetic defects in offspring. In addition, ICSI may result in the transmission from father to son of infertility-causing Y chromosome defects.

IVF, GIFT, and ZIFT do have drawbacks. Success rates vary from about 15% to 38%. They cost between $8000 and $10,000 per procedure and may require five or more cycles to produce one live birth. They also increase the chance of multiple births.

Even more advanced techniques are under development. Researchers are exploring ways to freeze unfertilized eggs as means to extend their fertility or to protect eggs from fertility-damaging cancer treatments. Injecting the cytoplasm (the material in a cell that surrounds the nucleus) from a younger woman's egg into an older woman's egg is being studied as a possible means of reducing genetic errors in the older woman's egg. A related technique under study, known as nuclear transfer, uses **cloning** technology: The nucleus of an older woman's egg is transferred into an egg from a younger woman from which the nucleus has been removed.

Surrogate Motherhood

A controversial approach to infertility is surrogate motherhood. This practice involves a contract between an infertile couple and a fertile woman who agrees to carry a fetus. The surrogate mother agrees to be artificially inseminated by the father's sperm or to undergo IVF with the couple's embryo, to carry the baby to term, and to give it to the couple at birth. In return, the couple pays her for her services. There are thought to be several hundred births to surrogate mothers each year in the United States. Some people think that surrogate motherhood is essentially an arrangement to sell a baby, and they worry about the psychological consequences for children who learn that their mothers "sold" them. Experience has shown, too, that some surrogate mothers have a very difficult time giving up the baby and are unwilling to fulfill the contract after the birth, causing emotional trauma for themselves and the couple.

Ethical Challenges

Assisted reproductive technology is a scientific frontier, and legal and ethical issues loom large. The following are just a few of the difficult questions that have been raised:

- Who owns frozen embryos? Should "extra" embryos be donated to other infertile couples, used for research, or destroyed?

- Should ART be used to help men who are infertile due to Y chromosome defects have children, even if it means that any sons they have will inherit the defect and also be infertile?

- In the case of a multiple pregnancy, should the number of embryos the woman is carrying be reduced to increase the likelihood of a safe and successful pregnancy?

- In the case of IVF involving donor eggs and sperm and a surrogate mother, who are the legal parents of the child?

The potential use of cloning technology is another hotly debated area. Cloning is different from any of the techniques discussed here because it is a form of asexual reproduction: A clone carries the genes of only one person, not two. However, as described above, the cloning technique of nuclear transfer could potentially be used in the treatment of infertility. And although success is uncertain, nuclear transfer could theoretically be used to create a child that is the genetic offspring of two people of the same sex. As technology continues to advance, the ethical and legal issues are likely to become even more complex.

SOURCES: Annas, G. J. 2000. Ulysses and the fate of frozen embryos—reproduction, research, or destruction. *New England Journal of Medicine* 343(5): 373–376. Assisted reproductive technology in the United States. 2000. *Fertility and Sterility* 74: 641–653. Centers for Disease Control and Prevention. 2000. *1998 Assisted Reproductive Technology Success Rates.* Atlanta: CDC Division of Reproductive Health.

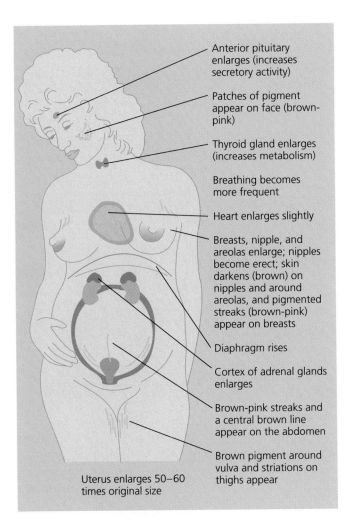

- Anterior pituitary enlarges (increases secretory activity)
- Patches of pigment appear on face (brown-pink)
- Thyroid gland enlarges (increases metabolism)
- Breathing becomes more frequent
- Heart enlarges slightly
- Breasts, nipple, and areolas enlarge; nipples become erect; skin darkens (brown) on nipples and around areolas, and pigmented streaks (brown-pink) appear on breasts
- Diaphragm rises
- Cortex of adrenal glands enlarges
- Brown-pink streaks and a central brown line appear on the abdomen
- Brown pigment around vulva and striations on thighs appear
- Uterus enlarges 50–60 times original size

Figure 8-2 Physiological changes during pregnancy.

who misses a period after having unprotected intercourse may be pregnant.

- *Slight bleeding.* Slight bleeding may follow implantation of the fertilized egg. Because this happens about the time a period is expected, the bleeding is sometimes mistaken for menstrual flow. It usually lasts only a few days.

- *Nausea.* About two-thirds of pregnant women feel nauseated, probably as a reaction to increased levels of progesterone and other hormones. Often called morning sickness, some women have it all day long. It frequently begins during the 3rd or 4th week and disappears by the 12th week. In some cases, it can last throughout a pregnancy.

- *Breast tenderness.* Some women experience breast tenderness, swelling, and tingling, usually described as different from the tenderness experienced before menstruation.

- *Sleepiness, fatigue, and emotional upset.* These symptoms result from hormonal changes.

The first reliable physical signs of pregnancy can be distinguished about 4 weeks after a woman misses her menstrual period. A softening of the uterus just above the cervix, called *Hegar's sign,* and other changes in the cervix and pelvis are apparent during a pelvic examination. The labia minora and the cervix may take on a purple color rather than their usual pink hue.

Four weeks after a woman misses her menstrual period, she would be considered to be about 8 weeks pregnant because pregnancy is calculated from the time of a woman's last menstrual period rather than from the time of actual fertilization. (The timing of ovulation and fertilization are often difficult to determine.) Although a woman should see her physician to determine her due date, due dates can be approximated by subtracting three months from the date of the last menstrual period and then adding 7 days. For example, a woman whose last menstrual period began on September 20th would have a due date of about June 27th.

Continuing Changes in the Woman's Body   The most obvious changes during pregnancy occur in the reproductive organs. During the first 3 months, the uterus enlarges to about three times its nonpregnant size, but it still cannot be felt in the abdomen. By the fourth month, it is large enough to make the abdomen protrude. By the seventh or eighth month, the uterus pushes up into the rib cage, which makes breathing slightly more difficult. The breasts enlarge and are sensitive; by week 8, they may tingle or throb. The pigmented area around the nipple, the areola, darkens and broadens. After the 10th week, **colostrum,** a yellowish fluid, may be squeezed from the mother's nipples, but the secretion of milk is prevented by high levels of estrogen and progesterone.

Other changes are going on as well. Early in pregnancy, the muscles and ligaments attached to bones begin to soften and stretch. The joints between the pelvic bones loosen and spread, making it easier to have a baby but

Terms

artificial (intrauterine) insemination The introduction of semen into the vagina by artificial means, usually by syringe.

in vitro fertilization (IVF) Combining egg and sperm outside of the body and inserting the fertilized egg into the uterus.

gamete intrafallopian transfer (GIFT) Surgically introducing eggs and sperm into the fallopian tube prior to fertilization.

zygote intrafallopian transfer (ZIFT) Surgically introducing a fertilized egg into the fallopian tube.

cloning Asexual reproduction in which offspring are genetically identical to one parent. DNA from the cell of one animal is transferred to an egg from which DNA has been removed; the egg is then placed in a surrogate and develops as though it were an embryo derived from two parents.

colostrum A yellowish fluid secreted by the mammary glands around the time of childbirth until milk comes in, about the third day.

harder to walk. The circulatory system becomes more efficient to accommodate the blood volume, which increases by 50%, and the heart pumps it more rapidly. Much of the increased blood flow goes to the uterus and placenta (the organ that exchanges nutrients and waste between mother and fetus). The mother's lungs also become more efficient, and her rib cage widens to permit her to inhale up to 40% more air. Much of the oxygen goes to the fetus. The kidneys become highly efficient, removing waste products from fetal circulation and producing large amounts of urine by midpregnancy.

Women of normal weight gain an average of 18–25% of their initial weight: 20–28 lb for a woman weighing 110; 23–32 lb for a woman weighing 128. About 60% of weight gained relates directly to the baby—about 6.8 lb for the baby and 7.5 lb for the placenta, amniotic fluid, heavier breasts and uterus—and 40% accumulates over the mother's entire body as fluid (blood, about 4 lb) and fat (4–8 lb). As the woman's skin stretches, small breaks may occur in the elastic fibers of the lower layer of skin, producing stretch marks on her abdomen, hips, breasts, or thighs. Increased pigment production darkens the skin in 90% of pregnant women, especially in places that have stretched.

Changes During the Later Stages of Pregnancy
By the end of the sixth month, the increased needs of the fetus place a burden on the mother's lungs, heart, and kidneys. Her back may ache from the pressure of the baby's weight and from having to throw her shoulders back to keep her balance while standing (Figure 8-3). Her body retains more water, perhaps up to 3 extra quarts of fluid. Her legs, hands, ankles, or feet may swell, and she may be bothered by leg cramps, heartburn, or constipation. Despite discomfort, both her digestion and her metabolism are working at top efficiency.

The uterus prepares for childbirth with preliminary contractions, called **Braxton Hicks contractions.** Unlike true labor contractions, these are usually short, irregular, and painless. The mother may only be aware that at times her abdomen is hard to the touch. These contractions become more frequent and intense as the delivery date approaches.

In the ninth month, the baby settles into the pelvic bones, usually head down, fitting snugly. This process, called **lightening,** allows the uterus to sink down about 2 inches, producing a visible change in the mother's profile. Pelvic pressure increases, and pressure on the diaphragm lightens. Breathing becomes easier; urination becomes more frequent. Sometimes, after a first pregnancy, the baby doesn't settle down into the pelvis until labor begins.

Emotional Responses to Pregnancy

A woman's feelings during pregnancy will depend on her circumstances—her self-image, how she feels about pregnancy and motherhood, whether the pregnancy was

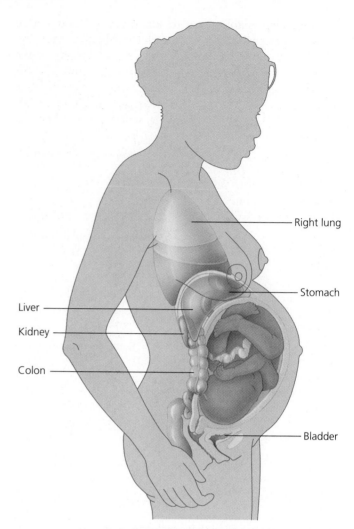

Figure 8-3 The woman and fetus during the third trimester of pregnancy. Pressure from the rapidly growing fetus on the mother's lungs, bladder, stomach, and other organs may cause shortness of breath, heartburn, and the need for frequent urination. The mother's uterus has expanded to 50–60 times its original size.

planned, what type of relationship she has with her partner, whether she has a secure home situation, and many other factors. A first pregnancy is especially important because it has traditionally symbolized the transition to maturity and is a major developmental milestone in the lives of mothers—and fathers as well.

Both partners may have fears about the approaching birth, their ability to be good parents, and the ways in which the baby will affect their own relationship. These concerns are normal, and sharing them can deepen and strengthen a relationship. For a woman without a partner or whose partner is not supportive, it's important that she find other sources of support, perhaps from friends, family members, or support groups. The relationships that parents-to-be have with their own parents may also undergo changes. Impending parenthood may encourage them to assert their independence from their parents, but it may also enable them to identify with their parents' own experience of pregnancy, childbirth, and parenting.

Rapid changes in hormone levels can cause a pregnant woman to experience unpredictable emotions. A great part of pregnancy is beyond the woman's control—her changing appearance, her energy level, her variable moods—and some women need extra support and reassurance to keep on an even keel. Hormonal changes can also make women feel exhilarated and euphoric, although for some women such moods are temporary.

Like the physical changes that accompany pregnancy, emotional responses also change as the pregnancy develops. During the first trimester, the pregnant woman may fear that she may miscarry or that the child will not be normal. Education about pregnancy and childbirth and support from her partner, friends, relatives, and health care professionals are important antidotes to these fears. During the second trimester, the pregnant woman can feel the fetus move within her, and worries about miscarriages usually begin to diminish. She may look and feel radiantly happy and be delighted as her pregnancy begins to show. However, she may also worry that her increasing size makes her unattractive. Reassurance from her partner can ease these fears.

The third trimester is the time of greatest physical stress during the pregnancy. A woman may find that her physical abilities are limited by her size. Because some women feel physically awkward and sexually unattractive, they may experience periods of depression. But many also feel a great deal of happy excitement and anticipation. The fetus may already be looked upon as a member of the family, and both parents may begin talking to the fetus and interacting with it by patting the mother's belly. The upcoming birth will probably be a focus for both the woman and her partner.

WW. Fetal Development

Now that we've seen what happens to the mother's body during pregnancy, let's consider the development of the fetus (Figure 8-4).

The First Trimester About 30 hours after the egg is fertilized, the cell divides, and this process of cell division repeats many times. As the cluster of cells drifts down the oviduct, several different kinds of cells emerge. The entire set of genetic instructions is passed to every cell, but each cell follows only certain instructions; if this were not the case, there would be no different organs or body parts. For example, all cells carry genes for hair color and eye color, but only the cells of the hair follicles and irises (of the eye) respond to that information.

On about the fourth day after fertilization, the cluster, now about 32–128 cells and hollow, arrives in the uterus; this is a **blastocyst.** On about the sixth or seventh day, the blastocyst attaches to the uterine wall, usually along the upper curve; over the next few days, it becomes firmly implanted and begins to draw nourishment from the endometrium, the uterine lining.

The blastocyst becomes an **embryo** by about the end of the second week after fertilization. The inner cells of the blastocyst separate into three layers. One layer becomes inner body parts, the digestive and respiratory systems; the middle layer becomes muscle, bone, blood, kidneys, and sex glands; and the third layer becomes the skin, hair, and nervous tissue.

The outermost shell of cells becomes the **placenta, umbilical cord,** and **amniotic sac** (Figure 8-5). A network of blood vessels called chorionic villi eventually forms the placenta. The human placenta is a two-way exchange of nutrients and waste materials between the mother and the fetus. The placenta brings oxygen and nutrients to the fetus and transports waste products out. The placenta does not provide a perfect barrier between the fetal circulation and the maternal circulation, however. Some blood cells are exchanged and certain substances, such as alcohol, pass freely from the maternal circulation through the placenta to the fetus.

The period between weeks 2 and 9 is a time of rapid differentiation and change. All the major body structures are formed during this time, including the heart, brain, liver, lungs, and sex organs; the eyes, nose, ears, arms, and legs also appear. Some organs begin to function—the heart begins to beat and the liver starts producing blood cells. Because body structures are forming, the developing organism is vulnerable to damage from environmental influences such as drugs and infections (discussed in detail in sections that follow).

By the end of the second month, the brain sends out impulses that coordinate the functioning of other organs. The embryo is now a fetus, and most further changes will be in the size and refinement of working body parts. In the third month, the fetus begins to be quite active. By the end of the first trimester, the fetus is about 4 inches long and weighs 1 ounce.

Braxton Hicks contractions Uterine contractions that occur during the third trimester of pregnancy, preparing it for labor. | Terms

lightening A process in which the uterus sinks down because the baby's head settles into the pelvic area.

blastocyst A stage of development, days 6–14, when the cell cluster becomes the embryo and placenta.

embryo The stage of development between blastocyst and fetus; about weeks 2–8.

placenta The organ through which the fetus receives nourishment and empties waste via the mother's circulatory system; after birth, the placenta is expelled from the uterus.

umbilical cord The cord connecting the placenta and fetus, through which nutrients pass.

amniotic sac A membranous pouch enclosing and protecting the fetus, containing amniotic fluid.

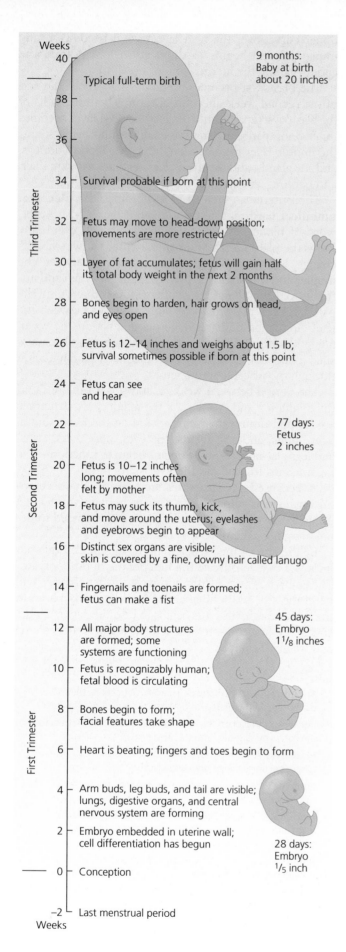

Weeks
40 ─ Typical full-term birth

9 months:
Baby at birth
about 20 inches

38

36

Third Trimester

34 ─ Survival probable if born at this point

32 ─ Fetus may move to head-down position; movements are more restricted

30 ─ Layer of fat accumulates; fetus will gain half its total body weight in the next 2 months

28 ─ Bones begin to harden, hair grows on head, and eyes open

26 ─ Fetus is 12–14 inches and weighs about 1.5 lb; survival sometimes possible if born at this point

24 ─ Fetus can see and hear

22

77 days:
Fetus
2 inches

Second Trimester

20 ─ Fetus is 10–12 inches long; movements often felt by mother

18 ─ Fetus may suck its thumb, kick, and move around the uterus; eyelashes and eyebrows begin to appear

16 ─ Distinct sex organs are visible; skin is covered by a fine, downy hair called lanugo

14 ─ Fingernails and toenails are formed; fetus can make a fist

12 ─ All major body structures are formed; some systems are functioning

45 days:
Embryo
1 1/8 inches

10 ─ Fetus is recognizably human; fetal blood is circulating

First Trimester

8 ─ Bones begin to form; facial features take shape

6 ─ Heart is beating; fingers and toes begin to form

4 ─ Arm buds, leg buds, and tail are visible; lungs, digestive organs, and central nervous system are forming

2 ─ Embryo embedded in uterine wall; cell differentiation has begun

28 days:
Embryo
1/5 inch

0 ─ Conception

−2 ─ Last menstrual period
Weeks

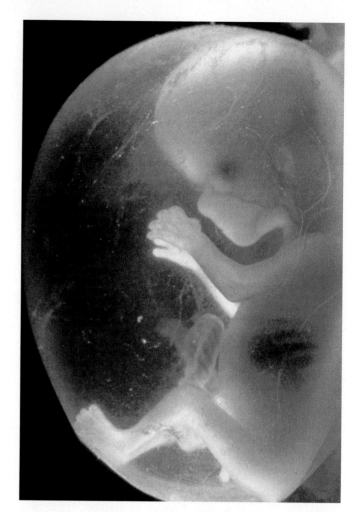

By the fourth month, the fetus is growing rapidly and is about 10 inches long. Weighing about 6 ounces, it moves vigorously in the uterus and can suck, frown, and turn its head.

The Second Trimester   To grow during the second trimester, to about 14 inches and 2 pounds, the fetus must have large amounts of food, oxygen, and water, which come from the mother through the placenta. All body systems are operating, and the fetal heartbeat can be heard with a stethoscope. Fetal movements can be felt by the mother beginning in the fourth or fifth month. Against great odds, a fetus born prematurely at the end of the second trimester might survive.

The Third Trimester   The fetus gains most of its birth weight during the last 3 months. Some of the weight is fatty tissue under the skin that insulates the fetus and supplies food. The fetus must obtain large amounts of calcium, iron, and nitrogen from the food the mother eats.

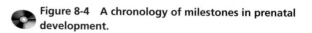

Figure 8-4   A chronology of milestones in prenatal development.

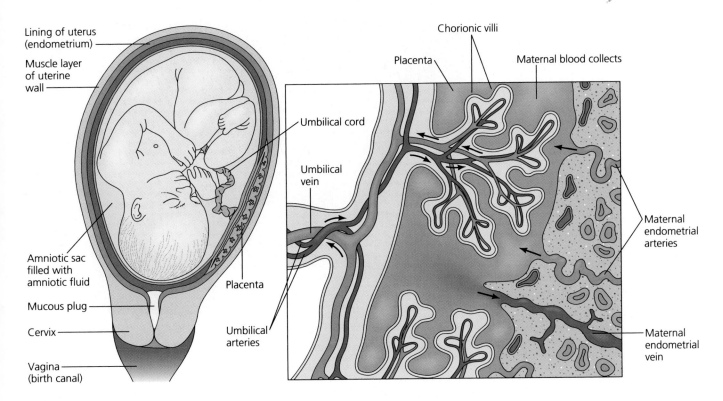

Lining of uterus (endometrium)

Muscle layer of uterine wall

Amniotic sac filled with amniotic fluid

Mucous plug

Cervix

Vagina (birth canal)

Umbilical cord

Umbilical vein

Placenta

Umbilical arteries

Chorionic villi

Placenta

Maternal blood collects

Maternal endometrial arteries

Maternal endometrial vein

Figure 8-5   A cross-sectional view of the fetus in the uterus and an enlargement of the placenta.

Some 85% of the calcium and iron she consumes goes into the fetal bloodstream.

Although the fetus may live if it is born during the seventh month, it needs the fat layer acquired in the eighth month and time for the organs, especially the respiratory and digestive organs, to develop. It also needs the immunity the mother's blood supplies during the final 3 months. Her blood protects the fetus against many of the diseases to which she has acquired immunity. These immunities wear off within 6 months after birth, but they can be replenished by the mother's milk if the baby is breastfed.

Diagnosing Fetal Abnormalities   Information about the health and sex of a fetus can be obtained prior to birth through prenatal testing. The most common tests now used are ultrasound, amniocentesis, chorionic villus sampling (CVS), and the triple marker screen.

Ultrasonography (also called *ultrasound*) uses high-frequency sound waves to create a visual image, or **sonogram**, of the fetus in the uterus. Sonograms show the position of the fetus, its size and gestational age, and the presence of certain anatomical problems. Sonograms can sometimes be used to determine the sex of the fetus.

Amniocentesis involves the removal of fluid from the uterus with a long, thin needle inserted through the abdominal wall. It is usually performed between 14 and 18 weeks into the pregnancy, although earlier amniocen-

tesis is becoming available at some centers. A genetic analysis of the fetal cells in the fluid can reveal the presence of chromosomal disorders, such as Down syndrome, and some genetic diseases, including Tay-Sachs disease. The sex of the fetus can also be determined. Most amniocentesis tests are performed on pregnant women over age 35, who have a greater risk of chromosomal abnormalities, or in cases where the fetus is known to be at risk for a particular chromosomal or genetic defect. Amniocentesis carries a slight risk (a 0.5–2% chance of miscarriage).

A newer alternative is **chorionic villus sampling (CVS)**, which can be performed earlier in pregnancy than amniocentesis, between week 10 and 12. This procedure involves removal through the cervix (by catheter) or abdomen (by needle) of a tiny section of chorionic villi, which contain fetal cells that can be analyzed. CVS carries a slightly higher risk of miscarriage than amniocentesis.

Terms

ultrasonography The use of high-frequency sound waves to view the fetus in the uterus; also known as *ultrasound*.

sonogram The visual image of the fetus produced by ultrasonography.

amniocentesis A process in which amniotic fluid is removed and analyzed to detect possible birth defects.

chorionic villus sampling (CVS) Surgical removal of a tiny section of chorionic villi to be analyzed for genetic defects.

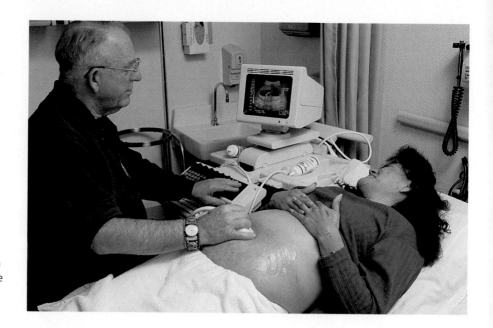

Ultrasonography provides information about the position, size, and physical condition of a fetus in the uterus. This mother-to-be can see her baby move and perhaps tell its sex by watching it on the screen.

The **triple marker screen (TMS)** is a maternal blood test that can be used to help identify fetuses with neural tube defects, Down syndrome, and other anomalies. Blood is taken from the mother at 16 to 19 weeks of pregnancy and analyzed for three hormone levels—human chorionic gonadotropin (HCG), unconjugated estriol, and alpha-fetoprotein (AFP). The three hormone levels are compared to appropriate standards, and the results are used to estimate the probability that the fetus has particular anomalies. In the case of abnormal TMS results, parents may choose further testing such as ultrasonography or amniocentesis.

Genetic counselors explain the results of the different tests so that parents can understand their implications. If a fetus is found to have a defect, it may be carried to term, aborted, or, in rare instances, treated while still in the uterus. Results of most current screening tests are not available until after week 12 of pregnancy; consequently, if abortion is chosen, it is likely to involve one of the more medically complex and physically difficult methods (see Chapter 7). Researchers are searching for new fetal screening techniques that are less invasive and that can be done earlier in pregnancy.

Fetal Programming Amniocentesis, CVS, and TMS look for chromosomal, genetic, and other anomalies that typically cause immediate problems. A new area of study known as fetal programming theory focuses on how conditions in the womb may influence the risk of adult diseases. For example, researchers have linked low birth weight to an increased risk of heart disease, obesity, diabetes, and schizophrenia; high birth weight in female infants, on the other hand, has been linked to an increased risk of breast cancer in later life.

How might conditions during gestation affect the risk of adult diseases? A number of studies have looked at groups of people born in areas of poverty or at times of famine, when pregnant women were unable to obtain an adequate diet. The poor prenatal conditions that stunt the growth of a developing fetus and lead to low birth weight may also affect specific organs. For example, if energy is limited, resources may be directed toward the developing fetal brain and away from other organs, including the liver and kidneys. Later in life, a small liver may be unable to clear cholesterol from the bloodstream, thereby increasing cholesterol levels and raising the risk of heart disease; undersized kidneys may be less able to regulate blood pressure. The fetus may also respond to limited resources by developing a permanently thrifty metabolism that triggers increased appetite and fat storage—leading to a greater risk of adult obesity and diabetes. Stress, both physical and emotional, increases maternal levels of the hormone cortisol, which in turn may permanently affect an infant's system of blood pressure regulation (see the box "Stress and Pregnancy").

Hormones may also be involved in the link between high birth weight and increased risk of breast cancer. Growth factors that contribute to high birth weight include leptin, insulin, and estrogen. Exposure to high lev-

Pregnancy is a time of great change for a pregnant woman, and these changes can increase her level of stress. High levels of stress can have the same adverse effects on a pregnant woman as they do on anyone else (see Chapter 2). However, recent research suggests that stress can also affect the course of pregnancy and the health of the fetus.

Researchers have linked high levels of stress to miscarriage, preterm labor, and low birth weight. In one study, women who reported high levels of job stress were found to have a risk of miscarriage two to three times higher than that of less-stressed women. Other studies have found that pregnant women who experience major life changes, traumatic experiences, or high levels of pregnancy-related anxiety are at greater risk for preterm labor and for having a low-birth-weight infant. Stress hormones may constrict blood flow to the placenta, depriving the fetus of the oxygen and nutrients needed for optimal growth and development. Stress hormones also play a role in triggering labor, so high hormone levels may also increase the risk of preterm labor. Stress may also affect the behavior of a pregnant woman; negative coping techniques such as use of tobacco, alcohol, and other drugs can adversely affect a developing fetus. On the flip side, social support during pregnancy has been linked to improved fetal growth and healthy birth weight.

The time in pregnancy in which stress is experienced may be important in determining its effects. A study of earthquake survivors found that women who were in their first trimester when the earthquake occurred were at increased risk for preterm labor; women further along in their pregnancies experienced no such increase in risk. Researchers hypothesize that hormones produced in the later stages of pregnancy may protect both mother and fetus from the effects of stress.

High levels of stress have also been linked to birth defects. Although the overall risk of birth defects is very low, women who experience severe emotional trauma around the time of conception or during the first trimester are more likely to have an infant with defects of the skull, spine, palate, or limbs. The relationship between stress and birth defects has been found to be significantly greater in women with lower levels of education, suggesting that chronic stressors and behaviors that go along with low educational attainment and low income may increase the impact of stressful life events on fetal development.

As described in the discussion of fetal programming, stress during pregnancy can have even longer-term effects. Stress leads to high maternal levels of the hormone cortisol; when maternal diet is also poor, more cortisol crosses the placenta and reaches the fetal brain. Prenatal exposure to high levels of cortisol may increase susceptibility to stress in adulthood and permanently raise blood pressure.

Researchers have studied the long-term effects of stress by looking at children of pregnant Dutch women who experienced high levels of physical and emotional stress during the "Hunger Winter" of 1944–1945, when the Nazis blockaded the western Netherlands. Fetuses exposed to the famine early in development were found to be at increased risk of central nervous system defects and, as adults, obesity and schizophrenia. Studies of English children born in areas of poverty in the early 1900s found links between poor prenatal conditions and high blood pressure and heart disease. Although most American women do not experience such extreme stressors during pregnancy, these studies reinforce the importance of adequate prenatal care, including stress management and social support.

els of these in the womb may alter developing breast tissue in such a way that when exposed to estrogen later in life, breast cells may be more likely to become malignant.

Although fetal programming theory is not yet embraced by all scientists, these studies emphasize that everything that occurs during pregnancy can have an impact on the developing fetus. For pregnant women, adequate nutrition and stress management are vital for both their own health and the health of the fetus (see the next section on prenatal care). In the future, people may be able to use information about their birth weight and other indicators of gestational conditions just as they can now use family history and genetic information—to alert them to special health risks they may face and to give them the opportunity to respond appropriately to maximize their health and well-being.

The Importance of Prenatal Care

Adequate prenatal care—a nutritious diet, exercise, adequate rest, avoidance of drugs, and regular medical evaluation—is essential to the health of both mother and baby. The pregnant woman cannot help but be responsible for the condition of the baby she carries. Everything she eats, drinks, and does affects the fetus in some respect. The fetus gets its nutrients and oxygen from the mother's bloodstream and has its wastes removed the same way. Many harmful substances can also be passed to the fetus via the placenta and umbilical cord. For these reasons, a mother's caring for her own health during pregnancy is a lifelong investment in her child's health.

Regular Checkups   In the woman's first visit to her obstetrician, she will be asked for a detailed medical history of herself and her family. The physician or midwife will note any hereditary conditions that may assume increased significance during pregnancy. The tendency to develop gestational diabetes (diabetes during pregnancy only), for example, can be inherited; appropriate treatment during pregnancy reduces the risk of serious harm.

The woman is given a complete physical exam and is informed about appropriate diet. She returns for regular checkups throughout the pregnancy, during which her blood pressure and weight gain are measured, her urine is analyzed, and the size and position of the fetus are monitored. Regular prenatal visits also give the mother a chance to discuss her concerns and assure herself that everything is proceeding normally. Early advice from physicians, midwives, health educators, and teachers of childbirth classes provides the mother with invaluable information.

Blood Tests A blood sample is taken during the initial prenatal visit to determine blood type and detect possible anemia or Rh incompatibilities. The Rh factor is a blood protein. If an Rh-positive father and an Rh-negative mother conceive an Rh-positive baby, the baby's blood will be incompatible with the mother's. If some of the baby's blood enters the mother's bloodstream during delivery, she will develop antibodies to it just as she would toward a virus. If she has subsequent Rh-positive babies, the antibodies in the mother's blood, passing through the placenta, will destroy the fetus's red blood cells, possibly leading to jaundice, anemia, mental retardation, or death. This condition is completely treatable with a serum called Rh-immune globulin, which destroys Rh-positive cells as they enter the mother's body and prevents her from forming antibodies to them. (Blood tests can also reveal the presence of some STDs, discussed later in the chapter.)

Prenatal Nutrition The saying that a pregnant woman needs to "eat for two" is true. A nutritious diet throughout pregnancy is essential for both the fetus and the mother. Not only does the baby get all its nutrients from the mother, but it also competes with her for nutrients not sufficiently available to meet both their needs. When a woman's diet is low in iron or calcium, the fetus receives most of it, and the mother may become deficient in the mineral. To meet the increased nutritional demands of her body, a pregnant woman shouldn't just eat more; she should make sure that her diet is adequate in all the basic nutritional categories (see the box "Healthy Eating During Pregnancy").

Adequate intake of the B vitamin folic acid before conception and in the early weeks of pregnancy has been shown to decrease the risk of neural tube defects, including spina bifida. It is recommended that any woman capable of becoming pregnant consume at least 400 µg (0.4 mg) of folic acid daily from fortified foods and/or supplements, in addition to folate from a varied diet. For women who have already had a pregnancy involving a fetus with a neural tube defect, the CDC recommends consulting with a physician about taking a much larger amount of folic acid (4 mg), starting one month before conception and continuing through the first trimester. Since 1998, enriched grain products have been fortified with small amounts of folic acid; folate is found naturally in leafy green vegetables, legumes, citrus fruits, and most berries.

Avoiding Drugs and Other Environmental Hazards In addition to the food the mother eats, the drugs she takes and the chemicals she is exposed to affect the fetus. Everything the mother ingests may eventually reach the fetus in some proportion. Some drugs harm the fetus but not the mother because the fetus is in the process of developing and because the proper dose for the mother is a massive dose for the fetus.

During the first trimester, when the major body structures are rapidly forming, the fetus is extremely vulnerable to environmental factors such as viral infections, radiation, drugs, and other **teratogens,** any of which can cause **congenital malformations,** or birth defects. The most susceptible body parts are those growing most rapidly at the time of exposure. The rubella (German measles) virus, for example, can cause a congenital malformation of a delicate system such as the eyes or ears, leading to blindness or deafness, if exposure occurs during the first trimester, but it does no damage later in the pregnancy. Similarly, the tranquilizer thalidomide taken early in pregnancy prevented the formation of arms and legs in fetuses, but taken later, when limbs were already formed, it caused no damage. Other drugs can cause damage throughout prenatal development.

ALCOHOL Alcohol is a potent teratogen. Getting drunk just one time during pregnancy may be enough to cause brain damage in a fetus. A high level of alcohol consumption during pregnancy is associated with miscarriages, stillbirths, and, in live babies, **fetal alcohol syndrome (FAS).** A baby born with FAS is likely to suffer from a small head and body size, unusual facial characteristics, congenital heart defects, defective joints, mental impairment, and abnormal behavior patterns. The Centers for Disease Control and Prevention (CDC) estimate that about 1 out of every 1000 infants born in the United States has FAS. The rate is highest among those of low socioeconomic status, African Americans, and Native Americans. Researchers now doubt that any level of alcohol consumption is safe, and they recommend total abstinence during pregnancy (see Chapter 10).

TOBACCO Pregnant women who smoke should quit, and nonsmoking pregnant women should avoid places where

---

Terms

teratogen An agent or influence that causes physical defects in a developing embryo.

congenital malformation A physical defect existing at the time of birth, either inherited or caused during gestation.

fetal alcohol syndrome (FAS) A combination of birth defects caused by excessive alcohol consumption by the mother during pregnancy.

A healthy diet is a key part of prenatal care. To maintain her own health and help the fetus grow, a woman needs to consume about 300 extra calories per day during pregnancy. Breastfeeding an infant requires even more energy—about 500 extra calories per day.

Healthy Choices

To ensure a balanced intake of key nutrients, pregnant women should follow the U.S. Department of Agriculture's Food Guide Pyramid. The Pyramid recommends a range of servings for the following six different food groups; the number of servings in parentheses is the minimum suggested by the American College of Obstetricians and Gynecologists for pregnant women:

- Bread, cereal, rice, and pasta group: 6–11 servings (9 servings)
- Vegetables: 3–4 servings (4 servings)
- Fruits: 2–4 servings (3 servings)
- Milk, yogurt, and cheese: 2–3 servings (3 servings)
- Meat, poultry, fish, dry beans, eggs, and nuts: 2–3 servings (3 servings or 6 oz total)
- Fats, oils, and sweets: use sparingly according to total energy needs

Finally, it is also important to consume an adequate amount of fluids, the equivalent of 6–8 glasses of water per day.

Supplements

Some physicians may prescribe vitamin and mineral supplements for women who are pregnant or lactating or who are trying to get pregnant. Supplements may be for a particular nutrient, such as folic acid or iron, or may be a multivitamin and mineral supplement. It is important that a pregnant woman not supplement beyond her physician's advice because some vitamins and minerals are harmful if taken in excess. It is also important not to take herbal dietary supplements without consulting a physician; few dietary supplements have been tested for safety during pregnancy, and some have been shown to be dangerous.

Food Safety

Pregnant women should give special attention to food safety because foodborne pathogens can be particularly dangerous during pregnancy. Two such pathogens are *Listeria monocytogenes* and *Toxoplasma gondii*. *Listeria* is a bacterium most often found in undercooked or ready-to-eat meat, poultry, or seafood; soft cheeses; products made with unpasteurized milk; and unpasteurized juice. Listeriosis causes flulike symptoms in pregnant women; if the fetus is infected, the result can be miscarriage, premature birth, or birth defects.

T. gondii, a parasite carried by cats, can also contaminate food or soil. Toxoplasmosis is typically caused by eating undercooked meat or poultry or unwashed fruits and vegetables, cleaning a litter box, or handling contaminated soil. Toxoplasmosis causes few symptoms in pregnant women, but if passed to the fetus, it may cause miscarriage or mental impairment.

To avoid foodborne illness, pregnant women should wash their hands thoroughly before preparing or eating food and after handling raw meats or using the bathroom. They should cook meat, poultry, and seafood thoroughly and reheat leftovers or ready-to-eat foods until steaming hot. Fruits and vegetables should be thoroughly washed under running water. Pregnant women may choose to avoid foods that are most likely to carry dangerous pathogens. (Interestingly, researchers have found that the types of foods that pregnant women with "morning sickness" tend to avoid—meat, fish, poultry, eggs, and strong-tasting vegetables—are those that have historically been most likely to carry dangerous microorganisms or natural toxins, suggesting that morning sickness may be a protective adaptation.)

One further food safety recommendation for pregnant women relates to fish. Most types of fish are good choices for a healthy diet, but a few types can be contaminated with mercury or industrial pollutants. The FDA advises pregnant women not to eat swordfish, shark, king mackerel, or tilefish. Pregnant women are also advised to check with their local health departments before consuming any game fish.

For a more detailed discussion of recommended food choices, servings sizes, and food safety guidelines, see Chapter 12.

people smoke. Smoking during pregnancy increases the risk of miscarriage, low birth weight, and infant death. If nicotine levels in a mother's bloodstream are high, fetal breathing rate and movement become more rapid; the fetus may also metabolize cancer-causing by-products of tobacco. Infants of women who smoke during pregnancy have poorer lung function at birth, and exposure to secondhand smoke after birth increases a baby's susceptibility to pneumonia and bronchitis. If a mother who smokes breastfeeds, her infant will be exposed to tobacco chemicals through breast milk. See Chapter 11 for more on the effects of smoking.

CAFFEINE Caffeine, a powerful stimulant, should be used conservatively by pregnant women. It puts both mother and fetus under stress by raising the level of the hormone epinephrine. Caffeine also reduces the blood supply to the uterus. One study found that consuming the amount of caffeine in five or more cups of coffee a day doubled the risk of miscarriage. Coffee, colas, strong black tea, and chocolate are high in caffeine, as are over-the-counter medications such as Excedrin and NoDōz (See Chapter 9). A pregnant woman should limit her caffeine intake to no more than the equivalent of about 2 cups of coffee per day.

DRUGS AND CHEMICALS Some prescription drugs can also harm the fetus, so they should be used only under medical supervision. Accutane, a popular anti-acne drug, is thought to have been responsible for over 1000 cases of severe birth defects in the 1980s. Vitamins, aspirin, and other over-the-counter drugs should be used only under a physician's direction. Large doses of vitamin A, for example, can cause birth defects. Chemicals and pollutants can also pose a danger to the fetus. Mercury, from fish contaminated by industrial pollution, is known to cause physical deformities. Continuous exposure to lead, found in some paint products and in water from lead pipes, has been implicated as a cause of a variety of learning disorders. Any product containing chemicals—including chemical fertilizers, solvents, and pesticides—should be avoided or used with extreme caution.

STDs AND OTHER INFECTIONS Infections, including those that are sexually transmitted, are another serious problem for the fetus. The most common cause of life-threatening infections in newborns is Group B streptococcus (GBS), a type of bacterium that can cause pneumonia, meningitis, and blood infections. Many pregnant women who carry GBS do not become ill, so routine screening close to the time of delivery is recommended. A woman who carries GBS and who has certain other conditions, such as fever during labor, may be given intravenous antibiotics at the time of labor to reduce the risk of passing GBS to her baby.

If a mother contracts rubella during the first trimester, her child may be born with physical or mental disabilities. Immunization against measles must take place before pregnancy, because the immunization is harmful to the fetus. Syphilis can infect and kill a fetus; if the baby is born alive, it will have syphilis. Penicillin taken by the mother during pregnancy cures syphilis in both mother and fetus. Gonorrhea can infect the baby during delivery and cause blindness. Because gonorrhea is often asymptomatic, in many states the eyes of newborns are routinely treated with silver nitrate or another antibiotic to destroy gonorrheal bacteria. All pregnant women should be tested for hepatitis B, a virus that can pass from the mother to the infant at birth. Infants of infected mothers can be immunized shortly after birth.

Herpes simplex can damage the baby's eyes and brain and cause death, and no cure has yet been discovered for it. Genital herpes can be transmitted to the baby during delivery if the mother's infection is in the active phase. If this is the case, the baby may be delivered by cesarean section. An initial outbreak of herpes can be dangerous if it occurs during pregnancy because the virus may pass through the placenta to the fetus. For this reason, testing for genital herpes is recommended for both expectant parents. Once the baby is born, any caregiver who is experiencing a herpes outbreak should wash his or her hands often and not permit contact between hands or contaminated objects and the baby's mucous membranes (inside of eyes, mouth, nose, penis, vagina, vulva, and rectum).

The human immunodeficiency virus (HIV), which causes AIDS, can be passed to the fetus by an HIV-infected mother during pregnancy, labor and delivery, or breastfeeding. Nationwide, about 9000 children under age 13 have been diagnosed with AIDS, and many more are infected with HIV. The babies most at risk are those whose mothers inject drugs or are the sex partners of men who inject drugs. HIV testing is critical for any woman at risk for HIV, and some physicians recommend routine testing for all pregnant women. Antiviral drugs, given to an HIV-infected mother during pregnancy and delivery and to her newborn immediately following birth, reduce the rate of HIV transmission from mother to infant from 25% to 5% or less. Of course, women should also take all the necessary precautions against HIV infection during pregnancy. (See Chapter 18 for more on HIV and other STDs.)

Environmental factors affecting fetal or infant development are summarized in Table 8-1.

Prenatal Activity and Exercise Physical activity during pregnancy contributes to mental and physical wellness. Women can continue working at their jobs until late in their pregnancy, provided the work isn't so physically demanding that it jeopardizes their health. At the same time, pregnant women need more rest and sleep to maintain their own well-being and that of the fetus.

A moderate exercise program during pregnancy does not adversely affect pregnancy or birth; in fact, regular exercise appears to improve a woman's chance of an on-time delivery. The amniotic sac protects the fetus, and normal activities will not harm it. A woman who exercised before becoming pregnant can often continue her program, with appropriate modifications to maintain her comfort and safety. A pregnant woman who hasn't been exercising and wants to start should first consult a physician. Regular cardiorespiratory endurance exercise is recommended. Walking, swimming, and stationary cycling are all good choices; more strenuous activities that could result in a fall, such as skiing, skating, or horseback riding, are best delayed until after the birth. Recommendations for exercising safely during pregnancy include the following:

- Exercise regularly (at least three times a week) rather than intermittently.

- After 20 weeks of pregnancy, avoid exercise that requires lying on your back. Research indicates that this position restricts blood flow to the uterus. Also avoid prolonged periods of motionless standing.

- Modify the intensity of your exercise according to how you feel. Stop exercising if you feel fatigued, and don't exercise to exhaustion. You may find that non-weight-bearing exercises such as swimming and cycling are more comfortable than weight-bearing

Table 8-1   Selected Environmental Factors Associated with Problems in a Fetus or Infant

Agent or Condition	Potential Effects
Accutane (acne medication)	Small head, mental impairment, deformed or absent ears, heart defects, cleft lip and palate
Alcohol	Unusual facial characteristics, small head, heart defects, mental impairment, defective joints
Chlamydia	Eye infections, pneumonia
Cigarette smoking	Miscarriage, stillbirth, low birth weight, respiratory problems, sudden infant death
Cocaine	Miscarriage, stillbirth, low birth weight, small head, defects of genital and urinary tract
Cytomegalovirus (CMV)	Small head, mental impairment, blindness
Diabetes (insulin-dependent)	Malformations of the brain, spine, and heart
Gonorrhea	Eye infection leading to blindness if untreated
Herpes	Brain damage, death
HIV infection	Impaired immunity, death
Lead	Reduced IQ, learning disorders
Marijuana	Impaired fetal growth; increase in alcohol-related fetal damage
Mercury	Brain damage
Propecia (hair loss medication)	Abnormalities of the male sex organs
Radiation (high dose)	Small head, growth and mental impairment, multiple birth defects
Rubella (German measles)	Malformation of eyes or ears causing deafness or blindness; small head; mental impairment
Syphilis	Fetal death and miscarriage, prematurity, physical deformities
Tetracycline	Pigmentation of teeth, underdevelopment of enamel
Vitamin A (excess)	Miscarriage; defects of the head, brain, spine, and urinary tract

activities in the later months of pregnancy; they also minimize the risk of injury.

- Avoid any type of exercise that has the potential for even mild abdominal trauma, and take care when performing any activity in which balance is important or in which losing balance would be dangerous. Pregnancy shifts your center of gravity.

- Avoid heat stress, particularly during the first trimester, by drinking an adequate amount of fluid, wearing appropriate clothing, and avoiding activity in hot and humid weather.

- Resume prepregnancy exercise routines gradually. Many of the changes of pregnancy persist for 4–6 weeks after delivery.

- If you experience any unusual symptoms, stop exercising and consult your physician. Warning signs include pain, vaginal bleeding, dizziness, rapid heartbeat, shortness of breath, and uterine contractions.

Kegel exercises, to strengthen the pelvic floor muscles, are also recommended for pregnant women. These exercises are performed by alternately contracting and releasing the muscles used to stop the flow of urine. Each contraction should be held for about 5 seconds. Kegel exercises should be done several times a day, for a total of about 50 repetitions daily.

Prenatal exercise classes are valuable because they teach exercises that tone the body muscles involved in birth, especially those of the abdomen, back, and legs. Toned-up muscles aid delivery and help the body regain its nonpregnant shape afterward.

Preparing for Birth   Childbirth classes are almost a routine part of the prenatal experience for both mothers and fathers these days. These classes typically teach the details of the birth process as well as relaxation techniques to help deal with the discomfort of labor and delivery. The mother learns and practices a variety of techniques so she will be able to choose what works best for her during labor, when the time comes. The father typically acts as a coach, supporting his partner emotionally and helping her with her breathing and relaxing. He remains with her throughout labor and delivery, even when a cesarean section is performed. It can be an important and fulfilling time for the parents to be together.

Complications of Pregnancy and Pregnancy Loss

Pregnancy usually proceeds without major complications. Sometimes, however, complications may prevent full-term development of the fetus or affect the health of the infant at birth. As discussed earlier in the chapter, exposure to harmful substances, such as alcohol or drugs, can harm the fetus. Other complications are caused by physiological problems or genetic abnormalities.

Ectopic Pregnancy   In an **ectopic pregnancy,** the fertilized egg implants and begins to develop outside of the uterus, usually in an oviduct. Ectopic pregnancies usually occur because the fallopian tube is blocked, most often as a result of pelvic inflammatory disease. The embryo may spontaneously abort, or the embryo and placenta may continue to expand until they rupture the oviduct. Sharp pain on one side of the abdomen or in the lower back, usually in about the 7th or 8th week, may signal an ectopic pregnancy, and there may be irregular bleeding. If bleeding from a rupture is severe, the woman may go into shock, characterized by low blood pressure, a fast pulse, weakness, and fainting. Surgical removal of the embryo and the oviduct may be necessary to save the mother's life, although microsurgery can sometimes be used to repair the damaged oviduct. The incidence of ectopic pregnancy has more than quadrupled in the past 25 years, and it is the leading cause of pregnancy-related death in the United States.

Spontaneous Abortion   A **spontaneous abortion,** or **miscarriage,** is the termination of pregnancy before the 20th week. It is estimated that 10–40% of pregnancies end this way, some without the woman's awareness that she was even pregnant. Most miscarriages occur between the 6th and 8th weeks of pregnancy, and most—about 60%—are due to chromosomal abnormalities in the fetus. Certain occupations that involve exposure to chemicals may increase the likelihood of a spontaneous abortion. Vaginal bleeding (spotting) is usually the first sign that a pregnant woman may miscarry. She may also develop pelvic cramps, and her symptoms of pregnancy may disappear. One miscarriage doesn't mean that later pregnancies will be unsuccessful, and about 70–90% of women who miscarry eventually become pregnant again. About 1% of women suffer three or more miscarriages, possibly because of anatomical, hormonal, genetic, or immunological factors.

Preeclampsia   A disease unique to human pregnancy, **preeclampsia** is characterized by high blood pressure, leaking of protein into urine, and edema (fluid retention), which typically causes swelling of the hands and face.

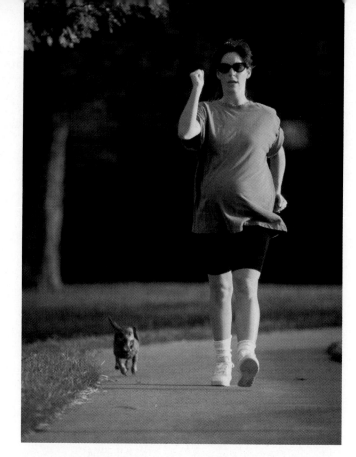

A woman's body changes drastically during pregnancy to accommodate and nourish the growing fetus. Prenatal exercise helps this woman stay healthy while her body works to sustain two lives.

Symptoms may include sudden weight gain, severe headache, abdominal pain, blurred vision, and swelling. If preeclampsia is not treated, it can cause seizures, a condition called **eclampsia.** Other potential problems from preeclampsia include liver and kidney damage, internal bleeding, poor fetal growth, and fetal death. Changes in blood pressure and the presence of excess protein in the urine are usually noticed and tracked during routine prenatal examinations.

The exact cause of preeclampsia is not known; however, the incidence is higher among first-time mothers, very young or very old mothers, women carrying multiple fetuses, or women with a history of this or other hypertensive diseases. Both men and women who were the product of a pregnancy complicated by preeclampsia are significantly more likely to have a pregnancy affected by preeclampsia, suggesting a genetic factor that is passed along to the fetus. Women with mild preeclampsia may be monitored and advised to rest in bed at home. Because more severe cases can be life-threatening for the woman and her fetus, patients may be hospitalized for close monitoring and treatment to prevent seizures. The only cure for preeclampsia is delivery.

Low Birth Weight   A **low-birth-weight (LBW)** baby is one that weighs less than 5.5 pounds at birth.

LBW babies may be premature (born before the 37th week of pregnancy) or full-term. Babies who are born small even though they're full-term are referred to as small-for-date babies. Most LBW babies will grow normally, but some will experience problems. Although they are at greater risk than bigger babies for complications during infancy, small-for-date babies tend to have fewer problems than premature infants. The most fundamental problem of prematurity is that many of the infant's organs are not sufficiently developed. Even mild prematurity increases an infant's risk of dying in the first month or year of life. Premature infants are subject to respiratory problems and infections. They may have difficulty eating because they may be too small to suck a breast or bottle, and their swallowing mechanism may be underdeveloped. As they get older, premature infants may have problems such as learning difficulties, poor hearing and vision, and physical awkwardness.

Low birth weight affects about 7.6% of infants born each year in the United States. About half of all cases of LBW are related to teenage pregnancy, cigarette smoking, poor nutrition, and poor health of the mother. One study found a sixfold increase in the risk of LBW if the mother had financial problems during the pregnancy. Adequate prenatal care is the best means of preventing LBW.

Infant Mortality   The U.S. rate of infant mortality, the death of a child of less than 1 year of age, is at its lowest point ever; however, it remains far higher than that of most of the developed world. The United States ranks twenty-sixth among the world's developed countries for low infant mortality, with 7.2 deaths for every 1000 live births in 1998. Poverty and inadequate health care are key causes; in some inner-city areas, the infant mortality rate approaches that of developing countries, with more than 20 deaths per 1000 births.

Other causes of infant death are congenital problems, infectious diseases, and injuries. In the United States, about 2800 infant deaths per year are due to **sudden infant death syndrome (SIDS)**, in which an apparently healthy infant dies suddenly while sleeping. The number of SIDS deaths has decreased since 1992, when the "Back to Sleep" campaign was instituted to make people aware that putting babies to bed on their backs rather than on their stomachs significantly reduces the risk of SIDS. Other risk factors for SIDS include abnormalities in heart rhythm or in brain receptors controlling breathing; exposing a fetus or infant to tobacco smoke, alcohol, or other drugs; and putting a baby to bed on a soft mattress or with fluffy bedding, pillows, or stuffed toys. Overbundling a baby or keeping a baby's room too warm also increases the risk of SIDS; because of this, the incidence of SIDS tends to rise in the colder months.

Coping with Loss   Parents form a deep attachment to their children even before birth, and those who lose an infant before or during birth usually experience deep grief. Initial feelings of shocked disbelief and numbness may give way to sadness, anger, crying spells, and preoccupation with the loss. Physical sensations such as tightness in the chest or stomach, loss of appetite, and sleeplessness may also occur. For the mother, physical exhaustion and hormone imbalances can compound the emotional and physical stress.

Experiencing the pain of loss is part of the healing process, which can take up to a year or more. Keeping active with work or travel can help renew interest in life. A support group or professional counseling is also often helpful. Planning the next pregnancy, with a physician's input, can be an important step toward recovery, as long as the mind and body are given time to heal. If future pregnancies are ruled out, couples can consider other options, such as adoption.

CHILDBIRTH

By the end of the ninth month of pregnancy, most women are tired of being pregnant; both parents are eager to start a new phase of their lives. Most couples find the actual process of birth to be an exciting and positive experience.

Choices in Childbirth

Many couples today can choose the type of practitioner and the environment they want for the birth of their child. A high-risk pregnancy is probably best handled by a specialist physician in a hospital with a nursery, but for low-risk births, many options are available.

Parents can choose to have their baby delivered by a physician (an obstetrician or family practitioner) or by a certified nurse-midwife. Certified nurse-midwives are registered nurses with special training in obstetrical techniques. They are usually much less expensive than physicians, and they are often part of a complete medical

ectopic pregnancy A pregnancy in which the embryo develops outside the uterus, usually in the fallopian tube.

spontaneous abortion (miscarriage) Termination of pregnancy at less than 20 weeks' gestation when the uterine contents are expelled; causes include an abnormal uterus, insufficient hormones, and genetic or physical fetal defects.

preeclampsia A condition of pregnancy characterized by high blood pressure, edema, and protein in the urine.

eclampsia A severe, potentially life-threatening form of preeclampsia, characterized by convulsions and coma.

low birth weight (LBW) Weighing less than 5.5 lb at birth, often the result of prematurity.

sudden infant death syndrome (SIDS) The sudden death of an apparently healthy infant during sleep.

Terms

A variety of birth situations can have positive physical and psychological outcomes. Parents should choose what is appropriate for their medical circumstances and what feels most comfortable to them. Prospective parents should discuss their preferences in the following areas with their physician or midwife:

1. Who will be present at the birth? The father? Friends? Children and other relatives? Will young siblings be allowed to visit the mother and new baby?

2. What type of room will the mother be in during labor, delivery, and recovery? How many times will she be moved?

3. What type of tables, beds, or birthing chairs are available? What type of environment can be created for the birth? Can specific music be played?

4. Will the mother receive any routine preparation, such as an enema, intravenous feeding, or shaving of the pubic area?

5. What is the policy regarding food and drink during labor? Will the mother have the option of walking around or taking a shower or bath during labor?

6. Under what circumstances does the physician or midwife administer drugs to induce or augment labor? The use of these drugs tends to change the course of labor and carries a small risk.

7. Is **electronic fetal monitoring (EFM)** typically used during labor? About 75% of all births are electronically monitored, but there is disagreement among medical authorities about the risks or benefits of EFM. The American College of Obstetricians and Gynecologists recommends periodic monitoring using a stethoscope rather than EFM for low-risk pregnancies.

8. Under what circumstances will an **episiotomy,** an incision at the base of the vaginal opening, be performed? Are any steps taken to avoid it?

9. Under what circumstances will forceps or vacuum extraction be used? In some cases of fetal distress, the use of forceps or vacuum extraction may be necessary to save the infant's life, but some authorities believe these techniques are overused.

10. What types of medications are typically used during labor and delivery? Some form of anesthetic is usually administered during most hospital deliveries, as are hormones that intensify the contractions and shrink the uterus after delivery. Different types of anesthetics, including short-acting narcotics, regional nerve blocks, and local anesthetics, may be available; each has different effects on the mother and the fetus.

11. Under what conditions or circumstances does the physician perform a cesarean section? If prospective parents are concerned, they should research the cesarean frequency rates of different physicians before they make their final choice.

12. Who will "catch" the baby as she or he is born? Who will cut the umbilical cord?

13. What will be done to the baby immediately after birth? What kinds of tests and procedures will be done on the baby, and when?

14. How often will the baby be brought to the mother while they remain in the hospital or birthing center? Can the baby stay in the mother's room rather than in the nursery? This practice is known as **rooming-in**.

15. How will the baby be fed—by breast or bottle? Will feeding be on a schedule or "on demand"? Is there someone with breastfeeding experience available to answer questions if necessary?

---

team that includes a backup physician in case of emergency. Nurse-midwives can usually participate in births in any setting, although this may vary according to hospital policy, state law, and the midwife's preferences. About 1 in 20 babies each year is delivered by a nurse-midwife.

Most babies in the United States are delivered in hospitals or in freestanding alternative birth centers; only about 2% of women choose to have their babies at home. Many hospitals have introduced alternative birth centers in response to criticisms of traditional hospital routines. Alternative birth centers provide a comfortable, emotionally supportive environment in close proximity to up-to-date medical equipment.

The impersonal, routine quality of hospital birth is increasingly being challenged, and many hospitals and physicians offer a variety of options to parents regarding many aspects of childbirth. It's important for prospective parents to discuss all aspects of labor and delivery with their physician or midwife beforehand, so they can learn what to expect and can state their preferences. For more information, see the box "Making a Birth Plan."

Labor and Delivery

The birth process occurs in three stages (Figure 8-6). **Labor** begins when hormonal changes in both the mother and the baby cause strong, rhythmic uterine **contractions** to begin. These contractions exert pressure on the cervix and cause the lengthwise muscles of the uterus to pull on the circular muscles around the cervix, causing effacement (thinning) and dilation (opening) of the

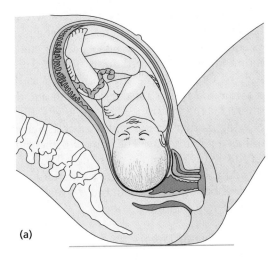

(a)

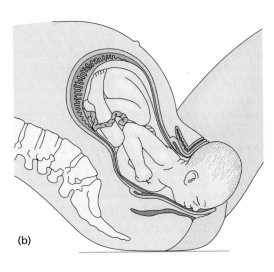

(b)

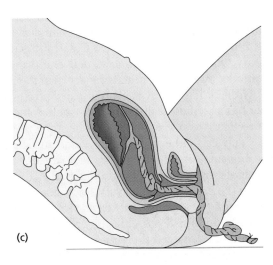

(c)

Figure 8-6   Birth: labor and delivery.   (a) The first stage of labor; (b) the second stage of labor: delivery of the baby; (c) the third stage of labor: expulsion of the placenta.

cervix. The contractions also pressure the baby to descend into the mother's pelvis, if it hasn't already. The entire process of labor and delivery usually takes between 2 and 36 hours, depending on the size of the baby, the baby's position in the uterus, the size of the mother's pelvis, and other factors. The length of labor is generally shorter for second and subsequent births.

The First Stage of Labor   The first stage of labor averages 13 hours for a first birth, although there is a wide variation among women. It begins with cervical effacement and dilation and continues until the cervix is completely dilated (10 centimeters). Contractions usually last about 30 seconds and occur every 15–20 minutes at first, more often later. The prepared mother relaxes as much as possible during these contractions to allow labor to proceed without being blocked by tension. Early in the first stage, a small amount of bleeding may occur as a plug of slightly bloody mucus that blocked the opening of the cervix during pregnancy is expelled. In some women, the amniotic sac ruptures and the fluid rushes out; this is sometimes referred to as the "water breaking."

The last part of the first stage of labor, called **transition,** is characterized by strong and frequent contractions, much more intense than in the early stages of labor. Contractions may last 60–90 seconds and occur every 1–3 minutes. During transition the cervix opens completely, to a diameter of about 10 centimeters. Since the head of the fetus usually measures 9–10 centimeters, once the cervix has dilated completely, the head can pass through. Many women report that transition, which normally lasts about 30 minutes to an hour, is the most difficult part of labor.

The Second Stage of Labor   The second stage of labor begins with complete cervical dilation and ends with the delivery of the baby. The baby is slowly pushed down, through the bones of the pelvic ring, past the cervix, and

Terms

electronic fetal monitoring (EFM) The use of an external or internal electronic monitor during labor to measure uterine contractions and fetal heart rate.

episiotomy An incision made to widen the vaginal opening to facilitate childbirth and prevent uncontrolled tearing during delivery.

rooming-in The practice of allowing the mother and baby to remain together in the hospital or birth center after delivery.

labor The act or process of giving birth to a child, expelling it with the placenta from the mother's body by means of uterine contractions.

contraction Shortening of the muscles in the uterine wall, which causes effacement and dilation of the cervix and assists in expelling the fetus.

transition The last part of the first stage of labor, during which the cervix becomes fully dilated; characterized by intense and frequent contractions.

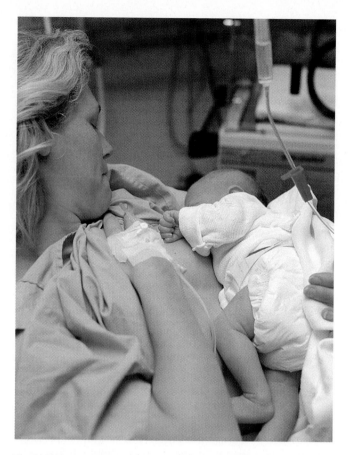

The bond between a mother and her child begins immediately after birth. After having her physical condition checked, this newborn is returned to her mother and begins to breastfeed for the first time.

into the vagina, which it stretches open. The mother bears down with the contractions to help push the baby down and out. Some women find this the most difficult part of labor, while others find that the contractions and bearing down bring a sense of euphoria. The baby's back bends, the head turns to fit through the narrowest parts of the passageway, and the soft bones of the baby's skull move together and overlap as it is squeezed through the pelvis. When the top of the head appears at the vaginal opening, the baby is said to be crowning.

As the head of the baby emerges, the physician or midwife will remove any mucus from the mouth and nose, wipe the baby's face, and check to ensure that the umbil-

ical cord is not around the neck. With a few more contractions, the baby's shoulders and body emerge. As the baby is squeezed through the pelvis, cervix, and vagina, the fluid in the lungs is forced out by the pressure on the baby's chest. Once this pressure is released as the baby emerges from the vagina, the chest expands and the lungs fill with air for the first time. The baby will still be connected to the mother via the umbilical cord, which is not cut until it stops pulsating. The baby will appear wet and often is covered with a milky substance. The baby's head may be oddly shaped at first, due to the molding of the soft plates of bone during birth, but it usually takes on a normal appearance within 24 hours.

The Third Stage of Labor In the third stage of labor, the uterus continues to contract until the placenta is expelled. This stage usually takes 5–20 minutes. If the placenta does not come out on its own, the physician or midwife may exert gentle pressure on the abdomen to help with its delivery. It is important that the entire placenta be expelled; if part remains in the uterus, it may cause infection or bleeding. Breastfeeding soon after delivery helps control uterine bleeding because it stimulates the secretion of a hormone that makes the uterus contract; massaging the abdomen may also help.

In the meantime, the physical condition of the baby will be assessed with the **Apgar score**, a formalized system for assessing the baby's need for medical assistance during the first few minutes of life. Heart rate, respiration, color, reflexes, and muscle tone are individually rated with a score of 0–2, and a total score between 0 and 10 is given at 1 and 5 minutes after birth. A score of 7–10 at 5 minutes is considered normal. The baby is then usually wrapped tightly in a blanket and returned to the mother, who may begin to nurse the baby right away.

Cesarean Deliveries About 22% of the babies born in the United States are delivered by **cesarean section**, in which the baby is removed through a surgical incision in the abdominal wall and uterus. Cesarean sections are necessary when a baby cannot be delivered vaginally—for example, if the baby's head is bigger than the mother's pelvic girdle or if the baby is in an unusual position. If the mother has a serious health condition such as high blood pressure, a cesarean may be safer for her than labor and a vaginal delivery. Other reasons for cesarean delivery include abnormal or difficult labor, fetal distress, and the presence of a dangerous infection like herpes that can be passed to the baby during delivery. Repeat cesarean deliveries are also very common; about 75% of American women who have had one child by cesarean have subsequent children delivered the same way.

A cesarean section is major surgery and carries some risk, but it is relatively safe. A regional anesthetic may be used so the woman can remain conscious during the operation, and the father may be present.

Some people believe cesareans are often performed unnecessarily in the United States. Other countries that have rates of maternal and infant death as low as those in the United States have much lower rates of cesarean section, particularly repeat cesareans. The *Healthy People 2010* report sets a goal for reducing the rate of cesarean delivery to no more than 15% for women giving birth for the first time and 63% of women with a prior cesarean birth. Several strategies have been suggested to help lower this rate: addressing physician malpractice concerns; eliminating the financial incentives for cesareans, which are currently more lucrative than vaginal deliveries; publishing cesarean rates of individual physicians and hospitals; and increasing training in normal vaginal deliveries.

The Postpartum Period

The **postpartum period,** a stage of about 3 months following childbirth, is a time of critical family adjustments. Parenthood—a job that goes on around the clock without relief—begins literally overnight, and the transition can cause considerable physical and emotional stress.

Following a vaginal delivery, mothers usually leave the hospital within 1–3 days (after a cesarean section, they usually stay 3–5 days). Uterine contractions will occur from time to time for several days after delivery, as the uterus begins to return to its prebirth size. It usually takes 6–8 weeks for a woman's reproductive organs to return to their prebirth condition. She will have a bloody discharge called *lochia* for several weeks after the birth.

Currently, just over 60% of mothers breastfeed their infants, up from about 10% in 1970. **Lactation,** the production of milk, begins about 3 days after childbirth. Prior to that time (sometimes as early as the second trimester), colostrum is secreted by the nipples. Colostrum contains antibodies that help protect the newborn from infectious diseases and is also high in protein.

The American Academy of Pediatricians recommends breastfeeding for at least the first year of a baby's life and for as long after that as a mother and baby desire. Human milk is perfectly suited to the baby's nutritional needs and digestive capabilities, and it supplies the baby with antibodies. Breastfeeding decreases the incidence of infant ear infections, allergies, anemia, diarrhea, and bacterial meningitis. One study has even suggested that children who are breastfed do better in school and score higher on standardized tests. Breastfeeding is also beneficial to the mother: It stimulates contractions that help the uterus return to normal more rapidly, contributes to postpregnancy weight loss, and may reduce the risk of ovarian cancer, breast cancer, and postmenopausal hip fracture. Nursing also provides a sense of closeness and emotional well-being for mother and child. For women who want to breastfeed but who have problems, help is available from support groups, books, or a lactation consultant.

For some women, physical problems such as tenderness or infection of the nipples can make breastfeeding difficult. If a woman has an illness or requires drug treatment, she may have to bottlefeed her baby because drugs and infectious agents may show up in breast milk. Breastfeeding can be restrictive, making it especially difficult for working mothers. Employers rarely provide nursing breaks, so bottlefeeding or the use of a breast pump (to express milk for use while the mother is away from her infant) may be the only practical alternatives. Bottlefeeding makes it easier to tell how much milk an infant is taking in, and bottlefed infants tend to sleep longer. Bottlefeeding also allows the father or other caregiver to share in the nurturing process. Both breastfeeding and bottlefeeding can be part of loving, secure parent-child relationships.

When a mother doesn't nurse, menstruation usually begins within about 10 weeks. Breastfeeding can prevent the return of menstruation for as long as 6 months because the hormone prolactin, which aids milk production, suppresses hormones vital to the development of mature eggs. However, ovulation—and pregnancy—can occur before menstruation returns, so breastfeeding is not a highly reliable contraceptive method; if a woman wishes to avoid pregnancy, she should use a more reliable method. If the mother becomes pregnant while still nursing, she needs to make sure that she is receiving adequate nutrition, since the energy requirement for both breastfeeding and gestating is immense. With proper counseling, breastfeeding can continue until near delivery.

Many women experience fluctuating emotions during the postpartum period as hormone levels change. The physical stress of labor, as well as dehydration, blood loss, and other physical factors, contributes to lowering the woman's stamina. About 50–80% of new mothers experience "baby blues," characterized by episodes of sadness, weeping, anxiety, headache, sleep disturbances, and irritability. A mother may feel lonely and anxious about caring for her infant. About 10% of new mothers experience **postpartum depression,** a more disabling syndrome characterized by despondency, mood swings, guilt, and occasional hostility. Rest, sharing feelings and concerns with others, and relying on supportive relatives and friends for assistance are usually helpful in dealing with mild cases of the baby blues or postpartum depression, which generally lasts only a few weeks. If the depression is serious, professional treatment may be needed. Some men also seem to get a form of postpartum depression, characterized by anxiety about their changing roles and feelings of inadequacy. Both mothers and fathers need time to adjust to their new roles as parents.

Another feature of the postpartum period is the development of attachment—the strong emotional tie that grows between the baby and the adult who cares for the baby. Parents can foster secure attachment relationships in the early weeks and months by responding sensitively to the baby's true needs. Parents who respond appropriately to the baby's signals of gazing, looking away, smiling, and crying establish feelings of trust in their child. They feed the baby when she's hungry, for example; respond when she cries; interact with her when she gazes, smiles, or babbles; and stop stimulating her when she frowns or looks away. A secure attachment relationship helps the child develop and function well socially, emotionally, and mentally.

For most people, the arrival of a child provides a deep sense of joy and accomplishment. However, adjusting to parenthood requires effort and energy. Talking with friends and relatives about their experiences during the first few weeks or months with a baby can help prepare new parents for the period when the baby's needs may require all the energy that both parents have to expend. But the pleasures of nurturing a new baby are substantial, and many parents look back on this time as one of the most significant and joyful of their lives.

COMMUNICATE! The transition to parenthood occurs overnight and creates tremendous physical and emotional stress for the parents, no matter how many books they read or how well prepared they are. During the period of adjustment, many couples who were quite egalitarian before the birth find themselves falling into more conventional gender roles. The woman may take a larger role in "mothering" the baby—feeding, diapering, soothing, nurturing—and the man may start thinking of himself more as "the provider." Rather than becoming entrenched in these roles, partners can discuss their wants and needs with each other and negotiate differences. By remaining aware of their actions and by communicating with each other, partners can make conscious decisions about how much they will share the child-rearing roles in their new family.

Tips for Today

Having a child is one of life's most important events. It transforms people as individuals, as partners in a relationship, and as members of a family. Preparation for being a parent begins long before pregnancy; it includes healthy lifestyle choices in all the areas of wellness.

Right now you can

- Take some time to think about whether *you* want to have children; try to cut through the cultural, societal, family, and personal expectations that may stand in the way of your making the decision you really want to make.

- Think of one thing your mother or father did as a parent that you particularly disliked; if you become a parent, how can you keep from repeating that behavior with your own children?

- Think of one thing your mother or father did as a parent that you particularly liked; if you become a parent, how

can you make sure you do the same thing with your own children?

- If you are sexually active, consider your sexual behavior and your contraceptive choice (or lack of one). Are you taking any chances that would jeopardize your future fertility or reproductive options? If so, resolve to change that behavior.

- If you smoke, start thinking about how to quit.

- If you are sedentary, start thinking about a form of moderate exercise that you can continue throughout your life, such as swimming or walking. Make a plan to begin the activity today or tomorrow.

SUMMARY

- Factors to consider when deciding if and when to have a child include physical health and age; financial circumstances; relationship with your partner; educational, career, and child care plans; emotional readiness for parenthood; social support system; personal qualities, attitudes toward children, and aptitude for parenting; and philosophical or religious beliefs.

- Preconception care examines factors such as preexisting medical conditions, current medications, past history of pregnancy, age of the mother, lifestyle behaviors, infections, nutritional status, and family history of genetic disease.

- Fertilization is a complex process culminating when a sperm penetrates the membrane of the egg released from the woman's ovary.

- Infertility affects about 10% of the reproductive-age population of the United States. The leading causes of infertility in women are blocked oviducts and ovulation disorders. Exposure to toxic substances, the use of certain drugs, injury to the testicles, and infection can all cause infertility in men.

- One way to avoid some forms of infertility is to protect oneself against STDs and to get treatment for any disease contracted.

- Early signs and symptoms of pregnancy include a missed menstrual period; slight bleeding; nausea; breast tenderness; sleepiness, fatigue, and emotional upset; and a softening of the uterus just above the cervix.

- During pregnancy, the uterus enlarges until it pushes up into the rib cage; the breasts enlarge and may secrete colostrum; the muscles and ligaments soften and stretch; and the circulatory system, lungs, and kidneys become more efficient.

- The fetal anatomy is almost completely formed in the first trimester and is refined in the second; during the third trimester, the fetus grows and gains most of its weight, storing nutrients in fatty tissues.

- Information about the health and sex of a fetus can be obtained through prenatal tests such as ultrasound, amniocentesis, chorionic villus sampling, and triple marker screening.

- Health care during pregnancy includes a complete history and physical at the beginning, followed by regular checkups for blood pressure, weight gain, and size and position of the fetus. Blood tests reveal blood type, anemia, STDs, and Rh incompatibilities.

- Important elements of prenatal care include good nutrition; avoiding drugs, alcohol, tobacco, infections, and other harmful environmental agents or conditions; regular physical activity; and childbirth classes.

- Pregnancy usually proceeds without major complications. Problems that can occur include ectopic pregnancy, spontaneous abortion, preeclampsia, and low birth weight. The loss of a fetus or infant is deeply felt by most parents, who need time to experience their grief and to heal.

- Couples preparing for childbirth may have many options to choose from, including type of practitioner and facility.

- The first stage of labor begins with contractions that exert pressure on the cervix, causing effacement and dilation. The second stage begins with complete cervical dilation and ends when the baby emerges. The third stage of labor is expulsion of the placenta.

- During the postpartum period, the mother's body begins to return to its prepregnancy state, and she may begin to breastfeed. Both mother and father must adjust to their new roles as parents, as they develop a strong emotional tie to their baby.

TAKE ACTION

1. Interview your parents to find out what your birth was like. What were the cultural conditions like at the time, and what were their personal preferences? Find out as much as you can about hospital procedure, the use of anesthetics, length of hospital stay, and so on. Did your father have a role in your birth? If possible, interview your grandparents or someone of their generation. How was their experience different from that of your parents'?

2. Investigate the childbirth facilities in your community. If possible, visit the maternity wing of a hospital and an alternative birth center. What do you like about them, and what do you not like? What types of childbirth preparation classes do they offer? Which of these do you feel most comfortable with? Why?

JOURNAL ENTRY

1. Would you take advantage of a prenatal diagnostic tool like amniocentesis to find out ahead of time if your child had a genetic abnormality? If such an abnormality was discovered, would you choose to terminate the pregnancy? Write an essay describing what you would do and why. What criteria would you use to make your decision?

2. Do you think you are ready to become a parent? Make a list of the qualities you possess that you think would make you a good parent. Then list those qualities that might be a hindrance to good parenting. Do you think your partner (if you have one) is ready to become a parent? Create the same type of lists based on his or her personal qualities.

3. *Critical Thinking* There have been many legal cases involving the status of sperm or embryos frozen as part of an infertility treatment such as artificial insemination or in vitro fertilization. Research one or more of these cases, and write an essay outlining some of the moral and legal implications of this technology. What guidelines would you suggest for regulating the use and status of frozen sperm and embryos? What evidence can you give to support your position?

Books

Andrews, L. B. 2000. *The Clone Age: Adventures in the New World of Reproductive Technology.* New York: Henry Holt. *Examines the medical, legal, and ethical implications of recent advances in reproductive technology.*

Appelbaum, A., and S. Ilse. 2000. *Empty Arms: Coping After Miscarriage, Stillbirth, and Infant Death,* rev. ed. Maple Plain, Minn.: Wintergreen Press. *A sensitive guide to the experience of pregnancy loss.*

Brothers, B. J., ed. 2000. *Couples and Pregnancy: Welcome, Unwelcome, and In-Between.* Binghamton, N.Y.: Haworth. *Looks at the psychological effects of pregnancy and birth on a couple's relationship.*

Glazer, E. S., and S. L. Cooper. 1999. *Choosing Assisted Reproduction: Social, Emotional, and Ethical Considerations.* Indianapolis: Perspectives Press. *Support, information, and advice for couples considering assisted reproduction.*

Massimini, K. 2000. *Genetic Disorders Sourcebook: Basic Consumer Health Information About Hereditary Diseases and Disorders,* 2nd ed. Detroit: Omnigraphics. *Provides up-to-date information on the workings of genes, the ethics of genetic testing, and the causes and treatments of common genetic disorders.*

Nathanielsz, P. W. 1999. *Life in the Womb: The Origin of Health and Disease.* Ithaca, N.Y.: Promethean Press. *Provides information about how gestational conditions may affect health later in life.*

Nilsson, L., and L. Hamberger. 1993. *A Child Is Born.* New York: DPT/Seymour Lawrence. *The story of birth, beginning with fertilization, told in text and with stunning photographs.*

The following are a few of the many excellent guides to conception, pregnancy, and birth:

American College of Obstetricians and Gynecologists. 2000. *Planning Your Pregnancy and Birth,* 3rd ed. Washington, D.C.: ACOG.

Fairview Health Services. 2000. *Caring for You and Your Baby: From Pregnancy Through the First Year of Life.* Minneapolis: Fairview Press.

Heinowitz, J. 2000. *Fathering Right from the Start: Straight Talk About Pregnancy, Birth, and Beyond.* San Diego: Parents as Partners Press.

Lieberman, A. B., and L. H. Holt. 2000. *Nine Months and a Day: A Pregnancy, Labor, and Delivery Companion.* Boston: Harvard Common Press.

Stoppard, M. 2000. *Conception, Pregnancy, and Birth.* New York: DK.

WW. Organizations and Web Sites

American Academy of Family Physician: Provides information about many aspects of pregnancy and childbirth.
  http://familydoctor.org

American College of Obstetricians and Gynecologists (ACOG). Provides written materials relating to many aspects of preconception care, pregnancy, and childbirth.
  202-863-2518
  http://www.acog.org

The American Society for Reproductive Medicine. Provides up-to-date information on all aspects of infertility.
  205-978-5000
  http://www.asrm.org

Centers for Disease Control and Prevention, Division of Birth Defects, Child Development, and Disability and Health. Provides information about a variety of topics related to birth defects, including fetal alcohol syndrome and the importance of folic acid.
  http://www.cdc.gov/nceh/cddh

Childbirth.Org. Contains medical information and personal stories about all phases of pregnancy and birth.
  http://www.childbirth.org

Generational Health. Helps you create a family health tree online and provides information about detection and screening for any conditions that are common in your family history.
  http://healthygenerations.com

International Council on Infertility Information Dissemination. A Web site that includes information on current research and treatments for infertility.
  http://www.inciid.org

La Leche League International. Provides advice and support for breastfeeding mothers.
  800-LaLeche
  http://www.lalecheleague.org

The March of Dimes. Provides public education materials on many pregnancy-related topics, including preconception care, genetic screening, diet and exercise, and the effects of smoking and drinking during pregnancy.
  888-MODIMES; 914-428-7100
  http://www.modimes.org

National Institute of Child Health and Human Development. Provides information about reproductive and genetic problems; sponsors the "Back to Sleep" campaign to fight SIDS.
  800-505-CRIB (Back to Sleep hotline)
  http://www.nichd.nih.gov

National Maternal and Child Health Clearinghouse. Distributes publications, posters, and videos relating to maternal, infant, and family health; most items are available free-of-charge.
  888-434-4MCH; 703-356-1964
  http://www.nmchc.org

ParentsPlace.com Pregnancy Department. Includes a pregnancy calendar, a due date calculator, and lots of advice on preparing a birth plan and other pregnancy topics.
  http://www.parentsplace.com/pregnancy

Resolve. Provides information, support, and referrals for people facing infertility.
  617-623-0744 (National Helpline)
  http://www.resolve.org

SHARE. Provides information, support, and referrals to parents who have experienced miscarriage, stillbirth, or infant death.
  800-821-6819

The following sites include information, graphics, and video clips of fetal development:

Nova/Odyssey of Life
  http://www.pbs.org/wgbh/nova/odyssey/clips

University of Pennsylvania Basic Embryology Review
  http://www.med.upenn.edu/meded/public/berp

Visible Embryo
  http://visembryo.com

SELECTED BIBLIOGRAPHY

Acacio, B. D., et al. 2000. Evaluation of a large cohort of men presenting for a screening semen analysis. *Fertility and Sterility* 73(3): 595–597.

American Academy of Pediatrics Task Force on Infant Sleep Position and Sudden Infant Death Syndrome. 2000. Changing concepts of sudden infant death syndrome: Implications for infant sleeping environment and sleep position. *Pediatrics* 105(3 Pt 1): 650–656.

American College of Obstetricians and Gynecologists. 1998. *Exercise During Pregnancy*. Washington, D.C.: ACOG.

American College of Obstetricians and Gynecologists. 2000. *HIV Tests Urged for All Pregnant Women* (http://www.acog.org/from_home/publications/press_releases/nr05-23-00-2.htm; retrieved September 27, 2000).

Baeten, J. M., E. A. Bukusi, and M. Lambe. 2001. Pregnancy complications and outcomes among overweight and obese nulliparous women. *American Journal of Public Health* 91(3): 436–440.

Barton, J. C., and R. T. Acton. 2000. Population screening for hemochromatosis: Has the time finally come? *Current Gastroenterology Reports* 2(1): 18–26.

Breastfeeding. 2001. *Journal of the American Medical Association* 285(4): 490.

Campbell, M. K., and M. F. Mottola. 2001. Recreational exercise and occupational activity during pregnancy and birth weight: A case-control study. *American Journal of Obstetrics and Gynecology* 184(3): 403–408.

Carmichael, S. L., and G. M. Shaw. 2000. Maternal life event stress and congenital anomalies. *Epidemiology* 11(1): 30–35.

Centers for Disease Control and Prevention. 2000. Entry into prenatal care—United States, 1989–1997. *Morbidity and Mortality Weekly Report* 49(18): 393–398.

Centers for Disease Control and Prevention, Division of Birth Defects and Developmental Disabilities. 2000. *Preventing Neural Tube Birth Defects: A Prevention Model and Resource Guide*. Atlanta: CDC.

Centers for Disease Control and Prevention. 2001. Knowledge and use of folic acid among women of reproductive age. *Morbidity and Mortality Weekly Report* 50(10): 185–189.

Cook, A. J., et al. 2000. Sources of toxoplasma infection in pregnant women. *British Medical Journal* 321(7254): 142–147.

De Celis, R., et al. 2000. Semen quality of workers occupationally exposed to hydrocarbons. *Fertility and Sterility* 73(2): 221–228.

Down syndrome. 2001. *Journal of the American Medical Association* 285(8): 1112.

Esplin, M. S., et al. 2001. Paternal and maternal components of the predisposition to preeclampsia. *New England Journal of Medicine* 344(12): 867–872.

Feeding your newborn. 2000. *Journal of the American Medical Association Patient Page* 283(9).

Feldman, P. J., et al. 2000. Maternal social support predicts birth weight and fetal growth in human pregnancy. *Psychosomatic Medicine* 62(5): 715–725.

Flaxman, S. M., and P. W. Sherman. 2000. Morning sickness: A mechanism for protecting mother and embryo. *Quarterly Review of Biology* 75(2): 113–148.

Food and Drug Administration. 2001. FDA Announces Advisory on Methyl Mercury in Fish (http://fda.gov/bbs/topics/ANSWERS/2001/ANS01065.html; retrieved January 15, 2001).

Godfrey, K. M., and D. J. Barker. 2000. Fetal nutrition and adult disease. *American Journal of Clinical Nutrition.* 71(5 Suppl): 1344S–1352S.

Hansen, D., H. C. Lou, and J. Olsen. 2000. Serious life events and congenital malformations: A national study with complete follow-up. *Lancet* 356: 875–880.

Ikonomidou, C., et al. 2000. Ethanol-induced apoptotic neurodegeneration and fetal alcohol syndrome. *Science* 287(5455): 1056–1060.

Karmer, M. S., et al. 2001. Promotion of Breastfeeding Intervention Trial (PROBIT). *Journal of the American Medical Association* 285(4): 413–320.

Klebanoff, M. A., et al. 1999. Maternal serum paraxanthine, a caffeine metabolite, and the risk of spontaneous abortion. *New England Journal of Medicine* 341(22): 1639–1644.

Kramer, M. S., et al. 2000. The contribution of mild and moderate preterm birth to infant mortality. *Journal of the American Medical Association* 284(7): 843–849.

March of Dimes. 1999. *Food-Borne Risks in Pregnancy* (http://www.modimes.org/HealthLibrary2/FactSheets/Food_Born_Risks.htm; retrieved September 25, 2000).

March of Dimes. 1999. *Stress and Pregnancy* (http://www.modimes.org/HealthLibrary2/FactSheets/Stress_and_Pregnancy.htm; retrieved September 25, 2000).

Mortaz, M., et al. 2001. Birth weight, subsequent growth, and cholesterol metabolism in children 8-12 years old born preterm. *Archives of Disease in Childhood* 84(3): 212–217.

National Center for Health Statistics. 2000. Births: Preliminary data for 1999. *National Vital Statistics Reports* 48(14).

National Center for Health Statistics. 2000. *Health, United States, 2000, with Adolescent Health Chartbook*. Hyattsville, Md.: National Center for Health Statistics.

National Center for Health Statistics. 2000. Infant mortality statistics from the 1998 period linked birth/infant death data set. *National Vital Statistics Reports* 48(12).

Newman, R. B., et al. 2001. Occupational fatigue and preterm premature rupture of membranes. *American Journal of Obstetrics and Gynecology* 184(3): 438–446.

Nielsen, G. L., et al. 2001. Risk of adverse birth outcome and miscarriage in pregnant users of non-steroidal anti-inflammatory drugs. *British Medical Journal* 322: 266–270.

Nybo Andersen, A. M., et al. 2000. Maternal age and fetal loss: Population based register linkage study. *British Medical Journal* 320(7251): 1708–1712.

Pribila, B. A., et al. 2000. Improved lactose digestion and intolerance among African-American adolescent girls fed a dairy-rich diet. *Journal of the American Dietetic Association* 100(5): 524–528.

Roseboom, T. J., et al. 2001. Maternal nutrition during gestation and blood pressure in later life. *Journal of Hypertension* 19(1): 29–34.

Schrag, S. J., et al. 2000. Group B streptococcal disease in the era of intrapartum antibiotic prophylaxis. *New England Journal of Medicine* 342: 15–20.

Seng, J. S., et al. 2001. Posttraumatic stress disorder and pregnancy complications. *Obstetrics and Gynecology* 97(1): 17–22.

U.S. Department of Agriculture, Center for Nutrition Policy and Promotion. 2000. *Expenditures on Children by Families. 1999 Annual Report.* Washington, D.C.: CNPP.

Wahlbeck, K., et al. 2001. Association of schizophrenia with low maternal body mass index, small size at birth, and thinness during childhood. *Archives of General Psychiatry* 58(1): 48–52.

Wisborg, K., et al. 2000. A prospective study of smoking during pregnancy and SIDS. *Archives of Disease in Childhood* 83(3): 203–206.

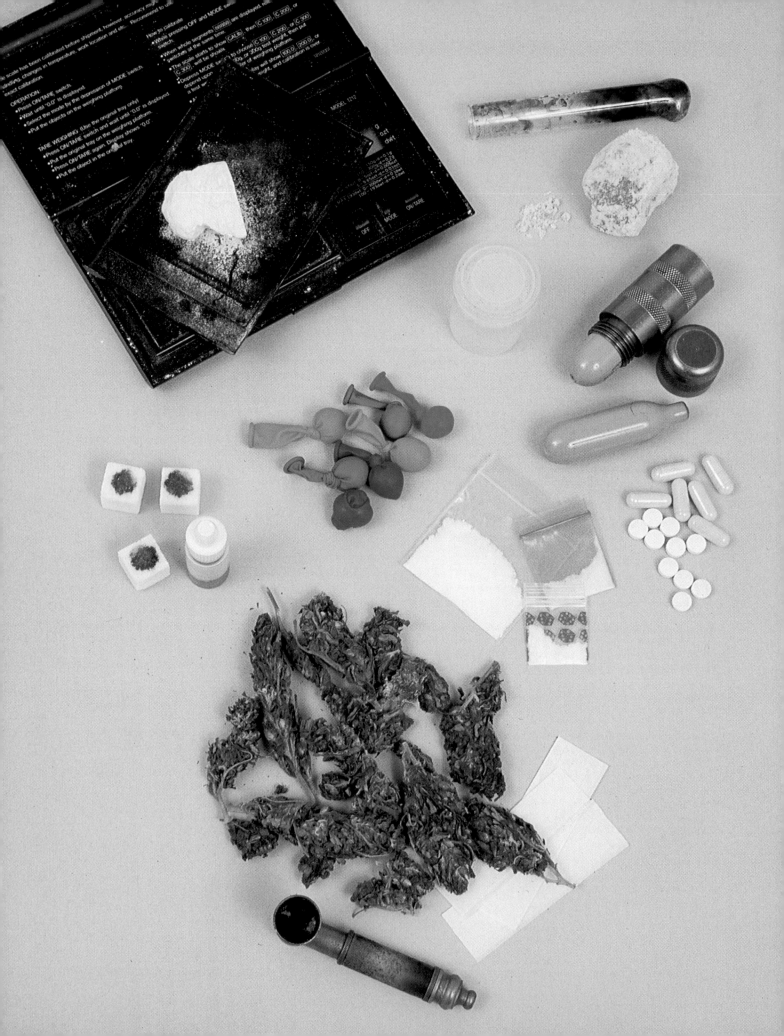

After reading this chapter, you should be able to

- Define and discuss the concepts of addictive behavior, substance abuse, and substance dependence

- Explain factors contributing to drug use and dependence

- List the major categories of psychoactive drugs and describe their effects, methods of use, and potential for abuse and dependence

- Discuss social issues related to psychoactive drug use and its prevention and treatment

- Evaluate the role of drugs and other addictive behaviors in your life and identify your risk factors for abuse or dependence

The Use and Abuse of Psychoactive Drugs

TEST YOUR KNOWLEDGE

1. Which of the following is the most widely used illegal drug among college students?
   a. cocaine
   b. hallucinogens
   c. marijuana
   d. heroin

2. Caffeine use can produce physical dependence.
   True or false?

3. Which of the following drugs is most addictive?
   a. marijuana
   b. nicotine
   c. Valium
   d. LSD

4. About what percentage of street drugs contain the promised primary ingredient?
   a. 50%
   b. 66%
   c. 75%

5. Among illegal drugs, cocaine is responsible for the greatest number of emergency room visits each year.
   True or false?

ANSWERS

1. **C.** Marijuana ranks first, with hallucinogens a distant second. In surveys, the vast majority of college students (80%) report no drug use in the previous month; only about 6% report using any drug other than marijuana.

2. **TRUE.** Regular users of caffeine develop physical tolerance, needing more caffeine to produce the same level of alertness. Many also experience withdrawal symptoms, such as headaches and irritability, when they decrease their intake.

3. **B.** Valium is also addictive, LSD and marijuana less so. Nicotine is believed to be the most highly addictive psychoactive drug.

4. **A.** This figure is even lower for drugs that are difficult to obtain or manufacture. Street drugs may be sold in unsafe dosages and are typically mixed ("cut") with cheaper and often more hazardous substances.

5. **TRUE.** Marijuana/hashish ranks second, followed by heroin. Cocaine is also responsible for the greatest number of drug-related deaths. Using combinations of drugs, including alcohol, is particularly dangerous.

The use of **drugs** for both medical and social purposes is widespread in American society (Table 9-1). Many people believe that every problem, no matter how large or small, has or should have chemical solutions. For fatigue, many of us turn to caffeine; for insomnia, sleeping pills; for anxiety or boredom, alcohol or other recreational drugs. Advertisements, social pressures, and the human desire for quick fixes to life's difficult problems all contribute to the prevailing attitude that drugs can ease all pain. Unfortunately, using drugs can—and often does—have serious consequences.

The most serious consequences are abuse and addiction. The drugs most often associated with abuse are **psychoactive drugs**—those designed to alter a person's experiences or consciousness. In the short term, psychoactive drugs can cause **intoxication,** a state in which sometimes unpredictable physical and emotional changes occur. A person who is intoxicated may experience potentially serious changes in physical functioning; his or her emotions and judgment may be affected in ways that lead to uncharacteristic and unsafe behavior. In the long term, recurrent drug use can have profound physical, emotional, and social effects.

This chapter focuses primarily on psychoactive drugs: their short- and long-term effects and their potential for abuse and addiction. Two of the most widely used psychoactive drugs—alcohol and nicotine—will be treated in detail in Chapters 10 and 11. Before turning to the specific types of psychoactive drugs, let's take a closer look at addictive behavior in general.

VITAL STATISTICS

Table 9-1 Nonmedical Drug Use Among Americans

	Percentage Using Substance in the Past 30 Days	
	College Students	All Americans
Alcohol	63.2	47.3
Tobacco (all forms)[a]	39.6	30.2
Cigarettes	*33.8*	*25.8*
Cigars	*11.4*	*5.5*
Spit tobacco	*5.4*	*3.4*
Pipes	*1.4*	*1.1*
Marijuana/hashish	17.3	5.1
Pain relievers	2.5	1.2
Hallucinogens	2.3	0.4
Cocaine	1.4	0.7
Stimulants	1.2	0.4
Inhalants	1.1	0.5
Tranquilizers	0.9	0.5
Sedatives	0.1	0.1
Heroin	0.0	0.1

[a]Some people use more than one form of tobacco, so the sum of the percentages for different forms of tobacco exceeds the total percentage of tobacco users.

SOURCE: Substance Abuse and Mental Health Services Administration. 2000. *National Household Survey on Drug Abuse, 1999—Appendix G: Detailed National Tables* (http://www.samhsa.gov/oas/NHSDA/1999/Appendixg.htm; retrieved October 4, 2000).

ADDICTIVE BEHAVIOR

Although addiction is most often associated with drug use, many experts now extend the concept of addiction to other areas. **Addictive behaviors** are habits that have gotten out of control, with a resulting negative impact on a person's health. Looking at the nature of addiction and a range of addictive behaviors can help us understand similar behaviors when they involve drugs.

What Is Addiction?

The word *addiction* tends to be a highly charged one for most people. We may jokingly say we're "addicted to" fudge swirl ice cream or our morning jog, but most of us think of true addiction as a habitual and uncontrollable behavior, usually involving the use of a drug. Some people think of addiction as a moral flaw or a personal weakness. Others think addictions arise from certain personality traits, genetic factors, or socioeconomic influences. Views on the causes of addictions have an impact on our attitudes toward people with addictive disorders, as well as on the approaches to treatment.

Historically, the term *addiction* was applied only when the habitual use of a drug produced chemical changes in the user's body. One such change is physical tolerance, in which the body adapts to a drug so that the initial dose no longer produces the original emotional or psychological effects. This process, caused by chemical changes, means the user has to take larger and larger doses of the drug to achieve the same "high." (Tolerance will be discussed in greater detail later in the chapter.) The concept of addiction as a disease process, one based in brain chemistry, rather than a moral failing, has led to many advances in the understanding and treatment of drug addiction.

Some scientists think that other behaviors may share some of the chemistry of drug addiction. They suggest that activities like gambling, eating, exercising, and sex trigger the release of brain chemicals that cause a pleasurable "rush" in much the same way that psychoactive drugs do. The brain's own chemicals thus become the "drug" that can cause addiction. These theorists suggest that drug addiction and addiction to other pleasurable behaviors have a common mechanism in the brain. In this view, addiction is partly the result of our own natural "wiring."

However, and very importantly, the view that addiction is based in our own brain chemistry does *not* imply that an individual bears no responsibility for his or her addictive behavior. Many experts believe that it is inaccurate and counterproductive to think of all bad habits and excessive behaviors as diseases. They point to other factors, especially lifestyle and personality traits, that play key roles in the development of addictive behaviors. Before we consider what those factors are, let's first look in more detail at what constitutes addictive behavior.

Characteristics of Addictive Behavior

It is often difficult to distinguish between a healthy habit and one that has become an addiction. Experts have identified some general characteristics typically associated with addictive behaviors:

- *Reinforcement.* Addictive behaviors are physically and/or psychologically reinforcing. Some aspect of the behavior produces pleasurable physical and/or emotional states or relieves negative ones.

- *Compulsion or craving.* The individual feels a strong compulsion—a compelling need—to engage in the behavior, often accompanied by obsessive planning for the next opportunity to perform it.

- *Loss of control.* The individual loses control over the behavior and cannot block the impulse to engage in it. He or she may deny that the behavior is problematic or may have tried but failed to control it.

- *Escalation.* Addiction often involves a pattern of escalation, in which more and more of a particular substance or activity is required to produce its desired effects. This escalation typically means that a person must give an increasing amount of his or her time, attention, and resources to the behavior.

- *Negative consequences.* The behavior has serious negative consequences, such as problems with academic or job performance, personal relationships, and health; legal or financial troubles are also typical.

The Development of Addiction

There is no single cause of addiction. Instead, characteristics of an individual person, of the environment in which the person lives, and of the substance or behavior he or she abuses combine in an addictive behavior. Although addictive behaviors share many common characteristics, the importance of these different factors varies from one case to another, even when the addiction is to the same substance or behavior.

We all engage in activities that are potentially addictive. Some of these activities can be part of a wellness lifestyle if they are done appropriately and in moderation, but if a behavior starts to be excessive, it may become an addiction. An addiction often starts when a person does something he or she thinks will bring pleasure or help avoid pain. The activity may be drinking a beer, going on the Internet, playing the lottery, or going shopping. If it works, and the behavior does bring pleasure or dull pain, the person is likely to repeat it. He or she becomes in-

creasingly dependent on the behavior, and tolerance develops—that is, the person needs more of the behavior to feel the same effect. Eventually, the behavior becomes a central focus of the person's life, and there is a deterioration in other areas, such as school performance or relationships. The behavior no longer brings pleasure, but it is necessary to avoid the pain of going without it. What started as a seemingly innocent way of feeling good can become a prison.

Many common behaviors are potentially addictive, but most people who engage in them do not develop problems. The reason, again, lies in the combination of factors that are involved in the development of addiction, including personality, lifestyle, heredity, the social and physical environment, and the nature of the substance or behavior in question. For a behavior to become an addiction, these diverse factors must come together in a certain way. For example, nicotine, the psychoactive drug in tobacco, has a very high potential for physical addiction; but a person who doesn't choose to try cigarettes, perhaps because of family influence or a tendency to develop asthma, will never develop nicotine addiction.

Characteristics of People with Addictions

The causes and course of an addiction are extremely varied, but people with addictions do seem to share some characteristics. Many use the substance or activity as a substitute for other, healthier, coping strategies. People vary in their ability to manage their lives, and those who have the most trouble dealing with stress and painful emotions may be more susceptible to addiction.

Some people may have a genetic predisposition to addiction to a particular substance; such predispositions may involve variations in brain chemistry. People with addictive disorders usually have a distinct preference for a particular addictive behavior, and they typically expect to have a positive experience with it even before they try it. They also often have problems with impulse control and self-regulation and tend to be risk takers.

Ww. Examples of Addictive Behaviors

The use and abuse of psychoactive drugs will be explored in detail later in the chapter. In this section, we'll examine some behaviors that are not related to drugs and that can become addictive for some people.

---

drug Any chemical other than food intended to affect the structure or function of the body.

psychoactive drug A drug that can alter a person's consciousness or experience.

intoxication The state of being mentally affected by a chemical (literally, a state of being poisoned).

addictive behavior Any habit that has gotten out of control, resulting in a negative effect on one's health.

Terms

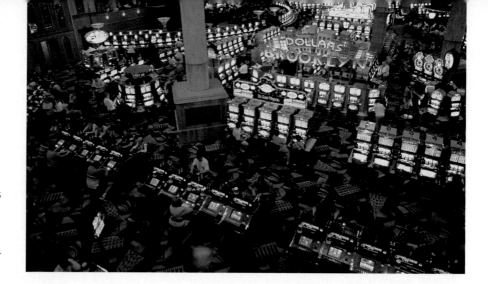

Most people who gamble do so casually and occasionally, but for a few, the habit spins out of control and becomes the central focus of their life. A variety of factors appear to influence whether a habit becomes an addiction, including personality, lifestyle, heredity, social environment, and the nature of the activity.

Compulsive or Pathological Gambling   Many people gamble casually by putting a dollar in the office football pool, buying a lottery ticket, or going to the races. But a few become compulsive gamblers, unable to resist or control the urge to gamble, even in the face of financial and personal ruin. Most compulsive gamblers say they are seeking excitement even more than money. Increasingly larger bets are necessary to produce the desired level of excitement. A series of losses can lead to a perceived need to keep placing bets to win back the money. When financial resources become strained, the person may lie or steal to pay off debts. The consequences of compulsive gambling are not just financial; the suicide rate of compulsive gamblers is 20 times higher than that of the general population.

Compulsive gamblers may gamble to relieve negative feelings and become restless and irritable when they are unable to gamble. As with many addictive behaviors, compulsive gambling may begin or flare up in times of stress. The earlier one starts to gamble, the more likely one is to become a pathological gambler. Gambling is often linked to other risky behaviors, and many compulsive gamblers also have drug and alcohol abuse problems.

The American Psychiatric Association (APA) recognizes pathological gambling as a mental disorder and lists ten characteristic behaviors, including preoccupation with gambling, unsuccessful efforts to cut back or quit, using gambling to escape problems, and lying to family members to conceal the extent of involvement with gambling. Compulsive gambling shares many of these traits with other addictive behaviors, including drug use. An estimated 1.1 million adolescents and 1.9 million adults in the United States may be compulsive gamblers. These numbers may increase due to the spread of legalized gambling, both on the Internet and on American Indian tribal reservations.

Sex and Love Addiction   More controversial is the notion of addiction to sex or love. Some researchers believe that the initial rush of arousal and erotic or romantic "chemistry" produces an effect in the brain comparable to that of taking amphetamines or morphine. After a time, the brain becomes desensitized to those chemicals, and the addict must then seek his or her next "fix" by pursuing a new partner. According to this view, cheating on a partner, having many partners, and sexually victimizing others are behaviors parallel to drug-seeking behavior. Behaviors associated with so-called sex addicts include an extreme preoccupation with sex, a compulsion to have sex repeatedly within a short period of time, spending a great deal of time and energy looking for partners or engaging in sex, using sex as a means of relieving painful feelings, and suffering negative emotional, personal, and professional consequences as a result of sexual activities.

Some experts are reluctant to call compulsive sexual activity a true addiction. However, even therapists who challenge the concept of sex addiction recognize that some people become overly preoccupied with sex, cannot seem to control their sex drive, and act in potentially harmful ways in order to obtain satisfaction. This pattern of sexual behavior does seem to meet the criteria for addictive behaviors discussed earlier.

Compulsive Spending or Shopping   Nearly everyone splurges at the mall or goes into debt once in a while. But a compulsive spender repeatedly gives in to the impulse to buy much more than he or she needs or can afford. For the compulsive shopper, spending may serve to relieve painful feelings like depression or anxiety, or it may produce positive emotions like excitement or happiness. Compulsive spenders usually buy luxury items rather than daily necessities. Men tend to buy cars, exercise equipment, and sporting gear; women are more likely to buy clothes, jewelry, and perfume. Some experts link compulsive shopping with neglect or abuse during childhood; it also seems to be associated with eating disorders, depression, and bipolar disorder. Some compulsive shoppers are helped by antidepressant medications.

Compulsive shoppers are usually significantly distressed by their behavior and its social, personal, and financial consequences. Characteristics of out-of-control spending include shopping in order to "feel better," using money or time that had been set aside for other purposes, hiding spending from others, and spending so much that one goes into debt or engages in illegal activities such as shoplifting or writing bad checks. Like other addictive behaviors, compulsive shopping is characterized by a loss of control over the behavior and significant negative consequences.

Internet Addiction Some recent research has indicated that surfing the World Wide Web can also be addictive. In order to spend more time online, Internet addicts skip important social, school, or recreational activities, thereby damaging personal relationships and jeopardizing academic and job performance. Despite the negative consequences they are experiencing, they don't feel able to stop. The Internet addicts identified in one study averaged 38 online hours per week. Internet addicts may feel uncomfortable or be moody when they are not online. They may be preoccupied with getting back online and may stay there longer than they intend. As with other addictive behaviors described here, online addicts may be using their behavior to alleviate stress or avoid painful emotions.

Activities by Internet addicts may take many forms, some of which, such as e-mail and chat rooms, are specific to the online format. However, widespread access to the Internet may expose many more people to other potentially addictive behaviors, including gambling, shopping, and sex. There are thousands of online gambling sites and millions of online stores that allow people to gamble or shop from their homes at all times of the day or night; in addition, sites featuring online auctions or stock trading offer activities that are very similar to gambling. As described in Chapter 5, easy access to sexually oriented Web sites can lead to cybersex addiction for some people. It remains to be seen whether increasing access to the Internet among Americans will lead to more problems with many types of addictive behaviors.

COMMUNICATE! Ample opportunities for "addiction" are offered by computers in general and the Internet in particular, through games, gambling, shopping, stock trading, pornography, and chat rooms. Many people "binge" on computer activities once or twice and then never do it again, while others seem to lose control. If a friend or roommate is spending more and more time in front of the computer and doesn't seem to be able to set limits, you might want to talk to him or her about it. For example, "You've been spending so much time online that I'm getting worried about you. You seem to feel more connected to your online friends and activities than your real-life ones. I wonder if you'd consider cutting back on your computer time—I miss your company! If you can't do it, maybe you should talk to a counselor about it."

Other behaviors that can become addictive include eating, watching TV, and working. Any substance or activity that becomes the focus of a person's life at the expense of other needs and interests can be damaging to health.

We turn now to the substances most commonly associated with addiction: psychoactive drugs.

DRUG USE, ABUSE, AND DEPENDENCE

Drugs are chemicals other than food that are intended to affect the structure or function of the body. They include prescription medicines, such as antibiotics and antidepressants; nonprescription, or over-the-counter (OTC), substances, such as alcohol, tobacco, and caffeine products; and illegal substances, such as cocaine and heroin. The use of drugs is not a new phenomenon in our society; in fact, drug use has a long history.

The Drug Tradition

Using drugs to alter consciousness is an ancient and universal pursuit. People have used alcohol to celebrate and intoxicate for thousands of years. People in all parts of the world have discovered and exploited the psychoactive properties of various local plants, such as the coca plant in South America and the opium poppy in the Middle East and Far East.

In the nineteenth century, chemists were successful in extracting the active chemicals from medicinal plants, such as morphine from the opium poppy and cocaine from the coca leaf. This was the beginning of modern *pharmacy,* the art of compounding drugs, and of *pharmacology,* the science and study of drugs. From this point on, a variety of drugs began to be produced, including morphine, cocaine, codeine, and heroin (Figure 9-1).

Initially, the manufacture and sale of these new drugs were not regulated. Pure morphine or cocaine could be purchased by mail order, and the makers of patent medicines and tonics included potentially addictive drugs in their products without informing the consumer of the ingredients or the dangers. The earliest version of the soft drink Coca-Cola contained cocaine, which accounted for the "lift" it provided.

Drug addiction among middle-class Europeans and North Americans was more common by 1900 than at any time before or since. Concerns about drug addiction and the need to regulate drug sales and manufacture led in the early 1900s to the passage of U.S. federal drug regulations. Middle-class use of the regulated drugs dropped, and drug use became restricted to, and increasingly identified with, criminal subcultures.

Nonmedical (recreational) drug use expanded in the general U.S. population during the 1960s and 1970s, reaching a peak in 1979. After a 12-year decline, marijuana use rose between 1991 and 1997 and then

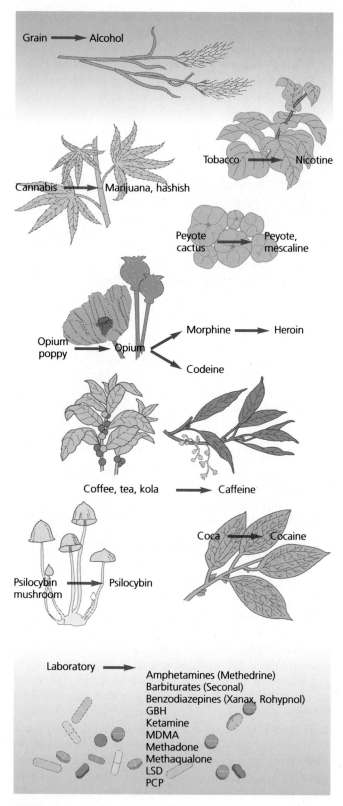

Grain → Alcohol

Tobacco → Nicotine

Cannabis → Marijuana, hashish

Peyote cactus → Peyote, mescaline

Opium poppy → Opium → Morphine → Heroin
→ Codeine

Coffee, tea, kola → Caffeine

Coca → Cocaine

Psilocybin mushroom → Psilocybin

Laboratory → Amphetamines (Methedrine)
Barbiturates (Seconal)
Benzodiazepines (Xanax, Rohypnol)
GBH
Ketamine
MDMA
Methadone
Methaqualone
LSD
PCP

Figure 9-1 Sources of selected psychoactive drugs.

appeared to level off. The use of some other drugs by young people also increased during the 1990s. While it is appropriate for us to be concerned about these increases,

no one should lose sight of the fact that the vast majority of young people still do not use marijuana or other illicit drugs.

Drug Abuse and Dependence

The APA's *Diagnostic and Statistical Manual of Mental Disorders* is the authoritative reference for defining all sorts of behavioral disorders, including those related to drugs. The APA has chosen not to use the term *addiction*, in part because it is so broad and has so many connotations. Instead, the APA refers to two forms of substance (drug) disorders: substance abuse and substance dependence. Both are maladaptive patterns of substance use that lead to significant impairment or distress. Although the APA's definitions are more precise and more directly related to drug use, they clearly encompass the general characteristics of addictive behavior described in the last section.

Drug Abuse   As defined by the APA, **substance abuse** involves one or more of the following:

- Recurrent drug use, resulting in a failure to fulfill major responsibilities at work, school, or home
- Recurrent drug use in situations in which it is physically hazardous, such as before driving a car
- Recurrent drug-related legal problems
- Continued drug use despite persistent social or interpersonal problems caused or exacerbated by the effects of the drug

The pattern of use may be constant or intermittent, and **physical dependence** may or may not be present. For example, a person who smokes marijuana once a week but cuts classes because he or she is high is abusing marijuana, even though he or she is not physically dependent.

Drug Dependence   **Substance dependence** is a more complex disorder and is what many people associate with the idea of addiction. The seven specific criteria the APA uses to diagnose substance dependence are listed below. The first two are associated with physical dependence; the final five are associated with compulsive use. To be considered dependent, an individual must experience a cluster of three or more of these seven symptoms during a 12-month period.

1. *Developing tolerance to the substance.* When a person requires increased amounts of a substance to achieve the desired effect or notices a markedly diminished effect with continued use of the same amount, he or she has developed **tolerance**. For example, heavy heroin users may need to take ten times the amount they took at the beginning in order to achieve the desired effect; such a large dose would be lethal to a nonuser. The degree to

which tolerance develops varies widely depending on the drug.

2. *Experiencing withdrawal.* In an individual who has maintained prolonged, heavy use of a substance, a drop in its concentration within the body can result in unpleasant physical and cognitive **withdrawal** symptoms. The person is likely to take the substance to relieve or avoid those symptoms. Withdrawal symptoms are different for different drugs. For example, nausea, vomiting, and tremors are common for alcohol, opioids, and sedatives; for stimulants like amphetamines, cocaine, and caffeine, fatigue and irritability may occur. Other drugs have no significant withdrawal symptoms.

3. *Taking the substance in larger amounts or over a longer period than was originally intended.*

4. *Expressing a persistent desire to cut down or regulate substance use.* This desire is often accompanied by many unsuccessful efforts to reduce or discontinue use of the substance.

5. *Spending a great deal of time obtaining the substance, using the substance, or recovering from its effects.*

6. *Giving up or reducing important social, school, work, or recreational activities because of substance use.* A dependent person may withdraw from family activities and hobbies in order to use the substance in private or to spend more time with substance-using friends.

7. *Continuing to use the substance in spite of recognizing that it is contributing to a psychological or physical problem.* For example, a person might continue to use cocaine despite recognizing that she is suffering from cocaine-induced depression.

If a drug-dependent person experiences either tolerance or withdrawal, he or she is considered physically dependent. However, not everyone who experiences tolerance or withdrawal is drug dependent. For example, a hospital patient who is prescribed therapeutic doses of morphine to relieve pain may develop a tolerance to the drug and experience withdrawal symptoms when the prescription is discontinued. But without showing any signs of compulsive use, this individual would not be considered dependent. Dependence can occur without a physical component, based solely on compulsive use. For example, people with at least three symptoms of compulsive use of marijuana who show no signs of tolerance or withdrawal are suffering from substance dependence. In general, dependence problems that involve physical dependence carry a greater risk of immediate general medical problems and have higher relapse rates.

Who Uses Drugs?

The use and abuse of drugs occur at all income and education levels, among all ethnic groups, and at all ages.

One reason for our society's concern with the casual or recreational use of illegal drugs is that it is not really possible to know when drug use will lead to abuse or dependence. Some casual users develop substance-related problems; others do not. Some psychoactive drugs are more likely than others to lead to dependence (Table 9-2). But some users of even heroin or cocaine do not meet the APA's criteria for substance dependence. However, people who begin to use drugs at very young ages have a greater risk for dependence and serious health consequences.

Although we can't accurately predict which drug users will become drug abusers, researchers have identified some characteristics that place young people at higher-than-average risk for *trying* illicit drugs. Being male is one risk factor: Although gender differences in drug use are gradually narrowing, males are still about twice as likely as females to use illicit drugs. An adolescent who has a poor self-image; lacks self-control; is aggressive, impulsive, or moody; or suffers from attention-deficit/hyperactivity disorder (ADHD) may be at increased risk for trying drugs. A thrill-seeking or risk-taking personality is another factor. People who drive too fast or who don't wear safety belts may have this personality type, which is characterized by a sense of invincibility. Such people find it easy to dismiss warnings of danger, whether about drugs or safety belts—"That only happens to other people; it could never happen to me."

Belonging to a peer group or family that accepts or rewards drug use is a significant risk factor for trying illicit drugs. One survey of people in drug treatment found that 20% had used drugs with their parents, usually before age 18. Chaotic home environments, dysfunctional families, and parental abuse also increase risk. Children with no parental monitoring after school are more likely to try illicit drugs than those with regular adult supervision. Young people who live in disadvantaged areas are more

Terms

substance abuse A maladaptive pattern of use of any substance that persists despite adverse social, psychological, or medical consequences. The pattern may be intermittent, with or without tolerance and physical dependence.

physical dependence The result of physiological adaptation that occurs in response to the frequent presence of a drug; typically associated with tolerance and withdrawal.

substance dependence A cluster of cognitive, behavioral, and physiological symptoms that occur in an individual who continues to use a substance despite suffering significant substance-related problems, leading to significant impairment or distress; also known as *addiction.*

tolerance Lower sensitivity to a drug so that a given dose no longer exerts the usual effect and larger doses are needed.

withdrawal Physical and psychological symptoms that follow the interrupted use of a drug on which a user is physically dependent; symptoms may be mild or life-threatening.

	Psychoactive Drugs and Their Potential for Producing Dependence		
Table 9-2			

	Potential for Dependence	
Drug	**Physical**	**Psychological**
Nicotine	Very high	Very high
Heroin	Very high	Very high
Methamphetamine smoked ("ice")	Very high	Very high
Crack cocaine	Possible	Very high
Alcohol	High	High
Barbiturates	High	High
Methaqualone (Quaalude)	High	High
Amphetamine	Possible	High
Cocaine	Possible	High
Diazepam (Valium)	Low	High
PCP	Unknown	High
Chloral hydrate ("mickey")	Moderate	Moderate
Codeine	Moderate	Moderate
Marijuana/ hashish	Unknown	Moderate
Inhalants	Unknown	Moderate
Steroids	Possible	Possible
LSD	None	Unknown

SOURCES: National Clearinghouse for Alcohol and Drug Information. 2000. *Drugs of Abuse* (http://www.health.org/govpubs/rpo926; retrieved October 3, 2000). Beers, M. H., and R. Berkow, eds. 1999. *Merck Manual of Diagnosis and Therapy*, 17th ed. Rahway, N.J.: Merck. Food and Drug Administration. 1995. Nicotine in cigarettes and smokeless tobacco products is a drug and these products are nicotine delivery devices under the Federal Food, Drug, and Cosmetic Act. *Federal Register* 60(155): 41454–41459.

likely to be offered drugs at a young age, thereby increasing their risk of drug use. Especially at younger ages, the risk of using drugs is higher for people who come from a single-parent family, for those whose parents failed to complete high school, and for those who are uninterested in school and earn poor grades. However, drug use rates among middle-class youths with college-educated parents tend to catch up with, and in some cases outstrip, those of other groups by the time students reach the twelfth grade.

What about people who *don't* use drugs? As a group, nonusers also share some characteristics. Not surpris-

ingly, people who perceive drug use as risky and who disapprove of it are less likely to use drugs than those who believe otherwise. Drug use is also less common among people who have positive self-esteem and self-concept and who are assertive, independent thinkers who are not controlled by peer pressure. Self-control, social competence, optimism, academic achievement, and regular church attendance are also linked to lower rates of drug use (see the box "Spirituality and Drug Abuse").

Home environments are also influential: Coming from a strong family, one that has a clear policy on drug use, is another characteristic of people who don't use drugs. Young people who communicate openly with their parents and feel supported by them are also less likely to use drugs. Although parents may feel they have little effect on their children's drug-related attitudes and behaviors, evidence suggests that they can be a major influence. Some parents may wait too long to express a clear drug policy. Recent surveys indicate that attitudes about drugs and access and exposure to drugs change most dramatically between the ages of 12 and 13. Compared to a 12-year-old, a 13-year-old is about three times more likely to know teens who use and sell drugs and to know where and how to buy drugs. Yet nearly half of 13-year-olds report that their parents have never seriously discussed the dangers of illegal drugs with them.

Why Do People Use Drugs?

The answer to this question depends on both the user and the drug. Young people, especially those from middle-class backgrounds, are frequently drawn to drugs by the allure of the exciting and illegal. They may be curious, rebellious, or vulnerable to peer pressure. They may want to appear to be daring and to be part of the group. Young people may want to imitate adult models in their lives or in the movies. Most people who have taken illicit drugs have done so on an experimental basis, typically trying the drug one or more times but not continuing. The main factors in the initial choice of a drug are whether it is available and whether other people around are already using it.

Although some people use drugs because they have a desire to alter their mood or are seeking a spiritual experience, others are motivated primarily by a desire to escape boredom, anxiety, depression, feelings of worthlessness, or other distressing symptoms of psychological problems. They use drugs as a way to cope with the difficulties they are experiencing in life. The common practice in our society of seeking a drug solution to every problem is a factor in the widespread reliance on both illicit and prescription drugs.

For people living in poverty in the inner cities, many of these reasons for using drugs are magnified. The problems are more devastating, the need for escape more compelling. Furthermore, the buying and selling of drugs pro-

The use of alcohol and other drugs is intertwined with spirituality and religion. Some religions use drugs in the quest for spiritual transcendence: American Indian, Polynesian, African, and other indigenous religions have used psychoactive drugs such as peyote, khat, alcohol, and hashish for expanding consciousness and developing personal spirituality. For other religions, the use of psychoactive drugs is seen as a threat to spirituality. In Islam, for example, the consumption of alcohol and certain other drugs is strictly forbidden. Although there are diverse religious viewpoints on drug use, many religions infer some link between psychoactive drugs and spirituality.

In studies of American teens and adults, spiritual or religious involvement is generally associated with a lower risk of trying psychoactive drugs and, for those who do use drugs, a lower risk of heavy use and dependence. The mechanism for this protective effect is unclear; possibilities include the adoption of a strict code of behavior or set of principles that forbids drug use; the presence of a social support system for abstinence or moderation; and the promotion of a large, complex set of values that includes avoidance of drug use. The relationship between religious faith and avoidance of drug use appears to be even stronger in teens than in adults. One recent study found that teens who felt they had a personal relationship with the divine and/or who belonged to a more fundamentalist religious denomination were less likely to engage in substance use and abuse than other teens. Overall, people who spend time regularly engaging in spiritual practices such as prayer and transcendental meditation have lower rates of drug abuse.

People with current substance abuse problems tend to have lower rates of religious affiliation and involvement and lower levels of spiritual wellness, characterized by a lack of a sense of meaning in life. One of the hallmarks of drug dependence is spending increasing amounts of time and energy obtaining and using drugs; such a pattern of behavior inevitably reduces the resources an individual puts toward developing physical, emotional, and spiritual wellness.

What about those seeking to break their dependence on drugs? Among people in treatment for substance abuse, higher levels of religious faith and spirituality may contribute to the recovery process. A study of people recovering from alcohol or other drug abuse found that spirituality and religiosity were associated with increased coping skills, greater optimism about life, greater resilience to stress, and greater perceived social support. If, for a particular individual, there is a spiritual aspect to his or her substance abuse problem, then it is likely that spirituality may also play a role in recovery.

More research is needed to clarify the relationship among spirituality, religion, drug use, and recovery. One of the difficulties in conducting research in this area is the difficulty in defining and measuring spirituality and religious involvement. Spirituality is a complex part of human nature, involving behavior, belief, and experience. And although behaviors such as the spiritual practices of prayer or meditation can be measured, it is more difficult to determine what such practices mean to an individual and her or his overall sense of self.

SOURCES: Plante, T. G., and D. A. Pardini. 2000. Religious denomination affiliation and psychological health: Results from a substance abuse population. Presented at the American Psychological Association Annual Convention, August 7. Miller, L., M. Davies, and S. Greenwald. 2000. Religiosity and substance use and abuse among adolescents in the national comorbidity survey. *Journal of the American Academy of Child and Adolescent Psychiatry* 39(9): 1190–1197. Miller, W. R. 1998. Researching the spiritual dimensions of alcohol and other drug problems. *Addiction* 93(7): 979–990.

vide access to an unofficial, alternative economy that may seem like an opportunity for success.

Risk Factors for Dependence

Why do some people use psychoactive drugs without becoming dependent, while others aren't as lucky? The answer seems to be a combination of physical, psychological, and social factors. Research indicates that some people may be born with certain characteristics of brain chemistry or metabolism that make them more vulnerable to drug dependence. Other research suggests that people who were exposed to drugs while still in the womb may have an increased risk of abusing drugs themselves later in life. People who suffer from chronic pain, such as those with back injuries, also risk becoming dependent on the medications they take to relieve pain.

Psychological risk factors for drug dependence include difficulty in controlling impulses and a strong need for excitement, stimulation, and immediate gratification.

Feelings of rejection, hostility, aggression, anxiety, or depression are also associated with drug dependence. People may turn to drugs to blot out their emotional pain.

People with mental illnesses have a very high risk of substance dependence. Research shows that about one-third of people with psychological disorders also have a substance-dependence problem and about one-third of those have another mental disorder. People with two or more coexisting mental disorders are referred to as having **dual disorders.** Diagnosis of psychological problems among people with substance dependence can be very difficult because drug intoxication and withdrawal can mimic the symptoms of a mental illness.

dual disorder The presence of two or more mental disorders simultaneously in the same person; for example, drug dependence and depression.

Terms

Answer yes (Y) or no (N) to the following questions:

_____ **1.** Do you take the drug regularly?

_____ **2.** Have you been taking the drug for a long time?

_____ **3.** Do you always take the drug in certain situations or when you're with certain people?

_____ **4.** Do you find it difficult to stop using the drug? Do you feel powerless to quit?

_____ **5.** Have you tried repeatedly to cut down or control your use of the drug?

_____ **6.** Do you need to take a larger dose of the drug in order to get the same high you're used to?

_____ **7.** Do you feel specific symptoms if you cut back or stop using the drug?

_____ **8.** Do you frequently take another psychoactive substance to relieve withdrawal symptoms?

_____ **9.** Do you take the drug to feel "normal"?

_____ **10.** Do you go to extreme lengths or put yourself in dangerous situations to get the drug?

_____ **11.** Do you hide your drug use from others? Have you ever lied about what you're using or how much you use?

_____ **12.** Do people close to you ask you about your drug use?

_____ **13.** Are you spending more and more time with people who use the same drug as you?

_____ **14.** Do you think about the drug when you're not high, figuring out ways to get it?

_____ **15.** If you stop taking the drug, do you feel bad until you can take it again?

_____ **16.** Does the drug interfere with your ability to study, work, or socialize?

_____ **17.** Do you skip important school, work, social, or recreational activities in order to obtain or use the drug?

_____ **18.** Do you continue to use the drug despite a physical or mental disorder or despite a significant problem that you know is made worse by drug use?

_____ **19.** Have you developed a mental or physical condition or disorder because of prolonged drug use?

_____ **20.** Have you done something dangerous or that you regret while under the influence of the drug?

The more times you answer yes, the more likely it is that you are developing a dependence on the drug. If your answers suggest dependence, talk to someone at your school health clinic or to your physician about taking care of the problem before it gets worse.

Social factors that may influence drug dependence include growing up in a family in which a parent or sibling abused drugs, belonging to a peer group that emphasizes and encourages drug abuse, and living in poverty. Because they have easy access to drugs, health care professionals also have a higher risk. To determine whether you are at risk, take the quiz in the box "Do You Have a Problem with Drugs?"

Other Risks of Drug Use

Dependence is not the only serious potential consequence of drug use. People who are under the influence of drugs—intoxicated—may act in uncharacteristic and unsafe ways because both their physical and mental functioning are impaired. They are more likely to be injured from a variety of causes, including falls, drowning, and automobile crashes; to engage in unsafe sex, increasing their risk for sexually transmitted diseases and unin-

tended pregnancy; and to be involved in incidents of aggression and violence, including sexual assault.

Psychoactive drugs have many physical and psychological effects beyond the alteration of consciousness. These effects range from nausea and constipation to paranoia, depression, and heart failure; some drugs also carry the risk of potentially fatal overdose. Certain methods of drug administration are inherently dangerous; injecting drugs, for example, increases one's risk of HIV infection, hepatitis C, and gangrene (see the box "Injection Drug Use"). There is no quality control in the illegal drug market, so the composition, dosage, and toxicity of street drugs is highly variable. Studies of samples indicate that many street drugs don't contain their promised primary ingredient; in some cases, a drug may be present in unsafe dosages or mixed with other drugs to boost the effects. Careless manufacturing practices can result in the presence of toxic contaminants. Finally, many psychoactive drugs are illegal, so using them can result in large fines and/or imprisonment.

Different methods of administering drugs are associated with different risks—dangers beyond the actual effects of the drug being used. The method of drug use most frequently linked to serious health problems is injection drug use. Many injection drug users (IDUs) share or reuse needles, syringes, and other injection equipment, which can easily become contaminated with the user's blood. In addition, IDUs typically prepare drugs using unsterile water and equipment, and they do not clean injection sites before injecting drugs, giving disease-causing microorganisms easy access to the body.

Small amounts of blood can carry enough human immunodeficiency virus (HIV) and hepatitis C virus (HCV) to be infectious, and injection drug use accounts for almost a third of all AIDS cases and half of all hepatitis C cases reported in the United States. (Hepatitis C infection can cause chronic liver disease, liver cancer, and death; hepatitis and HIV/AIDS are discussed in more detail in Chapters 17 and 18.) It's estimated that about 15% of current IDUs are infected with HIV, and as many as 80% may carry HCV. Unsterile injection practices can cause skin and soft tissue infections, which can progress to gangrene and be fatal if untreated. IDUs are also at greater risk for endocarditis (microbial infection of the heart valves), tuberculosis, human herpesvirus 8, tetanus, the collapse of veins, and scarring at the site of injections.

Heroin and other injectable opiates are the drugs most often used by IDUs, but cocaine, amphetamines, and other drugs may also be injected. Concerns have also recently been raised about steroids: Steroid users who inject the drug face the same health risks as other IDUs, and steroids have been found to be a gateway to the use of other drugs. A study of steroid users who progressed to heroin use found that the steroid users typically obtained heroin from the same dealer who provided the steroids; they also originally used heroin in an effort to blunt some of the side effects of steroid use and withdrawal, including insomnia, irritability, and depression. (Steroid use is discussed further in Chapter 13.)

The surest way to prevent diseases related to injection drug use is never to inject drugs. Those who do inject drugs should use a new needle and syringe with each injection and should use sterile water and other equipment to prepare drugs. Bleach or boiling water may kill some viruses and bacteria, but they are not foolproof sterilization methods. Many viruses can survive in a syringe for a month or more.

Some public health experts believe free syringe exchange programs (SEPs)—in which IDUs can turn in a used syringe and get a new, clean one back—could help slow the spread of HIV and reduce the rates of other health problems associated with injection drug use. Opponents of SEPs argue that supplying addicts with syringes gives them the message that illegal drug use is acceptable and could thus exacerbate the nation's drug program. However, studies have shown that well-implemented programs do not increase the use of illegal drugs. Most current SEPs offer AIDS counseling and testing and provide referrals to drug-treatment programs. Despite funding bans and legal problems, local SEPs are proliferating and are exchanging more than 20 million syringes per year. However, with more than 1.5 million IDUs in the United States, each injecting about 1000 times per year, many more SEPs would be needed. Other strategies include distribution of new syringes through physician prescriptions or through local pharmacies. Getting people off drugs is clearly the best solution, but there are far more IDUs than treatment facilities can currently handle.

SOURCES: Centers for Disease Control and Prevention. 2000. *Fact Sheet: Access to Sterile Syringes.* Washington, D.C.: Academy for Educational Development. Arvary, D., and H. G. Pope. 2000. Anabolic-androgenic steroids as a gateway to opioid dependence. *New England Journal of Medicine* 342(20): 1532. Centers for Disease Control and Prevention. 1998. Update: Syringe-exchange programs. *Morbidity and Mortality Weekly Report* 47(31): 652–655.

In the following sections of the chapter, you'll learn more about how drugs affect the body and how drug use and abuse affect individuals, families, and society as a whole.

COMMUNICATE!   As a college student, you will probably sooner or later find yourself in a situation where drugs are being used or abused. Anticipate such situations and think ahead about how you will respond. Remember that you are entitled to make your own decisions about your life, even in the face of peer pressure. Sometimes, all you have to do is say, "No thanks." Other times, it's best to use nonverbal communication—leave the situation as soon as you can and go home.

HOW DRUGS AFFECT THE BODY

The psychoactive drugs discussed in this chapter have complex and variable effects, many of which can be traced to changes in brain chemistry. However, the same drug may affect different people differently or the same person in different ways under different circumstances. Beyond a fairly predictable general change in brain chemistry, the effects of a drug may vary depending on three general categories of factors: drug factors, user factors, and social factors.

Changes in Brain Chemistry

How can different drugs produce such different effects— making a person alert and wired or putting her or him to

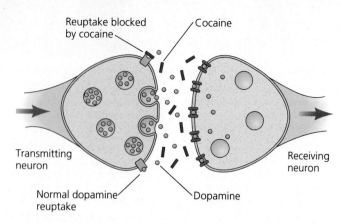

Figure 9-2 Effect of cocaine on brain chemistry. Under normal circumstances, the amount of dopamine at a synapse is controlled in part by the re-uptake of dopamine by the transmitting neuron. Cocaine blocks the removal of dopamine from a synapse; the resulting buildup of dopamine causes continuous stimulation of the receiving neurons.

sleep? Psychoactive drugs produce most of their key effects by acting on brain chemistry in a characteristic fashion. Before any changes in brain chemistry can occur, however, molecules of the drug have to be carried to the brain through the bloodstream. A drug that is taken by mouth has to dissolve in the stomach, be absorbed into the bloodstream through the lining of the small intestine, and then pass through the liver, heart, and lungs before returning to the heart to be carried via arteries to the brain. A drug that is already dissolved and is injected directly into the bloodstream will reach the brain in much less time, and drugs that are inhaled and absorbed by the lungs travel to the brain even more rapidly.

Once a psychoactive drug reaches the brain, it acts on one or more neurotransmitters, either increasing or decreasing their concentration and actions. Cocaine, for example, affects dopamine, a neurotransmitter thought to play a key role in the process of reinforcement—the brain's way of telling itself, "that's good; do the same thing again." As described in Chapter 3, when a neurotransmitter is released by one neuron to signal another neuron, its level or concentration is controlled in part by the reuptake or resorption of the neurotransmitter by the releasing neuron. Cocaine inhibits the resorption of dopamine, thereby increasing the concentration of dopamine in the synapse and lengthening the time of its action (Figure 9-2). The euphoria produced by cocaine is thought to be a result of its effect on dopamine. Heroin, nicotine, and amphetamines also affect dopamine levels.

The duration of a drug's effect depends on many factors and may range from 5 minutes (crack cocaine) to 12 or more hours (peyote). As drugs circulate through the body, they are metabolized by the liver and eventually excreted by the kidneys in urine. Small amounts may also

be eliminated in other ways, including in sweat, in breast milk, and via the lungs.

Drug Factors

When different drugs or dosages produce different effects, the differences are usually caused by one or more of five different drug factors:

1.   The **pharmacological properties** of a drug are its overall effects on a person's body chemistry, behavior, and psychology. The pharmacological properties also include the amount of a drug required to exert various effects, the time course of these effects, and other characteristics, such as a drug's chemical composition.

2.   The **dose-response function** is the relationship between the amount of drug taken and the type and intensity of the resulting effect. Many psychological effects of drugs reach a plateau in the dose-response function, so that increasing the dose does not increase the effect any further. With LSD, for example, the maximum changes in perception occur at a certain dose, and no further changes in perception take place if higher doses are taken. However, all drugs have more than one effect, and the dose-response functions usually are different for different effects. This means that increasing the dose of any drug may begin to result in additional effects, which are likely to be increasingly unpleasant or dangerous at high doses.

3.   The **time-action function** is the relationship between the time elapsed since a drug was taken and the intensity of its effect. The effects of a drug are greatest when concentrations of the drug in body tissues are changing the fastest, especially if they are increasing.

4.   The person's *drug use history* may influence the effects of a drug. A given amount of alcohol, for example, will generally affect a habitual drinker less than an occasional drinker. Tolerance to some drugs, such as LSD, builds rapidly. To experience the same effect, a user has to abstain from the drug for a period of time before that dosage will again exert its original effects.

5.   The *method of use* has a direct effect on how strong a response a drug produces. Methods of use include ingestion, inhalation, injection, and absorption through the skin or tissue linings. Drugs are usually injected one of three ways: intravenously (IV, or mainlining), intramuscularly (IM), or subcutaneously (SC, or "skin popping"). If a drug is taken by a method that allows the drug to enter the bloodstream and reach the brain rapidly, the effects are usually stronger and the potential for dependence greater than when the method involves slower absorption. For example, injecting a drug intravenously produces stronger effects than swallowing the same drug. Inhaling a drug, such as when tobacco or crack cocaine is smoked, produces very rapid effects on the brain.

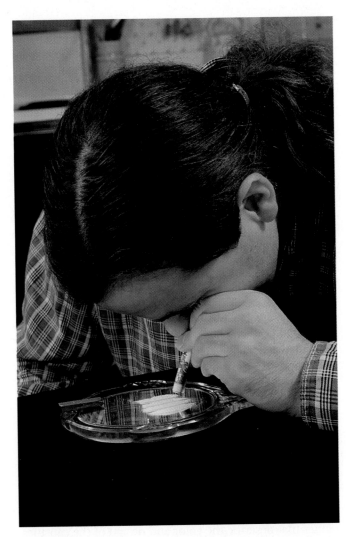

Method of use is one variable in the overall effect of a drug on the body. Sniffing or "snorting" cocaine produces effects in 2–3 minutes. With other methods, such as injecting it intravenously, inhaling vapors, or smoking crack, the effects of cocaine are felt within seconds.

User Factors

The second category of factors that determine how a person will respond to a particular drug involves certain physical and psychological characteristics. Body mass is one variable. The effects of a certain dose of a drug on a 100-pound person will be twice as great as on a 200-pound person. Other variables include general health and genetic factors. For example, some people have an inherited ability to rapidly metabolize a cough suppressant called dextromethorphan, which also has psychoactive properties. These people must take a higher-than-normal dose to get a given cough-suppressant effect.

If a person's biochemical state is already altered by another drug, this too can make a difference. Some drugs intensify the effects of other drugs, as is the case with alcohol and sedatives. Some drugs block the effects of other drugs, such as when a tranquilizer is used to relieve anxiety caused by cocaine. Interactions between drugs, including many prescription and OTC medications, can be unpredictable and dangerous.

One physical condition that requires special precautions is pregnancy. It can be risky for a woman to use any drugs at all during pregnancy, including alcohol and common OTC preparations like cough medicine. The risks are greatest during the first trimester, when the fetus's body is rapidly forming and even small biochemical alterations in the mother can have a devastating effect on fetal development. Even later, the fetus is more susceptible than the mother to the adverse effects of any drugs she takes. The fetus may even become physically dependent on a drug being taken by the mother and suffer withdrawal symptoms after birth.

Sometimes a person's response to a drug is strongly influenced by the user's expectations about how he or she will react. With large doses, the drug's chemical properties do seem to have the strongest effect on the user's response. But with small doses, psychological (and social) factors are often more important. When people strongly believe that a given drug will affect them a certain way, they are likely to experience those effects regardless of the drug's pharmacological properties. In one study, regular users of marijuana reported a moderate level of intoxication (**high**) after using a cigarette that smelled and tasted like marijuana but contained no THC, the active ingredient in marijuana. This is an example of the **placebo effect**—when a person receives an inert substance yet responds as if it were an active drug. (The placebo effect is discussed in more detail in Chapter 21.) In other studies, subjects who smoked low doses of real marijuana that they believed to be a placebo experienced no effects from the drug. Clearly, the user's expectations had greater effects on the smokers than the drug itself.

Social Factors

The *setting* is the physical and social environment surrounding the drug use. If a person uses marijuana at home with trusted friends and pleasant music, the effects are likely to be different from the effects if the same dose is taken in an austere experimental laboratory with an

pharmacological properties The overall effects of a drug on a person's behavior, psychology, and chemistry.

dose-response function The relationship between the amount of a drug taken and the intensity or type of the resulting effect.

time-action function The relationship between the time elapsed since a drug was taken and the intensity of its effect.

high The subjectively pleasing effects of a drug, usually felt quite soon after the drug is taken.

placebo effect A response to an inert or innocuous medication given in place of an active drug.

Terms

impassive research technician. Similarly, the dose of alcohol that produces mild euphoria and stimulation at a noisy, active cocktail party might induce sleepiness and slight depression when taken at home while alone.

WW. REPRESENTATIVE PSYCHOACTIVE DRUGS

What are the major psychoactive drugs, and how do they produce their effects? We discuss six different representative groups in this chapter: (1) opioids, (2) central nervous system depressants, (3) central nervous system stimulants, (4) marijuana and other cannabis products, (5) hallucinogens, and (6) inhalants. Some of these drugs are classified according to how they affect the body; others—the opioids and the cannabis products—are classified according to their chemical makeup. (For the sources of selected psychoactive drugs, see Figure 9-1.)

Opioids

Also called *narcotics,* **opioids** are natural or synthetic (laboratory-made) drugs that relieve pain, cause drowsiness, and induce **euphoria.** Opium, morphine, heroin, methadone, codeine, meperidine, and fentanyl are examples of drugs in this category. Opioids tend to reduce anxiety and produce lethargy, apathy, and an inability to concentrate. Opioid users become less active and less responsive to frustration, hunger, and sexual stimulation. These effects are more pronounced in novice users; with repeated use, many effects diminish.

Opioids are typically injected or absorbed into the body from the stomach, intestines, nasal membranes (from snorting or sniffing), or lungs (from smoking). Effects depend on the method of administration. If tissue levels of the drug change rapidly, more immediate effects will result. Although the euphoria associated with opioids is an important factor in their abuse, many people experience a feeling of uneasiness when they first use these drugs. Users also often feel nauseated and vomit, and they may have other unpleasant sensations. Even so, the abuse of opioids often results in dependence. Tolerance can de-

velop rapidly and be pronounced. Withdrawal symptoms include cramps, chills, sweating, nausea, tremors, irritability, and feelings of panic.

Rates of heroin use have always been low, but there are periodic episodes of increased use among some groups. Use among college students remains below 1%, but between 1991 and 2000, heroin use among high school seniors more than doubled, mostly due to increased rates of sniffing or smoking the drug. Although these users avoid the special disease risks of injection drug use, including HIV infection, dependence can readily result from sniffing and smoking heroin. In addition, the potentially high but variable purity of street heroin poses a risk of unintentional overdose. Symptoms of overdose include respiratory depression, coma, and constriction of the pupils; death can result.

Central Nervous System Depressants

Central nervous system **depressants,** also known as **sedative-hypnotics,** slow down the overall activity of the **central nervous system (CNS).** The result can range from mild **sedation** to death, depending on the various factors involved—which drug is used, how it's taken, how tolerant the user is, and so on. CNS depressants include alcohol (discussed in Chapter 10), barbiturates, and other sedatives.

Types The various types of barbiturates are similar in chemical composition and action, but they differ in how quickly and how long they act. Drug users call barbiturates "downers" or "downs" and refer to specific brands by names that describe the color and design of the capsules: "reds" or "red devils" for Seconal; "yellows" or "yellow jackets" for Nembutal. People usually take barbiturates in capsules, but they may also inject them.

Antianxiety agents, also called sedatives or **tranquilizers,** include the benzodiazepines such as Xanax, Valium, Librium, clonazepam (Klonopin), and flunitrazepam (Rohypnol, also called "roofies"). Other CNS depressants include methaqualone (Quaalude), ethchlorvynol (Placidyl), chloral hydrate ("mickey"), and gamma hydroxy butyrate (GHB, or "liquid ecstasy").

Effects CNS depressants reduce anxiety and cause mood changes, impaired muscular coordination, slurring of speech, and drowsiness or sleep. Mental functioning is also affected, but the degree varies from person to person and also depends on the kind of task the person is trying to do. Most people become drowsy with small doses, although a few become more active.

Medical Uses Barbiturates, antianxiety agents, and other sedative-hypnotics are widely used to treat insomnia and anxiety disorders and to control seizures. Some CNS depressants are used for their calming properties in com-

Terms

opioid Any of several natural or synthetic drugs that relieve pain and cause drowsiness and/or euphoria; examples are opium, morphine, and heroin; also called *narcotic.*

euphoria An exaggerated feeling of well-being.

depressant or sedative-hypnotic A drug that decreases nervous or muscular activity, causing drowsiness or sleep.

central nervous system (CNS) The brain and spinal cord.

sedation The induction of a calm, relaxed, often sleepy state.

tranquilizer A CNS depressant that reduces tension and anxiety.

anesthetic A drug that produces a loss of sensation with or without a loss of consciousness.

In the United States and elsewhere, euphoria-inducing drugs known as club drugs have gained popularity in recent years. Club drugs include a variety of very different drugs that are part of the popular dance culture of clubs and "raves"—all-night dance parties held in fields or abandoned buildings. Some people refer to club drugs as "soft" drugs because they see them as recreational—more for the casual, weekend user—rather than as addictive. But club drugs have many potential negative effects and are particularly potent and unpredictable when mixed with alcohol. Substitute drugs are often sold in place of club drugs, putting users at risk for taking dangerous combinations of unknown drugs.

MDMA *(ecstasy, E, X, XTC, Adam, clarity, lover's speed):* Taken in pill form, MDMA (methylenedioxymethamphetamine) is a stimulant with mildly hallucinogenic and amphetamine-like effects. In club settings, using it can produce dangerously high body temperature and potentially fatal dehydration; some users experience confusion, depression, anxiety, or paranoia. Even low doses may affect concentration and driving ability. Chronic use of MDMA may produce long-lasting, perhaps permanent, damage to the neurons that release serotonin; this may explain why heavy use is associated with persistent problems with verbal and visual memory. At high doses or mixed with other drugs, MDMA is extremely dangerous; several deaths in 2000 were traced to pills containing a combination of MDMA and the related drug PMA or PMAA. Research suggests that pregnant women who use MDMA are at increased risk for having a baby with congenital malformations.

LSD *(acid, boomers, yellow sunshines, red dragon):* A popular and potent hallucinogen, LSD (lysergic acid diethylamide) is sold in tablets or capsules, in liquid form, or on small squares of paper called blotters. LSD increases heart rate and body temperature and may cause nausea, tremors, sweating, numbness, and weakness. (See p. 244 for more on LSD.)

Ketamine *(special K, vitamin K, K, cat valium):* A veterinary anesthetic that can be taken in powdered or liquid form, ketamine may cause hallucinations and impaired attention and memory. At higher doses, ketamine can cause delirium, amnesia, high blood pressure, and potentially fatal respiratory problems. Tolerance to ketamine develops rapidly.

GHB *(Georgia home boy, G, grievous bodily harm, liquid ecstasy):* GHB (gamma hydroxybutyrate) can be produced in clear liquid, white powder, tablet, and capsule form; it is often made in basement chemistry labs, where toxic substances may unintentionally be added or produced. GHB is a CNS depressant that in large doses can cause sedation, loss of consciousness, respiratory arrest, and death. In 2000, three teens were convicted of manslaughter after they gave a female party guest a soda laced with GHB; the young woman lost consciousness and died from choking on her own vomit. Evidence suggests that GHB is addictive and that it may cause prolonged and potentially life-threatening withdrawal symptoms. Some products sold as dietary supplements for bodybuilding, weight loss, or insomnia contain the chemically similar compounds GBL (gamma butyrolactone) or BD (butanediol); the FDA considers these products dangerous and is working to remove them from the market.

Rohypnol *(roofies, roche, forget-me pill):* Taken in tablet form, Rohypnol (flunitrazepam) is a sedative that is 10 times more potent than Valium. Its effects, which are magnified by alcohol, include reduced blood pressure, dizziness, confusion, gastrointestinal disturbances, and loss of consciousness. Users of Rohypnol may develop physical and psychological dependence on the drug.

An additional problem associated with Rohypnol, GHB, and several other club drugs is their potential use as "date rape drugs." Because they can be added to beverages surreptitiously, these drugs may be unknowingly consumed by intended rape victims. In addition to depressant effects, some drugs also cause *anterograde amnesia,* the loss of memory of things occurring while under the influence of the drug. Because of concern about Rohypnol, GHB, and other similarly abused drugs, Congress passed the "Drug-Induced Rape Prevention and Punishment Act," which increased federal penalties for use of any controlled substance to aid in sexual assault (see Chapter 23).

---

bination with **anesthetics** before operations and other medical or dental procedures.

From Use to Abuse   People are usually introduced to CNS depressants either through a medical prescription or through drug-using peers. The use of Rohypnol and GHB is often associated with dance clubs and raves (see the box "Club Drugs"). The abuse of CNS depressants by a medical patient may begin with repeated use for insomnia and progress to dependence through increasingly larger doses at night, coupled with a few capsules at stressful times during the day.

Most CNS depressants, including alcohol, can lead to classical physical dependence. Tolerance, sometimes for up to 15 times the usual dose, can develop with repeated use. Tranquilizers have been shown to produce physical dependence even at ordinary prescribed doses. Withdrawal symptoms can be more severe than those accompanying opioid dependence and are similar to the DTs of alcoholism (see Chapter 10). They may begin as anxiety, shaking, and weakness but may turn into convulsions and possibly cardiovascular collapse and death.

While intoxicated, people on depressants cannot function very well. They are mentally confused and are frequently obstinate, irritable, and abusive. Even prescription use of benzodiazepines has been associated with an increased risk of automobile crashes. After long-term use, depressants like alcohol can lead to generally poor health and brain damage, with impaired ability to reason and make judgments.

Overdosing with CNS Depressants Too much depression of the central nervous system slows respiration and may stop it entirely. CNS depressants are particularly dangerous in combination with another depressant, such as alcohol. People who combine depressants with alcohol account for thousands of emergency room visits and hundreds of overdose deaths each year. Rohypnol is ten times more potent than Valium and can be fatal if combined with alcohol. GHB is often produced clandestinely, resulting in widely varying degrees of purity; it has been responsible for many poisonings and several deaths.

In recent surveys, about 1.5% of college students report having used a CNS depressant (other than alcohol) within the past month.

Central Nervous System Stimulants

CNS **stimulants** speed up the activity of the nervous or muscular system. Under their influence, the heart rate accelerates, blood pressure rises, blood vessels constrict, the pupils of the eyes and the bronchial tubes dilate, and gastric and adrenal secretions increase. There is greater muscular tension and sometimes an increase in motor activity. Small doses usually make people feel more awake and alert, less fatigued and bored. The most common CNS stimulants are cocaine, amphetamine, nicotine (discussed in Chapter 11), ephedrine, and caffeine.

Cocaine Usually derived from the leaves of coca shrubs that grow high in the Andes Mountains in South America, cocaine is a potent CNS stimulant. For centuries, natives of the Andes have chewed coca leaves both for pleasure and to increase their endurance. For a short time during the nineteenth century, some physicians were enthusiastic about the use of cocaine to cure alcoholism and addiction to the painkiller morphine: Enthusiasm waned after the adverse side effects became apparent.

Cocaine—also known as "coke" or "snow"—quickly produces a feeling of euphoria, which makes it a popular recreational drug. Cocaine use surged in popularity during the early 1980s, when the drug's high price made it a "status" drug. The introduction of "crack" cocaine during the 1980s made the drug available in smaller quantities and at lower prices to more people. The typical recreational user shifted rapidly from the wealthy professional snorting (inhaling) powdered cocaine to poor inner-city smokers of crack cocaine. In the general population,

cocaine use peaked in 1985 with an estimated 3% of adult Americans reporting use. In recent surveys, about 0.7% of all adults and 1.4% of college students surveyed reported using cocaine in the previous month.

METHODS OF USE Cocaine is usually inhaled or injected intravenously, providing rapid increases of the drug's concentration in the blood and therefore fast, intense effects. Another method of use involves processing cocaine with baking soda and water, yielding the ready-to-smoke form of cocaine known as crack. Crack is typically available as small beads or pellets smokable in glass pipes. The tiny but potent beads can be handled more easily than cocaine powder and marketed in smaller, less expensive doses.

EFFECTS The effects of cocaine are usually intense but short-lived. The euphoria lasts from 5 to 20 minutes and ends abruptly, to be replaced by irritability, anxiety, or slight depression. When cocaine is absorbed via the lungs, by either smoking or inhalation, it reaches the brain in about 10 seconds, and the effects are particularly intense. This is part of the appeal of smoking crack. The effects from IV injections occur almost as quickly—in about 20 seconds. Since the mucous membranes in the nose briefly slow absorption, the onset of effects from snorting takes 2–3 minutes. Heavy users may inject cocaine intravenously every 10–20 minutes to maintain the effects.

The larger the cocaine dose and the more rapidly it is absorbed into the bloodstream, the greater the immediate—and sometimes lethal—effects. Sudden death from cocaine is most commonly the result of excessive CNS stimulation that causes convulsions and respiratory collapse, irregular heartbeat, blood clots, and possibly heart attack or stroke. Although rare, fatalities can occur in healthy young people; among people ages 18–59, cocaine users are seven times more likely than nonusers to have a heart attack. Chronic cocaine use produces inflammation of the nasal mucosa, which can lead to persistent bleeding and ulceration of the septum between the nostrils. The use of cocaine may also cause paranoia and/or aggressiveness.

Although the use of cocaine decreased in the general U.S. population after 1985, cocaine is responsible for more deaths and emergency room visits than any other illicit drug. This presumably reflects the fact that smoking crack is more toxic than snorting powdered cocaine. Most deaths result from people using cocaine in combination with another substance, such as alcohol or heroin.

ABUSE AND DEPENDENCE When steady cocaine users stop taking the drug, they experience a sudden "crash," characterized by depression, agitation, and fatigue, followed by a period of withdrawal. Their depression can be temporarily relieved by taking more cocaine, so its continued use is reinforced. Cocaine use follows different patterns in

Terms **stimulant** A drug that increases nervous or muscular activity.

state dependence A situation in which information learned in a drug-induced state is difficult to recall when the effect of the drug wears off.

psychosis A severe mental disorder characterized by a distortion of reality; symptoms might include delusions or hallucinations.

different individuals. A binge cocaine user may go for weeks or months without using any cocaine and then take large amounts repeatedly. Although not physically dependent, a binge cocaine user who misses work or school and risks serious health consequences is clearly abusing the drug.

COCAINE USE DURING PREGNANCY   Cocaine rapidly passes from the mother's bloodstream into the placenta and can have serious effects on the fetus. A woman who uses cocaine during pregnancy is at higher risk for miscarriage, premature labor, and stillbirth. She is more likely to deliver a low-birth-weight baby who has a small head circumference. Her infant may be at increased risk for defects of the genitourinary tract, cardiovascular system, central nervous system, and extremities. It is difficult to pinpoint the effects of cocaine because many women who use cocaine also use tobacco and/or alcohol.

Infants whose mothers use cocaine may also be born intoxicated. They are typically irritable and jittery and do not eat or sleep normally. These characteristics may affect their early social and emotional development because it may be more difficult for adults to interact with them. Cocaine also passes into breast milk, from where it can intoxicate a breastfeeding infant.

Research on the long-term effects of prenatal exposure to cocaine has been inconclusive. Initial findings of devastating effects have not been borne out. Recent studies suggest that prenatal cocaine exposure may cause subtle changes in the brain that affect IQ, language skill, and motor development; behavioral problems—disorganization, poor social skills, and hyperactivity—have also been reported. Although fetal cocaine exposure is an important issue, the type and magnitude of effects produced by nicotine are similar, and there are nearly 20 times more infants exposed to cigarettes than to cocaine.

Amphetamines
Amphetamines are a group of synthetic chemicals that are potent CNS stimulants. Some common drugs in this family are amphetamine (Benzedrine), dextroamphetamine (Dexedrine), and methamphetamine (Methedrine). Popular names for these drugs include "speed," "crank," "chalk," "crystal," and "meth," and users refer to them all as "uppers."

"Ice," a smokable, high-potency form of methamphetamine, is popular in some cities. Easy to manufacture, ice is cheaper than crack and produces a similar but longer-lasting euphoria. The use of ice can quickly lead to dependence. In a recent survey of high school students, about 4% reported having tried ice at least once.

EFFECTS   Small doses of amphetamines usually make people feel more alert and wide-awake and less fatigued or bored. Amphetamines generally increase motor activity but do not measurably alter a normal, rested person's ability to perform tasks calling for challenging motor skills or complex thinking. When amphetamines do improve performance, it is primarily by counteracting fatigue and boredom. Amphetamines in small doses also increase heart rate and blood pressure and change sleep patterns.

Amphetamines are sometimes used to curb appetite, but after a few weeks the user develops tolerance, and higher doses are necessary. When people stop taking the drug, their appetite usually returns, and they gain back the weight they lost unless they have made permanent changes in eating behavior.

FROM USE TO ABUSE   Much amphetamine abuse begins as an attempt to cope with a temporary situation. A student cramming for an exam or an exhausted long-haul truck driver can go a little longer by taking amphetamines, but the results can be disastrous. The likelihood of making bad judgments significantly increases. The stimulating effects may also wear off suddenly, and the user may precipitously feel exhausted or fall asleep ("crash").

Another problem is **state dependence**, the phenomenon whereby information learned in a certain drug-induced state is difficult to recall when the person is not in that same physiological state. Test performance may deteriorate when students use drugs to study and then take tests in their normal, nondrug state. (Users of antihistamines may also experience state dependence.)

DEPENDENCE   Repeated use of amphetamines, even in moderate doses, often leads to tolerance and the need for increasingly larger doses. The result can be severe disturbances in behavior, including a temporary state of paranoid **psychosis,** with delusions of persecution and unprovoked violence. If injected in large doses, amphetamines produce a feeling of intense pleasure, followed by sensations of vigor and euphoria that last for several hours. As these feelings wear off, they are replaced by feelings of irritability and vague uneasiness. Long-term use of amphetamines at high doses can cause paranoia, hallucinations, delusions, and incoherence. Researchers have also identified signs of brain damage in methamphetamine users that appear to persist even after drug use ceases, causing impaired memory and motor coordination. Withdrawal symptoms may include muscle aches and tremors, along with profound fatigue, deep depression, despair, and apathy. Chronic high-dose amphetamine use is often associated with pronounced psychological cravings and obsessive drug-seeking behavior.

Women who use amphetamines during pregnancy risk premature birth, stillbirth, and early infant death. Babies born to amphetamine-using mothers have a higher incidence of cleft palate, cleft lip, and deformed limbs. They may also be born dependent on amphetamines.

Ritalin
A stimulant with effects similar to amphetamines, Ritalin (methylphenidate) is used to treat attention-deficit/hyperactivity disorder. When taken orally at

prescribed levels, it has little potential for abuse. When injected or snorted, however, dependence and tolerance can rapidly result. Ritalin abuse among high school and college students began to be reported in the 1990s.

Ephedrine   Amphetamine was made in the 1920s by modifying the chemical ephedrine, which was originally isolated from a Chinese herbal tea. Although somewhat less potent than amphetamine, ephedrine does produce stimulant effects. It is found in OTC weight-loss preparations, energy-boosting supplements, and a product known as "herbal ecstasy." Uncontrolled use of ephedrine has been associated with some deaths. The FDA recently banned the chemically similar compound phenyl-propanolamine (PPA) because it increases the risk of stroke.

Caffeine   Caffeine is probably the most popular psychoactive drug and also one of the most ancient. It is found in coffee, tea, cocoa, soft drinks, headache remedies, and OTC preparations like No-Dōz. In ordinary doses, caffeine produces greater alertness and a sense of well-being. It also decreases feelings of fatigue or boredom, and using caffeine may enable a person to keep at physically exhausting or repetitive tasks longer. Such use is usually followed, however, by a sudden letdown. Caffeine does not noticeably influence a person's ability to perform complex intellectual tasks unless fatigue, boredom, alcohol, or other factors have already affected normal performance.

Caffeine mildly stimulates the heart and respiratory system, increases muscular tremor, and enhances gastric secretion. Higher doses may cause nervousness, anxiety, irritability, headache, disturbed sleep, and gastric irritation or peptic ulcers. In people with high blood pressure, caffeine can cause blood pressure to rise even further above normal. Some people, especially children, are quite vulnerable to the adverse effects of caffeine. They become "wired"—hyperactive and overly sensitive to any stimulation in their environment. In rare instances, the disturbance is so severe that there is misperception of their surroundings—a toxic psychosis.

Drinks containing caffeine are rarely harmful for most individuals, but some tolerance develops, and withdrawal symptoms of irritability, headaches, and even mild depression do occur. Thus, although we don't usually think of caffeine as a dependence-producing drug, for some people it is. People can usually avoid problems by simply decreasing their daily intake of caffeine (Figure 9-3).

Marijuana and Other Cannabis Products

Marijuana is the most widely used illegal drug in the United States (cocaine is second). More than 30% of Americans—more than 70 million—have tried marijuana at least once; among 18–25-year-olds, more than 45% have tried marijuana. Recent surveys of college stu-

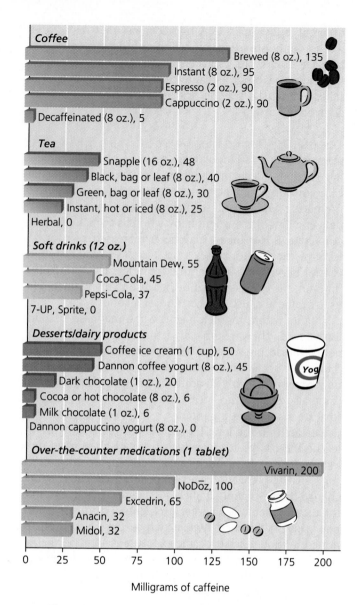

Figure 9-3   Common sources of caffeine.   The caffeine content of products varies with the brand and preparation method; the values shown here are averages. Among Americans, the average daily intake of caffeine is about 230 milligrams.   SOURCES: Become a bean counter. 2000. *Prevention*, July. International Food Information Council. 1998. *IFIC Review: Caffeine and Health* (http://ificinfo.health.org/review/ircaffh.htm; retrieved October 8, 2000). Caffeine content of foods and drugs. 1996. *Nutrition Action Healthletter*, December.

dents indicate that about 17% used marijuana within the past month.

Marijuana is a crude preparation of various parts of the Indian hemp plant *Cannabis sativa*, which grows in most parts of the world. THC (tetrahydrocannabinol) is the main active ingredient in marijuana. Based on THC content, the potency of marijuana preparations varies widely. Marijuana plants that grow wild often have less than 1% THC in their leaves, whereas when selected strains are cultivated by separation of male and female plants

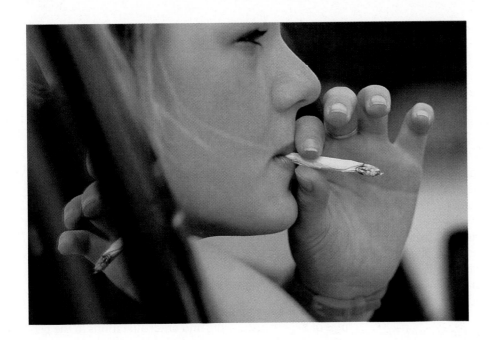

Marijuana is the most widely used illegal drug in the United States. At low doses, marijuana users typically experience euphoria and a relaxed attitude. Further research is needed to determine its precise physiological and psychological effects, particularly for chronic use.

(*sinsemilla*), the bud leaves from the flowering tops may contain 7–8% THC. Hashish, a potent preparation made from the thick resin that exudes from the leaves, may contain up to 14% THC. These various preparations have all been known and used for centuries, so the frequently heard claim that today's marijuana is more potent than the marijuana of the 1970s is not strictly true. However, a greater proportion of the marijuana sold today may be the higher potency (and more expensive) sinsemilla.

Marijuana is usually smoked, but it can also be ingested. The classification of marijuana is a matter of some debate. For this reason, it is treated separately here.

Short-Term Effects and Uses

As is true with most psychoactive drugs, the effects of a low dose of marijuana are strongly influenced both by the user's expectations and by past experiences. At low doses, marijuana users typically experience euphoria, a heightening of subjective sensory experiences, a slowing down of the perception of passing time, and a relaxed, "laid-back" attitude. These pleasant effects are the reason this drug is so widely used. With moderate doses, these effects become stronger, and the user can also expect to have impaired memory function, disturbed thought patterns, lapses of attention, and feelings of **depersonalization,** in which the mind seems to be separated from the body. Decreased driving and workplace safety can also be expected.

The effects of marijuana in higher doses are determined mostly by the drug itself rather than by the user's expectations and setting. Very high doses produce feelings of depersonalization, as well as marked sensory distortion and changes in body image (such as a feeling that the body is very light). Inexperienced users sometimes think these sensations mean they are going crazy and be-

come anxious or even panicky. Such reactions resemble a bad trip on LSD, but they happen much less often, are less severe, and do not last as long. However, unexpected reactions are the leading reason for emergency room visits by users of marijuana or hashish. And marijuana/hashish is now cited more frequently than heroin as a reason for emergency room visits, although heroin is involved in far more deaths than marijuana each year.

Physiologically, marijuana increases heart rate and dilates certain blood vessels in the eyes, which creates the characteristic bloodshot eyes. The user also feels less inclined toward physical exertion.

The question of whether marijuana has any medical uses has been hotly debated. Cannabis preparations were once medically prescribed for a variety of illnesses, but most such uses are no longer supported by research. A legal, prescription form of THC called dronabinol has been available in a capsule for some patients since 1985; however, many patients argue that oral THC is not as effective as smoked marijuana. A 1999 government-commissioned report from the Institute of Medicine concluded that substances in marijuana have potential therapeutic value for pain relief, for control of nausea and vomiting in chemotherapy patients, and for stimulating appetite in people with AIDS-related wasting. Although effective drugs already exist for these conditions, marijuana may be suitable for patients who do not respond to other therapies. The report recommends further studies and the

---

depersonalization A state in which a person loses the sense of his or her own reality or perceives his or her own body as unreal.

Terms

development of alternative methods of drug delivery—inhalers or patches—that would safely deliver set doses of specific compounds in marijuana.

Long-Term Effects The most probable long-term effect of smoking marijuana is respiratory damage, including chronic bronchial irritation and precancerous changes in the lungs. People who smoke marijuana may be at increased risk for emphysema and cancer of the head and neck. (These negative effects from smoking marijuana are key reasons why the Institute of Medicine report on medical marijuana recommended the development of alternative methods of delivering the potentially beneficial compounds in marijuana.) Heavy users who are frequently intoxicated experience subtle impairments of attention and memory that may or may not be reversible following long-term abstinence. Long-term use may also decrease testosterone levels and sperm counts and increase sperm abnormalities.

Heavy marijuana use during pregnancy may cause impaired fetal growth and development and low birth weight. Marijuana may act synergistically with alcohol to increase the damaging effects of alcohol on the fetus. THC rapidly enters breast milk and may impair an infant's early motor development.

When we consider the long-term effects of marijuana (and of any other drugs), we should keep in mind the time-lag factor. Tobacco, for example, was long thought to be a "harmless" drug. Widespread marijuana use has been common for only about 30 years, and some effects may take longer than that to appear and be linked to marijuana.

Dependence Regular users of marijuana can develop tolerance; a few develop dependence. Withdrawal symptoms are generally mild and short-lived; they include restlessness, irritability, insomnia, nausea, and cramping. As with all drugs that relieve "bad" feelings and produce "good" feelings, marijuana can become the focus of the user's life, to the exclusion of other activities. Drug uses appear to be related, and the chronic marijuana user is more likely to be a heavy user of tobacco, alcohol, and other dangerous drugs.

Hallucinogens

Hallucinogens are a group of drugs whose predominant pharmacological effect is to alter the user's perceptions, feelings, and thoughts. Hallucinogens include LSD (lysergic acid diethylamide), mescaline, psilocybin, STP (dimethoxymethyl amphetamine), DMT (dimethyltryptamine), MDMA (3,4-methylene-dioxymethamphetamine), ketamine, and PCP (phencyclidine). These drugs are most commonly ingested or smoked.

LSD LSD is one of the most powerful psychoactive drugs. Tiny doses will produce noticeable effects in most people, such as an altered sense of time, visual disturbances, an improved sense of hearing, mood changes, and distortions in how people perceive their bodies. Dilation of the pupils and slight dizziness, weakness, and nausea may also occur. With larger doses, users may experience a phenomenon known as **synesthesia**, feelings of depersonalization, and other alterations in the perceived relationship between self and external reality.

Many hallucinogens induce tolerance so quickly that after only one or two doses, their effects decrease substantially. The user must then stop taking the drug for several days before his or her system can be receptive to it again. These drugs cause little drug-seeking behavior and no physical dependence or withdrawal symptoms.

The immediate effects of low doses of hallucinogens are largely determined by expectations and setting. Many effects are hard to describe because they involve subjective and unusual dimensions of awareness—the **altered states of consciousness** for which these drugs are famous. For this reason, hallucinogens have acquired a certain aura not associated with other drugs. People have taken LSD in search of a religious or mystical experience or in the hope of exploring new worlds. During the 1960s, some psychiatrists gave LSD to their patients to help them talk about their repressed feelings.

A severe panic reaction, which can be terrifying in the extreme, can result from taking any dose of LSD. It is impossible to predict when a panic reaction will occur. Some LSD users report having hundreds of pleasurable and ecstatic experiences before having a "bad trip," or "bummer." If the user is already in a serene mood and feels no anger or hostility and if he or she is in secure surroundings with trusted companions, a bad trip may be less likely, but a tranquil experience is not guaranteed.

Even after the drug's chemical effects have worn off, spontaneous flashbacks and other psychological disturbances can occur. **Flashbacks** are perceptual distortions and bizarre thoughts that occur after the drug has been entirely eliminated from the body. Although they are relatively rare phenomena, flashbacks can be extremely distressing. They are often triggered by specific psychological cues associated with the drug-taking experience, such as certain mood states or even types of music.

Terms

hallucinogen Any of several drugs that alter perception, feelings, or thoughts; examples are LSD, mescaline, and PCP.

synesthesia A condition in which a stimulus evokes not only the sensation appropriate to it but also another sensation of a different character; such as when a color evokes a specific smell.

altered states of consciousness Profound changes in mood, thinking, and perception.

flashback A perceptual distortion or bizarre thought that recurs after the chemical effects of a drug have worn off.

proprioception The sensation of body position and movement, from muscles, joints, and skin.

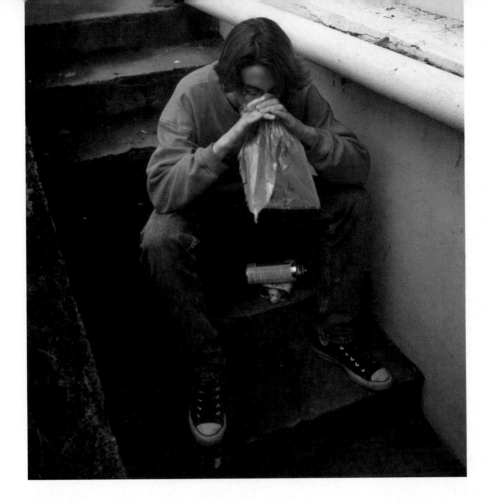

Inhalant use is difficult to monitor and control because inhalants are found in many inexpensive and legal products. Low doses of inhalants may cause a user to feel slightly stimulated; higher concentrations can cause a loss of consciousness, heart failure, and death.

During the 1970s, researchers claimed that LSD damages chromosomes. But later evidence indicates that LSD in moderate doses, at least the pure LSD produced in the laboratory, does not damage chromosomes, cause detectable genetic damage, or produce birth defects.

Other Hallucinogens Most other hallucinogens have the same general effects as LSD, but there are some variations. For example, a DMT or ketamine high does not last as long as an LSD high; an STP high lasts longer. MDMA has both hallucinogenic and amphetamine-like properties. Tolerance to MDMA develops quickly, and high doses can cause anxiety, delusions, and paranoia. (See the box on "Club Drugs" on p. 239 for more on MDMA.)

PCP, also known as "angel dust," "hog," and "peace pill," reduces and distorts sensory input, especially **proprioception,** the sensation of body position and movement; it creates a state of sensory deprivation. PCP was initially used as an anesthetic but was unsatisfactory because it caused agitation, confusion, and delirium (loss of contact with reality). Because it can be easily made, PCP is often available illegally and is sometimes used as an inexpensive replacement for other psychoactive drugs. The effects of ketamine are similar to those of PCP—confusion, agitation, aggression, and lack of coordination—

but tend to be less predictable. Tolerance to either drug can develop rapidly.

Mescaline (peyote), the ceremonial drug of the Native North American Church, produces an experience different from that caused by LSD. Obtaining mescaline costs far more than making LSD, however, so most street mescaline is LSD that has been highly diluted. Hallucinogenic effects can be obtained from certain mushrooms (*Psilocybe mexicana,* or "magic mushrooms"), certain morning glory seeds, nutmeg, jimsonweed, and other botanical products, but unpleasant side effects, such as dizziness, have limited the popularity of these products.

Inhalants

Inhaling certain chemicals can produce effects ranging from heightened pleasure to delirium. Inhalants fall into three major groups: (1) volatile solvents, which include adhesives and aerosols; (2) nitrites, such as butyl nitrite and amyl nitrite; and (3) anesthetics, which include nitrous oxide, or "laughing gas." About 14% of all high school seniors have reported using inhalants.

Inhalant use is difficult to control because inhalants are easy to obtain. They are present in a variety of seemingly harmless products, from dessert-topping sprays to underarm deodorants, that are both inexpensive and legal.

Using the drugs also requires no illegal or suspicious paraphernalia. Inhalant users get high by "sniffing," "snorting," "bagging" (inhaling fumes from a plastic bag), or "huffing" (placing an inhalant-soaked rag in the mouth).

Although different in makeup, nearly all inhalants produce effects similar to those of anesthetics, which slow down body functions. Low doses may cause users to feel slightly stimulated; at higher doses, users may feel less inhibited and less in control. Sniffing high concentrations of the chemicals in solvents or aerosol sprays can cause a loss of consciousness, heart failure, and death. High concentrations of any inhalant can also cause death from suffocation by displacing the oxygen in the lungs and central nervous system. Deliberately inhaling from a bag or in a closed area greatly increases the chances of suffocation. Other possible effects of the excessive or long-term use of inhalants include damage to the nervous system (impaired perception, reasoning, memory, and muscular coordination); hearing loss; and damage to the liver, kidneys, and bone marrow.

> **COMMUNICATE!** One of the hallmarks of drug dependence is denial—the firm belief that one is still in control of one's life or can "quit anytime." Some people don't see their own behavior as matching what they think of as "addiction." If you have not yet answered the questions in the self-assessment on p. 234, do so now. Do your answers suggest that you have a dependency? If so, the best response is honesty with yourself. Only after you admit to yourself that you have a problem with a drug can you begin to figure out how to solve it.

DRUG USE: THE DECADES AHEAD

Drug research will undoubtedly provide new information, new treatments, and new chemical combinations in the decades ahead. New psychoactive drugs may present unexpected possibilities for therapy, social use, and abuse. Making honest and unbiased information about drugs available to everyone, however, may cut down on their abuse. Misinformation about the dangers of drugs— "scare tactics"—can lead some people to disbelieve any reports of drug dangers, no matter how soundly based and well documented they are.

Although the use of some drugs, both legal and illegal, has declined dramatically since the 1970s, the use of others has held steady or increased. Mounting public concern has led to great debate and a wide range of opinions about what should be done. Efforts to combat the problem include workplace drug testing, tougher law enforcement and prosecution, and treatment and education. With drugs entering the country on a massive scale from South America, Southeast Asia, and elsewhere and distributed through tightly controlled drug-smuggling organizations and street gangs, it remains to be seen how effective any program will be.

Drugs, Society, and Families

The economic cost of drug use is staggering. Each year, Americans spend over $50 billion on illegal drugs, with an additional $100 billion going to cover enforcement, prevention, treatment, lost wages, and drug-related injuries and crime. But the costs are more than just financial; they are also paid in human pain and suffering

The relationship between drugs and crime is complex. The criminal justice system is inundated with people accused of crimes related to drug possession, sale, or use. More than 2 million arrests are made each year for drug and alcohol violations, and over 100,000 people are in jail for violating drug laws. Many assaults and murders occur when people try to acquire or protect drug territories, settle disputes about drugs, or steal from dealers. Violence and the use of guns are more common in neighborhoods where drug trafficking is prevalent. Addicts commit more robberies and burglaries than criminals not on drugs. People under the influence of drugs, especially alcohol, are more likely to commit violent crimes like rape and murder than people who do not use drugs. Although often associated with poor inner-city areas, drug-related problems affect every area of the country (see the box "Drug Use in Rural America").

Drug use is also a health care issue for society. In the United States, illegal drug use leads to more than 500,000 emergency room admissions and about 20,000 deaths annually. While it is in the best interest of society to treat addicts who want help, there is not nearly enough space in treatment facilities to help the estimated 5 million Americans in need of immediate treatment. Drug addicts who want to quit, especially those among the urban poor, often have to wait a year or more for acceptance into a residential care or other treatment program.

Drug abuse also takes a toll on individuals and families. Children born to women who use drugs like alcohol, tobacco, or cocaine may have long-term health problems. Drug use in families can become a vicious cycle. Observing adults around them using drugs, children assume it is an acceptable way to deal with problems. Other problems like abuse, neglect, lack of opportunity, and unemployment become contributing factors to drug use and serve to perpetuate the cycle.

Legalizing Drugs

Pointing out that many of the social problems associated with drugs are related to prohibition rather than to the effects of the drugs themselves, some people have argued for various forms of drug legalization. Proposals range from making such drugs as marijuana and heroin available by prescription to allowing licensed dealers to sell

Most people associate drug abuse problems with big cities. However, a recent report that examined drug use patterns in the United States found that small cities and rural areas have rates of drug abuse and related problems that are as high as or even higher than the rates in large cities. Adults in rural areas are just as likely as those in urban centers to use and abuse illegal drugs, alcohol, and tobacco. Young teens in small cities and rural areas are even more likely to abuse substances than teens in large metropolitan areas. Eighth-graders living in rural America are

- 104% more likely to use amphetamines
- 83% more likely to use crack
- 50% more likely to use cocaine
- 34% more likely to smoke marijuana
- 29% more likely to drink alcohol, and 70% more likely to get drunk

In addition, rural eighth-graders are more than twice as likely to smoke cigarettes and nearly five times as likely to use spit tobacco. The trend continues for older teens: Among tenth-graders living in rural areas, rates of drug use exceed those for tenth-graders in large urban areas for every drug except MDMA (ecstasy) and marijuana. One group at particular risk for drug use and related problems is Native American teens living on reservations. A high rate of drug use among young teens is of particular concern because the earlier people begin to use drugs, the more likely they are to suffer serious medical and social consequences.

Along with higher rates of drug use come higher rates of drug-related problems—legal, medical, and social. In the 1990s, the smaller the community, the faster the rate of increase in drug-related crimes. Arrest rates for DUIs in small cities and rural areas are more than double those of large cities. The proportion of teens and young adults who have used drugs intravenously is greatest in rural areas; related to this, AIDS cases since 1994 have increased at a greater rate in rural areas (82%) than in large metropolitan areas (59%). In addition, more workers in rural areas test positive for drugs, which can lead to higher rates of absenteeism, unemployment, and job-related injuries.

Small cities and rural areas also face greater challenges in dealing with substance abuse problems. Drugs are equally available in all areas of the United States: In surveys, the percentage of people in rural towns, small cities, and large urban areas who report that drugs are "very easy" or "fairly easy" to obtain is essentially the same. However, rural areas must tackle drug-related problems with less information and fewer resources. Due to stereotypes about drug abuse patterns in the United States, there has been little research examining the drug problem in rural areas. Rural communities have a smaller tax base, making it difficult for substance abuse service providers to achieve the economies of scale needed to provide effective treatment services. Thus, most people in rural areas who need services must travel long distances for treatment or go without help. Smaller cities and rural areas also lack the money, personnel, and expertise to deal with drug trafficking organizations.

SOURCE: National Center on Addiction and Substance Abuse. 2000. *No Place to Hide: Substance Abuse in Mid-Size Cities and Rural America.* New York: National Center on Addiction and Substance Abuse.

---

some of these drugs to adults. Proponents argue that crimes by drug users are usually committed to buy drugs that cost relatively more than alcohol and tobacco because they are produced illegally. By making some currently illicit drugs legal—but putting controls on them similar to those used for alcohol, tobacco, and prescription drugs—many of the problems related to drug use could be eliminated.

Opponents of drug legalization argue that allowing easier access to drugs would expose many more people to possible abuse and dependence. Drugs would be cheaper and easier to obtain, and drug use would be more socially acceptable. Legalizing drugs could cause an increase in drug use among children and teenagers. Opponents point out that alcohol and tobacco are major causes of disease and death in our society and that they should not be used as models for other practices.

Drug Testing

One of the most controversial issues in American politics is drug testing in the workplace. It has been estimated that as many as 10% of workers use psychoactive drugs on the job. For some occupations, such as air traffic controllers, truck drivers, and train engineers, drug use can create significant hazards, sometimes involving hundreds of people. Some people believe that the dangers are so great that all workers should be tested and that anyone found with traces of drugs in the blood or urine should be either fired or treated. Others insist that this would violate people's right to privacy and to freedom from unreasonable search, guaranteed by the Fourth Amendment. Opponents point out that most jobs do not involve hazards, so employees who take drugs are not any more dangerous than employees who do not.

Despite the expense, many employers now test their employees, and the U.S. armed forces test military personnel regularly. People in jobs involving transportation—truck drivers, bus drivers, train engineers, airline pilots—are required by federal law to be tested regularly to ensure public safety. The primary criterion leading most companies to use drug testing is the company's liability if an employee under the influence of a drug makes a mistake that could potentially harm others.

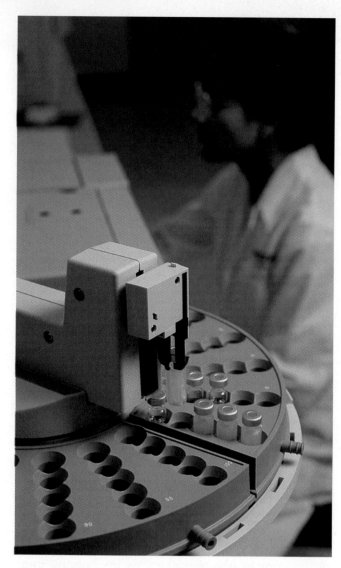

Many companies test current and prospective employees for drug use. Most drug testing involves a urine test that can detect recent use of marijuana, heroin, cocaine, amphetamines, codeine, and many other psychoactive drugs.

Most drug testing involves a urine test; a test for alcohol uses a blood test or a breath test. The accuracy of these tests has been improved in recent years, so there are fewer opportunities for people to cheat or for the tests to yield inaccurate results. If a person tests positive for drugs, the employer may provide drug counseling or treatment, suspend the employee until he or she tests negative, or fire the individual.

The FDA has approved several over-the-counter home drug testing kits designed to allow parents to check their children for drug use. For one type, a urine sample is collected at home and sent to a laboratory for analysis; results are available by phone. Another type provides preliminary results in 10 minutes, but final results also require follow-up laboratory testing.

Treatment for Drug Dependence

A variety of programs are available to help people break their drug habits, but there is no single best method of treatment. The relapse rate is high for all types of treatment but is similar to the rate of relapse seen in people being treated for diabetes, high blood pressure, and asthma. Numerous studies have shown that being treated is better than not being treated. To be successful, a treatment program must deal with the reasons behind people's drug abuse and help them develop behaviors, attitudes, and a social support system that will help them remain drug-free.

Drug Substitution Programs Sometimes a less debilitating drug can be substituted for one with many damaging effects, thus reducing the risks of the drug use. Methadone is a synthetic drug used as a substitute for heroin. When methadone is used, addicts can stop taking heroin without experiencing severe withdrawal reactions. Although methadone is addictive, it decreases the craving for heroin and enables the individual to function normally in social and vocational activities. Methadone maintenance treatment allows many former heroin abusers to live more useful lives. Other heroin substitutes in use or being studied include LAAM (levo-alpha-acetylmethadol), buprenorphine, and naltrexone.

Because they are relatively inexpensive to administer, drug substitution programs are a popular form of treatment. However, the relapse rate is high. Combining drug substitution with psychological and social services improves success rates, underscoring the importance of psychological factors in drug dependence.

Treatment Centers Treatment centers offer a variety of short-term and long-term services, including hospitalization, detoxification, counseling, and other mental health services. A specific type of center is the therapeutic community, a residential program run in a completely drug-free atmosphere. Administered by ex-addicts, these programs use confrontation, strict discipline, and unrelenting peer pressure to attempt to resocialize the addict with a different set of values. "Halfway houses," transitional settings between a 24-hour-a-day program and independent living, are an important phase of treatment for some people. Strategies for evaluating programs are given in the box "Choosing a Drug-Treatment Program."

Self-Help Groups and Peer Counseling Groups such as Alcoholics Anonymous (AA) and Narcotics Anonymous (NA) have helped many people. People treated in drug substitution programs or substance-abuse treatment centers are often urged or required to join a self-help group as part of their recovery. These groups follow a 12-step program. Group members' first step is to acknowledge that they have a problem over which they have

When evaluating different facilities or programs for drug treatment, consider the following issues:

- *What type of treatment or facility is most appropriate?* Intensive outpatient treatment is available through many community mental health centers, as well as through specialized drug-treatment facilities. Such programs typically require several sessions per week, combining individual therapy, group counseling, and attendance at 12-step meetings. Residential, or inpatient, facilities may be associated with a medical facility such as a hospital, or they may be free-standing programs that focus solely on substance-abuse treatment. Some residential treatment programs last longer or cost more per week than many health insurance plans will cover.

- *How will treatment be paid for?* Many health insurance plans limit residential treatment to a maximum of 3 weeks or less. They may also require that you first attempt a less expensive form of treatment before they will approve coverage for a residential facility.

- *Is there likely to be a need for medical support?* Chronic alcoholics or abusers of other CNS depressants may experience life-threatening seizures or other withdrawal symptoms during the first few days of detoxification. Malnutrition is common among substance abusers, and injection drug users may suffer from local infections and bloodborne diseases such as hepatitis or HIV infection. Medical problems such as these are best handled in an inpatient program with good medical support.

- *What is the level of professional training of the staff?* Is there a medical doctor on-site or making frequent visits? Are there trained nurses? Licensed psychologists or social workers? Many successful programs are staffed primarily by recovering alcoholics or drug users. Do those staff members have training and certification as addiction specialists or some other license or certificate?

- *Can the program provide the names of previous clients who would be willing to talk to you?* The best way to learn about the true nature of a program is to talk with someone who has been through it.

- *Does the program provide related services, such as family and job counseling and post-treatment follow-up?* These types of services are extremely important for the long-term success of drug-abuse treatment.

- *Can you visit the facility and speak with the staff and clients?* A prospective client and his or her family should be allowed to visit any treatment center or program. There used to be a small number of restricted-access programs that isolated clients from their families and demanded total dedication.

---

no control. Peer support is a critical ingredient of these programs, and members usually meet at least once a week. Each member is paired with a sponsor to call on for advice and support if the temptation to relapse becomes overwhelming. With such support, thousands of substance-dependent people have been able to recover, remain abstinent, and reclaim their lives. Chapters of AA and NA meet on some college campuses; community-based chapters are listed in the phone book and local newspapers. (Also see the For More Information section at the end of the chapter.)

Many colleges also have peer counseling programs, in which students are trained to help other students who have drug problems. A peer counselor's role may be as limited as referring a student to a professional with expertise in substance dependence for an evaluation or as involved as helping arrange a leave of absence from school for participation in a drug-treatment program. Most peer counseling programs are founded on principles of strict confidentiality. Peer counselors may also be able to help students who are concerned about a classmate or loved one with an apparent drug problem (see the box "If Someone You Know Has a Drug Problem . . . "). Information about peer counseling programs is usually available from the student health center.

Codependency   Many treatment programs also offer counseling for those who are close to drug abusers. Drug abuse takes a toll on friends and family members, and counseling can help people work through painful feelings of guilt and powerlessness. Sometimes people close to a drug abuser develop patterns of behavior, known as **codependency,** that help or enable the person to remain drug dependent. Codependency, also called *enabling,* removes or softens the effects of the drug use on the user. People often become enablers spontaneously and naturally. When someone they love becomes dependent on a drug, they want to help, and they may assume that their good intentions will persuade the drug user to stop.

However, the habit of enabling may actually inhibit a drug-dependent person's recovery because the person never has to experience the consequences of his or her behavior. Often, the enabler is dependent, too—on the patterns of interaction in the relationship. People who need to take care of people often marry people who need to be

codependency A relationship in which a non–substance-abusing partner or family member enables the other's substance abuse.

Terms

If you notice changes in behavior and mood in someone you know, they may signal a growing dependence on drugs. Signs that a person's life is beginning to focus on drugs include the following:

- Sudden withdrawal or emotional distance
- Rebellious or unusually irritable behavior
- A loss of interest in usual activities or hobbies
- A decline in school performance
- A sudden change in the chosen group of friends
- Changes in sleeping or eating habits
- Frequent borrowing of money or stealing
- Secretive behavior about personal possessions, such as a backpack or the contents of a drawer
- Deterioration of physical appearance

If you believe a family member or friend has a drug problem, obtain information about resources for drug treatment available on your campus or in your community. Communicate your concern, provide him or her with information about treatment options, and offer your support during treatment. If the person continues to deny having a problem, you may want to talk with an experienced counselor about setting up an "intervention"— a formal, structured confrontation designed to end denial by having family, friends, and other caring individuals present their concerns to the drug user. Participants in an intervention would indicate the ways in which the individual is hurting others as well as himself or herself. If your friend or family member agrees to treatment, encourage him or her to attend a support group such as Narcotics Anonymous or Alcoholics Anonymous. And finally, examine your relationship with the abuser for signs of codependency. If necessary, get help for yourself; friends and family of drug users can often benefit from counseling.

taken care of. Children in these families often develop the same behavior pattern as one of their parents, by either becoming helpless or becoming a caregiver. For this reason, many treatment programs involve the whole family.

Have you ever been an enabler in a relationship? You may have, if you've ever done any of the following:

- Given someone one more chance to stop abusing drugs, then another, and another . . .
- Made excuses or lied for someone to his or her friends, teachers, or employer
- Joined someone in drug use and blamed others for your behavior
- Loaned money to someone to continue drug use
- Stayed up late waiting for or gone out searching for someone who uses drugs
- Felt embarrassed or angry about the actions of someone who uses drugs
- Ignored the drug use because the person got defensive when you brought it up
- Not confronted a friend or relative who was obviously intoxicated or high on a drug

If you come from a codependent family or see yourself developing codependency relationships, consider acting now to make changes in your patterns of interaction.

Preventing Drug Abuse

Obviously, the best solution to drug abuse is prevention. Government attempts at controlling the drug problem tend to focus on stopping the production, importation, and distribution of illegal drugs. Creative effort also has to be put

into stopping the demand for drugs. Developing persuasive antidrug educational programs offers the best hope for solving the drug problem in the future. Indirect approaches to prevention involve building young people's self-esteem, improving their academic skills, and increasing their recreational opportunities. Direct approaches involve giving information about the adverse effects of drugs and teaching tactics that help students resist peer pressure to use drugs in various situations. Developing strategies for resisting peer pressure is one of the more effective techniques.

Prevention efforts need to focus on the different motivations individuals have for using and abusing specific drugs at different ages. For example, grade school children seem receptive to programs that involve their parents or well-known adults like professional athletes. Adolescents in junior or senior high school are often more responsive to peer counselors. Many young adults tend to be influenced by efforts that focus on health education. For all ages, it is important to provide nondrug alternatives that speak to the individual's or group's specific reasons for using drugs, such as recreational facilities, counseling, greater opportunities for leisure activities, and places to socialize. Reminding young people that most people, no matter what age, are *not* users of illegal drugs, do *not* smoke cigarettes, and do *not* get drunk frequently is a critical part of preventing substance abuse.

The Role of Drugs in Your Life

Where do you fit into this complex picture of drug use and abuse? Chances are that you've had experience with OTC and prescription drugs, and you may or may not have had experience with one or more of the drugs described in this chapter. You probably know someone who has used or abused a psychoactive drug. Whatever your experience has been up to now, it's likely that you will encounter drugs at some point in your life. To make sure you'll have the inner resources to resist peer pressure and make your own decision, cultivate a variety of activities you enjoy doing, realize that you are entitled to have your own opinion, and don't neglect your self-esteem.

Issues to Consider   Before you try a psychoactive drug, consider the following questions:

- *What are the risks involved?* Many drugs carry an immediate risk of injury or death. Almost all involve the longer-term risk of abuse and dependence.

- *Is using the drug compatible with your goals?* Consider how drug use will affect your education and career objectives, your relationships, your future happiness, and the happiness of those who love you.

- *What are your ethical beliefs about drug use?* Consider whether using a drug would cause you to go against your personal ethics, religious beliefs, social values, or family responsibilities.

- *What are the financial costs?* Many drugs are expensive, especially if you become dependent on them.

- *Are you trying to solve a deeper problem?* Drugs will not make emotional pain go away; in the long run, they will only make it worse. If you are feeling depressed or anxious, seek help from a mental health professional instead of self-medicating with drugs.

Like all aspects of health-related behavior, making responsible decisions about drug use depends on information, knowledge, and insight into yourself. Many choices are possible; making the ones that are right for you is what counts.

What to Do Instead of Drugs   If you have used or considered using drugs, think carefully about your reasons for doing so. Consider trying healthier strategies for dealing with difficult emotions and peer pressure. For ideas, look over the following list of reasons for drug use and suggested alternative activities:

- *Bored?* Go for a walk or a run; stimulate your senses at a museum or a movie; challenge your mind with a new game or book; introduce yourself to someone new.

- *Stressed?* Practice relaxation or visualization; try to slow down and open your senses to the natural world; get some exercise.

- *Shy or lonely?* Talk to a counselor; enroll in a shyness clinic; learn and practice communication techniques.

- *Feeling low on self-esteem?* Focus on the areas in which you are competent; give yourself credit for the things you do well. A program of regular exercise can also enhance self-esteem.

- *Depressed or anxious?* Talk to a friend, parent, or counselor.

- *Apathetic or lethargic?* Force yourself to get up and get some exercise to energize yourself; assume responsibility for someone or something outside yourself; volunteer.

- *Searching for meaning?* Try yoga or meditation; explore spiritual experiences through religious groups, church, prayer, or reading.

- *Afraid to say no?* Take a course in assertiveness training; get support from others who don't want to use drugs; remind yourself that you have the right and the responsibility to make your own decisions.

- *Still feeling peer pressure?* Begin to look for new friends or roommates. Take a class or join an organization that attracts other health-conscious people.

Tips for Today

The essence of wellness is taking charge of your life. Dependence on drugs or compulsive activities is the very opposite of wellness, since it involves relinquishing control over your life to chemical substances or forces outside yourself. The best treatment for dependence is prevention—not starting in the first place—but it's never too late to regain control of your life.

Right now you can

- Go outside and sit on a park bench, or walk around outside at half your normal pace, opening all your senses to the beauty of nature. If you can't get to a beautiful place, close your eyes and visualize one. See if you can experience a "natural high."

- Substitute some bottled water for your caffeinated soda, and make your next cup of coffee half decaf.

- Consider whether someone you love has a drug problem; if so, consider how you can best help that person face and solve the problem.

- Plan to get enough sleep this week, so you won't feel the need for stimulants to be awake and alert.

- Examine what you've been doing lately to see if you are truly making your own decisions—or if some substance or out-of-control behavior has you in its power; if so, start thinking about how to regain control.

SUMMARY

- Addictive behaviors are reinforcing. Addicts experience a strong compulsion for the behavior and a loss of control over it; an escalating pattern of abuse with serious negative consequences may result.

- The sources or causes of addiction include heredity,

This behavior change strategy focuses on one of the most commonly used drugs—caffeine. If you are concerned about your use of a different drug or another type of addictive behavior, you can devise your own plan based on this one and on the steps outlined in Chapter 1.

Because caffeine supports certain behaviors that are characteristic of our culture, such as sedentary, stressful work, you may find yourself relying on coffee (or tea, chocolate, or cola) to get through a busy schedule. Such habits often begin in college. Fortunately, it's easier to break a habit before it becomes entrenched as a lifelong dependency.

When you are studying for exams, the forced physical inactivity and the need to concentrate even when fatigued may lead you to overuse caffeine. But caffeine doesn't "help" unless you are already sleepy. And it does not relieve any underlying condition (you are just more tired when it wears off). How can you change this pattern?

Self-Monitoring

Keep a log of how much caffeine you eat or drink. Use a measuring cup to measure coffee or tea. Using Figure 9-3, convert the amounts you eat or drink into an estimate expressed in milligrams of caffeine. Be sure to include all forms, such as chocolate bars and OTC medications, as well as caffeine candy, colas, cocoa or hot chocolate, chocolate cake, tea, and coffee.

Self-Assessment

At the end of the week, add up your daily totals and divide by 7 to get your daily average in milligrams. How much is too much? At more than 250 mg per day, you may well be experiencing some adverse symptoms. If you are experiencing at least five of the following symptoms, you may want to cut down.

- Restlessness
- Nervousness
- Excitement
- Insomnia
- Flushed face
- Excessive sweating

- Gastrointestinal problems
- Muscle twitching
- Rambling thoughts and speech
- Irregular heartbeat
- Periods of inexhaustibility
- Excessive pacing or movement

Set Limits

Can you restrict your caffeine intake to a daily total, and stick to this contract? If so, set a cutoff point, such as one cup of coffee. Pegging it to a specific time of day can be helpful, because then you won't confront a decision at any other point (and possibly fail). If you find you cannot stick to your limit, you may want to cut out caffeine altogether; abstinence can be easier than moderation for some people. If you experience caffeine withdrawal symptoms (headache, fatigue), you may want to cut your intake more gradually.

Find Other Ways to Keep Your Energy Up

If you are fatigued, it makes sense to get enough sleep or exercise more, rather than drowning the problem in coffee or tea. Different people need different amounts of sleep; you may also need more sleep at different times, such as during a personal crisis or an illness. Also, exercise raises your metabolic rate for hours afterward—a handy fact to exploit when you want to feel more awake and want to avoid an irritable caffeine jag. And if you've been compounding your fatigue by not eating properly, try filling up on complex carbohydrates such as whole-grain bread or crackers instead of candy bars.

Tips on Cutting Out Caffeine Here are some more ways to decrease your consumption of caffeine:

- Keep some noncaffeinated drinks on hand, such as decaffeinated coffee, herbal teas, mineral water, bouillon, or hot water.
- Alternate between hot and very cold liquids.
- Fill your coffee cup only halfway.
- Avoid the office or school lunchroom or cafeteria and the chocolate sections of the grocery store. (Often people drink coffee or tea and eat chocolate simply because they're available.)
- Read labels of over-the-counter medications to check for hidden sources of caffeine.

---

personality, lifestyle, and environmental factors. People may use an addictive behavior as a means of alleviating stress or painful emotions.

- Many common behaviors are potentially addictive, including gambling, shopping, sexual activity, Internet use, eating, and working.
- Drug abuse is a maladaptive pattern of drug use that persists despite adverse social, psychological, or medical consequences.
- Drug dependence involves taking a drug compulsively, which includes neglecting constructive activities because of it and continuing to use it despite

experiencing adverse effects resulting from its use. Tolerance and withdrawal symptoms are often present.

- Risk factors for drug use include being male, being young, having frequent exposure to drugs, and having a risk-taking personality.
- Reasons for using drugs include the lure of the illicit; curiosity; rebellion; peer pressure; and the desire to alter one's mood or escape boredom, anxiety, depression, or other psychological problems.
- Psychoactive drugs affect the mind and body by altering brain chemistry. The effect of a drug depends

on the properties of the drug and how it's used (drug factors), the physical and psychological characteristics of the user (user factors), and the physical and social environment surrounding drug use (social factors).

- Opioids relieve pain, cause drowsiness, and induce euphoria; they reduce anxiety and produce lethargy, apathy, and an inability to concentrate.

- CNS depressants slow down the overall activity of the nerves; they reduce anxiety and cause mood changes, impaired muscular coordination, slurring of speech, and drowsiness or sleep.

- CNS stimulants speed up the activity of the nerves, causing acceleration of the heart rate, a rise in blood pressure, dilation of the pupils and bronchial tubes, and an increase in gastric and adrenal secretions.

- Marijuana usually causes euphoria and a relaxed attitude at low doses; very high doses produce feelings of depersonalization and sensory distortion. The long-term effects may include chronic bronchi-

tis and cancer; use during pregnancy may impair fetal growth.

- Hallucinogens alter perception, feelings, and thought and may cause an altered sense of time, visual disturbances, and mood changes.

- Inhalants are present in a variety of harmless products; they can cause delirium. Their use can lead to loss of consciousness, heart failure, suffocation, and death.

- Economic and social costs of drug abuse include the financial costs of law enforcement, treatment, and health care and the social costs of crime, violence, and family problems. Drug testing and drug legalization have been proposed to address some of the problems related to drug abuse.

- Approaches to treatment include drug substitution programs, treatment centers, self-help groups, and peer counseling; many programs also offer counseling to family members.

TAKE ACTION

1. Find out what types of services are available on your campus or in your community to handle drug dependence and other addictive behaviors. If there are none, what services are needed? Locate the school official and public health agency responsible for your campus and community, and ask why these needs aren't being met.

2. Survey three older adults and three young students about their attitudes toward legalizing marijuana.

Are there any differences? If so, what accounts for these differences? What kinds of reasons do they give for their positions?

3. Look at a current movie or television program, paying special attention to how drug use is portrayed. What messages are being conveyed? If possible, compare a recent movie with a movie made 10–20 years ago. Has the presentation of drug use changed? If so, how?

JOURNAL ENTRY

1. Keep track of your own drug use for a week, noting in your health journal the name of the drug, the approximate dosage, the time of day, and what you think your reasons were for taking each dose. Don't forget to include coffee, soft drinks, and OTC medications. What types of drugs are you taking? Are there any patterns? Are there any signs of abuse or dependence? If you'd like to cut down, begin by making a list of alternative behaviors you could substitute for drug use.

2. *Critical Thinking* Does a woman have an obligation to avoid alcohol and other drugs during pregnancy? What about smoking cigarettes and eating junk food? If she doesn't follow her physician's advice,

should she be held legally responsible for the effects on her child? What rights do the mother and child have in this situation? In your health journal, write an essay stating your opinion; be sure to defend your position.

3. *Critical Thinking* Do you think there is such a thing as the responsible use of illegal psychoactive drugs? Are they a legitimate recreational activity? Would you change any of the current laws governing drugs? If so, how would you draw the line between legitimate and illegitimate use? Write an essay explaining your position.

Books

Dupont, R. L. 2000. *The Selfish Brain: Learning from Addiction.* Center City, Minn.: Hazelden Information and Educational Services. *Explores the biological roots of addiction and various approaches to treatment.*

Escohotado, A. 1999. *A Brief History of Drugs: From the Stone Age to the Stoned Age.* Rochester, Vt.: Inner Traditions. *A history of human involvement with psychoactive plants and drugs that explores the cultural, spiritual, and social effects of drug use.*

Hardiman, M., and M. Russell. 2000. *Overcoming Addiction: A Common Sense Approach.* Freedom, Calif.: Crossing Press. *A practical guide to the nature of addiction and how to find help.*

Hurley, J. A. 2000. *Addiction: Opposing Viewpoints.* San Diego: Greenhaven Press. *Explores contrasting views about the roots, contributory factors, and treatment of addiction.*

Julien, R. M. 2001. *A Primer of Drug Action,* 9th ed. New York: Freeman. *A guide to the actions, uses, and side effects of psychoactive drugs.*

Kuhn, C., et al. 1998. *Buzzed: The Straight Facts About the Most Used and Abused Drugs from Alcohol to Ecstasy.* New York: Norton. *An accurate, straightforward guide to commonly used drugs.*

Weinberg, B. A., and B. K. Bealer. 2001. *The World of Caffeine: The Science and Culture of the World's Most Popular Drug.* New York: Routledge. *An interesting history of the use of caffeine.*

WW. Organizations, Hotlines, and Web Sites

Addiction: Close to Home. Created to accompany a PBS television series on addiction, this site provides information about prevention, treatment, and public policy; it also includes animated illustrations of how drugs affect the brain.

http://www.pbs.org/wnet/closetohome/home.html

Center for On-Line Addiction. Contains information about Internet and cybersex addiction.

http://netaddiction.com

ClubDrugs.Org. Provides information on drugs commonly classified as "club drugs."

http://www.clubdrugs.org

Do It Now Foundation. Provides youth-oriented information about drugs.

http://www.doitnow.org

Drug Enforcement Administration: Drugs of Abuse. Provides basic facts about major drugs of abuse, including penalties for drug trafficking.

http://www.usdoj.gov/dea/concern/abuse/contents.htm

DrugHelp Hotlines. A 24-hour service that provides confidential information and referrals.

800-DRUGHELP; 800-COCAINE; 800-HEROIN; 888-MARIJUANA; 800-RELAPSE

http://www.drughelp.org

Gamblers Anonymous. Includes questions to help diagnose gambling problems and resources for getting help.

http://www.gamblersanonymous.org

Habitsmart. Contains information about addictive behavior, including tips for effectively managing problematic habitual behaviors, a self-scoring alcohol check-up, and links.

http://www.habitsmart.com

Higher Eduction Center for Alcohol and Other Drug Prevention. Gives information about alcohol and drug abuse on campus and links to related sites; it includes an area designed specifically for students.

http://www.edc.org/hec

Indiana Prevention Resource Center. A clearinghouse of information and links on substance-abuse topics, including specific psychoactive drugs and issues such as drug testing and drug legalization.

http://www.drugs.indiana.edu

Narcotics Anonymous (NA). Similar to Alcoholics Anonymous, NA sponsors 12-step meetings and provides other support services for drug abusers.

818-773-9999

http://www.na.org

There are also 12-step programs that focus on specific drugs:

Cocaine Anonymous

http://www.ca.org

Marijuana Anonymous

http://www.marijuana-anonymous.org

National Center on Addiction and Substance Abuse (CASA) at Columbia University. Provides information about the costs of substance abuse to individuals and society.

http://www.casacolumbia.org

National Clearinghouse for Alcohol and Drug Information. Provides statistics, information, and publications on substance abuse, including resources for people who want to help friends and family members overcome substance-abuse problems.

800-729-6686; 301-468-2600

http://www.health.org

National Drug Information, Treatment, and Referral Hotlines. Sponsored by the SAMHSA Center for Substance Abuse Treatment, these hotlines provide information on drug abuse and on HIV infection as it relates to substance abuse; referrals to support groups and treatment programs are available.

800-662-HELP

800-729-6686 (Spanish)

800-487-4889 (TDD for hearing impaired)

National Institute on Drug Abuse. Develops and supports research on drug abuse prevention programs; fact sheets on drugs of abuse are available on the Web site or via recorded phone messages, fax, or mail.

888-644-6432 (Infofax)

http://www.nida.nih.gov; http://www.drugabuse.gov

Office of National Drug Control Policy (ONDCP). Provides information on national and international drug-related topics, including U.S. policies relating to prevention, education, treatment, and enforcement.

http://www.whitehousedrugpolicy.gov

Substance Abuse and Mental Health Services Administration (SAMHSA). Provides statistics, information, and other resources relating to substance-abuse prevention and treatment.

301-443-8956

http://www.samhsa.gov

Web of Addictions. Provides a wealth of information about substance abuse and dependence, including fact sheets, contact information for relevant agencies and organizations, and links to related sites.

http://www.well.com/user/woa

See also the listings for Chapters 10 and 11.

After reading this chapter, you should be able to

- Explain how alcohol is absorbed and metabolized by the body

- Describe the immediate and long-term effects of drinking alcohol

- Define alcohol abuse, binge drinking, and alcoholism and discuss their effects on the drinker and others

- Evaluate the role of alcohol in your life, and list strategies for using it responsibly

The Responsible Use of Alcohol

10

TEST YOUR KNOWLEDGE

1. "Moderate drinking" is having three or fewer drinks per day.
   True or false?

2. How many adults in the United States do not drink any alcohol?
   a. 1 in 10
   b. 1 in 5
   c. 1 in 3

3. If a man and a woman of the same weight drink the same amount of alcohol, the woman will become intoxicated more quickly than the man.
   True or false?

4. Drinking too much alcohol in too short a time can cause death from alcohol poisoning.
   True or false?

5. Drinking coffee will help you sober up.
   True or false?

6. If you are under the influence of alcohol, you are so relaxed that you are less likely to get hurt in a car crash or fall.
   True or false?

ANSWERS

1. FALSE. Moderate drinking is no more than one drink per day for women and no more than two drinks per day for men.

2. C. Most other adults drink lightly and occasionally; a small number of heavy drinkers, about 8.5% of adults, consume more than half of all the alcohol in the United States.

3. TRUE. Women usually have a higher percentage of body fat than men and a less active form of a stomach enzyme that breaks down alcohol. Both factors cause them to become intoxicated more quickly and to a greater degree.

4. TRUE. Drinking rate is very important: Consuming a number of drinks over a period of several hours is likely to cause intoxication, followed by a hangover; chugging the same amount in an hour or less can be lethal.

5. FALSE. Once alcohol has been absorbed by the body, nothing speeds its metabolism.

6. FALSE. Alcohol slows reflexes and impairs coordination. People under the influence have a much greater risk of injury and death from car crashes and falls.

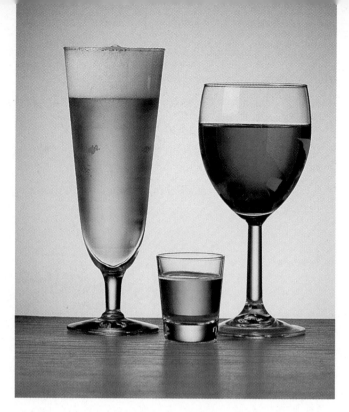

Alcohol has been used in religious ceremonies, in feasts and celebrations, and as a medicine for thousands of years. Throughout history, alcohol has been more popular than any other drug in the Western world, despite numerous prohibitions against it. Alcohol has a somewhat contradictory role in human life. Most of us think of alcohol the way it is portrayed in advertisements, on television, and in movies—as part of good times at the beach, social occasions, and elegant gatherings. Used in moderation, alcohol can enhance social occasions by loosening inhibitions and creating a pleasant feeling of relaxation. But the use of alcohol can also be an unhealthy adaptation. Like other drugs, alcohol has definite physiological effects on the body that can impair functioning in the short term and cause devastating damage in the long term. For some people, alcohol becomes an addiction, leading to a lifetime of recovery or, for a few, to debilitation and death. Many of our slang expressions for intoxication reflect its less positive aspects; we say we're "smashed," "bombed," "wasted."

About 64% of Americans over the age of 12 drink alcohol in some form. If the total amount of alcohol consumed in the United States in a year were evenly divided among drinkers, each would consume the equivalent of 4 gallons of whiskey, 20 gallons of wine, or 50 gallons of beer. But heavy drinkers, who constitute about 8.5% of the American drinking population, account for over half of all the alcohol consumed, as well as a disproportionate amount of the social, economic, and medical costs of alcohol abuse (estimated at over $180 billion per year). And through unintentional injuries, especially automobile crashes, alcohol is the leading cause of death among people between the ages of 15 and 24.

The use of alcohol is a complex issue, one that demands conscious thought and informed decisions. In our society, some people choose to drink in moderation, some choose not to drink at all, and others realize too late that they've made an unwise choice—when they become dependent on alcohol, are involved in an alcohol-related car crash, or simply wake up to discover they've done something they regret. This chapter discusses the complexities of alcohol use and provides information that will help you make the choices that are right for you.

Ethyl alcohol is the common psychoactive drug found in all alcoholic beverages. One drink—a 12-ounce beer, a 1.5-ounce cocktail, or a 5-ounce glass of wine—contains about 0.6 ounce of ethyl alcohol.

THE NATURE OF ALCOHOL

How does alcohol affect people? Does it affect some people differently than others? Can some people "handle" alcohol? Is it possible to drink a safe amount of alcohol? Many of the misconceptions about the effects of alcohol can be cleared up by taking a closer look at the chemistry of alcohol and how it is absorbed and metabolized by the body.

The Chemistry of Alcohol

Ethyl alcohol is the psychoactive ingredient in all alcoholic beverages. Beer, a mild intoxicant brewed from a mixture of grains, usually contains 3–6% alcohol by volume. Ales and malt liquors are 6–8% alcohol by volume. Wines are made by *fermenting* the juices of grapes or other fruits. The concentration of alcohol in table wines is about 9–14%. *Fortified wines,* so named because alcohol has been added to them, contain about 20% alcohol; these include sherry, port, and Madeira. Stronger alcoholic beverages, called *hard liquors,* are made by *distilling* brewed or fermented grains or other products. These beverages, including gin, whiskey, brandy, rum, tequila, vodka, and liqueurs, usually contain 35–50% alcohol.

The concentration of alcohol in a beverage is indicated by the **proof value,** which is two times the percentage

Terms
proof value Two times the percentage of alcohol by volume; a beverage that is 50% alcohol by volume is 100 proof.

alcohol The intoxicating ingredient in fermented liquors; a colorless, pungent liquid.

metabolism The chemical transformation of food and other substances in the body into energy and wastes.

Do you notice that you react differently to alcohol than some of your friends do? If so, you may be noticing genetic differences in alcohol metabolism that are associated with gender or ethnicity. Alcohol is metabolized mainly in the liver, but some alcohol is broken down in the stomach before it can be sent into the bloodstream and on to the liver. Once it's circulating in the bloodstream, alcohol produces the well-known feelings of intoxication. Studies have shown that women metabolize less alcohol in the stomach than men do, so they release more unmetabolized alcohol into the bloodstream. (The stomach enzyme that breaks down alcohol before it enters the bloodstream is less active in women than in men.) The same amount of alcohol will have more effect on a woman than on a man—she will feel the effects sooner and more strongly.

Other differences in alcohol metabolism are associated with ethnicity. Alcohol is broken down in the liver by an enzyme called alcohol dehydrogenase, producing a by-product called acetaldehyde (see the figure). Acetaldehyde is responsible for many of the unpleasant effects of alcohol abuse. Another enzyme, acetaldehyde dehydrogenase, breaks this product down further. Some people, including many of Asian descent, have genetic information that causes them to produce somewhat different forms of the two enzymes that metabolize alcohol. The result is high concentrations of acetaldehyde in the brain and other tissues, producing a host of unpleasant symptoms. When people with these enzymes drink alcohol, they experience a physiological reaction referred to as *flushing syndrome*. Their skin feels hot, their heart and respiration rates increase, and they may get a headache, vomit, or break out in hives. Drinking makes some people so uncomfortable that it's unlikely they

could ever become addicted to alcohol. The body's response to acetaldehyde is the basis for treating alcohol abuse with the drug disulfiram (Antabuse), which inhibits the action of acetaldehyde dehydrogenase. When a person taking disulfiram ingests alcohol, acetaldehyde levels increase rapidly, and he or she develops an intense flushing reaction along with weakness, nausea, vomiting, and other disagreeable symptoms.

How people behave in relation to alcohol is influenced in complex ways by many factors, including social and cultural ones. But in these two cases at least, individual choices and behavior are strongly influenced by a specific genetic characteristic.

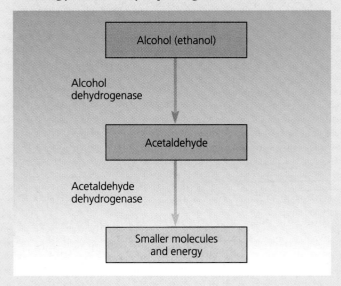

concentration. For example, if a beverage is 100 proof, it contains 50% alcohol. Two ounces of 100-proof whiskey contain 1 ounce of pure alcohol. The proof value of hard liquors can usually be found on the bottle labels. When alcohol consumption is discussed, "one drink" refers to a 12-ounce bottle of beer, a 5-ounce glass of table wine, or a cocktail with 1.5 ounces of 80-proof liquor. Each of these different drinks contains approximately the same amount of alcohol: 0.6 ounce.

There are a number of different kinds of alcohol. In this book, the term **alcohol** refers to ethyl alcohol, which is the only kind of alcohol that can be consumed. Other kinds of alcohol such as methanol (wood alcohol) and isopropyl alcohol (rubbing alcohol) are highly toxic and can cause blindness and other serious problems when consumed even in low doses.

Absorption

When a person ingests alcohol, about 20% is rapidly absorbed from the stomach into the bloodstream. About 75% is absorbed through the upper part of the small intestine. Any remaining alcohol enters the bloodstream further along the gastrointestinal tract. The rate of absorption is affected by a variety of factors. For example, the carbonation in a beverage like champagne increases the rate of alcohol absorption. Food in the stomach slows the rate of absorption, as does the drinking of highly concentrated alcoholic beverages such as hard liquor. But remember: *All* alcohol a person consumes is eventually absorbed.

Metabolism and Excretion

Alcohol is quickly transported throughout the body by the blood. Because alcohol easily moves through most biological membranes, it is rapidly distributed throughout most body tissues. The main site of alcohol **metabolism** is the liver, though a small amount of alcohol is metabolized in the stomach. (See the box "Metabolizing Alcohol: Our Bodies Work Differently" for more information.)

About 2–10% of ingested alcohol is not metabolized in the liver or other tissues but is excreted unchanged by the lungs, kidneys, and sweat glands. Excreted alcohol causes the telltale smell on a drinker's breath and is the basis of breath and urine analyses for alcohol levels. Although such analyses do not give precise measurements

	The Effects of Alcohol	
Table 10-1		
BAC (%)	Common Behavioral Effects	Hours Required to Metabolize Alcohol
0.00–0.05	Slight change in feelings, usually relaxation and euphoria. Decreased alertness.	2–3
0.05–0.10	Emotional instability, with exaggerated feelings and behavior. Reduced social inhibitions. Impairment of reaction time and fine motor coordination. Increasingly impaired during driving. Legally drunk at 0.08% in many states and 0.10% in others.	3–6
0.10–0.15	Unsteadiness in standing and walking. Loss of peripheral vision. Driving is extremely dangerous.	6–10
0.15–0.30	Staggering gait. Slurred speech. Pain and other sensory perceptions greatly impaired.	10–24
More than 0.30	Stupor or unconsciousness. Anesthesia. Death possible at 0.35% and above. Can result from rapid or binge drinking with few earlier effects.	More than 24

of alcohol concentrations in the blood, they do provide a reasonable approximation if done correctly.

Alcohol Intake and Blood Alcohol Concentration

Blood alcohol concentration (BAC), a measure of intoxication, is determined by the amount of alcohol consumed in a given amount of time and by individual factors such as body weight and amount of body fat. In most cases, a smaller person develops a higher BAC than a larger person after drinking the same amount of alcohol. This is because a smaller person has less overall body tissue into which alcohol can be distributed. A person with a higher percentage of body fat will usually develop a higher BAC than a more muscular person who weighs the same. This is because alcohol does not concentrate as much in fatty tissue as in muscle and most other tissues, in part because fat has fewer blood vessels. Women generally have higher BACs than men after consuming the same amount of alcohol because they usually have a higher percentage of body fat than men and because the stomach enzyme that breaks down alcohol before it enters the bloodstream is four times more active in men than in women.

BAC also depends on the balance between the rate of alcohol absorption and the rate of alcohol metabolism. A man who weighs 154 pounds and has normal liver function metabolizes about 0.3–0.5 ounce of alcohol per hour, the equivalent of slightly less than a 12-ounce bottle of beer or a 5-ounce glass of wine.

The rate of alcohol metabolism varies among individuals and is largely determined by genetic factors and drinking behavior. (Chronic drinking activates enzymes that metabolize alcohol in the liver, so people who drink frequently metabolize alcohol at a more rapid rate than nondrinkers.) Contrary to popular myths, this metabolic rate cannot be influenced by exercise, breathing deeply, eating, drinking coffee, or taking other drugs. The rate of alcohol metabolism is the same whether a person is asleep or awake.

If a person absorbs slightly less alcohol each hour than he or she can metabolize in an hour, the BAC remains low. People can drink large amounts of alcohol this way over a long period of time without becoming noticeably intoxicated; however, they do run the risk of significant long-term health hazards (described later in the chapter). If a person is absorbing alcohol more quickly than it can be metabolized, the BAC will steadily increase, and he or she will become more and more drunk (Table 10-1). How fast you drink makes a big difference in how high your BAC will be. Consuming several drinks over a period of 2 or 3 hours is likely to cause intoxication, followed on the next day by a hangover; chugging the same amount of alcohol in an hour or less could be lethal.

ALCOHOL AND HEALTH

The effects of alcohol consumption on health depend on the individual, the circumstances, and the amount of alcohol consumed.

Terms

blood alcohol concentration (BAC) The amount of alcohol in the blood in terms of weight per unit volume; used as a measurement of intoxication.

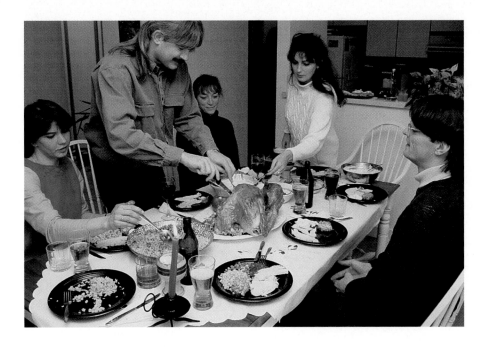

Alcoholic beverages like beer and wine are an integral part of social occasions for many people. A central nervous system depressant, alcohol loosens inhibitions; when used in moderation, it tends to make people feel more relaxed and sociable.

The Immediate Effects of Alcohol

BAC is a primary factor determining the effects of alcohol (see Table 10-1). At low concentrations, alcohol tends to make people feel relaxed and jovial, but at higher concentrations people are more likely to feel angry, sedated, or sleepy. Alcohol is a CNS depressant, and its effects vary because body systems are affected to different degrees at different BACs. At any given BAC, the effects of alcohol are more pronounced when the BAC is rapidly increasing compared to when it is slowly increasing, steady, or decreasing. The effects of alcohol are more pronounced if a person drinks on an empty stomach, because alcohol is absorbed more quickly and the BAC rises more quickly.

Low Concentrations of Alcohol The effects of alcohol can first be felt at a BAC of about 0.03–0.05%. These effects may include light-headedness, relaxation, and a release of inhibitions. Most drinkers experience mild euphoria and become more sociable. When people drink in social settings, alcohol often seems to act as a stimulant, enhancing conviviality or assertiveness. This apparent stimulation occurs because alcohol depresses inhibitory centers in the brain.

Higher Concentrations of Alcohol At higher concentrations, the pleasant effects tend to be replaced by more negative ones: interference with motor coordination, verbal performance, and intellectual functions. The drinker often becomes irritable and may be easily angered or given to crying. When the BAC reaches 0.1%, most sensory and motor functioning is reduced, and many people become sleepy. Vision, smell, taste, and hearing become less acute. At 0.2%, most drinkers are completely unable to function,

either physically or psychologically, because of the pronounced depression of the central nervous system, muscles, and other body systems. Coma usually occurs at a BAC of 0.35%, and any higher level can be fatal.

Shakespeare accurately described the effects of alcohol on sexual functioning. He said (in *Macbeth*) that "it stirs up desire, but it takes away the performance." Small doses may improve sexual functioning for individuals who are especially anxious or self-conscious, but higher doses usually have a negative effect. Excessive alcohol use can result in reduced erection response and reduced vaginal lubrication. Testicular atrophy (shrinking) may result from the long-term overuse of alcohol.

Alcohol causes blood vessels near the skin to dilate, so drinkers often feel warm; their skin flushes, and they may sweat more. Flushing and sweating contribute to heat loss, and so the internal body temperature falls. High doses of alcohol may impair the body's ability to regulate temperature, causing it to drop sharply, especially if the surrounding temperature is low. Drinking alcoholic beverages to keep warm in cold weather does not work, and it can even be dangerous.

Drinking alcohol, particularly in large amounts, disturbs normal sleep patterns. Alcohol may facilitate falling asleep more quickly, but the sleep is often light, punctuated with awakenings, and unrefreshing. Even after the habitual drinker stops drinking, his or her sleep may be altered for weeks or months.

Alcohol Hangover Despite all the jokes about hangovers, anyone who has experienced a severe hangover knows they are no laughing matter. The symptoms include headache, shakiness, nausea, diarrhea, fatigue, and impaired mental functioning. It is estimated that hangovers

Remember: Being very drunk is potentially life-threatening. Helping a drunken friend could save a life.

- Be firm but calm. Don't engage the person in an argument or discuss her drinking behavior while she is intoxicated.

- Get the person out of harm's way—don't let her drive or wander outside. Don't let her drink any more alcohol.

- If the person is unconscious, don't assume she is just "sleeping it off." Place her on her side with her knees up. This position will help prevent choking if the person should vomit.

- Stay with the person—you need to be ready to help if she vomits or stops breathing.

- Don't try to give the person anything to eat or drink, including coffee or other drugs. Don't give cold showers or try to make her walk around. None of these things help sober someone up, and they can be dangerous.

Call 911 immediately in any of the following instances:

- You can't wake the person up even with shouting or shaking.

- The person is taking fewer than 8 breaths per minute or her breathing seems shallow or irregular.

- You think the person took other drugs in addition to alcohol.

- The person has had an injury, especially a blow to the head.

- The person drank a large amount of alcohol within a short period of time and then became unconscious. Death due to alcohol poisoning most often occurs when the blood alcohol level rises very quickly due to rapid ingestion of alcohol.

If you aren't sure what to do, call 911. You may be saving a life.

---

cost the U.S. economy about $148 billion each year because of absenteeism and poor job performance. Hangovers represent a substantial portion of the money lost to society as a result of alcohol use.

A hangover is probably caused by a combination of the toxic products of alcohol breakdown, dehydration, and hormonal effects. During a hangover, heart rate and blood pressure increase, making some individuals more vulnerable to heart attack. Electroencephalography (brain wave testing) shows diffuse slowing of brain waves for up to 16 hours after BAC drops to zero. Studies of pilots, drivers, and skiers all indicate that coordination and cognition are impaired in a person with a hangover, increasing the risk of injury.

The best treatment for hangover is prevention. Nearly all men can expect a hangover if they drink more than 5 or 6 drinks; for women, the number is 3 to 4 drinks. Drinking less, drinking more slowly, and consuming plenty of nonalcoholic liquids decrease the risk of hangover. If you do get a hangover, remember that your ability to drive is definitely impaired, even after your BAC has returned to zero.

Alcohol Poisoning   Acute alcohol poisoning occurs much more frequently than most people realize, and all too often it can cause death. Drinking large amounts of alcohol over a short period of time can rapidly raise the BAC into the lethal range. Alcohol, either alone or in combination with other drugs, is responsible for more toxic overdose deaths than any other drug. A common scenario for alcohol poisoning occurs when inexperienced drinkers try to outdo each other by consuming glass after glass of alcohol as rapidly as possible. Coma and death can result before the participants in this game have any awareness of how dangerous this can be. Children are at especially high risk for alcohol poisoning. Even a partially empty glass of liquor carelessly left out after a party can result in serious poisoning, or even death, if consumed by a toddler or small child.

Death from alcohol poisoning may be caused either by central nervous system and respiratory depression or by inhaling fluid or vomit into the lungs. The amount of alcohol it takes to make a person unconscious is dangerously close to a fatal dose. Special care should be taken to ensure the safety of anyone who has been drinking heavily, especially if the person becomes unconscious (see the box "Dealing with an Alcohol Emergency").

Using Alcohol with Other Drugs   Alcohol-drug combinations are the number one cause of drug-related deaths in this country. Using alcohol while taking any other drug that can cause CNS depression increases the effects of both drugs, potentially leading to coma, respiratory depression, and death. Examples of common drugs that can result in oversedation when combined with alcohol include barbiturates, Valium-like drugs, narcotics such as codeine, antidepressants such as Prozac, and OTC antihistamines like Benadryl. For people who consume three or more drinks per day, use of OTC pain relievers like aspirin, ibuprofen, or acetaminophen increases the risk of stomach bleeding or liver damage. Some antibiotics and diabetes medications can also interact dangerously with alcohol.

Many illegal drugs are especially dangerous when combined with alcohol. Life-threatening overdoses occur at much lower doses when heroin and other narcotics are combined with alcohol. When cocaine and alcohol are used together, a toxic substance called cocaethylene is formed; this substance is responsible for more than half of all cocaine-related deaths.

The safest strategy is to avoid combining alcohol with any other drug—prescription, over-the-counter, or illegal. If in doubt, ask your pharmacist or physician before using any drug in combination with alcohol, or just don't do it.

Alcohol-Related Injuries and Violence   The combination of impaired judgment, weakened sensory perception, reduced inhibitions, impaired motor coordination, and, often, increased aggressiveness and hostility that characterize alcohol intoxication can be dangerous or even deadly. Through homicide, suicide, automobile crashes (discussed in the next section), and other incidents, alcohol kills over 100,000 Americans each year. Alcohol use contributes to over 50% of all murders, assaults, and rapes, and alcohol is frequently found in the bloodstream of both perpetrators and victims. Nearly 80% of people who attempt suicide have been drinking, and about half of all successful suicides are alcoholics. Alcohol use more than triples the chances of fatal injuries during leisure activities such as swimming and boating, and more than half of all fatal falls and serious burns happen to people who have been drinking. Being drunk is clearly hazardous to your health.

Alcohol and Sexual Decision Making   Alcohol seriously affects a person's ability to make wise decisions about sex. A recent survey of college students revealed that frequent binge drinkers were five times more likely to engage in unplanned sexual activity and five-and-a-half times more likely to have unprotected sex than non–binge drinkers. Heavy drinkers are also more likely to have multiple sex partners and to engage in other forms of high-risk sexual behavior. For all these reasons, rates of sexually transmitted diseases and unwanted pregnancy are higher among people who drink heavily than among people who drink moderately or not at all. A study comparing rates of gonorrhea (a sexually transmitted disease) in states with varying minimum drinking ages and beer taxes found that gonorrhea rates dropped significantly among young people when beer taxes were increased and the minimum drinking age was raised.

Women who binge-drink are at increased risk for rape and other forms of nonconsensual sex. The laws regarding sexual consent are clear: A person who is very drunk or passed out cannot consent to sex. If you have sex with a person who is drunk or unconscious, you are committing sexual assault. Claiming that you were drunk at the time won't absolve you of your legal and moral responsibility for this serious crime.

WWW. Drinking and Driving

Despite recent improvements, drunk driving continues to be one of the most serious public health and safety

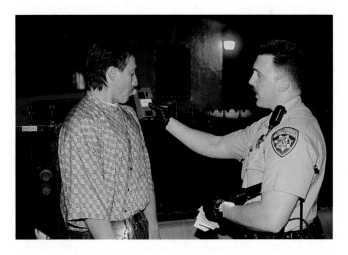

Figure 10-1   The dose-response relationship between BAC and automobile crashes.

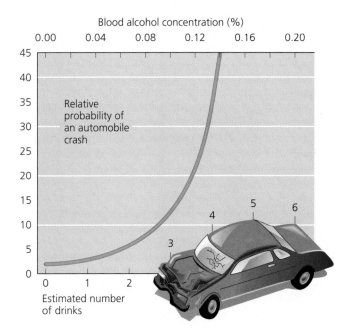

Alcohol interferes with judgment, perception, coordination, and other areas of mental and physical functioning, and it is a factor in a majority of all fatal automobile crashes. This driver is lucky that he was stopped by a suspicious police officer before a crash occurred. He is being given a breath test to determine his blood alcohol concentration.

problems in the United States. Every year, more than 800,000 people are injured in alcohol-related automobile crashes—an average of *one person every 40 seconds* (Figure 10–1). About 40% of the more than 40,000 crash fatalities in 1998 were alcohol-related, down from about 50% ten years ago. Increased public education about drunk driving and stiffer drunk driving laws are primarily responsible for this improvement. Still, in surveys, more than 1 in 4 of U.S. drivers admit to having used alcohol or another drug within 2 hours before driving a vehicle.

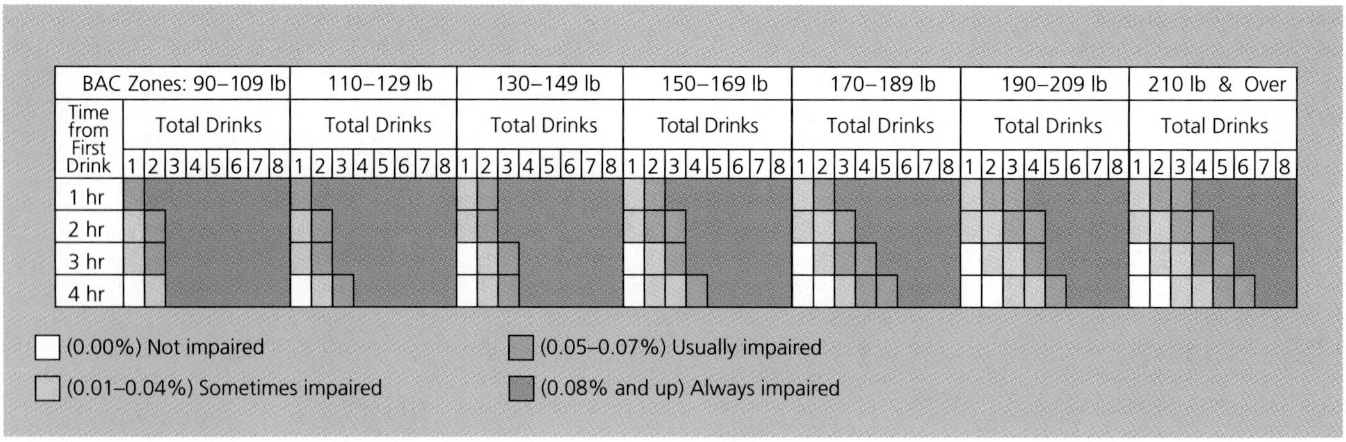

BAC Zones: 90–109 lb								110–129 lb								130–149 lb								150–169 lb								170–189 lb								190–209 lb								210 lb & Over							
Time from First Drink	Total Drinks								Total Drinks								Total Drinks								Total Drinks								Total Drinks								Total Drinks								Total Drinks							
	1	2	3	4	5	6	7	8	1	2	3	4	5	6	7	8	1	2	3	4	5	6	7	8	1	2	3	4	5	6	7	8	1	2	3	4	5	6	7	8	1	2	3	4	5	6	7	8	1	2	3	4	5	6	7	8
1 hr																																																								
2 hr																																																								
3 hr																																																								
4 hr																																																								

☐ (0.00%) Not impaired   ☐ (0.05–0.07%) Usually impaired

☐ (0.01–0.04%) Sometimes impaired   ■ (0.08% and up) Always impaired

Figure 10-2 Approximate blood alcohol concentration and body weight. This chart illustrates the BAC an average person of a given weight would reach after drinking the specified number of drinks in the time shown. The legal limit for BAC is 0.08% in some states and 0.10% in others. For drivers under 21 years of age, many states have "zero tolerance" laws that set BAC limits of 0.01% or 0.02%.

The *dose-response function* (see Chapter 9) is the relationship between the amount of alcohol or drug consumed and the type and intensity of the resulting effect. Higher doses of alcohol are associated with a much greater probability of automobile crashes. A person driving with a BAC of 0.14% is more than 40 times more likely to be involved in a crash than someone with no alcohol in his or her blood. For those with a BAC above 0.14%, the risk of a fatal crash is estimated to be 380 times higher. The risks for young drivers are even greater than indicated in Figure 10-1, especially at very low BACs. Younger drivers have less experience with both driving and alcohol, which results in significant impairment even with BACs as low as 0.02%.

In addition to an increased risk of injury and death, driving while intoxicated can have serious legal consequences. Drunk driving is against the law. In 2000, the legal limit for BAC was 0.08% in 18 states and the District of Columbia and 0.10% in 31 other states (in Massachusetts, a BAC of 0.08% is evidence of alcohol impairment but not illegal per se). Under a law signed in 2000, states must lower their BAC limits to 0.08% by 2004 to avoid federal penalties. Under current "zero tolerance" laws in many states, drivers under age 21 who have consumed *any* alcohol may have their licenses suspended. There are stiff penalties for drunk driving, including fines, loss of license, confiscation of vehicle, and jail time. Many cities have checkpoints where drivers are stopped and checked for intoxication.

Numerous studies have shown that alcohol-related highway deaths fall when states lower the legal BAC. It is estimated that when all states lower their BAC limits to 0.08%, alcohol-related traffic fatalities will decrease by about 500 deaths per year. Many developed countries have lower BAC limits than the United States. The most common BAC limit is 0.05%, a level used by Australia, Belgium, Denmark, France, Germany, Greece, Spain, and many other countries; Sweden and Russia have BAC limits of 0.02%.

People who drink and drive are unable to drive safely because their judgment is impaired, their reaction time is slower, and their coordination is reduced. The number of drinks it takes the average person to reach various BACs is shown in Figure 10-2. However, some driving skills are affected at BACs of 0.02% and lower; at 0.05%, visual perception, reaction time, and certain steering tasks are all impaired. Any amount of alcohol impairs your ability to drive safely, and fatigue augments alcohol's effects.

If you are out of your home and drinking, find an alternative means of transportation or follow the practice of having a *designated driver,* an individual who refrains from drinking in order to provide safe transportation home for others in the group. The responsibility can be rotated for different occasions. Remember, you risk more than your own life when you drink and drive. Causing serious injury or death results in lifelong feelings of sadness and guilt for the driver and tremendous grief for the friends and families of victims.

It's more difficult to protect yourself against someone else who drinks and drives. Learn to be alert to the erratic driving that signals an impaired driver. Warning signs include wide, abrupt, and illegal turns; straddling the center line or lane marker; driving on the shoulder; weaving, swerving, or nearly striking an object or another vehicle; following too closely; erratic speed; driving with headlights off at night; and driving with the window down in very cold weather. If you see any of these signs, try the following strategies:

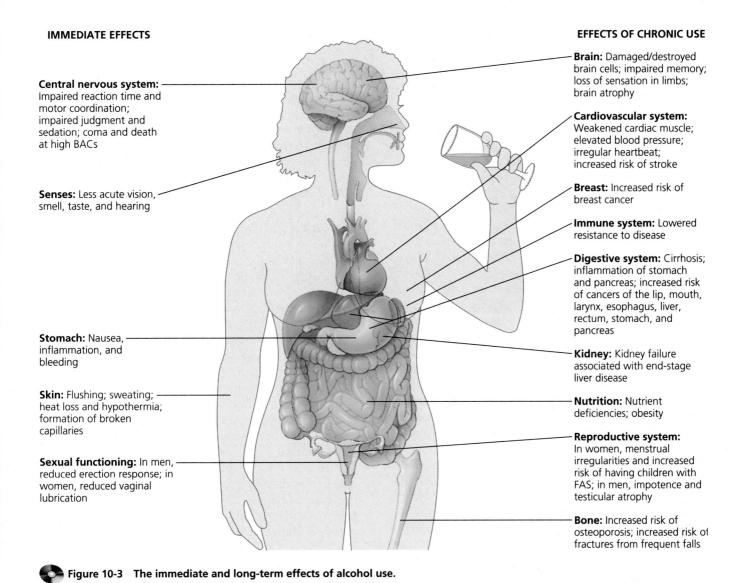

Central nervous system: Impaired reaction time and motor coordination; impaired judgment and sedation; coma and death at high BACs

Senses: Less acute vision, smell, taste, and hearing

Stomach: Nausea, inflammation, and bleeding

Skin: Flushing; sweating; heat loss and hypothermia; formation of broken capillaries

Sexual functioning: In men, reduced erection response; in women, reduced vaginal lubrication

Brain: Damaged/destroyed brain cells; impaired memory; loss of sensation in limbs; brain atrophy

Cardiovascular system: Weakened cardiac muscle; elevated blood pressure; irregular heartbeat; increased risk of stroke

Breast: Increased risk of breast cancer

Immune system: Lowered resistance to disease

Digestive system: Cirrhosis; inflammation of stomach and pancreas; increased risk of cancers of the lip, mouth, larynx, esophagus, liver, rectum, stomach, and pancreas

Kidney: Kidney failure associated with end-stage liver disease

Nutrition: Nutrient deficiencies; obesity

Reproductive system: In women, menstrual irregularities and increased risk of having children with FAS; in men, impotence and testicular atrophy

Bone: Increased risk of osteoporosis; increased risk of fractures from frequent falls

Figure 10-3   The immediate and long-term effects of alcohol use.

- If the driver is ahead of you, maintain a safe following distance. Don't try to pass.
- If the driver is behind you, turn right at the nearest intersection, and let the driver pass.
- If the driver is approaching your car, move to the shoulder and stop. Avoid a head-on collision by sounding your horn or flashing your lights.
- When approaching an intersection, slow down and stay alert for vehicles that don't appear to be slowing in preparation for stopping at a stop sign or red light.
- Make sure your safety belt is fastened and children are in approved safety seats.
- Report suspected impaired drivers to the nearest police station by phone. Give a description of the vehicle, license number, location, and direction the vehicle is headed.

> **COMMUNICATE!**   To avoid dangerous alcohol-related situations, such as riding with a driver who has been drinking, you may need to use assertive communication. Try stating specifically what you want, using a firm but neutral tone. For example, "I don't feel comfortable riding with you after you've been drinking, and I don't think it's safe for you either. I'd feel better if we used a designated driver. I'll volunteer for tonight, and in the future we can all take turns."

The Effects of Chronic Use

Because alcohol is distributed throughout most of the body, it can affect many different organs and tissues (Figure 10-3). Problems associated with chronic, or habitual, use of alcohol include diseases of the digestive and cardiovascular systems and some cancers. Drinking during pregnancy risks the health of both the woman and the developing fetus.

The Digestive System   Even in relatively small amounts, alcohol can alter the normal functioning of the liver. Within just a few days of heavy alcohol consumption, fat begins to accumulate in liver cells, resulting in the development of "fatty liver." If drinking continues, inflammation of the liver can occur, resulting in alcoholic hepatitis, a frequent cause of hospitalization and death in alcoholics. Both fatty liver and alcoholic hepatitis are potentially reversible if the person stops drinking. With continued alcohol use, however, liver cells are progressively damaged and then permanently destroyed. The destroyed cells are replaced by fibrous scar tissue, a condition known as **cirrhosis.** As cirrhosis develops, a drinker may gradually lose his or her capacity to tolerate alcohol, because there are fewer and fewer healthy cells remaining in the liver to metabolize it. Alcohol-precipitated cirrhosis is the tenth leading cause of death in the United States.

As with most health hazards, the risk of cirrhosis depends on an individual's susceptibility, largely genetically determined, and the amount of alcohol consumed over time. Some people show signs of cirrhosis after a few years of consuming three or four drinks per day. Women generally develop cirrhosis at lower levels of alcohol consumption than men. Alcoholics are especially susceptible to infection with hepatitis C virus (HCV); the combination of alcohol abuse and HCV infection greatly increases the risk for cirrhosis and liver cancer.

Signs of cirrhosis can include jaundice (a yellowing of the skin and white part of the eyes) and the accumulation of fluid in the abdomen and lower extremities. Some people with cirrhosis have no obvious outward signs of the disease. Treatment for cirrhosis includes a balanced diet and complete abstinence from alcohol. People with cirrhosis who continue to drink have only a 50% chance of surviving 5 or more years.

Alcohol can inflame the pancreas, causing nausea, vomiting, abnormal digestion, and severe pain. Acute alcoholic pancreatitis generally occurs in binge drinkers. Unlike cirrhosis, which usually occurs after years of fairly heavy alcohol use, pancreatitis can occur after just one or two severe binge-drinking episodes. Acute pancreatitis is often fatal and can also develop into a chronic condition.

Overuse of alcohol is a common cause of bleeding in the gastrointestinal tract. Vomiting after an alcohol binge can result in tearing of esophageal blood vessels. Chronic alcohol use with cirrhosis frequently results in the development of enlarged, fragile esophageal and rectal veins, which can easily burst with potentially fatal results. Even a relatively small amount of alcohol can cause painful irritation of the lining of the stomach.

The Cardiovascular System   The effects of alcohol on the cardiovascular system depend on the amount of alcohol consumed. Moderate doses of alcohol—less than one drink a day for women and two drinks a day for men—may reduce the risk of heart disease and heart attack in some people. (The possible health benefits of alcohol are discussed later in this chapter.) However, higher doses of alcohol have harmful effects on the cardiovascular system. In some people, more than two drinks a day will elevate blood pressure, making stroke and heart attack more likely. Some alcoholics show a weakening of the heart muscle, a condition known as **cardiac myopathy.** Binge drinking can cause "holiday heart," a syndrome characterized by serious abnormal heart rhythms, which usually appear within 24 hours of a binge episode.

Although the relationships between alcohol and cardiovascular disease are multiple and complex, it is clear that excessive drinking increases the risk of disease. These health risks progressively increase as the amount of excessive drinking increases.

Cancer   Alcoholics have a cancer rate about ten times higher than that of the general population. They are particularly vulnerable to cancers of the throat, larynx, esophagus, upper stomach, liver, and pancreas. Drinking three or more alcoholic beverages per day doubles a woman's risk of developing breast cancer. Some studies have linked even moderate drinking to increased risk for cancers of the breast, mouth, throat, and esophagus. In May 2000, the U.S. Department of Health and Human Services added alcoholic beverages to the list of known human carcinogens.

Mortality   As an ancient proverb states, "Those who worship Bacchus [the god of wine] die young." Excessive alcohol consumption is a factor in five of the ten leading causes of death for Americans. Average life expectancy among alcoholics is about 58 years; heavy drinkers may die in their 20s or 30s.

The Effects of Alcohol Use During Pregnancy

Alcohol ingested during pregnancy is harmful to the developing fetus. Alcohol and its metabolic product, ac-

---

Terms

cirrhosis A disease in which the liver is severely damaged by alcohol, other toxins, or infection.

cardiac myopathy Weakening of the heart muscle through disease.

fetal alcohol syndrome (FAS) A characteristic group of birth defects caused by excessive alcohol consumption by the mother, including facial deformities, heart defects, and physical and mental impairments.

alcohol-related neurodevelopmental disorder (ARND) Cognitive and behavioral problems seen in people whose mothers drank alcohol during pregnancy.

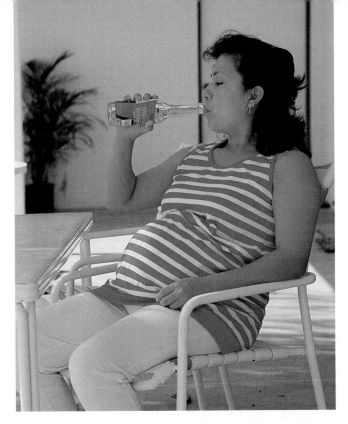

A high level of alcohol consumption during pregnancy is associated with miscarriage, stillbirth, and a cluster of birth defects known as fetal alcohol syndrome. Total abstinence from alcohol during pregnancy is recommended.

etaldehyde, readily cross the placenta. The damage to the fetus depends on the stage of pregnancy and the amount of alcohol consumed. Alcohol use in early pregnancy can cause a miscarriage. Moderate to heavy alcohol use in pregnancy can cause a collection of birth defects known as **fetal alcohol syndrome (FAS).** Children with FAS have a characteristic mixture of deformities that include a small head, abnormal facial structure, heart defects, and other physical abnormalities; most are mentally impaired and their physical and mental growth is slower than normal.

FAS is a permanent, incurable condition that causes lifelong disability; it is by far the most common preventable cause of mental retardation in the Western world. Full-blown FAS occurs in about 1 or 2 out of every 1000 live births in the United States. Many more babies are born with **alcohol-related neurodevelopmental disorder (ARND).** Children with ARND appear physically normal, but they often have significant learning and behavioral disorders and are, as adults, more likely to develop substance abuse problems and to have criminal records.

Heavy drinking early in pregnancy is responsible for most of the physical abnormalities associated with FAS. Binge drinking among women of childbearing age is thus of particular concern because women may drink heavily during the first few days and weeks of gestation before they become aware that they are pregnant. Fetal alcohol exposure later in pregnancy is more likely to cause brain damage without obvious external signs. A recent study found that getting drunk just one time during the final 3 months of pregnancy, when brain cells are developing rapidly, can cause fetal brain damage.

No one is sure exactly how much alcohol is required to cause FAS, but no amount of alcohol during pregnancy is considered safe. Despite this, more than half of pregnant women do consume alcohol, and rates of drinking among pregnant women have recently increased. Researchers speculate that publicity regarding the potential health benefits of alcohol may have given some women the false impression that light or moderate drinking poses no risk during pregnancy. Experts agree that the safest course of action is complete abstinence from alcohol during pregnancy.

Any alcohol consumed by a nursing mother quickly enters the breast milk. What impact this has on the child or on the mother's milk production is a matter of controversy. Dosage may again be the key issue. However, many physicians advise nursing mothers to abstain from drinking alcohol because of the belief that any amount may have negative effects on the baby's brain development.

Possible Health Benefits of Alcohol

The relationship between alcohol use and health is complex and still under investigation. Both abstainers and light to moderate drinkers live longer than heavy drinkers, but people who drink moderately—no more than one drink a day for women and two drinks a day for men— live longer than those who abstain completely. According to the *Dietary Guidelines for Americans,* published by the U.S. Department of Agriculture, drinking in moderation may lower risk of coronary heart disease, mainly among men over age 45 and women over age 55; moderate drinking provides little if any health benefits for younger people. Moderate drinking appears to affect heart health by raising blood levels of HDL, the beneficial form of cholesterol, and reducing inflammation and the risk of dangerous blood clots; people with a particular gene variation that affects alcohol metabolism may benefit most. Some evidence also suggests that moderate drinkers may be less likely to develop a variety of other conditions, including diabetes, arterial blockages in the legs, Alzheimer's disease, and benign prostate enlargement.

Moderate drinking is not without risk, however. It increases the risk of dying from unintentional injuries, violence, and certain types of cancer. In women, even moderate drinking may increase the risk of breast cancer; those who are at risk for breast cancer should discuss the potential risks and benefits of alcohol with their physician. There is also a risk that moderate drinking will not stay moderate. People who avoid alcohol because they or family members have had problems with dependence in the past should not start drinking for their health. People with conditions such as diabetes or depression that are worsened by alcohol use should probably avoid even moderate drinking. Nor should drinkers use this information as an excuse to overindulge; any health benefits of alcohol are negated by heavy use. In addition, there are many situations in which consuming any amount of alcohol is unwise, including during pregnancy, while taking medication that may interact with alcohol, and when driving or engaging in another activity that requires alertness. Sexually active women who are not consistently using effective contraception should not drink, since fetal damage due to alcohol use frequently occurs in the first days and weeks of pregnancy, before most women are aware that they are pregnant.

The bottom line is that limited, regular consumption of alcohol appears to be beneficial for some adults, but there is a narrow window of benefit, and excessive drinking causes serious health problems. The *Dietary Guidelines for Americans* recommend that if you drink alcoholic beverages, do it in moderation, with meals, at times when consumption does not put you or others at risk.

ALCOHOL ABUSE AND DEPENDENCE

Abuse and dependence on alcohol affect more than just the drinker. Friends, family members, coworkers, strangers that drinkers encounter on the road, and society as a whole pay the physical, emotional, and financial costs of the misuse of alcohol.

Alcohol Abuse

As explained in Chapter 9, the American Psychiatric Association's *Diagnostic and Statistical Manual of Mental Disorders* makes a distinction between substance abuse and substance dependence. **Alcohol abuse** is recurrent alcohol use that has negative consequences, such as drinking in dangerous situations (before driving, for instance), or drinking patterns that result in academic, professional, interpersonal, or legal difficulties. **Alcohol dependence, or alcoholism,** involves more extensive problems with alcohol use, usually involving physical tolerance and withdrawal. Alcoholism is discussed in greater detail later in the chapter.

Other authorities use different definitions to describe problems associated with drinking. The important point is that one does not have to be an alcoholic to have problems with alcohol. The person who drinks only once a month, perhaps after an exam, but then drives while intoxicated is an alcohol abuser.

How can you tell if you are beginning to abuse alcohol or if someone you know is doing so? Look for the following warning signs:

- Drinking alone or secretively
- Using alcohol deliberately and repeatedly to perform or get through difficult situations
- Feeling uncomfortable on certain occasions when alcohol is not available
- Escalating alcohol consumption beyond an already established drinking pattern
- Consuming alcohol heavily in risky situations, such as before driving
- Getting drunk regularly or more frequently than in the past
- Drinking in the morning or at other unusual times

Ww. Binge Drinking

A common form of alcohol abuse on college campuses is known as **binge drinking.** In surveys of students on over 100 college campuses, 44% reported binge drinking, defined as having five drinks in a row for men or four in a row for women on at least one occasion in the 2 weeks prior to the survey. Some 23% of all students were found to be frequent binge drinkers, defined as having at least three binges during the 2-week period. Students living at fraternity or sorority houses had the highest rate of binge drinking, 80%. Men were more likely to binge than women, and white students had higher rates of binge drinking than students of other ethnicities. Nineteen percent of students abstained from alcohol (Figure 10-4).

Binge drinking has a profound effect on students' lives. Frequent binge drinkers were found to be 3–7 times more likely than non–binge drinkers to engage in unplanned or unprotected sex, to drive after drinking, and to get hurt or injured (Table 10-2). Binge drinkers were also more likely to miss classes, get behind in schoolwork, and argue with friends. The more frequent the binges, the more problems the students encountered. Despite their experiences, fewer than 1% of the binge drinkers identified themselves as problem drinkers.

Terms

alcohol abuse The use of alcohol to a degree that causes physical damage, impairs functioning, or results in behavior harmful to others.

alcohol dependence A pathological use of alcohol or impairment in functioning due to alcohol; characterized by tolerance and withdrawal symptoms; alcoholism.

alcoholism A chronic psychological disorder characterized by excessive and compulsive drinking.

binge drinking Periodically drinking alcohol to the point of severe intoxication.

hallucination A false perception that does not correspond to external reality, such as seeing visions or hearing voices that are not there.

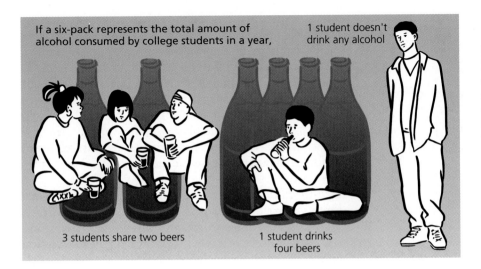

If a six-pack represents the total amount of alcohol consumed by college students in a year,

1 student doesn't drink any alcohol

3 students share two beers

1 student drinks four beers

Figure 10-4   Alcohol consumption by college students.   Alcohol consumption by students varies considerably, with some abstaining and some drinking large amounts. Only one in five college students is a frequent binge drinker, but this group accounts for two-thirds of all the alcohol consumed by college students each year and causes or experiences the majority of alcohol-related problems.   SOURCE: Wechsler, H., et al. 2000. *From Knowledge to Action: How Harvard's College Alcohol Study Can Help Your Campus Design a Campaign Against Student Alcohol Abuse* (http://www.hsph.harvard.edu/cas/test/articles/change2.html; retrieved July 17, 2000).

Binge drinking kills dozens of American college students each year. Some die from acute alcohol poisoning. The typical scenario involves a hazing ritual, a competition, or a bet that involves drinking a large amount of alcohol very quickly. This kind of fast, heavy drinking can result in unconsciousness and death very quickly, before anyone realizes that something is seriously wrong. Many other students die from alcohol-related injuries, including those from motor vehicle crashes.

Binge drinking also affects nonbingeing students. At schools with high rates of binge drinking, the nonbingers were up to twice as likely to report being bothered by the alcohol-related behaviors of others than students at schools with lower rates of binge drinking. These problems included having sleep or studying disrupted; having to take care of a drunken student; being insulted or humiliated; experiencing unwanted sexual advances; and being pushed, hit, or assaulted.

The *Healthy People 2010* report sets the goal of reducing the rate of binge drinking to 20% among college students. Binge drinking is a difficult problem to address because many students arrive at college with drinking patterns already established (binge drinking during high school is a strong predictor of binge drinking during the college years). The National Institutes of Health estimate that 3 million children between the ages of 14 and 17 are already problem drinkers. Many colleges have drinking "cultures" that perpetuate the pattern of binge drinking. On many campuses, drinking behavior that would be classified as abuse in another setting may be viewed as socially acceptable or even attractive. This is despite the evidence that such behavior leads to automobile crashes, injuries, violence, suicide, and high-risk sexual behavior (see the box "Facts About Drinking Among College Students").

COMMUNICATE!   Responsible drinking typically involves saying no to alcoholic beverages—either because you choose not to drink at all or because you want to limit your drinks. Because it's much more difficult to say no once you're in a social situation, it's a good idea to plan ahead and even rehearse what you'll say. Some possible responses are "No thanks—I've had enough for now," "I'm going to wait for a while," "I have to get up early," and "I think I'll switch to soda." Develop responses that are comfortable for you and that work in your social situations.

Alcoholism

As mentioned earlier, alcoholism, or alcohol dependence, is usually characterized by tolerance to alcohol and withdrawal symptoms. Everyone who drinks—even nonalcoholics—develops tolerance after repeated alcohol use. As described in Chapter 9, *tolerance* means that a drinker needs more alcohol to achieve intoxication or the desired effect, that the effects of continued use of the same amount of alcohol are diminished, or that the drinker can function adequately at doses or a BAC that would produce significant impairment in a casual user. Heavy users of alcohol may need to consume about 50% more than they originally needed in order to experience the same degree of intoxication.

Withdrawal occurs when someone who has been using alcohol heavily for several days or more suddenly stops drinking or markedly reduces her or his intake. Symptoms of withdrawal include trembling and nervousness and sometimes even **hallucinations** and seizures.

Table 10-2	The Effects of Binge Drinking on College Students	
	Percentage of Students Experiencing Problems	
Alcohol-Related Problem	Non–Binge Drinkers	Frequent Binge Drinkers
Drove after drinking alcohol	19	57
Did something they regretted	18	62
Got behind in schoolwork	10	46
Argued with friends	10	43
Missed a class	9	63
Engaged in unplanned sex	8	42
Had unprotected sex	4	20
Got hurt or injured	4	27
Got into trouble with police	1	13
Had five or more of these problems since school year began	4	48

SOURCE: Wechsler, H., et al. 2000. College binge drinking in the 1990s: A continuing problem. *Journal of American College Health* 48: 199–210.

Patterns and Prevalence   Alcoholism occurs among people of all ethnic groups and at all socioeconomic levels. The stereotype of the alcoholic skid row bum actually accounts for fewer than 5% of all alcohol-dependent people and usually represents the final stage of a drinking career that began years earlier. There are different patterns of alcohol dependence, including these four common ones:

1. *Regular daily intake of large amounts.* This continuous pattern is the most common adult pattern of excessive consumption in most countries.

2. *Regular heavy drinking limited to weekends.* This pattern of binge drinking is often followed by teenagers and college students.

3. *Long periods of sobriety interspersed with binges of daily heavy drinking lasting for weeks or months.* This episodic, or "bender," pattern is common in the United States but quite uncommon in France, although the per capita consumption of alcohol is higher in France.

4. *Heavy drinking limited to periods of stress.* This "reactive" pattern is associated with periods of anxiety or depression, such as at times of test anxiety or during other performance fears, interpersonal problems, or school or work pressures.

Once established, alcoholism often exhibits a pattern of exacerbations and remissions. The person may stop drinking and abstain from alcohol for days or months after a frightening problem develops. After a period of abstinence, an alcoholic often attempts controlled drinking, which almost inevitably leads to an escalation in drinking and more problems. Alcoholism is not hopeless, however; many alcoholics do achieve permanent abstinence.

According to the National Household Survey on Drug Abuse about 12.4 million Americans are heavy drinkers and 45 million are binge drinkers. Studies suggest that the lifetime risk of alcoholism in the United States is about 10% for men and about 3% for women. The risk for women has been increasing in recent years, as women's roles in our society have expanded.

Health Effects   Tolerance and withdrawal can have a serious impact on health. An alcoholic requires increasingly larger amounts to produce the desired effects, and these larger doses increase the chance of adverse physical effects. When alcoholics stop drinking or sharply decrease their intake, they experience withdrawal. Symptoms include trembling hands ("shakes" or "jitters"), a rapid pulse and accelerated breathing rate, insomnia, nightmares, anxiety, and gastrointestinal upset. These symptoms usually begin 5–10 hours after alcohol intake is decreased and improve after 4–5 days. After a week, most people feel much better, but occasionally anxiety, insomnia, and other symptoms persist for 6 months or more.

More severe withdrawal symptoms occur in about 5% of alcoholics. These include seizures (sometimes called "rum fits"), confusion, and hallucinations. Still less common is **DTs (delirium tremens),** a medical emergency characterized by severe disorientation, confusion, multiple seizures, and vivid hallucinations, often of vermin and small animals. The mortality rate from DTs can be as high as 15%, especially in very debilitated people with preexisting medical illnesses.

Because alcohol is distributed throughout the body's organs and tissues, alcoholism takes a heavy physical and psychological toll. Alcoholics face all the physical health risks associated with intoxication and chronic drinking described earlier in the chapter. Some of the damage is worsened by nutritional deficiencies that often accompany alcoholism. Some people develop alcoholic **paranoia,** characterized by delusions, jealousy, suspicion, and mistrust. Other mental problems associated with alcoholism include profound memory gaps (commonly known as "blackouts"), which are sometimes filled by conscious or unconscious lying.

The specific health effects of alcoholism tend to vary from person to person. One individual may suffer primarily from problems with memory and CNS defects while having no liver or gastrointestinal problems. Another person with a similar drinking and nutritional history may have advanced liver disease but no memory gaps.

Social and Psychological Effects   Alcohol use causes more serious social and psychological problems than all other forms of substance abuse combined. For every person who is an alcoholic, another three or four people are

- About 20% of students do not use any alcohol, and a large majority (66%) do not binge-drink. About 23% of college students are frequent binge drinkers.

- Students who do well academically tend to drink less than those who do poorly. About 40% of students' academic problems and 28% of dropouts are related to alcohol use.

- Among students at 2-year colleges, those with an A average have about 2.5 drinks per week; B students have 3.5; C students, 4; and D or F students, 6. A similar pattern is seen among students at 4-year colleges.

- Students who drink moderately or not at all are less likely to be victims of crime. Between 50% and 80% of all violence on college campuses is alcohol-related, with both perpetrators and victims likely to have been drinking. Nearly 70% of perpetrators and 80% of victims of sexual assault are under the influence of alcohol at the time of the attack.

- College students who abstain or drink moderately are less likely to acquire sexually transmitted diseases or have an unwanted pregnancy.

- One in ten female frequent binge drinkers reports having engaged in nonconsensual sexual intercourse while drunk.

- Binge drinking is especially common in fraternities and sororities and among athletes. Enrollment in Greek organizations has been flat or down during the past few years on most campuses, in part due to negative publicity about alcohol abuse, hazing, violence, and poor academics.

- Seven in eight nonbingeing students have been negatively affected by the drinking of others. In surveys, more than half of all students favor more college intervention to stop excessive student drinking.

- Nearly 90% of college students support the policy of providing alcohol-free dormitories on campus. Three of five non–binge drinkers either currently live in an alcohol-free dorm or would like to live in one.

- College students sometimes turn to alcohol because it is one of the least expensive forms of "entertainment" available. A recent survey of college communities showed that students could binge-drink for well under five dollars, making drinking much cheaper than going to the movies or to a concert. Many large campuses are surrounded by a high density of stores and bars that sell alcohol at very low cost.

SOURCES: Wechsler, H., et al. 2000. College binge drinking in the 1990s: A continuing problem. *Journal of American College Health* 48: 199–210. Wechsler, H., et al. 2000. Environmental correlates of underage alcohol use and related problems of college students. *American Journal of Preventive Medicine* 19(1): 24–29. Elgin, L. D. 1991. *Alcohol Practices, Policies, and Potentials of American Colleges and Universities.* Washington, D.C.: U.S. Department of Health and Human Services.

---

directly affected (see the box "Children of Alcoholics"). In a 2000 Gallup poll, 36% of Americans reported that alcohol had been a source of trouble in their family—the highest rate recorded since Gallup began asking the question in 1950.

Alcoholics frequently suffer from *dual disorders,* mental disorders in addition to their substance dependence. Alcoholics are much more likely than nonalcoholics to suffer from clinical depression, panic disorder, schizophrenia, and antisocial personality disorders. People with anxiety or panic attacks may try to use alcohol to lessen their anxiety, even though alcohol often makes these disorders worse. Alcoholics also often have other substance-abuse problems.

An estimated 3 million Americans age 14–17 show signs of potential alcohol dependence. These numbers are far greater than those associated with cocaine, heroin, or marijuana use. The social and psychological consequences of excessive drinking in young people are more difficult to measure than the risks to physical health. One of the consequences is that excessive drinking interferes with learning the interpersonal and job-related skills required for adult life. Excessive drinkers sometimes narrow their circle of friends to other heavy drinkers and thus limit the range of people they can learn from. Per-

haps most important is that people who were excessive drinkers in college are more likely to have social, occupational, and health problems 20 years later. Despite media attention on cocaine and other drugs, alcohol abuse remains our society's number one drug problem.

Causes of Alcoholism   The precise causes of alcoholism are unknown, but many factors are probably involved. Recent studies of twins and adopted children clearly demonstrate the importance of genetics. If one of a pair of fraternal twins is alcoholic, then the other has about twice the chance of becoming alcoholic. For the identical twin of an alcoholic, the risk of alcoholism is about four times that of the general population. These risks persist even when the twins have little contact with each other or their biological parents. Similarly, adoption studies show an increased risk

DTs (delirium tremens) A state of confusion brought on by the reduction of alcohol intake in an alcohol-dependent person; other symptoms are sweating, trembling, anxiety, hallucinations, and seizures.

paranoia A mental disorder characterized by persistent delusions—fixed, false beliefs that would not be accepted by the individual's culture.

Terms

About one out of eight Americans grows up in an alcoholic household. For these children, life is a struggle to deal with constant stress, anxiety, and embarrassment. They may be victims of violence, abuse, or neglect in the home. Family life centers on the drinking parent, and children's needs are often ignored.

Children in alcoholic households often cope by learning patterns of interaction that help them survive childhood but that don't support their own healthy development. Many adult children of alcoholics fear losing control, and they try to control their own feelings and behavior and those of people around them. They may fear emotions, even pleasant feelings such as happiness and joy. They avoid conflict and are easily upset by criticism from authority figures. Other common traits include an overdeveloped sense of responsibility and hypersensitivity to the needs of others. Children of alcoholics often feel guilty if they stand up for themselves and acknowledge their own needs. All these characteristics can be stumbling blocks to forming healthy relationships.

Children of alcoholics are more likely than other children to become alcoholic themselves and to marry alcoholics. An estimated 13–25% of children of alcoholics will become alcoholic at some point in their lives. They are more likely to abuse other

drugs and develop an eating disorder. They are also particularly prone to stress-related medical illnesses.

If you are the child of an alcoholic, be aware, first, that you are not alone. Millions of people have been through the same problem and have dreamed of having a happy family life in which drinking is not an issue. Realize, too, that other people can understand what you have been through and can help. Find a person you can trust, and confide in her or him. It may seem safer to keep your feelings secret, but talking about the problem is the first step toward a healthy readjustment. Many adult children of alcoholics benefit greatly from therapy with a counselor who is experienced in treating people who have been affected by an alcoholic family. Individual or group therapy can be a critical step in recovery. (The For More Information section at the end of this chapter lists agencies that can provide help and referrals.)

Finally, acknowledge that your parent's alcoholism is not your fault. Many children of alcoholics carry a burden of guilt from early childhood, when they could not understand that they weren't the cause of their parent's behavior. This unexamined assumption is often part of the emotional pain experienced by children of alcoholics.

for children of alcoholics, even if they were adopted at birth into nondrinking families. Alcoholism in adoptive parents, on the other hand, doesn't make individuals more or less likely to become alcoholic. Some studies suggest that as much as 50% of a person's risk for alcoholism is determined by genetic factors.

Not all children of alcoholics become alcoholic, however, and it is clear that other factors are involved. A person's risk of developing alcoholism may be increased by certain personality disorders, having been subjected as a child to destructive child-rearing practices, and imitating the alcohol abuse of peers and other role models. People who begin drinking excessively in their teens are especially prone to alcoholism later in life. Common psychological features of individuals who abuse alcohol are denial ("I don't have a problem") and rationalization ("I drink because I need to socialize with my customers"). Certain social factors have also been linked with alcoholism, including urbanization, disappearance of the extended family, a general loosening of kinship ties, increased mobility, and changing values.

Treatment   Some alcoholics recover without professional help. How often this occurs is unknown, but possibly as many as 25% stop drinking on their own or reduce their drinking enough to eliminate problems. Often these spontaneous recoveries are linked to an alcohol-related crisis, such as a health problem or the threat of being fired. Not all alcoholics must "hit bottom" before they are motivated to stop. People vary markedly in what induces them

to change their behavior. For some, the first blackout or alcohol-related automobile crash fosters abstinence.

Most alcoholics, however, require a treatment program of some kind in order to stop drinking. Many different kinds of programs exist. No single treatment works for everyone, so a person may have to try different programs before finding the right one. Over 1 million Americans enter treatment for alcoholism every year.

Although treatment is not successful for all alcoholics, considerable optimism has replaced the older view that nothing could be done. Many alcoholics have patterns of drinking that fluctuate widely over time. These fluctuations indicate that their alcohol abuse is a response to environmental factors, such as life stressors or social pressures, and therefore may be influenced by treatment.

One of the oldest and best-known recovery programs is Alcoholics Anonymous (AA). AA consists of self-help groups that meet several times each week in most communities and follow a 12-step program. Important steps for people in these programs include recognizing that they are "powerless over alcohol" and must seek help from a "higher power" in order to regain control of their lives. By verbalizing these steps, the alcoholic directly addresses the denial that is often prominent in alcoholism and other addictions. Many AA members have a sponsor of their choosing who is available by phone 24 hours a day for individual support and crisis intervention. AA convincingly shows the alcoholic that abstinence can be achieved and also provides a sober peer group of people who share the same identity—that of recovering alcoholics.

Nearly all alcohol treatment and support groups stress abstinence as the only option for problem drinkers. An exception is Moderation Management (MM), a recovery program and national support group network formed in the early 1990s as an alternative to typical AA-style 12-step programs. MM encourages people in the early stages of alcohol problems to learn to manage their drinking behaviors to avoid negative consequences, either by limiting alcohol intake or by abstaining. MM is quick to point out that it is not intended for alcoholics, chronic drinkers, or people who experience withdrawal symptoms when they stop drinking. Part of the MM program is a 30-day abstinence period during which people can assess for themselves whether abstinence may be preferable or easier than attempting to drink in moderation.

Many alcohol treatment experts and alcoholics in recovery have been alarmed by the MM program. They fear that it is unrealistic for people with significant alcohol problems to expect that they will ever be able to drink in moderation. According to this point of view, it is only a matter of time before the problem drinker will lose control and drink excessively. MM came under extra criticism in 2000 because Audrey Kishline, the founder of MM, killed two people in an alcohol-related car crash. Her BAC at the time was 0.26%, more than three times the legal limit. She pled guilty to charges of vehicular homicide and was sentenced to four-and-a-half years in prison.

It is tempting but perhaps unfair to blame this tragedy on MM. For one thing, Kishline had recognized several months before the crash that moderate drinking was not working for her and had joined AA. Unfortunately, she also failed at abstinence, with tragic results. MM's critics point out that a problem drinker may not be a good judge of whether he or she has a "mild" problem with alcohol and perhaps could learn to drink in moderation or has a more severe alcohol problem, where abstinence would be the only reasonable option. Considering that denial is a major aspect of alcohol addiction, alcoholics may be most likely to underestimate the severity of their difficulties with alcohol. Critics also point to MM's rather liberal drinking limits, which allow a higher level of alcohol intake than suggested by the *Dietary Guidelines for Americans*. (MM suggests that people abstain from drinking alcohol at least 3 or 4 days per week, that women limit themselves to no more than 3 drinks on any day and 9 drinks total per week, and that men limit themselves to no more than 4 drinks on any day and 14 drinks total per week. The limits set by the *Dietary Guidelines* are no more than 2 drinks per day for men and 1 drink per day for women.) Critics fear that MM's drinking limits may attract alcoholics looking for an excuse to leave AA and abstinence.

The flip side of this argument is that AA and similar programs may not appeal to people in the beginning stages of problem drinking. These individuals may opt to do nothing about their problem if they feel that their only alternative is a program that prescribes lifetime abstinence. MM may seem like a less-threatening first step. A recent study of former alcoholics and alcohol abusers who had been in remission for at least 1 year found that two-thirds of the subjects still drank alcohol occasionally, while the remaining one-third did not drink at all. (In this study, remission was defined as cessation of the negative consequences of drinking, and participants had been in remission for an average of 11 years.) Other studies have also shown that many people who were once problem drinkers have successfully altered their drinking patterns to avoid the negative consequences of alcohol use—without totally abstaining. MM and similar programs may provide support for people who have just begun to have problems with drinking and who want to control their use of alcohol without abstaining.

Alcoholics Anonymous is generally recognized as an effective mutual help program, but not everyone responds to its style and message, and other recovery approaches are available. Some, like Rational Recovery and Women for Sobriety, deliberately avoid any emphasis on higher spiritual powers. Even people who are helped by AA often find that it works best in combination with counseling and medical care. A more controversial approach to problem drinking is offered by the group Moderation Management, which encourages people to manage their drinking behavior by limiting intake or abstaining (see the box "Does Moderation Work for Problem Drinkers?").

A companion program to AA is Al-Anon, which consists of groups for families and friends of alcoholics. In Al-Anon, spouses and others explore how they enabled the alcoholic to drink by denying, rationalizing, or covering up his or her drinking and how they can change this codependent behavior.

Employee assistance programs and school-based programs represent another approach to alcoholism treatment that works for some people. One of the advantages of these programs is that they can deal directly with work and campus issues, often important sources of stress for the alcohol abuser. These programs sometimes encourage learning effective coping responses for internal and external sources of distress. Individuals might also benefit from learning new cognitive concepts, such as a self-identity that does not involve drinking.

Inpatient hospital rehabilitation is useful for some alcoholics, especially if they have serious medical or mental problems or if life stressors threaten to overwhelm them. When the person returns to the community, however, it is critical that there be some form of active, continuing, long-term treatment. Patients who return to a spouse or family often require ongoing treatment on issues involving those significant others, such as establishing new routines and planning shared recreational activities that do not involve drinking.

There are also some pharmacological treatments for alcoholism. One involves the use of disulfiram (trade name

Antabuse), which inhibits the metabolic breakdown of acetaldehyde (see the box "Metabolizing Alcohol: Our Bodies Work Differently"). Disulfiram causes patients to become violently ill when they drink and thus theoretically prevents impulse drinking. However, it is potentially dangerous and must be combined with ongoing therapy to be useful over time. In contrast to Antabuse, naltrexone reduces the craving for alcohol and decreases the pleasant, reinforcing effects of alcohol without making the user ill. Naltrexone works most effectively in combination with counseling and other forms of psychosocial treatment. Research is currently underway on other medications, including nalmefene, acamprosate, and ondansetron.

In people who abuse alcohol and have significant depression or anxiety, the use of antidepressant or antianxiety medication can improve both mental health and drinking behavior. In addition, drugs such as diazepam (Valium) are sometimes prescribed to replace alcohol during initial stages of withdrawal. Most therapists feel that such chemical substitutes are useful for only a week or so, because alcoholics are at particularly high risk for developing dependence on Valium and other similar medications. Drug therapy is usually only a small component of an alcohol-treatment plan. Counseling and peer-group support are generally the most essential elements of alcoholism treatment.

Alcohol-treatment programs are successful in achieving an extended period of sobriety for about half of those who participate. Success rates of conventional treatment programs are about the same for men and women and for people from different ethnic groups. Women, minorities, and the poor often face major economic and social barriers to receiving treatment. Most inpatient treatment programs are financially out of reach for people of low income or those without insurance coverage. AA remains the mainstay of treatment for most people and is often a component of even the most expensive treatment programs. Special AA groups exist in many communities for young people, women, gay men and lesbians, non–English speakers, and a variety of interest groups. You can find out about AA meetings in your community by looking in the phone book or consulting the For More Information section at the end of the chapter.

Gender and Ethnic Differences

Alcohol abusers come from all socioeconomic levels and cultural groups, but there are notable differences in patterns of drinking between men and women and among different ethnic groups.

Men Among white American men, excessive drinking often begins in the teens or twenties and progresses gradually through the thirties, until the individual is clearly identifiable as an alcoholic by the time he is in his late thirties or early forties. Other men remain controlled drinkers until later in life, sometimes becoming alcoholic in association with retirement, the inevitable losses of aging, boredom, illness, or psychological disorders.

Women The progression of alcoholism in women is usually different. Women tend to become alcoholic at a later age and with fewer years of heavy drinking. It is not unusual for women in their forties or fifties to become alcoholic after years of controlled drinking. Women alcoholics develop cirrhosis and other medical complications somewhat more often than men. Women alcoholics may have more medical problems because they are less likely to seek early treatment. In addition, there may be an inherently greater biological risk for women who drink (see the box "Women and Alcohol").

African Americans Alcohol abuse is a serious problem for African Americans. Although as a group they use less alcohol than most other groups (including whites), they face disproportionately high levels of alcohol-related birth defects, cirrhosis, cancer, hypertension, and other medical problems. In addition, blacks are more likely than members of other ethnic groups to be victims of alcohol-related homicides, criminal assaults, and injuries. African American women are more likely to abstain from alcohol use than white women, but among black women who drink, there is a higher percentage of heavy drinkers. Urban black males commonly start drinking excessively and develop serious neurological illnesses at an earlier age than urban white males. They also have a higher rate of alcoholism-related suicide.

AA groups of predominantly African Americans have been shown to provide effective treatment, perhaps because essential elements of AA—sharing common experiences, mutual acceptance of one another as human beings, and trusting a higher power—are already a part of African American culture. Treatment efforts that use the extended family and include occupational training are also especially effective.

Latinos Drinking patterns among Latinos vary significantly, depending on their specific cultural background and how long they and their families have lived in the United States. Drunk driving and cirrhosis are the most common causes of alcohol-related death and injury among Hispanic men. Hispanic women are more likely to abstain from alcohol than white or black women, but those who do drink are at special risk for problems. Treating the entire family as a unit is an important part of treatment because family pride, solidarity, and support are important aspects of Latino culture. Some Hispanics do better during treatment if treatment efforts are integrated with the techniques of *curanderos* (folk healers) and *espiritistas* (spiritists).

Asian Americans As a group, Asian Americans have lower-than-average rates of alcohol abuse. However, ac-

Whether a woman is a "social drinker," a binge drinker, or a heavy daily user, the impact of alcohol on her will be different from and generally greater than for comparable use in a man. Women become intoxicated at lower doses of alcohol because of their smaller size, greater proportion of body fat, and less active form of an alcohol-metabolizing stomach enzyme. Hormonal fluctuations may also affect the rate of alcohol metabolism, making a woman more susceptible to high BACs at certain times during her menstrual cycle (usually just prior to the onset of menstruation).

Like men, women are more likely to be the perpetrator or victim of a crime when they have been drinking. Sexual assaults of all types, and date rape in particular, are more likely to occur if a woman has been drinking. Alcohol use makes women much less likely to practice safer sex, leaving them especially vulnerable to significant and lasting health problems as a result of sexually transmitted diseases and unintended pregnancy.

Women tend to experience the adverse physical effects of chronic drinking sooner and at lower levels of alcohol consumption than men. Female alcoholics have death rates 50–100% higher than those of male alcoholics. They develop alcohol liver disease after a comparatively shorter period of heavy drinking and at a lower level of daily drinking than men. They have higher death rates from cirrhosis. Other alcohol-related health problems that are unique to women include an increased risk for breast cancer, menstrual disorders, infertility, and, in pregnant women, giving birth to a child suffering from FAS. Because of the social stigma attached to problem drinking, women are also less likely to seek early treatment.

About one-third of all problem drinkers in the United States are women. Women from all walks of life and all ethnic groups can develop alcohol problems, but those who have never married or are divorced are more likely to drink heavily than married or widowed women. Women who have multiple life roles, such as parent, worker, and spouse, are less vulnerable to alcohol problems than women who have fewer roles.

culturation may somewhat weaken the generally strong Asian taboos and community sanctions against alcohol use. For many Asian Americans, though, the genetically based physiological aversion to alcohol remains a deterrent to abuse. For those needing treatment, ethnic agencies, health care professionals, and ministers seem to be the most effective sources.

American Indians and Alaska Natives   Alcohol abuse is one of the most widespread and severe health problems among American Indians and Alaska Natives, especially for adolescents and young adults. Excessive drinking varies from tribe to tribe but is generally high in both men and women. The rate of alcoholism among American Indians is twice that of the general population, and the death rate from alcohol-related causes is about eight times higher. Treatment programs may be more effective if they reflect tribal values. Some healers have incorporated aspects of American Indian religions into the therapeutic process, using traditional sweat houses, prayers, and dances.

Helping Someone with an Alcohol Problem

Helping a friend or relative with an alcohol problem requires skill and tact. One of the first steps is making sure you are not an enabler or codependent, perhaps unknowingly allowing someone to continue excessively using alcohol. Enabling takes many forms. One of the most common is making excuses or covering up for the alcohol abuser—for example, saying "he has the flu" when it is really a hangover. Whenever you find yourself minimizing or lying about someone's drinking behavior, a warn-

ing bell should sound. Another important step is open, honest labeling—"I think you have a problem with alcohol." Such explicit statements usually elicit emotional rebuttals and may endanger a relationship. In the long run, however, you are not helping your friends by allowing them to deny their problems with alcohol or other drugs. Taking action shows that you care.

Even when problems are acknowledged, there is usually reluctance to get help. You can't cure a friend's drinking problem, but you can guide him or her to appropriate help. Your best role might be to obtain information about the available resources and persistently encourage their use. Consider making an appointment for your friend at the student health center and then go with him or her to the appointment. Most student health centers will be able to recommend local options for self-help groups and formal treatment; the counseling center is another excellent source for help. You can also check the phone book and the Internet for local chapters of AA and other groups (see For More Information at the end of the chapter). And don't underestimate the power of families to help. An honest phone call to your friend's parents could save a life if your friend is in serious trouble with alcohol.

DRINKING BEHAVIOR AND RESPONSIBILITY

The responsible use of alcohol means drinking in such a way that you keep your BAC low, so that your behavior is always under your control. In addition to controlling your own drinking, there are things you can do to promote responsible alcohol use in others.

Examine Your Attitudes About Alcohol Use

Think about how you really feel about drinking. Is it of little consequence to you or perhaps even an intrusion into your college experience? Or is alcohol the key ingredient for any and all fun activities? Can you imagine having a good time at a party or at the beach without alcoholic beverages? How do you perceive nondrinkers at a party where others are drinking? Do they seem mature or odd? What do your answers to these questions say about your attitude about alcohol and the role of alcohol in your life?

Attitudes toward drinking are usually based on a multitude of experiences, including your family background. Consider how alcohol was used in your family when you were growing up. Was it used for family celebrations? Was alcohol a "big deal" in your family, or was it treated as a relatively unimportant occasional addition to dinner? Was alcohol a source of problems, with a parent or relative becoming dependent on alcohol and/or abusive when drunk? Do you think that alcohol problems run in your family? Understanding the source of some of your beliefs and feelings about alcohol may give you insight into your current drinking habits as well as your feelings about other people's use of alcohol.

Also examine your ideas about alcohol use on your college campus. Does it seem to you as if everyone at your college drinks? Do you feel pressure to drink or use drugs, even if you don't really feel like it? Who pressures you? Why do you think some people push others to engage in heavy drinking? A recent survey of college students found that over half felt pressured to use alcohol or illegal drugs and that this pressure hampered their schoolwork. Even though it may seem that "everyone" drinks, about 1 in 5 college students is a nondrinker, with a higher percentage of abstainers at many schools. Remember, too, that the majority of American adults drink moderately or not at all. Frequent binge drinking is far outside the norm in the adult world.

WW. Examine Your Drinking Behavior

When you want to drink responsibly, it's helpful to know, first of all, why you drink. The following are common reasons given by college students:

- "It lets me go along with my friends."
- "It makes me less self-conscious and more social."
- "It makes me less inhibited in thinking, saying, or doing certain things."
- "It relieves depression, anxiety, tension, or worries."
- "It enables me to experience a different state of consciousness."

If you drink alcohol, what are your reasons for doing so? Are you attempting to meet underlying needs that could best be addressed by other means?

After examining your reasons for drinking, take a closer look at your drinking behavior. Is it moderate and responsible? Or do you frequently overindulge and suffer negative consequences? The Behavior Change Strategy at the end of the chapter explains how to keep and analyze a record of your drinking. The so-called CAGE screening test can help you determine whether you, or someone close to you, may have a drinking problem. Answer yes or no to the following questions:

Have you ever felt you should
    Cut down on your drinking?
Have people
    Annoyed you by criticizing your drinking?
Have you ever felt bad or
    Guilty about your drinking?
Have you ever had an
    Eye-opener (a drink first thing in the morning to steady your nerves or get rid of a hangover)

One "yes" response suggests a possible alcohol problem; if you answered yes to more than one question, it is highly likely that a problem exists. For a more detailed evaluation of your drinking habits, complete the questionnaire in the box "Do You Have a Problem with Alcohol?" If the results of either assessment test indicate a potential problem, get help right away.

Drink Moderately and Responsibly

Sometimes people lose control when they misjudge how much they can drink. At other times, they set out deliberately to get drunk. Following are some strategies for keeping your drinking and your behavior under control.

Drink Slowly   Learn to sip your drinks rather than gulp them. Do not drink alcoholic beverages to quench your thirst. Avoid drinks made with carbonated mixers, especially if you're thirsty; you'll be more likely to gulp them down.

Space Your Drinks   Learn to drink nonalcoholic drinks at parties, or alternate them with alcoholic drinks. Learn to refuse a round: "I've had enough for right now." Parties are easier for some people if they hold a glass of something nonalcoholic that has ice and a twist of lime floating in it so it looks like an alcoholic drink.

Eat Before and While Drinking   Avoid drinking on an empty stomach. Food in your stomach will not prevent the alcohol from eventually being absorbed, but it will slow down the rate somewhat and thus often lower the peak BAC. In restaurants, order your food before you order a drink. Try to have something to eat before you go out to a party where alcohol will be served.

Know Your Limits and Your Drinks   Learn how different BACs affect you. In a safe setting such as your home, with your roommate or a friend, see how a set amount—

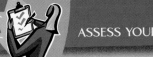

For each question, choose the answer that best describes your behavior. Then total your scores.

Questions	Points					Your Score
	0	1	2	3	4	
1. How often do you have a drink containing alcohol?	Never	Monthly or less	2–4 times a month	2–3 times a week	4 or more times a week	_____
2. How many drinks containing alcohol do you have on a typical day when you are drinking?	1 or 2	3 or 4	5 or 6	7 to 9	10 or more	_____
3. How often do you have six or more drinks on one occasion?	Never	Less than monthly	Monthly	Weekly	Daily or almost daily	_____
4. How often during the past year have you found that you were not able to stop drinking once you had started?	Never	Less than monthly	Monthly	Weekly	Daily or almost daily	_____
5. How often during the past year have you failed to do what was normally expected because of drinking?	Never	Less than monthly	Monthly	Weekly	Daily or almost daily	_____
6. How often during the past year have you needed a first drink in the morning to get yourself going after a heavy drinking session?	Never	Less than monthly	Monthly	Weekly	Daily or almost daily	_____
7. How often during the past year have you had a feeling of guilt or remorse after drinking?	Never	Less than monthly	Monthly	Weekly	Daily or almost daily	_____
8. How often during the past year have you been unable to remember what happened the night before because you had been drinking?	Never	Less than monthly	Monthly	Weekly	Daily or almost daily	_____
9. Have you or has someone else been injured as a result of your drinking?	No	Yes, but not in the past year (2 points)		Yes, during the past year (4 points)		_____
10. Has a relative, friend, doctor, or other health worker been concerned about your drinking or suggested you cut down?	No	Yes, but not in the past year (2 points)		Yes, during the past year (4 points)		_____

Total _____

A total score of 8 or more indicates a strong likelihood of hazardous or harmful alcohol consumption. Even if you score below 8, if you are encountering drinking-related problems with your academic performance, job, relationships, health, or the law, you should consider seeking help. The effects of alcohol abuse can be extremely serious—even fatal—both to you and to others.

SOURCE: Saunders, J. B., et al. 1993. Development of the Alcohol Use Disorders Identification Test (AUDIT): WHO collaborative project on early detection of persons with harmful alcohol consumption—II. *Addiction* 88: 791–804. Reprinted with permission from Carfax Publishing, a division of Taylor & Francis Ltd. (http://www.tandf.co.uk).

say, two drinks in an hour—affects you. A good test is walking heel to toe in a straight line with your eyes closed or standing with your feet crossed and trying to touch your finger to your nose with your eyes closed.

But be aware that in different settings your performance, and especially your ability to judge your behavior, may change. At a given BAC, you will perform less well when surrounded by activity and boisterous companions than you will in a quiet test setting with just one or two other people. This impairment results partially because

alcohol reduces your ability to perform when your brain is bombarded by multiple stimuli. It is useful to discover the rate at which you can drink without increasing your BAC. Be able to calculate the approximate amount a given drink increases your BAC.

Promote Responsible Drinking in Others

Although you cannot completely control the drinking behavior of others, there are things you can do to help promote responsible drinking.

To be a careful and informed health consumer, you need to consider the effects that advertisements have on you. Are alcohol ads, such as those featuring talking frogs or football games between beer bottles, harmless fun? Or can they have more serious effects? How do such ads affect you?

Alcohol manufacturers spend $2 billion every year on advertising. They claim that the purpose of their advertising is to persuade adults who already drink to choose a certain brand. But in reality, ads cleverly engage young people and children—never overtly suggesting that young people should drink, but clearly linking alcohol and good times. Alcohol ads are common during televised sporting events and other shows popular with teenagers. By age 18, the average American teen will have seen 100,000 TV beer commercials. Studies show that the more TV adolescents watch, the more likely they are to take up drinking in their teens.

Alcohol manufacturers also reach out to young people at youth-oriented activities like concerts and sporting events. Product logos are heavily marketed through sales of T-shirts, hats, and other items. Many colleges allow alcohol manufacturers to advertise at campus events in exchange for sponsorship.

What is the message of all these advertisements? Think about the alcohol ads you've seen. Many give the impression that drinking alcohol is a normal part of everyday life and good times. This message seems to work well on the young, many of whom believe that heavy-duty drinking at parties is normal and fun. The use of famous athletes or actors in commercials increases the appeal of alcohol by associating it with fame, wealth, and popularity. The "Whassup?!" Bud ads feature the humorous use of "guy talk" to portray beer drinking as a supposedly critical aspect of men's relationships. What ads don't show is the darker side of drinking. You never see hangovers, car crashes, slipping grades, or violence. Although some ads include a brief message such as "know when to say when," the impact of such cautions is small compared to that of the image of happy, attractive young people having fun while drinking.

The next time you see an advertisement for alcohol, take a critical look. What is the message of the ad? What audience is being targeted, and what is the ad implying about alcohol use? Be aware of its effect on you.

Encourage Responsible Attitudes   Our society teaches us attitudes toward drinking that contribute to alcohol-related problems. Many of us have difficulty expressing disapproval about someone who has drunk too much, and we are amused by the antics of the "funny" drunk. We accept the alcohol industry's linkage of drinking with virility or sexuality (see the box "Alcohol Advertising"). And many people treat nondrinkers as nonconformists in social settings.

We need to recognize that the choice to abstain is neither odd nor unusual. More than one-third of adults do not drink at all or drink very infrequently. Most adults are capable of enjoying their leisure time without alcohol or drugs. In hazardous situations, such as driving or operating complicated machinery, abstinence is the only appropriate choice.

Be a Responsible Host   When you are the host, serve nonalcoholic beverages as well as alcohol. Popular nonalcoholic choices include soft drinks, sparkling water, fruit juice, and alcohol-free wine, beer, and mixers. Serve only enough alcohol for each guest to have a moderate number of drinks. Don't put out large kegs of beer, as these invite people to overindulge. For parties hosted by a dorm, fraternity, or other campus group, don't allow guests to have unlimited drinks for a single admission fee, as this also encourages binge drinking.

Always serve food along with alcohol, and stop serving alcohol an hour or more before people will leave. If possible, arrange carpools with designated nondrinking drivers in advance. Remind your guests who are under 21

about the new "zero tolerance" laws in many states—even a single drink can result in an illegal BAC. Insist that a guest who drank too much take a taxi, ride with someone else, or stay overnight rather than drive.

Plan social functions with no alcohol at all. Outdoor parties, hikes, and practically every other type of social occasion can be enjoyable without alcohol. If that doesn't seem possible to you, then examine your drinking patterns and attitudes toward alcohol. If you can't have fun without drinking, you may have a problem with alcohol.

Hold the Drinker Responsible   When any alcohol is consumed, the individual must take full responsibility for his or her behavior. Pardoning unacceptable behavior fosters the attitude that the behavior is due to the drug. The drinker is thereby excused from responsibility and learns to expect minimal adverse consequences for his or her behavior. Research indicates that the opposite approach—holding the individual fully accountable for his or her behavior—is a more effective policy. For example, alcohol-impaired drivers who receive legal penalties have fewer subsequent rearrests than those who receive only mandatory treatment. Restrictions on public smoking gained momentum after nonsmokers learned about the dangers that environmental tobacco smoke posed to them. Other people's drunkenness can impinge on your living or study environment. Speak up against this behavior—and insist on your rights.

Learn About Prevention Programs   What alternatives are being developed on your campus or in your commu-

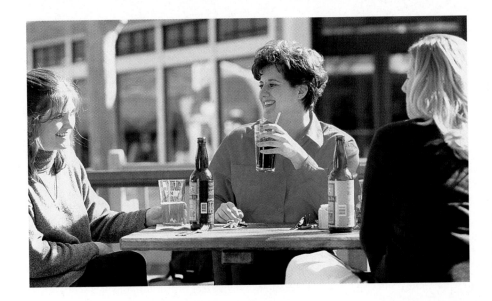

People who choose to drink should do so responsibly—in moderation and when doing so does not put themselves or others in danger. By choosing a designated driver, these women help ensure a safe trip home.

nity to "keg parties" and other events where heavy drinking occurs? Does your campus have dormitories, fraternities, or sororities where members agree to abstain from alcohol or drug use? Are programs available for students who are at high risk for alcohol abuse, such as those whose parents abused alcohol? Are counseling or self-help programs like AA available?

Take Community Action Consider joining an action group such as Students Against Destructive Decisions (SADD). The goal of SADD is to address the issues of drinking, impaired driving, drug use, and other destructive decisions and killers of young people. Lesson plans, peer counseling, and the promotion of better communication between students and parents are all used to help protect students from the dangers of drinking, drug use, and impaired driving.

COMMUNICATE! Holding drinkers accountable for their actions is a key step in promoting responsible drinking. If someone you know causes problems because of drinking, talk with her or him about it and insist on your own rights. Be honest and specific, and say how you are willing to help. Don't judge, blame, attack, or force. For example, "I'm really worried about your drinking, and I hope you won't get mad at me for saying so. You've come back to our room really drunk four times in the past week, and you woke me up when I had a big test the next morning. You've also been driving yourself home when you're drunk. I really wish you would talk to someone about your drinking. I know they have counselors at the health center, and I've heard some of them are pretty good. I'd be happy to go with you, if you want."

Tips for Today

Alcohol has a paradoxical place in our culture. Sometimes it's associated with pleasure and celebration, and sometimes it's associated with disease and death. The key is how people use or misuse it. The responsible use of alcohol means drinking in moderation or not at all.

Right now you can

- Consider whether you have a history of alcohol abuse or dependence in your family; if you do, ask yourself if you are making good decisions about alcohol right now, ones that will not cause you problems later in your life.

- If you drink, put some sodas in your refrigerator, and have one the next time you reach for a beer; offer your friends sodas too.

- If you drink, plan ahead for the next party you attend, figuring out how you can limit yourself to one or two drinks.

- Ask your roommates or friends if they know that binge drinking can be fatal; if they don't know, give them the facts about it; also share with them the information in this chapter about dealing with an alcohol emergency.

SUMMARY

- Although alcohol has been a part of human celebrations for a long time, it is a psychoactive drug capable of causing addiction.

- After being absorbed into the bloodstream in the stomach and small intestine, alcohol is transported throughout the body. The liver metabolizes alcohol as blood circulates through it.

How much do you drink? Is it the right amount for you? You may know the answer to this question already, or you may not have given it much thought. Many people learn through a single unpleasant experience how alcohol affects them. Others suffer ill effects but choose to ignore or deny them.

To make responsible, informed choices about using alcohol, consider, first, whether there is any history of alcohol abuse in your family. If someone in your family is dependent on alcohol, you have a higher-than-average likelihood of becoming dependent too. Second, consider whether you are dependent on other substances or behaviors. Do you smoke, drink strong coffee every day, or use other drugs regularly? Does some habit control your life? Some people have more of a tendency to become addicted than others, and a person with one addiction is often likely to have other addictions as well. If this is the case for you, again, you may need to be more cautious with alcohol.

Keep a Record

Once you have answered these questions, find out more about your alcohol-related behavior by keeping track of your drinking for 2 weeks in your health journal. Keep a daily alcohol behavior record like the one illustrated in Chapter 1 for eating behavior. Include information on

- *The drinking situation,* including type of drink, time of day, how fast you drank it, where you were, and what else you were doing.

- *Your internal state,* including what made you want to drink and your feelings, thoughts, and concerns at the time. Note how others influenced you.

- *The consequences of drinking,* including any changes in your feelings or behavior while or after you were drinking, such as silliness, assertiveness, aggressiveness, or depression.

Analyze Your Record

Next, analyze your record to detect patterns of feelings and environmental cues. Do you always drink when you're at a certain place or with certain people? Do you sometimes drink just to be sociable, when you don't really want a drink and would be satisfied with a nonalcoholic beverage? Refer to the list of warning signs of alcohol abuse given in the text. Are any of them true for you? For example, do you feel uncomfortable in a social situation if alcohol is *not* available?

Set Goals

Now that you've analyzed your record, think about whether you want to change any of your behaviors. Would you do better academically if you drank less? Has drinking had a negative impact on any of your relationships? Have you risked infection and unplanned pregnancy by having unprotected sex while drunk? Do you depend on alcohol in order to have a good time? Have you been injured while drinking? If you drink and drive or if you feel you are becoming dependent on alcohol, it is time

---

- If people drink more alcohol each hour than their body can metabolize, blood alcohol concentration (BAC) increases. The rate of alcohol metabolism depends on a variety of individual factors, including gender, body weight, and percentage of body fat.

- Alcohol is a CNS depressant. At low doses, it tends to make people feel relaxed.

- At higher doses, alcohol interferes with motor and mental functioning; at very high doses, alcohol poisoning, coma, and death can occur. Effects may be increased if alcohol is combined with other drugs.

- Alcohol use increases the risk of injury and violence; drinking before driving is particularly dangerous, even at low doses.

- Continued alcohol use has negative effects on the digestive and cardiovascular systems and increases cancer risk and overall mortality.

- Pregnant women who drink risk giving birth to children with a cluster of birth defects known as fetal alcohol syndrome (FAS). Even occasional drinking during pregnancy can cause brain injury in the fetus.

- Moderate drinking may decrease the risk of coronary heart disease in some people.

- Alcohol abuse involves drinking in dangerous situations or drinking to a degree that causes academic, professional, interpersonal, or legal difficulties.

- Alcohol dependence, or alcoholism, is characterized by more extensive problems with alcohol, usually involving tolerance and withdrawal.

- Binge drinking is a common form of alcohol abuse on college campuses that has negative effects on both drinking and nondrinking students.

- Physical consequences of alcoholism include the direct effects of tolerance and withdrawal, as well as all the problems associated with chronic drinking. Psychological problems include paranoia, memory loss, and dual disorders.

- Treatment approaches include mutual support groups like AA, job- and school-based programs, inpatient hospital programs, and pharmacological treatments.

- Helping someone who abuses alcohol means avoid-

to change your drinking behavior. Decide on goals that will give you the best health and safety returns, such as a beer or a glass of wine with dinner, one drink per hour at a party, or no alcohol at all.

Devise a Plan

Refer to your health journal to see what kinds of patterns your drinking falls into and where you can intervene to break the behavior chain. If you have determined that your life would be improved if you changed your drinking habits, now is the time to make changes. For some people, simple changes in the environment such as stocking the refrigerator with alternative beverages like juices or sparkling water can be helpful. If you feel self-conscious about ordering a nonalcoholic drink when you're out with a group, try recruiting a friend to do the same. If it's too difficult to avoid drinking in some situations, such as at a bar or beer party, you may decide to avoid those situations for a period of time.

Examine your friendships. If drinking is becoming a problem for you and some of your friends drink heavily, you may need to think about letting those relationships go. If you find support groups helpful, check with your college counseling center or health clinic; most schools sponsor peer group activities for those who are working to change their drinking habits. Local chapters of AA and other organizations may have groups geared toward college-age people.

Instead of drinking, you can try other activities that produce the same effect. For example, if you drink to relieve anxiety or tension, try adding 20–30 minutes of exercise to your schedule to help you manage stress. Or try doing a relaxation exercise or going for a brisk walk to help reduce anxiety before a party or date. If you drink to relieve depression or to stop worrying, consider finding a trustworthy person (perhaps a professional counselor) to talk to about the problem that's bothering you. If you drink to feel more comfortable sexually, consider ways to improve communication with your partner so you can deal with sexual issues more openly. When these activities are successful, they will reinforce your responsible drinking decisions and make it more likely that you'll make the same decisions again in the future.

For other ways to monitor and control your drinking behavior, see the suggestions in the section "Drinking Behavior and Responsibility."

Reward Yourself and Monitor Your Progress

If changing your drinking behavior turns out to be difficult, it may be a clue that drinking was becoming a problem for you— all the more reason to get it under control now. Be sure to reward yourself as you learn to drink responsibly (or not at all). You may lose weight, look better, feel better, and have higher self-esteem as a result of limiting your drinking. Keep track of your progress in your health journal, and use the strategies described in Chapter 1 for maintaining your program. Remember, when you establish sensible drinking habits, you're planning not just for this week or month—but for your whole life.

- ing being an enabler and obtaining information about available resources and persistently encouraging their use.
- Strategies for keeping drinking under control include examining attitudes about drinking and drinking behavior, drinking slowly, spacing drinks, eating before and while drinking, and knowing one's limits.

- Strategies for promoting responsible drinking in others include encouraging responsible attitudes, being a responsible host, holding the drinker responsible for his or her actions, learning about prevention programs, and taking community action.

TAKE ACTION

1. Interview some of your fellow students about their drinking habits. How much do they drink, and how often? Are they more likely to drink on certain days or in certain circumstances? Are there any habits that seem to be common to most students? How do your own drinking habits compare to those of people you interviewed?

2. Some AA groups encourage visitors. If your local chapter does so, attend a meeting to see how the organization functions. What behavioral techniques are used to help people stop drinking? How effective do these techniques seem to be? If there is a local codependent or Al-Anon group, attend one of their meetings. What themes are emphasized? Do any themes apply to your relationships?

3. Plan an alcohol-free party. What would you serve to eat and drink? What would you tell people about the party when you invite them?

1. In your health journal, list the positive behaviors that help you drink responsibly. Consider how you can strengthen these behaviors. Then list the behaviors that interfere with responsible drinking for you. Which ones can you change?

2. Write a list of statements or questions you might use to talk with (1) a person you think is developing a drinking problem; (2) a person planning to drive under the influence of alcohol, with and without you in the car; and (3) a person you want to ask about your own behavior when you drink. Consider using statements from your list when an appropriate situation arises.

3. Critical Thinking Look at advertisements for alcoholic beverages in magazines and on billboards. Analyze several of these ads. What psychological techniques are used to sell the products? What are the hidden messages? Write an essay outlining your opinion of alcohol advertising and marketing. Do you think it's ethical to sell a potentially dangerous substance by appealing to people's desires and vulnerabilities? Do you think liquor manufacturers ought to be held responsible for the damage alcohol inflicts on some people? Explain your reasoning.

FOR MORE INFORMATION

Books

Alcoholics Anonymous, 3rd ed. 1976. New York: Alcoholics Anonymous World Services. *The "Big Book," the basic text for AA; includes the founding tenets of AA and vivid histories of recovering alcoholics.*

Dimeff, L. A., et al. 1999. *Brief Alcohol Screening and Interventions for College Students (BASICS). A Harm Reduction Approach.* New York: Guilford Press. *Presents a model designed to help students reduce their alcohol consumption and the risks they face from heavy drinking; includes handouts and assessment forms.*

From Survival to Recovery: Growing Up in an Alcoholic Home. 1994. New York: Al-Anon Family Group Headquarters. *First-person accounts of life with an alcoholic and the 12-step healing process.*

Goodwin, D. W. 2000. *Alcoholism: The Facts.* Oxford University Press. *Provides information and advice about alcoholism, including causes and treatment.*

Jerslid, D. 2001. *Happy Hours: Alcohol in a Woman's Life.* New York: Cliff Street Books. *Provides facts about the effects of drinking on women along with personal stories of recovery.*

Ketcham, K., and W. F. Asbury. 2000. *Beyond the Influence: Understanding and Defeating Alcoholism.* New York: Bantam. *Presents a wealth of information about how alcohol affects the body and mind and about treatment for alcohol abuse and alcoholism.*

Kinney, J., and G. Leaton. 2000. *Loosening the Grip: A Handbook of Alcohol Information,* 6th ed. St. Louis: Mosby. *A fascinating book about alcohol, including information on physical effects, abuse, alcoholism, and cultural aspects of alcohol use.*

Ogilvie, H. 2001. *Alternatives to Abstinence: Controlled Drinking and Other Approaches to Managing Alcoholism.* New York: Hatherleigh Press. *Examines the controversy around the concept of controlled drinking.*

WW Organizations, Hotlines, and Web Sites

Al-Anon Family Group Headquarters. Provides information and referrals to local Al-Anon and Alateen groups. The Web site includes a self-quiz to determine if you are affected by someone's drinking.
888-4AL-ANON
http://www.al-anon.alateen.org

Alcohol and Drug Helpline. Provides referrals to local treatment facilities.
800-821-4357

Alcoholics Anonymous (AA) World Services. Provides general information on AA, literature on alcoholism, and information about AA meetings and related 12-step organizations.
212-870-3400
http://www.alcoholics-anonymous.org

Alcohol Treatment Referral Hotline. Provides referrals to local intervention and treatment providers.
800-ALCOHOL

Bacchus and Gamma Peer Education Network. An association of college- and university-based peer education programs that focus on prevention of alcohol abuse.
http://www.bacchusgamma.org

The College Alcohol Study. Harvard School of Public Health. Provides information about and results from the recent studies of binge drinking on college campuses.
http://www.hsph.harvard.edu/cas

Facts on Tap. Provides information about alcohol and college life, sex and alcohol, and children of alcoholics, as well as suggestions for students who have been negatively affected by other students' alcohol use.
http://www.factsontap.org

Habitsmart. Contains an online self-scoring alcohol-use assessment, tips for outsmarting cravings, and links to related sites.
http://www.habitsmart.com

Had Enough.Org. Provides information and a self-quiz on binge drinking among college students.
http://www.hadenough.org

Higher Education Center for Alcohol and Other Drug Prevention. Provides support for campus alcohol and illegal drug prevention efforts; a Web site gives information about alcohol and drug abuse on campus and links to related sites and also has an area designed specifically for students.
http://www.edc.org/hec

Intoximeters Drink Wheel Blood Alcohol Test. Calculate your approximate BAC based on body weight, gender, and amount of alcohol consumed.
http://www.intox.com

Moderation Management Network. Controversial self-help program designed to help early problem drinkers limit their drinking; not intended for serious alcohol abusers or alcoholics.
http://www.moderation.org

Mothers Against Drunk Driving (MADD). Supports efforts to develop solutions to the problems of drunk driving and underage drinking; provides news, information, and brochures about many topics, including a guide for giving a safe party.

http://www.madd.org

National Association for Children of Alcoholics (NACoA). Provides information and support for children of alcoholics.

888-554-COAS; 301-468-0985

http://www.nacoa.net

National Clearinghouse for Alcohol and Drug Information/Prevention Online. Provides statistics, information, and publications on alcohol abuse, including resources for people who want to help friends and family members overcome alcohol-abuse problems.

800-729-6686; 301-468-2600

http://www.health.org

National Council on Alcoholism and Drug Dependence (NCADD). Provides information on alcoholism and counseling referrals.

212-269-7797; 800-NCA-CALL (24-hour Hope Line)

http://www.ncadd.org

National Institute on Alcohol Abuse and Alcoholism (NIAAA). Provides booklets and other publications on a variety of alcohol-related topics, including fetal alcohol syndrome, alcoholism treatment, and alcohol use and minorities.

301-443-3860

http://www.niaaa.nih.gov

Rational Recovery. A free self-help program that offers an alternative to 12-step programs; the emphasis is on learning the skill of abstinence.

http://www.rational.org

Women for Sobriety. A self-help program for women that offers an alternative to 12-step programs; the program includes positive thinking, meditation, group activities, and diet and exercise.

http://www.womenforsobriety.org

See also the listings for Chapter 9.

SELECTED BIBLIOGRAPHY

Austin, E. W., B. E. Pinkleton, and Y. Fujioka. 2000. The role of interpretation processes and parental discussion in the media's effects on adolescents' use of alcohol. *Pediatrics* 105(2): 343–349.

Center for Science in the Public Interest. 1999. *Fact Sheet: Fetal Alcohol Syndrome* (http://www.cspinet.org/booze/fas.htm; retrieved July 22, 2000).

Centers for Disease Control and Prevention. 2000. Alcohol policy and sexually transmitted disease rates—United States 1981–1995. *Morbidity and Mortality Weekly Report* 49: 346–349.

Dawson, D. A. 2000. Alcohol consumption, alcohol dependence, and all-cause mortality. *Alcoholism: Clinical and Experimental Research* 24(1): 72–81.

Drug Strategies. 1999. *Millennium Hangover: Keeping Score on Alcohol —Treatment for Alcohol Problems* (http://www.drugstrategies.org/keepingscore1999/treatment.html; retrieved July 21, 2000).

Foundation for Academic Standards and Tradition. 2000. *Student Life Survey* (http://www.gofast.org/studentlifesurvey.htm; retrieved June 24, 2000).

Gallup Organization. 2000. *One in Six Americans Admit to Drinking Too Much* (http://www.gallup.com/poll/releases/pr001204.asp; retrieved February 4, 2001).

Goldberg, I. J., et al. 2001. Wine and your heart: A science advisory for healthcare professionals from the Nutrition Committee, Council on Epidemiology and Prevention, and Council on Cardiovascular Nursing of the American Heart Association. *Circulation* 103: 472–475.

Green, G. A., et al. 2001. NCAA study of substance use and abuse habits of college student-athletes. *Clinical Journal of Sports Medicine* 11(1): 51–56.

Hines, L. S., et al;. 2001. Genetic variation in alcohol dehydrogenase and the beneficial effect of moderate alcohol consumption on myocardial infarction. *New England Journal of Medicine* 344(8): 549–555.

Hingson, R. W., et al. 2000. Age of drinking onset and unintentional injury involvement after drinking. *Journal of the American Medical Association* 284(12): 1527–1533.

Ikonomidou, C. 2000. Ethanol-induced apoptotic neurodegeneration and fetal alcohol syndrome. *Science* 287(5455): 1056–1060.

Imhof, A., et al. 2001. Effect of alcohol consumption on systemic markers of inflammation. *Lancet* 357(9258): 763–767.

Lacoste, L., J. Hung, and J. Y. Lam. 2001. Acute and delayed antithrombotic effects of alcohol in humans. *American Journal of Cardiology* 87(1): 82–85.

Malarcher, A. M., et al. 2001. Alcohol intake, type of beverage, and the risk of cerebral infarction in young women. *Stroke* 32(1): 77–83.

Margolis, L. H., et al. 2000. Alcohol and motor vehicle–related deaths of children as passengers, pedestrians, and bicyclists. *Journal of the American Medical Association* 283(17): 2245–2248.

National Highway Traffic Safety Administration. 2000. *Impaired Driving in the United States* (http://www.nhtsa.dot.gov/people/injury/alcohol/US.htm; retrieved October 12, 2000).

National Highway Traffic Safety Administration. 2000. *On DWI Laws in Other Countries* (http://www.nhtsa.dot.gov/people/injury/research/pub/DWIothercountries/dwiothercountries.html; retrieved July 22, 2000).

National Highway Traffic Safety Administration. 2000. *Presidential Initiative for Making. 08 BAC the National Legal Limit: A Progress Report* (http://www.nhtsa.dot.gov/people/injury/alcohol/limit.08/08progressreport/info.html; retrieved July 21, 2000).

National Institute on Alcohol Abuse and Alcoholism. 2000. *10th Special Report to the U.S. Congress on Alcohol and Health.* Washington, D.C.: U.S. Department of Health and Human Services.

National Toxicology Program. 2000. *Ninth Report on Carcinogens.* Research Triangle Park, N.C.: U.S. Department of Health and Human Services.

Philip, P., et al. 2001. Fatigue, alcohol, and serious road crashes in France: Factorial study of national data. *British Medical Journal* 322(7290): 829–830.

Reynaud, M., et al. 2001. Patients admitted to emergency services for drunkenness: Moderate alcohol users or harmful drinkers? *American Journal of Psychiatry* 158(1): 96–99.

Robinson, T. N., H. L. Chen, and J. D. Killen. 1998. Television and music video exposure and risk of adolescent alcohol use. *Pediatrics* 102(5): e54 (http://www.pediatrics.org/cgi/content/abstract/102/5/e54; retrieved November 2, 1998).

Substance Abuse and Mental Health Services Administration. 2000. *National Household Survey on Drug Abuse, 1999.* Rockville, Md.: Substance Abuse and Mental Health Services Administration.

U.S. Department of Agriculture. 2000. *Dietary Guidelines for Americans, 2000.* USDA Home and Garden Bulletin No. 232.

Verhovek, S. 2000. Moderate-drinking advocate learns sobering lesson. *Sacramento Bee,* July 9.

Wechsler, H. 2000. College binge drinking in the 1990s: A continuing problem. Results of the Harvard School of Public Health 1999 College Alcohol Study. *Journal of American College Health* 48: 199–210.

Wechsler, H., et al. 2001. Drinking levels, alcohol problems, and second-hand effects in substance-free college residences: Results of a national study. *Journal of Studies on Alcohol* 62(1): 23–31.

Weiss, J., et al. 2000. The alcohol hangover. *Annals of Internal Medicine* 132(11): 897–902.

Zhang, Y., et al. 1999. Alcohol consumption and risk of breast cancer: The Framingham Study revisited. *American Journal of Epidemiology* 149(2): 93–101.

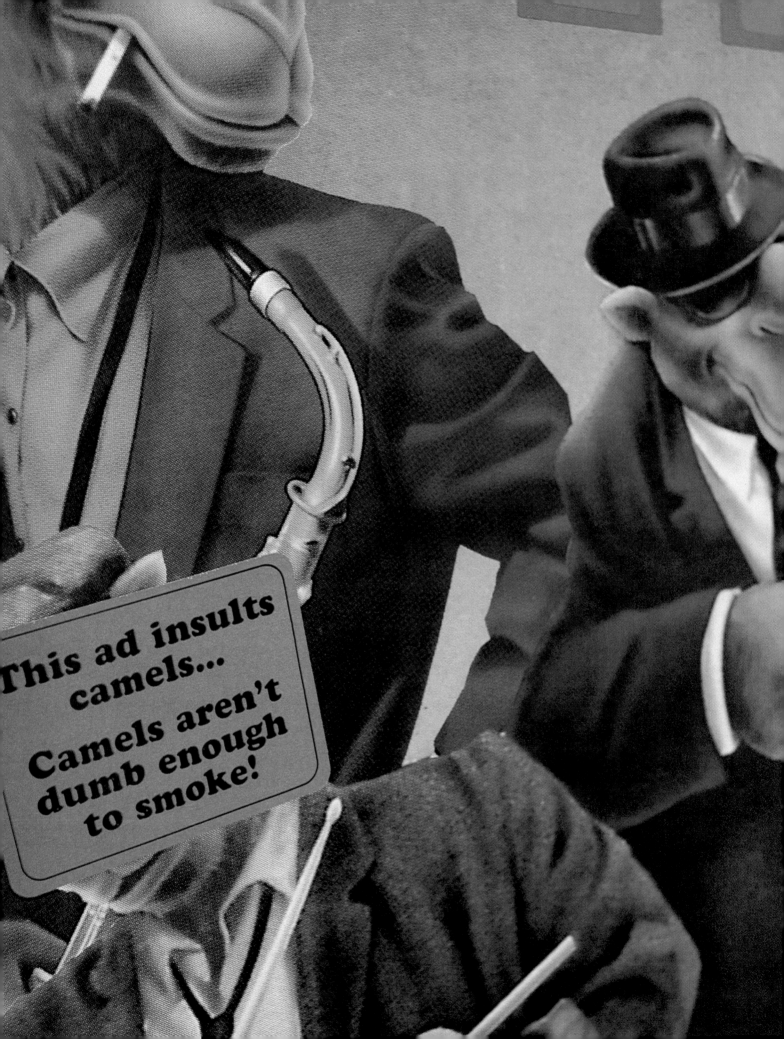

After reading this chapter, you should be able to

- List the reasons people start using tobacco and why they continue to use it

- Explain the short- and long-term health risks associated with tobacco use

- Discuss the effects of environmental tobacco smoke on nonsmokers

- Describe the social costs of tobacco, and list actions that have been taken to combat smoking in the public and private sectors

- Prepare plans to stop using tobacco and to avoid environmental tobacco smoke

Toward a Tobacco-Free Society

11

TEST YOUR KNOWLEDGE

1. Male and female college students use tobacco at about the same rate.
True or false?

2. Which of the following substances is found in tobacco smoke?
a. acetone (nail polish remover)
b. ammonia (cleaner)
c. hexamine (lighter fluid)
d. toluene (industrial solvent)

3. The health care costs associated with smoking work out to about $0.40 per pack of cigarettes, the average tax collected by states to offset these costs.
True of false?

4. Cigarette smoking increases the risk for which of the following conditions?
a. facial wrinkling
b. miscarriage
c. impotence
d. automobile crashes

5. A person who quits smoking now will reduce her risk of lung cancer within 10 years.
True or false?

6. Every cigarette a person smokes reduces life expectancy by about 1 minute.
True or false?

ANSWERS

1. **FALSE.** About 38% of men and 30% of women in college are tobacco users, a difference caused by men's much higher use of cigars.

2. **ALL FOUR.** Tobacco contains thousands of chemical substances, including many that are poisonous or linked to the development of cancer.

3. **FALSE.** States collect about $0.40 per pack in taxes, but total health care costs are close to $125 billion a year, or $5 per pack.

4. **ALL FOUR.** Cigarette smoking reduces the quality of life and is the greatest preventable cause of death in the United States.

5. **TRUE.** The lung cancer rate of a former smoker is 50% of that of a continuing smoker within 10 years of quitting.

6. **FALSE.** Every cigarette reduces life expectancy by about 11 minutes; one carton represents a day and a half of lost life.

Once considered a glamorous and sophisticated habit, smoking is now viewed with increasing disapproval. The recognition of the health risks of smoking is a primary cause of this change in public opinion, and it has led to significant changes in the behavior of many Americans. Over the past four decades, the proportion of cigarette smoking among adults in the United States has dropped 30%. Private businesses and all levels of government have jumped on the nonsmoking bandwagon: Almost every state now restricts smoking in public places, and several have introduced statewide smoking bans for indoor workplaces. The U.S. Surgeon General has proposed that America become completely smoke-free.

Despite such progress, tobacco use remains widespread. About one in four American adults smokes, and each year more than 400,000 Americans die from the effects of cigarette smoking (Figure 11-1). This is equivalent to three fully loaded 747s crashing every day with no survivors. Nonsmokers also suffer: Exposure to environmental tobacco smoke (ETS) causes more than 60,000 deaths annually among nonsmokers. Smoking by pregnant women is responsible for about 10% of all infant deaths in this country. Spit (smokeless) tobacco and cigars are regaining popularity: The use of spit tobacco products has tripled since 1972, and cigar smoking has increased 50% since 1993; (see the box "Uncovering Tobacco Use on Campus").

Given the overwhelming evidence against tobacco, why would anyone today begin using it? How does it exercise its hold over users? What can smokers and nonsmokers do to help achieve a tobacco-free society? In this chapter, we explore answers to these and other questions about nicotine addiction.

WHY PEOPLE USE TOBACCO

About 48 million American adults and 4 million adolescents smoke. Two-thirds of adult smokers believe that they'll die of tobacco-related causes if they don't quit. Yet each day, 6000 young people try cigarettes and 3000 become regular smokers. This section examines the personal and societal forces that induce people to start smoking and encourage them to continue.

Nicotine Addiction

The primary reason people continue to use **tobacco** despite the health risks is that they have become addicted to a powerful psychoactive drug: **nicotine.** Although the tobacco industry long maintained that there was insufficient evidence about the addictiveness of nicotine, scientific evidence overwhelmingly supports the conclusion that nicotine is highly addictive. In fact, many researchers consider nicotine to be the most physically addictive of all the psychoactive drugs.

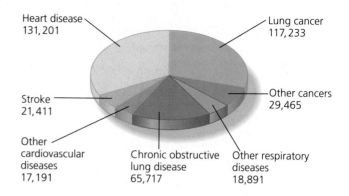

VITAL STATISTICS

Figure 11-1   Annual deaths among smokers attributable to smoking-related diseases.   SOURCE: Thun, M. J., L. F. Apicella, and S. J. Henley. 2000. Smoking vs. other risk factors as the cause of smoking-attributable deaths. *Journal of the American Medical Association* 284(6): 706–712.

Recent neurological studies indicate that nicotine acts on the brain in much the same way as cocaine and heroin. Nicotine reaches the brain via the bloodstream seconds after it is inhaled or, in the case of spit tobacco, absorbed through membranes of the mouth or nose. It triggers the release of powerful chemical messengers in the brain, including epinephrine, norepinephrine, and dopamine. But unlike street drugs, most of which are used to achieve a high, nicotine's primary attraction seems to lie in its ability to modulate everyday emotions.

At low doses, nicotine acts as a stimulant: It increases heart rate and blood pressure and can enhance alertness, concentration, rapid information processing, memory, and learning. People type faster on nicotine, for instance. At high doses, on the other hand, nicotine appears to act as a sedative; it can reduce aggressiveness and alleviate the stress response. Tobacco users may be able to fine-tune nicotine's effects and regulate their moods by increasing or decreasing their intake of the drug. Studies have shown that smokers experience milder mood variation than nonsmokers while performing long, boring tasks or while watching emotional movies, for example.

All tobacco products contain nicotine, and the use of any of them can lead to addiction (see the box "Nicotine Dependence: Are You Hooked?"). Nicotine addiction fulfills the criteria for substance dependence described in Chapter 9, including loss of control, tolerance, and withdrawal.

Loss of Control   Three out of four smokers want to quit but find they cannot. Of the 60–80% of people who kick cigarettes at stop-smoking clinics, 75% start smoking again within a year—a relapse rate similar to rates for alcoholics and heroin addicts. Some evidence suggests quitting is even harder for smokeless users: In one study,

A 2000 study revealed that rates of tobacco use among college students are even higher than previously suspected. Earlier surveys looked solely at cigarette smoking; however, this survey of students at over 100 college campuses looked at all forms of tobacco use. When cigarette smoking alone was measured, the percentage of college students who had ever used tobacco was 53%. But when cigar, pipe, and spit tobacco users were also counted, the percentage rose to 61%.

According to the survey, nearly half of all college students used tobacco in the past year—one-third within the past month. Cigarettes were the most common form of tobacco used, followed by cigars. Despite nearly identical smoking rates for men (28.5%) and women (28.4%), *total* tobacco use was higher among men (38%) than women (30%) due to greater use of cigars and spit tobacco among men. More than one-third of college students have smoked a cigar, including more than half of the men and one-quarter of the women; 16% of men and 4% of women report cigar use within the past month. Surprisingly, unlike patterns of use for other tobacco products, cigar use by first- and second-year students exceeds that of juniors and seniors. This may indicate that cigar use is a relatively new phenomenon on college campuses and reflect the growing popularity of cigars among adolescents, who bring their habit with them to college.

Most college students who have used tobacco used more than one product; the most frequent combinations are cigarettes and cigars (20% of tobacco users), cigarettes and pipes (12% of users), and cigarettes, cigars, and spit tobacco (6% of users). Men were much more likely than women to have used more than one kind of tobacco product; 37% of men but only 11% of women had used more than one product in the past month.

Although many students report smoking, most do not smoke in large quantities. Of those who had smoked in the past 30 days, 32% smoke less than 1 cigarette per day, 44% smoke 1 to 10 cigarettes per day, and 13% smoke 1 or more packs per day. Of course, smoking in any quantity has health risks and also lays the groundwork for increased nicotine dependence.

The results of this survey indicate that more needs to be done to highlight the dangers of all forms of tobacco use. Although cigarette use among college students, which increased dramatically between 1993 and 1997, does seem to have stabilized since 1997, use of other forms of tobacco is high and possibly increasing. Although college is a time of experimentation, it can be hoped that fewer students will start using tobacco in any form in years to come.

SOURCE: Rigotti, N. A., J. E. Lee, and H. Wechsler. 2000. U.S. college students' use of tobacco products. *Journal of the American Medical Association* 284(6): 699–705.

---

only 1 of 14 spit tobacco users who participated in a tobacco-cessation clinic was able to stop for more than 4 hours.

Regular tobacco users live according to a rigid cycle of need and gratification. On average, they can go no more than 40 minutes between doses of nicotine; otherwise, they begin feeling edgy and irritable and have trouble concentrating. If ignored, nicotine cravings build until getting a cigarette or some spit tobacco becomes a paramount concern, crowding out other thoughts. Tobacco users may plan their daily schedule around opportunities to satisfy their nicotine cravings; this loss of control and personal freedom can affect all the dimensions of wellness (see the box "Tobacco Use and Religion: Global Views").

Tobacco users become adept, therefore, at keeping a steady amount of nicotine circulating in the blood and going to the brain. In one experiment, smokers were given cigarettes that looked and tasted alike but varied in nicotine content. The subjects automatically adjusted their rate and depth of inhalation so that they absorbed their usual amount of nicotine. In other studies, heavy smokers were given nicotine without knowing it, and they cut down on their smoking without a conscious effort. Spit tobacco users maintain blood nicotine levels as high as those of cigarette smokers.

Tolerance and Withdrawal   Using tobacco builds up tolerance. Where one cigarette may make a beginning smoker nauseated and dizzy, a long-term smoker may have to chain-smoke a pack or more to experience the same effects. For most regular tobacco users, sudden abstinence from nicotine produces predictable withdrawal symptoms as well. These symptoms, which come on several hours after the last dose of nicotine, can include severe cravings, insomnia, confusion, tremors, difficulty concentrating, fatigue, muscle pains, headache, nausea, irritability, anger, and depression. Users undergo measurable changes in brain waves, heart rate, and blood pressure, and they perform poorly on tasks requiring sustained attention. While most of these symptoms pass in 2–3 days, many ex-smokers report intermittent, intense urges to smoke for years after quitting.

Addiction occurs at an early age, despite many teenagers' beliefs that they will be able to stop when they wish to. Nicotine addiction can start within a few days of

tobacco The leaves of cultivated tobacco plants prepared for smoking, chewing, or use as snuff.

nicotine A poisonous, addictive substance found in tobacco and responsible for many of the effects of tobacco.

Terms

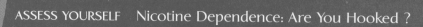

Answer each question in the list below, giving yourself the appropriate number of points.

_____ 1. How soon after you wake up do you have your first cigarette?
   a. within 5 minutes (3)
   b. 6–30 minutes (2)
   c. 31–60 minutes (1)
   d. After 60 minutes (0)

_____ 2. Do you find it difficult to refrain from smoking in places where it is forbidden, such as the library, a theater, or a doctor's office?
   a. yes (1)
   b. no (0)

_____ 3. Which cigarette would you most hate to give up?
   a. the first one in the morning (1)
   b. any other (0)

_____ 4. How many cigarettes a day do you smoke?
   a. 10 or less (0)
   b. 11–20 (1)
   c. 21–30 (2)
   d. 31 or more (3)

_____ 5. Do you smoke more frequently during the first hours after waking than during the rest of the day?
   a. yes (1)
   b. no (0)

_____ 6. Do you smoke if you are so ill that you are in bed most of the day?
   a. yes (1)
   b. no (0)

_____ TOTAL

A total score of 7 or more indicates that you are very dependent on nicotine and are likely to experience withdrawal symptoms when you stop smoking. A score of 6 or less indicates low to moderate dependence.

SOURCE: Heatherton, T. F., et al. 1991. The Fagerstrom Test for Nicotine Dependence: A revision of the Fagerstrom Tolerance Questionnaire. *British Journal of Addictions* 86(9): 1119–1127.

smoking and after just a few cigarettes. Over half of teenagers who try cigarettes progress to daily use, and about half of those who ever smoke daily progress to nicotine dependence. In polls, about 75% of smoking teens state they wish they had never started. Another survey revealed that only 5% of high school smokers predicted they would definitely be smoking in 5 years; in fact, close to 75% were smoking 7–9 years later.

Social and Psychological Factors

Why do tobacco users have such a hard time quitting even when they want to? Social and psychological forces combine with physiological addiction to maintain the tobacco habit. Many people, for example, have established habits of smoking while doing something else—while talking, working, drinking, and so on. The spit tobacco habit is also associated with certain situations—studying, drinking coffee, or playing sports. It is difficult for these people to break their habits because the activities they associate with tobacco use continue

to trigger their urge. Such activities are called **secondary reinforcers;** they act together with the physiological addiction to keep the user dependent on tobacco.

Why Start in the First Place?

A junior high school girl takes up smoking in an attempt to appear older. A high school boy uses spit tobacco in the bullpen, emulating the major league ball players he admires. An overweight first-year college student turns to cigarettes, hoping they will curb her appetite. Smoking rates among American youth declined throughout the 1980s but rose steadily during the 1990s. The largest increase was among 13- and 14-year-olds, and the prevalence of current smoking among college students increased from 22% in 1993 to 29% in 1999. Children and teenagers constitute 90% of all new smokers in this country: Every day, an estimated 3000 adolescents become regular cigarette smokers, while hundreds of others take up snuff or chewing tobacco. The average age for starting smokers is 13; for spit tobacco users, 10. Meanwhile, children—especially girls—are beginning to experiment with tobacco at ever-younger ages. The trends are particularly worrisome because the earlier people begin smoking, the more likely they are to become heavy smokers—and to die of tobacco-related disease.

Terms   **secondary reinforcers** Stimuli that are not necessarily pleasurable in themselves, but that are associated with other stimuli that are pleasurable.

What contributions can the world's religions make to efforts to limit tobacco use? This was the question behind a meeting convened in May 1999 at the headquarters of the World Health Organization (WHO) in Geneva, Switzerland. The meeting was in support of the Tobacco Free Initiative, a WHO project, and was attended by representatives of the major religions of the world. Participants explained how tobacco use was viewed by their religion and discussed ways they could collaborate with public health programs to help control its use.

Tobacco Use as a Violation of Religious Principles

A primary thread among all the religions is a condemnation of tobacco use for its damaging effects on the body. Most religions regard the human body as the dwelling place of the spirit; as such, it deserves care and respect. Tobacco use is clearly contrary to this principle. The Baha'i faith, for example, strongly discourages smoking as unclean and unhealthy. Some Protestant churches, including Quakers, Mormons, and Seventh-Day Adventists, consider tobacco use a violation of the body. For Hindus, smoking goes against one of the primary spiritual practices, the care of the body. The Roman Catholic Church endorses the age-old adage "a sound mind in a sound body." For Muslims, one of the five essential principles on which religious law is based is the protection of the integrity of the individual. All forms of consumption that might jeopardize the life or health of an individual are contrary to the spirit of Islam. In Judaism, people are urged to "choose life" and to choose whatever strengthens the capacity to live. Tobacco use is clearly something that jeopardizes life. Buddhists believe that the body doesn't belong to the person at all—even suicide is considered murder—and one must do nothing to harm it.

A second thread common to most religions is the notion that dependence and addiction run counter to ideas of freedom, choice, and human dignity. Buddhism teaches a path of freedom—a way of life without dependence on anything. Hindus regard tobacco use as a *vyasana,* a dependence that is not necessary for the preservation of health. Protestant churches caution that any form of dependence is contrary to the notion of Christian freedom.

A third argument against tobacco use is the immorality of imposing secondhand smoke on nonsmokers, which is seen as inflicting harm on others. In Hinduism, harming others is sinful, so people should not smoke out of consideration for others. In the Jewish tradition, those who force nonsmokers to breathe smoke jeopardize the lives of others; according to Scripture, to jeopardize the life of another person is to jeopardize the whole universe.

Addressing the Problem: The Role of Individual Responsibility

Most religions focus on the role of individual responsibility in overcoming dependence on tobacco. Baha'is support the use of strategies that encourage individuals to find solutions to their problems within themselves, often with the help of a supportive group. In Buddhism, people must assume responsibility for their habits; they practice introspection to understand the cause of problems within themselves and the effects of their actions on others. Once the cause is deeply understood, the problem is already, to a great extent, solved.

The principles of Islam are based on notions of responsibility and protection. When believers obey a rule prohibiting consumption of a harmful substance, they do so as responsible beings who appreciate the need to protect the body and keep it in good health. A fundamental message of Islam is that you are responsible for your body and for your health.

What Can Religions Do to Support the Tobacco Free Initiative?

Common threads again emerged in discussions of how the problem of tobacco use should be approached, with a primary focus on prevention and education rather than prohibition. The Islamic view is that the campaign to control tobacco use must be based on awareness, responsibility, and justice. Developing awareness means providing information on the global problem, from tobacco cultivation to marketing, from consumption to its effects, from the impact of fashion to the effects of advertising. Fostering responsibility means helping people understand what they need to do to attain well-being; such a message has nothing to do with inducing guilt or denigrating people who smoke. Emphasizing social and human justice means helping the farmers and societies that depend on tobacco cultivation to find alternative crops.

According to the representative from the Geneva Inter-religious Platform (a project involving Hindus, Buddhists, Jews, Christians, Muslims, and Baha'is), it is morally legitimate to restrict tobacco consumption, but outright prohibition comes up against two major obstacles: In terms of effectiveness, it has been shown that it doesn't work, and in terms of principle, it is an infringement of freedom of choice, which a democratic and pluralistic state must allow its adult citizens.

The next approach, then, is prevention, according to the Inter-religious representative. Here, the rights of nonsmokers not to be subjected to passive smoking must be protected because they clearly prevail over the freedom of smokers. In support of this position, the common religious exhortation not to do unto others what you would not have them do unto you can be invoked. Further, adequate information should be provided to counter the deceptive images projected by tobacco industry advertising, especially where minors are concerned. Protection of the weak and denunciation of dishonesty are underlying values of all religious traditions.

Finally, in the Inter-religious view, for adult smokers who are conscious of their choice and whose smoking does not infringe on the rights of others, ideals of good health can be proposed but not imposed. The religious traditions can best assist adult smokers by reminding them of two principles: one, the value of liberation from any form of slavery, and two, respect for life out of deference to the source of all life, which religions call by different names—God, ultimate reality, and so on—but which is the supreme value of any religious commitment.

SOURCE: World Health Organization Tobacco Free Initiative. 1999. *Meeting Report: Meeting on Tobacco and Religion* (3 May 1999). Geneva: World Health Organization.

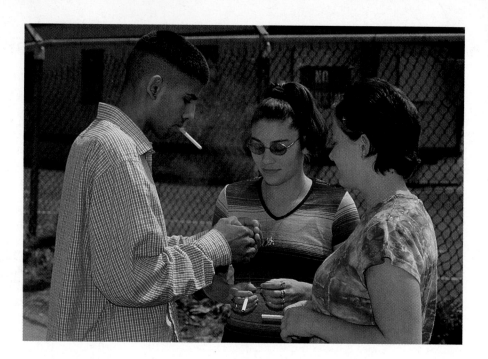

The average age of new smokers is 13, and most adult smokers began as teenagers. In polls, about 75% of teen smokers state they wish they had never started.

Rationalizing the Dangers   Making the decision to smoke requires minimizing or denying both the health risks of tobacco use and the tremendous pain, disability, emotional trauma, family stress, and financial expense involved in tobacco-related diseases such as cancer and emphysema. A sense of invincibility, characteristic of many adolescents and young adults, also contributes to the decision to use tobacco. These young people may persuade themselves they are too intelligent, too lucky, or too robustly healthy to be vulnerable to tobacco's dangers (see the box "Building Motivation to Quit Smoking"). "I'm not dumb enough to get hooked," they may argue. "I'll be able to quit before I do myself any real harm." Other typical rationalizations: "My grandmother smoked and she lived to be 80" and "You can get killed just by crossing the street."

Listening to Advertising   Advertising is another influence. The tobacco industry spends nearly $6 billion each year on ads—more than the entire annual budget for Puerto Rico. These ads link tobacco products with desirable traits such as confidence, popularity, sexual attractiveness, and slenderness. Young people are a prime target of these ads. Once a teen begins smoking, nicotine addiction can lead to a lifetime of smoking. As one teenager said, "It may have been my decision to smoke my first cigarette, and maybe even my second. But now *needing* to smoke is no longer a choice."

One measure of the effectiveness of advertising can be seen in the fact that 86% of teens prefer the three most heavily advertised brands (Marlboro, Camel, Newport); these three are preferred by just 32% of adults, who tend to favor cheap generic brands. Joe Camel, the former advertising image of Camel cigarettes, had become more familiar to children than Mickey Mouse. In surveys, more than 90% of 6-year-olds recognized him and associated him with cigarettes. In the 3 years following the introduction of the Joe Camel ad campaign, the Camel market share among underage smokers quadrupled. In part because of criticism and a lawsuit brought by the Federal Trade Commission, the R. J. Reynolds Tobacco Company discontinued the Joe Camel campaign in July 1997.

Young people are not the only group targeted. Certain brands are designed to appeal primarily to men, women, or particular ethnic groups. For example, Virginia Slims tries to appeal to women by associating the brand with confidence and sexual attractiveness. Magazines that are targeted at African American audiences receive proportionately more revenues from cigarette advertising than do other consumer magazines. Billboards advertising tobacco products are placed in African American communities four or five times more often than in primarily white communities.

Tobacco advertising extends beyond magazines and billboards. Sponsorship of sports or racing events may result in millions of people, many of them children, viewing the name of a brand or company for hours. Brand names are also advertised on free caps, gym bags, and other products that appeal to youths. Virginia Slims introduced a line of clothing designed to appeal to young women and girls that can be purchased with proofs of purchase from cigarette packages.

The government began regulating tobacco advertising in 1967. Under the Fairness Doctrine, the Federal Com-

A common misconception among smokers is that a few cigarettes a day aren't enough to cause harm. Perhaps this is why a recent survey showed that among college students who smoke, 75% smoke 10 or fewer cigarettes a day. These smokers are ignoring the very real health risks of even one cigarette. The U.S. Public Health Service suggests a "5 R's" strategy to enhance motivation to quit. If you are a smoker or are trying to help one, think about these areas of concern and see if they help develop a desire and readiness to make a real attempt at quitting.

Relevance: Think about the personal relevance of quitting tobacco use. What would the effects be on your family and friends? How would your daily life improve? What is the most important way that quitting would change your life?

Risks: There are immediate risks, such as shortness of breath, infertility, and impotence, and long-term risks, including cancer, heart disease, and respiratory problems. Remember, smoking is harmful both to you and to anyone exposed to your smoke.

Rewards: The list of rewards of quitting is almost endless, including improving immediate and long-term health, saving money, and feeling better about yourself. You can also stop worrying about quitting and set a good example for others.

Roadblocks: What are the potential obstacles to quitting? Are you worried about withdrawal symptoms, weight gain, or lack of support? How can these barriers be overcome?

Repetition: Revisit your reasons for quitting and strengthen your resolve until you are ready to prepare a plan. Most people make several attempts to quit before they succeed. Relapsing once does not mean that you will never succeed.

SOURCES: Rigotti, N. A., J. E. Lee, and H. Wechsler. 2000. U.S. college students' use of tobacco products. *Journal of the American Medical Association* 284(6): 699–705. Fiore, M. C., et al. 2000. *Treating Tobacco Use and Dependence.* Clinical Practice Guidelines. Rockville, Md.: U.S. Department of Health and Human Services.

munications Commission (FCC) required broadcasters to air anti-smoking messages along with industry-sponsored cigarette advertisements on television and radio. Anti-smoking ad campaigns can be extremely effective. Ads featuring unattractive older people smoking or cigarettes used as coffin nails counteract the glamorous images that appear in tobacco ads. Between 1967 and 1971, when anti-smoking messages were first broadcast, per capita cigarette consumption declined by 7%—one of the largest declines ever. Cigarette advertising on television and radio was banned altogether in 1971. In 1996, the FDA issued strict advertising regulations designed to reduce minors' exposure and access to tobacco advertising and products; however, the Supreme Court ruled in March 2000 that the FDA does not have the authority to regulate tobacco. Debate continues over legislation that would give the FDA regulatory authority.

In November 1998, controls on advertising were enacted as part of the $206 billion deal to settle lawsuits brought against the tobacco industry by the attorneys general of 39 states (see pp. 301–302 for more information). This settlement limits or bans billboard and transit advertising of tobacco products; cartoon characters in advertisements and packaging; tobacco logos on T-shirts, hats, and other promotional items; brand-name sponsorship of sporting events; and payments for product placement in movies, television, and concerts. Some health officials are worried about potential loopholes in the settlement deal, and even if the deal results in a dramatic change in advertising patterns, it will be many years before the positive image of smoking promoted in tobacco ads fades from the public's mind. For current information on the tobacco settlement deal and other legal actions, call or visit the Web site of one of the tobacco control advocacy groups listed in the For More Information section at the end of the chapter.

COMMUNICATE!   Many people are not aware of the power cigarette advertising has to influence their attitudes toward smoking. A good way to resist the influence of ads is to critically evaluate them. Try analyzing a cigarette ad, looking at the image of smokers the ad communicates. Are they attractive, young, confident, successful, sexy, sophisticated, adventurous, rich, satisfied? Do you want to be like them or have the same lifestyle they have? Based on what you learn in this chapter about tobacco, do you think smoking can deliver what the ad promises?

Who Uses Tobacco?

Not all young people are equally vulnerable to the lure of tobacco. Research suggests that the more of the following characteristics that apply to a child or adolescent, the more likely he or she is to use tobacco:

- A parent or sibling uses tobacco.
- Peers use tobacco.
- The child comes from a blue-collar family.
- The child comes from a low-income home.
- The family is headed by a single parent.
- The child performs poorly in school.

Table 11-1	Who Smokes?		

| | Percentage of Smokers | | |
	Men	Women	Total
Ethnic group (age ≥ 18)			
White	27	24	25
Black	29	21	25
Asian/Pacific Islander	18	10	14
American Indian/ Alaska Native	42	38	40
Latino	25	13	19
Education, in years (age ≥ 25)			
≤8	28	17	22
9–11	40	34	37
12	32	24	27
13–15	27	23	25
≥16	12	11	11
Total	26	22	24

SOURCE: Centers for Disease Control and Prevention. 2000. Cigarette smoking among adults—United States, 1998. *Morbidity and Mortality Weekly Report* 49(39): 880–884.

- The child drops out of school.
- The child has positive attitudes about tobacco use.

In 1998, about 26% of men and 22% of women smoked cigarettes (Table 11-1). Rates of smoking varied, based on gender, age, ethnicity, and education level. Adults with less than a twelfth-grade education were three times as likely to smoke cigarettes as those with a college degree. The reverse is true for cigars: Cigar smoking is most common among the affluent and those with high educational attainment.

Although all states ban the sale of tobacco to anyone under 18 years of age, at least 500 million packs of cigarettes and 26 million containers of chewing tobacco are consumed by minors each year. About 13% of middle school students use some form of tobacco. Among high school students, about 28% smoke cigarettes at least occasionally and 15% smoke cigars. An estimated 7%, including 19% of white male students, use spit tobacco. Male college athletes and professional baseball players report even higher rates of spit tobacco use.

Drug addicts are another major group of tobacco users. Some studies have found that over 90% of heroin addicts and 80% of alcoholics are heavy cigarette smokers. Other recent studies suggest that smokers are more likely than nonsmokers to have suffered from depression. Such findings lead some researchers to suggest that underlying psychological or physiological traits may predispose people to drug use, including tobacco.

HEALTH HAZARDS

Tobacco adversely affects nearly every part of the body, including the brain, stomach, mouth, and reproductive organs.

Tobacco Smoke: A Poisonous Mix

Tobacco smoke contains hundreds of damaging chemical substances, including acetone (nail polish remover), ammonia, hexamine (lighter fluid), and toluene (industrial solvent). Smoke from a typical unfiltered cigarette contains about 5 billion particles per cubic millimeter— 50,000 times as many as are found in an equal volume of smoggy urban air. These particles, when condensed, form the brown, sticky mass called **cigarette tar.**

At least 43 chemicals in tobacco smoke are linked to the development of cancer. Some, such as benzo(a)pyrene and urethane, are **carcinogens;** that is, they directly cause cancer. Other chemicals, such as formaldehyde, are **cocarcinogens;** they do not themselves cause cancer but combine with other chemicals to stimulate the growth of certain cancers, at least in laboratory animals. Other substances in tobacco cause health problems because they damage the lining of the respiratory tract or decrease the lungs' ability to fight off infection.

Tobacco also contains poisonous substances, including arsenic and hydrogen cyanide. In addition to being an addictive psychoactive drug, nicotine is also a poison and can be fatal in high doses. Many cases of nicotine poisoning occur each year in toddlers and infants who pick up and eat cigarette butts they find at home or on the playground.

Cigarette smoke contains carbon monoxide, the deadly gas in automobile exhaust, in concentrations 400 times greater than is considered safe in industrial workplaces. Not surprisingly, smokers often complain of breathlessness when they require a burst of energy to run across campus for their next class. Carbon monoxide displaces oxygen in red blood cells, depleting the body's supply of life-giving oxygen for extra work. Carbon monoxide also impairs visual acuity, especially at night.

All smokers absorb some gases, tar, and nicotine from cigarette smoke, but smokers who inhale bring most of these substances into their bodies and keep them there. In 1 year, a typical pack-a-day smoker takes in 50,000– 70,000 puffs. Smoke from a cigarette, pipe, or cigar directly assaults the mouth, throat, and respiratory tract. The nose, which normally filters about 75% of foreign matter we breathe, is completely bypassed.

In a cigarette, the unburned tobacco itself acts as a filter. As a cigarette burns down, there is less and less filter. Thus, more chemicals are absorbed into the body during the last third of a cigarette than during the first. A smoker can cut down on the absorption of harmful chemicals by not smoking cigarettes down to short butts. Any gains, of

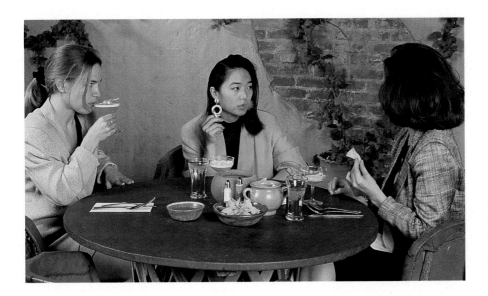

Cigarette smoke contains many toxic and carcinogenic chemicals that affect both the person smoking and the people breathing the environmental tobacco smoke. A growing body of evidence links ETS with lung cancer and respiratory and cardiovascular diseases.

course, will be offset by smoking more cigarettes, inhaling more deeply, or puffing more frequently.

Some smokers switch to low-tar, low-nicotine, or filtered cigarettes because they believe them to be healthier alternatives. But there is no such thing as a "safe" cigarette, and smoking behavior is a more important factor in tar and nicotine intake than the type of cigarette smoked. Smokers who switch to a low-nicotine brand often compensate by smoking more cigarettes, inhaling more deeply, taking larger or more frequent puffs, or blocking ventilation holes with lips or fingers to offset the effects of filters. Studies have found that people who smoke "light" cigarettes inhale up to eight times as much tar and nicotine as printed on the label.

Concerns have also been raised about menthol cigarettes. About 76% of African American smokers smoke these cigarettes, as compared to 23% of whites. Studies have found that blacks absorb more nicotine than other groups and metabolize it more slowly. The anesthetizing effect of menthol, which may allow smokers to inhale more deeply and hold smoke in their lungs for a longer period, may be partly responsible for this difference. Further research is needed to determine if chemical effects of menthol and differences in smoking behavior can help explain the higher rates of smoking-related diseases seen among blacks.

The Immediate Effects of Smoking

The beginning smoker often has symptoms of mild nicotine poisoning: dizziness; faintness; rapid pulse; cold, clammy skin; and sometimes nausea, vomiting, and diarrhea. The seasoned smoker occasionally suffers these effects of nicotine poisoning, particularly after quitting and returning to a previous level of consumption. The effects of nicotine on smokers vary, depending greatly on the size of the nicotine dose and how much tolerance previous smoking has built up. Nicotine can either excite or tranquilize the nervous system, depending on dosage.

Nicotine has many other immediate effects. It stimulates the part of the brain called the **cerebral cortex.** It also stimulates the adrenal glands to discharge adrenaline. And it inhibits the formation of urine; constricts the blood vessels, especially in the skin; accelerates the heart rate; and elevates blood pressure. Higher blood pressure, faster heart rate, and constricted blood vessels require the heart to pump more blood. In healthy people, the heart can usually meet this demand, but in people whose coronary arteries are damaged enough to interfere with the flow of blood, the heart muscle may be strained.

Smoking depresses hunger contractions and dulls the taste buds; smokers who quit often notice that food tastes much better. Smoking is not useful for weight loss, however. (Smoking for decades may lessen or prevent age-associated weight gain for some smokers, but for people under 30, smoking is not associated with weight loss.) Figure 11-2 summarizes these immediate effects.

Terms

cigarette tar A brown, sticky mass created when the chemical particles in tobacco smoke condense.

carcinogen Any substance that causes cancer.

cocarcinogen A substance that works with a carcinogen to cause cancer.

cerebral cortex The outer layer of the brain, which controls complex behavior and mental activity.

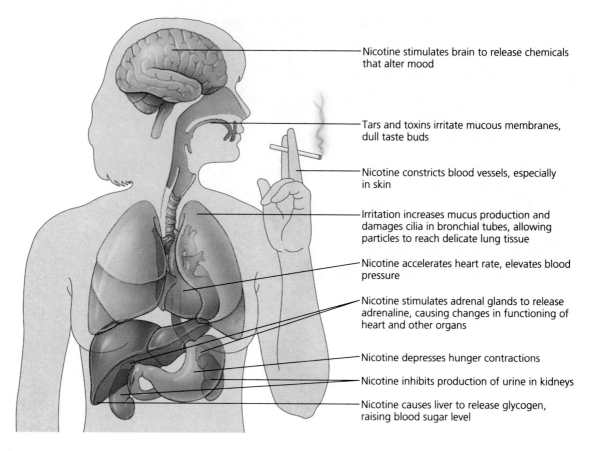

Nicotine stimulates brain to release chemicals that alter mood

Tars and toxins irritate mucous membranes, dull taste buds

Nicotine constricts blood vessels, especially in skin

Irritation increases mucus production and damages cilia in bronchial tubes, allowing particles to reach delicate lung tissue

Nicotine accelerates heart rate, elevates blood pressure

Nicotine stimulates adrenal glands to release adrenaline, causing changes in functioning of heart and other organs

Nicotine depresses hunger contractions

Nicotine inhibits production of urine in kidneys

Nicotine causes liver to release glycogen, raising blood sugar level

Figure 11-2   The short-term effects of smoking a cigarette.

The Long-Term Effects of Smoking

Smoking is a dangerous habit that is linked to many deadly and disabling diseases. Research indicates that the total amount of tobacco smoke inhaled is a key factor contributing to disease. People who smoke more cigarettes per day, inhale deeply, puff frequently, smoke cigarettes down to the butts, or begin smoking at an early age run a greater risk of disease than do those who smoke more moderately or who do not smoke at all. Many diseases have already been linked to smoking, and as more research is done, even more diseases associated with smoking are being uncovered. The most costly ones—to society as well as to the individual—are cardiovascular diseases, respiratory diseases such as emphysema and lung cancer, and other cancers.

Cardiovascular Disease   Although cancer tends to receive the most publicity, one form of cardiovascular disease, **coronary heart disease (CHD),** is actually the most widespread single cause of death for cigarette smokers. CHD often results from **atherosclerosis,** a condition in which fatty deposits called **plaques** form on the inner walls of heart arteries, causing them to narrow and stiffen. Smoking and exposure to environmental tobacco smoke

(ETS) permanently accelerate the rate of plaque accumulation in the coronary arteries—50% for smokers, 25% for ex-smokers, and 20% for people regularly exposed to ETS. The crushing chest pain of **angina pectoris,** a primary symptom of CHD, results when the heart muscle, or *myocardium,* does not get enough oxygen. Sometimes a plaque forms at a narrow point in a main coronary artery. If the plaque completely blocks the flow of blood to a portion of the heart, that portion may die. This type of heart attack is called a **myocardial infarction.**

CHD can also interfere with the heart's electrical activity, resulting in disturbances of the normal heartbeat rhythm. Sudden and unexpected death is a common result of CHD, particularly among smokers. (See Chapter 15 for a more extensive discussion of cardiovascular disease.)

Smokers have a death rate from CHD that is 70% higher than that of nonsmokers. Deaths from CHD associated with cigarette smoking are most common in people age 40–50. (By contrast, deaths from lung cancer caused by smoking are most likely to occur in 60–70-year-olds.) Cigar and pipe smokers run a lower risk than cigarette smokers.

We do not completely understand how cigarette smoking increases the risk of CHD, but researchers are beginning to shed light on the process. Smoking reduces the amount of "good" cholesterol (high-density lipoprotein, or HDL) in the blood, thereby promoting plaque formation in artery walls. Smoking may also increase tension in heart muscle walls, speeding up the rate of muscular contraction and accelerating the heart rate. The workload of the heart thus increases, as does its need for oxygen and other nutrients. Carbon monoxide produced by cigarette smoking combines with hemoglobin in the red blood cells, displacing oxygen and thus providing less oxygen to the heart. A recent study showed that the additional blood supply available to the heart during stress was 21% less in smokers than in nonsmokers. This reduced blood flow is an early indicator of future heart attacks or strokes.

The risks of CHD decrease rapidly when a person stops smoking; this is particularly true for younger smokers, whose coronary arteries have not yet been extensively damaged. Cigarette smoking has also been linked to other cardiovascular diseases, including

- *Stroke,* a sudden interference with the circulation of blood in a part of the brain, resulting in the destruction of brain cells

- *Aortic aneurysm,* a bulge in the aorta caused by a weakening in its walls

- *Pulmonary heart disease,* a disorder of the right side of the heart, caused by changes in the blood vessels of the lungs

Lung Cancer and Other Cancers   Cigarette smoking is the primary cause of lung cancer. A recent study identified the precise mechanism: Benzo(a)pyrene, a chemical found in tobacco smoke, causes genetic mutations in lung cells that are identical to those found in many patients with lung cancer. Those who smoke two or more packs of cigarettes a day have lung cancer death rates 12–25 times greater than those of nonsmokers. The dramatic rise in lung cancer rates among women in the past 40 years clearly parallels the increase of smoking in this group; lung cancer now exceeds breast cancer as the leading cause of cancer deaths among women. The risk of developing lung cancer increases with the number of cigarettes smoked each day, the number of years smoking, and the age at which the person started smoking.

While cigar and pipe smokers have a higher risk of lung cancer than nonsmokers do, the risk is lower than that for cigarette smokers. Smoking filter-tipped cigarettes slightly reduces health hazards, unless the smoker compensates by smoking more, as is often the case.

Evidence suggests that after 1 year without smoking, the risk of lung cancer decreases substantially. After 10 years, the risk of lung cancer among ex-smokers is 50% of that of continuing smokers. The sooner one quits, the better: If smoking is stopped before cancer has started, lung tissue tends to repair itself, even if cellular changes that can lead to cancer are already present.

Research has also linked smoking to cancers of the trachea, mouth, pharynx, esophagus, larynx, pancreas, bladder, kidney, cervix, stomach, liver, colon, and skin. For more information on cancer, see Chapter 16.

Chronic Obstructive Lung Disease   The lungs of a smoker are constantly exposed to dangerous chemicals and irritants, and they must work harder to function adequately. The stresses placed on the lungs by smoking can permanently damage lung function and lead to *chronic obstructive lung disease (COLD),* also known as chronic obstructive pulmonary disease. COLD is the fourth leading cause of death in the United states. This progressive and disabling disorder consists of several different but related diseases; emphysema and chronic bronchitis are two of the most common.

Cigarette smokers are up to 18 times more likely than nonsmokers to die from emphysema and chronic bronchitis. (Pipe and cigar smokers are more likely to die from COLD than are nonsmokers, but they have a smaller risk than cigarette smokers.) The risk of developing COLD rises with the number of cigarettes smoked and falls when smoking ceases. For most Americans, cigarette smoking is a more important cause of COLD than air pollution, but exposure to both is more dangerous than exposure to either by itself.

EMPHYSEMA   Smoking is the primary cause of **emphysema,** a particularly disabling condition in which the walls of the air sacs in the lungs lose their elasticity and are gradually destroyed. The lungs' ability to obtain oxygen and remove carbon dioxide is impaired. A person with emphysema is breathless, is constantly gasping for air, and has the feeling of drowning. The heart must pump harder and may become enlarged. People with emphysema often die from a damaged heart. There is no known way to reverse this disease. In its advanced stage, the victim is bedridden and severely disabled.

coronary heart disease (CHD) Cardiovascular disease caused by hardening of the arteries that supply oxygen to the heart muscle; also called *coronary artery disease.*

atherosclerosis Cardiovascular disease caused by the deposit of fatty substances in the walls of the arteries.

plaque A deposit on the inner wall of blood vessels; blood can coagulate around plaque and form a clot.

angina pectoris Chest pain due to coronary heart disease.

myocardial infarction A heart attack caused by the complete blockage of a main coronary artery.

emphysema A disease characterized by a loss of lung tissue elasticity and breakup of the air sacs, impairing the lungs' ability to obtain oxygen and remove carbon dioxide.

Terms

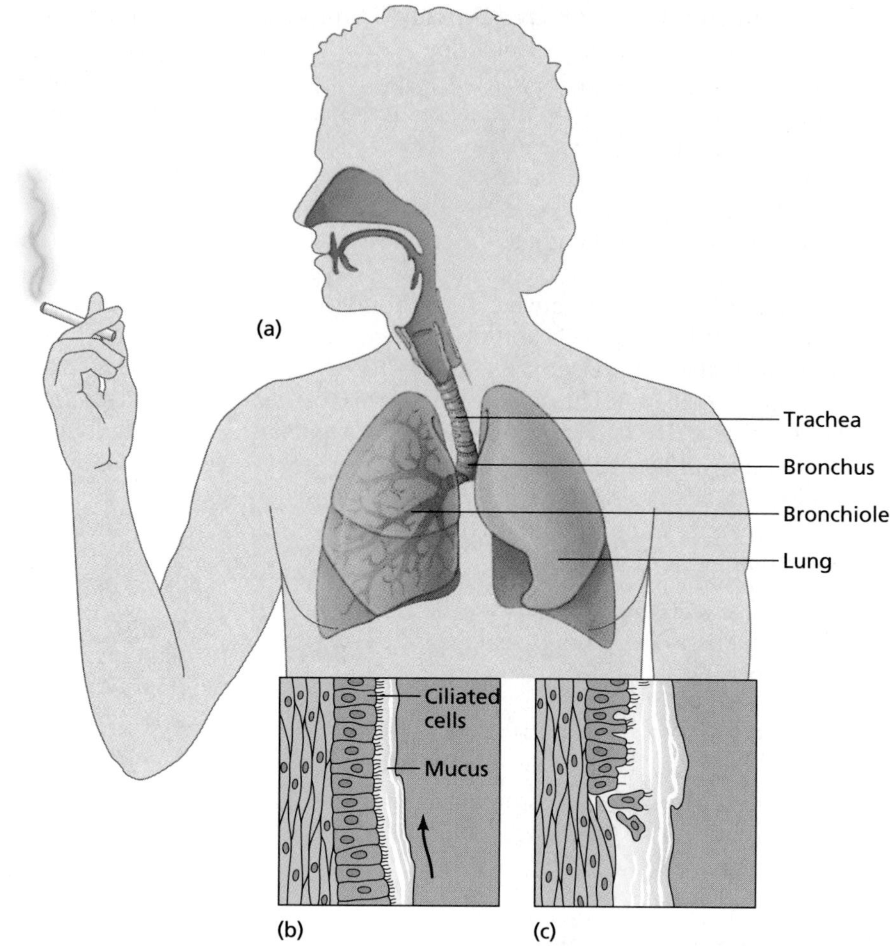

Figure 11-3 Damage to the lungs caused by smoking. (a) The respiratory system. (b) The inside of a bronchiole of a nonsmoker. Foreign particles are collected by a thin layer of sticky mucus and transported out of the lungs, up toward the mouth, by the action of cilia. (c) The inside of a bronchiole of a smoker. Smoking irritates the lung tissue and causes increased mucus production, which can overwhelm the action of the cilia. A smoker develops a chronic cough as the lungs try to rid themselves of foreign particles and excess mucus. Eventually the cilia are destroyed, leaving the delicate lung tissue exposed to injury from foreign substances.

CHRONIC BRONCHITIS   Persistent, recurrent inflammation of the bronchial tubes characterizes **chronic bronchitis**. When the cell lining of the bronchial tubes is irritated, it secretes excess mucus. Bronchial congestion is followed by a chronic cough, which makes breathing more and more difficult. If smokers have chronic bronchitis, they face a greater risk of lung cancer, no matter how old they are or how many (or few) cigarettes they smoke. Chronic bronchitis seems to be a shortcut to lung cancer.

Other Respiratory Damage   Even when the smoker shows no signs of lung impairment or disease, cigarette smoking damages the respiratory system. Normally the cells lining the bronchial tubes secrete mucus, a sticky fluid that collects particles of soot, dust, and other substances in inhaled air. Mucus is carried up to the mouth by the continuous motion of the cilia, hairlike structures that protrude from the inner surface of the bronchial tubes (Figure 11-3). If the cilia are destroyed or impaired, or if the pollution of inhaled air is more than the system can remove, the protection provided by cilia is lost.

Cigarette smoke first slows and then stops the action of the cilia. Eventually it destroys them, leaving delicate membranes exposed to injury from substances inhaled in cigarette smoke or from the polluted air in which the person lives or works. Special cells, *macrophages,* a type of white blood cell, also work to remove foreign particles from the respiratory tract by engulfing them. Smoking appears to make macrophages work less efficiently. This interference with the functioning of the respiratory system often leads rapidly to the conditions known as smoker's throat and smoker's cough, as well as to shortness of breath. Even smokers of high school age show impaired respiratory function, compared with nonsmokers of the same age. Other respiratory effects of smoking include a worsening of allergy and asthma symptoms and an increase in the smoker's susceptibility to colds.

Although cigarette smoking can cause many respiratory disorders and diseases, the damage is not always permanent. Once a person stops smoking, steady improvement in overall lung function usually takes place. Chronic coughing subsides, mucus production returns to normal, and breathing becomes easier. The likelihood of lung disease drops sharply. People of all ages, even those who have been smoking for decades, improve after they stop smoking. If given a chance, the human body has remarkable powers of restoring itself.

Additional Health, Cosmetic, and Economic Concerns

- *Ulcers.* People who smoke are more likely to develop peptic ulcers and are more likely to die from them (especially stomach ulcers), because smoking impairs the body's healing ability.

- *Impotence.* Smoking affects blood flow in the veins and arteries of the penis, and it is an independent risk factor for impotence. In one recent study, smokers were twice as likely as nonsmokers to experience erectile dysfunction (impotence).

- *Reproductive health problems.* Smoking is linked to reduced fertility in both men and women. A study of 18-year-old smoking men found that they had a significantly higher proportion of abnormally shaped sperm and sperm with genetic defects than nonsmokers. In women, smoking can contribute to menstrual disorders, early menopause, and complications of pregnancy (see p. 301).

- *Dental diseases.* Smokers are at increased risk for tooth decay and gum and periodontal diseases, with symptoms appearing by the mid-20s.

- *Diminished physical senses.* Smoking dulls the senses of taste and smell. Over time, it increases the risk for hearing loss and cataracts (a serious eye condition that can result in partial or total blindness).

- *Injuries.* Smokers have higher rates of motor vehicle crashes, fire-related injuries, and back pain.

- *Cosmetic concerns.* Smoking can cause premature skin wrinkling, premature baldness, stained teeth, discolored fingers, and a persistent tobacco odor in clothes and hair.

- *Economic costs.* A pack-a-day habit costs an average of $1000 per year. Other financial costs include higher health and home insurance premiums; more frequent cleaning of clothes, teeth, home, office, and car; and repair of burnt clothing, upholstery, and carpeting.

In addition, smoking contributes to osteoporosis, increases the risk of complications from diabetes, and accelerates the course of multiple sclerosis. Further research may link tobacco use to still other disorders.

Cumulative Effects   The cumulative effects of tobacco use fall into two general categories. The first category is reduced life expectancy. A male who takes up smoking before age 15 and continues to smoke is only half as likely to live to age 75 as a male who never smokes. If he inhales deeply, he risks losing a minute of life for every minute of smoking. Females who have similar smoking habits also have a reduced life expectancy. On average, smokers live 8 years less than nonsmokers.

The second category involves quality of life. A national health survey begun in 1964 shows that smokers spend one-third more time away from their jobs because of illness than nonsmokers. Female smokers spend 17% more days sick in bed than female nonsmokers. Lost work days due to smoking number in the millions.

Both men and women smokers show a greater rate of acute and chronic disease than those who have never smoked. Smokers become disabled at younger ages than nonsmokers and have more years of unhealthy life in addition to a shorter life span. The U.S. Public Health Service estimates that if all people had the same rate of disease as those who never smoked, there would be 1 million fewer cases of chronic bronchitis, 1.8 million fewer cases of **sinusitis**, and 1 million fewer cases of peptic ulcers in the country every year.

WWW. Other Forms of Tobacco Use

Many smokers have switched from cigarettes to other forms of tobacco, such as cigars, pipes, clove cigarettes, and spit (smokeless) tobacco. However, each of these alternatives is far from safe.

Spit (Smokeless) Tobacco   More than 5 million adults and about 7% of all high school students are current spit tobacco users. Spit tobacco use has increased in recent years and is especially common among Native Americans, adolescent males (especially white males), male college athletes, and professional baseball players. About 80% of users start by the ninth grade.

Spit tobacco comes in two major forms—snuff and chewing tobacco ("chew"). In snuff, the tobacco leaf is processed into a coarse, moist powder and mixed with flavorings. Snuff is usually sold in small tins. Users place a "pinch," "dip," or "quid" between the lower lip or cheek and gum and suck on it. In chewing tobacco, the tobacco leaf may be shredded ("leaf"), pressed into bricks or cakes ("plugs"), or dried and twisted into ropelike strands ("twists"). Chew is usually sold in pouches. Users place a wad of tobacco in their mouth and then chew or suck it to release the nicotine. All types of smokeless tobacco cause an increase in saliva production, and resulting tobacco juice is spit out or swallowed.

The nicotine in spit tobacco—along with flavorings and additives—is absorbed through the gums and lining of the mouth. Holding an average-size dip in the mouth for 30 minutes delivers about the same amount of nicotine as two or three cigarettes. Because of its nicotine content, spit tobacco is highly addictive. Some users keep it in their mouth even while sleeping.

Although not as dangerous as smoking cigarettes, the use of spit tobacco carries many health risks. Changes can occur in the mouth after only a few weeks of use: Gums and lips become dried and irritated and may bleed. White or red patches may appear inside the mouth; this condition, known as *leukoplakia,* can lead to oral cancer (see below). A study of major league baseball players found dangerous mouth lesions in 83 out of the 141 spit tobacco–using players who were examined. Other studies have found even higher rates of oral sores. About 25% of regular spit tobacco users have *gingivitis* (inflammation) and recession of the gums and bone loss around the teeth, especially where the tobacco is usually placed. The senses of taste and smell are usually dulled. In addition, many people find the presence of wads of tobacco in the mouth, stained teeth, bad breath, and behaviors such as frequent spitting to be unpleasant.

One of the most serious effects of spit tobacco is an increased risk of oral cancer—cancers of the lip, tongue, cheek, throat, gums, roof and floor of the mouth, and larynx. Spit tobacco contains at least 28 chemicals known to cause cancer, and long-term snuff use may increase the risk of oral cancer by as much as 50 times. Surgery to treat oral cancer is often disfiguring and may involve removing parts of the face, tongue, cheek, or lip.

Data on the incidence of heart disease among spit tobacco users have not yet been collected. But it is known that dipping and chewing tobacco produce blood levels of nicotine similar to those in cigarette smokers. High blood levels of nicotine have dangerous effects on the cardiovascular system, including elevation of blood pressure, heart rate, and blood levels of certain fats. Other chemicals in spit tobacco are believed to pose risks to developing fetuses.

Cigars and Pipes After more than two decades of decline, cigar smoking has increased by nearly 50% since 1993. The popularity of cigars is highest among white males age 18–44 with higher than average income and education, but women are also smoking cigars in record numbers. Cigar use is also growing among young people: In the latest government surveys, 15% of high school students reported having smoked at least one cigar in the previous month. An estimated 2% of Americans, mostly males who also smoke cigarettes, are pipe smokers.

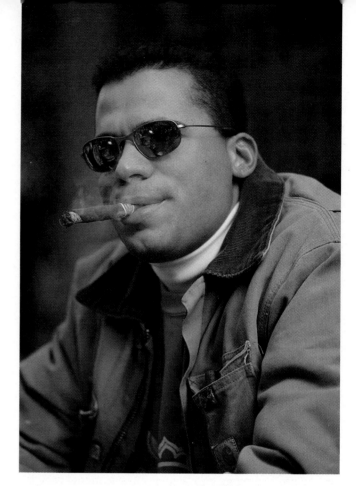

Cigars contain more tobacco than cigarettes and so produce more tar when smoked. Cigar smokers face an increased risk of cancer even if they don't inhale the smoke.

Cigars are made from rolled whole tobacco leaves; pipe tobacco is made from shredded leaves and often flavored. Because cigar and pipe smoke are more alkaline than cigarette smoke, users of cigars and pipes do not need to inhale in order to ingest nicotine; instead, they absorb nicotine through the gums and lining of the mouth. Cigars contain more tobacco than cigarettes and so contain more nicotine and produce more tar when smoked. Large cigars may contain as much tobacco as a whole pack of cigarettes and take 1–2 hours to smoke.

The smoke from cigars contains many of the same toxins and carcinogens as the smoke from cigarettes, some in much higher quantities. The health risks of cigars depend on the number of cigars smoked and whether or not the smoker inhales. Because most cigar and pipe users do not inhale, they have a lower risk of cancer and cardiovascular and respiratory diseases than cigarette smokers. However, their risks are substantially higher than those of nonsmokers. For example, compared to nonsmokers, people who smoke one or two cigars per day without inhaling have six times the risk of cancer of the larynx. The risks are much higher for cigar smokers who do inhale: They have 27 times the risk of oral cancer and 53 times the risk

Terms **environmental tobacco smoke (ETS)** Smoke that enters the atmosphere from the burning end of a cigarette, cigar, or pipe, as well as smoke that is exhaled by smokers; also called *secondhand smoke.*

mainstream smoke Smoke that is inhaled by a smoker and then exhaled into the atmosphere.

sidestream smoke Smoke that comes from the burning end of a cigarette, cigar, or pipe.

of cancer of the larynx compared to nonsmokers, and their risk of heart and lung diseases approaches that of cigarette smokers. Smoking a cigar immediately impairs the ability of blood vessels to dilate, reducing the amount of oxygen delivered to tissues, including heart muscle, especially during times of stress. Pipe and cigar smoking are also risk factors for pancreatic cancer, which is almost always fatal.

Nicotine addiction is another concern. Most adults who smoke cigars do so only occasionally, and there is little evidence that use of cigars by adults leads to addiction. The recent rise in cigar use among teens has raised concerns, however, because nicotine addiction almost always develops in the teen or young adult years. More research is needed to determine if cigar use by teens will develop into nicotine addiction and frequent use of either cigarettes or spit tobacco. In June of 2000 the FTC announced an agreement to put warning labels on cigar boxes, 34 years after warning labels first appeared on cigarette packages.

Clove Cigarettes and Bidis Clove cigarettes, also called "kreteks" or "chicartas," are made of tobacco mixed with chopped cloves; they are imported primarily from Indonesia and Pakistan. Clove cigarettes contain almost twice as much tar, nicotine, and carbon monoxide as conventional cigarettes and so have all the same health hazards. Some chemical constituents of cloves may also be dangerous. For example, eugenol, an anesthetic compound found in cloves, may impair the respiratory system's ability to detect and defend against foreign particles. There have been a number of serious respiratory injuries and deaths from the use of clove cigarettes.

Bidis, or "beadies," are small cigarettes imported from India that contain species of tobacco different from those used by U.S. cigarette manufacturers. The tobacco in bidis is hand-rolled in Indian ebony leaves (tendu) and then often flavored; clove, mint, chocolate, and fruit varieties are available. Bidis contain up to four times more nicotine than and twice as much tar as U.S. cigarettes. Use of bidis has been growing among teens, possibly because of the flavorings they contain or because they look and smell somewhat like marijuana cigarettes ("joints"); they do not have the same effects as marijuana, however.

Currently, an estimated 6% of high school students use clove cigarettes or bidis (Figure 11-4). Neither is a safe or healthy alternative to conventional tobacco cigarettes.

THE EFFECTS OF SMOKING ON THE NONSMOKER

In a watershed decision in 1993, the U.S. Environmental Protection Agency (EPA) designated **environmental tobacco smoke (ETS)** a Class A carcinogen—an agent known to cause cancer in humans. In 2000, the Depart-

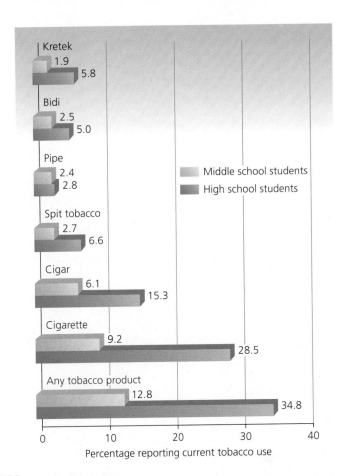

VITAL STATISTICS

Figure 11-4 Tobacco use among middle school and high school students. Although it is illegal for those under age 18 to purchase tobacco, 12.8% of middle school and 34.8% of high school students report having used some form of tobacco within the past month.
SOURCE: Centers for Disease Control and Prevention. 2000. CDC surveillance summaries: Youth tobacco surveillance—United States, 1998–1999. *Morbidity and Mortality Weekly Report* 49(SS-10): 7.

ment of Health and Human Services' National Toxicology Program classified ETS as a "known human carcinogen." These designations put ETS in the same category as notorious cancer-causing agents like asbestos. Every year, ETS causes thousands of deaths from lung cancer and heart disease and is responsible for hundreds of thousands of respiratory infections in young children. The health effects of ETS are the basis for efforts to limit or ban smoking in public and in the workplace.

Environmental Tobacco Smoke

Environmental tobacco smoke, commonly known as *secondhand smoke,* consists of mainstream smoke and sidestream smoke. Smoke exhaled by smokers is referred to as **mainstream smoke. Sidestream smoke** enters the atmosphere from the burning end of a cigarette, cigar, or pipe. Undiluted sidestream smoke, because it is not

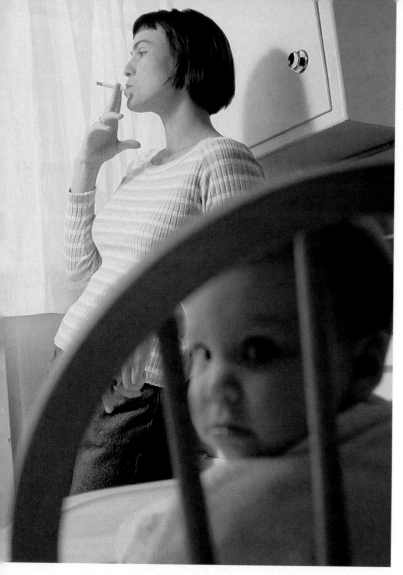

It is estimated that 9 million American infants and children are regularly exposed to environmental tobacco smoke. ETS can cause SIDS, trigger respiratory infections, cause or aggravate asthma, contribute to middle-ear infections, and impair development.

that the smoker does. Still, the concentrations can be considerable. In rooms where people are smoking, levels of carbon monoxide, for instance, can exceed those permitted by Federal Air Quality Standards for outside air. In a typical home with the windows closed, it takes about 6 hours for 95% of the airborne cigarette smoke particles to clear.

The secondhand smoke from a cigar can be even more dangerous than that from cigarettes. The EPA has found that the output of carcinogenic particles from a cigar exceeds that of three cigarettes, and cigar smoke contains up to 30 times more carbon monoxide.

ETS Effects   Studies show that up to 25% of nonsmokers subjected to ETS develop coughs, 30% develop headaches and nasal discomfort, and 70% suffer from eye irritation. Other symptoms range from breathlessness to sinus problems. People with allergies tend to suffer the most. The odor of tobacco smoke clings to skin and clothes—another unpleasant effect of ETS.

But ETS causes more than just annoyance and discomfort; it causes 3000 lung cancer deaths annually. People who live, work, or socialize among smokers face a 24–50% increase in lung cancer risk. ETS is also responsible for about 60,000 deaths from heart disease each year. As described earlier, exposure to ETS is associated with a 20% increase in the progression of atherosclerosis. ETS also aggravates asthma, an increasing cause of sudden death in otherwise healthy adults. Scientists have been able to measure changes that contribute to lung tissue damage and potential tumor promotion in the bloodstreams of healthy young test subjects who spend just 3 hours in a smoke-filled room. And nonsmokers can still be affected by the harmful effects of ETS hours after they have left a smoky environment. Carbon monoxide, for example, lingers in the bloodstream 5 hours later.

Infants, Children, and ETS   Recent studies have shown that infants exposed to smoke from more than 21 cigarettes a day are more than 23 times more likely to die of sudden infant death syndrome (SIDS) than babies not exposed to ETS. The National Cancer Institute recently estimated that ETS causes up to 2700 SIDS deaths and up to 18,600 cases of low birth weight each year. Children under 5 whose primary caregiver smokes 10 or more cigarettes per day have measurable blood levels of nicotine and tobacco carcinogens. Chemicals in tobacco smoke also show up in breast milk, and breastfeeding may pass more chemicals to the infant of a smoking mother than direct exposure to ETS.

ETS triggers 150,000–300,000 cases of bronchitis, pneumonia, and other respiratory infections in infants and toddlers up to 18 months of age each year, resulting in 7500–15,000 hospitalizations. Older children suffer, too. ETS is a risk factor for asthma in children who have not previously displayed symptoms of the disease, and it

filtered through either a cigarette filter or a smoker's lungs, has significantly higher concentrations of the toxic and carcinogenic compounds found in mainstream smoke. For example, compared to mainstream smoke, sidestream smoke has (1) twice as much tar and nicotine; (2) three times as much benzo(a)pyrene, a carcinogen; (3) almost three times as much carbon monoxide, which displaces oxygen from red blood cells and forms *carboxyhemoglobin,* a dangerous compound that seriously limits the body's ability to use oxygen; and (4) three times as much ammonia.

Nearly 85% of the smoke in a room where someone is smoking comes from sidestream smoke. Of course, sidestream smoke is diffused through the air, so nonsmokers don't inhale the same concentrations of toxic chemicals

aggravates the symptoms of the 200,000 to 1 million children who already have asthma. ETS is also linked to reduced lung function and fluid buildup in the middle ear, a contributing factor in middle-ear infections, a leading reason for childhood surgery.

Why are infants and children so vulnerable? Because they breathe faster than adults, they inhale more air—and more of the pollutants in the air. Because they also weigh less, they inhale three times more pollutants per unit of body weight than adults do. And because their young lungs are still growing, this intake can impair optimal development. The problem is widespread. The American Academy of Pediatrics estimates that some 9 million American children are exposed to ETS.

Avoiding ETS Given the health risks of exposure to ETS, try these strategies to keep the air around you safe:

- *Speak up tactfully.* Smokers may not know the dangers they are causing or may not know it bothers you.
- *Display reminders.* Put up signs asking smokers to refrain in your home, work area, and car.
- *Don't allow smoking in your home or room.* Get rid of ashtrays and ask smokers to light up outside.
- *Open a window.* If you cannot avoid being in a room with a smoker, at least try to provide some ventilation.
- *Sit in the nonsmoking section in restaurants and other public areas.* Complain to the manager if none exists.
- *Fight for a smoke-free work environment.* Join with your coworkers to either eliminate all smoking indoors or to confine it to certain areas.
- *Discuss quitting strategies.* Social pressure is a major factor in many former smokers' decision to quit. Help the smokers in your life by sharing quitting strategies with them.

COMMUNICATE! Nonsmokers have the right to breathe clean air; this right takes precedence over the freedom of smokers to smoke. If you find yourself in a situation where you are forced to breathe cigarette smoke against your will, you have the right to speak up politely but firmly. For example, "Would you mind putting your cigarette out [or moving to another spot]? The smoke is bothering me." If you are courteous and appropriately assertive without being judgmental or insulting, chances are good the smoker will comply.

Smoking and Pregnancy

Smoking almost doubles a pregnant woman's chance of having a miscarriage, and it significantly increases her risk of ectopic pregnancy (see the box "Special Risks for Women Who Smoke"). Maternal smoking causes an estimated 4600 infant deaths in the United States each year, primarily due to premature delivery and smoking-related problems with the placenta. Maternal smoking is a major factor in low birth weight, which puts newborns at high risk for infections and other serious problems. If a nonsmoking mother is regularly exposed to ETS, her infant is also at greater risk for low birth weight. Recent studies have also shown that babies whose mothers smoked during pregnancy had higher rates of colic, clubfoot, cleft lip and palate, and impaired lung function.

Babies born to mothers who smoke more than two packs a day perform poorly on developmental tests in the first hours after birth, compared to babies of nonsmoking mothers. Later in life, hyperactivity, short attention span, and lower scores on spelling and reading tests all occur more frequently in children whose mothers smoked during pregnancy than in those born to nonsmoking mothers. Prenatal tobacco exposure has also been associated with behavioral problems in children, including immaturity, emotional instability, physical aggression, and hyperactivity. Males born to smoking mothers have higher rates of adolescent and adult criminal activity, suggesting that maternal smoking may cause brain damage that increases the risk of criminal behavior. Nevertheless, only about 14% of female smokers quit while pregnant; *Healthy People 2010* sets a goal of increasing this to 30%.

The Cost of Tobacco Use to Society

The health care costs associated with smoking exceed $70 billion per year. If the cost of lost productivity from sickness, disability, and premature death is included, the total is closer to $125 billion. This works out to $5 per pack of cigarettes, far more than the average $0.39 per pack tax collected by states to offset tobacco-related medical costs.

In order to recoup public health care expenditures, 43 state attorneys general filed suit against tobacco companies. In March 1997, Liggett Group settled its part of the suit by agreeing to turn over internal documents and to pay a portion of its profits to cover tobacco-related medical expenses and anti-smoking campaigns. In November 1998, an agreement was reached that settled 39 state lawsuits and applied to seven states that never filed suit. (Four states—Florida, Minnesota, Mississippi, and Texas—settled their suits separately for a total of $40 billion.) The 1998 settlement requires the tobacco companies to pay states $206 billion over 25 years; it also limits or bans certain types of advertising, promotions, and lobbying. Many of the provisions of the deal are designed to limit youth exposure and access to tobacco. In exchange, the tobacco industry settles the state lawsuits and is protected from future suits by states, counties, towns, and other public entities. Tobacco companies passed the costs of the settlement on to smokers, increasing the average price of a pack of cigarettes by approximately 45 cents.

Everyone knows that smoking shortens life expectancy and increases the risk of cancer, lung disease, and heart disease. But did you know that smoking carries special risks for women? Many of these risks are associated with reproduction and the reproductive organs. Rates of cervical cancer and vulvar cancer, for example, are higher in women who smoke than in women who don't. Smoking diminishes fertility, and for pregnant women, smoking increases the risk of ectopic pregnancy, miscarriage, preterm birth, preeclampsia, and stillbirth.

The combination of smoking and taking oral contraceptives is dangerous; women who smoke and take the pill have a higher risk of potentially fatal blood clots, heart attacks, and strokes than other women. Women smokers are also at increased risk for irregular and painful menstruation, early menopause, and more menopause symptoms.

Smoking increases a woman's chance of developing osteoporosis, a disease in which bones become thinner and more brittle. Older women who smoke are thus more likely to suffer hip fractures from falls. Women who smoke are also at increased risk for thyroid-related diseases and depression.

For the first time in U.S. history, teenage girls are taking up smoking in greater numbers than teenage boys. Female smokers are expected to soon outnumber male smokers in the adult population. We can expect to see a corresponding increase in tobacco-related diseases among women. Already, lung cancer has surpassed breast cancer as the most common cause of cancer death in American women. According to several recent studies, female smokers are more vulnerable than male smokers to lung cancer and bladder cancer. Unless smoking rates decline significantly, we can expect to see more of these life-threatening and debilitating tobacco-related diseases affecting women.

SOURCE: Centers for Disease Control and Prevention. 2001. *Women and Smoking: A Report of the Surgeon General.* Atlanta, GA.: CDC Office on Smoking and Health.

Legal action also continues on other fronts. In March 2000 the Supreme Court ruled that the FDA lacks the authority to regulate tobacco products, stopping the FDA's efforts to prevent tobacco sales and marketing aimed at minors. Among the FDA's guidelines affected by the ruling is the requirement that retailers ask for identification from tobacco purchasers who appear to be under age 27. In July 2000, a Florida jury ordered tobacco companies to pay a $145 billion penalty in a class action suit filed on behalf of sick Florida smokers, the largest penalty in U.S. history (the verdict is under appeal). The Justice Department also continued a lawsuit alleging that tobacco companies violated racketeering laws by conspiring to mislead the public about the dangers of smoking. This case is scheduled for trial in early 2003. For current information on political and legal activities, call or visit the Web site of one of the tobacco control advocacy groups listed in the For More Information section at the end of the chapter.

W. WHAT CAN BE DONE?

Every hour, 60 Americans die from preventable smoking-related diseases. Today there are more avenues than ever before for individual and group action against this major public health threat.

Action at the Local Level

Before the EPA issued its report declaring ETS to be a carcinogen, most efforts to limit smoking focused on enacting local laws and ordinances. Tobacco interests have been able to block actions at the national and state levels through lobbying and political contributions. However, during the 1980s and 1990s, tobacco restrictions were passed by local school boards, town councils, and county boards of supervisors, over which the tobacco industry has little or no influence.

There are now thousands of local ordinances across the nation that restrict or ban smoking in restaurants, stores, and workplaces. Since the EPA classification of environmental tobacco smoke as a carcinogen, local governments and businesses have become bolder about protecting nonsmokers. Even public outdoor areas are not exempt from regulations: Sharon, Massachusetts, has banned smoking at all beaches and playgrounds. Honolulu, Hawaii, has also banned smoking at the beach, but for a different reason—to protect sea turtles from being poisoned by eating cigarette butts.

As local no-smoking rules proliferate, evidence is mounting that such restrictions encourage smokers to quit. The smoking rate dropped from one in three adults in 1980 to one in four in 1998.

Action at the State and Federal Levels

The EPA report fundamentally changed the politics of tobacco by declaring that smokers not only shorten their own lives but also kill innocent bystanders. It became harder for politicians who are sympathetic to the tobacco industry—and who often accept sizable contributions from tobacco interests—to argue that anti-tobacco laws constitute unwarranted intrusions into voters' private lives.

State legislatures have passed many tough new anti-tobacco laws. California has one of the most aggressive—

The United States has made some gains since the days when cigarettes were advertised on TV and women smoked throughout their pregnancies. Much of the public is aware of the dangers of tobacco use, and, although still too high, the rate of smoking has declined. There are now about as many ex-smokers in the United States as there are current smokers. To compensate for the loss in revenue, the U.S. tobacco industry has increased its efforts to sell to foreign markets, especially those in developing nations. Worldwide, about 1.1 billion people smoke, with this number expected to increase to 1.6 billion by 2025. Smoking currently causes about 4 million deaths per year, but the annual toll is expected to rise to 10 million by 2025, with 70% of deaths occurring in developing countries.

China presents an especially striking case. About two-thirds of Chinese men become smokers by the age of 25, and few quit before dying. The number of male deaths alone from tobacco is expected to be about 3 million annually by the middle of the twenty-first century. About 100 million of the 300 million Chinese men now alive under the age of 29 will die from tobacco-related causes, with 50 million of those men dying before leaving middle age.

It is not only adults who have been vulnerable to the tobacco industry. At the Eleventh Global Conference on Tobacco or Health, the director-general of the World Health Organization (WHO) reported the results of a survey of 50,000 children age 13 to 15 in developing or transitional countries. Twenty-four percent of the children had tried smoking and 9% were current smokers. A quarter of those who smoked said they started before they were 11 years old. One encouraging note is that 68% of the children wanted to kick the habit.

WHO has taken steps to address tobacco's global impact, establishing the Tobacco Free Initiative in 1998 to coordinate its anti-tobacco efforts. In October 2000, WHO began drafting the Framework Convention on Tobacco Control (FCTC), the first international treaty for public health ever proposed by WHO. This treaty will have the force of international law in those countries that sign it and will allow those countries to regulate advertising, pursue smugglers, and otherwise cooperate in tobacco control efforts. Nations differ in their approach to such issues as advertising to minors, taxation, and wording of warning labels. Many countries have few, if any, restrictions on advertising, and tobacco companies can use marketing techniques long banned in the United States. In Poland, for example, cigarette billboards can be found adjacent to elementary schools; in Japan, tobacco ads appear even during children's TV shows. It is hoped that the treaty will be completed by May 2002 and adopted by the 191 WHO member states no later than May 2003.

Another international activity has been the annual commemoration of World No Tobacco Day, May 31, on which smokers are encouraged to stop smoking for one day. If a smoker successfully takes the first step of quitting for a day, he or she may be encouraged enough to follow through on the commitment and become a permanent nonsmoker. On World No Tobacco Day in Thailand, a giant digital "death clock" was unveiled to show that at least eight people die every minute worldwide from smoking. With international efforts and cooperation increasing, strides are being made to lessen tobacco's global impact.

and successful—tobacco control programs, combining taxes on cigarettes, graphic advertisements, and bans on smoking in bars and restaurants. In the past decade, per capita cigarette consumption fell by 50% in California, lung cancer cases dropped 14%, and heart disease deaths were reduced by more than 30,000.

The federal government is also acting to protect nonsmokers from environmental tobacco smoke. Smoking has been banned on virtually all domestic airplane flights, and the U.S. Defense Department has banned smoking at all military work sites. And the U.S. Occupational Safety and Health Administration considered nationwide rules that would, in effect, ban smoking on the job except in specially ventilated areas.

International Action

Many countries are following the United States' lead in restricting smoking. Smoking is now banned on many international air flights, as well as in many restaurants and hotels and on public transportation in some countries. The World Health Organization has taken the lead in international anti-tobacco efforts; see the box "Tobacco Control Around the World."

Action in the Private Sector

The EPA report also shook up the private sector, giving employers reason to fear worker's compensation claims based on exposure to workplace smoke. The year after the report was issued, businesses including McDonald's and Taco Bell banned smoking in thousands of their restaurants across the country. The number of smoke-free restaurants has increased dramatically in recent years, and the vast majority of the nation's shopping malls now prohibit smoking.

Such local, state, national, and international efforts represent progress, but health activists warn that tobacco industry influence remains strong. The tobacco industry contributes heavily to sympathetic legislative officeholders and candidates. Many states have relatively weak anti-smoking laws that are backed by the tobacco industry and include clauses that prevent the passage of stricter local ordinances. Since 1997, tobacco interests have spent more than $120 million on federal lobbying activities.

The U.S. Public Health Service recommends a "Five A's" approach for physicians to help patients quit tobacco use. If someone you care about uses tobacco, you can try the same strategies to help them quit.

1. **Ask** about tobacco use. How many cigarettes does your girlfriend smoke each day? How long has your roommate been dipping snuff?

2. **Advise** tobacco users to stop. Express your concern over the tobacco user's habit. "When we're close, the smell of smoke on your hair and breath bothers me. I've noticed you cough a lot and your voice is raspy. I'm worried about your health. You should stop."

3. **Assess** the tobacco user's willingness to quit. "Next week would be a good time to try to quit. Would you be willing to give it a try?"

4. **Assist** the tobacco user who is willing to stop. To coincide with your partner's quit date, take him away for a romantic weekend far from the places he associates with smoking. Offer to be an exercise partner. Call once a day to offer support and help. Bring gifts of low-calorie snacks or projects that occupy the hands. If the quitter lapses, be encouraging. A lapse doesn't have to become a relapse.

5. **Arrange** follow-up. Maintaining abstinence is an ongoing process. Celebrate milestones of 1 week, 1 month, 1 year without tobacco. Note how much better your friend's or partner's car, room, and person smell, how much healthier he or she is, and how much you appreciate not having to breathe tobacco smoke.

Keep in mind the special influence that a partner or loved one can have on someone who is trying to quit using tobacco. Recent research has shown that certain kinds of behavior by a partner are consistently related to successful quitting, while other behaviors are related to relapse. Behaviors linked to success include expressing pleasure at the smoker's efforts to quit, actively rewarding the smoker's efforts (for example, giving a small gift), helping to calm the smoker when he or she is feeling stressed or irritable, and actively sharing in an activity such as dancing, jogging, or hiking that serves as a distraction from smoking.

Sometimes a tobacco user's partner does things that are intended to be helpful but actually interfere with the user's efforts to quit. These behaviors include hiding ashtrays, keeping track of the amount of tobacco used, hiding or throwing out the smoker's cigarettes, frequently mentioning the health risks associated with tobacco, ignoring the smoker during efforts to quit, downplaying the difficulty of quitting, and complaining about the partner's irritability during attempts to quit.

If your partner is trying to quit and you are uncertain how to help, ask what would be most helpful. Recognize that tobacco use is your partner's problem, and while there may be things you can do to help, your partner is ultimately in control of his or her own body. If your partner asks you to back off, then do so within the limits you have established in your relationship. If your partner gets angry or irritable, recognize that this hypersensitivity is a normal but temporary side effect of nicotine withdrawal and remind yourself that it will pass. Listen to your partner, communicate your own feelings as clearly as possible, and do what you can to reduce your partner's stress level, such as temporarily taking over a household chore. If you smoke yourself, you can help your partner by not smoking in open view and by providing positive support. Even better, take inspiration from your partner's efforts and quit yourself.

SOURCE: "Five A's" from Fiore, E. M. C., et al. 2000. *Treating Tobacco Use and Dependence.* Clinical Practice Guideline. Rockville, Md.: U.S. Department of Health and Human Services.

Individual Action

When a smoker violates a no-smoking designation, complain. If your favorite restaurant or shop doesn't have a nonsmoking policy, ask the manager to adopt one. If you see children buying tobacco, report this illegal activity to the facility manager or the police. Learn more about addiction and tobacco cessation so you can better support the tobacco users you know (see the box "Helping a Friend or Partner Stop Using Tobacco"). Vote for candidates who support anti-tobacco measures; contact local, state, and national representatives to express your views.

Cancel your subscriptions to magazines that carry tobacco advertising; send a letter to the publisher explaining your decision. Voice your opinion about other positive representations of tobacco use. (A recent study found that more than two-thirds of children's animated feature films have featured tobacco or alcohol use with no clear message that such practices were unhealthy.) Volunteer with the American Lung Association, the American Cancer Society, or the American Heart Association.

These are just some of the many ways individuals can help support tobacco prevention and stop-smoking efforts. Nonsmokers not only have the right to breathe clean air but also have the right to take action to help solve one of society's most serious public health threats.

> **COMMUNICATE!**   Does someone you care about smoke— a parent, sibling, friend, partner? This chapter is full of ideas about how to help someone quit, including recommendations from the U.S. Public Health Service and suggestions from representatives of the world's religions. Perhaps the simplest and most straightforward thing you can say is "I love you very much, and I worry about your smoking. I wish you would quit."

Table 11-2	Benefits of Quitting Smoking

Within 20 minutes of your last cigarette:
- You stop polluting the air
- Blood pressure drops to normal
- Pulse rate drops to normal
- Temperature of hands and feet increases to normal

8 hours:
- Carbon monoxide level in blood drops to normal
- Oxygen level in blood increases to normal

24 hours:
- Chance of heart attack decreases

48 hours:
- Nerve endings start regrowing
- Ability to smell and taste things is enhanced

2–3 months:
- Circulation improves
- Walking becomes easier
- Lung function increases up to 30%

1–9 months:
- Coughing, sinus congestion, fatigue, and shortness of breath all decrease
- Cilia regrow in lungs, reduce infection

1 year:
- Heart disease death rate is half that of a smoker

5 years:
- Stroke risk drops nearly to the risk for nonsmokers

10 years:
- Lung cancer death rate drops to 50% of that of continuing smokers
- The incidence of other cancers (mouth, throat, larynx, esophagus, bladder, kidney, and pancreas) decreases

15 years:
- Risk of lung cancer is about 25% of that of continuing smokers
- Risks of heart disease and stroke are close to those for nonsmokers.

SOURCES: American Cancer Society. 2000. *Quitting Smoking* (http://www.cancer.org/tobacco/quitting.html; retrieved July 10, 2000). American Lung Association. 1999. *Benefits of Quitting* (http://www.lungusa.org/tobacco/quit_ben.html; retrieved October 14, 2000).

Controlling the Tobacco Companies

With their immensely profitable industry shrinking, tobacco companies are concentrating on appealing to narrower and narrower market segments with an ever-increasing array of brands and styles—over 350 in all. As tobacco use has declined among better-educated, wealthier segments of the American population, tobacco companies have redirected their marketing efforts toward minorities, the poor, and young women, populations among whom smoking rates are still high. This practice of targeting specific segments of the market has become controversial, especially when the segment has an unusually high risk for fatal diseases caused by tobacco use.

With cigarette sales falling in the United States, tobacco companies have begun focusing on increasing the export of cigarettes, particularly to developing nations. As companies compete for customers in the years ahead, the need to exercise public pressure to keep the powerful tobacco companies in check will persist.

WW. HOW A TOBACCO USER CAN QUIT

Since 1964, over 50% of all adults who have ever smoked have quit. Giving up tobacco is a long-term, intricate process. Heavy smokers who say they have just stopped "cold turkey" don't tell of the thinking and struggling and other mental processes that contributed to their final conquest over this powerful addiction. Olympic diver Greg Louganis, who began smoking at the age of 8, has said that he considers quitting, at the age of 23, the greatest accomplishment of his life.

Research shows that tobacco users move through predictable stages—from being uninterested in stopping, to thinking about change, to making a concerted effort to stop, to finally maintaining abstinence. But most attempt to quit several times before they finally succeed. Relapse is a normal part of the process.

The Benefits of Quitting

Giving up tobacco provides immediate health benefits to men and women of all ages (Table 11-2). People who quit smoking find that food tastes better. Their sense of smell is sharper. Circulation improves, heart rate and blood pressure drop, and lung function and heart efficiency increase. Ex-smokers can breathe more easily, and their capacity for exercise improves. Many ex-smokers report feeling more energetic and alert. They experience fewer headaches. Even their complexion may improve. Quitting also has a positive effect on long-term disease risk. From the first day without tobacco, ex-smokers begin to decrease their risk of cancer of the lung, larynx, mouth, pancreas, bladder, cervix, and other sites. Risk of heart attack, stroke, and other cardiovascular diseases drops quickly, too.

The younger people are when they stop smoking, the more pronounced the health improvements. And these improvements gradually but invariably increase as the

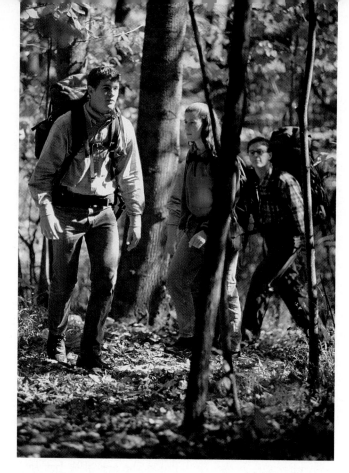

Quitting smoking improves the quality of life. In addition to reducing their long-term disease risks, these ex-smokers have more energy and an improved capacity for exercise.

Support can come from friends and family and/or formal group programs sponsored by organizations such as the American Cancer Society, the American Lung Association, and the Seventh-Day Adventist Church or by your college health center or community hospital. Programs that combine group support with nicotine replacement therapy have rates of continued abstention as high as 35% after one year.

Most smokers in the process of quitting experience both physical and psychological effects of nicotine withdrawal, and exercise can help with both. For many smokers, their tobacco use is associated with certain times and places—following a meal, for example. Resolving to walk after dinner instead of lighting up provides a distraction from cravings and eliminates the cues that trigger a desire to smoke. In addition, many people worry about weight gain associated with quitting. Although most ex-smokers do gain a few pounds, at least temporarily, incorporating exercise into a new tobacco-free routine lays the foundation for healthy weight management. The health risks of adding a few pounds are far outweighed by the risks of continued smoking; it's estimated that a smoker would have to gain 75–100 pounds to equal the health risks of smoking a pack a day.

As with any significant change in health-related behavior, giving up tobacco requires planning, sustained effort, and support. It is an ongoing process, not a one-time event. The Behavior Change Strategy at the end of the chapter describes the steps that successful quitters follow.

period of nonsmoking lengthens. It's never too late to quit, though. According to a U.S. Surgeon General's report, people who quit smoking, regardless of age, live longer than people who continue to smoke. Even smokers who have already developed chronic bronchitis or emphysema show some improvement when they quit.

Options for Quitting

Most tobacco users—76% in a recent survey—want to quit, and half of those who want to quit will make an attempt this year. What are their options? No single method works for everyone, but each does work for some people some of the time. In June 2000, the U.S. Public Health Service issued new guidelines for medical professionals on how to help their patients quit smoking, emphasizing the benefits of both behavioral and pharmacological interventions.

Choosing to quit requires developing a strategy for success. Some people quit "cold turkey," while others taper off more slowly. There are over-the-counter and prescription products that help many people (see the box "Smoking Cessation Products" for more on these options). Behavioral factors that have been shown to increase the chances of a smoker's permanent smoking cessation are support from others and regular exercise.

Tips for Today

Smoking is the leading preventable cause of death in the United States. Most smokers get hooked before they realize it, providing a market of millions to the tobacco industry. For most smokers, quitting is one of the hardest things they'll ever do. The best choice is never to start.

Right now you can

- If you smoke, put your cigarette out and go brush your teeth. Throw the pack and matches away.

- If you smoke, think about the next time you'll want a cigarette, such as while taking on the phone this afternoon or relaxing after dinner tonight. Visualize yourself enjoying this activity without a cigarette in your hand. Imagine yourself as a healthier, more robust person. See if you get pleasure or satisfaction from thinking of yourself as a nonsmoker, an ex-smoker, or someone liberated from dependence on cigarettes.

- If you use tobacco, go outside for a short walk or a stretch to limber up. Breathe deeply. Tell a friend you've just decided to quit.

- Resolve to talk to someone you know who uses tobacco, offering support and assistance if the person is interested in quitting.

Nicotine Replacement Therapy

As the name suggests, nicotine replacement therapy involves supplying the tobacco user with nicotine from a source other than standard tobacco products. This allows a user to overcome the psychological and behavioral aspects of a tobacco habit without having to simultaneously endure the physical symptoms of withdrawal. Although still harmful, nicotine replacement provides a cleaner form of nicotine. It avoids the thousands of poisons and tars that are found in burning tobacco and delivers a lower dose of nicotine than most smokers receive. After a few weeks or months of use, the reforming tobacco user begins to taper off use of the replacement, alleviating withdrawal symptoms.

There are several types of nicotine replacements, each with advantages and disadvantages. None of them are safe to use if the smoker plans to continue using tobacco; nicotine is a powerful stimulant, and an overdose can cause serious health complications. Studies have shown that combining nicotine replacement therapy with behavioral counseling can double the number of smokers who quit.

Nicotine patches can be purchased in varying strengths without a prescription. The patches release a controlled and steady supply of nicotine through the skin for 16 or 24 hours, depending on the type selected. Smokers often begin using a full-strength patch and then switch to a weaker one to decrease the nicotine dosage. The most common side effects of the patch are skin irritation and redness, which can often be cleared up by switching to another brand.

Another nonprescription option is *nicotine gum*. When chewed, the gum releases nicotine that is absorbed through the mucous membranes of the mouth. Most users chew one to two pieces per hour. An advantage of the gum versus the patch is that it allows the user to control the nicotine doses, so that the smoker can chew more during a craving. Long-term dependence seems to be a problem for some gum users. Research has shown that 15–20% of gum users who successfully quit smoking continued using the gum for a year or longer, despite the recommended 6-month limit on use.

Nicotine nasal spray and *nicotine inhalers* are available only by prescription. The nasal spray immediately relieves withdrawal symptoms by delivering nicotine to the bloodstream through the nose. The most common side effects are nasal irritation and sinus problems. Inhalers are plastic rods with a nicotine plug. When the smoker puffs on the rod, the plug produces a nicotine vapor that goes to the mouth instead of the lungs. A benefit of the inhaler is that it mimics hand and mouth actions of smoking.

Non-Nicotine Medications

One of the most exciting developments in smoking cessation has been the recent use of bupropion (Zyban), a prescription antidepressant that affects neurotransmitters related to nicotine cravings. In one study of quitting success, 36% of nicotine patch users quit for at least the month, 49% of bupropion users quit, and 58% of users of both the patch and bupropion quit. Another study found that quitters who use bupropion tend to gain less weight than quitters who do not; an especially significant difference was seen among women. Bupropion has also been shown to be successful in helping even the most hardened smokers quit. If bupropion is not effective, there are two other drugs that may be prescribed, clonidine and nortriptyline; however, neither has been approved by the FDA specifically for nicotine dependence.

Each smoking cessation product may be successful for some people, but any attempt to quit must address both the psychological and the physical aspects of nicotine dependence. Plan carefully how you will quit, to maximize your chance of conquering this powerful addiction.

SUMMARY

- Smoking is the largest preventable cause of ill health and death in the United States. Nevertheless, millions of Americans continue to use tobacco.

- Regular tobacco use causes physical dependence on nicotine, characterized by loss of control, tolerance, and withdrawal. Habits can become associated with tobacco use and trigger the urge for a cigarette.

- People who begin smoking are usually imitating others or responding to seductive advertising. Smoking is associated with low education level and the use of other drugs.

- Tobacco smoke is made up of several hundred different chemicals, including some that are carcinogenic or poisonous or that damage the respiratory system.

- Nicotine acts on the nervous system as a stimulant or a depressant. It can cause blood pressure and heart rate to increase, straining the heart.

- Cardiovascular disease is the most widespread cause of death for cigarette smokers. It is the primary cause of lung cancer and is linked to many other cancers. Smoking can permanently damage lung function.

- Cigarette smoking is linked to ulcers, impotence, reproductive health problems, dental diseases, and other conditions. Tobacco use leads to lower life expectancy and to a diminished quality of life.

- The use of spit tobacco leads to nicotine addiction and is linked to oral cancers.

- Cigars, pipes, clove cigarettes, and bidis are not safe alternatives to cigarettes.

You can look forward to a longer and healthier life if you join the 47 million Americans who have quit using tobacco. The steps for quitting described below are discussed in terms of the most popular tobacco product in the United States—cigarettes—but they can be adapted for all forms of tobacco.

Gather Information

Collect personal smoking information in a detailed journal about your smoking behavior. Write down the time you smoke each cigarette of the day, the situation you are in, how you feel, where you smoke, and how strong your craving for the cigarette is, plus any other information that seems relevant. Part of the job is to identify patterns of smoking that are connected with routine situations (for example, the coffee break smoke, the after-dinner cigarette, the tension-reduction cigarette). Use this information to discover the behavior patterns involved in your smoking habit.

Make the Decision to Quit

Choose a date in the near future when you expect to be relatively stress-free and can give quitting the energy and attention it will require. Don't choose a date right before or during finals week, for instance. Consider making quitting a gift: Choose your birthday as your quit date, for example, or make quitting a Father's Day or Mother's Day present. You might also want to coordinate your quit date with a buddy—a fellow tobacco user who wants to quit or a nonsmoker who wants to give up another bad habit or begin an exercise program. Tell your friends and family when you plan to quit. Ask them to offer encouragement and help hold you to your goal.

Decide what approach to quitting will work best for you. Will you go cold turkey, or will you taper off? Will you use nicotine patches or gum? Will you join a support group or enlist the help of a buddy? Prepare a contract for quitting, as discussed in Chapter 1. Set firm dates and rewards, and sign the contract. Post it in a prominent place.

Prepare to Quit

One of the most important things you can do to prepare to quit is to develop and practice nonsmoking relaxation techniques. Many smokers find that they use cigarettes to help them unwind in tense situations or to relax at other times. If this is true for you, you'll need to find and develop effective substitutes. It takes time to become proficient at relaxation techniques, so begin practicing before your quit date. Refer to the detailed discussion of relaxation techniques in Chapter 2.

Other things you can do to help prepare for quitting include the following:

- Make an appointment to see your physician. Ask about OTC and prescription aids for tobacco cessation and whether one or more might be appropriate for you.

- Make a dentist's appointment to have your teeth cleaned the day after your target quit date.

- Start an easy exercise program, if you're not exercising regularly already.

- Buy some sugarless gum. Stock your kitchen with low-calorie snacks.

- Clean out your car, and air out your house. Send your clothes out for dry cleaning.

- Throw away all your cigarette-related paraphernalia (ashtrays, lighters, etc.).

- The night before your quit day, get rid of all your cigarettes. Have fun with this—get your friends or family to help you tear them up.

- Make your last few days of smoking inconvenient: Smoke only outdoors and when alone. Don't do anything else while you smoke.

Quitting

Your first few days without cigarettes will probably be the most difficult. It's hard to give up such a strongly ingrained habit, but remember that millions of Americans have done it—and you can too. Plan and rehearse the steps you will take when you experience a powerful craving. Avoid or control situations that you know from your journal are powerfully associated with your smoking (see the table). If your hands feel empty without a cigarette, try holding or fiddling with a small object such as a paper clip or pencil.

Social support can also be a big help. Arrange with a buddy to help you with your weak moments, and call him or her whenever you feel overwhelmed by an urge to smoke. Tell people you've just quit. You may discover many inspiring former smokers who can encourage you and reassure you that it's possible to quit and lead a happier, healthier life. Find a formal support group to join if you think it will help.

Maintaining Nonsmoking

The lingering smoking urges that remain once you've quit should be carefully tracked and controlled because they can cause

- Environmental tobacco smoke (ETS) contains high concentrations of toxic chemicals and can cause headaches, eye and nasal irritation, and sinus problems. Long-term exposure to ETS can cause lung cancer and heart disease.

- Infants and young children take in more pollutants than adults do; children whose parents smoke are especially susceptible to respiratory diseases.

- Smoking during pregnancy increases the risk of miscarriage, stillbirth, congenital abnormalities, prema-

relapses if left unattended. Keep track of these urges in your journal to help you deal with them. If certain situations still trigger the urge for a cigarette, change something about the situation to break past associations. If stress or boredom causes strong smoking urges, use a relaxation technique, take a brisk walk, have a stick of gum, or substitute some other activity for smoking.

Don't set yourself up for a relapse. If you allow yourself to get overwhelmed at school or work or to gain weight, it will be easier to convince yourself that now isn't the right time to quit. This is the right time. Continue to practice time-management and relaxation techniques. Exercise regularly, eat sensibly, and get enough sleep. These habits will not only ensure your success at remaining tobacco-free but also serve you well in stressful times throughout your life. In fact, former smokers who have quit for at least 3 months report reduced stress levels, probably because quitting smoking lowers overall arousal.

Watch out for patterns of thinking that can make nonsmoking more difficult. Focus on the positive aspects of not smoking, and give yourself lots of praise—you deserve it. Stick with the schedule of rewards you developed for your contract.

Keep track of the emerging benefits that come from having quit. Items that might appear on your list include improved stamina, an increased sense of pride at having kicked a strong addiction, a sharper sense of taste and smell, no more smoker's cough, and so on. Keep track of the money you're saving by not smoking, and spend it on things you really enjoy. And if you do lapse, be gentle with yourself. Lapses are a normal part of quitting. Forgive yourself, and pick up where you left off.

Strategies for Dealing with High-Risk Smoking Situations

Cues and High-Risk Situations	Suggested Strategies
Awakening in morning	Brush your teeth as soon as you wake up. Take a shower or bath.
Drinking coffee	Do something else with your hands. Drink tea or another beverage instead.
Eating meals	Sit in nonsmoking sections of restaurants. Get up from the table right away after eating, and start another activity. Brush your teeth right after eating.
Driving a car	Have the car cleaned when you quit smoking. Chew sugarless gum or eat a low-calorie snack. Take public transportation or ride your bike. Turn on the radio and sing along.
Socializing with friends who smoke	Suggest nonsmoking events (movies, theater, shopping). Tell them you've quit and ask them not to smoke around you, offer you cigarettes, or give you cigarettes if you ask for them.
Drinking at a bar, restaurant, or party	Try to take a nonsmoker with you, or associate with nonsmokers. Let friends know you've just quit. Moderate your intake of alcohol (it can weaken your resolve).
Encountering stressful situations	Practice relaxation techniques. Take some deep breaths. Get out of your room or house. Go somewhere that doesn't allow smoking. Take a shower, chew gum, call a friend, or exercise.

SOURCES: Strategies adapted with permission from *Postgraduate Medicine* 90(1), July 1991. Antonuccio, D.O. 1993. *Butt Out, The Smoker's Book: A Compassionate Guide to Helping Yourself Quit Smoking, With or Without a Partner.* Saratoga, Calif.: R & E.

ture birth, and low birth weight. SIDS, behavior problems, and long-term impairments in development are also risks.

- The overall cost of tobacco use to society includes the cost of both medical care and lost worker productivity.

- There are many avenues individuals and groups can take to act against tobacco use. Nonsmokers can use social pressure and legislative channels to assert their rights to breathe clean air.

- Giving up smoking is a difficult and long-term process. Although most ex-smokers quit on their own, some smokers benefit from stop-smoking programs, OTC and prescription medications, and support groups.

1. Interview one or two former tobacco users about their experiences with tobacco and the methods they used to quit. Why did they start smoking or using tobacco, how old were they when they started, and how long did their habit continue? What made them decide to quit? How did they quit? What could a current tobacco user learn from their experience of quitting?

2. Make a tour of the public facilities in your community and on your campus, such as movie theaters, auditoriums, business and school offices, and classrooms. What kinds of restrictions on smoking do these places have? In your opinion, are they appropriate? If you feel more or different restrictions are in order, write a letter to the editor of your school or local newspaper, and state your case. Support it with convincing arguments and appropriate facts.

WW. JOURNAL ENTRY

1. *Critical Thinking* Examine advertisements for cigarettes and smokeless tobacco products. What markets are they targeting? How do they try to appeal to their audience? How do the advertisers deal with the mandatory warning labels? Write a short essay describing your findings.

2. *Critical Thinking* Restrictions on smoking are increasing in our society. Do you think they're fair? Do they infringe on people's rights? Do they go too far or not far enough? Write a brief essay stating your position on smoking restrictions. Be sure to explain your reasoning. What are the most important factors in your decision? Why do you think you have the opinion you do?

3. *Critical Thinking* Research the roles the U.S. government plays in tobacco use and sales. Describe these roles and their effects. Do you think the government is acting appropriately? In your opinion, what role should the government have regarding tobacco use and sales?

FOR MORE INFORMATION

Books

Brigham, J. 1998. *Dying to Quit: Why We Smoke and How We Stop.* Washington, D.C.: National Academy Press. *A discussion of the process and nature of nicotine addiction from both the scientific and personal perspectives.*

Kessler, D. 2001. *A Question of Intent: A Great American Battle with a Deadly Industry.* New York: Public Affairs. *A description of the federal government's attempts to regulate tobacco, written by the former head of the FDA.*

Parker-Pope, T. 2001. *Cigarettes: Anatomy of an Industry from Seed to Smoke.* New York: New Press. *An entertaining history of cigarettes, with information on the industry and on individual smokers.*

Watson, R. R., and M. L. Witten, eds. 2001. *Environmental Tobacco Smoke.* Boca Raton, Fla.: CRC Press. *A scientific look at the health effects of environmental tobacco smoke.*

Self-help books designed to help smokers quit:

Antonuccio, D. O. 1993. *Butt Out, The Smoker's Book: A Compassionate Guide to Helping Yourself Quit Smoking, With or Without a Partner.* Saratoga, Calif.: R & E.

Chenoweth, B. 2000. *Changing Your Mind About Smoking.* New Plymouth, Idaho: A. B.

Dodds, B. 2000. *1,440 Reasons to Quit Smoking: 1 for Every Minute of the Day.* Minnetonka, Minn.: Meadowbrook Press.

Kleinman, L. 2000. *The Complete Idiot's Guide to Quitting Smoking.* Indianapolis, Ind.: Macmillan.

WW. Organizations, Hotlines, and Web Sites

Action on Smoking and Health (ASH). An advocacy group that provides statistics, news briefs, and other information.
202-659-4310
http://ash.org

American Cancer Society (ACS). Sponsor of the annual Great American Smokeout; provides information on the dangers of tobacco, as well as tools for prevention and cessation for both smokers and users of spit tobacco.
800-ACS-2345
http://www.cancer.org

American Lung Association. Provides information on lung diseases, tobacco control, and environmental health.
800-LUNG-USA; 212-315-8700
http://www.lungusa.org

CDC's Tobacco Information and Prevention Source (TIPS). Provides research results, educational materials, and tips on how to quit smoking; Web site includes special sections for kids and teens.
800-CDC-1311
http://www.cdc.gov/tobacco

Environmental Protection Agency Indoor Air Quality/ETS. Provides information and links about secondhand smoke.
800-438-4318
http://www.epa.gov/iaq/ets.html

National Cancer Institute: Smoking and Cancer. Provides fact sheets and other publications on the health effects of smoking and strategies for quitting.

http://rex.nci.nih.gov/PREV_AND_ERLYDETC/PREV_SMOKE. HTM

Nicotine Anonymous. A 12-step program for tobacco users.

http://www.nicotine-anonymous.org

Quitnet. Provides interactive tools and questionnaires, support groups, a library, news on tobacco issues, and quitting programs for both smokers and spit tobacco users.

http://www.quitnet.org

Tobacco BBS. A resource center on tobacco and smoking issues that includes news and information, assistance for smokers who want to quit, and links to related sites.

http://www.tobacco.org

Tobacco Control Resource Center and Tobacco Products Liability Project (TPLP). Provides current information about tobacco-related court cases and legislation; based at the Northeastern School of Law.

http://www.tobacco.neu.edu

World Health Organization Tobacco Free Initiative. Promotes the goal of a tobacco-free world.

http://www.who.int/toh

World No Tobacco Day (WNTD). Provides information on the annual worldwide event to encourage people to quit smoking; includes general information about tobacco use and testimonials of ex-smokers.

http://www.worldNoTobaccoDay.com

See also the listings for Chapters 9, 15, and 16.

SELECTED BIBLIOGRAPHY

American Cancer Society. 2000. *Quitting Smoking* (http://www.cancer.org/tobacco/quitting.html; retrieved July 10, 2000).

Brook, J. S., D. W. Brook, and M. Whiteman. 2000. The influence of maternal smoking during pregnancy on the toddler's negativity. *Archives of Pediatric and Adolescent Medicine* 154(4): 381–385.

Brundtland, G. H. 2000. Achieving worldwide tobacco control. *Journal of the American Medical Association* 284(6): 750–751.

Brundtland, G. H. 2000. *Keynote Address at the Opening of the 11th Global Conference on Tobacco or Health* (http://www.who.int/director-general/speeches/2000/20000807_chicago.html; retrieved October 14, 2000).

Centers for Disease Control and Prevention. 2000. Cigarette smoking among adults—United States, 1998. *Morbidity and Mortality Weekly Report* 49(39): 881–884.

Centers for Disease Control and Prevention. 2000. Declines in lung cancer rates—California, 1988–1997. *Morbidity and Mortality Weekly Report* 49(47): 1066–1069.

Chung, K. C., et al. 2000. Maternal cigarette smoking during pregnancy and the risk of having a child with cleft lip/palate. *Plastic and Reconstructive Surgery* 105(2): 485–491.

Common Cause. 2000. *How Special Interests Block Common Sense Solutions* (http://commoncause.org/publications/price/tobacco.htm; retrieved October 19, 2000).

DeHertog, S. A., et al. 2001. Relation between smoking and skin cancer. *Journal of Clinical Oncology* 19(1): 231–238.

Differences in weight gain evaluated in smokers who quit using Zyban vs. placebo. 2000. *EurekAlert,* August 4 (http://www.eurekalert.org/releases/cwg-diw080400.html; retrieved August 11, 2000).

DiFranza, J. R., et al. 2000. Initial symptoms of nicotine dependence in adolescents. *Tobacco Control* 9(3): 313–319.

Feldman, H. A., et al. 2000. Erectile dysfunction and coronary risk factors: Prospective results from the Massachusetts male aging study. *Preventive Medicine* 30(4): 328–338.

Fichtenberg, C. M., and S. A. Glantz. 2000. Association of the California Tobacco Control Program with declines in cigarette consumption and mortality from heart disease. *New England Journal of Medicine* 343(24): 1772–1777.

Fiore, M. C., et al. 2000. *Treating Tobacco Use and Dependence.* Clinical Practice Guidelines. Rockville, Md.: U.S. Department of Health and Human Services.

Gallup Organization. 1999. *Majority of Smokers Want to Quit, Consider Themselves Addicted* (http://www.gallup.com/poll/releases/pr991118.asp; retrieved May 18, 2000).

Gilliland, F. D., et al. 2000. Maternal smoking during pregnancy, environmental tobacco smoke exposure and childhood lung function. *Thorax* 55(4): 271–276.

Honein, M. A., L. J. Paulozzi, and C. A. Moore. 2000. Family history, maternal smoking, and clubfoot: An indication of a gene-environment interaction. *American Journal of Epidemiology* 152(7): 658–665.

Ismail, K., A. Sloggett, and B. DeStavola. 2000. Do common mental disorders increase cigarette smoking? *American Journal of Epidemiology* 152(7): 651–657.

Jarvis, M. J., et al. 2001. Nicotine yield from machine-smoked cigarettes and nicotine intakes in smokers: Evidence from a representative population survey. *Journal of the National Cancer Institute* 93(2): 134–138.

Kaufmann, P. A., et al. 2000. Coronary heart disease in smokers: Vitamin C restores coronary microcirculatory function. *Circulation* 102(11): 1233–1238.

Mannino, D. M., et al. 2001. Health effects related to environmental tobacco smoke exposure in children in the United States. *Archives of Pediatrics and Adolescent Medicine* 155: 36–41.

Mitka, M. 2000. Antitobacco forces seek first international treaty. *Journal of the American Medical Association* 284(12): 1502–1503.

National Cancer Institute. 1999. *Health Effects of Exposure to Environmental Tobacco Smoke.* Smoking and Tobacco Control Monograph No. 10. Washington, D.C.: National Cancer Institute.

Nusselder, W., et al. 2000. Smoking and the compression of morbidity. *Journal of Epidemiology and Community Health* 54(8): 566–574.

Rigotti, N. A., J. E. Lee, and H. Wechsler. 2000. U.S. college students' use of tobacco products: Results of a national survey. *Journal of the American Medical Association* 284(6): 699–705.

Sargent, J. D., et al. 2001. Brand appearances in contemporary cinema films and contribution to global marketing of cigarettes. *Lancet* 357(9249): 29–32.

Shaw, M., R. Mitchell, and D. Dorling. 2000. Time for a smoke? One cigarette reduces your life by 11 minutes. *British Medical Journal* 320(7226): 53.

Smoking and Health Action Foundation. 2000. *Global Cigarette Taxes and Prices* (http://www.nsra-adnf.ca/english/staxratesus.html; retrieved October 19, 2000).

Tashkin, D. P., et al. 2000. An evaluation of the effects of bupropion versus placebo in a population of smokers with COPD. Presented September 1 at the World Congress on Lung Health (Abstract 1405).

Treating tobacco dependence. 2000. *Journal of the American Medical Association* 283(24): 3334.

Wakefield, M. A., et al. 2000. Effects of restrictions on smoking at home, at school, and in public places on teenage smoking. *British Medical Journal* 321: 333–337.

Wenger, L., R. Malone, and L. Bero. 2001. The cigar revival and the popular press: A content analysis, 1987–1999. *American Journal of Public Health* 91: 288–291.

World Health Organization. 2000. *Tobacco Free Initiative: Burden of Disease* (http://tobacco.who.int/en/health/burden.html; retrieved October 14, 2000).

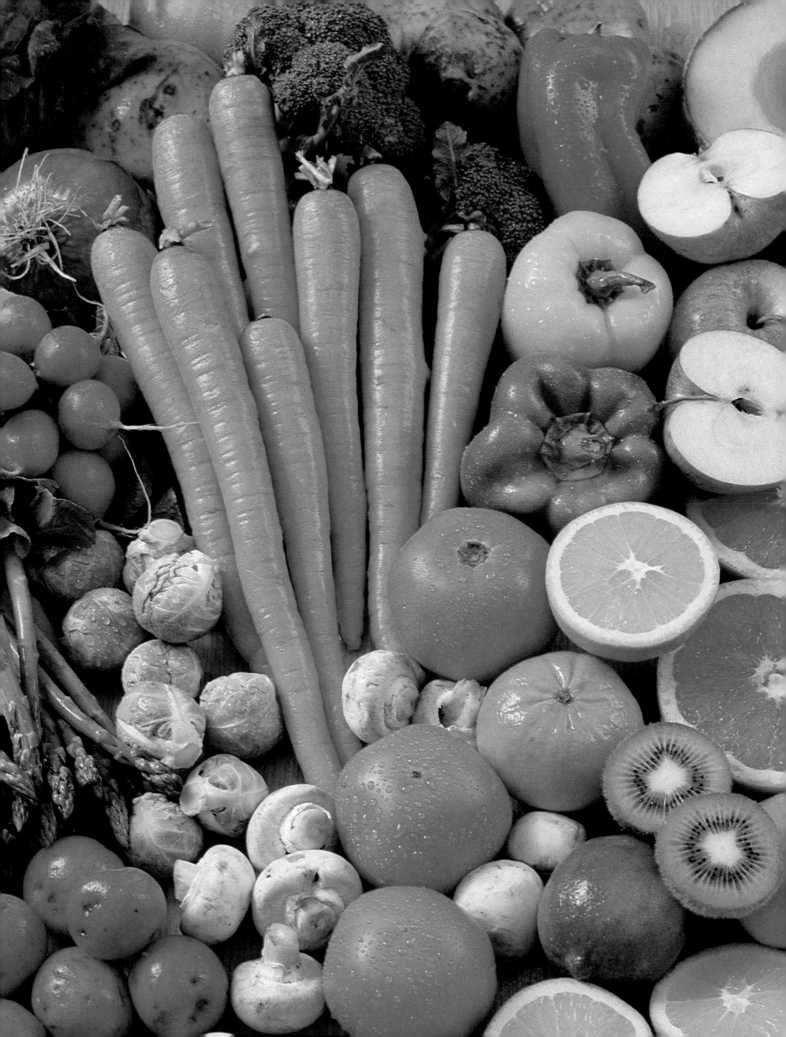

After reading this chapter, you should be able to

- List the essential nutrients, and describe the functions they perform in the body

- Describe the guidelines that have been developed to help people choose a healthy diet, avoid nutritional deficiencies, and protect themselves from diet-related chronic diseases

- Discuss nutritional guidelines for vegetarians and for special population groups

- Explain how to use food labels and other consumer tools to make informed choices about foods

- Put together a personal nutrition plan based on affordable foods that you enjoy and that will promote wellness, today as well as in the future

Nutrition Basics

12

TEST YOUR KNOWLEDGE

1. It is recommended that all adults consume one to two servings each of fruits and vegetables every day.
   True or false?

2. Three ounces of chicken or meat, the amount considered to be one serving, is approximately the size of which of the following?
   a. a domino
   b. a deck of cards
   c. a small paperback book

3. Candy is the leading source of added sugars in the American diet.
   True or false?

4. Which of the following is not a whole grain?
   a. brown rice
   b. wheat flour
   c. popcorn

5. Nutritionists advise reduced intake of saturated fat for which of the following reasons?
   a. It increases levels of low-density lipoproteins (LDL), or "bad" cholesterol.
   b. It provides more calories than other types of fat.
   c. It increases the risk of heart disease.

ANSWERS

1. FALSE. A minimum of five servings per day—two of fruits and three of vegetables—is recommended. The majority of Americans fail to meet this goal; half of all the vegetables we *do* eat are potatoes—and half of those are french fried.

2. B. Many people underestimate the size of the servings they eat, leading to overconsumption of calories and fat.

3. FALSE. Regular (nondiet) sodas are the leading source, with an average of 54 gallons consumed per person per year. Each 12-ounce soda supplies about 10 teaspoons of sugar, the total recommended daily limit for a 2000-calorie diet.

4. B. Unless labeled "*whole wheat*," wheat flour is processed to remove the bran and the germ and is not a whole grain. Brown rice and popcorn are whole grains, as are whole-grain corn, oatmeal, and whole-grain rye.

5. A AND C. High intake of saturated fat raises LDL levels and the risk of heart disease. However, saturated fat provides the same number of calories as other types of fat—9 calories per gram (compared to 4 calories per gram for protein and carbohydrate).

In your lifetime, you'll spend about 6 years eating—about 70,000 meals and 60 tons of food. What you choose to eat can have profound effects on your health and well-being. Of particular concern is the connection between lifetime nutritional habits and the risk of major chronic diseases, including heart disease, cancer, stroke, and diabetes. Choosing foods that provide adequate amounts of the nutrients you need while limiting the substances linked to disease should be an important part of your daily life. The food choices you make will significantly influence your health—both now and in the future.

Choosing a healthy diet that supports maximum wellness and protects against disease is a two-part process. First, you have to know which nutrients are necessary and in what amounts. Second, you have to translate those requirements into a diet consisting of foods you like to eat that are both available and affordable. Once you have an idea of what constitutes a healthy diet for you, you may want to make adjustments in your current diet to bring it into line with your goals.

This chapter provides the basic principles of **nutrition.** It introduces the six classes of essential nutrients, explaining their roles in the functioning of the body. It also provides different sets of guidelines that you can use to design a healthy diet plan. Finally, it offers practical tools and advice to help you apply the guidelines to your own life. Diet is an area of your life in which you have almost total control. Using your knowledge and understanding of nutrition to create a healthy diet plan is a significant step toward wellness.

WW. NUTRITIONAL REQUIREMENTS: COMPONENTS OF A HEALTHY DIET

When you think about your diet, you probably do so in terms of the foods you like to eat—a turkey sandwich and a glass of milk or a steak and a baked potato. What's important for your health, though, are the nutrients contained in those foods. Your body requires proteins, fats, carbohydrates, vitamins, minerals, and water—about 45 **essential nutrients.** The word *essential* in this context means that you must get these substances from food because your body is unable to manufacture them at all, or at least not fast enough to meet your physiological needs. Plants obtain all the chemicals they need from air, water, soil, and sunlight. Animals, including humans, must eat foods to obtain the nutrients necessary to keep their bodies growing and functioning properly. Your body obtains these nutrients through the process of **digestion,** in which the foods you eat are broken down into compounds your gastrointestinal tract can absorb and your body can use (Figure 12-1). A diet containing adequate amounts of all essential nutrients is vital because various nutrients provide energy, help build and maintain body tissues, and help regulate body functions.

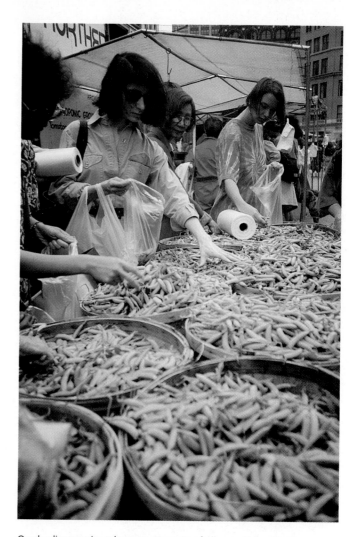

Our bodies require adequate amounts of all essential nutrients—water, proteins, carbohydrates, fats, vitamins, and minerals—in order to grow and function properly. Choosing foods to satisfy these nutritional requirements is an important part of a healthy lifestyle.

The energy in foods is expressed as **kilocalories.** One kilocalorie represents the amount of heat it takes to raise the temperature of 1 liter of water 1°C. A person needs about 2000 kilocalories per day to meet his or her energy needs. In common usage, people usually refer to kilocalories as *calories,* which is a much smaller energy unit: 1 kilocalorie contains 1000 calories. We'll use the familiar word *calorie* in this chapter to stand for the larger energy unit.

Three classes of nutrients supply energy: protein, carbohydrates, and fats. Fats provide the most energy, at 9 calories per gram; protein and carbohydrates each provide 4 calories per gram. The high caloric content of fat is one reason experts continually advise against high fat consumption; most of us do not need the extra calories. Alcohol, though it is not an essential nutrient and has no nutritional value, also supplies energy—7 calories per gram.

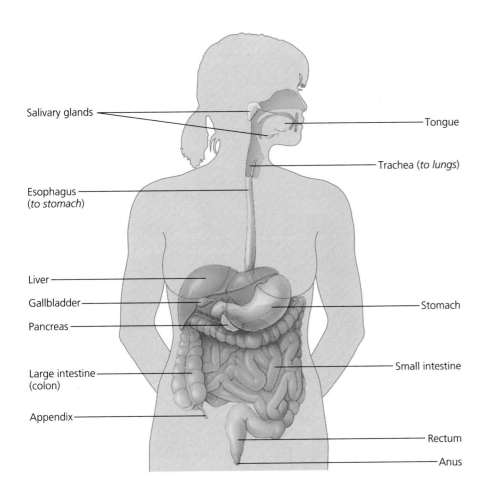

Salivary glands

Tongue

Trachea (*to lungs*)

Esophagus
(*to stomach*)

Liver

Gallbladder

Pancreas

Stomach

Large intestine
(colon)

Small intestine

Appendix

Rectum

Anus

Figure 12-1   The digestive system. Food is partially broken down by being chewed and mixed with saliva in the mouth. As food moves through the digestive tract, it is mixed by muscular contractions and broken down by chemicals. After traveling to the stomach via the esophagus, food is broken down further by stomach acids. Most absorption of nutrients occurs in the small intestine, aided by secretions from the pancreas, gallbladder, and intestinal lining. The large intestine reabsorbs excess water; the remaining solid wastes are collected in the rectum and excreted through the anus.

But just meeting energy needs is not enough; our bodies require adequate amounts of all the essential nutrients to grow and function properly. Practically all foods contain mixtures of nutrients, although foods are commonly classified according to the predominant nutrient; for example, spaghetti is thought of as a "carbohydrate" food. Let's take a closer look at the function and sources of each class of nutrients.

Proteins—The Basis of Body Structure

Proteins form important parts of the body's main structural components: muscles and bones. Proteins also form important parts of blood, enzymes, some hormones, and cell membranes. As mentioned above, proteins can provide energy for the body (4 calories per gram).

Amino Acids   The building blocks of proteins are called **amino acids.** Twenty common amino acids are found in food; nine of these are essential: histidine, isoleucine, leucine, lysine, methionine, phenylalanine, threonine, tryptophan, and valine. The other 11 amino acids can be produced by the body, given the presence of the needed components supplied by foods.

Complete and Incomplete Proteins   Individual protein sources are considered "complete" if they supply all the

essential amino acids in adequate amounts and "incomplete" if they do not. Meat, fish, poultry, eggs, milk, cheese, and soy provide complete proteins. Incomplete proteins, which come from other plant sources such as **legumes** and nuts, are good sources of most essential amino acids but are usually low in one or two.

Combining two vegetable proteins, such as wheat and peanuts in a peanut butter sandwich, allows each vegetable protein to make up for the amino acids missing in the other protein. The combination yields a complete protein. Your concern with amino acids and complete protein in your diet should focus on what you consume throughout the day, rather than at each meal. It was once believed that vegetarians had to "complement" their proteins at each meal in order to receive the benefit of a complete protein. It is now known, however, that proteins consumed throughout the course of the day can complement each other to form a pool of amino acids the body can draw from to produce the necessary proteins. (Healthy vegetarian diets are discussed later in the chapter.)

Recommended Protein Intake

The leading sources of protein in the American diet are (1) beef, steaks, and roasts; (2) hamburger and meatloaf; (3) white bread, rolls, and crackers; (4) milk; and (5) pork. About two-thirds of the protein in the American diet comes from animal sources; therefore, the American diet is rich in essential amino acids. Most Americans consume more protein than they need each day. Protein consumed beyond what the body needs is synthesized into fat for energy storage or burned for energy requirements. Consuming somewhat above our needs is not harmful but it can contribute fat to the diet because protein-rich foods are often fat-rich as well. The amount of protein you eat should represent 10–15% of your total daily calorie intake.

Fats—Essential in Small Amounts

Fats, also known as *lipids,* are the most concentrated source of energy, at 9 calories per gram. The fats stored in your body represent usable energy; they help insulate your body, and they support and cushion your organs. Fats in the diet help your body absorb fat-soluble vitamins, as well as add important flavor and texture to foods. Fats are the major fuel for the body during rest and light activity. Two fats—linoleic acid and alpha-linolenic acid —are essential components of the diet. They are key regulators of such body functions as the maintenance of blood pressure and the progress of a healthy pregnancy.

Types and Sources of Fats

Most of the fats in food are in the form of triglycerides, which are composed of a glycerol molecule (an alcohol) plus three fatty acids. A fatty acid is made up of a chain of carbon atoms with oxygen attached at one end and hydrogen atoms attached along the length of the chain. Fatty acids differ in the length of their carbon atom chains and in their degree of saturation (the number of hydrogens attached to the chain). If every available bond from each carbon atom in a fatty acid chain is attached to a hydrogen atom, the fatty acid is said to be **saturated** (Figure 12-2). If not all the available bonds are taken up by hydrogens, the carbon atoms in the chain will form double bonds with each other. Such fatty acids are called unsaturated fats. If there is only one double bond, the fatty acid is called **monounsaturated.** If there are two or more double bonds, the fatty acid is

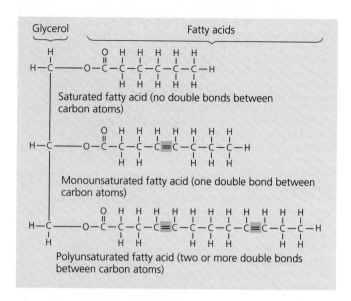

Figure 12-2 Chemical structures of saturated and unsaturated fatty acids. This example of a triglyceride consists of a molecule of glycerol with three fatty acids attached. Fatty acids can differ in the length of their carbon chains and their degree of saturation.

called **polyunsaturated.** The essential fatty acids, linoleic and alpha-linolenic acids, are both polyunsaturated. The different types of fatty acids have different characteristics and different effects on your health.

Food fats are often composed of both saturated and unsaturated fatty acids; the dominant type of fatty acid determines the fat's characteristics. Food fats containing large amounts of saturated fatty acids are usually solid at room temperature; they are generally found naturally in animal products. The leading sources of saturated fat in the American diet are red meats (hamburger, steak, roasts), whole milk, cheese, hot dogs, and lunch meats. Food fats containing large amounts of monounsaturated and polyunsaturated fatty acids are usually from plant sources and are liquid at room temperature. Olive, canola, safflower, and peanut oils contain mostly monounsaturated fatty acids. Soybean, corn, and cottonseed oils contain mostly polyunsaturated fatty acids.

There are notable exceptions to these generalizations. When unsaturated vegetable oils undergo the process of **hydrogenation,** a mixture of saturated and unsaturated fatty acids is produced. Hydrogenation turns many of the double bonds in unsaturated fatty acids into single bonds, increasing the degree of saturation and producing a more solid fat from a liquid oil. Hydrogenation also changes some unsaturated fatty acids to **trans fatty acids,** unsaturated fatty acids with an atypical shape that affects their behavior in the body. Food manufacturers use hydrogenation to increase the stability of an oil so it can be reused for deep frying; to improve the texture of certain foods (to make pastries and pie crusts flakier, for example); and to extend the shelf life of foods made with oil.

Hydrogenation is also used to transform a liquid oil into margarine or vegetable shortening.

Many baked and fried foods are prepared with hydrogenated vegetable oils, so they can be relatively high in saturated and trans fatty acids. Leading sources of trans fats in the American diet are deep-fried fast foods such as french fries and fried chicken (typically fried in vegetable shortening rather than oil); baked and snack foods such as pot pies, cakes, cookies, pastries, doughnuts, and chips; and stick margarine. In general, the more solid a hydrogenated oil is, the more saturated and trans fats it contains; for example, stick margarines typically contain more saturated and trans fats than do tub or squeeze margarines. Small amounts of trans fatty acids are found naturally in meat and milk.

Hydrogenated vegetable oils are not the only plant fats that contain saturated fats. Palm and coconut oils, although derived from plants, are also highly saturated. On the other hand, fish oils, derived from an animal source, are rich in polyunsaturated fats.

Fats and Health   Different types of fats have very different effects on health. Many studies have examined the effects of dietary fat intake on blood **cholesterol** levels and the risk of heart disease. Saturated and trans fatty acids raise blood levels of **low-density lipoprotein (LDL),** or "bad" cholesterol, thereby increasing a person's risk of heart disease. Unsaturated fatty acids, on the other hand, lower LDL. Monounsaturated fatty acids, such as those found in olive and canola oils, may also increase levels of **high-density lipoproteins (HDL),** or "good" cholesterol, providing even greater benefits for heart health. In large amounts, trans fatty acids may lower HDL. Thus, to reduce the risk of heart disease, it is important to substitute unsaturated fats for saturated and trans fats. (See Chapter 15 for more on cholesterol and a heart-healthy diet.)

Most Americans consume more saturated fat than trans fat (11% versus 2–4% of total daily calories). However, health experts are particularly concerned about trans fats because of their double negative effect on heart health—they both raise LDL and lower HDL—and because there is less public awareness of trans fats. The saturated fat content of prepared foods has been listed on nutrition labels since 1994. The FDA has proposed that information on trans fat content also be listed on food labels, included with the amount of saturated fat. Consumers would thus be able to determine the total amount of unhealthy fats that a food contains. Until trans fat content appears on food labels, consumers can check for the presence of trans fats by examining the ingredient list of a food: If a food contains "partially hydrogenated oil" or "vegetable shortening," it contains trans fat.

For heart health, it's important to limit your consumption of both saturated and trans fats. The best way to reduce saturated fat in your diet is to lower your intake of meat and full-fat dairy products (whole milk, cream, butter, cheese, ice cream). To lower trans fats, decrease your intake of deep-fried foods and baked goods made with hydrogenated vegetable oils; use liquid oils rather than margarine or shortening for cooking; and favor tub or squeeze margarines or those labeled low-trans or trans-free over standard stick margarines. Remember, the softer or more liquid a fat is, the less saturated and trans fat it is likely to contain.

Although saturated and trans fats pose health hazards, other fats are beneficial. Monounsaturated fatty acids, as found in avocados, most nuts, and olive, canola, peanut, and safflower oils, improve cholesterol levels and may help protect against some cancers. **Omega-3 fatty acids,** a form of polyunsaturated fat found primarily in fish, may be even more healthful. Omega-3s are produced when the endmost double bond of a polyunsaturated fat occurs three carbons from the end of the fatty acid chain. (The polyunsaturated fatty acid shown in Figure 12-2 is an omega-3 form.) Omega-3s have a number of heart-healthy effects: They reduce the tendency of blood to clot, inhibit inflammation and abnormal heart rhythms, and reduce blood pressure and risk of heart attack and stroke in some people. Because of these benefits, nutritionists recommend that Americans increase the proportion of omega-3s in their diet by eating fish two or more times a week. Salmon, tuna, trout, mackerel, herring, sardines, and anchovies are all good sources of omega-3s; lesser

Terms

saturated fat A fat with no carbon-carbon double bonds; usually solid at room temperature.

monounsaturated fat A fat with one carbon-carbon double bond; liquid at room temperature.

polyunsaturated fat A fat containing two or more carbon-carbon double bonds; liquid at room temperature.

hydrogenation A process by which hydrogens are added to unsaturated fats, increasing the degree of saturation and turning liquid oils into solid fats. Hydrogenation produces a mixture of saturated fatty acids and standard and trans forms of unsaturated fatty acids.

trans fatty acid A type of unsaturated fatty acid produced during the process of hydrogenation; trans fats have an atypical shape that affects their chemical activity.

cholesterol A waxy substance found in the blood and cells and needed for cell membranes, vitamin D, and hormone synthesis.

low-density lipoprotein (LDL) Blood fat that transports cholesterol to organs and tissues; excess amounts result in the accumulation of deposits on artery walls.

high-density lipoprotein (HDL) Blood fat that helps transport cholesterol out of the arteries, thereby protecting against heart disease.

omega-3 fatty acids Polyunsaturated fatty acids commonly found in fish oils that are beneficial to cardiovascular health; the endmost double bond occurs three carbons from the end of the fatty acid chain.

Type of Fatty Acid	Found In[a]	Possible Effects on Health
SATURATED *(Keep Intake Low)*	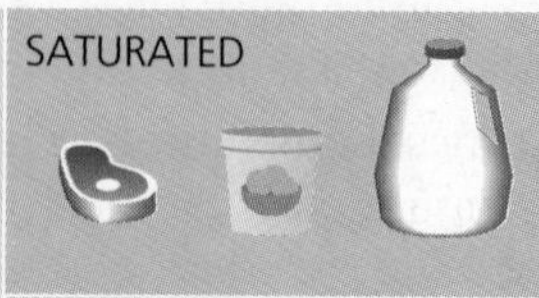 Animal fats (especially fatty meats and poultry fat and skin) Butter, cheese, and other high-fat dairy products Palm and coconut oils	Raises total cholesterol and "bad" (LDL) cholesterol levels Increases risk of heart disease May increase risk of colon and prostate cancers
TRANS *(Keep Intake Low)*	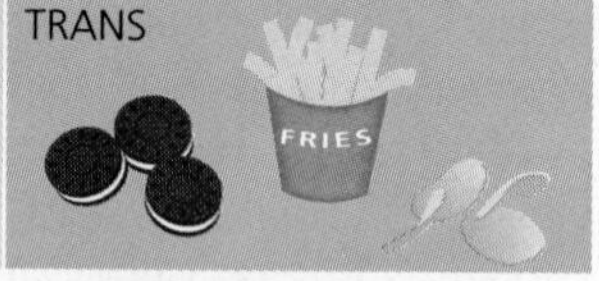 French fries and other deep-fried fast foods Stick margarines, shortening Packaged cookies and crackers Processed snacks and sweets	Raises total cholesterol and "bad" (LDL) cholesterol levels Lowers "good" (HDL) cholesterol levels May increase risk of heart disease and breast cancer
MONOUNSATURATED *(Choose Moderate Amounts)*	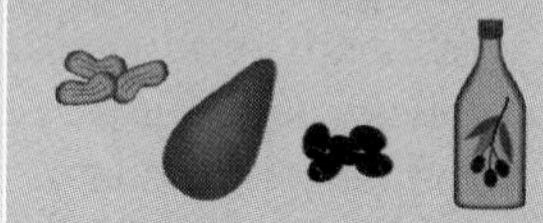 Olive, canola, and safflower oils Avocados, olives Peanut butter (without added fat) Many nuts, including almonds, cashews, pecans, pistachios	Lowers total cholesterol and "bad" (LDL) cholesterol levels May reduce blood pressure and lower triglyceride levels (a risk factor for CVD) May reduce risk of heart disease, stroke, and some cancers
POLYUNSATURATED (two groups)[b]		
Omega-3 fatty acids 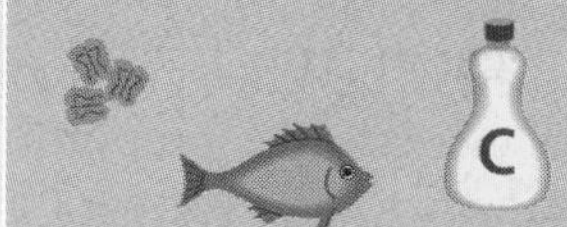	Fatty fish, including salmon, white albacore tuna, mackerel, anchovies, and sardines Lesser amounts in walnut, flaxseed, canola, and soybean oils; tofu; walnuts; flaxseeds; and dark-green, leafy vegetables	Reduces blood clotting and inflammation and inhibits abnormal heart rhythms Lowers triglyceride levels (a risk factor for CVD) May lower blood pressure in some people May reduce risk of fatal heart attack, stroke and some cancers
Omega-6 fatty acids 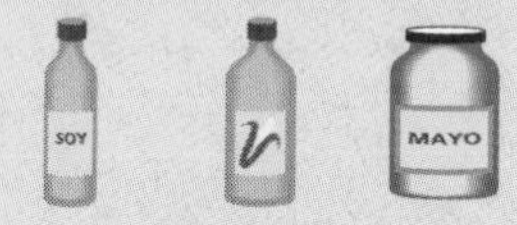	Corn, soybean, and cottonseed oils (often used in margarine, mayonnaise, and salad dressing)	Lowers total cholesterol and "bad" (LDL) cholesterol levels May lower "good" (HDL) cholesterol levels May reduce risk of heart disease May slightly increase risk of cancer if omega-6 intake is high and omega-3 intake is low

[a] Food fats contain a combination of types of fatty acids in various proportions; for example, canola oil is composed mainly of monounsaturated fatty acids (62%) but also contains polyunsaturated (32%) and saturated (6%) fatty acids. Food fats are categorized here according to their predominant fatty acid.

[b] The essential fatty acids are polyunsaturated: Linoleic acid is an omega-6 fatty acid and alpha-linolenic acid is an omega-3 fatty acid.

Figure 12-3   Types of fatty acids and their possible effects on health.   The health effects of dietary fats are still being investigated. In general, nutritionists recommend that we consume a diet moderate in fat overall and that we substitute unsaturated fats for saturated and trans fats. Monounsaturated fats and omega-3 polyunsaturated fats may be particularly good choices for promoting health. Eating lots of fat of any type can provide excess calories because all types of fats are rich sources of energy (9 calories per gram).

amounts are found in plant sources, including dark-green leafy vegetables; walnuts; flaxseeds; and canola, walnut, and flaxseed oils.

Another form of polyunsaturated fat, omega-6 fatty acid, is produced if the endmost double bond occurs at the sixth carbon atom. Most of the polyunsaturated fats currently consumed by Americans are omega-6s, primarily from corn oil and soybean oil. Foods rich in omega-6s are important because they contain the essential nutrient linoleic acid. However, some nutritionists recommend that people reduce the proportion of omega-6s they consume in favor of omega-3s. To make this adjustment, use canola oil rather than corn oil in cooking, and check for corn, soybean, or cottonseed oil in products such as mayonnaise, margarine, and salad dressing.

In addition to its effects on heart disease risk, dietary fat can affect health in other ways. Diets high in fatty red meat are associated with an increased risk of certain forms of cancer, especially colon cancer. A high-fat diet can also make weight management more difficult. Because fat is a concentrated source of calories (9 calories per gram versus 4 calories per gram for protein and carbohydrate), a high-fat diet is often a high-calorie diet that can lead to weight gain. In addition, there is some evidence that calories from fat are more easily converted to body fat than calories from protein or carbohydrate.

Although more research is needed on the precise effects of different types and amounts of fat on overall health, a great deal of evidence points to the fact that most people benefit from lowering their overall fat intake to

Table 12-1

Recommended Daily Intake for Fat, Protein, and Carbohydrate

Recommended Daily Nutrient Intake Goal or Limit

	Energy/Gram	Percent of Total Calories	Calories and Grams for Three Levels of Energy Intake		
			1600 Calories	2200 Calories	2800 Calories
Fat	9 calories/gram	30% or less	480 calories = 53 grams	660 calories = 73 grams	840 calories = 93 grams
Saturated fat	*9 calories/gram*	*less than 10%*	*160 calories = 18 grams*	*220 calories = 24 grams*	*280 calories = 31 grams*
Protein	4 calories/gram	15%	240 calories = 60 grams	330 calories = 83 grams	420 calories = 105 grams
Carbohydrate	4 calories/gram	55%	880 calories = 220 grams	1210 calories = 303 grams	1540 calories = 385 grams
Added sugars	*4 calories/gram*		*6 teaspoons = 24 grams*	*12 teaspoons = 48 grams*	*18 teaspoons = 72 grams*

recommended levels and substituting unsaturated fats for saturated and trans fats. The types of fatty acids and their effects on health are summarized in Figure 12-3.

Recommended Fat Intake   You need only about 1 tablespoon (15 grams) of vegetable oil per day incorporated into your diet to supply the essential fats. The average American diet supplies considerably more than this amount; in fact, fats make up about 33% of our total calorie intake. (This is the equivalent of about 75 grams, or 5 tablespoons, of fat per day for someone who consumes 2000 calories.) Although the percentage of calories from fat has declined in the American diet in recent years, the simultaneous increase in total calorie intake means that we're actually consuming more total grams of fat.

The 2000 Dietary Guidelines for Americans recommend that most people limit their total fat intake to 30% or less of total calories, with less than 10% coming from saturated fat. A 2001 report by the National Cholesterol Education Program (NCEP) suggests total fat intake of 25–35%, with less than 7% coming from saturated fat, up to 10% from polyunsaturated fat, and up to 20% from monounsaturated fat. The NCEP diet also recommends that trans fat intake be kept low and that total calorie intake allow for the maintenance of a healthy weight.

The number of calories and grams of fat that correspond to the 30% (total fat) and 10% (saturated fat) limits are shown in Table 12-1 for diets consisting of 1600, 2200, and 2800 calories per day. For example, if you consume about 2200 calories per day, you should limit your total fat intake to 73 grams per day, of which no more than 24 grams should be saturated fat; recommended intakes for protein and carbohydrate are also provided in Table 12-1. To determine how close you are to meeting these intake goals for fat, keep a running total over the course of the day. For prepared foods, food labels list the number of grams of fat, protein, and carbohydrate;

the breakdown for popular fast-food items can be found in Appendix A. Nutrition information is also available in many grocery stores, published in inexpensive nutrition guides, and online (see For More Information at the end of the chapter). By checking these resources, you can keep track of the total grams of fat, protein, and carbohydrate you eat and assess how close your current diet is to the recommended intake goals.

In reducing fat intake to recommended levels, the emphasis should be on lowering saturated and trans fats (see Figure 12-3). You can still eat high-fat foods, but it makes good sense to limit the size of your portions and to balance your intake with low-fat foods. For example, peanut butter is high in fat, with 8 grams (72 calories) of fat in each 90-calorie tablespoon. Two tablespoons of peanut butter eaten on whole-wheat bread and served with a banana, carrot sticks, and a glass of nonfat milk makes a nutritious lunch—high in protein and carbohydrate, relatively low in fat (500 calories, 18 grams of total fat, 4 grams of saturated fat). Four tablespoons of peanut butter on high-fat crackers with potato chips, cookies, and whole milk is a less healthy combination (1000 calories, 62 grams of total fat, 15 grams of saturated fat). So although it's important to evaluate individual food items for their fat content, it is more important to look at them in the context of your overall diet.

COMMUNICATE! Fast-food restaurants are convenient, fast, and inexpensive—but feature many high-fat, high-sodium options. The next time your friends or family want to go get a burger, try persuading them to make a different choice. Engage both their minds and their emotions by pointing out the facts about fat and salt and appealing to their desire to be fit and active. End with specific suggestions, such as going to a salad bar or an ethnic restaurant or cooking a meal together at home.

Carbohydrates—An Ideal Source of Energy

Carbohydrates are needed in the diet primarily to supply energy for body cells. Some cells, such as those found in the brain and other parts of the nervous system and in blood, use only carbohydrates for fuel. During high-intensity exercise, muscles also use primarily carbohydrates for fuel. When we don't eat enough carbohydrates to satisfy the needs of the brain and red blood cells, our bodies synthesize carbohydrates from proteins. In situations of extreme deprivation, when the diet lacks a sufficient amount of both carbohydrates and proteins, the body turns to its own organs and tissues, breaking down proteins in muscles, the heart, kidneys, and other vital organs to supply carbohydrate needs. This rarely occurs, however, because consuming the equivalent of just three or four slices of bread supplies the body's daily minimum need for carbohydrates.

Simple and Complex Carbohydrates   Carbohydrates are classified into two groups: simple and complex. Simple carbohydrates contain only one or two sugar units in each molecule; they include sucrose (table sugar), fructose (fruit sugar), maltose (malt sugar), and lactose (milk sugar). Simple carbohydrates provide much of the sweetness in foods and are found naturally in fruits and milk and are added to soft drinks, fruit drinks, candy, and sweet desserts. There is no evidence that any type of simple sugar is more nutritious than others.

Complex carbohydrates consist of chains of many sugar molecules; they include starches and most types of dietary fiber. Starches are found in a variety of plants, especially grains (wheat, rye, rice, oats, barley, millet), legumes (dry beans, peas, and lentils), and tubers (potatoes and yams). Most other vegetables contain a mixture of starches and simple carbohydrates. Dietary fiber, discussed in the next section, is found in grains, fruits, and vegetables.

During digestion in the mouth and small intestine, your body breaks down starches and double sugars into single sugar molecules, such as **glucose,** for absorption. Once glucose is in the bloodstream, the pancreas releases the hormone insulin, which allows cells to take up glu-

cose and use it for energy. The liver and muscles also take up glucose to provide carbohydrate storage in the form of **glycogen.** Some people have problems controlling blood glucose levels, a disorder called diabetes mellitus (see Chapter 14 for more on diabetes).

Refined Carbohydrates Versus Whole Grains   Complex carbohydrates can be further divided between refined, or processed, carbohydrates and unrefined carbohydrates, or whole grains. Before they are processed, all grains are **whole grains,** consisting of an inner layer of germ, a middle layer called the endosperm, and an outer layer of bran. During processing, the germ and bran are often removed, leaving just the starchy endosperm. The refinement of whole grains transforms whole-wheat flour to white flour, brown rice to white rice, and so on.

Refined carbohydrates usually retain all the calories of their unrefined counterparts, but they tend to be much lower in fiber, vitamins, minerals, and other beneficial compounds. Unrefined carbohydrates tend to take longer to chew and digest than refined ones; they also enter the bloodstream more slowly. This slower digestive pace tends to make people feel full sooner and for a longer period, lessening the chance that they will overeat. Also, a slower rise in blood glucose levels following consumption of complex carbohydrates may help in the management of diabetes. Whole grains are also high in dietary fiber and so have all the benefits of fiber. Consumption of whole grains has been linked to reduced risk for heart disease, diabetes, high blood pressure, stroke, and certain forms of cancer. For all these reasons, whole grains are recommended over those that have been refined. This does not mean that you should never eat refined carbohydrates such as white bread or white rice, simply that whole-wheat bread, brown rice, and other whole grains are healthier choices. See the box "Choosing More Whole-Grain Foods" for tips on increasing your intake of whole grains.

Recommended Carbohydrate Intake   On average, Americans consume over 250 grams of carbohydrate per day, well above the minimum of 50–100 grams of essential carbohydrate required by the body. However, health experts recommend that most Americans increase their consumption of carbohydrates to 55–60% of total daily calories, or about 275–300 grams of carbohydrate for someone consuming 2000 calories per day. The focus should be on consuming a variety of foods rich in complex carbohydrates, especially whole grains.

Experts also recommend that Americans alter the proportion of simple and complex carbohydrates in the diet, lowering simple carbohydrate intake from about 25% to 10–15% of total daily calories. To accomplish this change, reduce your intake of foods like soft drinks, candy, sweet desserts, and sweetened fruit drinks, which are high in simple sugars but low in other nutrients. The

Terms   **carbohydrate** An essential nutrient; sugars, starches, and dietary fiber are all carbohydrates.

glucose A simple sugar that is the body's basic fuel.

glycogen An animal starch stored in the liver and muscles.

whole grain The entire edible portion of a grain such as wheat, rice, or oats, including the germ, endosperm, and bran. During milling or processing, parts of the grain are removed, often leaving just the endosperm.

dietary fiber Carbohydrates and other substances in plants that are indigestible by humans.

Whole-grain foods are good weapons against heart disease, diabetes, high blood pressure, stroke, and certain cancers. They are also low in fat and so can be a good choice for managing weight. Federal dietary guidelines recommend 6–11 total servings of grain products every day, with at least several of these servings from whole grains. However, Americans currently average less than one serving of whole grains per day.

What Are Whole Grains?

The first step in increasing your intake of whole grains is to correctly identify them. The following are whole grains:

whole wheat	whole-grain corn
whole rye	popcorn
whole oats	brown rice
oatmeal	barley

More unusual choices include bulgur (cracked wheat), millet, kasha (roasted buckwheat kernels), quinoa, wheat and rye berries, amaranth, graham flour, whole-grain kamut, whole-grain spelt, and whole-grain triticale.

Wheat flour, unbleached flour, enriched flour, and degerminated corn meal are not whole grains. Wheat germ and wheat bran are also not whole grains, but they are the constituents of wheat typically left out when wheat is processed and so are healthier choices than regular wheat flour, which typically contains just the endosperm.

Reading Food Packages to Find Whole Grains

To find packaged foods rich in whole grains, read the list of ingredients and check for special health claims related to whole grains. The *first* item on the list of ingredients should be one of the whole grains listed above. In addition, the FDA allows manufacturers to include special health claims for foods that contain 51% or more whole-grain ingredients. Such products may contain a statement such as the following on their packaging: "Rich in whole grain," "Made with 100% whole grain," or "Diets rich in whole-grain foods may help reduce the risk of heart disease and certain cancers." However, many whole-grain products will not carry such claims.

Don't be misled by a food's name or description. Products named or described as 9-grain, stoned wheat, wheat bran, cracked wheat, wheat berry, rye, oatmeal, or multigrain or as being *made with* whole wheat or whole grains often contain mostly refined grains. Color can also be misleading: Although many whole-grain breads and cereals are darker than their refined counterparts, manufacturers may use ingredients such as molasses or caramel coloring to darken a product. *When in doubt, always check the list of ingredients, looking for "whole" as the first word on the list.*

Incorporating Whole Grains into Your Daily Diet

There are many opportunities to choose whole-grain foods. For maximum nutrition, look for whole-grain foods that are also low in fat.

- *Bread:* Look for sandwich breads, bagels, English muffins, buns, and pita breads with a whole grain listed as the first ingredient.
- *Breakfast cereals:* Check the ingredient list for whole grains. Whole-grain choices include oatmeal, muesli, shredded wheat, and some types of raisin bran, bran flakes, wheat flakes, toasted oats, and granola.
- *Rice:* Choose brown rice or rice blends that include brown rice.
- *Pasta:* Look for whole-wheat, whole-grain kamut, or whole-grain spelt pasta.
- *Tortillas:* Choose whole-wheat or whole-corn tortillas.
- *Crackers and snacks:* Some varieties of crackers are made from whole grains, including some flatbreads or crispbreads, woven wheat crackers, and rye crackers. Other whole-grain snack possibilities include popcorn, popcorn cakes, brown rice cakes, whole-corn tortilla chips, and whole-wheat fig cookies. Be sure to check food labels for fat content, as many popular snacks are also high in fat.
- *Mixed-grain dishes:* Combine whole grains with other foods to create healthy mixed dishes. Possibilities include tabouli; soups made with hulled barley or wheat berries; and pilafs, casseroles, and salads made with brown rice, whole-wheat couscous, kasha, millet, wheat bulgur, and quinoa.

If your grocery store doesn't carry all of these items, try your local health food store.

---

bulk of the simple carbohydrates in your diet should come from fruits, which are excellent sources of vitamins and minerals, and milk, which is high in protein and calcium.

Athletes in training can especially benefit from high-carbohydrate diets (60–70% of total daily calories), which enhance the amount of carbohydrates stored in their muscles (as glycogen) and therefore provide more carbohydrate fuel for use during endurance events or long workouts. In addition, carbohydrates consumed during prolonged athletic events can help fuel muscles and extend the availability of the glycogen stored in muscles. Caution is in order, however, because overconsumption of carbohydrates can lead to feelings of fatigue and underconsumption of other nutrients.

Dietary Fiber—A Closer Look

Dietary fiber consists of carbohydrate plant substances that are difficult or impossible for humans to digest. Instead, fiber passes through the intestinal tract and provides bulk for feces in the large intestine, which in turn facilitates elimination. In the large intestine, some types of fiber are broken down by bacteria into acids and gases, which explains why consuming too much fiber can lead to intestinal gas. Because humans cannot digest dietary fiber, fiber is not a source of carbohydrate in the diet; however, the consumption of dietary fiber is necessary for good health.

Types of Dietary Fiber Nutritionists classify fibers as soluble or insoluble. **Soluble fiber** slows the body's absorption of glucose and binds cholesterol-containing compounds in the intestine, lowering blood cholesterol levels and reducing the risk of cardiovascular disease. **Insoluble fiber** binds water, making the feces bulkier and softer so they pass more quickly and easily through the large intestine.

Both kinds of fiber contribute to disease risk reduction and management. A diet high in soluble fiber can help people manage diabetes and high blood cholesterol levels. A diet high in insoluble fiber can help prevent a variety of health problems, including constipation, hemorrhoids, and **diverticulitis.** Some studies have linked high-fiber diets with a reduced risk of colon and rectal cancer; more recent evidence suggests that other characteristics of diets rich in fruits, vegetables, and whole grains may be responsible for this reduction in risk (see Chapter 16 for more on cancer and diet).

Sources of Dietary Fiber All plant foods contain some dietary fiber. Fruits, legumes, oats (especially oat bran), barley, and psyllium (found in some cereals and laxatives) are particularly rich in soluble fiber. Wheat (especially wheat bran), cereals, grains, and vegetables are all good sources of insoluble fiber. However, the processing of packaged foods can remove fiber, so it's important to depend on fresh fruits and vegetables and foods made from whole grains as sources of dietary fiber.

Recommended Intake of Dietary Fiber Although it is not yet clear precisely how much and what types of fiber

are ideal, most experts believe the average American would benefit from an increase in daily fiber intake. Currently, most Americans consume about 16 grams of dietary fiber a day, whereas the recommended daily amount is 20–35 grams of fiber. However, too much fiber—more than 40–60 grams a day—can cause health problems, such as excessively large stools or the malabsorption of important minerals. Fiber should come from foods, not supplements, which should only be used under medical supervision. In fiber intake, as in all aspects of nutrition, balance and moderation are key principles.

To increase the amount of fiber in your diet, try the following:

- Choose whole-grain foods instead of those made from processed grains. Select high-fiber breakfast cereals (those with 5 or more grams of fiber per serving).
- Eat whole, unpeeled fruits rather than drinking fruit juice. Top cereals, yogurt, and desserts with berries, unpeeled apple slices, or other fruit.
- Include legumes in soups and salads. Combine raw vegetables with pasta, rice, or beans in salads.
- Substitute bean dip for cheese-based or sour cream–based dips or spreads. Use raw vegetables rather than chips for dipping.

Vitamins—Organic Micronutrients

Vitamins are organic (carbon-containing) substances required in very small amounts to regulate various processes within living cells (Table 12-2). Humans need 13 vitamins. Four are fat-soluble (A, D, E, and K), and nine are water-soluble (C, and the eight B-complex vitamins: thiamin, riboflavin, niacin, vitamin B-6, folate, vitamin B-12, biotin, and pantothenic acid). Solubility affects how a vitamin is absorbed, transported, and stored in the body. The water-soluble vitamins are absorbed directly into the bloodstream, where they travel freely; excess water-soluble vitamins are detected and removed by the kidneys and excreted in urine. Fat-soluble vitamins require a more complex absorptive process; they are usually carried in the blood by special proteins and are stored in the body in fat tissues rather than excreted.

Functions of Vitamins Many vitamins help chemical reactions take place. They provide no energy to the body directly but help unleash the energy stored in carbohydrates, proteins, and fats. Vitamins are critical in the production of red blood cells and the maintenance of the nervous, skeletal, and immune systems. Some vitamins act as **antioxidants,** which help preserve healthy cells in the body. Key vitamin antioxidants include vitamin E, vitamin C, and the vitamin A precursor beta-carotene. (The actions of antioxidants will be described in greater detail later in the chapter.)

Terms

soluble fiber Fiber that dissolves in water or is broken down by bacteria in the large intestine.

insoluble fiber Fiber that does not dissolve in water and is not broken down by bacteria in the large intestine.

diverticulitis A digestive disorder in which abnormal pouches form in the walls of the intestine and become inflamed.

vitamins Carbon-containing substances needed in small amounts to help promote and regulate chemical reactions and processes in the body.

antioxidant A substance that can lessen the breakdown of food or body constituents by free radicals; actions include binding oxygen, donating electrons to free radicals, and repairing damage to molecules.

Table 12-2   Facts About Vitamins

Vitamin	Important Dietary Sources	Major Functions	Signs of Prolonged Deficiency	Toxic Effects of Megadoses
Fat-Soluble				
Vitamin A	Liver, milk, butter, cheese, and fortified margarine; carrots, spinach, and other orange and deep-green vegetables and fruits	Maintenance of vision, skin, linings of the nose, mouth, digestive and urinary tracts, immune function	Night blindness; dry, scaling skin; increased susceptibility to infection; loss of appetite; anemia; kidney stones	Headache, vomiting and diarrhea, vertigo, double vision, bone abnormalities, liver damage, miscarriage and birth defects
Vitamin D	Fortified milk and margarine, fish liver oils, butter, egg yolks (sunlight on skin also produces vitamin D)	Development and maintenance of bones and teeth, promotion of calcium absorption	Rickets (bone deformities) in children; bone softening, loss, and fractures in adults	Kidney damage, calcium deposits in soft tissues, depression, death
Vitamin E	Vegetable oils, whole grains, nuts and seeds, green leafy vegetables, asparagus, peaches	Protection and maintenance of cellular membranes	Red blood cell breakage and anemia, weakness, neurological problems, muscle cramps	Relatively nontoxic, but may cause excess bleeding or formation of blood clots
Vitamin K	Green leafy vegetables; smaller amounts widespread in other foods	Production of factors essential for blood clotting	Hemorrhaging	Anemia, jaundice
Water-Soluble				
Vitamin C	Peppers, broccoli, spinach, brussels sprouts, citrus fruits, strawberries, tomatoes, potatoes, cabbage, other fruits and vegetables	Maintenance and repair of connective tissue, bones, teeth, and cartilage; promotion of healing; aid in iron absorption	Scurvy, anemia, reduced resistance to infection, loosened teeth, joint pain, poor wound healing, hair loss, poor iron absorption	Urinary stones in some people, acid stomach from ingesting supplements in pill form, nausea, diarrhea, headache, fatigue
Thiamin	Whole-grain and enriched breads and cereals, organ meats, lean pork, nuts, legumes	Conversion of carbohydrates into usable forms of energy, maintenance of appetite and nervous system function	Beriberi (symptoms include muscle wasting, mental confusion, anorexia, enlarged heart, nerve changes)	None reported
Riboflavin	Dairy products, enriched breads and cereals, lean meats, poultry, fish, green vegetables	Energy metabolism; maintenance of skin, mucous membranes, and nervous system structures	Cracks at corners of mouth, sore throat, skin rash, hypersensitivity to light, purple tongue	None reported
Niacin	Eggs, poultry, fish, milk, whole grains, nuts, enriched breads and cereals, meats, legumes	Conversion of carbohydrates, fats, and protein into usable forms of energy	Pellagra (symptoms include diarrhea, dermatitis, inflammation of mucous membranes, dementia)	Flushing of the skin, nausea, vomiting, diarrhea, liver dysfunction, glucose intolerance
Vitamin B-6	Eggs, poultry, fish, whole grains, nuts, soybeans, liver, kidney, pork	Protein and neurotransmitter metabolism; red blood cell synthesis	Anemia, convulsions, cracks at corners of mouth, dermatitis, nausea, confusion	Neurological abnormalities and damage
Folate	Green leafy vegetables, yeast, oranges, whole grains, legumes, liver	Amino acid metabolism, synthesis of RNA and DNA, new cell synthesis	Anemia, weakness, fatigue, irritability, shortness of breath, swollen tongue	Masking of vitamin B-12 deficiency
Vitamin B-12	Eggs, milk, meats, other animal foods	Synthesis of blood cells; other metabolic reactions	Anemia, fatigue, nervous system damage, sore tongue	None reported
Biotin	Cereals, yeast, egg yolks, soy flour, liver; widespread in foods	Metabolism of fats, carbohydrates, and proteins	Rash, nausea, vomiting, weight loss, depression, fatigue, hair loss	None reported
Pantothenic acid	Animal foods, whole grains, broccoli, legumes; widespread in foods	Metabolism of fats, carbohydrates, and proteins	Fatigue, numbness and tingling of hands and feet, gastrointestinal disturbances	None reported

SOURCES: Food and Nutrition Board, National Academy of Sciences. 2000. *Dietary Reference Intakes for Vitamin C, Vitamin E, Selenium, and Carotenoids*. Washington, D.C.: National Academy Press. Food and Nutrition Board, National Academy of Sciences. 1998. *Dietary Reference Intakes for Thiamin, Riboflavin, Niacin, Vitamin B6, Folate, Vitamin B12, Pantothenic Acid, and Choline*. Washington, D.C.: National Academy Press. National Research Council. 1989. *Recommended Dietary Allowances*, 10th ed. Washington, D.C.: National Academy Press. Shils, M. E., et al., eds. 1998. *Modern Nutrition in Health and Disease*, 9th ed. Baltimore: Williams & Wilkins.

Sources of Vitamins The human body does not manufacture most of the vitamins it requires and must obtain them from foods. Vitamins are abundant in fruits, vegetables, and grains. In addition, many processed foods, such as flour and breakfast cereals, contain added vitamins. A few vitamins are made in certain parts of the body: The skin makes vitamin D when it is exposed to sunlight, and intestinal bacteria make vitamin K. Nonetheless, you still need to obtain vitamin D and vitamin K from foods.

Vitamin Deficiencies and Excesses If your diet lacks sufficient amounts of a particular vitamin, characteristic symptoms of deficiency develop (see Table 12-2.) For example, vitamin A deficiency can cause blindness, and vitamin B-6 deficiency can cause seizures. The best-known deficiency disease is probably **scurvy**, caused by vitamin C deficiency. In the eighteenth century, it killed many sailors on long ocean voyages, until people realized that eating citrus fruits could prevent it. Even today people develop scurvy; its presence suggests a very poor intake of fruits and vegetables, which are rich sources of vitamin C.

Vitamin deficiency diseases are most often seen in developing countries; they are relatively rare in the United States because vitamins are readily available from our food supply. People suffering from alcoholism and malabsorption disorders probably run the greatest risk of vitamin deficiencies. However, intakes below recommended levels can have adverse effects on health even if they are not low enough to cause a deficiency disease. For example, low intake of folate and vitamins B-6 and B-12 has been linked to increased heart disease risk. Many Americans consume less-than-recommended amounts of several vitamins, including vitamins A, C, and B-6; vitamin E intake is also low among some groups, especially African Americans. Table 12-2 lists good food sources of vitamins.

Extra vitamins in the diet can be harmful, especially when taken as supplements. High doses of vitamin A are toxic and increase the risk of birth defects, for example. Vitamin B-6 can cause irreversible nerve damage when taken in large doses. Megadoses of fat-soluble vitamins are particularly dangerous because the excess will be stored in the body rather than excreted, increasing the risk of toxicity. Even when vitamins are not taken in excess, relying on supplements for an adequate intake of vitamins can be a problem. There are many substances in foods other than vitamins and minerals, and some of these compounds may have important health effects. Later in the chapter we will discuss specific recommendations for vitamin intake and when a vitamin supplement is advisable. For now, keep in mind that it's best to obtain most of your vitamins from foods rather than supplements.

Keeping the Nutrient Value in Food Vitamins and minerals can be lost or destroyed during the storage and cooking of foods. To retain nutrients, consume or process vegetables as soon as possible after purchasing. Store fruits and vegetables in the refrigerator in covered containers or plastic bags to minimize moisture loss; freeze foods that won't be eaten within a few days. (Frozen and canned vegetables are usually as high in nutrients as fresh vegetables because nutrients are "locked in" when produce is frozen or canned.) To reduce nutrient losses during food preparation, minimize the amount of water used and the total cooking time. Develop a taste for a crunchier texture in cooked vegetables. Baking, steaming, broiling, and microwaving are all good methods of preparing vegetables.

Minerals—Inorganic Micronutrients

Minerals are inorganic (non–carbon-containing) elements you need in relatively small amounts to help regulate body functions, aid in the growth and maintenance of body tissues, and help release energy (Table 12-3). There are about 17 essential minerals. The major minerals, those that the body needs in amounts exceeding 100 milligrams, include calcium, phosphorus, magnesium, sodium, potassium, and chloride. The essential trace minerals, those that you need in minute amounts, include copper, fluoride, iodide, iron, selenium, and zinc.

Characteristic symptoms develop if an essential mineral is consumed in a quantity too small or too large for good health. The minerals most commonly lacking in the American diet are iron, calcium, zinc, and magnesium. Focus on good food choices for these (see Table 12-3). Lean meats are rich in iron and zinc, while low-fat or fat-free dairy products are excellent choices for calcium. Plant foods such as whole grains and leafy vegetables are good sources of magnesium. Iron-deficiency **anemia** is a problem in many age groups, and researchers fear poor calcium intakes are sowing the seeds for future **osteoporosis**, especially in women. See Chapter 19 for more information on osteoporosis; the box "Eating for Healthy Bones" has tips for building and maintaining bone density.

Water—Vital but Often Ignored

Water is the major component in both foods and the human body: You are composed of about 60% water. Your need for other nutrients, in terms of weight, is much less than your need for water. You can live up to 50 days without food, but only a few days without water.

Terms

scurvy A disease caused by a lack of vitamin C, characterized by bleeding gums, loosening teeth, and poor wound healing.

minerals Inorganic compounds needed in relatively small amounts for regulation, growth, and maintenance of body tissues and functions.

anemia A deficiency in the oxygen-carrying material in the red blood cells.

osteoporosis A condition in which the bones become extremely thin and brittle and break easily.

| *Table 12-3* | **Facts About Selected Minerals** |

Mineral	Important Dietary Sources	Major Functions	Signs of Prolonged Deficiency	Toxic Effects of Megadoses
Calcium	Milk and milk products, tofu, fortified orange juice and bread, green leafy vegetables, bones in fish	Maintenance of bones and teeth, control of nerve impulses and muscle contraction	Stunted growth in children, bone mineral loss in adults; urinary stones	Constipation, calcium deposits in soft tissues, inhibition of mineral absorption
Fluoride	Fluoride-containing drinking water, tea, marine fish eaten with bones	Maintenance of tooth and bone structure	Higher frequency of tooth decay	Increased bone density, mottling of teeth, impaired kidney function
Iodine	Iodized salt, seafood	Essential part of thyroid hormones, regulation of body metabolism	Goiter (enlarged thyroid), cretinism (birth defect)	Depression of thyroid activity, hyperthyroidism in susceptible people
Iron	Meat, legumes, eggs, enriched flour, dark-green vegetables, dried fruit, liver	Component of hemoglobin, myoglobin, and enzymes	Iron-deficiency anemia, weakness, impaired immune function, gastrointestinal distress	Liver and kidney damage, joint pains, sterility, disruption of cardiac function, death
Magnesium	Widespread in foods and water (except soft water); especially found in grains, legumes, nuts, seeds, green vegetables	Transmission of nerve impulses, energy transfer, activation of many enzymes	Neurological disturbances, cardiovascular problems, kidney disorders, nausea, growth failure in children	Nausea, vomiting, diarrhea, central nervous system depression, coma; death in people with impaired kidney function
Phosphorus	Present in nearly all foods, especially milk, cereal, legumes, meat, poultry, fish	Bone growth and maintenance, energy transfer in cells	Impaired growth, weakness, kidney disorders, cardiorespiratory and nervous system dysfunction	Drop in blood calcium levels, calcium deposits in soft tissues, bone loss
Potassium	Meats, milk, fruits, vegetables, grains, legumes	Nerve function and body water balance	Muscular weakness, nausea, drowsiness, paralysis, confusion, disruption of cardiac rhythm	Cardiac arrest
Selenium	Seafood, meat, eggs, whole grains	Protection of cells from oxidative damage, immune response	Muscle pain and weakness, heart disorders	Hair and nail loss, nausea and vomiting, weakness, irritability
Sodium	Salt, soy sauce, salted foods, tomato juice	Body water balance, acid-base balance, nerve function	Muscle weakness, loss of appetite, nausea, vomiting; deficiency is rarely seen	Edema, hypertension in sensitive people
Zinc	Whole grains, meat, eggs, liver, seafood (especially oysters)	Synthesis of proteins, RNA, and DNA; wound healing; immune response; ability to taste	Growth failure, loss of appetite, impaired taste acuity, skin rash, impaired immune function, poor wound healing	Vomiting, impaired immune function, decline in blood HDL levels, impaired copper absorption

SOURCES: Food and Nutrition Board, National Academy of Sciences, 2001. *Dietary Reference Intakes for Vitamin A, Vitamin K, Arsenic, Boron, Chromium, Copper, Iodine, Iron, Manganese, Molybdenum, Nickel, Silicon, Vanadium, and Zinc*. Washington, D.C.: © 2000 by the National Academy of Sciences. Courtesy of the National Academy Press. Food and Nutrition Board. *Dietary Reference Intakes for Vitamin C, Vitamin E, Selenium, and the Carotenoids*. Washington, D.C.: National Academy Press. Food and Nutrition Board, National Academy of Sciences. 1997. *Dietary Reference Intakes for Calcium, Phosphorus, Magnesium, Vitamin D, and Fluoride*. Washington, D.C.: Shils, M. E., et al., eds. 1998. *Modern Nutrition in Health and Disease*, 9th ed. Baltimore: Williams & Wilkins.

Water is distributed all over the body, among lean and other tissues and in blood and other body fluids. Water is used in the digestion and absorption of food and is the medium in which most of the chemical reactions take place within the body. Some water-based fluids like blood transport substances around the body, while other fluids serve as lubricants or cushions. Water also helps regulate body temperature.

Water is contained in almost all foods, particularly in liquids, fruits, and vegetables. The foods and fluids you consume provide 80–90% of your daily water intake; the remainder is generated through metabolism. You lose

Osteoporosis is a condition in which bones become dangerously thin and fragile over time. It currently afflicts over 28 million Americans, 80% of them women, and results in over 1.5 million bone fractures each year. Most bone mass is built by age 18, and after bone density peaks between the ages of 25 and 35, bone mass is slowly lost over time. To prevent osteoporosis, the best strategy is to build as much bone as possible during your young years and then do everything you can to maintain it as you age. Up to 50% of bone loss is determined by controllable lifestyle factors, especially diet and exercise habits. Key nutrients include the following:

Calcium   Consuming an adequate amount of calcium is important throughout life to build and maintain bone mass. Americans average 600–800 mg of calcium per day, only about half of what is recommended. Milk, yogurt, and calcium-fortified orange juice, bread, and cereals are all good sources. Nutritionists suggest that you obtain calcium from foods first and then take supplements only if needed to make up the difference.

Vitamin D   Vitamin D is necessary for bones to absorb calcium; a daily intake of 400–800 IU is recommended by the National Osteoporosis Foundation. Vitamin D can be obtained from foods and is manufactured by the skin when exposed to sunlight. Candidates for vitamin D supplements include people who don't eat many foods rich in vitamin D; those who don't expose their face, arms, and hands to the sun (without sunscreen) for 5–15 minutes a few times each week; and people who live north of an imaginary line roughly between Boston and the Oregon–California border (the sun is weaker in northern latitudes).

Vitamin K   Recent studies have linked high vitamin K intake to a lower risk of fractures. Vitamin K promotes the synthesis of proteins that help keep bones strong. Broccoli and leafy green vegetables are rich in vitamin K.

Other Nutrients   Several other nutrients may play an important role in bone health.

- *Vitamin C* works with calcium and other minerals to build bone; it also helps produce the connective tissue collagen, which forms the scaffolding in bones.

- *Magnesium* aids in bone formation.
- *Potassium* helps bones retain calcium.
- *Manganese* may help lessen calcium losses.
- *Zinc* and *copper* help maintain collagen.
- *Boron* may increase calcium absorption.

Several dietary substances may have a *negative* effect on bone health. Alcohol reduces the body's ability to absorb calcium and may interfere with the bone-protecting effects of the hormone estrogen. A high intake of protein and sodium has been shown to increase calcium loss in the urine, especially when calcium intake is low, and thus may lead to loss of calcium from the skeleton. Caffeine may also cause small losses of urinary calcium, and experts often recommend that heavy caffeine consumers take special care to include calcium-rich foods in their diet. Adding milk to coffee or tea may offset the effect of caffeine on calcium loss. Chronic excess intake of retinol, one form of vitamin A, is associated with decreased bone density; if you consume a vitamin supplement or vitamin A–fortified foods, try to limit your daily intake of retinol to no more than 100% of the RDA. (You may need to check labels to determine what form of vitamin A is present; beta-carotene, which the body can convert to vitamin A, is not associated with problems.) Drinking lots of soda, which often replaces milk in the diet and which is high in phosphorus (a mineral that may interfere with calcium absorption), has been shown to increase the risk of bone fracture in teenage girls. For healthy bones, then, it is important to be moderate in your consumption of alcohol, protein, sodium, caffeine, retinol, and sodas.

Finally, it is important to combine a healthy diet with regular exercise. Weight-bearing aerobic activities, if performed regularly, help build and maintain bone mass throughout life. Strength training improves bone density, muscle mass, strength, and balance, protecting against both bone loss and falls, a major cause of fractures. See Chapter 13 for tips on creating a complete, personalized exercise program.

---

water each day in urine, feces, and sweat and through evaporation from your lungs. To maintain a balance between water consumed and water lost, you need to take in about 1 milliliter of water for each calorie you burn—about 2 liters, or 8 cups, of fluid per day—more if you live in a hot climate or engage in vigorous exercise. Many Americans fall short of this recommended intake.

Thirst is one of the body's first signs of dehydration that we can actually recognize. However, by the time we are thirsty, our cells have been needing fluid for quite some time. A good motto to remember, especially when exercising, is: Drink *before* you're thirsty. Severe dehydration causes weakness and can lead to death.

Other Substances in Food

Many substances in food are not essential nutrients but may influence health.

Antioxidants   When the body uses oxygen or breaks down certain fats or proteins as a normal part of metabolism, it gives rise to substances called **free radicals**. Environmental factors like cigarette smoke, exhaust fumes, radiation, excessive sunlight, certain drugs, and stress can increase free radical production. A free radical is a chemically unstable molecule that is missing an electron; it will react with any molecule it encounters from which it can

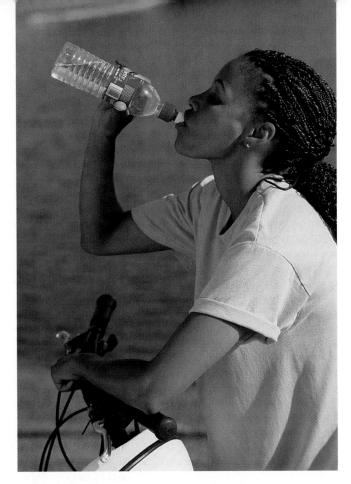

Often overlooked but absolutely crucial to life, water is an essential part of the diet. You need to drink about 8 cups of fluid per day—more if you live in a hot climate or exercise vigorously.

begun to identify and study all the different compounds found in foods, and many preliminary findings are promising. For example, certain substances found in soy foods may help lower cholesterol levels. Sulforaphane, a compound isolated from broccoli and other **cruciferous vegetables,** may render some carcinogenic compounds harmless. Allyl sulfides, a group of chemicals found in garlic and onions, appear to boost the activity of cancer-fighting immune cells. Further research on phytochemicals may extend the role of nutrition to the prevention and treatment of many chronic diseases.

If you want to increase your intake of phytochemicals, it is best to obtain them by eating a variety of fruits, vegetables, and grains rather than relying on supplements. Like many vitamins and minerals, isolated phytochemicals may be harmful if taken in high doses. In addition, it is likely that their health benefits are the result of chemical substances working in combination. The role of phytochemicals in disease prevention is discussed further in Chapters 15 and 16.

COMMUNICATE! Changing our eating and cooking habits is hard work, and getting others to change is even harder. If your parents, roommates, or friends could be preparing food in healthier ways, you may want to suggest some changes. For example, "I saw some pump sprays for cooking oil at the store. You spray oil on the frying pan instead of pouring the oil in. It cuts back on the amount of oil you have to use. Would you try it if I picked one up?" Or, "Some people I know have stopped cooking with salt, mostly because they're worried about high blood pressure, which extra salt can sometimes make worse. They have salt at the table; they just don't cook with it. Since we have high blood pressure in our family, I'm wondering if you'd consider using less salt when you cook." You might also offer to cut up some fresh fruit, prepare a green salad, or buy whole-grain bread.

NUTRITIONAL GUIDELINES: PLANNING YOUR DIET

The second part of putting together a healthy food plan—after you've learned about necessary nutrients—is choosing

take an electron. In their search for electrons, free radicals react with fats, proteins, and DNA, damaging cell membranes and mutating genes. Because of this, free radicals have been implicated in aging, cancer, cardiovascular disease, and other degenerative diseases like arthritis.

Antioxidants found in foods can help protect the body from damage by free radicals in several ways. Some dietary antioxidants prevent or reduce the formation of free radicals; others remove free radicals from the body by reacting with them directly by donating electrons. Antioxidants can also repair some types of free radical damage after it occurs. Some antioxidants, such as vitamin C, vitamin E, and selenium, are also essential nutrients; others, such as carotenoids, found in yellow, orange, and deep-green vegetables, are not. Obtaining a regular intake of these nutrients is vital for maintaining the health of the body. Many fruits and vegetables are rich in antioxidants.

Phytochemicals Antioxidants are a particular type of **phytochemical,** a substance found in plant foods that may help prevent chronic disease. Researchers have just

free radical An electron-seeking compound that can react with fats, proteins, and DNA, damaging cell membranes and mutating genes in its search for electrons; produced through chemical reactions in the body and by exposure to environmental factors such as sunlight and tobacco smoke.

phytochemical A naturally occurring substance found in plant foods that may help prevent and treat chronic diseases like cancer and heart disease; *phyto* means plant.

cruciferous vegetables Vegetables of the cabbage family, including cabbage, broccoli, brussels sprouts, kale, and cauliflower; the flower petals of these plants form the shape of a cross, hence the name.

Terms

foods that satisfy nutritional requirements and meet your personal criteria. Various tools have been created by scientific and government groups to help people design healthy diets. The **Dietary Reference Intakes (DRIs)** are standards for nutrient intake designed to prevent nutritional deficiencies and reduce the risk of chronic disease. The **Food Guide Pyramid** translates these nutrient recommendations into a balanced food-group plan that includes all essential nutrients. To provide further guidance, **Dietary Guidelines for Americans** have been established to address the prevention of diet-related chronic diseases. Together, these tools make up a complete set of resources for dietary planning.

Dietary Reference Intakes (DRIs)

How much vitamin C, iron, calcium, and other nutrients do you need to stay healthy? The Food and Nutrition Board of the National Academy of Sciences establishes dietary standards, or recommended intake levels, for Americans of all ages. The current set of standards, called Dietary Reference Intakes (DRIs), is relatively new, having been introduced in 1997. An earlier set of standards, called the **Recommended Dietary Allowances (RDAs)**, focused on preventing nutritional deficiency diseases such as anemia; the RDAs were established in 1941 and updated periodically, most recently in 1989. The newer DRIs have a broader focus because recent research has looked not just at the prevention of nutrient deficiencies but also at the role of nutrients in promoting optimal health and preventing chronic diseases such as cancer, osteoporosis, and heart disease.

The DRIs include standards for both recommended intakes and maximum safe intakes. The recommended intake of each nutrient is expressed as either a *Recommended Dietary Allowance (RDA)* or *Adequate Intake (AI)*. An AI is set when there is not enough information available to set an RDA value; regardless of the type of standard used,

however, the DRI represents the best available estimate of intake for optimal health. The *Tolerable Upper Intake Level (UL)* sets the maximum daily intake by a healthy person that is unlikely to cause health problems. For example, the RDA for calcium for an 18-year-old female is 1300 mg per day; the UL is 2500 mg per day. Because of lack of data, ULs have not been set for all nutrients. This does not mean that people can tolerate chronic intakes of these vitamins and minerals above recommended levels. Like all chemical agents, nutrients can produce adverse effects if intakes are excessive. There is no established benefit from consuming nutrients at levels above the RDA or AI.

The DRIs are being issued in stages, and, by early 2001, they had been set for most vitamins and minerals. By 2002, the remaining nutrients will have DRI values set, and other substances such as fiber will also be considered by the Food and Nutrition Board. The DRIs established to date can be found in the Nutrition Resources section at the end of the chapter (pp. 356–357); there you can also find an abridged version of the 1989 RDAs, which includes recommended intakes for nutrients for which DRIs have not yet been set. (For more on updates and additions to the DRIs, visit the Web site of the Food and Nutrition Board; see For More Information at the end of the chapter.)

Should You Take Supplements? The aim of the DRIs is to guide you in meeting your nutritional needs primarily with food, rather than with vitamin and mineral supplements. This goal is important because recommendations have not yet been set for some essential nutrients. Many supplements contain only nutrients with established recommendations, so using them to meet nutrient needs can leave you deficient in other nutrients. Supplements also lack potentially beneficial phytochemicals that are found only in whole foods. Nutrition scientists generally agree that most Americans can obtain most of the vitamins and minerals they need to prevent deficiencies by consuming a varied, nutritionally balanced diet. The use of supplements of antioxidants to reduce heart disease or cancer risk remains controversial; intake levels above the UL should be avoided.

The question of whether or not to take supplements is a serious one. Some vitamins and minerals are dangerous when ingested in excess, as shown in Tables 12-2 and 12-3. Large doses of particular nutrients can also cause health problems by affecting the absorption of other vitamins and minerals. For all these reasons, you should think carefully about whether or not to take supplements; consider consulting a physician or registered dietitian.

In setting the DRIs, the Food and Nutrition Board recommended supplements of particular nutrients for the following groups:

- Women who are capable of becoming pregnant should take 400 µg per day of folic acid (the synthetic form of the vitamin folate) from fortified foods

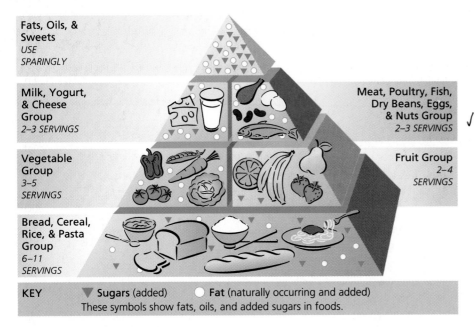

**Fats, Oils, &
Sweets**
*USE
SPARINGLY*

**Milk, Yogurt,
& Cheese
Group**
2–3 SERVINGS

**Vegetable
Group**
*3–5
SERVINGS*

**Bread, Cereal,
Rice, & Pasta
Group**
*6–11
SERVINGS*

**Meat, Poultry, Fish,
Dry Beans, Eggs,
& Nuts Group**
2–3 SERVINGS

Fruit Group
*2–4
SERVINGS*

KEY ▼ **Sugars** (added) ○ **Fat** (naturally occurring and added)
These symbols show fats, oils, and added sugars in foods.

**Figure 12-4 The Food Guide Pyra-
mid: a guide to daily food choices.**
The Pyramid is an outline of what to eat each
day—not a rigid prescription, but a general
guide that lets you choose a healthful diet
that's right for you. It calls for eating a variety
of foods to get the nutrients you need and at
the same time the right amount of calories to
maintain a healthy weight. The Pyramid also
focuses on fat because many Americans
eat too much fat, especially saturated fat.
SOURCE: U.S. Department of Agriculture, Center
for Nutrition Policy and Promotion. 1996. *The Food
Guide Pyramid.* Home and Garden Bulletin No. 252.

and/or supplements in addition to folate from a varied diet. Research indicates that this level of folate
intake will reduce the risk of neural tube defects.
(This defect occurs early in pregnancy, before most
women know they are pregnant; therefore, the recommendation for the folate intake applies to all
women of reproductive age rather than only to pregnant women.) Since 1998, enriched breads, flours,
corn meals, rice, noodles, and other grain products
have been fortified with small amounts of folic acid.
Folate is found naturally in leafy green vegetables,
legumes, oranges and orange juice, and strawberries.

• People over age 50 should consume foods fortified
with vitamin B-12, B-12 supplements, or a combination of the two in order to meet the majority of the
DRI of 2.4 mg of B-12 daily. Up to 30% of people
over 50 may have problems absorbing protein-
bound B-12 in foods. Vitamin B-12 in supplements
and fortified foods is more readily absorbed and can
help prevent a deficiency.

Because of the oxidative stress caused by smoking, the
Food and Nutrition Board also recommends that smokers
consume 35 mg *more* vitamin C per day than the DRI
intake level set for their age and sex (for adults, recommended daily vitamin C intakes for nonsmokers are 90 mg
for men and 75 mg for women). However, supplements are
not usually needed because this extra vitamin C can easily be obtained from foods. For example, one cup of orange juice has about 100 mg of vitamin C.

Supplements may also be recommended in other
cases. Women with heavy menstrual flows may need extra iron to compensate for the monthly loss. Some vegetarians may need supplemental calcium, iron, zinc, and
vitamin B-12, depending on their food choices. New-

borns need a single dose of vitamin K, which must be administered under the direction of a physician. People who
consume few calories, who have certain diseases, or who
take certain medications may need specific vitamin and
mineral supplements; such supplement decisions must
be made by a physician because some vitamins and minerals counteract the actions of certain medications.

In deciding whether to take a vitamin and mineral supplement, consider whether you already regularly consume a fortified breakfast cereal. Many breakfast cereals
contain almost as many nutrients as a vitamin pill! If you
do decide to take a supplement, choose a balanced for-
mulation that contains 50–100% of the Daily Value for
vitamins and minerals. Avoid supplements containing
large doses of particular nutrients. See p. 343 for more on
choosing and using supplements.

Daily Values   Because the DRIs are far too cumbersome
to use as a basis for food labels, the U.S. Food and Drug
Administration developed another set of dietary standards, the **Daily Values.** The Daily Values are based on
several different sets of guidelines and include standards
for fat, cholesterol, carbohydrate, dietary fiber, and selected vitamins and minerals. The Daily Values represent
appropriate intake levels for a 2000-calorie diet. The percent Daily Value shown on a food label shows how well
that food contributes to your recommended daily intake.
Food labels are described in more detail later in the
chapter.

The Food Guide Pyramid

The Food Guide Pyramid is a food-group plan developed
by the U.S. Department of Agriculture that gives a recom-

Studies have shown that most people underestimate the size of their food portions, in many cases by as much as 50%. If you need to retrain your eye, try using measuring cups and spoons and an inexpensive kitchen scale when you eat at home. With a little practice, you'll learn the difference between 3 and 8 ounces of chicken or meat, and what a half-cup of rice really looks like. For quick estimates, use the following equivalents:

- 1 teaspoon of margarine = the tip of your thumb
- 1 ounce of cheese = your thumb, four dice stacked together, or an ice cube
- 3 ounces of chicken or meat = a deck of cards or an audio-cassette tape
- 1 cup of pasta = a small fist or a tennis ball

- ½ cup of rice or cooked vegetables = an ice cream scoop or one-third of a can of soda
- 2 tablespoons of peanut butter = a ping pong ball or large marshmallow
- 1 medium potato = a computer mouse
- 1–2-ounce muffin or roll = plum or large egg
- 1-ounce bagel = hockey puck or yo-yo
- 1 medium fruit (apple or orange) = baseball
- ¼ cup nuts = golf ball
- Small cookie or cracker = poker chip

---

mended number of servings for five different major food groups (Figure 12-4). A range of servings is given for each group: The smaller number is for people who consume about 1600 calories a day, such as many sedentary women; the larger number is for those who consume about 2800 calories a day, such as active men. Serving sizes and examples of foods are described below for each group. The fundamental principles of the Food Guide Pyramid are moderation, variety, and balance—a theme echoed throughout this chapter. A diet is balanced if it contains appropriate amounts of each nutrient, and choosing foods from each of the food groups helps ensure that balance.

It is important to choose a variety of foods within each group because different foods have different combinations of nutrients: for example, within the vegetable group, potatoes are high in vitamin C, while spinach is a rich source of vitamin A. Foods also vary in their amount of calories and nutrients, and people who do not need many calories should focus on nutrient-dense foods within each group (foods that are high in nutrients relative to the number of calories they contain). For example, whole-grain bread is more nutrient-dense than white bread, and 100% orange juice is more nutrient-dense than an orange-flavored drink. Many foods you eat contain servings from more than one food group.

For more on the basic pyramid and alternative pyramids for special populations such as young children and people choosing particular ethnic diets, contact the USDA's Center for Nutrition Policy and Promotion (see For More Information at the end of the chapter).

Bread, Cereals, Rice, and Pasta (6–11 Servings)

Foods from this group are usually low in fat and rich in complex carbohydrates, dietary fiber (if grains are unrefined), and many vitamins and minerals, including thi-

amin, riboflavin, iron, niacin, folate, and zinc. Although 6–11 servings may seem like a large amount of food, many people eat several servings at a time. A single serving is the equivalent of the following:

- 1 slice of bread or half of a hamburger bun, English muffin, or bagel
- 1 small roll, biscuit, or muffin
- 1 ounce of ready-to-eat cereal
- ½ cup cooked cereal, rice, or pasta
- 5–6 small or 2–3 large crackers

If you are one of the many people who have trouble identifying an ounce of cereal or half a cup of rice, see the strategies in the box "Judging Serving Sizes." Choose foods that are typically made with little fat or sugar (bread, rice, pasta) over those that are high in fat and sugar (croissants, chips, cookies, doughnuts). For maximum nutrition, choose whole-grain breads, high-fiber cereals, whole-wheat pasta, and brown rice.

Vegetables (3–5 Servings)

Vegetables are rich in carbohydrates, dietary fiber, vitamin A, vitamin C, folate, magnesium, and other nutrients. They are also naturally low in fat. A serving of vegetables is equivalent to the following:

- 1 cup raw leafy vegetables
- ½ cup raw or cooked vegetables
- ¾ cup vegetable juice
- ½ cup tomato sauce
- ½ cup cooked dry beans

Good choices from this group include dark-green leafy vegetables such as spinach, chard, and collards; deep-orange and red vegetables such as carrots, winter squash, red bell peppers, and tomatoes; broccoli, cauliflower, and other cruciferous vegetables; peas; green beans; potatoes; and corn. Dry beans (legumes) such as pinto, navy, kidney, and black beans can be counted as servings of vegetables or as alternatives to meat.

Fruits (2–4 Servings)   Like vegetables, fruits are rich in carbohydrates, dietary fiber, and many vitamins, especially vitamin C. The serving sizes used in the Pyramid are as follows:

- 1 medium (apple, banana, peach, orange, pear) or 2 small (apricot, plum) whole fruit(s)
- 1 melon wedge
- ½ cup berries, cherries, or grapes
- ½ grapefruit
- ¼ cup dried fruit
- ½ cup chopped, cooked, canned, or frozen fruit
- ¾ cup fruit juice (100% juice)

Good choices from this group are citrus fruits and juices, melons, pears, apples, bananas, and berries. Choose whole fruits often—they are higher in fiber and ofen lower in calories than fruit juices. Fruit *juices* typically contain more nutrients than fruit *drinks*. For canned fruits, choose those packed in fruit juice or water rather than in syrup.

Milk, Yogurt, and Cheese (2–3 Servings)   Foods from this group are high in protein, carbohydrate, calcium, riboflavin, and vitamin D. To limit the fat in your diet, it is best to choose servings of low-fat or nonfat items from this group:

- 1 cup milk or yogurt
- 1½ ounces cheese
- 2 ounces processed cheese

Cottage cheese is lower in calcium than most other cheeses, and 1 cup of cottage cheese counts as only half a serving for this food group. Ice cream is also lower in calcium than many other dairy products (½ cup is equivalent to ⅓ serving); in addition, it is high in sugar and fat.

Meat, Poultry, Fish, Dry Beans, Eggs, and Nuts (2–3 Servings)   This group of foods provides protein, niacin, iron, vitamin B-6, zinc, and thiamin; the animal foods in the group also provide vitamin B-12. The Pyramid recommends 2–3 servings each day of foods from this group. The total amount of these servings should be the equivalent of 5–7 ounces of cooked lean meat, poultry, or fish per day. Many people misjudge what makes up a single serving for this food group:

- 2–3 ounces cooked lean meat, poultry, or fish (an average hamburger or a medium chicken breast half is about 3 ounces; 4 thin slices of bologna, 6 slices of hard salami, or ½ cup of drained canned tuna counts as about 2 ounces)

- The following portions of nonmeat foods are equivalent to 1 ounce of lean meat:
  ½ cup cooked dry beans (if not counted as a vegetable)
  1 egg
  2 tablespoons peanut butter
  ⅓ cup nuts
  ¼ cup seeds
  ½ cup tofu

One egg at breakfast, a cup of pinto beans at lunch, and a hamburger at dinner would add up to the equivalent of 6 ounces of lean meat for the day. To limit your intake of fat and saturated fat, choose lean cuts of meat and skinless poultry, and watch your serving sizes carefully. Nuts and seeds are high in fat, so eat them in moderation. Choose at least one serving of plant proteins, such as black beans, lentils, or tofu, every day.

Fats, Oils, and Sweets   The tip of the Pyramid includes fats, oils, and sweets—foods such as salad dressings, oils, butter, margarine, gravy, mayonnaise, soft drinks, sugar, candy, jellies and jams, syrups and sweet desserts. Foods from the tip of the Pyramid provide calories but few nutrients; they should not replace foods from the other groups. The total amount of fats, oils, and sweets you consume should be determined by your overall energy needs.

The colored triangles and circles in the Pyramid appear in all the other food groups to remind you that food choices in those groups can also be high in fats and added sugars (see Figure 12-4). ("Added sugars" are sugars added to foods in processing or at the table, not the sugars found naturally in fruits and milk.) Foods that come from animals (the meat and milk groups) are naturally higher in fat than foods that come from plants, which is why it's important to choose lean meats and low-fat dairy products. Fruits, vegetables, and grain products are naturally low in fat, but they can be prepared in ways that make them higher-fat choices—for example, potatoes served as french fries and pasta served as fettucini alfredo. Added sugars are common in the milk group (ice cream, sweetened yogurt), the fruit group (canned fruit in syrup), and the grain group (bakery goods). Reduced-fat versions of foods such as cookies and ice cream are often *very* high in added sugars and just as high in calories as their full-fat versions.

The average American diet currently includes more fat and added sugars than recommended. The Pyramid suggests that Americans limit the fat in their diets to 30% of total calories. You can moderate your fat intake by making low-fat choices from each group and minimizing the use of fat in cooking or as toppings such as sour cream and heavy sauces. Added sugars are less of a concern to health than fat, but consumption of large amounts of sugars adds

	Recommended Diets at Three Calorie Levels[a]			Average American Diet	
				Women (1600 calories)	Men (2400 calories)
	1600	2200	2800		
Grain group (servings)	6	9	11	5.5	7.9
Vegetable group (servings)	3	4	5	3.1	4.1
Fruit group (servings)	2	3	4	1.5	1.5
Dairy group (servings)[b]	2–3	2–3	2–3	1.1	1.5
Meat group (ounces)[c]	5	6	7	3.9	6.4
Total fat (grams)[d]	53	73	93	58.1	90.1
Total added sugars (teaspoons)[d,e]	6	12	18	15.4	22.3

Table 12-4   Food Guide Pyramid Recommendations Compared with the Average American Diet

[a]The bottom of the recommended range of servings (1600 calories) is about right for many sedentary women and older adults. The middle range (2200 calories) is about right for most children, teenage girls, active women, and many sedentary men. The top of the range (2800 calories) is about right for teenage boys, many active men, and some very active women.
[b]Women who are pregnant or lactating, teenagers, and young adults to age 24 need 3 servings.
[c]The Pyramid recommends 2–3 servings a day, the equivalent of 5–7 ounces of cooked lean meat, poultry, or fish (see p. 329).
[d]Values for total fat and added sugars include fat and added sugars that are in food choices from the five major food groups as well as fat and added sugars from foods in the Fats, Oils, and Sweets group. The total for added sugars does not include sugars that occur naturally in foods such as fruit and milk. The recommended fat totals are based on a limit of 30% of total calories as fat.
[e]A teaspoon of sugar is equivalent to 4 grams (16 calories).

SOURCES: U.S. Department of Agriculture, Agricultural Research Service. 1999. *Pyramid Servings Data: Results from USDA's Continuing Survey of Food Intakes by Individuals.* Beltsville, Md.: U.S. Department of Agriculture, Food Surveys Research Group. Shaw, A., et al. 1997. *Using the Food Guide Pyramid: A Resource for Nutrition Educators.* Washington, D.C.: U.S. Department of Agriculture, Center for Nutrition Policy and Promotion.

empty calories to the diet and can make weight management more difficult.

Analysis of the average diet of Americans has revealed that the number of servings from the fruit, dairy, and meat groups is below the recommended ranges, and servings from the grain and vegetable groups are near the bottom of the recommended ranges (Table 12-4). Overconsumption of fat and added sugars leaves fewer calories available for healthier food choices from the five major food groups. For example, the average daily diet among American women includes about 9 teaspoons (36 grams) of added sugars and 5 grams of fat above recommended limits. The 200 calories in these extra sugars and fats could be better used to increase the number of servings from the food groups for which women typically fall short of Pyramid recommendations.

General strategies for controlling intake of fat and added sugars include choosing lower-fat foods within each food group, eating fewer foods that are high in sugar and fat and low in other nutrients, and limiting the amount of fats and sugars added to foods during cooking or at the table. Consider the nutrient density of your food choices, and favor foods that are rich in nutrients relative to the number of calories they contain.

The Food Guide Pyramid is a general guide to what you should eat every day. By eating a balanced variety of foods from each of the five major food groups and including some plant proteins, you can ensure that your daily diet is adequate in all nutrients. A diet using low-fat food choices contains only about 1600 calories but meets all known nutritional needs, except possibly for iron in some women who have heavy menstrual periods. For these women, foods fortified in iron, such as breakfast cereals, can usually make up the deficit. To see how your current diet stacks up against the Pyramid, complete the analysis in the box "Your Diet Versus the Food Guide Pyramid." Table 4 in the Nutrition Resources section at the end of the chapter (p. 359) has a sample day's menu at three calorie levels (1600, 2200, and 2800 calories) that follows the Food Guide Pyramid.

COMMUNICATE! Maintaining a healthy diet when eating out may involve making special requests. Many people request that certain items be left off their selections (for example, "I'd like that without the cheese," "I'd like the dressing on the side"), ask for substitutions ("Could I have a baked potato instead of the fries?"), request information about menu items ("Do you know if the crab cakes are made with mayonnaise?"), or ask for different preparations ("May I have the halibut broiled instead of fried?"). The next time you're eating out, make sure you're getting the healthiest meal you can. If you feel awkward making such requests, explain your concern to your dining partners and ask for their support.

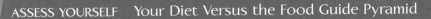

1.   **Keep a food record:** To evaluate your daily diet, begin by keeping a record of everything you eat on a typical day. To help with your analysis, break down each food item into its component parts and note your serving sizes; for example, a turkey sandwich might be listed as 2 slices sourdough bread, 3 ounces turkey, 1 tomato, 1 tablespoon mayonnaise, and so on.

2.   **Compare your servings to the recommendations of the Food Guide Pyramid:** Complete the chart below to compare your daily diet to the Pyramid. See Table 12-4 for the recommended number of servings for your calorie intake. Your portion sizes may have been smaller or larger than the serving sizes given in the Pyramid; translate your intake into actual Pyramid servings as you complete the chart. For example, if you consumed 1½ cups of spaghetti, you would count it as three servings.

Food Group	Pyramid Serving Sizes	Recommended Servings	Actual Servings
Bread, Cereal, Rice, and Pasta	• 1 slice bread • 1 oz ready-to-eat cereal • ½ cup cooked cereal, rice, or pasta		
Vegetable	• 1 cup raw leafy vegetables • ½ cup other cooked or raw vegetables • ¾ cup vegetable juice		
Fruit	• 1 medium apple, banana, or orange • ½ cup chopped, cooked, or canned fruit • ¾ cup fruit juice		
Milk, Yogurt, and Cheese	• 1 cup milk or yogurt • 1½ oz natural cheese • 2 oz processed cheese		
Meat, Poultry, Fish, Dry Beans, Eggs, and Nuts	• 2–3 oz cooked lean meat, poultry, or fish • 1 oz meat = ½ cup cooked dry beans, 1 egg, 2 tablespoons peanut butter, or ⅓ cup nuts		

Below, list the foods you consumed that don't fit into the major food groups (fats such as mayonnaise, butter, margarine, salad dressings, and sour cream; added sugars such as candy, jam, and regular soda; and alcoholic beverages).

_____   _____   _____

_____   _____   _____

_____   _____   _____

3.   **Evaluate your food choices within the groups:** Some choices within each food group are particularly healthy, while others should be eaten only in moderation. To further evaluate your current diet, indicate the number of servings you consumed of the following foods.

Foods to emphasize:

____ whole grains

____ dark-green leafy vegetables

____ orange fruits and vegetables

____ legumes

____ citrus, melon, berries

____ cruciferous vegetables

____ low-fat or nonfat dairy products

Foods to limit:

____ processed, sweetened grains

____ high-fat meats, poultry skin

____ deep-fried foods

____ full-fat dairy products

____ regular soda, sweetened teas, fruit drinks

____ foods from the Pyramid tip (fats, added sugars)

____ alcoholic beverages

4.   **Make healthy changes:** Bring your diet in line with the Pyramid by adding servings of food groups for which you fall short of the recommendations. To maintain a healthy weight, you may need to balance these additions by reductions in other areas—by eliminating some of the fats, oils, sweets, and alcohol you consume; by cutting extra servings from food groups for which your intake is more than adequate; or by making healthier choices within the food groups. Make a list of foods to add and a list of foods to eliminate; post your lists in a prominent location.

Dietary Guidelines for Americans

To provide further guidance for choosing a healthy diet, the U.S. Department of Agriculture (USDA) and the U.S. Department of Health and Human Services (DHHS) have issued Dietary Guidelines for Americans, most recently in 2000. These guidelines are intended for healthy children ages 2 years and older and adults of all ages. Following these guidelines promotes health and reduces risk for chronic diseases, including heart disease, cancer, diabetes, stroke, osteoporosis, and obesity. Ten guidelines are provided, organized under three messages, the "ABCs for Health":

Aim for fitness.

Build a healthy base.

Choose sensibly.

What follows is a brief summary of the guidelines.

Aim for Fitness The two guidelines in this category emphasize that a lifestyle combining sensible eating with regular physical activity promotes long-term health and fitness and enables people to enjoy life and feel their best.

AIM FOR A HEALTHY WEIGHT Evaluate your body weight in terms of body mass index (BMI), a measure of relative body weight that also takes height into account. (See Chapter 14 for instructions on how to determine your BMI.) If your current weight is healthy, aim to avoid weight gain. Do so by eating vegetables, fruits, and whole grains with little added fat or sugar; also focus on selecting sensible portion sizes. If you are overweight, first aim to prevent further weight gain, and then lose weight to improve your health. Plan to lose weight gradually—about 10% of your weight over about 6 months—through a combination of sensible eating, physical activity, and behavior change. Loss of $1/2$ to 2 pounds a week is usually safe. Your health is more likely to improve over the long term if you achieve and maintain a healthy weight than if you lose and regain weight several times. But even if you have regained weight in the past, it's worthwhile to try again.

BE PHYSICALLY ACTIVE EVERY DAY Regular physical activity improves fitness, helps manage weight, promotes psychological well-being, and reduces risk of heart disease, cancer, and diabetes. Become active if you are inactive, and maintain or increase physical activity if you are already active. Aim to accumulate at least 30 minutes (adults) or 60 minutes (children) of moderate physical activity on most days, preferably every day. Moderate physical activity is any activity that requires about as much energy as walking 2 miles in 30 minutes. You can do the activity all at once or spread it out over two to three periods during the day. Choose activities that you enjoy and can do regularly. If you already get 30 minutes of physical activity daily, you can gain even more health benefits by increasing the intensity or duration of your activity. Aerobic activities and activities for strength and flexibility are especially beneficial. (See Chapter 13 for advice on increasing daily physical activity and creating a complete exercise program.)

Physical activity and nutrition work together for better health. For example, physical activity increases the amount of calories you use, which in turn makes it easier to get the nutrients you need. For those who have intentionally lost weight, being active makes it easier to maintain the weight loss. However, to maintain a healthy weight after weight loss, adults will likely need more than 30 minutes of activity daily.

Build a Healthy Base The four guidelines in this category provide a foundation for healthy eating.

LET THE PYRAMID GUIDE YOUR FOOD CHOICES To ensure that you get all the nutrients and other substances you need, choose the recommended number of daily servings from each of the five major food groups shown in the Food Guide Pyramid (see Figure 12-4). Healthy eating patterns start with plant foods, represented in the three food groups at the base of the Pyramid: grains, vegetables, and fruits. Plan your meals around a variety of foods from these groups, keeping a close eye on serving sizes. Be flexible and adventurous—try new choices in place of some of the less nutritious foods you usually eat. Everyone, especially adolescent girls and women, should take special care to meet their recommended intakes for calcium, iron, and folic acid.

People's food choices are affected by culture, family background, religion, moral beliefs, the cost and availability of food, life experience, food intolerances, and allergies. The Pyramid provides a good guide to healthy eating no matter how the foods are prepared or combined. However, if you avoid all foods from any of the five major groups, be sure to get enough nutrients from other groups. For example, if you eat few dairy products because of intolerance to lactose, choose other foods that are good sources of calcium, and make sure you get enough vitamin D. If you avoid animal products, be sure you get enough iron, vitamin B-12, calcium, and zinc. Some people may need to consume fortified foods or take a vitamin or mineral supplement to meet a specific nutrient need; however, you should not depend on supplements to meet your usual nutritional needs.

CHOOSE A VARIETY OF GRAINS DAILY, ESPECIALLY WHOLE GRAINS Grains such as wheat, oats, corn, and rice are rich in complex carbohydrates and tend to be low in fat; whole grains provide more fiber and nutrients than refined grains. Make grains the foundation of your diet—eat six or more servings daily. If your calorie needs are low, eat only six servings of a sensible size. Include several

Your overall goal is to limit total fat intake to no more than 30% of total calories. Within that limit, favor unsaturated fats from vegetable oils, nuts, and fish over saturated and trans fats from animal products and foods made with hydrogenated vegetable oils or shortening. Limit saturated fat to less than 10% of total calories.

- Be moderate in your consumption of foods high in fat, including fast food, commercially prepared baked goods and desserts, deep-fried foods, meat, poultry, nuts and seeds, and regular dairy products.

- When you do eat high-fat foods, limit your portion sizes, and balance your intake with foods low in fat.

- Choose lean cuts of meat, and trim any visible fat from meat before and after cooking. Remove skin from poultry before or after cooking.

- Drink fat-free or low-fat milk instead of whole milk, and use lower-fat varieties in puddings, soups, and baked products. Substitute plain low-fat yogurt, blender-whipped low-fat cottage cheese, or buttermilk in recipes that call for sour cream.

- To reduce saturated and trans fat, use vegetable oil instead of butter or margarine. Use tub or squeeze margarine instead of stick margarine. Look for margarines that are free of trans fats.

- Season vegetables, seafood, and meats with herbs and spices rather than with creamy sauces, butter, or margarine.

- Try lemon juice on salad, or use a yogurt-based salad dressing instead of mayonnaise or sour cream dressings.

- Steam, boil, bake, or microwave vegetables, or stir-fry them in a small amount of vegetable oil.

- Roast, bake, or broil meat, poultry, or fish so that fat drains away as the food cooks.

- Use a nonstick pan for cooking so that added fat will be unnecessary; use a vegetable spray for frying.

- Chill broths from meat or poultry until the fat becomes solid. Spoon off the fat before using the broth.

- Substitute egg whites for whole eggs when baking; limit the number of egg yolks when scrambling eggs.

- Choose fruits as desserts most often.

- Eat a low-fat vegetarian main dish at least once a week.

---

servings of whole grains daily, choosing a variety of grains, such as whole wheat, brown rice, oats, and whole corn. Prepare or choose grain products with little added saturated fat and moderate or low amounts of added sugar.

EAT A VARIETY OF FRUITS AND VEGETABLES DAILY   Different fruits and vegetables are rich in different nutrients, so it's important to choose a variety. For example, carrots, dark-green leafy vegetables, and cantaloupe are excellent sources of carotenoids; citrus fruits, potatoes, and broccoli are rich in vitamin C; spinach, legumes, and orange juice are high in folate; and bananas, winter squash, and dried fruits are good sources of potassium. Fresh fruits and vegetables, especially when eaten with the peel, are also good sources of dietary fiber.

Eat at least two servings of fruit and three servings of vegetables daily. Choose fresh, frozen, dried, or canned forms and a variety of colors and kinds. Favor dark-green leafy vegetables, bright orange fruits and vegetables, and cooked dried peas and beans.

KEEP FOOD SAFE TO EAT   Safe foods are those that pose little risk from harmful bacteria, viruses, parasites, or chemical contaminants. It is especially important to be careful with perishable foods such as eggs, meats, poultry, fish, shellfish, milk products, and fresh fruits and vegetables. If food has been left out for too long or refrigerated for too long, it may not be safe to eat even if it looks and smells fine. Refer to the section "Protecting Yourself Against Foodborne Illness" (p. 345) for specific food safety tips.

Choose Sensibly   The four guidelines in this category help you make food choices that promote health and reduce the risk of certain chronic diseases.

CHOOSE A DIET LOW IN SATURATED FAT AND CHOLESTEROL AND MODERATE IN TOTAL FAT   This guideline echoes the advice of the American Heart Association and other health organizations. A diet low in saturated fat (less than 10% of daily calories) and cholesterol (less than 300 milligrams per day) helps keep blood cholesterol levels low and reduces the risk of cardiovascular disease. Moderate fat intake (no more than 30% of total calories) also helps with weight control.

To control your intake of saturated and total fat, choose lean meat, fish, and poultry and dry beans as protein sources; use nonfat or low-fat milk and milk products; and limit your consumption of high-fat foods. Choose vegetable oils rather than solid fats like those in meat, butter, margarine, and shortening. Refer to the box "Reducing the Fat in Your Diet" for specific suggestions.

Cholesterol is found only in animal foods. To limit your cholesterol intake, follow the Pyramid recommendations for consumption of animal foods, and pay particular attention to serving sizes. In addition, limit your intake of foods that are particularly high in cholesterol, including

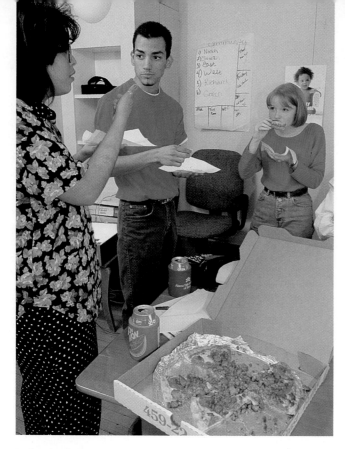

Eating on the run is a common—but not always healthy—habit among college students. After a lunch of pizza and soda, these students should complete their day's diet with a low-fat, nutrient-rich dinner.

egg yolks, dairy fats, and liver and other organ meats. Food labels provide the fat, saturated fat, and cholesterol content of foods.

CHOOSE BEVERAGES AND FOODS TO MODERATE YOUR INTAKE OF SUGARS   Sugar doesn't cause hyperactivity, but it does promote tooth decay. In addition, many foods high in sugar are relatively high in calories but low in other nutrients; consuming excess calories from added sugars may contribute to weight gain or lower consumption of more nutritious foods. The Pyramid recommends no more than about 6 teaspoons (24 g) of added sugars a day if you eat 1600 calories, 12 teaspoons (48 g) at 2200 calories, or 18 teaspoons (72 g) at 2800 calories. Most Americans consume much more than this—one can of regular soda, the leading source of added sugars in the American diet, supplies about 10 teaspoons of sugar (Figure 12-5). On average, Americans consume over 50 gallons of soda and 25 pounds of candy per year.

To reduce sugar consumption, cut back on soft drinks, candies, sweet desserts (cakes, cookies, pies), fruit drinks, and other foods high in added sugars. A food is likely high in sugar if one of the following ingredients appears first or second in the list of ingredients or if several are listed: sugar (any type, including beet, brown, raw, and cane), corn syrup or sweetener, fruit juice concentrate, honey, malt syrup, molasses, syrup, cane juice, or dextrose, fructose, glucose, lactose, maltose, mannitol, or sucrose. Try drinking water rather than sweetened drinks, and don't let sodas and other sweets crowd out more nutritious foods, such as low-fat milk. Keep your teeth and gums healthy by limiting consumption of sweet or starchy foods between meals and brushing and flossing regularly (see Chapter 21 for more on dental care).

CHOOSE AND PREPARE FOODS WITH LESS SALT   Many people can reduce their chance of developing high blood pressure by consuming less salt. Salt is made up of the minerals sodium and chloride, and while sodium is essential for normal body function, we need only small amounts, the equivalent of less than ¼ teaspoon of salt daily. It is recommended that you limit sodium intake to no more than 2400 mg per day, the equivalent of about 1 teaspoon of salt.

Salt is found mainly in processed and prepared foods and may also be added during cooking or at the table. To lower your intake of salt, choose fresh or plain frozen meat, poultry, seafood, and vegetables most often; they are lower in salt than more processed forms. Check and compare the sodium content in processed foods, including frozen dinners, cheeses, soups, salad dressings, sauces, and canned mixed dishes. Add less salt during cooking and at the table, and limit your use of high-sodium condiments like soy sauce, ketchup, mustard, pickles, and olives. Use lemon juice, herbs, and spices instead of salt to enhance the flavor of foods.

IF YOU DRINK ALCOHOLIC BEVERAGES, DO SO IN MODERATION   Alcoholic beverages supply calories but few nutrients; excess alcohol alters judgment and can lead to dependency and other serious health problems (see Chapter 10). Drinking in moderation is defined as no more than one drink a day for women and no more than two drinks a day for men. People who should not drink at all include individuals who cannot restrict their drinking to moderate levels, women who are or may become pregnant, individuals who plan to drive or operate machinery, and individuals taking medications that can interact with alcohol. If you choose to drink alcoholic beverages, do so sensibly, moderately, and with meals; never drink in situations where it may put you or others at risk.

Other organizations, such as the American Cancer Society, have additional recommendations to reduce cancer risk, including not smoking and limiting intake of salt-cured, smoked, and nitrate-cured foods such as bacon or sausage. Curing and smoking of foods help prevent the growth of certain harmful bacteria. However, nitrates have been associated with an increased risk of colon and other gastrointestinal cancers in some people. The addi-

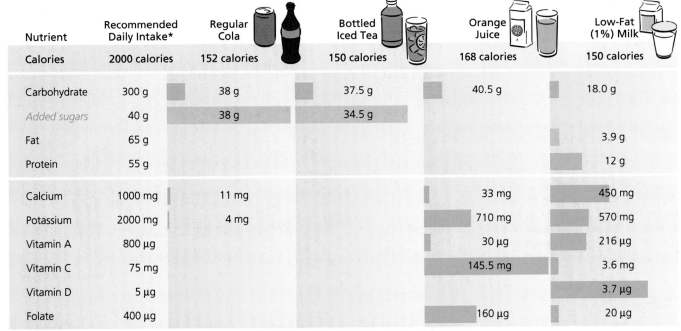

Nutrient	Recommended Daily Intake*	Regular Cola 152 calories	Bottled Iced Tea 150 calories	Orange Juice 168 calories	Low-Fat (1%) Milk 150 calories
Calories	2000 calories	152 calories	150 calories	168 calories	150 calories
Carbohydrate	300 g	38 g	37.5 g	40.5 g	18.0 g
Added sugars	40 g	38 g	34.5 g		
Fat	65 g				3.9 g
Protein	55 g				12 g
Calcium	1000 mg	11 mg		33 mg	450 mg
Potassium	2000 mg	4 mg		710 mg	570 mg
Vitamin A	800 µg			30 µg	216 µg
Vitamin C	75 mg			145.5 mg	3.6 mg
Vitamin D	5 µg				3.7 µg
Folate	400 µg			160 µg	20 µg

*Recommended intakes and limits for a 20-year-old woman consuming 2000 calories per day.

Figure 12-5 Nutrient density of 12-ounce portions of selected beverages. The four beverages shown have approximately the same number of calories in a 12-ounce serving. However, regular cola and iced tea provide few nutrients besides added sugars; both contain nearly the total daily recommended limit of added sugars (10 teaspoons). Orange juice is rich in potassium, vitamin C, and folate; low-fat milk is an excellent source of protein, calcium, potassium, vitamin A, and vitamin D. (Color bars represent percentage of recommended daily intake or limit for each nutrient.)

tion of vitamin C and other antioxidants to cured meats decreases the number of carcinogens, but salt-cured, smoked, and nitrate-cured foods should still be consumed in moderation because they are often high in saturated fat, cholesterol, and sodium.

Although the Dietary Guidelines apply to healthy Americans over the age of 2 years, not everyone has the same risk of developing high cholesterol, high blood pressure, obesity, cancer, and other health problems. You should consider your own health status and family history and apply these guidelines appropriately to address current or potential health problems.

The Vegetarian Alternative

Some people choose a diet with one essential difference from the diets we've already described—foods of animal origin (meat, poultry, fish, eggs, milk) are eliminated or restricted. Many do so for health reasons; vegetarian diets tend to be lower in saturated fat, cholesterol, and animal protein and higher in complex carbohydrates, dietary fiber, folate, vitamins C and E, carotenoids, and phytochemicals. Some people adopt a vegetarian diet out of concern for the environment, for financial considerations, or for reasons related to ethics or religion.

Types of Vegetarian Diets   There are various vegetarian styles; the wider the variety of the diet eaten, the easier it is to meet nutritional needs. **Vegans** eat only plant foods. **Lacto-vegetarians** eat plant foods and dairy products. **Lacto-ovo-vegetarians** eat plant foods, dairy products, and eggs. According to recent polls, about 5 million American adults never eat meat, poultry, or fish and fall into one of these three groups. Others can be categorized as **partial vegetarians, semivegetarians,** or **pescovegetarians;** these individuals eat plant foods, dairy products, eggs, and usually a small selection of poultry, fish, and other seafood. Many other people choose vegetarian meals frequently but are not strictly vegetarian. Including some animal protein (such as dairy products) in a vegetarian diet makes planning easier, but it is not necessary.

vegan A vegetarian who eats no animal products at all.

lacto-vegetarian A vegetarian who includes milk and cheese products in the diet.

lacto-ovo-vegetarian A vegetarian who eats no meat, poultry, or fish, but does eat eggs and milk products.

partial vegetarian, semivegetarian, or pescovegetarian A vegetarian who includes eggs, dairy products, and small amounts of poultry and seafood in the diet.

Terms

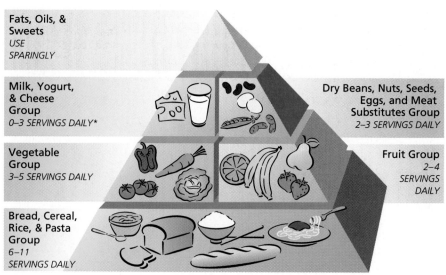

Figure 12-6 Food Guide Pyramid for Vegetarian Meal Planning. A healthy vegetarian diet includes a variety of foods, including whole grains, vegetables, fruits, legumes, nuts, seeds, and, if desired, dairy products and eggs.   SOURCE: American Dietetic Association. 1997. Vegetarian diets—position of ADA. *Journal of the American Dietetic Association* 97: 1317–1321. Copyright © the American Dietetic Association. Reprinted with permission.

Fats, Oils, & Sweets
USE SPARINGLY

Milk, Yogurt, & Cheese Group
0–3 SERVINGS DAILY*

Dry Beans, Nuts, Seeds, Eggs, and Meat Substitutes Group
2–3 SERVINGS DAILY

Vegetable Group
3–5 SERVINGS DAILY

Fruit Group
2–4 SERVINGS DAILY

Bread, Cereal, Rice, & Pasta Group
6–11 SERVINGS DAILY

*Vegetarians who choose not to use milk, yogurt, or cheese need to select other food sources rich in calcium.

A Food Pyramid for Vegetarians   Several organizations have adapted the USDA Food Guide Pyramid for vegetarian diets; the version shown in Figure 12-6 was created by the American Dietetic Association. At its base are the same three plant-based food groups found on the USDA Pyramid. The basic dairy group is also the same in this vegetarian pyramid; however, vegans and other vegetarians who do not consume any dairy products must find other rich sources of calcium (see below). The Dry Beans, Nuts, Seeds, Eggs, and Meat Substitutes group includes such foods as soy milk, legumes, eggs or egg whites, nuts, seeds, tofu (soybean curd), tempeh (a cultured soy product), and peanut butter.

A healthy vegetarian diet emphasizes a wide variety of plant foods. Although plant proteins are generally of lower quality than animal proteins, choosing a variety of plant foods will supply all of the essential amino acids. Choosing minimally processed and unrefined foods will maximize nutrient value and provide ample dietary fiber. Daily consumption of a variety of plant foods in amounts that meet total energy needs can provide all needed nutrients, except vitamin B-12 and possibly vitamin D. Strategies for obtaining these and other nutrients of concern include the following:

- *Vitamin B-12* is found naturally only in animal foods; if dairy products and eggs are limited or avoided, B-12 can be obtained from fortified foods such as ready-to-eat cereals, soy beverages, meat substitutes, and special yeast products or from supplements.

- *Vitamin D* can be obtained by spending 5–15 minutes a day out in the sun, by consuming vitamin D–fortified products like ready-to-eat cereals and soy or rice milk, or by taking a supplement.

- *Calcium* is found in legumes, tofu processed with calcium, dark-green leafy vegetables, nuts, tortillas

made from lime-processed corn, and fortified orange juice, soy milk, bread, and other foods.

- *Iron* can be obtained from whole grains, fortified bread and breakfast cereals, dried fruits, green leafy vegetables, nuts and seeds, legumes, and soy foods. The iron in plant foods is more difficult for the body to absorb than the iron from animal sources; consuming a good source of vitamin C with most meals is helpful because vitamin C improves iron absorption.

- *Zinc* is found in whole grains, nuts, legumes, and soy foods.

It takes a little planning and common sense to put together a good vegetarian diet. If you are a vegetarian or are considering becoming one, devote some extra time and thought to your diet. It's especially important that you eat as wide a variety of foods as possible to ensure that all your nutritional needs are satisfied. Consulting with a registered dietitian will make your planning even easier. Vegetarian diets for children, teens, and pregnant and lactating women warrant individual professional guidance.

Dietary Challenges for Special Population Groups

The Food Guide Pyramid and Dietary Guidelines for Americans provide a basis that everyone can use to create a healthy diet. However, some population groups face special dietary challenges.

Women   Women tend to be smaller and weigh less than men, meaning they have lower energy needs and therefore consume fewer calories. Because of this, women have more difficulty getting adequate amounts of all essential nutrients and need to focus on nutrient-dense foods. Two nutrients of special concern are calcium and iron, minerals of which many women have low intakes. Low calcium intake may be linked to the development of osteoporosis in later life. The *Healthy People 2010* report sets a goal of increasing from 40% to 75% the proportion of women age 20–49 who meet the dietary recommendation for calcium. Nonfat and low-fat dairy products and fortified cereal, bread, and orange juice are good choices. Iron is also a concern: Menstruating women have higher iron requirements than other groups, and a lack of iron in the diet can lead to iron-deficiency anemia. Lean red meat, green leafy vegetables, and fortified breakfast cereals are good sources of iron. As discussed earlier, all women capable of becoming pregnant should consume adequate folic acid from fortified foods and/or supplements.

Men Men are seldom thought of as having nutritional deficiencies because they generally have high-calorie diets. However, many men have a diet that does not follow the Food Guide Pyramid but that includes more red meat and fewer fruits, vegetables, and grains than recommended. This dietary pattern is linked to heart disease and some types of cancer. A high intake of calories can lead to weight gain in the long term if a man's activity level decreases as he ages. Men should use the Food Guide Pyramid as a basis for their overall diet and focus on increasing their consumption of fruits, vegetables, and grains to obtain vitamins, minerals, dietary fiber, and phytochemicals.

Children and Teenagers Young people often simply need to be encouraged to eat. Perhaps the best thing a parent can do for younger children is to provide them with a variety of foods. Add vegetables to casseroles and fruit to cereal; offer fruit and vegetable juices or homemade yogurt or fruit shakes instead of sugary drinks. Allowing children to help prepare meals is another good way to increase overall food consumption and variety. Many children and teenagers enjoy eating at fast-food restaurants; they should be encouraged to select the healthiest choices from fast-food menus (see Appendix A) and to complete the day's diet with low-fat, nutrient-rich foods.

College Students Foods that are convenient for college students are not always the healthiest choices. It is easy for students who eat in buffet-style dining halls to overeat, and the foods offered are not necessarily high in essential nutrients and low in fat. The same is true of meals at fast-food restaurants, another convenient source of quick and inexpensive meals for busy students. Although no food is entirely "bad," consuming a wide variety of foods is critical for a healthy diet. See the box "Eating Strategies for College Students" for tips on making healthy eating convenient and affordable.

Older Adults Nutrient needs do not change much as people age; but because they tend to become less active, older adults require fewer calories to maintain their body weight. At the same time, the absorption of nutrients tends to be lower in older adults because of age-related changes in the digestive tract. Thus, they must consume nutrient-dense foods in order to meet their nutritional requirements. As discussed earlier, foods fortified with vitamin B-12 and/or B-12 supplements are recommended for people over age 50. Because constipation is a common problem, consuming foods high in dietary fiber and getting adequate fluids are important goals. Social and economic factors such as isolation and low income can profoundly influence the eating habits of older Americans. (For more on healthy aging, refer to Chapter 19.)

Athletes Key dietary concerns for athletes are meeting their increased energy requirements and drinking enough fluids during practice and throughout the day to remain fully hydrated. Endurance athletes may also benefit from increasing the amount of carbohydrate in the diet to 60–70% of total daily calories; this increase should come in the form of complex, rather than simple, carbohydrates. Athletes for whom maintaining low body weight and body fat is important—such as skaters, gymnasts, and wrestlers—should consume adequate nutrients and avoid falling into unhealthy patterns of eating. Eating for exercise is discussed in more detail in Chapter 13; refer to Chapter 14 for information on eating disorders.

People with Special Health Concerns Many Americans have special health concerns that affect their dietary needs. For example, women who are pregnant or breast-feeding require extra calories, vitamins, and minerals (see Chapter 8). People with diabetes benefit from a well-balanced diet that is low in simple sugars, high in complex carbohydrates, and relatively rich in monounsaturated fats. People with high blood pressure need to control their weight and limit their sodium consumption. If you have a health problem or concern that may require a special diet, discuss your situation with a physician or registered dietitian (R.D.).

COMMUNICATE! Fast-food restaurants spend millions of advertising dollars to get you to eat their food. What appeals do you find most memorable and difficult to resist? What subtle messages do the ads send? The next time you see a TV ad for a fast-food restaurant, examine it carefully. What are the verbal and visual messages of the ad and what do they convey? Who do you think is being targeted by the ad? What does the ad suggest about people who eat at the restaurant—in terms of lifestyle or personality characteristics?

General Guidelines

- Eat slowly, and enjoy your food. Set aside a separate time to eat, and don't eat while you study.

- Eat a colorful, varied diet. The more colorful your diet is, the more varied and rich in fruits and vegetables it will be. Many Americans eat few fruits and vegetables, despite the fact that these foods are typically inexpensive, delicious, rich in nutrients, and low in fat and calories.

- Eat breakfast. You'll have more energy in the morning and be less likely to grab an unhealthy snack later on.

- Choose healthy snacks—fruits, vegetables, grains, and cereals—as often as you can.

- Drink water more often than soft drinks or other sweetened beverages. Rent a mini-refrigerator for your dorm room and stock up on healthy beverages.

- Pay attention to portion sizes.

- Combine physical activity with healthy eating. You'll feel better and have a much lower risk of many chronic diseases. Even a little exercise is better than none.

Eating in the Dining Hall

- Choose a meal plan that includes breakfast, and don't skip it.

- Accept that dining hall food is not going to be as good as home cooking. Find dishes that you like that are nutritious.

- If menus are posted or distributed, decide what you want to eat before you get in line, and stick to your choices. Consider what you plan to do and eat for the rest of the day before making your choices.

- Ask for large servings of vegetables and small servings of meat and other high-fat main dishes. Build your meals around grains and vegetables.

- Try whole grains like brown rice, whole-wheat bread, and whole-grain cereals.

- Choose leaner poultry, fish, or bean dishes rather than high-fat meats and fried entrees.

- Ask that gravies and sauces be served on the side; limit your intake.

- Choose broth-based or vegetable soups rather than cream soups.

- At the salad bar, load up on leafy greens, beans, and fresh vegetables. Avoid mayonnaise-coated salads, bacon, croutons, and high-fat dressings. Put dressing on the side, and dip your fork into it rather than pouring it over the salad.

- Drink nonfat milk, water, mineral water, or 100% fruit juice rather than heavily sweetened fruit drinks, whole milk, soft drinks, or beer.

- Choose fruit for dessert rather than pastries, cookies, or cakes.

- Do some research about the foods and preparation methods used in your dining hall or cafeteria. Discuss any suggestions you have with your food-service manager.

Eating in Fast-Food Restaurants

- Most fast-food chains can provide a brochure with a nutritional breakdown of the foods on the menu. Ask for it. (See also the information in Appendix A.)

- Order small single burgers with no cheese instead of double burgers with many toppings. If possible, ask for them broiled instead of fried.

- Ask for items to be prepared without mayonnaise, tartar sauce, sour cream, or other high-fat sauces. Ketchup, mustard, and fat-free mayonnaise or sour cream are better choices and are available at many fast-food restaurants.

- Choose whole-grain buns or bread for burgers and sandwiches.

- Choose chicken items made from chicken breast, not processed chicken.

- Order vegetable pizzas.

- If you order french fries or onion rings, get the smallest size, and/or share them with a friend.

Eating on the Run

Are you chronically short of time? The following healthy and filling items can be packed for a quick snack or meal: fresh or dried fruit, fruit juices, raw fresh vegetables like carrots, plain bagels, bread sticks, whole-wheat fig bars, low-fat cheese sticks or cubes, low-fat crackers or granola bars, nonfat or low-fat yogurt, snack-size cereal boxes, pretzels, rice or corn cakes, plain popcorn, soup (if you have access to a microwave), or water.

WWW. A PERSONAL PLAN: MAKING INFORMED CHOICES ABOUT FOOD

Now that you understand the basis of good nutrition and a healthy diet, you can put together a diet that works for you. Focus on the likely causes of any health problems in your life, and make specific dietary changes to address them. You may also have some specific areas of concern, such as interpreting food labels and dietary supplement labels, avoiding foodborne illnesses and environmental contaminants, and understanding food additives. We turn to these and other topics next.

Reading Food Labels

Consumers can get help in applying the principles of the Food Guide Pyramid and the Dietary Guidelines for Americans from food labels. Since 1994, all processed foods regulated by either the FDA or the USDA have included standardized nutrition information on their labels. Every food label shows serving sizes and the amount of fat, saturated fat, cholesterol, sodium, total carbohydrate, dietary fiber, sugars, and protein in each serving. To make intelligent choices about food, learn to read and *understand* food labels (see the box "Using Food Labels"). Research has shown that people who read food labels consume less fat.

Fresh meat, poultry, fish, fruits, and vegetables are not required to have food labels, and many of these products are not packaged. You can obtain information on the nutrient content of these items from basic nutrition books, registered dietitians, nutrient analysis computer software, the World Wide Web, and the companies that produce or distribute these foods. Also, supermarkets often have large posters or pamphlets listing the nutrient contents of these foods. The USDA is planning regulations for nutrition labels on fresh meat.

Reading Dietary Supplement Labels

Dietary supplements include vitamins, minerals, amino acids, herbs, glandular extracts, enzymes, and other compounds. They may come in the form of tablets, capsules, liquids, or powders. Surveys indicate that over half of American adults use dietary supplements at least occasionally, and sales have more than quadrupled since 1990, to over $14 billion per year. Although dietary supplements are often thought to be safe and "natural," they do contain powerful, bioactive chemicals that have the potential for harm. About one-quarter of all pharmaceutical drugs are derived from botanical sources—morphine from poppies and digoxin from foxglove, for example. And as described earlier, even essential vitamins and minerals can have toxic effects if consumed in excess.

In the United States, supplements are not legally considered drugs and are not regulated the way drugs are. Before they are approved by the FDA and put on the market, drugs undergo clinical studies to determine safety, effectiveness, side effects and risks, possible interactions with other substances, and appropriate dosages. The FDA does not authorize or test dietary supplements, and supplements are not required to demonstrate either safety or effectiveness prior to marketing. Supplement manufacturers have to supply only a single scientific report as supporting evidence for any health claims they make about a product—and then only after the product has been introduced and only if the FDA asks for the report. While dosage guidelines exist for some of the compounds in dietary supplements, dosages for many are not well established.

Although many ingredients in dietary supplements have been used for centuries in Eastern or European herbal medicine, some have been found to be dangerous or to interact with prescription or over-the-counter drugs in dangerous ways. Garlic supplements, for example, can cause bleeding if taken with anticoagulant ("blood thin-

ning") medications. Even products that are generally considered safe can have side effects—St. John's wort, for example, increases the skin's sensitivity to sunlight and may decrease the effectiveness of drugs used to treat HIV infection, oral contraceptives, and other medications.

There are also key differences between how drugs and supplements are manufactured. FDA-approved medications are standardized for potency, and quality control and proof of purity are required. Dietary supplement manufacture is not as closely regulated, and there is no guarantee that a product even contains a given ingredient, let alone in the appropriate amount. The potency of herbal supplements tends to vary widely due to differences in growing and harvesting conditions, preparation methods, and storage. (A 2000 test of seven brands of St. John's wort supplements found that only one had the potency level suggested for a key compound.) Some manufacturers attempt to standardize their products by isolating the compounds believed to be responsible for an herb's action. However, potency is often still highly variable, and when several compounds are thouht to be responsible for an herb's effect, often only one is standardized. In addition, herbs can be contaminated or misidentified at any stage from harvest to packaging. The FDA has recalled several products due to the presence of dangerous contaminants, including heavy metals and pharmaceutical drugs.

With increased consumer knowledge and demand, it is likely that both the research base and the manufacturing standards for dietary supplements will improve. In an effort to provide consumers with more reliable and consistent information about supplements, the FDA has developed new labeling regulations. Since March 1999, labels similar to those found on foods have been required for dietary supplements; label statements and claims about supplements are also regulated. See the box "Using Dietary Supplement Labels" for more information.

Finally, it is important to remember that dietary supplements are no substitute for a healthy diet. Supplements do not provide all the known—or yet-to-be-discovered—benefits of whole foods. Supplements should also not be used as a replacement for medical treatment for serious illnesses. (See Chapter 21 for more information on herbal remedies.)

Evaluating Functional Foods

Functional foods are foods and beverages that contain biologically active compounds that provide health benefits beyond basic nutrition. Technically, this definition

---

functional foods Foods and beverages that contain biologically active compounds that provide health benefits beyond basic nutrition.

Terms

Food labels are designed to help consumers make food choices based on the nutrients that are most important to good health. In addition to listing nutrient content by weight, the label puts the information in the context of a daily diet of 2000 calories that includes no more than 65 grams of fat (approximately 30% of total calories). For example, if a serving of a particular product has 13 grams of fat, the label will show that the serving represents 20% of the daily fat allowance. If your daily diet contains fewer or more than 2000 calories, you need to adjust these calculations accordingly (see Table 12-1).

Food labels contain uniform serving sizes. This means that if you look at different brands of salad dressing, for example, you can compare calories and fat content based on the serving amount. Regulations also require that foods meet strict definitions if their packaging includes the terms *light, low-fat,* or *high-fiber* (see below). Health claims such as "good source of dietary fiber" or "low in saturated fat" on packages are signals that those products can wisely be included in your diet. Overall, the food label is an important tool to help you choose a diet that conforms to the Food Guide Pyramid and the Dietary Guidelines.

Selected Nutrient Claims and What They Mean

Healthy   A food that is low in fat, is low in saturated fat, has no more than 360–480 mg of sodium and 60 mg of cholesterol, *and* provides 10% or more of the Daily Value for vitamin A, vitamin C, protein, calcium, iron, or dietary fiber.

Light or lite   One-third fewer calories or 50% less fat than a similar product.

Reduced or fewer   At least 25% less of a nutrient than a similar product; can be applied to fat ("reduced fat"), saturated fat, cholesterol, sodium, and calories.

Extra or added   10% or more of the Daily Value per serving when compared to what a similar product has.

Good source   10–19% of the Daily Value for a particular nutrient.

High, rich in, or excellent source of   20% or more of the Daily Value for a particular nutrient.

Low calorie   40 calories or less per serving.

High fiber   5 g or more of fiber per serving.

Good source of fiber   2.5–4.9 g of fiber per serving.

Fat-free   Less than 0.5 g of fat per serving.

Low-fat   3 g of fat or less per serving.

Saturated fat-free   Less than 0.5 g of saturated fat and 0.5 g of trans fatty acids per serving.

Low saturated fat   1 g or less of saturated fat per serving and no more than 15% of total calories.

Cholesterol-free   Less than 2 mg of cholesterol and 2 g or less of saturated fat per serving.

Low cholesterol   20 mg or less of cholesterol and 2 g or less of saturated fat per serving.

Low sodium   140 mg or less of sodium per serving.

Very low sodium   35 mg or less of sodium per serving.

Lean   Cooked seafood, meat, or poultry with less than 10 g of fat, 4.5 g or less of saturated fat, and less than 95 mg of cholesterol per serving.

Extra lean   Cooked seafood, meat, or poultry with less than 5 g of fat, 2 g of saturated fat, and 95 mg of cholesterol per

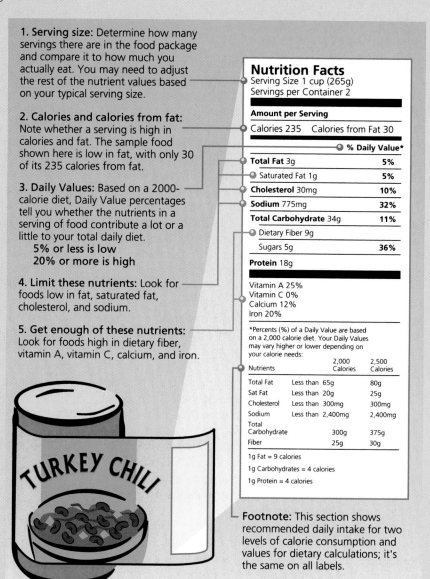

1. Serving size: Determine how many servings there are in the food package and compare it to how much you actually eat. You may need to adjust the rest of the nutrient values based on your typical serving size.

2. Calories and calories from fat: Note whether a serving is high in calories and fat. The sample food shown here is low in fat, with only 30 of its 235 calories from fat.

3. Daily Values: Based on a 2000-calorie diet, Daily Value percentages tell you whether the nutrients in a serving of food contribute a lot or a little to your total daily diet.
   5% or less is low
   20% or more is high

4. Limit these nutrients: Look for foods low in fat, saturated fat, cholesterol, and sodium.

5. Get enough of these nutrients: Look for foods high in dietary fiber, vitamin A, vitamin C, calcium, and iron.

Nutrition Facts
Serving Size 1 cup (265g)
Servings per Container 2

Amount per Serving

Calories 235   Calories from Fat 30

	% Daily Value*
Total Fat 3g	**5%**
Saturated Fat 1g	**5%**
Cholesterol 30mg	**10%**
Sodium 775mg	**32%**
Total Carbohydrate 34g	**11%**
Dietary Fiber 9g	
Sugars 5g	**36%**
Protein 18g	

Vitamin A 25%
Vitamin C 0%
Calcium 12%
Iron 20%

*Percents (%) of a Daily Value are based on a 2,000 calorie diet. Your Daily Values may vary higher or lower depending on your calorie needs:

Nutrients		2,000 Calories	2,500 Calories
Total Fat	Less than	65g	80g
Sat Fat	Less than	20g	25g
Cholesterol	Less than	300mg	300mg
Sodium	Less than	2,400mg	2,400mg
Total Carbohydrate		300g	375g
Fiber		25g	30g

1g Fat = 9 calories
1g Carbohydrates = 4 calories
1g Protein = 4 calories

Footnote: This section shows recommended daily intake for two levels of calorie consumption and values for dietary calculations; it's the same on all labels.

Since 1999, specific types of information have been required on the labels of dietary supplements. In addition to basic information about the product, labels include a "Supplement Facts" panel, modeled after the "Nutrition Facts" panel used on food labels (see the figure). Under the Dietary Supplement Health and Education Act (DSHEA) and food labeling laws, supplement labels can make three types of health-related claims.

- *Nutrient-content claims,* such as "high in calcium," "excellent source of vitamin C," or "high potency." The claims "high in" and "excellent source of" mean the same as they do on food labels. A "high potency" single-ingredient supplement must contain 100% of its Daily Value; a "high potency" multi-ingredient product must contain 100% or more of the Daily Value of at least two-thirds of the nutrients present for which Daily Values have been established.

- *Disease claims,* if they have been authorized by the FDA or another authoritative scientific body. The association between adequate calcium intake and lower risk of osteoporosis is an example of an approved disease claim.

- *Structure-function claims,* such as "antioxidants maintain cellular integrity" or "this product enhances energy levels." Because these claims are not reviewed by the FDA, they must carry a disclaimer (see the sample label).

Tips for Choosing and Using Dietary Supplements

- Check with your physician before taking a supplement. Many are not meant for children, elderly people, women who are pregnant or breastfeeding, people with chronic illnesses, or people taking prescription or OTC medications.

- Choose brands made by nationally known food and drug manufacturers or "house brands" from large retail chains.

Due to their size and visibility, such sources are likely to have higher manufacturing standards.

- Look for the *USP* or *NF* designation, indicating that the product meets some minimum safety and purity standard developed by the United States Pharmacopeia. (The United States Pharmacopeia develops standards for purity and potency for pharmaceutical drugs and has also set standards for vitamins, minerals, and some herbal products.) The designation *NNFA* indicates that the manufacturer has met the National Nutritional Foods Association standards for quality control and cleanliness. Other, smaller, associations and labs, including ConsumerLab.Com, also test and rate dietary supplements.

- Follow the cautions, instructions for use, and dosage given on the label.

- If you experience side effects, discontinue use of the product and contact your physician. Report any serious reactions to the FDA's MedWatch monitoring program (800-FDA-1088; http://www.fda.gov/medwatch).

For More Information About Dietary Supplements

ConsumerLab.Com: http://www.consumerlab.com

Food and Drug Administration: http://vm.cfsan.fda.gov/~dms/supplmnt.html

National Institutes of Health, Office of Dietary Supplements: http://dietary-supplements.info.nih.gov

National Nutritional Foods Association: http://www.nnfa.org

U.S. Department of Agriculture: http://www.nal.usda.gov/fnic/etext/000015.html

U.S. Pharmacopeia: http://www.usp.org/dietary

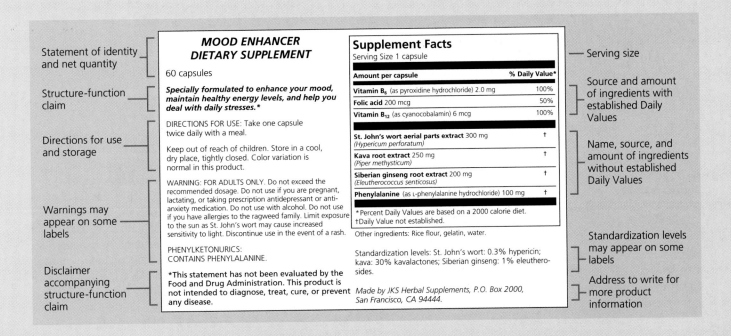

Genetic modification of foods, also frequently referred to as genetic engineering or biotechnology, has become a scientific, economic, and political issue around the world. Genetic engineering involves altering the characteristics of a plant, animal, or microorganism by adding, rearranging, or replacing genes in its DNA; the result is a **genetically modified (GM) organism.** New DNA may come from related species or organisms or from entirely different types of organisms. A number of genetically engineered products are already widely used, including insulin to treat diabetes and the enzyme chymosin to produce cheese. Over half of the current U.S. soybean crop has been genetically modified to be resistant to an herbicide used to kill weeds, and nearly a quarter of the U.S. corn crop carries genes for herbicide resistance or to produce a protein lethal to a destructive type of caterpillar. Products made with GM organisms include juice, soda, nuts, tuna, frozen pizza, spaghetti sauce, canola oil, chips, salad dressing, and soup; eating GM foods is virtually unavoidable in this country.

The potential benefits of GM foods cited by supporters include improved yields overall and in difficult growing conditions, increased disease resistance, improved nutritional content, lower prices, and less use of pesticides. For example, scientists have used genetic engineering to develop a new type of rice that is rich in beta-carotene. Introducing this plant in developing countries could reduce the incidence of vitamin A deficiency, a major worldwide health problem that causes a million deaths and over 300,000 cases of blindness among children each year. GM food supporters argue that all crops are genetically modified, either by traditional plant breeding or by newer biotechnology methods. Genetic engineering techniques are more effective than traditional breeding methods in developing desirable characteristics because the process is much quicker and more precise.

Critics of biotechnology argue that unexpected effects may occur. Gene manipulation could elevate levels of naturally oc-

curring toxins and allergens or could permanently change the gene pool and reduce biodiversity. Critics also fear that transfer of genes could result in pesticide-resistant insects, herbicide-resistant weeds, and antibiotic-resistant bacteria. In 2000, a form of GM corn approved for use only in animal feed was found to have co-mingled with other varieties of corn and to have been used in human foods; this mistake sparked fears of allergic reactions and led to recalls and the demand for better rules for segregating GM crops. Opposition to GM foods is particularly strong in Europe, where some countries have demanded GM-free imports; some U.S. food producers have echoed that sentiment. In many developing nations that face food shortages, responses to genetically engineered crops have tended to be more positive.

Another major concern has been labeling. Under current rules, the FDA requires special labeling only when a food's composition is changed significantly or when a known allergen is introduced. For example, soybeans that contain a gene from a peanut would have to be labeled because peanuts are a common allergen. Surveys indicate that most Americans don't have strong views about the safety of GM foods, but the majority want to know if their foods contain GM ingredients.

In April 2000, the National Academy of Sciences released a report stating that there is no proof that GM food on the market is unsafe but that regulatory changes are needed. The report called for better assessment of potential allergens in GM crops, more research into the spread of pest-resistant genes, and better coordination of regulatory agencies. The FDA is reconsidering how it reviews GM foods, and it may begin requiring new GM foods to undergo a mandatory (rather than the current voluntary) federal safety review. Further testing may help sort out the health and safety issues surrounding GM foods, while increased regulation, labeling, and consumer education may lead to more widespread acceptance of biotechnology.

covers all healthy whole foods like fruits, vegetables, and whole grains, but the term is most often used to refer to foods with added ingredients or foods in which one or more ingredients have been modified or enhanced. Added ingredients may be nutrients, such as calcium added to orange juice; herbs, such as St. John's wort added to soups; or other substances, such as plant sterols added to margarine. Functional foods can be created in other ways as well. Altering the feed of laying hens has allowed the development of eggs that are high in heart-healthy omega-3 fatty acids. Classic breeding techniques are being used to increase the concentration of carotenoids in carrots, for example, and the cancer-fighting compound sulforaphane in broccoli. Although controversial, genetic engineering could be used to create even more types of functional foods (see the box "Genetically Modified Foods"). Sales of functional foods have in-

creased rapidly in recent years and now top $10 billion annually.

Can functional foods help improve health? There is sound science behind some functional foods, including those with added calcium or fiber. However, many functional food claims are not supported by evidence. One strategy for consumers is to read labels carefully and check for different types of claims. Like labels for dietary supplements, labels for functional foods may carry disease claims or structure-function claims. A label that claims a link between a food substance and a disease, such as soy protein and reduced risk of heart disease, must be approved by the FDA and can therefore be considered scientifically valid. One of the most widely marketed and accepted types of functional foods is margarine spreads containing plant sterol or plant stanol esters. In 2000, the FDA approved a disease claim for these compounds, stating that they may reduce the risk of heart disease by reducing LDL.

Many functional foods are marketed as dietary supplements and carry structure-function claims, which do not require the same science base as disease claims. Statements such as "enhances immunity," "maintains heart health," and "boosts energy" are not evaluated by the FDA and so must be viewed with skepticism. Even when an ingredient, such as the herbal compound St. John's wort, has some research supporting its use, the functional foods that contain it are unlikely to have been tested. In addition, just as with dietary supplements, safe and effective intakes have not yet been determined for many compounds, and some may interact dangerously with prescription and over-the-counter drugs. Many functional foods contain very low concentrations of their added ingredients yet may be high in calories and expensive.

At this point, the best advice for consumers may be to read labels carefully and use common sense. Be alert to implied claims in product names such as "Think Drink." Consider the overall nutritional value and cost of a functional food before buying it; you may discover that it contains few nutrients overall. Functional foods cannot take the place of a varied diet rich in fruits, vegetables, and whole grains, which are naturally rich in disease-fighting compounds.

Protecting Yourself Against Foodborne Illness

Many people worry about additives or pesticide residues in their food. However, the greatest threat to the safety of the food supply comes from microorganisms that cause foodborne illnesses. Raw or undercooked animal products, such as chicken, hamburger, and oysters, pose the greatest risk for causing illness. The CDC estimates that 76 million illnesses, 325,000 hospitalizations, and 5,200 deaths occur each year in the United States due to foodborne illness. Your last bout of "stomach flu" may very well have been a foodborne illness. The symptoms of both are often the same: diarrhea, vomiting, fever, and weakness. Although the effects of foodborne illnesses are usually not serious, some groups, such as children, pregnant women, and the elderly, are more at risk for severe complications like rheumatic diseases, seizures, blood poisoning, other ailments, and death.

Causes of Foodborne Illnesses   Most cases of foodborne illness are caused by **pathogens,** disease-causing microorganisms. Food can be contaminated with pathogens through improper handling; pathogens can grow if food is prepared or stored improperly. Causes of foodborne illness in the United States include the following pathogens:

• *Campylobacter jejuni* causes more cases of foodborne illness than any other bacteria. It is most commonly found in contaminated water, raw milk, and raw or undercooked poultry, meat, or shellfish; the majority of chickens sold in the United States test positive for the

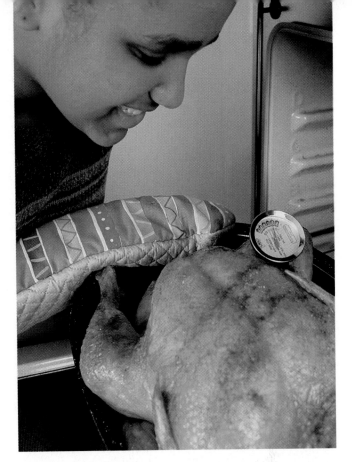

Careful food handling greatly reduces the risk of foodborne illness. Helpful strategies include washing all fruits and vegetables, using separate cutting boards for meat and for foods that will be eaten raw, cooking meat thoroughly, and refrigerating leftovers promptly.

presence of *C. jejuni.* Symptoms of infection include diarrhea, fever, abdominal and muscle pain, and headache, which resolve in 7–10 days. However, in about 1 in 1000 cases, *Campylobacter* infection triggers Guillain-Barré syndrome, a neurological disease that can cause numbness, weakness, and (usually temporary) paralysis.

• *Salmonella* bacteria are most often found in raw or undercooked eggs, poultry, and meat; milk and dairy products; seafood; fruits and vegetables, including sprouts; and inadequately refrigerated and reheated leftovers. The recent identification of an antibiotic-resistant strain of *Salmonella* has raised concerns about a potential increase in serious illness from *Salmonella.*

• *Shigella* bacteria are found in the human intestinal tract and usually transmitted via fecal contamination of food and water. Outbreaks are typically traced to foods,

Terms

especially salads, that have been handled by people using poor personal hygiene. Contaminated water, milk, and dairy products are other possible sources of infection.

- *Escherichia coli,* found in the intestinal tracts of humans and animals, most commonly contaminate water, raw milk, raw to rare ground beef, unpasteurized juices, and fruits and vegetables. A certain strain, known as *E. coli* O157:H7, is of particular concern because it produces a toxin that causes serious illness and up to 100 deaths annually. (Children are particularly at risk for developing hemolytic uremic syndrome, which causes kidney failure.) In 1992, a shipment of Jack-in-the-Box hamburgers that were contaminated with *E. coli* O157: H7 and not cooked thoroughly caused hundreds of cases of illness and several deaths. In 2000, an outbreak in Walkerton, Canada, that was traced to contaminated water sickened over 2000 people and killed 9.

- *Listeria monocytogenes* sickens about 1200–1800 Americans a year, causing death in about 20% of cases. It is found in soft cheeses, raw milk, improperly processed ice cream, raw leafy vegetables, hot dogs and lunch meats, and other meat, poultry, and processed foods. *Listeria* is particularly dangerous for pregnant women and their fetuses, babies and children, older adults, and people with weakened immune systems. A multistate outbreak in 1998–1999 sickened more than 1000 people, killing 15 adults and causing 6 miscarriages or stillbirths; it was traced to contaminated hot dogs and deli meats produced under many brand names by one manufacturer.

- *Staphylococcus aureus* lives mainly in nasal passages and skin sores; it is transferred to food when people handle food or sneeze or cough over food. Foods contaminated with *S. aureus* may include cooked hams, egg and potato salads, cheese, seafood, whipped cream, and milk. *S. aureus* multiplies rapidly at room temperature to produce a toxin that causes illness.

- *Clostridium botulinum* is widely distributed in nature, but it grows only in environments with little or no oxygen; it produces a toxin that causes illness. Potential sources of *C. botulinum* include improperly canned foods, garlic in oil, sausages and other meat products, and vacuum-packed and tightly wrapped foods. Although rare, botulism is potentially fatal if untreated because the toxin affects the nervous system.

- Norwalk viruses are the most common viral cause of foodborne illness; they may be found in contaminated water, raw or insufficiently cooked shellfish, and salad ingredients contaminated by food handlers. Norwalk viruses typically cause vomiting, diarrhea, and abdominal pain, lasting 1–3 days.

Other organisms that can cause types of foodborne illness include the bacteria *Clostridium perfringens, Vibrio vulnificus,* and *Yersinia enterocolytica;* the hepatitis A virus; the parasites *Trichinella spiralis* (found in pork and wild game), *Anisakis* (found in raw fish), *Giardia lamblia, Cyclospora cayetanensis,* and tapeworms; and certain molds.

Preventing and Treating Foodborne Illnesses Because every teaspoon of the soil that our food grows in contains about 2 billion bacteria (only some of them pathogenic), we are always exposed to the possibility of a foodborne illness. You can't tell by taste, smell, or sight whether a food is contaminated. Some studies have revealed high levels of contamination. In 1998, *Consumer Reports* tested 400 chickens purchased in grocery stores and found that 71% were contaminated with *Campylobacter,* and 10% with *Salmonella.*

Although pathogens are usually destroyed during cooking, the U.S. government is taking steps to bring down levels of contamination. New federal regulations require more precise national surveillance; inspectors at meat and poultry processing plants must also use microbiological testing methods, in addition to visual inspections, to check for the presence of pathogens. The new tests will not eliminate all contamination, however, and other regulations are designed to help prevent illness from contaminated foods that do make it to consumers. Raw meat and poultry products are now sold with safe handling and cooking instructions, and all packaged, unpasteurized fresh fruit and vegetable juices carry warnings about potential contamination. It is important to note that while foodborne illness outbreaks associated with food-processing plants make headlines, most cases of illness trace back to poor food handling in the home or in food-service establishments. To decrease your risk of foodborne illness, follow the guidelines in the box "Safe Food Handling."

If you think you may be having a bout of foodborne illness, drink plenty of clear fluids to prevent dehydration, and rest to speed recovery. To prevent further contamination, wash your hands often and always before handling food until the diarrhea disappears. A fever higher than 102°F, blood in the stool, or dehydration deserves a physician's evaluation, especially if the symptoms persist for more than 2–3 days. In cases of suspected botulism—characterized by symptoms such as double vision, paralysis, dizziness, and vomiting—consult a physician immediately, because the use of an antitoxin may help you recover sooner.

Terms

polychlorinated biphenyl (PCB) An industrial chemical used as an insulator in electrical transformers and linked to certain human cancers.

organic A designation applied to foods grown and produced according to strict guidelines limiting the use of pesticides, nonorganic ingredients, hormones, antibiotics, genetic engineering, irradiation, and other practices.

- Don't buy food in containers that leak, bulge, or are severely dented. Refrigerated foods should be cold, and frozen foods should be solid.

- Refrigerate perishable items as soon as possible after purchase. Use or freeze fresh meats within 3–5 days and fresh poultry, fish, and ground meat within 1–2 days.

- Store raw meat, poultry, fish, and shellfish in containers in the refrigerator so that the juices don't drip onto other foods. Keep these items away from other foods, surfaces, utensils, or serving dishes to prevent cross-contamination.

- Thaw frozen food in the refrigerator or in the microwave oven, not on the kitchen counter. Cook foods immediately after thawing.

- Thoroughly wash your hands with warm soapy water for 20 seconds before and after handling food, especially raw meat, fish, shellfish, poultry, or eggs.

- Make sure counters, cutting boards, dishes, utensils, and other equipment are thoroughly cleaned before and after use using hot soapy water. Wash dishcloths and kitchen towels frequently.

- If possible, use separate cutting boards for meat, poultry, and seafood and for foods that will be eaten raw, such as fruits and vegetables. Replace cutting boards once they become worn or develop hard-to-clean grooves.

- Thoroughly rinse and scrub fruits and vegetables with a brush, if possible, or peel off the skin.

- Cook foods thoroughly, especially beef, poultry, fish, pork, and eggs. Cooking kills most microorganisms, as long as an appropriately high temperature is reached. Use a food thermometer to ensure that foods are cooked to a safe temperature. If using a microwave, turn or stir the food to make sure it is heated evenly throughout. When eating out, order hamburger cooked "well-done" and make sure foods are served piping hot.

- Cook stuffing separately from poultry; or wash poultry thoroughly, stuff immediately before cooking, and transfer the stuffing to a clean bowl immediately after cooking. The temperature of cooked stuffing should reach 165°F.

- Keep hot foods hot (140°F or above) and cold foods cold (40°F or below); harmful bacteria can grow rapidly between these two temperatures. Refrigerate foods within 2 hours of purchase or preparation, and within 1 hour if the air temperature is above 90°F. Refrigerate foods at or below 40°F and freeze at or below 0°F. Use refrigerated leftovers within 3–4 days.

- Don't eat raw animal products, including raw eggs in homemade hollandaise sauce or eggnog. Use only pasteurized milk and juice, and look for pasteurized eggs, which are now available in some states.

- Cook eggs until they're firm, and fully cook foods containing eggs. Store eggs in the coldest part of the refrigerator, not in the door, and use them within 3–5 weeks.

- Because of possible contamination with *E. coli* O157:H7 and *Salmonella,* avoid raw sprouts. Even sprouts grown under clean conditions in the home can be risky because bacteria may be present in the seeds. Cook sprouts before eating them.

- Read the food label and package information, and follow safety instructions such as "Keep Refrigerated" and the "Safe Handling Instructions."

- According to the USDA, "When in doubt, throw it out." Even if a food looks and smells fine, it may not be safe. If you aren't sure that a food has been prepared, served, and stored safely, don't eat it.

Additional precautions are recommended for people at particularly high risk for foodborne illness—pregnant women, young children, older persons, and people with weakened immune systems or certain chronic illnesses. If you are a member of one of these groups, don't eat or drink any of the following products: unpasteurized juices; raw sprouts; raw (unpasteurized) milk and products made from unpasteurized milk; raw or undercooked meat, poultry, eggs, fish, and shellfish; and soft cheeses such as feta, Brie, Camembert, or blue-veined varieties. To protect against *Listeria,* it's also important to avoid ready-to-eat foods such as hot dogs, luncheon meats, and cold cuts unless they are reheated until they are steaming hot.

Environmental Contaminants and Organic Foods

Contaminants are also present in the food-growing environment, but few of them ever enter the food and water supply in amounts sufficient to cause health problems. Environmental contaminants include various minerals, antibiotics, hormones, pesticides, the industrial chemicals known as **PCBs (polychlorinated biphenyls),** and naturally occurring substances such as cyanogenic glycosides (found in lima beans and the pits of some fruits) and certain molds. Their effects depend on many factors, including concentration, length of exposure, and the age and health status of the person involved. Safety regulations attempt to keep our exposure to environmental contaminants at safe levels, but monitoring is difficult and many substances (such as pesticides) persist in the environment long after being banned from use.

Some people who are concerned about pesticides and other environmental contaminants choose to buy foods that are **organic.** In December 2000, the USDA enacted a new national standard for organic foods to replace the older system of local, state, and private standards. To be certified as organic, foods must meet strict production, processing, handling, and labeling criteria. Organic crops must meet limits on pesticide residues; for meat, milk, eggs, and other animal products to be certified organic, animals must be given organic feed and access to the outdoors and may not be given antibiotics or growth hormones. The use of genetic engineering, ionizing radiation, and sewage sludge are prohibited (see below for more on irradiated foods). Products can be labeled "100% organic" if they contain all organic ingredients and "organic" if they contain at least 95% organic ingredients; all such products may carry the new USDA organic seal. A product with at least 70% organic ingredients can be labeled "made with organic ingredients" but cannot use the USDA seal.

Foods that are organic are not chemical-free, however. They may be contaminated with pesticides used on neighboring lands or on foods transported in the same train or truck. However, they do tend to have lower levels of pesticide residues than conventionally grown crops. There are strict pesticide limits for all foods—organic and conventional—and the debate about the potential health effects of long-term exposure to small amounts of pesticide residues is ongoing. The benefits of a diet rich in fruits and vegetables far outweigh any potential long-term risks of exposure to pesticide residues. Some studies indicate that washing produce in a highly diluted liquid soap solution removes most pesticide residues, but many experts feel that the use of running water is sufficient.

Supporters of organic foods also note that practices associated with organic farming help maintain biodiversity of crops and are less likely to degrade soil, contaminate water, or expose farm workers to dangerous chemicals. Organic foods tend to be more expensive than those grown conventionally, however, and there is no evidence that they contain more nutrients or fewer foodborne pathogens. But some people choose to pay the higher prices for organic foods to support agricultural practices they believe promote a healthier environment. Since 1990, U.S. sales of organic foods have grown by 20% a year, reaching $6.5 billion in 2000. Similarly, sales of organic dairy products are increasing by more than 100% annually.

Additives in Food

Today, some 2800 substances are intentionally added to foods for one or more of the following reasons: (1) to maintain or improve nutritional quality, (2) to maintain freshness, (3) to help in processing or preparation, or (4) to alter taste or appearance. Additives make up less than 1% of our food. The most widely used are sugar, salt, and corn syrup; these three plus citric acid, baking soda, vegetable colors, mustard, and pepper account for 98% by weight of all food additives used in the United States.

Some additives may be of concern for certain people, because either they are consumed in large quantities or they cause some type of reaction. Additives having potential health concerns include the following:

- *Nitrates and nitrites:* Used to protect meats from contamination from the botulism pathogen. Their consumption is associated with the synthesis of cancer-causing agents in the stomach, but the cancer risk appears to be low, except for people with low stomach acid output (such as some elderly people). The use of nitrates or nitrites is allowed in small quantities.

- *BHA and BHT:* Used to help maintain the freshness of foods. Some studies indicate a potential link between BHT and an increased risk of certain cancers, but any risk from these agents is considered to be low. Some manufacturers have stopped using BHT and BHA.

- *Sulfites:* Used to keep vegetables from turning brown. They can cause severe reactions in some people. The FDA severely limits the use of sulfites and requires any foods containing sulfites to be clearly labeled.

- *Monosodium glutamate (MSG):* Typically used as a flavor enhancer. MSG may cause some people to experience episodes of increased blood pressure and sweating. If you are sensitive to MSG, check food labels when shopping, and ask to have it left out of dishes you order at restaurants.

Food additives pose no significant health hazard to most people because the levels used are well below any that could produce toxic effects. To avoid potential problems, eat a variety of foods in moderation. If you have a sensitivity to an additive, check food labels when you shop, and ask questions when you eat out.

Food Irradiation

Food irradiation is the treatment of foods with gamma rays, X rays, or high-voltage electrons to kill potentially harmful pathogens, including bacteria, parasites, insects, and fungi that cause foodborne illness. It also reduces spoilage and extends shelf life. For example, irradiated strawberries stay unspoiled in the refrigerator up to 3 weeks, versus only 3–5 days for untreated berries. Since 1963, the government has allowed the irradiation of certain foods; this growing list includes wheat and flour (1963); white potatoes (1964); pork, herbs and spices, and fruits and vegetables (1986); raw poultry (1992); and red meat (1999). The same irradiation process has also been used for decades on such items as plastic wrap, milk cartons, teething rings, contact lenses, and medical supplies.

Even though irradiation has been generally endorsed by agencies such as the World Health Organization, the Centers for Disease Control and Prevention, and the American Medical Association, few irradiated foods are currently on the market due to consumer resistance and skepticism. Opponents of irradiation say that essential nutrients in food may be destroyed, that eating irradiated foods may cause cancer or other debilitating conditions, and that irradiation may be hazardous to the employees and nearby residents of food irradiation sites. However, studies haven't conclusively identified any harmful effects of food irradiation. Some irradiated foods may taste slightly different, just as pasteurized milk tastes slightly different than unpasteurized milk. However, irradiated foods do not become radioactive, dangerous substances are not created, and the nutritional value of the food is essentially unchanged. In addition, the newer methods of irradiation involving electricity and X rays do not require the use of any radioactive materials.

Studies indicate that when consumers are given information about the process of irradiation and the benefits of irradiated foods, most want to purchase them. Without such information, many remain skeptical. All primary irradiated foods (meat, vegetables, and so on) are labeled with the flowerlike radura symbol and a brief information label; spices and foods that are merely ingredients do not have to be so labeled. It is important to remember that although irradiation kills most pathogens, it does not completely sterilize foods. Proper handling of irradiated foods is still critical for preventing foodborne illness.

Food Allergies and Food Intolerances

For some people, consuming a particular food causes symptoms such as itchiness, swollen lips, or abdominal pain. Adverse reactions like these may be due to a food allergy or a food intolerance, and symptoms may range from annoying to life-threatening. If you've had an adverse reaction to a food, it's important to determine whether your symptoms are due to an allergy or an intolerance so that you can take appropriate action.

Food Allergies   A true **food allergy** is a reaction of the body's immune system to a food or food ingredient, usually a protein. The immune system perceives the reaction-provoking substance, or allergen, as foreign and acts to destroy it. This immune reaction can occur within minutes of ingesting the food, resulting in symptoms that affect the skin (hives), gastrointestinal tract (cramps or diarrhea), respiratory tract (asthma), or mouth (swelling of the lips or tongue). The most severe response is a systemic reaction called anaphylaxis, which involves a potentially life-threatening drop in blood pressure.

Food allergies affect only about 2% of the adult population and about 4–6% of infants; many infants outgrow food allergies. Although numerous food allergens have been identified, just a few foods account for more than 90% of the food allergies in the United States: cow's milk, eggs, peanuts, tree nuts (walnuts, cashews, and so on), soy, wheat, fish, and shellfish. Individuals with food allergies, especially those prone to anaphylaxis, must diligently avoid trigger foods. This involves careful reading of food labels and asking questions about ingredients when eating out. People at risk are usually advised to carry medications to treat anaphylaxis, such as injectable epinephrine. Refer to Chapter 17 for more on allergies.

Food Intolerances   Many people who believe they have food allergies may actually suffer from a much more common source of adverse food reactions, a **food intolerance.** In the case of a food intolerance, the problem usually lies with metabolism rather than with the immune system. Typically, the body cannot adequately digest a food or food component, often because of some type of chemical deficiency; in other cases, the body reacts to a particular compound in a food. Lactose intolerance, described in Chapter 8, is a fairly common food intolerance; it occurs in people who are deficient in the enzyme lactase, which is needed to digest milk sugar (lactose). A more serious condition is intolerance of gluten, a protein component of some grains; in affected individuals, consumption of gluten damages the lining of the small intestine. Sulfite, a common food additive, can produce severe asthmatic reactions in sensitive individuals. Food intolerances have also been attributed to tartrazine (yellow food coloring), MSG, and the sweetener aspartame.

Food intolerance reactions often produce symptoms similar to food allergies, such as diarrhea or cramps, but reactions are typically localized and not life-threatening. Many people with food intolerances can consume small amounts of the food that affects them; exceptions are gluten and sulfite, which must be avoided by sensitive individuals. Through trial and error, most people with food intolerances can adjust their intake of the trigger food to an appropriate level.

If you suspect that you have a food allergy or intolerance, a good first step is to keep a food diary. Note everything you eat or drink, any symptoms you develop, and how long after eating the symptoms appear. Then make an appointment with your physician to go over your diary and determine if any additional tests are needed.

Staying Committed to a Healthy Diet

You've learned the basics of good nutrition, know how to interpret food and supplement labels, and have some guidelines for protecting yourself from food-related ill-

food irradiation The treatment of foods with gamma rays, X rays, or high-voltage electrons to kill potentially harmful pathogens and increase shelf life.

food allergy An adverse reaction to a food or food ingredient in which the immune system perceives a particular substance (allergen) as foreign and acts to destroy it.

food intolerance An adverse reaction to a food or food ingredient that doesn't involve the immune system; intolerances are often due to a problem with metabolism.

Terms

ness. With this foundation, you can now put together a diet that works for you. There is no single type of diet that provides optimal health for everyone, and many cultural dietary patterns can meet people's nutritional requirements (see the box "Ethnic Foods"). You can customize a food plan based on your age, sex, weight, activity level, medical risk factors—and, of course, personal tastes.

Sticking to a healthy diet is probably easiest when you choose and prepare your own food at home. For meals prepared at home, advance planning is the key: Map out meals and shop appropriately, cook in advance when possible, and prepare enough food for leftovers later in the week. A tight budget need not make it more difficult to eat healthy meals. It makes good health sense and good budget sense to use only small amounts of meat and to have a few meatless meals each week.

Healthy eating becomes more challenging when you dine out. Portion sizes in restaurants are often far larger than the serving sizes of the Food Guide Pyramid. Try eating only part of your meal and take the rest home for a meal later in the week. Don't hesitate to ask questions about how menu selections are prepared and to ask for adjustments, such as salad dressings or sauces served on the side. To limit your fat and calorie intake, order dishes that have been broiled or grilled rather than fried, choose rice or a plain baked potato over french fries, and select a clear soup rather than a creamy one. Desserts that are irresistible can, at least, be shared.

Strategies like these can be helpful, but small changes cannot change a fundamentally high-fat, high-calorie meal into a moderate, healthful one. Often, the best advice is to bypass a large steak with potatoes au gratin for a flavorful but low-fat entrée. Fast-food meals are often particularly high in calories, fat, sodium, and sugar and low in fiber and some vitamins and minerals. If you do eat at a fast-food restaurant, make sure the rest of your meals that day include healthier choices.

The information provided in this chapter should give you the tools you need to design and implement a diet that you enjoy and that promotes long-term health and well-being. If you need additional information or have questions about nutrition, be sure the source you consult is reliable.

Tips for Today

Eating is one of life's great pleasures. There are many ways to satisfy your nutrient needs, so you can create a healthy diet that takes into account your personal preferences and favorite foods. If your current eating habits are not as healthy as they could be, you can choose equally delicious foods that offer both short-term and long-term health benefits. Opportunities to improve your diet present themselves every day, and small changes add up.

Right now you can

- Substitute a healthy snack—an apple, a banana, or popcorn—for a bag of chips or cookies.

- Drink a glass of water, and put a bottle of water in your backpack for tomorrow.

- Plan to make healthy selections when you go to dinner, such as a baked potato instead of french fries or salmon instead of steak.

- Study the box on ethnic foods in this chapter and plan to order a healthy selection the next time you eat at your favorite ethnic restaurant. Do the same with the fast-food restaurants listed in Appendix A at the end of the book.

SUMMARY

- To function at its best, the human body requires about 45 essential nutrients in specific proportions. People get the nutrients needed to fuel their bodies and maintain tissues and organ systems from foods; the body cannot synthesize most of them.

- Proteins, made up of amino acids, form muscles and bones and help make up blood, enzymes, hormones, and cell membranes. Foods from animal sources provide complete proteins; plants provide incomplete proteins.

- Fats, a concentrated source of energy, also help insulate the body and cushion the organs; 1 tablespoon of vegetable oil per day supplies the essential fats. Dietary fat intake should be limited to 30% of total daily calories. Unsaturated fats should be favored over saturated and trans fats.

- Carbohydrates supply energy to the brain and other parts of the nervous system as well as to red blood cells. The body needs 50–100 grams of carbohydrates a day, but much more is recommended.

- Dietary fiber includes plant substances that are difficult or impossible for humans to digest. Insoluble fiber holds water and increases bulk in the stool. Soluble fiber binds cholesterol-containing compounds in the intestine and slows glucose absorption.

- The 13 vitamins needed in the diet are organic substances that promote specific chemical and cell processes within living tissue. Deficiencies or excesses can cause serious illnesses and even death.

- The approximately 17 minerals needed in the diet are inorganic substances that regulate body functions, aid in the growth and maintenance of body tissues, and help in the release of energy from foods.

- Water is used to digest and absorb food, transport substances around the body, lubricate joints and organs, and regulate body temperature.

There is no one ethnic diet that clearly surpasses all others in providing people with healthful foods. However, every diet has its advantages and disadvantages and, within each cuisine, some foods are better choices. The dietary guidelines described in this chapter can be applied to any ethnic cuisine. For additional guidance, refer to the table below.

	Choose More Often	Choose Less Often
Chinese	Dishes that are steamed, poached (jum), boiled (chu), roasted (kow), barbecued (shu), or lightly stir-fried Hoisin sauce, oyster sauce, wine sauce, plum sauce, velvet sauce, or hot mustard Fresh fish and seafood, skinless chicken, tofu Mixed vegetables, Chinese greens Steamed rice, steamed spring rolls, soft noodles	Fried wontons or egg rolls Crab rangoon Crispy (Peking) duck or chicken Sweet-and-sour dishes made with breaded and deep-fried meat, poultry, or fish Fried rice Fried or crispy noodles
French	Dishes prepared au vapeur (steamed), en brochette (skewered and broiled), or grillé (grilled) Fresh fish, shrimp, scallops, or mussels or skinless chicken, without sauces Clear soups	Dishes prepared à la crème (in cream sauce), au gratin or gratinée (baked with cream and cheese), or en croûte (in pastry crust) Drawn butter, hollandaise sauce, and remoulade (mayonnaise-based sauce)
Greek	Dishes that are stewed, broiled, or grilled, including shish kabobs (souvlaki) Dolmas (grape leaves) stuffed with rice Tzatziki (yogurt, cucumbers, and garlic) Tabouli (bulgur-based salad) Pita bread, especially whole wheat	Moussaka, saganaki (fried cheese) Vegetable pies such as spanakopita and tyropita Baba ghanoush (eggplant and olive oil) Deep-fried falafel (chickpea patties) Gyros stuffed with ground meat Baklava
Indian	Dishes prepared masala (curry), tandoori (roasted in a clay oven), or tikke (pan roasted); kabobs Raita (yogurt and cucumber salad) and other yogurt-based dishes and sauces Dal (lentils), pullao or pilau (basmati rice) Chapati (baked bread)	Ghee (clarified butter) Korma (meat in cream sauce) Samosas, pakoras (fried dishes) Molee and other coconut milk–based dishes Poori, bhatura, or paratha (fried breads)
Italian	Pasta primavera or pasta, polenta, risotto, or gnocchi with marinara, red or white wine, white or red clam, or light mushroom sauce Dishes that are grilled or prepared cacciatore (tomato-based sauce), marsala (broth and wine sauce), or piccata (lemon sauce) Cioppino (seafood stew) Vegetable soup, minestrone or fagioli (beans)	Antipasto (cheese, smoked meats) Dishes that are prepared alfredo, frito (fried), crema (creamed), alla panna (with cream), or carbonara Veal scaloppini Chicken, veal, or eggplant parmigiana Italian sausage, salami, and prosciutto Buttered garlic bread Cannoli
Japanese	Dishes prepared nabemono (boiled), shabu-shabu (in boiling broth), mushimono (steamed), nimono (simmered), yaki (broiled), or yakimono (grilled) Sushi or domburi (mixed rice dish) Steamed rice or soba (buckwheat), udon (wheat), or rice noodles	Tempura (battered and fried) Agemono (deep fried) Katsu (fried pork cutlet) Sukiyaki Fried tofu
Mexican	Soft corn or wheat tortillas Burritos, fajitas, enchiladas, soft tacos, and tamales filled with beans, vegetables, or lean meats Refried beans, nonfat or low-fat, rice and beans Ceviche (fish marinated in lime juice) Salsa, enchilada sauce, and picante sauce Gazpacho, menudo, or black bean soup Fruit or flan for dessert	Crispy, fried tortillas Dishes that are fried, such as chile relleños, chimichangas, flautas, and tostadas Nachos and cheese, chili con queso, and other dishes made with cheese or cheese sauce Guacamole, sour cream, and extra cheese Refried beans made with lard Fried ice cream
Thai	Dishes that are barbecued, sautéed, broiled, boiled, steamed, braised, or marinated Sâté (skewered and grilled meats) Fish sauce, basil sauce, chili or hot sauces Bean thread noodles, Thai salad	Coconut milk soup Peanut sauce or dishes topped with nuts Mee-krob (crispy noodles) Red, green, and yellow curries, which typically contain coconut milk

SOURCES: National Heart, Lung, and Blood Institute. 1998. Tips for Healthy Multicultural Dining Out. In *Clinical Guidelines on the Identification, Evaluation, and Treatment of Overweight and Obesity in Adults*. Bethesda, Md.: National Institutes of Health. Duyff, R. L. 1998. *The American Dietetic Association's Complete Food and Nutrition Guide*. Minneapolis, Minn.: Chronimed. Kirby, J. 1998. *Dieting for Dummies*. Foster City, Calif.: IDG Books.

After reading this chapter and completing the dietary assessment on p. 333, you can probably identify several changes you could make to improve your diet. Here, we focus on choosing healthy beverages to increase intake of nutrients and decrease intake of empty calories from added sugars and fat. However, this model of dietary change can be applied to any modification you'd like to make to your diet. Additional specific plans for improving diet can be found in the Behavior Change Strategies in Chapter 15 (decreasing saturated and trans fat intake) and Chapter 16 (increasing intake of fruits and vegetables).

Gather Data and Establish a Baseline

Begin by tracking your beverage consumption in your health journal. Write down the types and amounts of beverage you drink, including water. Also note where you were at the time and whether you obtained the beverage on-site or brought it with you.

At the same time, investigate your options. Find out what other beverages you can easily obtain over the course of your daily routine. For example, what drinks are available in the dining hall where you eat lunch or at the student union where you often grab snacks? How many drinking fountains do you walk by over the course of the day? This information will help you put together a successful plan for change.

Analyze Your Data and Set Goals

Evaluate your beverage consumption by dividing your typical daily consumption between healthy and less healthy choices. Use the following guide as a basis, and add other beverages to the lists as needed.

Choose less often:

- Regular soda
- Sweetened bottled iced tea
- Fruit beverages made with little fruit juice (usually labeled fruit drinks, punches, beverages, blends, or ades)
- Whole milk

Choose more often:

- Water—plain, mineral, and sparkling
- Low-fat or nonfat milk
- Fruit juice (100% juice)
- Unsweetened herbal tea

How many beverages do you consume daily from each category? What would be a healthy and realistic goal for change? For example, if your beverage consumption is currently evenly divided between the "choose more often" and "choose less often" categories (four from each list), you might set a final goal for your behavior change program of increasing your healthy choices by two (six from the "more often" list and two from the "less often" list).

Develop a Plan for Change

Once you've set your goal, you need to develop strategies that will help you choose healthy beverages more often. Consider the following possibilities:

- Keep healthy beverages on hand; if you live in a student dorm, rent a small refrigerator or keep juice, nonfat milk, and other healthy choices in the dorm's kitchen refrigerator.
- Plan ahead, and put a bottle of water or 100% juice in your backpack every day.
- Check food labels on beverages for serving sizes, calories, and nutrients; comparison shop to find the healthiest choices, and watch your serving sizes. Use this information to make your "choose more often" list longer and more specific.
- If you eat out frequently, examine all the beverages available at the places you typically eat your meals. You'll probably find that healthy choices are available; if not, bring along your own drink or find somewhere else to eat.
- For a snack, try water and a piece of fruit rather than a heavily sweetened beverage.
- Create healthy beverages that appeal to you; for example, try adding slices of citrus fruit to water or mixing 100% fruit juice with sparkling water.

You may also need to make some changes in your routine to decrease the likelihood that you'll make unhealthy choices. For example, you might discover from your health journal that you always buy a soda after class when you pass a particular vending machine. If this is the case, try another route that allows you to avoid the machine. And try to guard against impulse buying by carrying water or a healthy snack with you every day.

To complete your plan, try some of the other behavior change strategies described in Chapter 1: Develop and sign a contract, set up a system of rewards, involve other people in your program, and develop strategies for challenging situations. Once your plan is complete, take action. Keep track of your progress in your health journal by continuing to monitor and evaluate your beverage consumption.

- Foods contain other substances such as phytochemicals, which may not be essential nutrients but which reduce chronic disease risk.
- Dietary Reference Intakes (DRIs) are recommended intakes for essential nutrients that meet the needs of healthy people.

- The Food Guide Pyramid contains six food groups; choosing foods from each group every day helps ensure the appropriate amounts of necessary nutrients. The fundamental principles of the Food Guide Pyramid are moderation, variety, and balance.
- The Dietary Guidelines for Americans address the

prevention of diet-related diseases like cardiovascular disease, cancer, and diabetes. The guidelines advise us to aim for a healthy weight through diet and physical activity; build a healthy base for our diets by following the Pyramid, choosing a variety of plant foods, and handling foods safely; and make sensible food choices that consider intake of fat, sugar, salt, and alcohol.

- A vegetarian diet can meet human nutritional needs.
- Different population groups may face special dietary challenges. Women need to focus on nutrient-dense foods; men should limit fat intake and increase their consumption of fruits, vegetables, and grains.

- Almost all foods have labels that show how much fat, cholesterol, protein, fiber, and sodium they contain. Serving sizes are standardized, and health claims are carefully regulated. Dietary supplements also have uniform labels.
- Foodborne illnesses are a greater threat to health than additives and environmental contaminants. Other dietary issues of concern to some people include organic foods, food irradiation, and food allergies and intolerances.

TAKE ACTION

1. Read the list of ingredients on three or four canned or packaged foods that you enjoy eating. If any ingredients are unfamiliar to you, find out what they are and why they have been used. A nutrition textbook from the library may be a helpful resource.

2. Investigate the nutritional and dietary guidelines that are used to prepare the food served in your school. Are they consistent with what you've learned in this

chapter? If not, try to find out more about the guidelines that have been used and why they were chosen.

3. Prepare a flavorful low-fat vegetarian and/or ethnic meal. (Use the suggestions in the chapter, and check your local library for appropriate cookbooks.) How do the foods included in the meal and the preparation methods differ from what you're used to?

JOURNAL ENTRY

1. In your health journal, keep track of everything you eat and drink for 3–4 days. Calculate the average number of servings from each food group you consume each day. Then see how well your average daily intake meets the guidelines in the Food Guide Pyramid.

2. Put together three sample daily menus that follow the Food Guide Pyramid. Keep the dietary guidelines in mind as you make your food selections from each group. Also, be sure to base your menus on foods you enjoy eating.

3. *Critical Thinking* Analyze patterns of food advertising on television by recording the number and types of ads that appear each hour. If possible, compare the number and types of products advertised during an hour of cartoons or other children's programs, an hour of daytime programs, and an hour of prime-time programs. What patterns do you see? What types of information do the ads present? Are they geared toward different segments of the population? Do they encourage healthy eating?

FOR MORE INFORMATION

For reliable nutrition advice, talk to a faculty member in the nutrition department on your campus, a registered dietitian (R.D.), or your physician. Many large communities have a telephone service called Dial-a-Dietitian. By calling this number, people can receive nutrition information from an R.D. free of charge.

Experts on quackery suggest that you steer clear of anyone who puts forth any of the following false statements:

- Most diseases are caused by faulty nutrition.

- Large doses of vitamins are effective against many diseases.
- Hair analysis can be used to determine a person's nutritional state.
- A computer-scored nutritional deficiency test is a basis for prescribing vitamins.

Any practitioner—licensed or not—who sells vitamins in his or her office should be thoroughly scrutinized.

Books

American Dietetic Association. 1999. *The Essential Guide to Nutrition and the Foods We Eat: Everything You Need to Know About the Foods You Eat.* New York: HarperCollins. *An excellent review of current nutrition information and issues.*

Insel, P., R. E. Turner, and D. Ross. 2001. *Nutrition.* Sudbury, Mass.: Jones & Bartlett. *A comprehensive review of major concepts in nutrition.*

Nelson, M., and S. Wernick. 2000. *Strong Women, Strong Bones.* New York: Putnam. *A guide to the prevention of osteoporosis, with an emphasis on diet and exercise.*

Selkowitz, A. 2000. *The College Student's Guide to Eating Well on Campus.* Bethesda, Md.: Tulip Hill Press. *Provides practical advice for students, including how to make healthy choices when eating in a dorm or restaurant and how to stock a first pantry.*

Wolfe, F. A. 2000. *The Complete Idiot's Guide to Being a Vegetarian,* 2nd ed. Indianapolis, Ind.: Macmillan. *Provides information on the health benefits of vegetarian diets and how to plan healthy meals; advice is given for vegetarian diets for special population groups, including children.*

Newsletters

Environmental Nutrition (800-829-5384)

Nutrition Action Health Letter (202-332-9110; http://www.cspinet.org).

Tufts University Health & Nutrition Letter (800-274-7581; http://www.healthletter.tufts.edu)

WW. Organizations, Hotlines, and Web Sites

American Dietetic Association. Provides a wide variety of nutrition-related educational materials.

   800-366-1655

   http://www.eatright.org

American Heart Association: Delicious Decisions. Provides basic information about nutrition, tips for shopping and eating out, and heart-healthy recipes.

   http://www.deliciousdecisions.org

Ask the Dietitian. Questions and answers on many topics relating to nutrition.

   http://www.dietitian.com

Consumer Information Center: Food. Provides online government publications about dietary fat, fiber, food safety, and other nutrition issues.

   http://www.pueblo.gsa.gov/food.htm

CyberDiet. Provides a variety of resources, including a profile that calculates calorie and nutrient needs and a database that provides nutrition information in food label format.

   http://www.CyberDiet.com

FDA Center for Food Safety and Applied Nutrition. Offers information about topics such as food labeling, food additives, dietary supplements, and foodborne illness.

   http://vm.cfsan.fda.gov

Food Safety Hotlines. Provide information on safe purchase, handling, cooking, and storage of food.

   888-SAFEFOOD (FDA)

   800-535-4555 (USDA)

Gateways to Government Nutrition Information. Provide access to government resources relating to nutrition and food safety.

   http://www.nutrition.gov

   http://www.foodsafety.gov

International Food Information Council. Provides helpful information on food safety and nutrition for consumers, journalists, and educators.

   http://ificinfo.health.org

National Academies' Food and Nutrition Board. Provides information about the Dietary Reference Intakes and related guidelines.

   http://www4.nationalacademies.org/IOM/IOMHome.nsf/Pages/Food+and+Nutrition+Board

National Cancer Institute: 5-A-Day. Provides tips and recipes to help consumers increase their intake of fruits and vegetables.

   http://5aday.nci.nih.gov

Tufts University Nutrition Navigator. Provides descriptions and ratings for many nutrition-related Web pages.

   http://navigator.tufts.edu

USDA Center for Nutrition Policy and Promotion. Includes information on the Dietary Guidelines and the Food Guide Pyramid; also provides the Healthy Eating Index, an individualized online assessment of overall dietary quality.

   http://www.usda.gov/cnpp

USDA Food and Nutrition Information Center. Provides a variety of materials and extensive links relating to the Dietary Guidelines, food labels, Food Guide Pyramid, and many other topics.

   http://www.nal.usda.gov/fnic

Other USDA Web sites and programs of interest include the *Animal and Plant Health Inspection Service,* which provides information on biotechnology (http://www.aphis.usda.gov/biotechnology); the *Food Safety and Inspection Service,* which provides consumer resources on food safety and irradiation (http://www.fsis.usda.gov); and the *Agricultural Marketing Service,* which provides information on food standards, including the National Organic Program, and has a helpful series of consumer "How to Buy . . ." publications (http://www.ams.usda.gov).

Vegetarian Resource Group. Information and links for vegetarians and people interested in learning more about vegetarian diets.

   http://www.vrg.org

You can obtain nutrient breakdowns of individual food items from the following sites:

Nutrition Analysis Tool, University of Illinois, Urbana/Champaign.

   http://www.nat.uiuc.edu

USDA Nutrient Data Laboratory

   http://www.nal.usda.gov/fnic/foodcomp

You can also obtain recipes at many Web sites; the following are a few of the large, searchable recipe sites:

   Kitchen Link: http://www.kitchenlink.com

   Meals for You: http://www.mealsforyou.com

   Meals Online: http://www.my-meals.com

See also the resources listed in the dietary supplements box on p. 343 and in the For More Information sections in Chapters 13–16 and 19.

A fresh look at chicken safety. 1998. *Consumer Reports,* October.

Allison, D. B., et al. 1999. Estimated intakes of trans fatty and other fatty acids in the U.S. population. *Journal of the American Dietetic Association* 99(2): 166–174.

A healthy diet. 2000. *Journal of the American Medical Association Patient Page* 283(16): 2198.

American Dietetic Association. 1999. Functional foods—Position of ADA. *Journal of the American Dietetic Association* 99: 1278–1285.

American Heart Association Nutrition Committee. 2000. AHA Dietary Guidelines: Revision 2000. *Circulation* 102: 2296–2311.

Bock, S. A., A. Munoz-Furlong, and H. A. Sampson. 2001. Fatalities due to anaphylactic reactions to foods. *Journal of Allergy and Clinical Immunology* 107(1): 191–193.

Booth, S. L., et al. 2000. Dietary vitamin K intakes are associated with hip fractures but not with bone mineral density in elderly men and women. *American Journal of Clinical Nutrition* 71: 1201–1208.

Centers for Disease Control and Prevention. 2001. Diagnosis and management of foodborne illnesses. *MMWR Recommendations and Reports* 50(RR-2).

Centers for Disease Control and Prevention. 2001. Preliminary FoodNet data on the incidence of foodborne illnesses—Selected sites, United States, 2000. *Morbidity and Mortality Weekly Report* 50(13): 241–246.

Cleveland, L. E., et al. 2000. Dietary intake of whole grains. *Journal of the American College of Nutrition* 19(3): 331S–338S.

Denke, M. A., B. Adams-Huet, and A. T. Nguyen. 2000. Individual cholesterol variation in response to a margarine- or butter-based diet. *Journal of the American Medical Association* 284(21): 2740–2747.

Food and Drug Administration. 2000. *FDA Authorizes New Coronary Heart Disease Health Claim for Plant Sterol and Plant Stanol Esters* (http://vm.cfsan.fda.gov/~lrd/tpsterol.html).

Food and Drug Administration, Center for Drug Evaluation and Research. 2000. *FDA Public Health Advisory: Risk of Drug Interactions with St. John's Wort and Indinavir and Other Drugs* (http://www.fda.gov/cder/drug/advisory/stjwort.htm; retrieved May 31, 2000).

Food and Drug Administration, Center for Food Safety and Applied Nutrition. 1999. *Questions and Answers on Trans Fat Proposed Rule* (http://vm.cfsan.fda.gov/~dms/qatrans.html; retrieved February 16, 2000).

Food and Drug Administration, Center for Food Safety and Applied Nutrition. 2000. *Guidance on How to Understand and Use the Nutrition Facts Panel on Food Labels* (http://vm.cfsan.fda.gov/~dms/foodlab.html; retrieved July 14, 2000).

Food and Nutrition Board. National Academy of Sciences. 2001. *Dietary Reference Intakes for Vitamin A, Vitamin K, Arsenic, Boron, Chromium, Copper, Iodine, Iron, Manganese, Molybdenum, Nickel, Silicon, Vanadium, and Zinc.* Washington, D.C.: National Academy Press.

Ford, E. S., and A. Sowell. 1999. Serum alpha-tocopherol status in the United States population: Findings from the Third National Health and Nutrition Examination Survey. *American Journal of Epidemiology* 150(3): 290–300.

Formanek, R. 2001. Proposed rules issued for bioengineered foods. *FDA Consumer,* March-April.

French, S. A., et al. 2001. Pricing and promotion effects on low-fat vending snack purchases. *American Journal of Public Health* 91: 112–117.

Fung, T. T., et al. 2001. Association between dietary patterns and plasma biomarkers of obesity and cardiovascular disease risk. *American Journal of Clinical Nutrition* 73: 61–67.

Haddad, E. H., J. Sabaté, and C. G. Whitten. 1999. Vegetarian food guide pyramid: A conceptual framework. *American Journal of Clinical Nutrition* 70(Suppl): 615S–619S.

Henkel, J. 2000. Soy: Health claims for soy protein, questions about other compounds. *FDA Consumer,* May/June.

IFT Expert Report on Biotechnology and Foods: Human food safety evaluation of rDNA biotechnology-derived foods. 2000. *Food Technology* 54(9): 53–61.

IFT Expert Report on Biotechnology and Foods: Introduction. 2000. *Food Technology* 54(8): 124–136.

Insel, P., R. E. Turner, and D. Ross. 2001. *Nutrition.* Sudbury, Mass.: Jones & Bartlett.

Iso, H., et al. 2001. Intake of fish and omega-3 fatty acids and risk of stroke in women. *Journal of the American Medical Association* 285(3): 304–312.

Jacobs, D. R., H. E. Meyer, and K. Solvoll. 2001. Reduced mortality among whole grain bread eaters in men and women in the Norwegian County Study. *European Journal of Clinical Nutrition* 55(2): 137–143.

Kant, A. K. 2000. Consumption of energy-dense, nutrient-poor foods by adult Americans: Nutritional and health implications. *American Journal of Clinical Nutrition* 72(4): 929–936.

Lewis, C. 2000. Health claim for foods that lower heart disease risk. *FDA Consumer,* November/December.

Liu, S., et al. 2000. Whole grain consumption and risk of ischemic stroke in women. *Journal of the American Medical Association* 284(12): 1534–1540.

Nash, J. M. 2000. Grains of hope. *Time,* July 31.

National Research Council. 2000. *Genetically Modified Pest-Protected Plants: Science and Regulation.* Washington, D.C.: National Academy Press.

Oomen, C. M., et al. 2001. Association between trans fatty acid intake and 10-year risk of coronary heart disease in the Zutphen Elderly Study: A prospective population-based study. *Lancet* 3·57(9258): 746–751.

Patterson, R. E., et al. 2001. Is there a consumer backlash against the diet and health message? *Journal of the American Dietetic Association* 101(1): 37–41.

Pew Initiative on Food and Biotechnology. 2001. *Public Sentiment About Genetically Modified Food* (http://pewagbiotech.org/research; retrieved April 18, 2001).

Thompson, L. 2000. Are bioengineered foods safe? *FDA Consumer,* January/February.

U.S. Department of Agriculture, Agricultural Marketing Service. 2000. *Organic Foods: Labeling and Marketing Information* (http://www.ams.usda.gov/nop/facts/labeling; retrieved January 8, 2001).

U.S. Department of Agriculture, Center for Nutrition Policy and Promotion. 2000. Is intake of added sugars associated with diet quality? *Nutrition Insights* No. 21.

U.S. Department of Agriculture, Food Safety and Inspection Service. 2000. *Irradiation of Raw Meat and Poultry: Questions and Answers* (http://www.fsis.usda.gov/OA/pubs/qa_irrad.htm; retrieved October 23, 2000).

U.S. Department of Agriculture, National Agricultural Statistics Service. 2000. *Acreage, June 2000* (http://usda.mannlib.cornell.edu/reports/nassr/field/pcp-bba/acrg0600.txt; retrieved October 24, 2000).

U.S. Department of Agriculture and U.S. Department of Health and Human Services. 2000. *Nutrition and Your Health: Dietary Guidelines for Americans,* 5th ed. Home and Garden Bulletin No. 232.

Wheelwright, J. 2001. Don't eat again until you read this. *Discover.* March.

Wyshak, G. 2000. Teenaged girls, carbonated beverage consumption, and bone fracture. *Archives of Pediatric and Adolescent Medicine* 154: 610–613.

Table 1 — Dietary Reference Intakes (DRIs): Recommended Levels for Individual Intake

Life Stage	Group	Calcium (mg/day)	Phosphorus (mg/day)	Magnesium (mg/day)	Vitamin D (µg/day)[a,b]	Fluoride (mg/day)	Thiamin (mg/day)	Riboflavin (mg/day)	Niacin (mg/day)[c]	Vitamin B-6 (mg/day)	Folate (µg/day)[d]	Vitamin B-12 (µg/day)	Pantothenic Acid (mg/day)	Biotin (µg/day)
Infants	0–5 months	210	100	30	5	0.01	0.2	0.3	2	0.1	65	0.4	1.7	5
	6–11 months	270	275	75	5	0.5	0.3	0.4	3	0.3	80	0.5	1.8	6
Children	1–3 years	500	460	80	5	0.7	0.5	0.5	6	0.5	150	0.9	2	8
	4–8 years	800	500	130	5	1	0.6	0.6	8	0.6	200	1.2	3	12
Males	9–13 years	1300	1250	240	5	2	0.9	0.9	12	1.0	300	1.8	4	20
	14–18 years	1300	1250	410	5	3	1.2	1.3	16	1.3	400	2.4	5	25
	19–30 years	1000	700	400	5	4	1.2	1.3	16	1.3	400	2.4	5	30
	31–50 years	1000	700	420	5	4	1.2	1.3	16	1.3	400	2.4	5	30
	51–70 years	1200	700	420	10	4	1.2	1.3	16	1.7	400	2.4[e]	5	30
	>70 years	1200	700	420	15	4	1.2	1.3	16	1.7	400	2.4[e]	5	30
Females	9–13 years	1300	1250	240	5	2	0.9	0.9	12	1.0	300	1.8	4	20
	14–18 years	1300	1250	360	5	3	1.0	1.0	14	1.2	400[f]	2.4	5	25
	19–30 years	1000	700	310	5	3	1.1	1.1	14	1.3	400[f]	2.4	5	30
	31–50 years	1000	700	320	5	3	1.1	1.1	14	1.3	400[f]	2.4	5	30
	51–70 years	1200	700	320	10	3	1.1	1.1	14	1.5	400[f]	2.4[e]	5	30
	>70 years	1200	700	320	15	3	1.1	1.1	14	1.5	400	2.4[e]	5	30
Pregnancy	≤18 years	1300	1250	400	5	3	1.4	1.4	18	1.9	600[g]	2.6	6	30
	19–30 years	1000	700	350	5	3	1.4	1.4	18	1.9	600[g]	2.6	6	30
	31–50 years	1000	700	360	5	3	1.4	1.4	18	1.9	600[g]	2.6	6	30
Lactation	≤18 years	1300	1250	360	5	3	1.5	1.6	17	2.0	500	2.8	7	35
	19–30 years	1000	700	310	5	3	1.5	1.6	17	2.0	500	2.8	7	35
	31–50 years	1000	700	320	5	3	1.5	1.6	17	2.0	500	2.8	7	35

NOTE: This table includes Dietary Reference Intakes for those nutrients for which DRIs had been set through June 2001. The table includes values for the type of DRI standard—Adequate Intake (AI) or Recommended Dietary Allowance (RDA)—that has been established for that particular nutrient and life stage. RDAs are shown in **bold type.**

[a] As cholecalciferol. 1 µg cholecalciferol = 40 IU vitamin D.

[b] In the absence of adequate exposure to sunlight.

[c] As niacin equivalents. 1 mg of niacin = 60 mg of tryptophan.

[d] As dietary folate equivalents (DFE). 1 DFE = 1 µg food folate = 0.6 µg of folate (from fortified food or supplement) consumed with food = 0.5 µg of synthetic (supplemental) folic acid taken on an empty stomach.

[e] Since 10–30% of older people may malabsorb food-bound B-12, it is advisable for those older than 50 years to meet their RDA mainly by consuming foods fortified with B-12 or a B-12-containing supplement.

[f] In view of evidence linking folate intake with neural tube defects in the fetus, it is recommended that all women capable of becoming pregnant consume 400 µg of synthetic folic acid from fortified food and/or supplements in addition to intake of food folate from a varied diet.

[g] It is assumed that women will continue consuming 400 µg of folic acid until their pregnancy is confirmed and they enter prenatal care, which ordinarily occurs after the end of the periconceptional period—the critical time for formation of the neural tube.

Table 1

Dietary Reference Intakes (DRIs): Recommended Levels for Individual Intake (Continued)

Life Stage	Group	Choline (mg/day)[h]	Vitamin C (mg/day)	Vitamin E (mg/day)[i]	Selenium (µg/day)	Vitamin A (µg/day)[j]	Vitamin K (µg/day)	Chromium (µg/day)	Copper (µg/day)	Iodine (µg/day)	Iron (mg/day)[k]	Manganese (mg/day)	Molybdenum (µg/day)	Zinc (mg/day)[l]
Infants	0–5 months	125	40	4	15	400	2.0	0.2	200	110	0.27	0.003	2	2
	6–11 months	150	50	6	20	500	2.5	5.5	220	130	11	0.6	3	3
Children	1–3 years	200	15	6	20	300	30	11	340	90	7	1.2	17	3
	4–8 years	250	25	7	30	400	55	15	440	90	10	1.5	22	5
Males	9–13 years	375	45	11	40	600	60	25	700	120	8	1.9	34	8
	14–18 years	550	75[m]	15	55	900	75	35	890	150	11	2.2	43	11
	19–30 years	550	90[m]	15	55	900	120	35	900	150	8	2.3	45	11
	31–50 years	550	90[m]	15	55	900	120	35	900	150	8	2.3	45	11
	51–70 years	550	90[m]	15	55	900	120	30	900	150	8	2.3	45	11
	>70 years	550	90[m]	15	55	900	120	30	900	150	8	2.3	45	11
Females	9–13 years	375	45	11	40	600	60	21	700	120	8	1.6	34	8
	14–18 years	400	65[m]	15	55	700	75	24	890	150	15	1.6	43	9
	19–30 years	425	75[m]	15	55	700	90	25	900	150	18	1.8	45	8
	31–50 years	425	75[m]	15	55	700	90	25	900	150	18	1.8	45	8
	51–70 years	425	75[m]	15	55	700	90	20	900	150	8	1.8	45	8
	>70 years	425	75[m]	15	55	700	90	20	900	150	8	1.8	45	8
Pregnancy	≤18 years	450	80	15	60	750	75	29	1000	220	27	2.0	50	13
	19–30 years	450	85	15	60	770	90	30	1000	220	27	2.0	50	11
	31–50 years	450	85	15	60	770	90	30	1000	220	27	2.0	50	11
Lactation	≤18 years	550	115	19	70	1200	75	44	1300	290	10	2.6	50	14
	19–30 years	550	120	19	70	1300	90	45	1300	290	9	2.6	50	12
	31–50 years	550	120	19	70	1300	90	45	1300	290	9	2.6	50	12

[h]Although AIs have been set for choline, there are few data to assess whether a dietary supply of choline is needed at all stages of the life cycle, and it may be that the choline requirement can be met by endogenous synthesis at some of these stages.

[i]As α-Tocopherol.

[j]As retinol activity equivalents (RAE): 1 RAE = 1 µg retinol = 12 µg β-carotene = 24 µg of other provitamin A carotenoids. Preformed vitamin A (retinol) is abundant in animal-derived foods; provitamin A carotenoids are abundant in some dark-yellow, orange, red, and deep-green fruits and vegetables.

[k]Because the absorption of iron from plant foods is low compared to that from animal foods, the RDA for strict vegetarians is approximately 1.8 times higher than the values established for omnivores (14 mg/day for adult male vegetarians; 33 mg/day for premenopausal female vegetarians). Oral contraceptives (OCs) reduce menstrual blood losses, so women taking them need less daily iron; the RDA for premenopausal women taking OCs is 10.9 mg/day. For more on iron requirements for other special situations, refer to Dietary Reference Intakes for Vitamin A, Vitamin K, Arsenic, Boron, Chromium, Copper, Iodine, Iron, Manganese, Molybdenum, Nickel, Silicon, Vanadium, and Zinc.

[l]Vegetarians may need up to 50% more zinc because a chemical in plants (phytate) hinders zinc absorption in the body.

SOURCES: Food and Nutrition Board, National Academy of Sciences. 2000. Dietary Reference Intakes for Vitamin C, Vitamin E, Selenium, and Carotenoids. Washington, D.C.: National Academy Press. Food and Nutrition Board, National Academy of Sciences. 2001. Dietary Reference Intakes for Vitamin A, Vitamin K, Arsenic, Boron, Chromium, Copper, Iodine, Iron, Manganese, Molybdenum, Nickel, Silicon, Vanadium, and Zinc. Washington, D.C.: National Academy Press. Copyright © 1998 by the National Academy of Sciences. Reprinted with permission from National Academy Press, Washington, D.C.

Nutrition Resources

Table 2	Tolerable Nutrient Upper Intake Levels for Adults
Nutrient	**Upper Intake Level**
Calcium	2,500 mg/day
Phosphorus	4,000 mg/day
Magnesium (nonfood sources)	350 mg/day
Vitamin D	50 μg/day
Fluoride	10 mg/day
Niacin	35 mg/day
Vitamin B-6	100 mg/day
Folate	1,000 μg/day
Choline	3,500 mg/day
Vitamin C	2,000 mg/day
Vitamin E	1,000 mg/day
Selenium	400 μg/day
Vitamin A	3,000 μg/day
Boron	20 mg/day
Copper	10,000 μg/day
Iodine	1,100 μg/day
Iron	45 mg/day
Manganese	11 mg/day
Molybdenum	2,000 μg/day
Nickel	1.0 mg/day
Vanadium	1.8 mg/day
Zinc	40 mg/day

This table includes the adult Tolerable Upper Intake Level (UL) standard of the Dietary Reference Intakes (DRIs). For some nutrients, there is insufficient data on which to develop a UL. This does not mean that there is no potential for adverse effects from high intake, and when data about adverse effects are limited, extra caution may be warranted. In healthy individuals, there is no established benefit from nutrient intakes above the RDA or AI:

SOURCES: Food and Nutrition Board, National Academy of Sciences. 1997. *Dietary Reference Intakes for Calcium, Phosphorus, Magnesium, Vitamin D, and Fluoride.* Washington, D.C.: National Academy Press. Food and Nutrition Board, National Academy of Sciences. 1998. *Dietary Reference Intakes for Thiamin, Riboflavin, Niacin, Vitamin B₆, Folate, Vitamin B₁₂, Pantothenic Acid, Biotin, and Choline.* Washington, D.C.: National Academy Press. Food and Nutrition Board, National Academy of Sciences. 2000. *Dietary Reference Intakes for Vitamin C, Vitamin E, Selenium, and Carotenoids.* Washington, D.C.: National Academy Press. Food and Nutrition Board, National Academy of Sciences. 2001. *Dietary Reference Intakes for Vitamin A, Vitamin K, Arsenic, Boron, Chromium, Copper, Iodine, Iron, Manganese, Molybdenum, Nickel, Silicon, Vanadium, and Zinc.* Washington, D.C.: National Academy Press. Copyright © 1998 by the National Academy of Sciences. Reprinted with permission from National Academy Press, Washington, D.C.

Table 3	Recommended Dietary Allowances, Revised 1989[a,b] (Abridged)	
Category	**Age (years) or Condition**	**Protein (g/kg)[c]**
Infants	0.0–0.5	2.2
	0.5–1.0	1.6
Children	1–3	1.2
	4–6	1.1
	7–10	1.0
Males	11–14	1.0
	15–18	0.9
	19–24	0.8
	25–50	0.8
	51+	0.8
Females	11–14	1.0
	15–18	0.8
	19–24	0.8
	25–50	0.8
	51+	0.8
Pregnant		+10g
Lactating	1st 6 Months	+15g
	2nd 6 Months	+12g

[a]This table includes RDAs for those nutrients for which DRIs had not yet been established as of June 2001. The allowances, expressed as average daily intakes over time, are intended to provide for individual variations among most normal people as they live in the United States under usual environmental stresses. Diet should be based on a variety of common foods in order to provide other nutrients for which human requirements have been less well defined.
[b]Estimated Minimum Requirements of healthy adults: 500 mg sodium; 750 mg chloride; 2000 mg potassium. (For information on other age groups, see *Recommended Dietary Allowances*, 10th ed.)
[c]The RDA for protein is expressed as grams of protein per kilogram of body weight. To calculate the RDA, multiply body weight in kilograms (1 kilogram = 2.2 pounds) by the appropriate number from the protein column. For example, a 19-year-old male who weighs 165 pounds would calculate his protein RDA as follows: 165 lb ÷ 2.2 kg/lb = 75 kg × 0.8 g/kg (from table) = 60 g protein per day. For pregnant or lactating women, calculate RDA based on age and then add the appropriate number of additional grams listed in the table.

SOURCE: Reprinted with permission from *Recommended Dietary Allowances:* 10th Edition. Copyright © 1989 by the National Academy of Sciences. Courtesy of the National Academy Press, Washington, D.C.

Table 4	One Day's Menu and Food Group Servings at Three Calorie Levels

		Calorie Level		
		1600	**2200**	**2800**
Breakfast	Cantaloupe	¼ medium	¼ medium	¼ medium
	Whole-wheat pancakes	2	2	3
	Blueberry sauce	¼ cup	¼ cup	6 tablespoons
	Margarine		1 teaspoon	2 teaspoons
	Turkey patty		1½ ounces	1½ ounces
	Milk	skim, 1 cup	skim, 1 cup	2%, 1 cup
Lunch	Chili-stuffed baked potato	¾ cup chili, 1 potato	¾ cup chili, 1 potato	¾ cup chili, 1 potato
	Low-fat, low-sodium cheddar cheese		3 tablespoons	3 tablespoons
	Spinach-orange salad	1 cup	1 cup	1 cup
	Wheat crackers	6	6	6
	Grapes			12
	Fig bars			2
	Milk		skim, 1 cup	2%, 1 cup
Dinner	Apricot-glazed chicken	1 breast half	1 breast half	1 breast half
	Rice-pasta pilaf	¾ cup	¾ cup	¾ cup
	Steamed zucchini			½ cup
	Tossed salad	1 cup	1 cup	1 cup
	Reduced-calorie Italian dressing	1 tablespoon	1 tablespoon	
	Regular Italian dressing			1 tablespoon
	Hard roll(s)	1 small	2 small	2 small
	Margarine		2 teaspoons	2 teaspoons
	Vanilla ice milk	½ cup	½ cup	½ cup
Snacks	Fig bar	1		
	Skim milk	¾ cup		
	Apple		½ medium	½ medium
	Soft pretzel		1 large	1 large
	Lemonade			1 cup
	2% fat milk			1 cup
Number of Servings	Bread group	6	9	11
	Vegetable group	4¼	4¼	5¼
	Fruit group	2⅓	2¾	4
	Milk group	2	2⅔	3⅔
	Meat group (ounces)	5½	7	7
Nutrient Data	Calories	1,665	2,199	2,859
	Fat*, grams (percent calories)	38 (20%)	59 (24%)	87 (27%)
	Saturated fat*, grams (percent calories)	11 (6%)	17 (7%)	27 (8%)
	Cholesterol, mg	183	236	309
	Sodium, mg	1861	3138	3508
	Dietary fiber, g	23	25	31

*Values have been rounded to the nearest whole number.

SOURCE: Shaw, A., et al. 1997. *Using the Food Guide Pyramid: A Resource for Health Educators.* Washington, D.C.: U.S. Department of Agriculture.

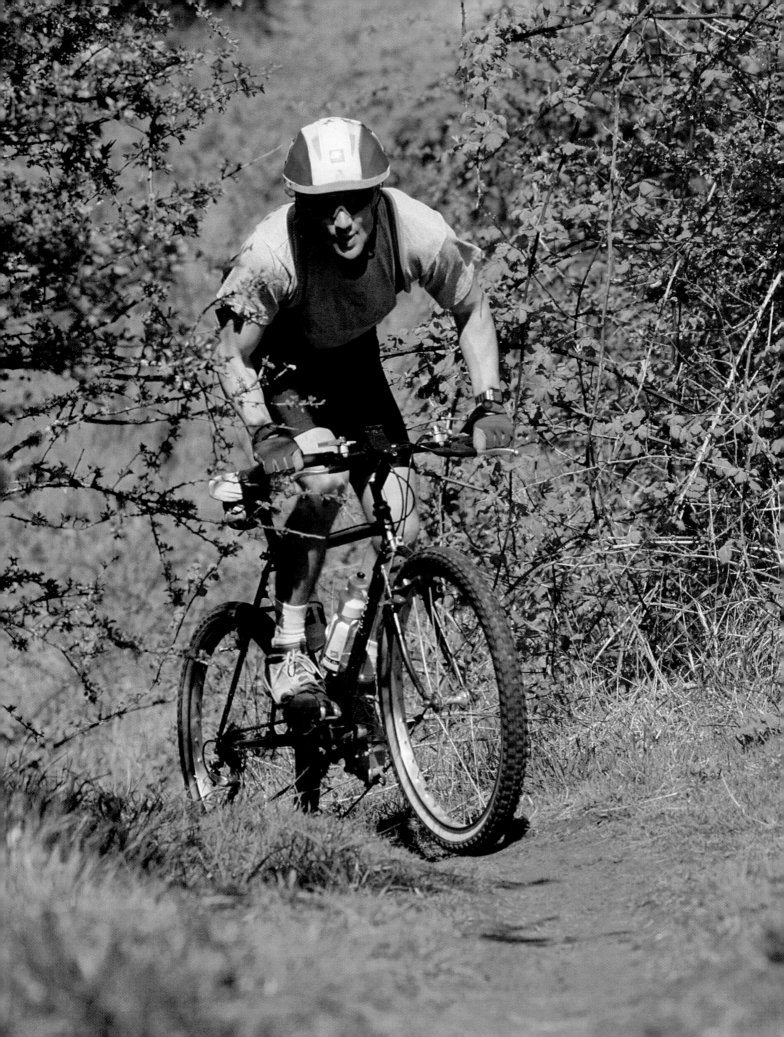

After reading this chapter, you should be able to

- Define physical fitness, and list the health-related components of fitness

- Explain the wellness benefits of physical activity and exercise

- Describe how to develop each of the health-related components of fitness

- Discuss how to choose appropriate exercise equipment, how to eat and drink for exercise, how to assess fitness, and how to prevent and manage injuries

- Put together a personalized exercise program that you enjoy and that will enable you to achieve your fitness goals

Exercise for Health and Fitness

13

TEST YOUR KNOWLEDGE

1. Among American adults, about what percentage of trips of less than 1 mile in length are made by walking?
   a. 15%
   b. 25%
   c. 50%

2. To improve your health, you must do high-intensity exercise.
   True or false?

3. The best time to do stretching exercises is after a workout.
   True or false?

4. If you want to lose fat around your middle to have a flat stomach, you should do sit-ups.
   True or false?

5. If you stop lifting weights, your muscles will turn to fat.
   True or False?

ANSWERS

1. **A.** The vast majority of short trips are made in automobiles. Most people have many opportunities to incorporate more physical activity into their daily routine.

2. **FALSE.** Even moderate physical activity—walking the dog or doing yard work—has significant health benefits.

3. **TRUE.** Your muscles can stretch farther with a lower risk of injury when they are warm, so it's best to do stretching as part of your cool-down after cardiorespiratory endurance exercise or strength training.

4. **FALSE.** The energy burned by sit-ups comes from fat stores throughout the body, not just from the abdomen, so sit-ups are no better at trimming fat from your stomach than any other calisthenic exercise.

5. **FALSE.** Muscles that aren't used become smaller, and body fat may increase if calorie intake exceeds calories burned. But fat and muscle are different tissues, and these changes are caused by two separate processes.

Your body is a wonderful moving machine. Your bones, joints, and ligaments provide a support system for movement; your muscles perform the motions of work and play; your heart and lungs nourish your cells as you move through your daily life. But your body is made to work best when it is physically active. It readily adapts to practically any level of activity and exercise: The more you ask of your body—your muscles, bones, heart, lungs—the stronger and more fit it becomes. The opposite is also true. Left unchallenged, bones lose their density, joints stiffen, muscles become weak, and cellular energy systems begin to degenerate. To be truly healthy, human beings must be active.

The benefits of physical activity are both physical and mental, immediate and far-reaching. Being physically fit makes it easier to do everyday tasks, such as lifting; it provides reserve strength for emergencies; and it helps people to look and feel good. Over the long term, physically fit individuals are less likely to develop heart disease, cancer, high blood pressure, diabetes, and many other degenerative diseases. Their cardiorespiratory systems tend to resemble those of people 10 or more years younger than themselves. As they get older, they may be able to avoid weight gain, muscle and bone loss, fatigue, memory loss, and other problems associated with aging. With a healthy heart, strong muscles, a lean body, and a repertoire of physical skills they can call on for recreation and enjoyment, fit people can maintain their physical and mental well-being throughout their entire lives.

Unfortunately, modern life for most Americans provides few built-in occasions for vigorous activity. Technological advances have made our lives increasingly sedentary: We drive cars, ride escalators, watch television, and push papers around at school and work. According to *Healthy People 2010,* levels of physical activity remain low for all populations of Americans (Figure 13-1). In 1996, the U.S. Surgeon General published *Physical Activity and Health,* a report designed to reverse these trends and get Americans moving. The report's conclusions include the following:

- People of all ages, both male and female, benefit from regular physical activity.

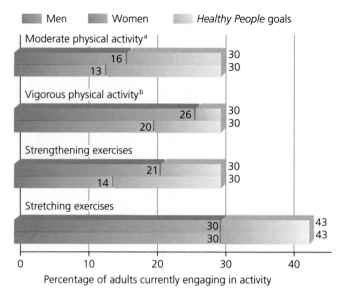

VITAL STATISTICS

Figure 13-1 Current levels of physical activity among American adults. SOURCE: U.S. Department of Health and Human Services. 2000. *Healthy People 2010.* Conference Edition. Washington, D.C.: DHHS.

- People can obtain significant health benefits by including a moderate amount of physical activity on most, if not all, days of the week. Through a modest increase in daily activity, most Americans can improve their health and quality of life.

- Additional health benefits can be gained through greater amounts of physical activity. People who can maintain a regular regimen of more vigorous or longer-duration activity are likely to obtain even greater benefits.

- Physical activity reduces the risk of premature mortality, improves psychological health, and is important for the health of muscle, bones, and joints.

Are you one of the 60% of Americans who are not regularly active? Or one of the 25% who are not active at all? This chapter will give you the basic information you need to put together a physical fitness program that will work for you. If approached correctly, physical activity can contribute immeasurably to overall wellness, add fun and joy to life, and provide the foundation for a lifetime of fitness.

WHAT IS PHYSICAL FITNESS?

Physical fitness is a set of physical attributes that allows the body to respond or adapt to the demands and stress of physical effort—that is, to perform moderate-to-vigorous levels of physical activity without becoming overly tired. Physical fitness has many components, some related to general health and others related more specifically to

Terms

physical fitness A set of physical attributes that allows the body to respond or adapt to the demands and stress of physical effort.

cardiorespiratory endurance The ability of the body to perform prolonged, large-muscle, dynamic exercise at moderate-to-high levels of intensity.

muscular strength The amount of force a muscle can produce with a single maximum effort.

muscular endurance The ability of a muscle or group of muscles to remain contracted or to contract repeatedly for a long period of time.

particular sports or activities. The five components of fitness most important for health are cardiorespiratory endurance, muscular strength, muscular endurance, flexibility, and body composition (proportion of fat to fat-free mass).

Cardiorespiratory Endurance

Cardiorespiratory endurance is the ability to perform prolonged, large-muscle, dynamic exercise at moderate-to-high levels of intensity. It depends on such factors as the ability of the lungs to deliver oxygen from the environment to the bloodstream, the heart's capacity to pump blood, the ability of the nervous system and blood vessels to regulate blood flow, the muscles' capacity to generate power, and the capability of the body's chemical systems to use oxygen and process fuels for exercise.

When levels of cardiorespiratory fitness are low, the heart has to work very hard during normal daily activities and may not be able to work hard enough to sustain high-intensity physical activity in an emergency. As cardiorespiratory fitness improves, the heart begins to function more efficiently. It doesn't have to work as hard at rest or during low levels of exercise. The heart pumps more blood per heartbeat, resting heart rate slows down, blood volume increases, blood supply to the tissues improves, the body is better able to cool itself, and resting blood pressure decreases. A healthy heart can better withstand the strains of everyday life, the stress of occasional emergencies, and the wear and tear of time. Endurance training also improves the functioning of biochemical systems, particularly in the muscles and liver, thereby enhancing the body's ability to use energy supplied by food and to do more exercise with less effort from the oxygen transport system.

Cardiorespiratory endurance is considered a critically important component of health-related fitness because the functioning of the heart and lungs is so essential to overall wellness. A person simply cannot live very long or very well without a healthy heart. Low levels of cardiorespiratory fitness are linked with heart disease, the leading cause of death in the United States. Cardiorespiratory endurance is developed by activities that involve continuous rhythmic movements of large-muscle groups like those in the legs—for example, walking, jogging, cycling, and aerobic dance.

Muscular Strength

Muscular strength is the amount of force a muscle can produce with a single maximum effort. Strong, powerful muscles are important for the smooth and easy performance of everyday activities, such as carrying groceries, lifting boxes, and climbing stairs, as well as for emergency situations. They help keep the skeleton in proper alignment, preventing back and leg pain and providing the support necessary for good posture. Muscular strength has obvious importance in recreational activities. Strong

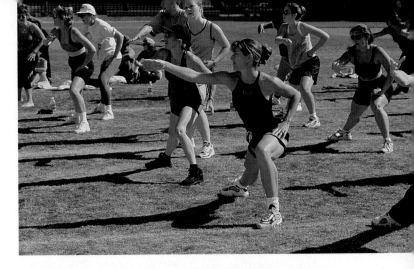

Cardiorespiratory endurance exercise conditions the heart, improves the function of the entire cardiorespiratory system, and has many other health benefits. An effective personal fitness program should be built around an activity like running, walking, biking, swimming, or group exercises such as aerobic dance or martial arts workouts.

people can hit a tennis ball harder, kick a soccer ball farther, and ride a bicycle uphill more easily.

Muscle tissue is an important element of overall body composition. Greater muscle mass makes possible a higher rate of metabolism and faster energy use, which help to maintain a healthy body weight. Maintaining strength and muscle mass is vital for healthy aging. Older people tend to lose muscle cells, and many of the remaining muscle cells become nonfunctional because they lose their attachment to the nervous system. Strength training helps maintain muscle mass and function in older people, which greatly enhances their quality of life and prevents life-threatening injuries. Strength training has also been shown to benefit cardiovascular health. Muscular strength can be developed by training with weights or by using the weight of the body for resistance during calisthenic exercises such as push-ups and sit-ups.

Muscular Endurance

Muscular endurance is the ability to sustain a given level of muscle tension—that is, to hold a muscle contraction for a long period of time, or to contract a muscle over and over again. Muscular endurance is important for good posture and for injury prevention. For example, if abdominal and back muscles are not strong enough to hold the spine correctly, the chances of low-back pain and back injury are increased. Muscular endurance helps people cope with the physical demands of everyday life and enhances performance in sports and work. It is also important for most leisure and fitness activities. Like muscular strength, muscular endurance is developed by stressing the muscles with a greater load (weight) than they are used to. The degree to which strength or endurance develops depends on the type and amount of stress that is applied.

Flexibility

Flexibility is the ability to move the joints through their full range of motion. Although range of motion is not a significant factor in everyday activities for most people, inactivity causes the joints to become stiffer with age. Stiffness often causes older people to assume unnatural body postures, and it can lead to back, shoulder, or neck pain. The majority of Americans experience low-back pain at some time in their lives, often because of stiff joints. Stretching exercises can help ensure a normal range of motion.

Body Composition

Body composition refers to the proportion of fat and fat-free mass (muscle, bone, and water) in the body. Healthy body composition involves a high proportion of fat-free mass and an acceptably low level of body fat. A person with excessive body fat is more likely to experience a variety of health problems, including heart disease, high blood pressure, stroke, joint problems, diabetes, gallbladder disease, cancer, and back pain. The best way to lose fat is through a lifestyle that includes a sensible diet and exercise. The best way to add muscle mass is through resistance training such as weight training. (Body composition is discussed in more detail in Chapter 14.)

In addition to these five health-related components of physical fitness, physical fitness for a particular sport or activity might include any or all of the following: coordination, speed, reaction time, agility, balance, and skill. Sport-specific skills are best developed through practice. The skill and coordination needed to play basketball, for example, are developed by playing basketball.

THE BENEFITS OF EXERCISE

As mentioned above, the human body is very adaptable. The greater the demands made on it, the more it adjusts to meet the demands—it becomes fit. Over time, immediate, short-term adjustments translate into long-term changes and improvements (Figure 13-2). For example, when breathing and heart rate increase during exercise, the heart gradually develops the ability to pump more blood with each beat. Then, during exercise, it doesn't have to beat as fast to meet the body's demand for oxygen.

Terms

flexibility The range of motion in a joint or group of joints; flexibility is related to muscle length.

body composition The proportion of fat and fat-free mass (muscle, bone, and water) in the body.

cardiovascular disease (CVD) A collective term for diseases of the heart and blood vessels.

The goal of regular physical activity is to bring about these kinds of long-term changes and improvements in the body's functioning.

Scientists have been actively studying these effects of exercise and their impact on health for over 40 years. They have found that exercise is one of the most important things you can do to improve your level of wellness. Regular exercise increases energy levels, improves emotional and psychological well-being, and boosts the immune system. It prevents heart disease, some types of cancer, stroke, high blood pressure, insulin resistance, Type 2 diabetes, obesity, and osteoporosis. At any age, people who exercise are less likely to die from all causes than their sedentary peers.

Improved Cardiorespiratory Functioning

Every time you take a breath, some of the oxygen in the air you take into your lungs is picked up by red blood cells and transported to your heart. From there, this oxygenated blood is pumped by the heart throughout the body to organs and tissues that use it. During exercise, the cardiorespiratory system (heart, lungs, and circulatory system) must work harder to meet the body's increased demand for oxygen. Regular endurance exercise improves the functioning of the heart and the ability of the cardiorespiratory system to carry oxygen to body tissues. It also reduces the risk of cardiovascular disease.

More Efficient Metabolism

Endurance exercise improves metabolism, the process by which food is converted to energy and tissue is built. This process involves oxygen, nutrients, hormones, and enzymes. A physically fit person is better able to generate energy, to use carbohydrates and fats for energy, and to regulate hormones. Physical training may also protect the body's cells from damage from free radicals, which are produced during normal metabolism (see Chapter 12). Training activates antioxidant enzymes that prevent free radical damage and maintain the health of the body's cells.

Improved Body Composition

Healthy body composition means that the body has a high proportion of fat-free mass (primarily composed of muscle) and a relatively small proportion of fat. Too much body fat is linked to a variety of health problems, including heart disease, cancer, and diabetes. Healthy body composition can be difficult to achieve and maintain because a diet that contains all essential nutrients can be relatively high in calories, especially for someone who is sedentary. Excess calories are stored in the body as fat.

Exercise can improve body composition in several ways. Endurance exercise significantly increases daily calorie expenditure; it can also slightly raise *metabolic*

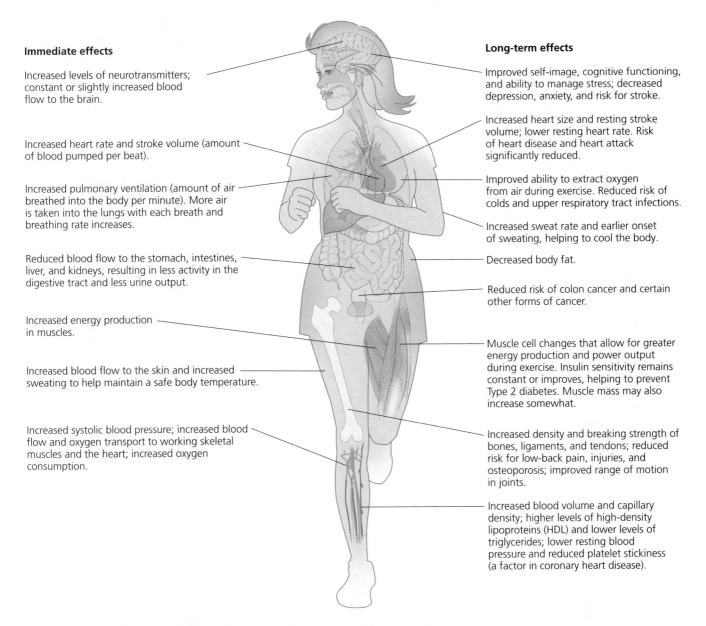

Immediate effects

Increased levels of neurotransmitters; constant or slightly increased blood flow to the brain.

Increased heart rate and stroke volume (amount of blood pumped per beat).

Increased pulmonary ventilation (amount of air breathed into the body per minute). More air is taken into the lungs with each breath and breathing rate increases.

Reduced blood flow to the stomach, intestines, liver, and kidneys, resulting in less activity in the digestive tract and less urine output.

Increased energy production in muscles.

Increased blood flow to the skin and increased sweating to help maintain a safe body temperature.

Increased systolic blood pressure; increased blood flow and oxygen transport to working skeletal muscles and the heart; increased oxygen consumption.

Long-term effects

Improved self-image, cognitive functioning, and ability to manage stress; decreased depression, anxiety, and risk for stroke.

Increased heart size and resting stroke volume; lower resting heart rate. Risk of heart disease and heart attack significantly reduced.

Improved ability to extract oxygen from air during exercise. Reduced risk of colds and upper respiratory tract infections.

Increased sweat rate and earlier onset of sweating, helping to cool the body.

Decreased body fat.

Reduced risk of colon cancer and certain other forms of cancer.

Muscle cell changes that allow for greater energy production and power output during exercise. Insulin sensitivity remains constant or improves, helping to prevent Type 2 diabetes. Muscle mass may also increase somewhat.

Increased density and breaking strength of bones, ligaments, and tendons; reduced risk for low-back pain, injuries, and osteoporosis; improved range of motion in joints.

Increased blood volume and capillary density; higher levels of high-density lipoproteins (HDL) and lower levels of triglycerides; lower resting blood pressure and reduced platelet stickiness (a factor in coronary heart disease).

Figure 13-2   Immediate and long-term effects of regular exercise.   When exercise is performed regularly, short-term changes in the body develop into more permanent adaptations; these long-term effects include improved ability to exercise, reduced risk of many chronic diseases, improved psychological and emotional well-being, and increased life expectancy.

rate, the rate at which the body burns calories, for several hours after an exercise session. Strength training increases muscle mass, thereby tipping the body composition ratio toward fat-free mass and away from fat. It can also help with losing fat because metabolic rate is directly proportional to fat-free mass: The more muscle mass, the higher the metabolic rate. (Metabolism, energy balance, and the role of exercise in improving body composition are discussed in detail in Chapter 14.)

Disease Prevention and Management

Regular physical activity lowers your risk of many chronic, disabling diseases. It can also help people with those diseases improve their health.

Cardiovascular Disease   A sedentary lifestyle is one of the six major risk factors for **cardiovascular disease (CVD)** (see Chapter 15). The others are smoking, unhealthy cholesterol levels, high blood pressure, diabetes, and obesity. People who are sedentary have CVD death rates significantly higher than those of fit individuals. There is a dose-response relationship between exercise and CVD: The benefit of physical activity occurs at moderate levels of activity and increases with increasing levels of activity. Many research studies have shown conclusively that exercise not only affects the risk factors for CVD but also directly interferes with the disease process itself.

BLOOD FAT LEVELS   Endurance exercise and strength training have a positive effect on the balance of lipids that circulate in the blood. High concentrations of lipids such as cholesterol and triglycerides are linked to heart disease because they contribute to the formation of fatty deposits on the linings of arteries. When such deposits block an artery, a heart attack or stroke can occur.

Cholesterol is carried in the blood by **lipoproteins,** which are classified according to size and density. Cholesterol carried by low-density lipoproteins (LDLs) tends to stick to the walls of coronary arteries. High-density lipoproteins (HDLs) tend to pick up excess cholesterol in the bloodstream and carry it back to the liver for excretion from the body. High LDL levels and low HDL levels are associated with a high risk of cardiovascular disease. High levels of HDL and low levels of LDL are associated with lower risk.

More information about cholesterol and heart disease is provided in Chapter 15. For our purposes in this chapter, it is important to know only that endurance exercise and strength training influence blood lipid, or fat, levels in a positive way, by increasing HDL and decreasing LDL and triglycerides—thereby helping to reduce the risk of CVD.

HIGH BLOOD PRESSURE   Regular endurance exercise tends to reduce high blood pressure, a contributing factor in diseases such as coronary heart disease, stroke, kidney failure, and blindness. People who exercise for a longer duration and at a higher intensity receive the greatest benefit, but even moderate exercise can produce significant improvements. Recent studies have found that strength training also reduces blood pressure.

CORONARY HEART DISEASE   Coronary heart disease (CHD) involves blockage of one of the coronary arteries. These blood vessels supply the heart with oxygenated blood, and an obstruction in one of them can cause a heart attack. Exercise directly interferes with the disease process that causes coronary artery blockage. It also enhances the

function of cells lining the arteries that help regulate blood flow. Finally, exercise minimizes other risk factors—such as obesity, high blood pressure, and blood fat levels—that contribute to CHD.

STROKE   A stroke occurs when a blood vessel leading to the brain is blocked, often through the same disease process that leads to heart attacks. Regular exercise reduces the risk of stroke.

Cancer   Some studies have shown a relationship between increased physical activity and a reduction in a person's risk of all types of cancer, but these findings are not conclusive. There is strong evidence that exercise reduces the risk of colon cancer, and promising data that it reduces the risk of cancer of the breast and reproductive organs in women and cancer of the prostate in men. Exercise may decrease the risk of colon cancer by speeding the movement of food through the gastrointestinal tract (quickly eliminating potential carcinogens), enhancing immune function, and reducing blood fats. The protective mechanism in the case of reproductive system cancers is less clear, but physical activity during the high school and college years may be particularly important for preventing breast cancer later in life.

Osteoporosis   A special benefit of exercise, especially for women, is protection against osteoporosis, a disease that results in loss of bone density and poor bone strength. Weight-bearing exercise, which includes almost everything except swimming, helps build bone during the teens and twenties. Older people with denser bones can better endure the bone loss that occurs with aging. Strength training can increase bone density throughout life. With stronger bones and muscles and better balance, fit people are less likely to experience debilitating falls and bone fractures. (But too much exercise can depress levels of estrogen, which helps maintain bone density, thereby leading to bone loss, even in young women.)

Diabetes   People with diabetes are prone to heart disease, blindness, and severe problems of the nervous and circulatory systems. Recent studies have shown that exercise actually prevents the development of Type 2 diabetes, the most common form. Exercise burns excess sugar and makes cells more sensitive to insulin. Exercise also helps keep body fat at healthy levels. (Obesity is a key risk factor for Type 2 diabetes.) For people who have diabetes, physical activity is an important part of treatment. (See Chapter 14 for more on diabetes.)

Improved Psychological and Emotional Wellness

The joy of a well-hit cross-court backhand, the euphoria of a walk through the park, or the rush of a downhill schuss through deep snow powder provides pleasure that transcends health benefits alone. People who are physi-

Terms   **lipoproteins** Substances in blood, classified according to size, density, and chemical composition, that transport fats.

endorphins Brain chemicals that seem to be involved in modulating pain and producing euphoria.

neurotransmitters Brain chemicals that transmit nerve impulses.

If you've ever gone for a long, brisk walk after a hard day's work, you know how refreshing exercise can be. Exercise can improve mood, stimulate creativity, clarify thinking, relieve anxiety, and provide an outlet for anger or aggression. But why does exercise make you feel good? Does it simply take your mind off your problems? Or does it cause a physical reaction that affects your mental state?

Current research indicates that exercise triggers many physical changes in the body that can alter mood. Scientists are now trying to explain how and why exercise affects the mind. One theory has to do with the physical structure of the brain. The area of the brain responsible for the movement of muscles is near the area responsible for thought and emotion. As muscles work vigorously, the resulting stimulation in the muscle center of the brain may also stimulate the thought and emotion center, producing improvements in mood and cognitive functions.

Other researchers suggest that exercise stimulates the release of **endorphins,** chemicals in the brain that can suppress fatigue, decrease pain, and produce euphoria. The "runner's high" often experienced after running several miles may be due to an increased production of endorphins.

A third area of research focuses on changes in brain activity during and after exercise. One change is an increase in alpha brain wave activity. Alpha waves indicate a highly relaxed state; meditation also induces alpha wave activity. A second change is an alteration in the levels of **neurotransmitters,** brain chemicals that increase alertness and reduce stress.

Higher levels of neurotransmitters such as serotonin may explain how exercise improves mild to moderate cases of depression. Researchers have found that exercise can be as effective as psychotherapy in treating depression, and even more effective when used in conjunction with other therapies. In addition to boosting neurotransmitter activity, exercise provides a distraction from stressful stimuli, enhances self-esteem, and may provide opportunity for positive social interactions.

Another benefit of regular exercise is improved self-esteem and body image. According to a recent study, women who worked out on a regular basis rated their bodies as more attractive and healthy than did sedentary women. They actually weighed an average of 11–12 pounds more than the less active women, suggesting that active women are more comfortable bucking cultural ideals of body shape. Other studies have found that athletes tend to have more positive images of their bodies than nonathletes, regardless of gender, sport, or level of expertise.

Although most people don't associate exercise with mental skills, physical activity has been shown to have positive effects on cognitive functioning in both the short term and the long term. Exercise improves alertness and memory and can help you perform cognitive tasks at your peak level. Exercise may also help boost creativity. In a study of college students, those who ran regularly or took aerobic dance classes scored significantly higher on standard psychological tests of creativity than sedentary students. Over the long term, exercise can slow and possibly even reverse certain age-related declines in cognitive performance, including slowed reaction time and loss of short-term memory and nonverbal reasoning skills.

The message from this research is that exercise is a critical factor in developing *all* the dimensions of wellness, not just physical health. Even moderate exercise like walking briskly a few times per week can significantly improve your well-being. A lifetime of physical activity can leave you with a healthier body and a sharper, happier, more creative mind.

---

cally active experience many social, psychological, and emotional benefits. For example:

- *Reduced stress.* In response to stressors, physically fit people experience milder physical responses and less emotional distress than sedentary individuals. Physical activity also provides protection against the effects of stress that have been linked to poor cardiorespiratory health. Psychological stress causes increased secretion of epinephrine and norepinephrine, the so-called fight-or-flight hormones, which are thought to speed the development of atherosclerosis, or hardening of the arteries. Excessive hostility is also associated with a risk of heart disease. Endurance exercise decreases the secretion of hormones triggered by emotional stress. It also can diffuse hostility and alleviate feelings of stress and anxiety by providing an emotional outlet and inducing feelings of relaxation. Regular exercise can also relieve sleeping problems.

- *Reduced anxiety and depression.* Sedentary adults have a much higher risk of feeling fatigue and depression than those who are physically active. Exercise is an effective treatment for people with depression and improves mood in nondepressed people who feel fine or who feel a little bit "down."

- *Improved self-image.* Performing physical activities provides proof of skill and self-control, thus enhancing self-concept. Exercise also helps you look and feel better, boosting self-confidence and body image.

- *Enjoyment.* Exercise is fun! It offers an arena for harmonious interaction with other people, as well as opportunities to strive and excel. Physically fit people can perform everyday tasks—such as climbing stairs and carrying books or groceries—with ease. They have plenty of energy and can lead lives that are full and varied.

For more on the psychological benefits of physical activity, see the box "Exercise and the Mind."

Improved Immune Function

Exercise can have either positive or negative effects on the immune system, the physiological processes that protect us from disease. It appears that moderate endurance exer-

Physical fitness and athletic achievement are not limited to the able-bodied. People with disabilities can also attain high levels of fitness and performance, as shown by the elite athletes who compete in the Paralympics. The premier event for athletes with disabilities, the Paralympics are held in the same year and city as the Olympics. The athletes who participate include people with cerebral palsy, people with visual impairments, paraplegics, quadriplegics, and others. They compete in wheelchair races and wheelchair basketball, tandem cycling, in which a blind cyclist pedals with a sighted athlete, and other events. The performance of these skilled athletes makes it clear that people with disabilities can be active, healthy, and extraordinarily fit; just like able-bodied athletes, athletes with disabilities strive for excellence and can serve as role models.

Currently, some 50 million Americans are estimated to have chronic, significant disabilities. Some disabilities are the result of injury, such as spinal cord injuries sustained in car crashes. Other disabilities result from illness, such as the blindness that sometimes occurs as a complication of diabetes or the joint stiffness that accompanies arthritis. And some disabilities are present at birth, as in the case of congenital limb deformities or cerebral palsy.

Exercise and physical activity are as important for people with disabilities as for able-bodied individuals—if not *more* important. Being active helps prevent secondary conditions that may result from prolonged inactivity, such as circulatory or muscular problems. It provides an emotional boost that helps support a positive attitude as well as opportunities to make new friends, increase self-confidence, and gain a sense of accomplishment. Currently, about 12% of people with disabilities engage in regular moderate activity.

People with disabilities don't have to be elite athletes to participate in sports and lead an active life. Some health clubs offer activities and events geared for people of all ages and types of disabilities. They may have modified aerobics classes, special weight training machines, classes involving mild exercise in warm water, and other activities adapted for people with disabilities. Popular sports and recreational activities include adapted horseback riding, golf, swimming, and skiing. Competitive sports are also available—for example, there are wheelchair versions of billiards, tennis, hockey, and basketball, as well as sports for people with hearing, visual, or mental impairments. For those who prefer to get their exercise at home, special videos are available geared to individuals who use wheelchairs or who have arthritis, hearing impairments, or many other disabilities.

If you have a disability and want to be more active, check with your physician about what's appropriate for you. Call your local community center, YMCA/YWCA, independent living center, or health club to locate potential facilities; look for a club or facility with experienced personnel and appropriate adaptive equipment. For specialized videos, check with hospitals and health associations that are geared to specific disabilities, such as the Arthritis Foundation. Remember that no matter what your level of ability or disability, it's possible to make physical activity an integral part of your life.

SOURCES: U.S. Department of Health and Human Services. 2000. *Healthy People 2010.* 2nd ed. Washington, D.C.: DHHS. National Center on Physical Activity and Disability. 2000. *White Paper: Spinal Cord Injury and Fitness.* Chicago: National Center on Physical Activity and Disability. U.S. Department of Health and Human Services. 1996. *Physical Activity and Health: A Report of the Surgeon General.* Atlanta, Ga.: DHHS.

---

cise boosts immune function, while excessive training depresses it. Physically fit people get fewer colds and upper respiratory tract infections than people who are not fit. The immune system—and ways to strengthen it—are discussed further in Chapter 17.

Prevention of Injuries and Low-Back Pain

Increased muscle strength provides protection against injury because it helps people maintain good posture and appropriate body mechanics when carrying out everyday activities like walking, lifting, and carrying. Strong muscles in the abdomen, hips, low back, and legs support the back in proper alignment and help prevent low-back pain, which afflicts over 85% of all Americans at some time in their lives.

Improved Wellness over the Life Span

Although people differ in the maximum levels of fitness they can achieve through exercise, the wellness benefits of

exercise are available to everyone (see the box "Fitness and Disability"). Exercising regularly may be the single most important thing you can do now to improve the quality of your life in the future. All the benefits of exercise continue to accrue but gain new importance as the resilience of youth begins to wane. Simply stated, exercising can help you live a longer and healthier life.

> **COMMUNICATE!**   Taking a walk at lunchtime can provide a healthful break from the mental stress and sedentary nature of many jobs, including the job of being a student. Try asking a colleague or fellow student to come along with you; it's usually easier to exercise with a friend. For example, "I need a break—want to go for a walk with me? We could walk to the park and back in about 15 minutes. Come on—it'll clear our heads and we'll work twice as hard when we get back!"

The best exercise program has two primary characteristics: It promotes your health, and it's fun for you to do. Exercise does not have to be a chore. On the contrary, it can provide some of the most pleasurable moments of your day, once you make it a habit. A little thought and planning will help you achieve these goals.

Physical Activity and Exercise for Health and Fitness

Physical activity can be defined as any body movement carried out by skeletal muscles and requiring energy. Different types of physical activity can be arranged on a continuum based on the amount of energy they require. Quick, easy movements such as standing up or walking down a hallway require little energy or effort; more intense, sustained activities such as cycling 5 miles or running in a race require considerably more.

The term *exercise* is usually used to refer to a subset of physical activity—planned, structured, repetitive movement of the body designed specifically to improve or maintain physical fitness. As described earlier, levels of fitness depend on physiological factors such as the heart's ability to pump blood. To develop fitness, a person must perform a sufficient amount of physical activity to stress the body and cause long-term physiological changes. The precise type and amount of activity required to develop fitness will be discussed in greater detail later in the chapter. For now, just remember that only some types of physical activity—what is commonly referred to as exercise—will develop fitness. This distinction is important for setting goals and developing a program.

Lifestyle Physical Activity for Health Promotion The Surgeon General's report recommends that all Americans include a moderate amount of physical activity on most, preferably all, days of the week. The report suggests a goal of expending 150 calories per day, or about 1000 calories per week, in physical activity. Because energy expenditure is a function of both intensity and duration of activity, the same amount of benefit can be obtained in longer sessions of moderate-intensity activities as in shorter sessions of more strenuous activities. Thus, 15 minutes of running is equivalent to 30 minutes of brisk walking (Figure 13-3).

In this lifestyle approach to physical activity, the daily total of activity can be accumulated in multiple short bouts—for example, two 10-minute bicycle rides to and from class and a brisk 15-minute walk to the post office. Everyday tasks at school, work, and home can be structured to contribute to the daily activity total (see the box "Becoming More Active"). In addition to recommending moderate-intensity physical activity, the Surgeon General's report recommends that people perform resistance training (exercising against an opposing force such as a weight) at least twice a week to build and maintain strength.

Washing and waxing a car for 45–60 minutes **Less Vigorous, More Time**
Washing windows or floors for 45–60 minutes
Playing volleyball for 45 minutes
Playing touch football for 30–45 minutes
Gardening for 30–45 minutes
Wheeling self in wheelchair for 30–40 minutes
Walking 1¾ miles in 35 minutes (20 min/mile)
Basketball (shooting baskets) for 30 minutes
Bicycling 5 miles in 30 minutes
Dancing fast (social) for 30 minutes
Pushing a stroller 1½ miles in 30 minutes
Raking leaves for 30 minutes
Walking 2 miles in 30 minutes (15 min/mile)
Water aerobics for 30 minutes
Swimming laps for 20 minutes
Wheelchair basketball for 20 minutes
Basketball (playing a game) for 15–20 minutes
Bicycling 4 miles in 15 minutes
Jumping rope for 15 minutes
Running 1½ miles in 15 minutes (10 min/mile)
Shoveling snow for 15 minutes **More Vigorous,**
Stairwalking for 15 minutes **Less Time**

Figure 13-3 Examples of moderate amounts of physical activity. A moderate amount of physical activity is roughly equivalent to physical activity that uses approximately 150 calories of energy per day, or 1000 calories per week. Some activities can be performed at various intensities; the suggested durations correspond to expected intensity of effort. SOURCE: U.S. Department of Health and Human Services. 1996. *Physical Activity and Health. A Report of the Surgeon General: At-a-Glance.* Washington, D.C.: U.S. Department of Health and Human Services.

By increasing lifestyle physical activity in accordance with the guidelines given in the Surgeon General's report, people can expect to significantly improve their health and well-being. Such a program may not, however, increase physical fitness.

Exercise Programs to Develop Physical Fitness The Surgeon General's report also summarized the benefits of more formal exercise programs. It concluded that people can obtain even greater health benefits by increasing the duration and intensity of activity. Thus a person who engages in a structured, formal exercise program designed to measurably improve physical fitness will obtain even greater improvements in quality of life and greater reductions in disease and mortality risk (Figure 13-4).

How Much Physical Activity Is Enough? Some experts feel that people get most of the health benefits of a formal exercise program simply by becoming more active over the course of the day. Others feel that the lifestyle approach sets too low an activity goal; they argue that people should exercise long and intensely enough to improve their body's capacity for exercise—that is, to improve

"Too little time" is a common excuse for not being physically active. Learning to manage your time successfully is crucial if you are to maintain a wellness lifestyle. You can begin by keeping a record of how you are currently spending your time; in your health journal, use a grid broken into blocks of 15, 20, or 30 minutes to track your daily activities. Then analyze your record: List each type of activity and the total time you engaged in it on a given day—for example, sleeping, 7 hours; eating, 1.5 hours, studying, 3 hours; and so on. Take a close look at your list of activities and prioritize them according to how important they are to you, from essential to somewhat important to not important at all.

Based on the priorities you set, make changes in your daily schedule by subtracting time from some activities in order to make time for physical activity. Look particularly carefully at your leisure time activities and your methods of transportation; these are areas where it is easy to build in physical activity. Make changes using a system of tradeoffs. For example, you may choose to reduce the total amount of time you spend playing computer games, listening to the radio, and chatting on the telephone in order to make time for an after-dinner bike ride or walk with a friend. You may decide to watch 10 fewer minutes of television in the morning in order to change your 5-minute drive to class into a 15-minute walk. In making these kinds of changes in your schedule, don't feel that you have to miss out on anything you enjoy. You can get more from less time by focusing on what you are doing and by combining activities.

The following are just a few ways to become more active:

- Take the stairs instead of the elevator or escalator.
- Walk to the mailbox, post office, store, bank, or library whenever possible.
- Park your car a mile or even just a few blocks from your destination, and walk briskly.
- Do at least one chore every day that requires physical activity: wash the windows or your car, clean your room or house, mow the lawn, rake the leaves.
- Take study or work breaks to avoid sitting for more than 30 minutes at a time. Get up and walk around the library, your office, or your home or dorm; go up and down a flight of stairs.
- Stretch when you stand in line or watch TV.
- When you take public transportation, get off one stop down the line and walk to your destination.
- Go dancing instead of to a movie.
- Walk to visit a neighbor or friend rather than calling him or her on the phone. Go for a walk while you chat.
- Put your remote controls in storage; when you want to change TV or radio stations, get up and do it by hand.
- Take the dog for a walk (or an extra walk) every day.
- Play actively with children or go for a walk pushing a stroller.
- Seize every opportunity to get up and walk around. Move more and sit less.

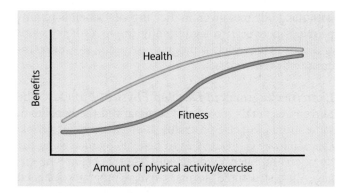

Figure 13-4   Relationship between amount of activity and health and fitness benefits.   The health benefits of physical activity and exercise exist along a continuum. A fairly low level of physical activity can provide substantial health benefits, although it does little to increase fitness. Engaging in exercise that is more intense or of longer duration leads to greater health benefits and significant increases in fitness.   SOURCE: American College of Sports Medicine. 1998. *ACSM's Resource Manual for Guidelines for Exercise Testing and Prescription,* 3rd ed. Baltimore, Md.: Williams & Wilkins, p. 440.

physical fitness. More research is needed to resolve this debate, but there is probably truth in both of these positions.

Regular physical activity, regardless of intensity, makes you healthier and can help protect you from many chronic diseases. However, exercising at low intensities does little to improve physical fitness. Although you get many of the health benefits of exercise by simply being more active, you obtain even more benefits when you are physically fit. In addition to long-term health benefits, fitness also significantly contributes to quality of life. Fitness can give you freedom—freedom to move your body the way you want. Fit people have more energy and better body control. They can enjoy a more active lifestyle—cycling, hiking, skiing, and so on—than their more sedentary counterparts. Even if you don't like sports, you need physical energy and stamina in your daily life and for many nonsport leisure activities—visiting museums, playing with children, gardening, and so on.

Where does this leave you? Most experts agree that some physical activity is better than none, but that more—as long as it does not result in injury or become

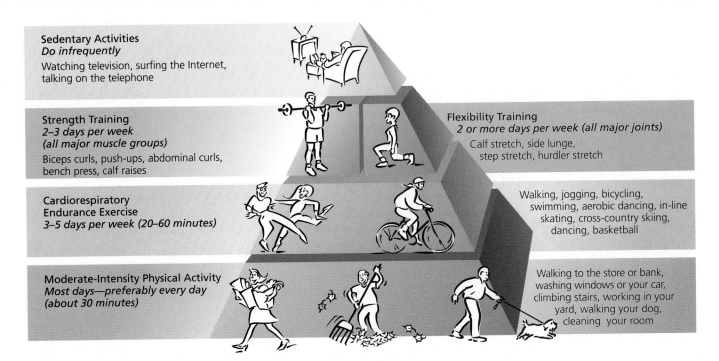

Sedentary Activities
Do infrequently
Watching television, surfing the Internet, talking on the telephone

Strength Training
2–3 days per week (all major muscle groups)
Biceps curls, push-ups, abdominal curls, bench press, calf raises

Flexibility Training
2 or more days per week (all major joints)
Calf stretch, side lunge, step stretch, hurdler stretch

Cardiorespiratory Endurance Exercise
3–5 days per week (20–60 minutes)

Walking, jogging, bicycling, swimming, aerobic dancing, in-line skating, cross-country skiing, dancing, basketball

Moderate-Intensity Physical Activity
Most days—preferably every day (about 30 minutes)

Walking to the store or bank, washing windows or your car, climbing stairs, working in your yard, walking your dog, cleaning your room

Figure 13-5 Physical activity pyramid. Similar to the Food Guide Pyramid, this physical activity pyramid is designed to help people become more active. If you are currently sedentary, begin at the bottom of the pyramid and gradually increase the amount of moderate-intensity physical activity in your life. If you are already moderately active, begin a formal exercise program that includes cardiorespiratory endurance exercise, flexibility training, and strength training to help you develop all the health-related components of fitness.

obsessive—is probably better than some. A physical activity pyramid to guide you in meeting these goals for physical activity is shown in Figure 13-5. If you are sedentary, start at the bottom of the pyramid and gradually increase the amount of moderate-intensity physical activity in your daily life. You don't have to exercise vigorously, but you should experience a moderate increase in your heart and breathing rates; appropriate activities include walking, climbing stairs, doing yard work, and washing your car. As described earlier, your activity time can be broken up into small blocks over the course of a day.

For even greater benefits, move up to the next two levels of the pyramid, which illustrate parts of a formal exercise program. The American College of Sports Medicine has established guidelines for creating an exercise program that includes **cardiorespiratory endurance (aerobic) exercise**, strength training, and flexibility training (Table 13-1). Such a program will develop all the health-related components of physical fitness. The following sections of this chapter will show you how to develop a personalized exercise program that is fun and that will enable you to enjoy all the physical and psychological benefits of physical fitness.

For a summary of the health and fitness benefits of different levels of physical activity, refer to Figure 13-6.

W. First Steps

Are you thinking about starting a formal exercise program? A little planning can help make it a success.

Medical Clearance Previously inactive men over 40 and women over 50 should get a medical examination before beginning an exercise program. Diabetes, asthma, heart disease, and extreme obesity are conditions that may call for a modified program. If you have an increased risk of heart disease because of smoking, high blood pressure, or obesity, have a physical checkup, including an **electrocardiogram (ECG or EKG)**, before beginning an exercise program. This checkup will help ensure that your program will be a benefit to your health, rather than a potential hazard.

cardiorespiratory endurance (aerobic) exercise Rhythmical, large-muscle exercise for a prolonged period of time; partially dependent on the ability of the cardiovascular system to deliver oxygen to tissues.

electrocardiogram (ECG or EKG) A recording of the changes in electrical activity of the heart.

Terms

Table 13-1   Exercise Recommendations for Healthy Adults

Exercise to Develop and Maintain Cardiorespiratory Endurance and Body Composition

Mode of activity	Any activity that uses large-muscle groups, can be maintained continuously, and is rhythmical and aerobic in nature; for example, walking-hiking, running-jogging, cycling-bicycling, cross-country skiing, aerobic dance and other forms of group exercise, rope skipping, rowing, stairclimbing, swimming, skating, and endurance game activities.
Frequency of training	3–5 days per week.
Intensity of training	55/65–90% of maximum heart rate or 40/50–85% of maximum oxygen uptake reserve. The lower intensity values (55–64% of maximum heart rate and 40–49% of maximum oxygen uptake reserve) are most applicable to individuals who are quite unfit. For average individuals, intensities of 75%–85% of maximum heart rate are appropriate; see p. 375 for instructions for determining target heart rate.
Duration of training	20–60 total minutes of continuous or intermittent (in sessions lasting 10 or more minutes) aerobic activity. Duration.is dependent on the intensity of activity; thus, lower-intensity activity should be conducted over a longer period of time (30 minutes or more). Lower-to-moderate-intensity activity of longer duration is recommended for the nonathletic adult.

Exercise to Develop and Maintain Muscular Strength and Endurance, Flexibility, and Body Composition

Resistance training	One set of 8–10 exercises that condition the major muscle groups should be performed 2–3 days per week. Most people should complete 8–12 repetitions of each exercise; for older and more frail people (approximately 50–60 years of age and above), 10–15 repetitions with a lighter weight may be more appropriate. Multiple-set regimens may provide greater benefits if time allows.
Flexibility training	Stretches for the major muscle groups should be performed a minimum of 2–3 days per week; at least four repetitions, held for 10–30 seconds, should be completed.

SOURCES: American College of Sports Medicine. 1998. ACSM position stand. The recommended quantity and quality of exercise for developing and maintaining cardiorespiratory and muscular fitness and flexibility in healthy adults. *Medicine and Science in Sports and Exercise* 30(6): 975–991.

Basic Principles of Physical Training As discussed earlier, fitness has many components; each has value and requires specific exercises. Lifting weights develops muscle strength, for example, but it does not do much to condition heart and lungs. Running is excellent for increasing cardiorespiratory capacity, but it contributes little to upper-body strength. Different sports and activities call for different skills, and to become proficient in them, you have to practice the specific movements they require. Therefore, to develop all the fitness components, you must participate in a variety of activities.

Your body adapts to the demands of exercise by improving its functioning. When the amount of exercise, also called **overload,** is progressively increased, fitness continues to improve. The amount of overload is very important. Too little exercise will have no effect on fitness; too much may cause injury. The amount of exercise needed depends on your current level of fitness, your fitness goals, and the fitness components being developed. A novice, for example, might experience fitness benefits from jogging a mile in 10 minutes, but this level of exercise would cause no physical adaptations in a trained distance runner.

The amount of overload needed to maintain or improve a particular level of fitness is determined in terms of three dimensions:

1. *Frequency, or how often.* Optimum exercise frequency, expressed in number of days per week, varies with the component being developed and your goals. A frequency of 3–5 days per week is recommended for cardiorespiratory endurance exercise, 2–3 days per week for strength training, and 2 or more days per week for stretching.

2. *Intensity, or how hard.* Fitness benefits occur when you exercise harder than your normal level of activity. To develop cardiorespiratory endurance, you must raise your heart rate above normal; to develop muscular strength, you must lift a heavier weight than you normally do; to develop flexibility, you must stretch your muscles beyond their normal length. A gradual increase in intensity is recommended to avoid injury.

3. *Duration, how long.* If fitness benefits are to occur, exercise sessions must last for an extended period of time. Depending on the component being devel-

	Lifestyle physical activity	Moderate exercise program	Vigorous exercise program
Description	Moderate physical activity—an amount of activity that uses about 150 calories per day	Cardiorespiratory endurance exercise (20–60 minutes, 3–5 days per week); strength training and stretching exercises (2–3 days per week)	Cardiorespiratory endurance exercise (20–60 minutes, 3–5 days per week); interval training; strength training (3–4 days per week); and stretching exercises (3–5 days per week)
Sample activities or program	*One of the following:* • Walking to and from work, 15 minutes each way • Cycling to and from class, 10 minutes each way • Raking leaves for 30 minutes • Dancing (fast) for 30 minutes • Playing basketball for 20 minutes	• Jogging for 30 minutes, 3 days per week • Weight training, 1 set of 8 exercises, 2 days per week • Stretching exercises, 3 days per week	• Running for 45 minutes, 3 days per week • Intervals: running 400 m at high effort 4 sets, 2 days per week • Weight training, 3 sets of 10 exercises, 3 days per week • Stretching exercises, 5 days per week
Health and fitness benefits	Better blood cholesterol levels, reduced body fat, better control of blood pressure, improved metabolic health, and enhanced glucose metabolism; improved quality of life; reduced risk of some chronic diseases	All the benefits of lifestyle physical activity, plus improved physical fitness (increased cardiorespiratory endurance, muscular strength and endurance, and flexibility) and even greater improvements in health and quality of life and reductions in chronic disease risk	All the benefits of lifestyle physical activity and a moderate exercise program, with greater increases in fitness and somewhat greater reductions in chronic disease risk Participating in a vigorous exercise program may increase risk of injury and overtraining

Figure 13-6   Health and fitness benefits of different amounts of physical activity and exercise.

oped and your intensity level, a duration of 20–60 minutes is usually recommended.

Each of these dimensions of overload will be described as it applies to the health-related components of fitness.

Selecting Activities   If you have been inactive, you should begin slowly by gradually increasing the amount of moderate physical activity in your life (the bottom of the activity pyramid). Once your body has adjusted to your new level of activity, you will be ready to choose additional activities for your exercise program.

Consider your choices carefully. First, be sure the activities you choose contribute to your overall wellness. Choose activities that make sense for you. Are you competitive? If so, try racquetball, basketball, or squash. Do you prefer to exercise alone? Then consider cross-country skiing or road running. Have you been sedentary? A walking program may be a good place to start.

If you think you may have trouble sticking with an exercise program, find a structured activity that you can do with a buddy or a group. If you don't have any favorite sports or activities, try something new. Take a physical education class, join a health club, or sign up for jazz danc-

ing. You're sure to find an activity that's both enjoyable and good for you.

Be realistic about the constraints presented by some sports, such as accessibility, expense, and time. For example, if you have to travel for hours to get to a ski area, skiing may not be a good choice for your regular exercise program. If you don't have large blocks of time available, you may have trouble squeezing in eighteen holes of golf. And if you've never played tennis, it will probably take you a fair amount of time to reach a reasonable skill level; you may be better off with a program of walking or jogging to get good workouts while you're improving your tennis game.

A general fitness program that supports an active lifestyle and promotes good health should contain the following components: cardiorespiratory endurance exercises, muscular strength and endurance exercises, flexibility exercises, and training in specific skills.

overload The amount of stress placed on the body; a gradual increase in the amount of overload causes adaptations that improve fitness.

Terms

Cardiorespiratory Endurance Exercises

Exercises that condition your heart and lungs should have a central role in your fitness program. The best exercises for developing cardiorespiratory endurance are those that stress a large portion of the body's muscle mass for a prolonged period of time. These include walking, jogging, running, swimming, bicycling, and aerobic dancing. Many popular sports and recreational activities such as racquetball, tennis, basketball, and soccer are also good if the skill level and intensity of the game are sufficient to provide a vigorous workout.

Frequency The optimal workout schedule for endurance training is 3–5 days per week. Beginners should start with 3 and work up to 5 days. Training more than 5 days a week often leads to injury for recreational athletes. While you do get health benefits from exercising very vigorously only 1–2 days per week, you risk injury because your body never gets a chance to adapt fully to regular exercise training.

Intensity The most misunderstood aspect of conditioning, even among experienced athletes, is training intensity. Intensity is the crucial factor in attaining a significant training effect—that is, in increasing the body's cardiorespiratory capacity. A primary purpose of endurance training is to increase **maximal oxygen consumption (MOC)**. MOC represents the maximum ability of the cells to use oxygen and is considered the best measure of car-

diorespiratory capacity. Intensity of training is the crucial factor in improving MOC.

However, it's not true that the harder you work, the better it is for you. Working too hard can cause injury, just as not working hard enough provides less benefit. One of the easiest ways to determine exactly how intensely you should work involves measuring your heart rate. It is not necessary or desirable to exercise at your maximum heart rate—the fastest heart rate possible before exhaustion sets in—in order to improve your cardiorespiratory capacity. Beneficial effects occur at lower heart rates with a much lower risk of injury. **Target heart rate** is the rate at which you should exercise to obtain cardiorespiratory benefits. To find out how you can determine the intensity at which you should exercise, refer to the box "Determining Your Target Heart Rate."

After you begin your fitness program, you may improve quickly because the body adapts readily to new exercises at first; the rate of improvement may slow after the first month or so. The more fit you become, the harder you will have to work to improve. By monitoring your heart rate, you will always know if you are working hard enough to improve, not hard enough, or too hard. For most people, a fitness program involves attaining an acceptable level of fitness and then maintaining that level. There is no need to keep working indefinitely to improve; doing so only increases the chance of injury. After you have reached the level you want, you can maintain fitness by exercising at the same intensity at least 3 nonconsecutive days per week.

Duration A total duration of 20–60 minutes is recommended; exercise can take place in a single session or in multiple bouts lasting 10 or more minutes. The total duration of exercise depends on its intensity. To improve cardiorespiratory endurance during a low- to moderate-intensity activity such as walking or slow swimming, you should exercise for 45–60 minutes. For high-intensity exercise performed at the top of your target heart rate zone, a duration of 20 minutes is sufficient. It is usually best to start off with less-vigorous activities and only gradually increase intensity.

You can use these three dimensions of cardiorespiratory endurance training—frequency, intensity, and duration—to develop a fitness program that strengthens your heart and lungs and provides all the benefits described earlier in this chapter. Build your program around at least 20 minutes of endurance exercise at your target heart rate three to five times a week. Then add exercises that develop the other components of fitness.

The Warm-Up and Cool-Down It is always important to warm up before you exercise and to cool down afterward. Warming up enhances your performance and decreases your chances of injury. Your muscles work better when

Terms

maximal oxygen consumption (MOC) The body's maximum ability to transport and use oxygen.

target heart rate The heart rate at which exercise yields cardiorespiratory benefits.

synovial fluid Fluid found within many joints that provides lubrication and nutrition to the cells of the joint surface.

resistance exercise Exercise that forces muscles to contract against increased resistance; also called *strength training*.

isometric exercise The application of force without movement; also called *static exercise*.

Your target heart rate is the rate at which you should exercise to experience cardiorespiratory benefits. Your target heart rate is based on your maximum heart rate, which can be estimated from your age. (If you are a serious athlete or face possible cardiovascular risks from exercise, you may want to have your maximum heart rate determined more accurately through a treadmill test in a physician's office, hospital, or sports medicine laboratory.) Your target heart rate is actually a range; the lower value corresponds to moderate-intensity exercise, while the higher value is associated with high-intensity activities. Target heart rates are shown in the accompanying table.

You can monitor the intensity of your workouts by measuring your pulse either at your wrist or at one of your carotid arteries, located on either side of your Adam's apple. Your pulse rate drops rapidly after exercise, so begin counting immediately after you have finished exercising. You will obtain the most accurate results by counting beats for 15 seconds and then multiplying by 4 to get your heart rate in beats per minute (bpm). The 15-second counts corresponding to each target heart rate range are also shown in the table at the right.

Age (years)	Target Heart Rate Range (bpm)*	15-Second Count (beats)*
20–24	127–182	32–46
25–29	124–176	31–44
30–34	121–171	30–43
35–39	118–167	30–42
40–44	114–162	29–41
45–49	111–158	28–40
50–54	108–153	27–38
55–59	105–149	26–37
60–64	101–144	25–36
65+	97–140	24–35

*Target heart rates lower than those shown here are appropriate for individuals who are quite unfit. Ranges are based on the following formula. Target heart rate = 0.65 to 0.90 of maximum heart rate, assuming maximum heart rate = 220 – age.

their temperature is elevated slightly above resting level. Warming up helps your body's physiology gradually progress from rest to exercise. Blood needs to be redirected to active muscles, and your heart needs time to adapt to the increased demands of exercise. A warm-up helps spread **synovial fluid** throughout the joints, which helps protect joint surfaces from wear and tear. (It's like warming up a car to spread oil through the engine parts before shifting into gear.)

A warm-up session should include low-intensity movements similar to those in the activity that will follow. Examples of low-intensity movements are hitting forehands and backhands before a tennis game and running a 12-minute mile before progressing to an 8-minute one. Some experts also recommend warm-up stretching exercises for flexibility after the general warm-up and before intense activity.

Cooling down after exercise is important to restore the body's circulation to its normal resting condition. When you are at rest, a relatively small percentage of your total blood volume is directed to muscles, but during exercise, as much as 85% of the heart's output is directed to them. During recovery from exercise, it is important to continue exercising at a low level to provide a smooth transition to the resting state. Cooling down helps regulate the return of blood to your heart.

Developing Muscular Strength and Endurance

Any program designed to promote health should include exercises that develop muscular strength and endurance.

Your ability to maintain correct posture and move efficiently depends in part on adequate muscle fitness. Strengthening exercises also increase muscle tone, which improves the appearance of your body. A lean, healthy-looking body is certainly one of the goals and one of the benefits of an overall fitness program.

Types of Strength Training Exercises Muscular strength and endurance can be developed in many ways, from weight training to calisthenics. Common exercises such as sit-ups, push-ups, pull-ups, and wall-sitting (leaning against a wall in a seated position and supporting yourself with your leg muscles) maintain the muscular strength of most people if they practice them several times a week. To condition and tone your whole body, choose exercises that work the major muscles of the shoulders, chest, back, arms, abdomen, and legs.

To increase strength, you must do **resistance exercise**—exercises in which your muscles must exert force against a significant amount of resistance. Resistance can be provided by weights, exercise machines, or your own body weight. **Isometric exercises** involve applying force without movement, such as when you contract your abdominal muscles. This static type of exercise is valuable for toning and strengthening muscles. Isometrics can be practiced anywhere and do not require any equipment. For maximum strength gains, hold an isometric contraction maximally for 6 seconds; do 5–10 repetitions. Don't hold your breath—that can restrict blood flow to your heart and brain. Within a few weeks, you will notice the

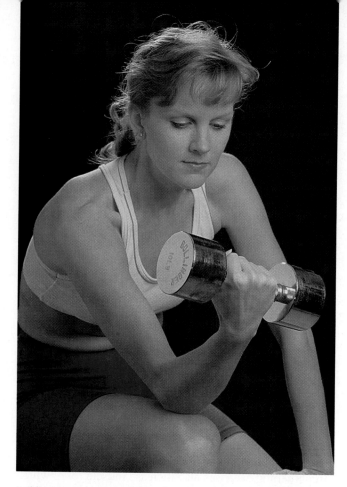

Building muscular strength is an important component of a fitness program. Weight training is just one way to increase strength, improve muscle tone, and enhance the overall appearance of the body.

effect of this exercise. Isometrics are particularly useful when recovering from an injury.

Isotonic exercises involve applying force with movement, as, for example, in weight training exercises such as the bench press. These are the most popular type of exercises for increasing muscle strength and seem to be most valuable for developing strength that can be transferred to other forms of physical activity. They include exercises using barbells, dumbbells, weight machines, and the body's own weight, as in push-ups or sit-ups.

Choosing Equipment   Weight machines are preferred by many people because they are safe, convenient, and easy to use. You just set the resistance (usually by placing a pin in the weight stack), sit down at the machine, and start

working. Machines make it easy to isolate and work specific muscles. Free weights require more care, balance, and coordination to use, but they strengthen your body in ways that are more adaptable to real life. For free weights, you need to use a spotter, someone who stands by to assist in case you lose control over a weight (see the box "Safe Weight Training").

Choosing Exercises   A complete weight training program works all the major muscle groups: neck, upper back, shoulders, arms, chest, abdomen, lower back, thighs, buttocks, and calves. Different exercises work different muscles, so it usually takes about 8–10 exercises to get a complete workout for general fitness—for example, bench presses to develop the chest, shoulders, and upper arms; pull-ups to work the biceps and upper back; squats to develop the legs and buttocks; toe raises to work the calves; and so on. If you are also training for a particular sport, include exercises to strengthen the muscles important for optimal performance and the muscles most likely to be injured. (A complete sample weight training program for general fitness can be found on the *Core Concepts Interactive* CD-ROM that accompanies the text.)

Intensity and Duration   The amount of weight (resistance) you lift in weight training exercises is equivalent to intensity in cardiorespiratory endurance training; the number of repetitions of each exercise is equivalent to duration. In order to improve fitness, you must do enough repetitions of each exercise to temporarily fatigue your muscles. The number of repetitions needed to cause fatigue depends on the amount of resistance: the heavier the weight, the fewer repetitions to reach fatigue. In general, a heavy weight and a low number of repetitions (1–5) build strength, while a light weight and a high number of repetitions (20–25) build endurance. For a general fitness program to build both strength and endurance, try to do 8–12 repetitions of each exercise; a few exercises, such as abdominal crunches and calf raises, may require more. (For people who are 50–60 years of age and older, 10–15 repetitions of each exercise using a lighter weight is recommended.)

Begin with a weight that you can lift fairly easily, and do 8–12 repetitions of each exercise. As you progress, add weight when you can do more than 12 repetitions of an exercise. By gradually increasing resistance over a period of weeks, you will increase your muscle strength and endurance without causing injury.

For developing strength and endurance for general fitness, a single set (group) of each exercise is sufficient, provided you use enough resistance (weight) to fatigue your muscles. Doing more than 1 set of each exercise may increase strength development, and most serious weight trainers do at least 3 sets of each exercise. If you do perform more than 1 set of an exercise, rest long enough between sets to allow your muscles to recover.

Terms   ✓**isotonic exercise** The application of force with movement.

General Strategies

- Lift weights from a stabilized body position. Protect your back from dangerous positions. Don't twist your body while lifting.

- Don't lift beyond the limits of your strength.

- Be aware of what's going on around you so that you don't bump into someone or get too close to a moving weight stack.

- Don't use defective equipment; report any equipment problems immediately.

- Don't hold your breath while doing weight training exercises. Exhale when exerting the greatest force, and inhale when moving the weight into position. (Holding your breath causes a decrease in blood returning to the heart and can make you become dizzy and faint.)

- Rest between lifts.

- Always warm up before training and cool down afterward.

Free Weights

- Use spotters to avoid injury. A spotter can help you if you cannot complete a lift or if the weight tilts.

- Secure weight plates to barbells with a collar to prevent them from sliding off.

- Keep weights as close to your body as possible. Do most of your lifting with your legs; keep your hips and buttocks tucked in.

- Lift weights smoothly and slowly; don't bounce or jerk them. Control the weight through the entire range of motion.

- When holding barbells and dumbbells, wrap your thumbs around the bar when gripping it.

Weight Machines

- Stay away from moving parts of the machine that could pinch your skin.

- Adjust each machine for your body so that you don't have to work in an awkward position.

- Beware of broken bolts, frayed cables, broken chains, or loose cushions that can give way and cause serious injury.

- Make sure the machines are clean. Carry a towel with you, and place it on the machine where you will sit or lie down.

As with cardiorespiratory endurance exercise, you should warm up before every weight training session and cool down afterward.

Frequency   For general fitness, the American College of Sports Medicine recommends a frequency of 2–3 days per week. Allow your muscles a day of rest between workouts to avoid soreness and injury. If you enjoy weight training and would like to train more often, try working different muscle groups on alternate days.

Gender Differences in Muscle Size and Strength   Men are generally stronger than women because they typically have larger bodies overall and larger muscles. But when the amount of muscle tissue is taken into account, men are only 1–2% stronger than women in the upper body and about equal to women in the lower body. (Men have a larger proportion of muscle tissue in the upper body, so it's easier for them to build upper-body strength than it is for women.) This disparity is probably due in large part to androgens, naturally occurring male hormones that are responsible for the development of secondary sex characteristics (facial hair, deep voice, and so on; see Chapter 5). Androgens also promote the growth of muscle tissue, and androgen levels are about 6–10 times higher in men than in women.

However, both men and women can increase strength through resistance training. Men tend to build larger, stronger muscles. Women tend to lose inches and increase strength without developing excessively bulky muscles. (Because of their lower levels of androgens, women do not develop large muscles from moderate strength training.) The lifetime wellness benefits of strength training are available to everyone.

A Caution About Supplements   No nutritional supplement or drug will change a weak, untrained person into a strong, fit person. Those changes require regular training that stresses the body and causes physiological adaptations. Supplements or drugs that promise quick, large gains in strength usually don't work and are often either dangerous or expensive, or both (see the box "Drugs and Supplements for Improved Athletic Performance"). The long-term effects of many supplements have not been studied. Use your critical thinking skills to evaluate claims made about supplements, and stay with the proven method of a steady, progressive fitness program to build strength.

Flexibility Exercises

Flexibility, or stretching, exercises are important for maintaining the normal range of motion in the major joints of

The 2000 Olympic Games in Sydney made headlines not just for athletic achievements but also for the number of athletes testing positive for performance-enhancing drugs. Some athletes were banned from competition before or during the games, while others had medals taken away after they failed postcompetition drug tests. The Olympic Movement Anti-Doping Code calls for the elimination of the use of performance-enhancing drugs in sports in order to both ensure respect for sports ethics and protect the health of athletes.

Drugs intended to enhance athletic performance are used not only by elite Olympic athletes but also by active individuals of all fitness levels. About 2–3% of high school and college students report having used steroids, and over-the-counter dietary supplements are much more popular. Many such substances are ineffective and expensive, and many are also dangerous. For example, supplements marketed to bodybuilders containing gamma butyrolactone or butanediol, CNS depressants related to the illegal drug gamma hydroxybutyrate (GHB), may cause vomiting, seizures, coma, and potentially fatal withdrawal reactions (see Chapter 9). A few of the most widely used compounds are described below.

Anabolic Steroids   These synthetic derivatives of testosterone are taken to increase strength, power, speed, endurance, muscle size, and aggressiveness. **Anabolic steroids** have dangerous side effects, including disruption of the body's hormone system, liver disease, acne, breast development and testicular shrinkage in males, masculinization in women and children, and increased risk of heart disease and cancer. Steroid use is also associated with an increased risk of drug abuse and HIV infection.

Adrenal Androgens   This group of drugs, which includes dehydroepiandrosterone (DHEA) and androstenedione, are typically taken to stimulate muscle growth and aid in weight control. The few studies of these agents done on humans show that they are of very little value in improving athletic performance, and they have side effects similar to those of anabolic steroids, especially when taken in high doses.

Erythropoietin (EPO)   A naturally occurring hormone that boosts the concentration of red blood cells, EPO is typically used by endurance athletes to improve their performance. EPO can cause blood clots and death.

Creatine Monohydrate   Use of creatine supplements may improve performance in short-term, high-intensity, repetitive exercise; however, in 2000, a panel of ACSM experts concluded that there is no evidence that creatine supplements increase the aerobic power of muscles. They may increase water retention in muscles, giving the feeling of increased muscularity without an actual increase in muscle size. The long-term effects of creatine use, especially among young people, are not well established.

Protein, Amino Acid, and Polypeptide Supplements   Little research supports the use of such supplements, even in athletes on extemely heavy training regimens. The protein requirements of athletes are not much higher than those of sedentary individuals, and most people take in more than enough protein in their diets. By substituting supplements for food sources of protein, people may risk deficiencies in other key nutrients typically found in such foods, including iron and B vitamins.

Chromium Picolinate   Sold over the counter, chromium picolinate is a more easily digested form of the trace mineral chromium. Although often marketed as a means to build muscle and reduce fat, most studies have found no positive effects. Long-term use of high dosages may have serious health consequences.

---

the body. Some exercises, such as running, can actually decrease flexibility because they require only a partial range of motion. Like a good weight training program, a good stretching program includes exercises for all the major muscle groups and joints of the body: neck, shoulders, back, hips, thighs, hamstrings, and calves. (A complete sample stretching program can be found on the *Core Concepts Interactive* CD-ROM that accompanies the text.)

Proper Stretching Technique   Stretching should be performed statically. "Bouncing" (known as ballistic stretching) is dangerous and counterproductive. Stretching can be either active or passive. In active stretching, a muscle is stretched by a contraction of opposing muscles. In passive stretching, an outside force or resistance provided by yourself, a partner, gravity, or a weight helps your joints move through their range of motion. You can achieve a greater range of motion and a more intense stretch using passive stretching, but there is a greater risk of injury. The safest and most convenient technique may be active static stretching with a passive assist. For example, you might do a seated stretch of your calf muscles both by contracting the muscles on the top of your shin and by grabbing your feet and pulling them toward you.

Intensity and Duration   For each exercise, stretch to the point of tightness in the muscle, and hold the position for 10–30 seconds. Rest for 30–60 seconds, and then repeat, trying to stretch a bit farther. Relax and breathe easily as you stretch. You should feel a pleasant, mild stretch as you let the muscles relax; stretching should not be painful. Do at least 4 repetitions of each exercise. A complete flexibility workout usually takes about 20–30 minutes.

Increase your intensity gradually over time. Improved flexibility takes many months to develop. There are large

Terms

anabolic steroids Synthetic male hormones used to increase muscle size and strength.

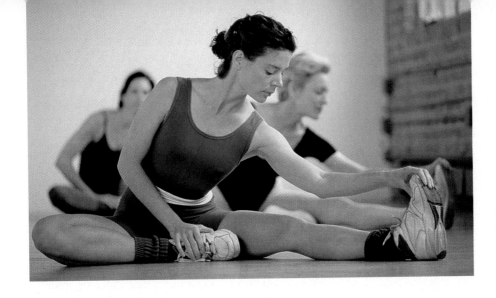

When performed regularly, stretching exercises help maintain or improve the range of motion in joints. For each exercise, stretch to the point of tightness in the muscle and hold the position for 10–30 seconds.

individual differences in joint flexibility. Don't feel you have to compete with others during stretching workouts.

Frequency   Do stretching exercises a minimum of 2–3 days per week. You can set apart a special time for these exercises or do them before or after cardiorespiratory endurance exercise or strength training. You may develop more flexibility if you do them after exercise, during your cool-down, because your muscles are warmer then and can be stretched farther.

Training in Specific Skills

The final component in your fitness program is learning the skills required for the sports or activities in which you choose to participate. Taking the time and effort to acquire competence means that instead of feeling ridiculous, becoming frustrated, and giving up in despair, you achieve a sense of mastery and add a new physical activity to your repertoire.

The first step in learning a new skill is getting help. Sports like tennis, golf, sailing, and skiing require mastery of basic movements and techniques, so instruction from a qualified teacher can save you hours of frustration and increase your enjoyment of the sport. Skill is also important in conditioning activities such as jogging, swimming, and cycling. Even if you learned a sport as a child, additional instruction now can help you refine your technique, get over stumbling blocks, and relearn skills that you may have learned incorrectly.

WW. Putting It All Together

Now that you know the basic components of a fitness program, you can put them all together in a program that works for you. Remember to include the following:

- *Cardiorespiratory endurance exercise:* Do at least 20 minutes of aerobic exercise at your target heart rate three to five times a week.

- *Muscular strength and endurance:* Work the major muscle groups (1 or more sets of 8–10 exercises) two to three times a week.

- *Flexibility exercise:* Do stretches at least two or three times a week.

- *Skill training:* Incorporate some or all of your aerobic or strengthening exercise into an enjoyable sport or physical activity.

A summary of the fitness benefits of a variety of activities is provided in Table 13-2 to help you plan your program.

COMMUNICATE!   Do you want to exercise more but find you just can't fit it into your day? Listen carefully to what you're telling yourself, perhaps by writing down your "self-talk" about exercise for a few days. Are you rationalizing, making excuses, procrastinating, or avoiding responsibility for your choices? For example, "I'm too busy with my classes this semester to fit exercise into my schedule," or "Right now I want to spend all my free time with my new girlfriend/boyfriend," or "I'll try to start running once the weather gets warmer." Can you think of ways to counter these statements and change your exercise habits? For example, "I see a lot of other busy people who are exercising, and I can probably do it too"; "I could ask my girlfriend/boyfriend to go for a hike in the hills with me"; "I can use the exercise equipment at the gym until the weather warms up." Remember that when you rationalize and make excuses, the only one who loses is you.

GETTING STARTED AND STAYING ON TRACK

Once you have a program that fulfills your basic fitness needs and suits your personal tastes, adhering to a few basic principles will help you improve at the fastest rate, have more fun, and minimize the risk of injury. These principles include buying appropriate equipment, eating

Table 13-2   **A Summary of Sports and Fitness Activities**

This table classifies sports and activities as high (H), moderate (M), or low (L) in terms of their ability to develop each of the five components of physical fitness: cardiorespiratory endurance (CRE), muscular strength (MS), muscular endurance (ME), flexibility (F), and body composition (BC). The skill level needed to obtain fitness benefits is noted: Low (L) means little or no skill is required to obtain fitness benefits; moderate (M) means average skill is needed to obtain fitness benefits; and high (H) means much skill is required to obtain fitness benefits. The fitness prerequisite, or conditioning needs of a beginner, is also noted: Low (L) means no fitness prerequisite is required; moderate (M) means some preconditioning is required; and high (H) means substantial fitness is required. The last two columns list the calorie cost of each activity when performed moderately and vigorously. To determine how many calories you burn, multiply the value in the appropriate column by your body weight and then by the number of minutes you exercise. Work up to using 300 or more calories per workout.

| Sports and Activities | Components | | | | | Skill Level | Fitness Prerequisite | Approximate Calorie Cost (cal/lb/min) | |
	CRE	MS*	ME*	F*	BC			Moderate	Vigorous
Aerobic dance	H	M	H	H	H	L	L	.046	.062
Backpacking	H	M	H	M	H	L	M	.032	.078
Badminton, skilled, singles	H	M	M	M	H	M	M	—	.071
Ballet (floor combinations)	M	M	H	H	M	M	L	—	.058
Ballroom dancing	M	L	M	L	M	M	L	.034	.049
Baseball (pitcher and catcher)	M	M	H	M	M	H	M	.039	—
Basketball, half court	H	M	H	M	H	M	M	.045	.071
Bicycling	H	M	H	M	H	M	L	.049	.071
Bowling	L	L	L	L	L	L	L	—	—
Calisthenic circuit training	H	M	H	M	H	L	L	—	.060
Canoeing and kayaking (flat water)	M	M	H	M	M	M	M	.045	—
Cheerleading	M	M	M	M	M	M	L	.033	.049
Fencing	M	M	H	H	M	M	L	.032	.078
Field hockey	H	M	H	M	H	M	M	.052	.078
Folk and square dancing	M	L	M	L	M	L	L	.039	.049
Football, touch	M	M	M	M	M	M	M	.049	.078
Frisbee, ultimate	H	M	H	M	H	M	M	.049	.078
Golf (riding cart)	L	L	L	M	L	L	L	—	—
Handball, skilled, singles	H	M	H	M	H	M	M	—	.078
Hiking	H	M	H	L	H	L	M	.051	.073
Hockey, ice and roller	H	M	H	M	H	M	M	.052	.078
Horseback riding	M	M	M	L	M	M	M	.052	.065
Interval circuit training	H	H	H	M	H	L	L	—	.062
Jogging and running	H	M	H	L	H	L	L	.060	.104

*Ratings are for the muscle groups involved.

and drinking properly, and managing your program so it becomes an integral part of your life.

Selecting Instructors, Equipment, and Facilities

Once you've chosen the activities for your program, you may need to obtain appropriate information, instruction, and equipment or find an appropriate facility.

Finding Help and Advice About Exercise   One of the best places to get help is an exercise class, where an expert instructor can help you learn the basics of training and answer your questions. A qualified personal trainer can also get you started on an exercise program or a new form

of training. Make sure that your instructor or trainer has proper qualifications, such as a college degree in exercise physiology or physical education and certification by the American College of Sports Medicine (ACSM), American Council on Exercise (ACE), or another professional organization. Don't seek out a person for advice simply because he or she looks fit. You can further your knowledge by reading articles by experts in fitness magazines. As with all types of health information, however, it's important to carefully consider the reliability of your sources.

Selecting Equipment   Try to purchase the best equipment you can afford. Good equipment will enhance your

Sports and Activities	Components					Skill Level	Fitness Prerequisite	Approximate Calorie Cost (cal/lb/min)	
	CRE	MS*	ME*	F*	BC			Moderate	Vigorous
Judo	M	H	H	M	M	M	L	.049	.090
Karate	H	M	H	H	H	L	M	.049	.090
Lacrosse	H	M	H	M	H	H	M	.052	.078
Modern dance (moving combinations)	M	M	H	H	M	L	L	—	.058
Orienteering	H	M	H	L	H	L	M	.049	.078
Outdoor fitness trails	H	M	H	M	H	L	L	—	.060
Popular dancing	M	L	M	M	M	M	L	—	.049
Racquetball, skilled, singles	H	M	M	M	H	M	L	.049	.078
Rock climbing	M	H	H	H	M	H	H	.033	.033
Rope skipping	H	M	H	L	H	M	M	.071	.095
Rowing	H	H	H	H	H	L	L	.032	.097
Rugby	H	M	H	M	H	M	M	.052	.097
Sailing	L	L	M	L	L	M	L	—	—
Skating, ice, roller, and in-line	M	M	H	M	M	H	M	.049	.095
Skiing, alpine	M	H	H	M	M	H	M	.039	.078
Skiing, cross-country	H	M	H	M	H	M	M	.049	.104
Soccer	H	M	H	M	H	M	M	.052	.097
Squash, skilled, singles	H	M	M	M	H	M	M	.049	.078
Stretching	L	L	L	H	L	L	L	—	—
Surfing (including swimming)	M	M	M	M	M	H	M	—	.078
Swimming	H	M	H	M	H	M	L	.032	.088
Synchronized swimming	M	M	H	H	M	H	M	.032	.052
Table tennis	M	L	M	M	M	M	L	—	.045
Tennis, skilled, singles	H	M	M	M	H	M	M	—	.071
Volleyball	M	L	M	M	M	M	M	—	.065
Walking	H	L	M	L	H	L	L	.029	.048
Water polo	H	M	H	M	H	H	M	—	.078
Water skiing	M	M	H	M	M	H	M	.039	.055
Weight training	L	H	H	H	M	L	L	—	—
Wrestling	H	H	H	H	H	H	H	.065	.094
Yoga	L	L	M	H	L	H	L	—	—

SOURCE: Kusinitz, I., and M. Fine. 1995. *Your Guide to Getting Fit*, 3rd ed. Mountain View, Calif.: Mayfield.

enjoyment and decrease your risk of injury. Appropriate safety equipment, such as pads and helmets for in-line skating, is particularly important. If you shop around, you can often find bargains through mail-order companies and discount or used equipment stores.

Before you invest in a new piece of equipment, investigate it. Is it worth the money? Does it produce the results its proponents claim for it? Is it safe? Does it fit properly, and is it in good working order? Does it provide a genuine workout? Will you really use it? Before you buy an expensive piece of equipment, try it out at a local gym to make sure that you'll use it regularly. Also check whether you have space to use and store it at home. Ask the experts (coaches, physical educators, and sports instructors) for their opinion. Better yet, educate yourself. Every sport, from running to volleyball, has its own magazine. A little effort to educate yourself will be well rewarded. Footwear is probably the most important piece of equipment for almost any activity; refer to the box "Choosing Exercise Footwear" for shopping strategies.

Choosing a Fitness Center Are you thinking of becoming a member of a health club or fitness center? Be sure to choose one that has the right programs and equipment available at the times you will use them. You should feel comfortable with the classes and activities available;

Footwear is perhaps the most important item of equipment for almost any activity. Shoes protect and support your feet and improve your traction. When you jump or run, you place as much as six times more force on your feet than when you stand still. Shoes can help cushion against the stress that this additional force places on your lower legs, thereby preventing injuries. Some athletic shoes are also designed to help prevent ankle rollover, another common source of injury.

General Guidelines

When choosing athletic shoes, first consider the activity you've chosen for your exercise program. Shoes appropriate for different activities have very different characteristics. For example, running shoes typically have highly cushioned midsoles, rubber outsoles with elevated heels, and a great deal of flexibility in the forefoot. The heels of walking shoes tend to be lower, less padded, and more beveled than those designed for running. For aerobic dance, shoes must be flexible in the forefoot and have straight, nonflared heels to allow for safe and easy lateral movements. Court shoes also provide substantial support for lateral movements; they typically have outsoles made from white rubber that will not damage court surfaces.

Also consider the location and intensity of your workouts. If you plan to walk or run on trails, you should choose shoes with water-resistant, highly durable uppers and more outsole traction. If you work out intensely or have a relatively high body weight, you'll need thick, firm midsoles to avoid bottoming-out the cushioning system of your shoes.

Foot type is another important consideration. If your feet tend to roll inward excessively, you may need shoes with additional stability features on the inner side of the shoe to counteract this movement. If your feet tend to roll outward excessively, you may need highly flexible and cushioned shoes that promote foot motion. For aerobic dancers with feet that tend to roll inward or outward, mid-cut to high-cut shoes may be more appropriate than low-cut aerobic shoes or cross-trainers (shoes designed to be worn for several different activities). Compared with men, women have narrower feet overall and narrower heels relative to the forefoot. Most women will get a better fit if they choose shoes that are specifically designed for women's feet rather than those that are downsized versions of men's shoes.

Successful Shopping

For successful shoe shopping, keep the following strategies in mind:

- Shop at an athletic shoe or specialty store that has personnel trained to fit athletic shoes and a large selection of styles and sizes.

- Shop late in the day or, ideally, following a workout. Your foot size increases over the course of the day and as a result of exercise.

- Wear socks like those you plan to wear during exercise. If you have an old pair of athletic shoes, bring them with you. The wear pattern on your old shoes can help you select a pair with extra support or cushioning in the places you need it the most.

- Ask for help. Trained salespeople know which shoes are designed for your foot type and your level of activity. They can also help fit your shoes properly.

- Don't insist on buying shoes in what you consider to be your typical shoe size. Sizes vary from shoe to shoe. In addition, foot sizes change over time, and many people have one foot that is larger or wider than the other. Try several sizes in several widths, if necessary. Don't buy shoes that are too small.

- Try on both shoes, and wear them around for 10 or more minutes. Try walking on a noncarpeted surface. Approximate the movements of your activity: walk, jog, run, jump, and so on.

- Check the fit and style carefully:

    Is the toe box roomy enough? Your toes will spread out when your foot hits the ground or you push off. There should be at least one thumb's width of space from the longest toe to the end of the toe box.

    Do the shoes have enough cushioning? Do your feet feel supported when you bounce up and down? Try bouncing on your toes and on your heels.

    Do your heels fit snugly into the shoe? Do they stay put when you walk, or do they rise up?

    Are the arches of your feet right on top of the shoes' arch supports?

    Do the shoes feel stable when you twist and turn on the balls of your feet? Try twisting from side to side while standing on one foot.

    Do you feel any pressure points?

- If the shoes are not comfortable in the store, don't buy them. Don't expect athletic shoes to stretch over time in order to fit your feet properly.

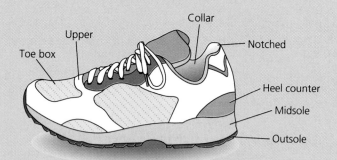

Toe box · Upper · Collar · Notched · Heel counter · Midsole · Outsole

the age, fitness level, and dress of others in the club; and the types of music used in classes. The facility and equipment should be clean and well maintained, including the showers and lockers; the staff should be well trained and helpful. Ask for a free trial workout, a 1-day pass, or an inexpensive 1- to 2-week trial membership before committing to a long-term contract. Be wary of promotional gimmicks and high-pressure sales tactics. Also make sure the facility is certified; look for the displayed names American College of Sports Medicine (ACSM), American Council on Exercise (ACE), or Aerobics and Fitness Association of America (AFAA). These trade associations have established standards to help protect consumer health, safety, and rights. Find a facility that you feel comfortable with and that meets your needs.

Eating and Drinking for Exercise

Most people do not need to change their eating habits when they begin a fitness program. Many athletes and other physically active people are lured into buying aggressively advertised vitamins, minerals, and protein supplements. But in almost every case, a well-balanced diet contains all the energy and nutrients needed to sustain an exercise program (see Chapter 12 for more information).

A balanced diet is also the key to improving your body composition when you begin to exercise more. One of the promises of a fitness program is a decrease in body fat and an increase in muscular body mass. As mentioned earlier, the control of body fat is determined by the balance of energy in the body. If more calories are consumed than are expended through metabolism and exercise, then fat increases. If the reverse is true, fat is lost. The best way to control body fat is to follow a diet containing adequate but not excessive calories and to be physically active.

One of the most important principles to follow when exercising is to drink enough water. Your body depends on water to sustain many chemical reactions and to maintain correct body temperature. Sweating during exercise depletes the body's water supply and can lead to dehydration if fluids are not replaced. Serious dehydration can cause reduced blood volume, accelerated heart rate, elevated body temperature, muscle cramps, heat stroke, and other serious problems. Drinking water before and during exercise is important to prevent dehydration and enhance athletic performance.

Thirst alone is not a good indication of how much you need to drink, because thirst is quickly depressed by drinking even small amounts of water. Most of the weight lost immediately after exercise is from the loss of fluids. If you rely on thirst, it can take 24 hours or more to replace these fluids. Ideally, you should restore your body fluids before you exercise vigorously again. As a rule of thumb, try to drink about 8 ounces of water (more in hot weather) for every 30 minutes of heavy exercise. Bring a water bottle with you when you exercise so you can replace your fluids while they're being depleted. For workouts lasting less than 60–90 minutes, cool water is an appropriate fluid replacement; for longer workouts or for exercise in especially hot and humid conditions, a commercial sports beverage that contains carbohydrates may be beneficial.

Managing Your Fitness Program

How can you tell when you're in shape? When do you stop improving and start maintaining? How can you stay motivated? If your program is going to become an integral part of your life, and if the principles behind it are going to serve you well in the years ahead, these are very important questions.

Consistency: The Key to Physical Improvement   It is important to be able to recognize when you have achieved the level of fitness that is appropriate for you. This level will vary, of course, depending on your goals, the intensity of your program, and your natural ability. Your body gets into shape by adapting to increasing levels of physical stress. If you don't push yourself by increasing the intensity of your workout—by adding weight or running a little faster or a little longer—no change will occur in your body.

But if you subject your body to overly severe stress, it will break down and become distressed, or injured. Overdoing exercise is just as bad as not exercising hard enough. No one can become fit overnight. Your body needs time to adapt to increasingly higher levels of stress. The process of improving fitness involves a countless number of stresses and adaptations. If you feel extremely sore and tired the day after exercising, then you have worked too hard. Injury will slow you down just as much as a missed workout.

Consistency is the key to getting into shape without injury. Steady fitness improvement comes when you overload your body consistently over a long period of time. The best way to ensure consistency is to keep a training journal in which you record the details of your workouts: how far you ran, how much weight you lifted, how many laps you swam, and so on. This record will help you evaluate your progress and plan your workout sessions intelligently. Don't increase your exercise volume by more than 5–10% per week.

Assessing Your Fitness   When are you "in shape"? It depends. One person may be out of shape running a mile in 5 minutes; another may be in shape running a mile in 12 minutes. As mentioned earlier, your ultimate level of fitness depends on your goals, your program, and your natural ability. The important thing is to set goals that make sense for you.

If you are interested in finding out exactly how fit you are before you begin a program, the best approach is to get an assessment from a modern sports medicine laboratory.

You can obtain a general rating of your cardiorespiratory fitness by taking the 1.5-mile run-walk test. Don't attempt this test unless you have completed at least 6 weeks of some type of conditioning activity. Also, if you are over age 35 or have questions about your health, check with your physician before taking this test.

You'll need a stopwatch, clock, or watch with a second hand and a running track or course that is flat and provides measurements of up to 1.5 miles. You may want to practice pacing yourself prior to taking the test to avoid going too fast at the start and becoming fatigued before you finish. Allow yourself a day or two to recover from your practice run before taking the test.

Warm up before taking the test with some walking, easy jogging, and stretching exercises. The idea is to cover the distance as fast as possible, at a pace that is comfortable for you. You can run or walk the entire distance, or use some combination of running and walking. If possible, monitor your own pace, or have someone call out your time at various intervals to help you determine whether your pace is correct. When you have completed the test, refer to the table for your cardiorespiratory fitness rating. Be sure to cool down by walking or jogging slowly for about 5 minutes.

Standards for the 1.5-Mile Run-Walk Test (minutes:seconds)

	Superior	Excellent	Good	Fair	Poor	Very Poor
Women						
Age: 18–29	11:00 or less	11:15–12:45	13:00–14:15	14:30–15:45	16:00–17:30	17:45 or more
30–39	11:45 or less	12:00–13:30	13:45–15:15	15:30–16:30	16:45–18:45	19:00 or more
40–49	12:45 or less	13:00–14:30	14:45–16:30	16:45–18:30	18:45–20:45	21:00 or more
50–59	14:15 or less	14:30–16:30	16:45–18:30	18:45–20:30	20:45–23:00	23:15 or more
60 and over	14:00 or less	14:15–17:15	17:30–20:15	20:30–22:45	23:00–24:45	25:00 or more
Men						
Age: 18–29	9:15 or less	9:30–10:30	10:45–11:45	12:00–12:45	13:00–14:00	14:15 or more
30–39	9:45 or less	10:00–11:00	11:15–12:15	12:30–13:30	13:45–14:45	15:00 or more
40–49	10:00 or less	10:15–11:45	12:00–13:00	13:15–14:15	14:30–16:00	16:15 or more
50–59	10:45 or less	11:00–12:45	13:00–14:15	14:30–15:45	16:00–17:45	18:00 or more
60 and over	11:15 or less	11:30–13:45	14:00–15:45	16:00–17:45	18:00–20:45	21:00 or more

SOURCES: Formula for maximal oxygen consumption taken from McArdle, W. D., F. I. Katch, and V. L. Katch. 1991. *Exercise Physiology: Energy, Nutrition, and Human Performance*. Philadelphia: Lea & Febiger, pp. 225–226. Ratings based on norms from the Cooper Institute for Aerobics Research, Dallas, Texas. *The Physical Fitness Specialist Manual*, revised 2000. Used with permission.

Such laboratories can be found in university physical education departments and medical centers. Here you will receive an accurate profile of your capacity to exercise. Typically, your endurance will be measured on a treadmill or bicycle, your body fat will be estimated, and your strength and flexibility will be tested. This evaluation will reveal whether your physical condition is consistent with good health, and the staff members at the laboratory can suggest an exercise program that will be appropriate for your level of fitness. To assess your own approximate level of cardiorespiratory endurance, take the test in the box "The 1.5-Mile Run-Walk Test."

Preventing and Managing Athletic Injuries

Although annoying, most injuries are neither serious nor permanent. However, an injury that is not cared for properly can escalate into a chronic problem. It is important to learn how to deal with injuries so they don't derail your fitness program (Table 13-3).

Some injuries require medical attention. Consult a physician for head and eye injuries, possible ligament injuries, broken bones, and internal disorders such as chest pain, fainting, and intolerance to heat. Also seek medical attention for apparently minor injuries that do not get better within a reasonable amount of time.

For minor cuts and scrapes, stop the bleeding and clean the wound with soap and water. Treat soft tissue injuries (muscles and joints) with the R-I-C-E principle:

Rest: Stop using the injured area as soon as you experience pain, and avoid any activity that causes pain.

Ice: Apply ice to the injured area to reduce swelling and alleviate pain. Apply ice immediately for 10–20 minutes, and repeat every few hours until the swelling disappears. Let the injured part return to normal temperature between icings, and do not apply ice to one area for more than 20 minutes (10 minutes if you are using a cold gel pack).

Compression: Wrap the injured area with an elastic or compression bandage between icings. If the area starts throbbing or begins to change color, the bandage may be wrapped too tightly. Do not sleep with the wrap on.

Table 13-3   Care of Common Exercise Injuries and Discomforts

Injury	Symptoms	Treatment
Blister	Accumulation of fluid in one spot under the skin	Don't pop or drain it unless it interferes too much with your daily activities. If it does pop, clean the area with antiseptic and cover with a bandage. Do not remove the skin covering the blister.
Bruise (contusion)	Pain, swelling, and discoloration	R-I-C-E: rest, ice, compression, elevation.
Joint sprain	Pain, tenderness, swelling, discoloration, and loss of function	R-I-C-E; apply heat after 36–48 hours if swelling has disappeared. Stretch and strengthen the affected area.
Muscle cramp	Painful, spasmodic muscle contractions	Gently stretch for 15–30 seconds at a time, and/or massage the cramped area. Drink fluids.
Muscle soreness or stiffness	Pain and tenderness in the affected muscle	Stretch the affected muscle gently; exercise at a low intensity; apply heat.
Muscle strain	Pain, tenderness, swelling, and loss of strength in the affected muscle	R-I-C-E; apply heat after 36–48 hours if swelling has disappeared. Stretch and strengthen the affected area.
Shin splints	Pain and tenderness on the front of the lower leg; sometimes also pain in the calf muscle	Rest; apply ice to the affected area several times a day and before exercise; wrap with tape for support. Stretch and strengthen muscles in the lower legs. Purchase good-quality footwear, and run on soft surfaces.
Side stitch	Pain on the side of the abdomen	Decrease the intensity of your workout, or stop altogether; bend over in the direction of the stitch.

SOURCE: Fahey, T. D., P. M. Insel, and W. T. Roth. 2001. *Fit and Well: Core Concepts and Labs in Physical Fitness and Wellness,* 4th ed. Mountain View, Calif.: Mayfield.

Elevation: Raise the injured area above heart level to decrease the blood supply and reduce swelling.

After about 36–48 hours, apply heat if the swelling has completely disappeared to help relieve pain, relax muscles, and reduce stiffness. Immerse the affected area in warm water or apply warm compresses, a hot water bottle, or a heating pad.

After a minor athletic injury, gradually reintroduce the stress of the activity until you are capable of returning to full intensity. Before returning to full exercise participation, you should have a full range of motion in your joints; normal strength and balance among your muscles; no injury-compensation movements, such as limping; and little or no pain.

To prevent injuries in the future, follow a few basic guidelines:

1. Stay in condition; haphazard exercise programs invite injury.
2. Warm up thoroughly before exercise.
3. Use proper body mechanics when lifting objects or executing sports skills.

4. Don't exercise when you're ill or overtrained (experiencing extreme fatigue due to overexercising).
5. Use the proper equipment.
6. Don't return to your normal exercise program until athletic injuries have healed.

Professional athletes appear to recover quickly from their injuries because they treat them promptly and correctly. You can keep your fitness program on track by doing the same.

Staying with Your Program   Once you have attained your desired level of fitness, you can maintain it by exercising regularly at a consistent intensity, three to five times a week. You must work at the intensity that brought you to your desired fitness level. If you don't, your body will become less fit because less is expected of it. In general, if you exercise at the same intensity over a long period, your fitness will level out and can be maintained easily.

What if you run out of steam? Although good health is an important *reason* to exercise, it's a poor *motivator* for consistent adherence to an exercise program. A variety of

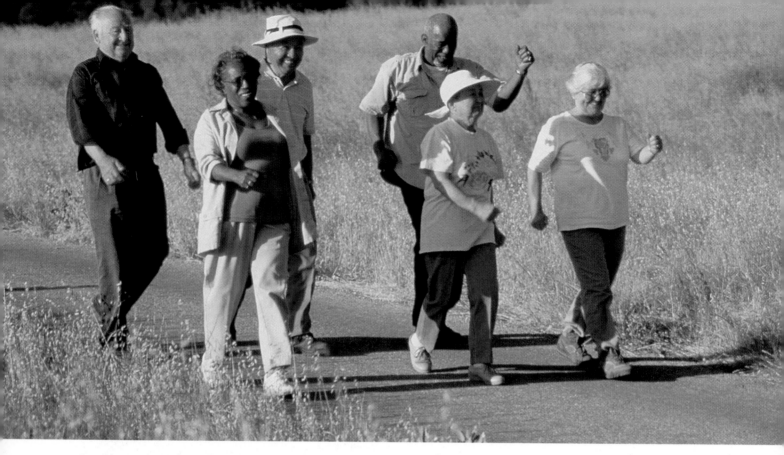

It makes sense to choose activities that will add enjoyment to your life for years to come. In this group of older people, we can see the rewards of a lifetime of fitness and smart exercise habits.

specific suggestions for staying with your program are given in the box "Maintaining Your Exercise Program" and in the Behavior Change Strategy at the end of the chapter. It's a good idea to have a meaningful goal, anything from fitting into the same-size jeans you used to wear to successfully skiing down a new slope.

Varying your program is another key strategy. Some people alternate two or more activities—swimming and jogging, for example—to improve a particular component of fitness. The practice, called **cross-training,** can help prevent boredom and overuse injuries. Explore many exercise options. Consider competitive sports at the recreational level: swimming, running, racquetball, volleyball, golf, and so on. Find out how you can participate in an activity you've never done before: canoeing, hang gliding, windsurfing, backpacking. Try new activities, especially ones that you will be able to do for the rest of your life. Get maps of the recreational or wilderness areas near you, and go exploring. Fill a canteen, pack a good lunch, and take along a wildflower or bird book. Every step you take will bring you closer to your ultimate goal—fitness and wellness that last a lifetime.

Terms   **cross-training** Participating in two or more activities to develop a particular component of fitness.

Tips for Today

Physical activity and exercise offer benefits in nearly every area of wellness, helping you generate energy, manage stress, control your weight, improve your mood, and, of course, become physically stronger and healthier. Building a program of regular exercise into your life is well worth the effort, even if it seems complicated or difficult at first. Even a low-to-moderate level of activity provides valuable health benefits. The important thing is to get moving: When in doubt, exercise!

Right now you can

- Get up and stretch.

- Go outside and take a brisk walk.

- Look at your calendar for the rest of the week and write in some physical activity—such as walking, running, biking, skating, swimming, hiking, or playing Frisbee—on as many days as you can; schedule the activity for a specific time, and stick to it.

- If you don't yet use the gym or fitness facility on your campus, go there now and begin planning how to use it.

- Call a friend and invite him or her to start a regular exercise program with you.

- *Set realistic goals.* Unrealistically high goals will only discourage you.
- *Sign a contract.* Also, keep records of your activities, and track your progress.
- *Start slowly, and increase your intensity and duration gradually.* Overzealous exercising can result in discouraging discomforts and injuries. Your program is meant to last a lifetime. The important first step is to break your established pattern of inactivity.
- *Make your program fun.* Participate in a variety of different activities that you enjoy. Vary the routes you take walking, running, or biking.
- *Exercise with a friend.* The social side of exercise is an important factor for many regular exercisers.
- *Focus on the positive.* Concentrate on the improvements you obtain from your program, how good you feel during and after exercise.
- *Revisit and revise.* If your program turns out to be unrealistic, revise it. Expect to make many adjustments in your program along the way.

- *Expect fluctuation.* On some days, your progress will be excellent, while on others, you'll barely be able to drag yourself through your scheduled activities.
- *Expect lapses.* Don't let them discourage you or make you feel guilty. Instead, feel a renewed commitment to your exercise program.
- *Reward yourself.* Give yourself frequent rewards for sticking with your program.
- *Renew your attitude.* If you notice you're slacking off, try to list the negative thoughts and behaviors that are causing noncompliance. Devise a strategy to decrease the frequency of negative thoughts and behaviors. Make changes in your program plan and reward system to help renew your enthusiasm and commitment.
- *Review your goals.* Visualize what it will be like to reach them, and keep these pictures in your mind as an incentive to stick to your program.

SUMMARY

- The five components of physical fitness most important to health are cardiorespiratory endurance, muscular strength, muscular endurance, flexibility, and body composition.
- Exercise improves the functioning of the heart and the ability of the cardiorespiratory system to carry oxygen to the body's tissues. It also increases the efficiency of the body's metabolism and improves body composition.
- Exercise lowers the risk of cardiovascular disease by improving blood fat levels, reducing high blood pressure, and interfering with the disease process that causes coronary artery blockage.
- Exercise reduces the risk of cancer, osteoporosis, and diabetes. It improves immune function and helps prevent injuries and low-back pain.
- Exercise can improve psychological health by reducing stress, anxiety, and depression; enhancing self-image; and providing opportunities for enjoyable social interaction.
- Everyone should accumulate at least 30 minutes per day of moderate endurance-type physical activity. Additional health and fitness benefits can be achieved through longer or more vigorous activity.
- Cardiorespiratory endurance exercises stress a large portion of the body's muscle mass. Endurance exercise should be performed 3–5 days per week for a total of 20–60 minutes per day. Intensity can be evaluated by measuring the heart rate.

- Warming up before exercising and cooling down afterward improve your performance and decrease your chances of injury.
- Exercises that develop muscular strength and endurance involve exerting force against a significant resistance. A strength training program for general fitness typically involves 1 set of 8–12 repetitions of 8–10 exercises, 2–3 days per week.
- A good stretching program includes exercises for all the major muscle groups and joints of the body. Do a series of active, static stretches (possibly with a passive assist) 2 or more days per week. Hold each stretch for 10–30 seconds; do at least 4 repetitions.
- Instructors, equipment, and facilities should be chosen carefully to enhance enjoyment and prevent injuries.
- A well-balanced diet contains all the energy and nutrients needed to sustain a fitness program. When exercising, remember to drink enough fluids.
- Rest, ice, compression, and elevation (R-I-C-E) are treatments for muscle and joint injuries.
- A desired level of fitness can be maintained by exercising three to five times a week at a consistent intensity.
- Strategies for maintaining an exercise program over the long term include having meaningful goals, varying the program, and trying new activities.

Although most people recognize the importance of incorporating exercise into their lives, many find it difficult to do. No single strategy will work for everyone, but the general steps outlined here should help you create an exercise program that fits your goals, preferences, and lifestyle. A carefully designed contract and program plan can help you convert your vague wishes into a detailed plan of action. And the strategies for program compliance outlined here and in Chapter 1 can help you enjoy and stick with your program for the rest of your life.

Step 1: Set Goals

Setting specific goals to accomplish by exercising is an important first step in a successful fitness program because it establishes the direction you want to take. Your goals might be specifically related to health, such as lowering your blood pressure and risk of heart disease, or they might relate to other aspects of your life, such as improving your tennis game or the fit of your clothes. If you can decide why you're starting to exercise, it can help you keep going.

Think carefully about your reasons for incorporating exercise into your life, and then fill in the goals portion of the Personal Fitness Contract.

Step 2: Select Activities

As discussed in the chapter, the success of your fitness program depends on the consistency of your involvement. Select activities that encourage your commitment: The right program will be its own incentive to continue; poor activity choices provide obstacles and can turn exercise into a chore.

When choosing activities for your fitness program, consider the following:

- Is this activity fun? Will it hold my interest over time?
- Will this activity help me reach the goals I have set?
- Will my current fitness and skill level enable me to participate fully in this activity?
- Can I easily fit this activity into my daily schedule? Are there any special requirements (facilities, partners, equipment, etc.) that I must plan for?
- Can I afford any special costs required for equipment or facilities?
- (If you have special exercise needs due to a particular health problem.) Does this activity conform to my special health needs? Will it enhance my ability to cope with my specific health problem?

Refer to Table 13-2, which summarizes the fitness benefits and other characteristics of many activities. Using the guidelines listed above, select a number of sports and activities. Fill in the Program Plan portion of the Fitness Contract, using Table 13-2 to include the fitness components your choices will develop and the intensity, duration, and frequency standard you intend to meet for each activity. Does your program meet the criteria of a complete fitness program discussed in the chapter?

Step 3: Make a Commitment

Complete your Fitness Contract and Program Plan by signing your contract and having it witnessed and signed by someone who can help make you accountable for your progress. By completing a written contract, you will make a firm commitment and will be more likely to follow through until you meet your goals.

Step 4: Begin and Maintain Your Program

Start out slowly to allow your body time to adjust. Be realistic and patient—meeting your goals will take time. The following guidelines may help you start and stick with your program:

- Set aside regular periods for exercise. Choose times that fit in best with your schedule, and stick to them. Allow an adequate amount of time for warm-up, cool-down, and a shower.
- Take advantage of any opportunity for exercise that presents itself (for example, walk to class, take the stairs instead of the elevator).
- Do what you can to avoid boredom. Do stretching exercises or jumping jacks to music, or watch the evening news while riding your stationary bicycle.
- Exercise with a group that shares your goals and general level of competence.
- Vary the program. Change your activities periodically. Alter your route or distance if biking or jogging. Change racquetball partners, or find a new volleyball court.
- Establish minigoals or a point system, and work rewards into your program. Until you reach your main goals, a system of self-rewards will help you stick with your program. Rewards should be things you enjoy that are easily obtainable.

TAKE ACTION

1. Go to your school's physical education office and ask for a comprehensive listing of all the exercise and fitness facilities available on your campus. Visit the facilities you haven't yet seen, and investigate the activities that are done there. If there are sports or activities you'd like to try, consider doing so.

2. Investigate the fitness clubs in your community. How do they compare with each other? How do they measure up in terms of the guidelines provided in this chapter?

Personal Fitness Contract

I, _____, am contracting with myself to follow an exercise program to work at the following goals. I will begin my program on _____ .

Fitness Goals

1. _____   4. _____
2. _____   5. _____
3. _____   6. _____

Program Plan

	Activities	Components (Check ✔)					Intensity	Duration	Frequency (Check ✔)						
		CRE	MS	ME	F	BC			M	Tu	W	Th	F	Sa	Su
1.															
2.															
3.															
4.															
5.															

Note: You should conduct activities for achieving CRE goals at your target heart rate.

I agree to maintain a record of my activity, assess my progress periodically, and, if necessary, revise my goals.

Signed _____   Date _____

Witness _____

Step 5: Record and Assess Your Progress

Keeping a record that notes the daily results of your program will help remind you of your ongoing commitment to your program and give you a sense of accomplishment. Create daily and weekly program logs that you can use to track your progress. Record the activity type, frequency, and duration. Keep your log handy, and fill it in immediately after each exercise session. Post it in a visible place to remind you of your activity schedule and provide incentive for improvement.

SOURCE: Adapted from Kusinitz, I., and M. Fine. 1995. *Your Guide to Getting Fit*, 3rd ed. Mountain View, Calif.: Mayfield.

JOURNAL ENTRY

1. In your health journal, list the positive behaviors and attitudes that help you avoid a sedentary lifestyle and stay fit. How can you strengthen these behaviors and attitudes? Then list the negative behaviors and attitudes that block a physically active lifestyle. Which ones can you change? How can you change them?

2. Habit helps us conserve energy as we go through our daily lives, but it also blinds us to areas we could change. Make a list of ten ways you can incorporate more physical activity into your life by changing a habit, such as walking instead of riding the bus, taking the stairs in a certain building instead of the elevator, and so on.

3. _Critical Thinking_ Study the ads for fitness products and clubs on television, in popular magazines, and in your local newspaper. What markets are they targeting? How do they try to appeal to their audience? What other messages are they sending? Write a short essay describing your findings.

FOR MORE INFORMATION

Books

Anderson, B., and J. Anderson. 2000. _Stretching,_ 20th anniv. ed. Bolinas, Calif.: Shelter Publications. _Updated edition of a classic, with more than 200 stretches for 60 sports and activities._

Fahey, T. 2000. _Basic Weight Training for Men and Women,_ 4th ed. Mountain View, Calif.: Mayfield. _A practical guide to developing training programs tailored to individual needs._

Fahey, T., P. Insel, and W. Roth. 2001. _Fit and Well: Core Concepts and Labs in Physical Fitness and Wellness,_ 4th ed. Mountain View, Calif.: Mayfield. _A comprehensive guide to developing a complete fitness program._

Nieman, D. C. 1999. _Exercise Testing and Prescription. A Health-Related Approach,_ 4th ed. Mountain View, Calif.: Mayfield. _A comprehensive discussion of the effects of exercise and exercise testing and prescription._

U.S. Department of Health and Human Services. 1996. _Physical Activity and Health: A Report of the Surgeon General._ Atlanta, Ga.: Department of Health and Human Services. (Also available online: http://www.cdc.gov/nccdphp/sgr/sgr.htm) _Provides a summary of the evidence for the benefits of physical activity as well as recommendations for activity and exercise._

Williams, M. H. 1998. _The Ergogenics Edge: Pushing the Limits of Sports Performance._ Champaign, Ill.: Human Kinetics. _An excellent review of the scientific basis of substances and techniques used to improve athletic performance._

WW. Organizations, Hotlines, and Web Sites

American College of Sports Medicine. Provides brochures, publications, and audio- and videotapes on the positive effects of exercise.
317-637-9200
http://www.acsm.org

American Council on Exercise. Promotes exercise and fitness for all Americans; the Web site features fact sheets on many consumer topics, including choosing shoes, cross-training, steroids, and getting started on an exercise program.
800-529-8227
http://www.acefitness.org

American Heart Association: Just Move. Provides practical advice for people of all fitness levels plus an online fitness diary.
http://www.justmove.org

Canada's Physical Activity Guide. Offers many suggestions for incorporating physical activity into everyday life; also includes the Physical Activity Readiness Questionnaire (PAR-Q) to assess safety of exercise.
http://www.hc-sc.gc.ca/hppb/paguide

CDC Physical Activity Information. Provides information on the benefits of physical activity and suggestions for incorporating moderate physical activity into daily life.
http://www.cdc.gov/nccdphp/phyactiv.htm

Exercise: A Guide from the National Institute on Aging and the National Aeronautics and Space Administration. Provides practical advice on fitness for seniors; includes animated instructions for specific weight training and flexibility exercises.
http://weboflife.arc.nasa.gov/exerciseandaging/index.html

Disabled Sports USA. Provides sport and recreation services to people with physical or mobility disorders.
http://www.dsusa.org

Federal Trade Commission: Consumer Protection—Diet, Health, and Fitness. Provides several brochures with consumer advice about purchasing exercise equipment.
http://www.ftc.gov/bcp/menu-health.htm

Georgia State University: Exercise and Physical Fitness Page. Provides information about the benefits of exercise and how to get started on a fitness program.
http://www.gsu.edu/~wwwfit

National Institute on Drug Abuse: Anabolic Steroid Abuse. Provides information and links about the dangers of anabolic steroids.
http://www.steroidabuse.org

Shape Up America! Fitness Center. Includes fitness assessments, information on the benefits of exercise, tips for overcoming barriers, and tracking forms.
http://shapeup.org/fitness

Workout.Com. A commercial site that includes a wide variety of illustrated exercises and fitness programs.
http://www.workout.com

Strong Women. Provides practical fitness advice for women, including sample programs and training tips.
http://www.strongwomen.com

Information on many specific sports, activities, and fitness issues is available on the Web; use the following sites that provide many links or use a search engine to locate appropriate sites (see Appendix C).

Fitness Find
http://www.fitnessfind.com

Fitness Link
http://www.fitnesslink.com

Fitness Partner Connection Jumpsite
http://www.primusweb.com/fitnesspartner

NetSweat: The Internet's Fitness Resource
http://www.sickbay.com/netsweat

Yahoo! Recreation and Sports
http://dir.yahoo.com/recreation/sports

See also the listings for Chapters 12, 14, and 15.

American College of Sports Medicine. 1998. ACSM position stand: The recommended quantity and quality of exercise for developing and maintaining cardiorespiratory and muscular fitness, and flexibility in healthy adults. *Medicine and Science in Sports and Exercise* 30(6): 975–991.

Andersen, L. B., et al. 2000. All-cause mortality associated with physical activity during leisure time, work, sports, and cycling to work. *Archives of Internal Medicine* 160(11): 1621–1628.

Babyak, M., et al. 2000. Exercise treatment for major depression: Maintenance of therapeutic benefit at 10 months. *Psychosomatic Medicine* 62(5): 633–638.

Boutelle, K. N., et al. 2000. Associations between exercise and health behaviors in a community sample of working adults. *Preventive Medicine* 30(3): 217–224.

Brooks, G. A., et al. 2000. *Exercise Physiology: Human Bioenergetics and Its Applications,* 3rd ed. Mountain View, Calif.: Mayfield.

Centers for Disease Control and Prevention. 2000. Compliance with physical activity recommendations by walking for exercise. *Morbidity and Mortality Weekly Report* 49(25): 560–565.

Centers for Disease Control and Prevention. 2000. Prevalence of leisure-time and occupational physical activity among employed adults—United States, 1990. *Morbidity and Mortality Weekly Report* 49(19): 420–424.

Centers for Disease Control and Prevention. 2001. Physical activity trends—United States, 1990–1998. *Morbidity and Mortality Weekly Report* 50(9): 166–169.

Centers for Disease Control and Prevention. 2001. Prevalence of disabilities and associated health conditions among adults—United States, 1999. *Morbidity and Mortality Weekly Report* 50(7): 120–125.

Chenowth, D., and S. Pfohl. 2000. The high cost of couch potatoes. *Business and Health* 18(1): 20–22.

Daley, M. J., and W. L. Spinks. 2000. Exercise, mobility and aging. *Sports Medicine* 29(1): 1–12.

Fahey, T., P. Insel, and W. Roth. 2001. *Fit and Well: Core Concepts and Labs in Physical Fitness and Wellness,* 4th ed. Mountain View, Calif.: Mayfield.

Galloway, M. T., and P. Jolk. 2000. Aging successfully: The importance of physical activity in maintaining health and function. *Journal of the American Academy of Orthopaedic Surgeons* 8(1): 37–44.

Geffken, D. F., et al. 2001. Association between physical activity and markers of inflammation in a healthy elderly population. *American Journal of Epidemiology* 153(3): 242–250.

Hu, F. B., et al. 2000. Physical activity and risk of stroke in women. *Journal of the American Medical Association* 283(22): 2961–2967.

Jakes, R. W., et al. 2001. Patterns of physical activity and ultrasound attenuation by heel bone among Norfolk cohort of European Prospective Investigation of Cancer (EPIC Norfolk). *British Medical Journal* 322: 140.

Kriketos, A. D., et al. 2000. Effects of aerobic fitness on fat oxidation and body fatness. *Medicine and Science in Sports and Exercise* 32(4): 805–811.

Lakka, T. A., et al. 2001. Cardiorespiratory fitness and the progression of carotid atherosclerosis in middle-aged men. *Annals of Internal Medicine* 134(1): 12–20.

Laukkanen, J. A., et al. 2001. Cardiovascular fitness as a predictor of mortality in men. *Archives of Internal Medicine* 161(6): 825–831.

Lee, I. M., and R. S. Paffenbarger. 2000. Associations of light, moderate, and vigorous intensity physical activity with longevity. The Harvard Alumni Health Study. *American Journal of Epidemiology* 151(3): 293–299.

McAuley, E., et al. 2000. Physical activity, self-esteem, and self-efficacy relationships in older adults: A randomized controlled trial. *Annals of Behavioral Medicine* 22(2): 131–139.

National Institute on Drug Abuse. 2001. *Steroids (Anabolic-Androgenic)* (http://www.drugabuse.gov/Infofax/steroids.html; retrieved April 16, 2001).

Paluska, S. A., and T. L. Schwenk. 2000. Physical activity and mental health: Current concepts. *Sports Medicine* 29(3): 167–180.

Pollock, M. L., et al. 2000. AHA Science Advisory. Resistance exercise in individuals with and without cardiovascular disease: Benefits, rationale, safety, and prescription. *Circulation* 101(7): 828–833.

Sader, M. A., et al. 2001. Androgenic anabolic steroids and arterial structure and function in male bodybuilders. *Journal of the American College of Cardiology* 37(1): 224–230.

Salmon, P. 2001. Effects of physical exercise on anxiety, depression, and sensitivity to stress. *Clinical Psychology Review* 21(1): 33–61.

Sharkey, N. A., N. I. Williams, and J. B. Guerin. 2000. The role of exercise in the prevention and treatment of osteoporosis and osteoarthritis. *Nursing Clinics of North America* 35(1): 209–221.

Stampfer, M. J., et al. 2000. Primary prevention of coronary heart disease in women through diet and lifestyle. *New England Journal of Medicine* 343(1): 16–22.

Tanji, J. L. 2000. The benefits of exercise for women. *Clinics in Sports Medicine* 19(2): 175–185, vii.

University of Florida News. 2001. *Study: Sports Participation Has Mental Perks for All* (http://www.napa.ufl.edu/2001news/bodyimag.htm; retrieved April 19, 2001).

Wallace, L. S., et al. 2000. Characteristics of exercise behavior among college students: Application of social cognitive theory to predicting stage of change. *Preventive Medicine* 31(5): 494–505.

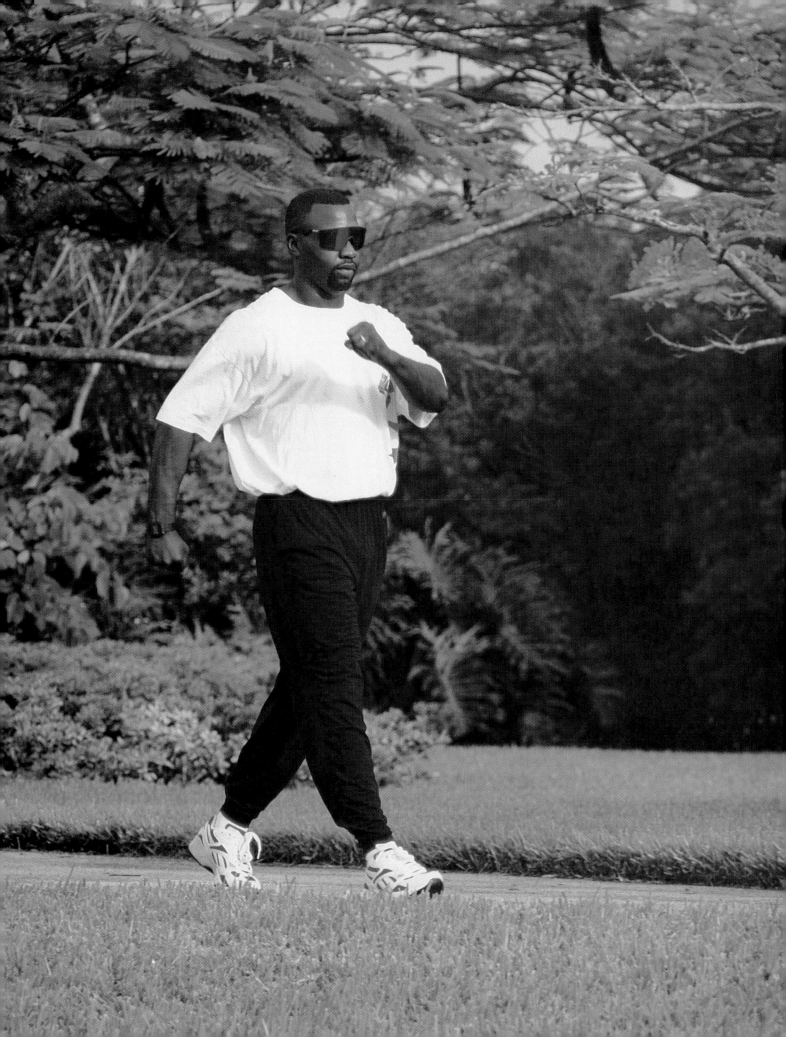

After reading this chapter, you should be able to

- Discuss different methods for assessing body weight and body composition

- Explain the health risks associated with overweight and obesity

- Explain factors that may contribute to a weight problem, including genetic, physiological, lifestyle, and psychosocial factors

- Describe lifestyle factors that contribute to weight gain and loss, including the role of diet, exercise, and emotional factors

- Identify and describe the symptoms of eating disorders and the health risks associated with them

- Design a personal plan for successfully managing body weight

Weight Management

14

TEST YOUR KNOWLEDGE

1. About what percentage of American adults are overweight?
   a. 10%
   b. 30%
   c. 60%

2. Genetic factors explain most cases of obesity.
   True or false?

3. The consumption of low-calorie sweeteners has helped Americans control their weight.
   True or false?

4. Approximately how many female high school and college students have either anorexia or bulimia?
   a. 1 in 250
   b. 1 in 100
   c. 1 in 30

5. Which of the following snacks contains the fewest calories—about 100 for the serving size listed?
   a. 8 ounces (⅔ of a can) of soda
   b. 2 fat-free sandwich cookies
   c. 4 pretzel twists
   d. 2 cups strawberries
   e. 20 baby carrots

ANSWERS

1. C. About 60% of American adults are overweight, including more than 20% who are obese. The rate of obesity among adults has increased more than 60% since 1990.

2. FALSE. Genetic factors may increase an individual's tendency for weight gain; however, lifestyle is the key contributing factor.

3. FALSE. Since the introduction of low-calorie sweeteners, both total calorie intake and total sugar intake have increased, as has the proportion of Americans who are overweight.

4. C. About 2–4% of female students suffer from bulimia or anorexia, and many more occasionally engage in behaviors associated with anorexia or bulimia.

5. ALL FIVE ARE EQUAL. Each of these snacks provides about 100 calories; however, the servings of strawberries and carrots are much larger because they are lower in energy (calorie) density.

A chieving and maintaining a healthy body weight is a serious public health challenge in the United States and a source of distress for many Americans. Under standards developed by the National Institutes of Health, about 60% of American adults are overweight, including more than 20% who are obese (Table 14-1). Lifestyle changes may be at the root of this increase (see the box "The Fattening of America"). And while millions struggle to lose weight, others fall into dangerous eating patterns such as binge eating or self-starvation.

Although not completely understood, managing body weight is not a mysterious process. The "secret" is balancing calories consumed with calories expended in daily activities—in other words, eating a moderate diet and exercising regularly. Unfortunately, this simple formula is not as exciting as the latest fad diet or "scientific breakthrough" that promises slimness without effort. Many people fail in their efforts to manage their weight because they emphasize short-term weight loss rather than permanent changes in lifestyle. Successful weight management requires the long-term coordination of many aspects of a wellness lifestyle, including proper nutrition, adequate physical activity, and stress management.

This chapter explores the factors that contribute to the development of overweight and obesity as well as to eating disorders. It also takes a closer look at weight management through lifestyle and suggests specific strategies for reaching and maintaining a healthy weight. This information is designed to provide the tools necessary for integrating effective weight management into a wellness lifestyle.

BASIC CONCEPTS OF WEIGHT MANAGEMENT

How many times have you or one of your friends said, "I'm too fat. I need to lose weight"? If you are like most people, you are concerned about what you weigh. But how do you decide if you are overweight? At what point does being overweight present a health risk? And how thin is too thin?

Terms

essential fat The fat in the body necessary for normal body functioning.

nonessential (storage) fat Extra fat or fat reserves stored in the body.

percent body fat The percentage of total body weight that is composed of fat.

overweight Body weight that falls above the range associated with minimum mortality.

obesity The condition of having an excess of nonessential body fat; having a body mass index of 30 or greater or having a percent body fat greater than 24% for men and 31% for women.

Table 14-1	The Prevalence of Obesity: Populations of Special Concern	
Group	**Estimated Prevalence of Obesity***	**Healthy People 2010 Target**
Children (age 6–11)	11%	5%
Adolescents (age 12–19)	10	5
Adults (age 20–74)	23	15
Men	20	15
Women	25	15
Low-income people	29	15
People with disabilities	30	15
Black women	38	15
Mexican American women	35	15

*Children and adolescents are classified as obese if they have a BMI at or above the appropriate 95th percentile for body mass index (BMI); adults are classified as obese if they have a BMI of 30 or above.

SOURCE: U.S. Department of Health and Human Services. 2000. *Healthy People 2010.* 2nd ed. Washington, D.C.: DHHS.

Body Composition

The human body can be divided into fat-free mass and body fat. Fat-free mass is composed of all the body's nonfat tissues: bone, water, muscle, connective tissue, organ tissues, and teeth. Body fat includes both essential and nonessential body fat. **Essential fat** includes lipids incorporated in the nerves, brain, heart, lungs, liver, and mammary glands. These fat deposits, crucial for normal body functioning, make up approximately 3% of total body weight in men and 12% in women. The larger percentage in women is due to fat deposits in the breasts, uterus, and other sites specific to females.

Nonessential (storage) fat exists primarily within fat cells, or *adipose tissue,* often located just below the skin and around major organs. The amount of storage fat varies from person to person based on many factors, including gender, age, heredity, metabolism, diet, and activity level. When we talk about wanting to "lose weight," most of us are referring to storage fat.

What is most important for health is not total weight but rather the proportion of the body's total weight that is fat—the **percent body fat.** For example, two women may both be 5 feet, 5 inches tall and weigh 130 pounds. But one woman, an endurance runner, may have only 15% of her body weight as fat, while the second, sedentary, woman could have 32% body fat. While 130 pounds is not considered "overweight" for women of this height by most standards, the second woman may be overfat. (Methods for measuring and evaluating percent body fat

Overweight and obesity are epidemic in the United States. More than half of all adults are overweight and nearly a quarter are obese. The rate of obesity has nearly doubled since 1960, and it continues to rise. If current rates of weight gain continue, *all* American adults will be overweight by 2030. The prevalence of overweight and obesity among children is also on the rise: One child in three is now either overweight or at risk for becoming so. The health problems associated with overweight have also increased, including a 33% rise in the rate of diabetes in just the past decade. It's estimated that inactivity and overweight account for more than 300,000 premature deaths annually in the United States, second only to tobacco-related deaths.

At the same time that Americans are getting fatter, more and more of them are becoming unhappy with their bodies and obsessed with their weight. In recent surveys, more than half of Americans have stated that they are dissatisfied with their weight, and only about 10% report being completely satisfied with their bodies. Dissatisfaction with body weight and shape is at the core of eating disorders, including anorexia, bulimia, and binge eating. Rising levels of overweight accompanied by increased body dissatisfaction have led to an increase in dieting. In surveys, about 30% of adult males and 55% of adult females report having tried to lose weight within the past year; the rate of dieting among adolescent girls and female college students is even higher.

Healthy People 2010 sets the goal of decreasing the number of people who are obese to no more than 15% of adults and 5% of children and adolescents. Despite widespread dieting, however, the trend has definitely been away from this goal, and many Americans appear to be losing the battle to manage their weight. In the hope of pinpointing solutions, researchers have looked at many possible explanations for increasing weight among Americans. At the root of the problem is energy balance: Americans currently consume about 160 more calories per day than they

did 20 years ago, and they engage in less physical activity. Some of the factors that may help explain this shift include the following:

- More meals eaten outside the home
- Greater consumption of fast food
- Increased portion sizes
- Increased consumption of soft drinks and convenience foods
- More time spent in sedentary activities (watching television, playing video games, surfing the Web, and so on)
- Greater numbers of labor-saving devices for household chores
- Fewer daily gym classes for children and adolescents
- Fewer short trips on foot and more by automobile

Public health officials have called for the development of a comprehensive national plan to address the obesity epidemic, one that targets both behavior and environment. Goals include preventing weight gain in adults who are at a healthy weight or who are overweight, promoting weight loss for the obese, and increasing physical activity for Americans of all ages. Proposed strategies include government subsidies for fruits and vegetables and a "sin tax" on high-calorie foods, with the proceeds going to create bike paths, parks, and other facilities that promote physical activity. As officials debate different solutions, there are many actions that individuals can take to manage their own weight and to promote healthy eating and activity habits among others. At the 2000 National Nutrition Summit, Secretary of Health and Human Services Donna Shalala stressed the importance of good nutrition and exercise and challenged everyone to turn off the television and get off the couch.

are presented later in this chapter.) Since most people use the word "overweight" to describe the condition of having too much body fat, we'll use it in this chapter, although "overfat" is actually a more accurate term.

Energy Balance

The key to keeping a healthy ratio of fat to fat-free mass is maintaining an energy balance (Figure 14-1). You take in energy (calories) from the food you eat. Your body uses energy (calories) to maintain vital body functions (resting metabolism), to digest food, and to fuel physical activity. When energy in equals energy out, you maintain your current weight. To change your weight and body composition, you must tip the energy balance equation in a particular direction. If you take in more calories daily than your body burns, the excess calories will be stored as fat, and you will gain weight over time. If you eat fewer calo-

ries than you burn each day, you will lose some of that storage fat and probably lose weight.

The two parts of the energy balance equation over which you have the most control are the energy you take in as food and the energy you burn during physical activity. To lose weight and body fat, you can increase the amount of energy you burn by increasing your level of physical activity and/or decrease the amount of energy you take in by consuming fewer calories. Specific strategies for altering energy balance are discussed later in the chapter.

Evaluating Body Weight and Body Composition

Overweight is usually defined as total body weight above the recommended range for good health (as determined by large-scale population surveys). **Obesity** is defined as a more serious degree of overweight. Many methods are

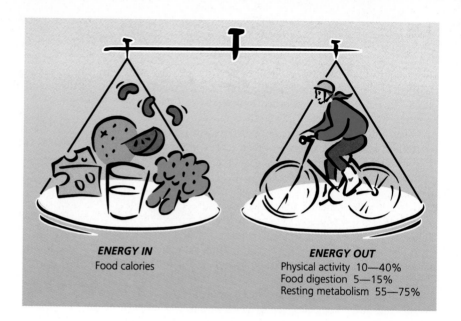

√ **Figure 14-1 The energy balance equation.** In order to maintain your current weight, you must burn up as many calories as you take in as food each day.

ENERGY IN
Food calories

ENERGY OUT
Physical activity 10—40%
Food digestion 5—15%
Resting metabolism 55—75%

available for measuring and evaluating body weight and percent body fat; the cutoff points for defining overweight and obesity vary with the method chosen.

Height-Weight Charts   In the past, many people relied on height-weight charts to evaluate their body weight. Based on insurance company statistics, these list a range of "ideal" or "recommended" body weights associated with the lowest mortality for people of a particular sex, age, and height. Although easy to use, height-weight charts can be highly inaccurate for some people, and they provide only an indirect measure of body fatness.

Body Mass Index   Although also based on the concept that a person's weight should be proportional to height, **body mass index (BMI)** is a more accurate assessment method than height-weight charts. BMI is easy to determine, correlates well with percent body fat for most people, and is a useful indicator of health. BMI is defined as body weight (in kilograms) divided by the square of height (in meters); you can determine your BMI by referring to Figure 14-2. Under standards issued by the National Institutes of Health, a BMI between 18.5 and 24.9 is considered healthy; a person with a BMI of 25 or above is classified as overweight; and a person with a BMI of 30 or above is classified as obese. A person with a BMI below 18.5 is classified as underweight, although low BMI values may be healthy in some cases if they are not the result of smoking, an eating disorder, or an underly-

ing disease; a BMI value of 17.5 or less is sometimes used as a diagnostic criterion for the eating disorder anorexia nervosa.

Like all measures, BMI has its limitations. BMI may classify as overweight a person who is very muscular, such as a football player. BMI may also classify as healthy a person with a relatively low weight but a high percent body fat, such as an older adult with little muscle mass due to inactivity or an underlying disease. BMI is also not particularly useful for tracking changes in an individual's body composition—gains in muscle mass and losses of fat.

Body Composition Analysis   The most accurate and direct way to evaluate body composition is to determine percent body fat; a variety of methods are available. Refer to Table 14-2 for body composition ratings based on percent body fat; as with BMI, the percent body fat ratings indicate cutoff points for health risks associated with underweight and obesity.

HYDROSTATIC (UNDERWATER) WEIGHING   One of the most accurate techniques is hydrostatic weighing. In this method, a person is submerged and weighed under water. Percent body fat can be calculated from body density. Muscle has a higher density and fat a lower density than water, so people with more fat tend to float and weigh less under water, while lean people tend to sink and weigh relatively more under water.

SKINFOLD MEASUREMENTS   The skinfold thickness technique measures the thickness of fat under the skin. A technician grasps a fold of skin at a predetermined location and measures it using an instrument called a caliper. Measurements are taken at several sites and plugged into formulas that predict body fat percentages.

Terms   **body mass index (BMI)** A measure of relative body weight that takes height into account and is highly correlated with more direct measures of body fat; calculated by dividing total body weight (in kilograms) by the square of height (in meters).

<18.5 Underweight		18.5–24.9 Normal						25–29.9 Overweight					30–34.9 Obesity (Class I)					35–39.9 Obesity (Class II)					≥40 Extreme obesity
BMI 17	18	19	20	21	22	23	24	25	26	27	28	29	30	31	32	33	34	35	36	37	38	39	40
Height												Body Weight (pounds)											
4' 10" — 81	86	91	96	101	105	110	115	120	124	129	134	139	144	148	153	158	163	168	172	177	182	187	192
4' 11" — 84	89	94	99	104	109	114	119	124	129	134	139	144	149	154	159	163	168	173	178	183	188	193	198
5' — 87	92	97	102	108	113	118	123	128	133	138	143	149	154	159	164	169	174	179	184	190	195	200	205
5' 1" — 90	95	101	106	111	117	122	127	132	138	143	148	154	159	164	169	175	180	185	191	196	201	207	212
5' 2" — 93	98	104	109	115	120	126	131	137	142	148	153	159	164	170	175	181	186	191	197	202	208	213	219
5' 3" — 96	102	107	113	119	124	130	136	141	147	153	158	164	169	175	181	186	192	198	203	209	215	220	226
5' 4" — 99	105	111	117	122	128	134	140	146	152	157	163	169	175	181	187	192	198	204	210	216	222	227	233
5' 5" — 102	108	114	120	126	132	138	144	150	156	162	168	174	180	186	192	198	204	210	216	222	229	235	241
5' 6" — 105	112	118	124	130	136	143	149	155	161	167	174	180	186	192	198	205	211	217	223	229	236	242	248
5' 7" — 109	115	121	128	134	141	147	153	160	166	173	179	185	192	198	204	211	217	224	230	236	243	249	256
5' 8" — 112	118	125	132	138	145	151	158	165	171	178	184	191	197	204	211	217	224	230	237	244	250	257	263
5' 9" — 115	122	129	136	142	149	156	163	169	176	183	190	197	203	210	217	224	230	237	244	251	258	264	271
5' 10" — 119	126	133	139	146	153	160	167	174	181	188	195	202	209	216	223	230	237	244	251	258	265	272	279
5' 11" — 122	129	136	143	151	158	165	172	179	187	194	201	208	215	222	230	237	244	251	258	265	273	280	287
6' — 125	133	140	148	155	162	170	177	184	192	199	207	214	221	229	236	243	251	258	266	273	280	288	295
6' 1" — 129	137	144	152	159	167	174	182	190	197	205	212	220	228	235	243	250	258	265	273	281	288	296	303
6' 2" — 132	140	148	156	164	171	179	187	195	203	210	218	226	234	242	249	257	265	273	281	288	296	304	312
6' 3" — 136	144	152	160	168	176	184	192	200	208	216	224	232	240	248	256	264	272	280	288	296	304	312	320
6' 4" — 140	148	156	164	173	181	189	197	206	214	222	230	238	247	255	263	271	280	288	296	304	312	321	329

Figure 14-2 Body mass index (BMI). To determine your BMI, find your height in the left column. Move across the appropriate row until you find the weight closest to your own. The number at the top of the column is the BMI at that height and weight. SOURCE: Ratings from National Heart, Lung, and Blood Institute. 1998. *Clinical Guidelines on the Identification, Evaluation, and Treatment of Overweight and Obesity in Adults: The Evidence Report.* Bethesda, Md.: National Institutes of Health.

Table 14-2	Percent Body Fat Standards for Men and Women	
	Men	Women
At risk[a]	≤5%	≤8%
Below average	6–14	9–22
Average	15	23
Above average	16–24	24–31
At risk[b]	≥25	≥32

[a]At risk for diseases and disorders associated with malnutrition
[b]At risk for diseases associated with obesity

Note: These percentages represent approximate standards for body composition; percent body fat associated with good health varies, depending on health status and risk factors for disease. For example, a man with high blood pressure and high cholesterol levels might want to reduce his percentage of body fat, even if it is average for the general population.

SOURCE: Heyward, V. H. 1998. *Advanced Fitness Assessment and Exercise Prescription.* Champaign, Ill.: Human Kinetics.

ELECTRICAL IMPEDANCE ANALYSIS   In this method, electrodes are attached to the body and a harmless electrical current is transmitted from electrode to electrode. The electrical conduction through the body favors the path of the fat-free tissues over the fat tissues. A computer can calculate fat percentages from current measurements.

SCANNING PROCEDURES   High-tech scanning procedures are highly accurate means of assessing body composition, but they require expensive equipment. These procedures include computed tomography (CT), magnetic resonance imaging (MRI), dual-energy X ray absorptiometry, and dual-photon absorptiometry.

Excess Body Fat and Wellness

The amount of fat in the body—and its location—can have profound effects on health.

The Health Risks of Excess Body Fat   Obese people have an overall mortality rate almost twice that of nonobese people. Obesity is associated with unhealthy cholesterol and triglyceride levels, impaired heart function, and death from cardiovascular disease. It is estimated that if all Americans had a healthy body composition, the incidence of coronary heart disease (CHD) would drop by more than 25%. Other health risks associated with obesity include hypertension, many kinds of cancer, impaired immune function, gallbladder and kidney diseases, skin problems, sleep disorders, arthritis, and other bone and joint disorders.

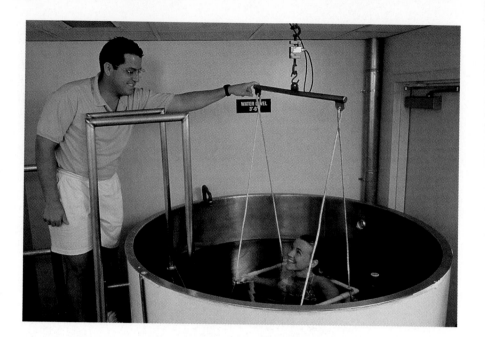

This woman is being submerged as part of a hydrostatic weighing procedure, one of several methods for measuring the percentage of body weight that is fat. A very high or very low percentage of body fat is associated with health problems.

Of particular note is the strong association between excess body fat and diabetes mellitus, a disease that causes a disruption of normal metabolism. The pancreas, a long, thin organ located behind the stomach, normally secretes the hormone insulin, which stimulates cells to take up glucose to produce energy (Figure 14-3). In a person with diabetes, this process is disrupted, causing a buildup of glucose in the bloodstream. Over the long term, diabetes is associated with kidney failure; nerve damage; circulation problems; retinal damage and blindness; and increased rates of heart attack, stroke, and hypertension. Excess body fat is a major risk factor for the most common form of diabetes (Type 2 diabetes). Obese people are more than three times as likely to develop diabetes, and the incidence of diabetes among Americans has increased dramatically as the rate of obesity has climbed. Diabetes is currently the seventh leading cause of death in the United States (see the box "Diabetes" for more information).

The risks from obesity increase with its severity, and they are much more likely to occur in people who are more than twice their desirable body weight. Controversy exists about the precise degree of risk at lower levels of overweight, particularly among overweight individuals who are physically active. The health risks associated with overweight depend in part on an individual's overall health and other risk factors, such as high blood pressure, unhealthy cholesterol levels, body fat distribution, and tobacco use. The National Institutes of Health recommends weight loss for people whose BMI places them in the obese category and for those who are overweight *and* have two or more major risk factors for disease. If your BMI is 25 or above, consult a physician for help in determining a healthy BMI for you.

Many people who are overweight do have at least some of the risk factors associated with obesity. The Nurses' Health Study, in which Harvard researchers have followed more than 120,000 women since 1976, has found that even mildly to moderately overweight women have an 80% increased risk of developing CHD compared to leaner women. This study also confirmed that to reduce the risk of dying prematurely of any cause, maintaining a desirable body weight is important.

Obesity can affect psychological as well as physical wellness. Being perceived as fat can be a source of ridicule, ostracism, and sometimes discrimination from others; it can contribute to psychological problems such as depression, anxiety, and low self-esteem (often caused by repeated failures at losing weight). For some, the stigma associated with obesity can give rise to a negative body image, body dissatisfaction, and eating disorders.

Body Fat Distribution and Health The distribution of body fat is also an important indicator of health. Men and postmenopausal women tend to store fat in the upper regions of their bodies, particularly in the abdominal area ("apples"). Premenopausal women usually store fat in hips, buttocks, and thighs ("pears"). Excess fat in the abdominal area, the apple shape, increases risk of high blood pressure, diabetes, early-onset heart disease, and certain types of cancer. The reason for this increase in risk is not entirely clear, but it appears that abdominal fat is more easily mobilized and sent into the bloodstream, increasing disease-related blood fat levels.

The risks from body fat distribution are usually assessed by measuring waist circumference or by calculating waist-to-hip ratio (the relative circumference of the waist and hips). More research is needed to determine the precise degree of risk associated with specific values for

Symptoms of diabetes:

- Frequent urination
- Extreme thirst and hunger
- Unexplained weight loss
- Extreme fatigue
- Blurred vision
- Frequent infections
- Slow wound healing
- Tingling or numbness inhands and feet
- Dry, itchy skin

Note: In the early stages, diabetes often has no symptoms.

Esophagus

Stomach

Pancreas

Small intestine

Normal:
Insulin binds to receptors on the surface of a cell and signals special transporters in the cell to transport glucose inside.

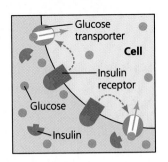

Glucose transporter

Cell

Insulin receptor

Glucose

Insulin

Type 1 diabetes:
The pancreas produces little or no insulin. Thus, no signal is sent instructing the cell to transport glucose, and glucose builds up in the bloodstream.

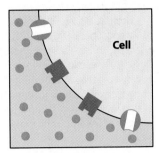

Cell

Type 2 diabetes:
The pancreas produces too little insulin and/or the body's cells are resistant to it. Some insulin binds to receptors on the cell's surface, but the signal to transport glucose is blocked. Glucose builds up in the bloodstream.

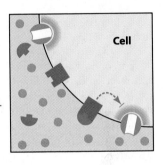

Cell

Figure 14-3   Diabetes mellitus. During digestion, carbohydrates are broken down in the small intestine into glucose, a simple sugar that enters the bloodstream. The presence of glucose signals the pancreas to release insulin, a hormone that helps cells take up glucose; once inside a cell, glucose can be converted to energy. In diabetes, this process is disrupted, resulting in a buildup of glucose in the bloodstream.

these two assessments of body fat distribution. However, a total waist measurement of more than 40 inches for men and 35 inches for women and a waist-to-hip ratio above 0.94 for young men and 0.82 for young women is associated with a significantly increased risk of disease.

A person doesn't have to be technically overfat to have fat distribution be a risk factor, nor do all overfat people face this increased risk. The National Institutes of Health BMI guidelines state that large waist circumference can be a marker for increased risk of diabetes, high blood pressure, and CVD even in people with a BMI in the normal range. And at any given level of overweight, people with a large waist circumference and/or additional disease risk factors are at greater risk for health problems. For example, a man with a BMI of 27, a waist circumference above 40 inches, and diabetes is at greater risk for health problems than another man who has a BMI of 27 but has a smaller waist and no other risk factors.

Weight Cycling   It has been hypothesized that repeatedly losing and regaining weight, known as weight cycling or yo-yo dieting, might be harmful to both overall health and to efforts at weight loss. Weight cycling, it was thought, might make the body more efficient at extracting and storing calories from food; thus, with each successive diet, it would become more difficult to lose weight. Most studies, however, have not supported this idea. Other studies have explored whether weight cycling might change body fat distribution, increase the body's preference for dietary fat, contribute to gallbladder disease and death from CVD, or lead to disordered eating habits. Studies have not yet conclusively shown weight cycling to be harmful to the health of an obese person, and most researchers believe that obese individuals should continue to try to control their weight. Losing even a few pounds brings substantial health benefits that appear to exceed any potential risks that might be incurred from weight loss or weight cycling.

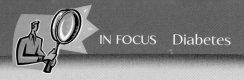

Types of Diabetes

Approximately 18 million Americans—nearly 7% of the population—have one of two major forms of diabetes. About 5–10% of people with diabetes have the more serious form, known as Type 1 diabetes. In this type of diabetes, the pancreas produces little or no insulin, so daily doses of insulin are required. (Without insulin, a person with Type 1 can lapse into a coma.) Type 1 diabetes usually strikes before age 30.

The remaining 90% of Americans with diabetes have Type 2 diabetes. This condition can develop slowly, and about half of affected individuals are unaware of their condition. In Type 2 diabetes, the pancreas doesn't produce enough insulin, cells are resistant to insulin, or both. This condition is usually diagnosed in people over age 40, although it is becoming more common at earlier ages. About one-third of people with Type 2 diabetes must take insulin; others may take medications that increase insulin production or stimulate cells to take up glucose.

A third type of diabetes occurs in about 2–3% of women during pregnancy. So-called *gestational diabetes* usually disappears after pregnancy, but more than half of women who experience it eventually develop Type 2 diabetes.

The major factors involved in the development of diabetes are age, obesity, physical inactivity, a family history of diabetes, and lifestyle. Excess body fat reduces cell sensitivity to insulin, and it is a major risk factor for Type 2 diabetes. Ethnic background also plays a role. African Americans and people of Hispanic background are 55% more likely than non-Hispanic whites to develop Type 2 diabetes; over 20% of Hispanics over age 65 have diabetes. Native Americans also have a higher-than-average incidence of diabetes.

Treatment

There is no cure for diabetes, but it can be successfully managed. Treatment involves keeping blood sugar levels within safe limits through diet, exercise, and, if necessary, medication. Blood sugar levels can be monitored using a home test; close monitoring and control of glucose levels can significantly reduce the rate of serious complications among people with diabetes. Nearly 90% of people with Type 2 diabetes are overweight when diagnosed, and an important step in treatment is to lose weight. Even a small amount of weight loss can be beneficial.

People with diabetes should eat regular meals with an emphasis on complex carbohydrates and ample dietary fiber; a dietitian can help design a healthy eating plan. Regular exercise and a healthy diet are often sufficient to control Type 2 diabetes.

Prevention

Exercise can help prevent the development of Type 2 diabetes, a benefit especially important in individuals with one or more risk factors for the disease. Exercise makes cells more sensitive to insulin and helps stabilize blood glucose levels. Exercise also helps keep body fat at healthy levels.

Eating a healthy diet to help control body fat is perhaps the most important dietary recommendation for the prevention of diabetes. However, there is some evidence that the composition of the diet may also be important. In a long-term study of over 65,000 nurses, a diet low in fiber and high in sugar and refined carbohydrates was found to increase risk for Type 2 diabetes. The foods most closely linked to higher diabetes risk were regular (nondiet) cola beverages, white bread, white rice, french fries, and potatoes; consumption of cereal fibers such as those found in cold breakfast cereals was associated with lower risk. (See Chapter 12 for more information on different types of carbohydrates and specific strategies for increasing fiber intake.)

Warning Signs and Testing

A wellness lifestyle that includes a healthy diet and regular exercise is the best strategy for preventing diabetes. If you do develop diabetes, the best way to avoid complications is to recognize the symptoms and get early diagnosis and treatment. Be alert for the warning signs listed in Figure 14-3.

Type 2 diabetes is often asymptomatic in the early stages, and routine screening is recommended for people over age 45 and anyone younger who is at high risk, including anyone who is obese. (The Web site for the American Diabetes Association, listed in the For More Information section at the end of the chapter, includes an interactive diabetes risk assessment.) Screening involves a blood test to check glucose levels after either a period of fasting or the administration of a set dose of glucose. If you are concerned about your risk for diabetes, talk with your physician about being tested.

Body Image   The collective picture of the body as seen through the mind's eye, **body image** consists of perceptions, images, thoughts, attitudes, and emotions. A negative body image is characterized by dissatisfaction with the body in general or some part of the body in particular. Recent surveys indicate that the majority of Americans, many of whom are not actually overweight, are unhappy with their body weight or with some aspect of their appearance.

This dissatisfaction can cause significant psychological distress. A person can become preoccupied by a perceived defect in appearance, thereby damaging self-esteem and interfering with relationships. Adolescents and adults who have a negative body image are more likely to diet restrictively, eat compulsively, or develop some other form of disordered eating. When dissatisfaction becomes extreme, the condition is called *body dysmorphic disorder;* people suffering from this disorder may desire and seek repeated cosmetic surgeries.

Losing weight or getting cosmetic surgery does not necessarily improve body image. On the other hand, improvements in body image may occur in the absence of changes in weight or appearance. Many experts now believe that body image issues must be dealt with as part of treating obesity and eating disorders. See pp. 416–419 for more information on body image and eating disorders.

Is It Possible to Be Too Lean? Health experts have generally viewed very low levels of body fat—less than 8% for women and 5% for men—as a threat to wellness. Extreme leanness has been linked with reproductive, circulatory, and immune system disorders. Extremely lean people may experience muscle wasting and fatigue; they are also more likely to suffer from dangerous eating disorders.

In physically active women and girls, particularly those involved in sports where weight and appearance are important (ballet, gymnastics, skating, and distance running, for example), a condition called the **female athlete triad** may develop. The triad consists of three interrelated disorders: abnormal eating patterns (and excessive exercising), followed by **amenorrhea** (absence of menstruation), followed by decreased bone density (premature osteoporosis). Prolonged amenorrhea can cause bone density to erode to a point that a woman in her twenties will have the bone density of a woman in her sixties. Left untreated, the triad can lead to decreased physical performance, increased incidence of bone fractures, disturbances of heart rhythm and metabolism, and even death.

> **COMMUNICATE!** The media often present images of tall, thin, young women as an ideal of female beauty. But the media communicate an ideal of male attractiveness as well. The next time you see male models in a magazine, examine the ad carefully to decode its verbal and visual messages. What attributes are being represented? What message is being communicated? Who is the intended target of the message? What effect do you think this message has on you and the people you know?

What Is the Right Weight for You?

For most of us, our body weight and percentage of body fat fall somewhere below the levels associated with significant health risks. For us, these assessment tests do not really answer the question: How much should I weigh? BMI, percent body fat, waist-to-hip ratio, and waist circumference measurement can best serve as general guides or estimates for body weight (see the box "Rate Your BMI and Body Fat Distribution").

To answer the question of what you "should" weigh, let your lifestyle be your guide. Don't focus on a particular weight as your goal. Instead, focus on living a lifestyle that includes eating moderate amounts of healthful foods, getting plenty of exercise, thinking positively, and learning to cope with stress. Then let the pounds fall where they may. For most people, the result will be close to the recommended weight ranges discussed earlier. For some, their weight will be somewhat higher than societal standards—but right for them. By letting a healthy lifestyle determine your weight, you can avoid developing unhealthy patterns of eating and a negative body image.

FACTORS CONTRIBUTING TO EXCESS BODY FAT

Much research has been done in an effort to pinpoint the cause of overweight and obesity. It appears, however, that body weight and body composition are determined by multiple factors that may vary with each individual. These factors can be grouped into genetic, physiological, lifestyle, and psychosocial factors.

Genetic Factors

Estimates of the genetic contribution to obesity vary widely, from about 5% to 40%. More than 20 genes have been linked to obesity, but their actions are still under study. Genes influence body size and shape, body fat distribution, and metabolic rate. Genetic factors also affect the ease with which weight is gained as a result of overeating and where on the body extra weight is added. If both parents are overweight, their children are twice as likely to be overweight as children who have only one overweight parent. In studies that compared adoptees and their biological parents, the weights of the adoptees were found to be more like those of the biological parents than the adoptive parents, again indicating a strong genetic link.

Research thus suggests a genetic component in the determination of body weight. However, hereditary influences must be balanced against the contribution of environmental factors. Not all children of obese parents become obese, and normal-weight parents also have overweight children. The incidence of obesity is rising rapidly in the United States, but not in all parts of the world. In a study comparing men born and raised in Ireland with their biological brothers who lived in the United States, the American men were found to weigh, on average, 6% more than their Irish brothers. Environmental factors like diet and exercise are probably responsible for this difference in weight. Thus, the *tendency* to develop obesity may be inherited, but the expression of this tendency is affected by environmental influences.

The message you should take from this research is that genes are not destiny. It is true that some people have a

Terms

body image The mental representation a person holds about his or her body at any given moment in time, consisting of perceptions, images, thoughts, attitudes, and emotions about the body.

female athlete triad A condition consisting of three interrelated disorders: abnormal eating patterns (and excessive exercising) followed by lack of menstrual periods (amenorrhea) and decreased bone density (premature osteoporosis).

amenorrhea The absence of menstruation.

1. Determine your BMI by referring to Figure 14-2, or calculate it more precisely by dividing your body weight (in kilograms) by the square of your height (in meters). To convert, multiply your height in inches by 0.0254 to get meters, and multiply your weight in pounds by 0.45 to get kilograms. For example, if you are 5 feet, 6 inches tall (66 inches) and weigh 150 pounds, you calculate your BMI as follows:

$$BMI = \frac{150 \times 0.45}{(66 \times 0.0254)^2} = \frac{67.5}{(1.676)^2} = 24.0$$

Then, refer to Table 1 for the appropriate rating of your BMI.

BMI:_____ Classification:_____

2. For information about the health risks associated with your body fat distribution, determine your waist circumference and your waist-to-hip ratio. Take measurements at your smallest waist circumference and largest hip circumference; if you don't have a natural waist, measure at the level of your navel. Calculate your waist-to-hip ratio by dividing your waist measurement by your hip measurement. For example, if your waist is 28 inches and your hips 38 inches, your waist-to-hip ratio is 28 ÷ 38 = 0.74.

Table 2 indicates values for waist circumference and waist-to-hip ratio above which the risk of health problems increases significantly. If your measurement or ratio is above either cutoff point, put a check on the appropriate line below.

Waist circumference:_____ High risk? (✓)_____

Waist-to-hip ratio: _____ High risk? (✓)_____

Table 1 **Body Mass Index (BMI) Classifications**

Classification	BMI (kg/m²)	Obesity class
Underweight*	<18.5	
Normal	18.5–24.9	
Overweight	25.0–29.9	
Obesity	30.0–34.9	I
	35.0–39.9	II
Extreme obesity	≥40.0	III

*Research suggests that a low BMI can be healthy in some cases, as long as it is not the result of smoking, an eating disorder, or an underlying disease process.

Table 2 **Body Fat Distribution: Cutoff Points for High Risk**

	Waist Circumference	Waist-to-Hip Ratio
Men	>40 inches	>0.94
Women	>35 inches	>0.82

SOURCES: National Heart, Lung, and Blood Institute. 1998. *Clinical Guidelines on the Identification, Evaluation, and Treatment of Overweight and Obesity in Adults: The Evidence Report.* Bethesda, Md.: National Institutes of Health. American College of Sports Medicine. 1998. *ACSM's Resource Manual for Guidelines for Exercise Testing and Prescription,* 3rd ed. Baltimore, Md.: Williams & Wilkins.

---

harder time losing weight and maintaining weight loss than others. However, with increased exercise and attention to diet, even those with a genetic tendency toward obesity can maintain a healthy body weight. And regardless of genetic factors, lifestyle choices remain the cornerstone of successful weight management.

Physiological Factors

Metabolism is a key physiological factor in the regulation of body fat and body weight; hormones also play a role. Other physiological factors that have been proposed as contributing to obesity include fat cells and carbohydrate craving.

Metabolism Metabolism is the sum of all the vital processes by which food energy and nutrients are made available to and used by the body. The largest component of metabolism, **resting metabolic rate (RMR),** is the energy required to maintain vital body functions, including respiration, heart rate, body temperature, and blood pressure, while the body is at rest. As shown in Figure 14-1, RMR accounts for 55–75% of daily energy expenditure. The energy required to digest food accounts for an addi-

tional 5–15% of daily energy expenditure. The remaining 10–40% is expended during physical activity.

Both heredity and behavior affect metabolic rate. Men, who have a higher proportion of muscle mass than women, have a higher RMR (muscle tissue is more metabolically active than fat). Also, some individuals inherit a higher or lower RMR than others. A higher RMR means that a person burns more calories while at rest and can therefore take in more calories without gaining weight.

Weight loss or gain also affects metabolic rate. When a person loses weight, both RMR and the energy required to perform physical tasks decrease. The reverse occurs when weight is gained.

Exercise has a positive effect on metabolism. When people exercise, they slightly increase their RMR—the number of calories their bodies burn at rest. They also increase their muscle mass, which is associated with a higher metabolic rate. The exercise itself also burns calories, raising total energy expenditure. The higher the energy expenditure, the more the person can eat without gaining weight. (The role of exercise in weight management is discussed in greater detail later in the chapter.)

Hormones Hormones clearly play a role in the accumulation of body fat, especially for females. Hormonal changes at puberty, during pregnancy, and at menopause contribute to the amount and location of fat accumulation. For example, during puberty, hormones cause the development of secondary sex characteristics, including larger breasts, wider hips, and a fat layer under the skin.

One hormone thought to be linked to obesity is leptin. Secreted by the body's fat cells, leptin is carried to the brain, where it appears to let the brain know how big or small the body's fat stores are. With this information, the brain can regulate appetite and metabolic rate accordingly. Other hormones that may be involved in the regulation of appetite are cholecystokinin (CCK), peptide YY, and gluconlike peptide-1 (GLP-1). Researchers hope to use these hormones to develop treatments for obesity based on appetite control; however, as most of us will admit, hunger is often *not* the primary reason we overeat. Cases of obesity based solely or primarily on hormone abnormalities do exist, but they are rare. Lifestyle choices still account for the largest proportion of the differences in body weight and body composition among individuals.

Fat Cells The amount of fat the body can store is a function of the number and size of fat cells. These fat cells are like little compartments that can be inflated to hold body fat; when all or nearly all the fat cells are filled, the body makes more, thereby increasing its ability to expand fat stores. Some people are born with an above-average number of fat cells and thus have the potential for storing more energy as body fat. Overeating at critical times, such as in childhood, can cause the body to expand the number of fat cells. It has been hypothesized that having more or larger fat cells creates biological pressure to keep eating to fill all the fat cells; however, this has not been substantiated by research. If a person loses weight, fat cell content is depleted, but it is unclear whether the number of fat cells can be decreased.

Carbohydrate Craving It has been hypothesized that carbohydrate craving may cause overeating and thus lead to overweight and obesity. Animal studies have suggested that consuming carbohydrates increases brain levels of serotonin, a neurotransmitter that induces calmness. People with low levels of serotonin thus might crave and consume carbohydrates because they experience improved mood and reduced fatigue after eating such foods as bread, pasta, and candy. However, research in humans supporting this hypothesis remains incomplete and unconvincing.

Lifestyle Factors

While genetic and physiological factors may increase risk for excess body fat, they are not sufficient to explain the increasingly high rate of obesity seen in the United States.

The gene pool has not changed dramatically in the past 40 years, during which time the rate of obesity among Americans has doubled. Clearly, other factors are at work—particularly lifestyle factors such as increased energy intake and decreased physical activity.

Eating Americans have access to an abundance of highly palatable and calorie-dense foods, and many have eating habits that contribute to weight gain. Most overweight adults will admit to eating more than they should of high-fat, high-sugar, high-calorie foods. Americans eat out more frequently now than in the past, and we rely more heavily on fast food and packaged convenience foods. Restaurant and convenience food portion sizes tend to be very large, and the foods themselves are more likely to be high in fat, sugar, and calories and low in nutrients. Studies have consistently found that people underestimate portion sizes by as much as 25%.

Many children and adolescents do not learn healthy eating habits. If parents make high-fat, high-calorie foods available to children, they are teaching them to prefer these foods—especially if such foods are used as rewards for good behavior. Studies have found that food choices of children as young as 2 years of age are influenced by television advertising. And many schools now offer not only soda and snack machines but also on-site outlets for fast-food chains. Parents need to practice good eating habits themselves, and both parents and schools should promote healthy habits in a way that is fun and inviting to young people.

According to the CDC, the average calorie intake by Americans has increased by 100–300 calories per day over the past two decades. Levels of physical activity did not increase during this period; in fact, they declined. The net result has been a substantial increase in the number of Americans who are overweight and obese. Healthy eating habits that are part of successful weight management are described later in this chapter.

Physical Activity Research has shown that activity levels among Americans are declining, beginning in childhood and continuing throughout the life cycle. Many schools have cut back on physical education classes and recess. Most adults drive to work, sit all day, and then relax in front of the TV at night. During leisure time, both children and adults surf the Internet, play video games, or watch TV rather than bicycle, participate in sports, or just do yardwork or chores around the house. One study found that 60% of the incidence of overweight can be linked to excessive television viewing. On average, Americans exercise 15 minutes per day and watch 150 minutes

resting metabolic rate (RMR) The energy required to maintain vital body functions, including respiration, heart rate, body temperature, and blood pressure, while the body is at rest.

Terms

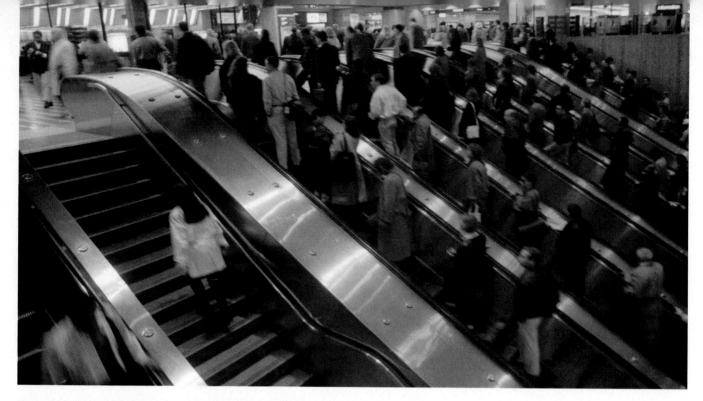

The typical American lifestyle does not lead naturally to healthy weight management. Labor-saving devices such as escalators help reinforce our sedentary habits.

of TV. Modern conveniences such as remote controls, elevators, and power mowers have also reduced daily physical activity.

Psychosocial Factors

Many people have learned to use food as a means of coping with stress and negative emotions. Eating can provide a powerful distraction from difficult feelings—loneliness, anger, boredom, anxiety, shame, sadness, inadequacy. It can be used to combat low moods, low energy levels, and low self-esteem (see the box "What Triggers Your Eating?"). When food and eating become the primary means of regulating emotions, binge eating or other disturbed eating patterns can develop.

Obesity is strongly associated with socioeconomic status. The prevalence of obesity goes down as income level goes up. More women are obese at lower income levels than men, but men are somewhat more obese at higher levels. These differences may reflect the greater sensitivity and concern for a slim physical appearance among upper-income women, as well as greater access to information about nutrition and to low-fat and low-calorie foods. It may also reflect the greater acceptance of obesity among certain ethnic groups, as well as different cultural values related to food choices.

In some families and cultures, food is used as a symbol of love and caring. It is an integral part of social gatherings and celebrations. In such cases, it may be difficult to change established eating patterns because they are linked to cultural and family values.

COMMUNICATE! When food is intertwined with cultural and social meanings, such as at a company picnic, a wedding banquet, or a holiday party, we often feel pressured to eat more than we need or even want. If you have such an event on your calendar, think ahead about how you can make healthy food and portion choices without breaking social norms. For example, instead of accepting seconds and thirds at Thanksgiving dinner, you could say simply, "Everything tastes wonderful, but I'm full!" If you're pressed, try saying, "Maybe I could take a piece of pie home with me for tomorrow."

ADOPTING A HEALTHY LIFESTYLE FOR SUCCESSFUL WEIGHT MANAGEMENT

When all the research has been assessed, it is clear that most weight problems are lifestyle problems. Even though more and more young people are developing weight problems, most arrive at early adulthood with the advantage of having a "normal" body weight—neither too fat nor too thin. In fact, many young adults get away

Hunger isn't the only reason people eat. Efforts to maintain a healthy body weight can be sabotaged by eating related to other factors, including emotions, environment, and patterns of thinking. This quiz is designed to provide you with a score for five factors that describe many people's eating habits. This information will put you in a better position to manage your eating behavior and control your weight. Circle the number that indicates to what degree each situation is likely to make you start eating.

				Very Unlikely						Very Likely

Social

	Very Unlikely									Very Likely
1. Arguing or having a conflict with someone	1	2	3	4	5	6	7	8	9	10
2. Being with others when they are eating	1	2	3	4	5	6	7	8	9	10
3. Being urged to eat by someone else	1	2	3	4	5	6	7	8	9	10
4. Feeling inadequate around others	1	2	3	4	5	6	7	8	9	10

Emotional

5. Feeling bad, such as being anxious or depressed	1	2	3	4	5	6	7	8	9	10
6. Feeling good, happy, or relaxed	1	2	3	4	5	6	7	8	9	10
7. Feeling bored or having time on my hands	1	2	3	4	5	6	7	8	9	10
8. Feeling stressed or excited	1	2	3	4	5	6	7	8	9	10

Situational

9. Seeing an advertisement for food or eating	1	2	3	4	5	6	7	8	9	10
10. Passing by a bakery, cookie shop, or other enticement to eat	1	2	3	4	5	6	7	8	9	10
11. Being involved in a party, celebration, or special occasion	1	2	3	4	5	6	7	8	9	10
12. Eating out	1	2	3	4	5	6	7	8	9	10

Thinking

13. Making excuses to myself about why it's OK to eat	1	2	3	4	5	6	7	8	9	10
14. Berating myself for being fat or unable to control my eating	1	2	3	4	5	6	7	8	9	10
15. Worrying about others or about difficulties I'm having	1	2	3	4	5	6	7	8	9	10
16. Thinking about how things should or shouldn't be	1	2	3	4	5	6	7	8	9	10

Physiological

17. Experiencing pain or physical discomfort	1	2	3	4	5	6	7	8	9	10
18. Experiencing trembling, headache, or light-headedness associated with no eating or too much caffeine	1	2	3	4	5	6	7	8	9	10
19. Experiencing fatigue or feeling overtired	1	2	3	4	5	6	7	8	9	10
20. Experiencing hunger pangs or urges to eat, even though I've eaten recently	1	2	3	4	5	6	7	8	9	10

Scoring

Total your scores for each category, and enter them below. Then rank the scores by marking the highest score 1, next highest score 2, and so on. Focus on the highest-ranked categories first, but any score above 24 is high and indicates that you need to work on that category.

Category	Total Score	Rank Order
Social (Items 1–4)	____	____
Emotional (Items 5–8)	____	____
Situational (Items 9–12)	____	____
Thinking (Items 13–16)	____	____
Physiological (Items 17–20)	____	____

What Your Score Means

Social   A high score here means you are very susceptible to the influence of others. Work on better ways to communicate more assertively, handle conflict, and manage anger. Challenge your beliefs about the need to be polite and the obligations you feel you must fulfill.

Emotional   A high score here means you need to develop effective ways to cope with emotions. Work on developing skills in stress management, time management, and communication. Practicing positive but realistic self-talk can help you handle small daily upsets.

Situational   A high score here means you are especially susceptible to external influences. Try to avoid external cues and respond differently to those you cannot avoid. Control your environment by changing the way you buy, store, cook, and serve food. Anticipate potential problems, and have a plan for handling them.

Thinking   A high score here means that the way you think—how you talk to yourself, the beliefs you hold, your memories, and your expectations—have a powerful influence on your eating habits. Try to be less self-critical, less perfectionistic, and more flexible in your ideas about the way things ought to be. Recognize when you're making excuses or rationalizations that allow you to eat.

Physiological   A high score here means that the way you eat, what you eat, or medications you are taking may be affecting your eating behavior. You may be eating to reduce physical arousal or deal with physical discomfort. Try eating three meals a day, supplemented with regular snacks if needed. Avoid too much caffeine. If any medication you're taking produces adverse physical reactions, switch to an alternative, if possible. If your medications may be affecting your hormone levels, discuss possible alternatives with your physician.

SOURCE: Adapted from Nash, J. D. 1997. *The New Maximize Your Body Potential*. Palo Alto, Calif.: Bull. Reprinted with permission from Bull Publishing Company.

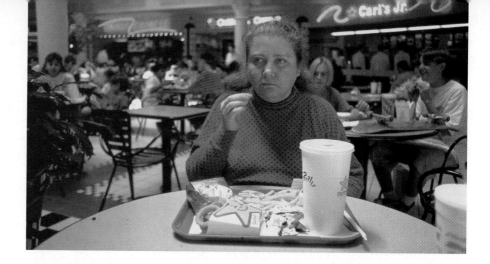

Large portions can make it more difficult to consume a moderate diet and manage weight. Many people significantly underestimate the amount of food they eat.

with terrible eating and exercise habits and don't develop a weight problem. But as the rapid growth of adolescence slows and family and career obligations increase, maintaining a healthy weight becomes a greater challenge. A good time to develop a lifestyle for successful weight management is during early adulthood, when healthy behavior patterns have a better chance of taking a firm hold.

Permanent weight loss is not something you start and stop. You need to adopt healthy behaviors that you can maintain throughout your life. Lifestyle factors that are critical for successful long-term weight management include eating habits, level of physical activity, an ability to think positively and manage your emotions effectively, and the coping strategies you use to deal with the stresses and challenges in your life.

Diet and Eating Habits

In contrast to "dieting," which involves some form of food restriction, "diet" refers to your daily food choices. Everyone has a diet, but not everyone is dieting. You need to develop a diet that you enjoy and that enables you to maintain a healthy body composition.

Use the Food Guide Pyramid as the basis for planning a healthy diet (see Chapter 12). For weight management, you may need to pay special attention to total calories, portion sizes, energy density, fat and sugar intake, and eating habits.

Total Calories The Food Guide Pyramid suggests the following approximate daily energy intakes:

- 1600 calories: Many sedentary women and some older adults

- 2200 calories: Most children, teenage girls, active women, and many sedentary men

- 2800 calories: Teenage boys, many active men, and some very active women

However, energy balance may be a more important consideration for weight management than total calories con-

sumed (see Figure 14-1). To maintain your current weight, the total number of calories you eat must equal the number you burn. To lose weight, you must decrease your calorie intake and/or increase the number of calories you burn; to gain weight, the reverse is true.

The best approach for weight loss is combining an increase in physical activity with moderate calorie restriction. Don't go on a "crash diet." You need to consume enough food to meet your need for essential nutrients. Also, to maintain weight loss, you will probably have to maintain some degree of the calorie restriction you used to lose the weight. Therefore, it is important that you adopt a level of food intake that you can live with over the long term.

Portion Sizes Overconsumption of total calories is closely tied to portion sizes. Many Americans are unaware that the portion sizes of packaged foods and of foods served at restaurants have increased in size, and most of us significantly underestimate the amount of food we eat. Limiting portion sizes to those recommended in the Food Guide Pyramid is critical for maintaining good health. For many people, concentrating on portion sizes is also a much easier method of monitoring and managing total food intake than counting calories.

To counteract portion distortion, weigh and measure your food at home for a few days every now and then. In addition, check the serving sizes listed on packaged foods. With practice, you'll learn to judge portion sizes more accurately. Refer to Chapter 12 for more information and hints on choosing appropriate portion sizes.

Energy (Calorie) Density Experts also recommend that you pay attention to "energy density"—the number of calories per ounce or gram of weight in a food. Studies suggest that it isn't consumption of a certain amount of fat or calories in food that reduces hunger and leads to feelings of fullness and satisfaction; rather, it is consumption of a certain weight of food. Foods that are low in energy density have more volume and bulk—that is, they are relatively heavy but have few calories. For example, for the same 100 calories, you could consume 21 baby carrots or 4 pretzel twists; you are more likely to feel full after eating the serving of carrots because it weighs 10 times that of the serving of pretzels (10 ounces versus 1 ounce).

To cut back on calories and still feel full, then, you should favor foods with a low energy density. Fresh fruits and vegetables, with their high water and fiber content, are low in energy density, as are whole-grain foods. Meat, ice cream, potato chips, croissants, crackers, and low-fat cakes and cookies are examples of foods high in energy density. Strategies for lowering the energy density of your diet include the following:

- Eat fruit with breakfast and for dessert.
- Add extra vegetables to sandwiches, casseroles, stir-fry dishes, pizza, pasta dishes, and fajitas.
- Start meals with a bowl of broth-based soup; include a green salad or fruit salad.
- Snack on fresh fruits and vegetables rather than crackers, chips, or other energy-dense snack foods.
- Limit serving sizes of energy-dense foods such as butter, mayonnaise, cheese, chocolate, fatty meats, croissants, and snack foods that are fried or high in added sugars (including reduced-fat products).

Fat Calories   Although some fat is needed in the diet to provide essential nutrients, you should avoid overeating fatty foods. There is some evidence that fat calories are more easily converted to body fat than calories from protein or carbohydrate. Limiting fat in the diet can also help you limit your total calories. As described in Chapter 12, fat should supply no more than 30% of your average total daily calories, which translates into no more than 66 grams of fat in a 2000-calorie diet each day. Foods rich in fat include oils, margarine, butter, cream, and lard, which are almost pure fat; meat and processed foods, which contain a great deal of "hidden" fat; and nuts, seeds, and avocados, which are plant sources of fats.

Some people are better fat burners than others; that is, they burn more of the fat they take in as calories and therefore have less fat to store. Low fat burners convert more dietary fat to stored body fat. This tendency to hoard fat calories may be an important part of the genetic tendency toward obesity. For low fat burners, restricting fat calories to a level even below 30% may be helpful in weight management.

As Chapter 12 made clear, moving toward a diet strong in complex carbohydrates and fresh fruits and vegetables, and away from a reliance on meat and processed foods, is an effective approach to reducing fat consumption. Watch out for processed foods labeled "fat-free" or "reduced fat," as they may be high in calories (see the box "Evaluating Fat and Sugar Substitutes"). In addition, researchers have found that many Americans compensate for a lower-fat diet by consuming more calories overall.

Complex Carbohydrates   It has long been the fashion among dieters to cut back on bread, pasta, and potatoes to control weight. But complex carbohydrates from these sources, as well as from vegetables, legumes, and whole grains, are precisely the nutrients that can help you achieve and maintain a healthy body weight. They help provide a feeling of satiety, or fullness, that can keep you from overeating. Carbohydrates should make up 55–65% of total daily calories for most people. Avoid high-fat toppings and sauces, however; try plain yogurt instead of sour cream on your baked potato and tomato-based sauces rather than cream sauces on your pasta.

Simple Sugars and Refined Carbohydrates   As described in Chapter 12, foods high in added sugar provide calories but few nutrients. Choose fresh fruits and whole grains instead of foods high in added sugars and refined carbohydrates. Avoid or minimize consumption of sugary soft drinks and fruit drinks, which are often high in calories.

Protein   The typical American consumes more than an adequate amount of protein. Special dietary supplements that provide extra protein are unnecessary for most people, and protein not needed by the body for growth and tissue repair will be stored as fat. Foods high in protein are often also high in fat. Stick to the recommended protein intake of 10–15% of total daily calories.

Eating Habits   Equally important to weight management is eating small, frequent meals—three or more a day plus snacks—on a dependable, regular schedule. Skipping meals leads to excessive hunger, feelings of deprivation, and increased vulnerability to binge eating or snacking on high-calorie, high-fat, or sugary foods. A regular pattern of eating, along with some personal "decision rules" governing food choices, is a way of thinking about and then internalizing the many details that go into a healthy, low-fat diet. Decision rules governing breakfast might be these, for example: Choose a sugar-free, high-fiber cereal with nonfat milk most of the time; once in a while (no more than once a week), have a hard-boiled egg; save pancakes and waffles for special occasions.

Decreeing some foods "off limits" generally sets up a rule to be broken. The better principle is "everything in moderation." If a particular food becomes troublesome, it might be placed off limits temporarily until control over it is regained. The ultimate goal for achieving a healthy diet that ensures successful weight management is to eat in moderation; no foods need to be entirely off limits, though some should be eaten judiciously. Making the healthier choice more often than not is the essence of moderation.

Physical Activity and Exercise

Regular physical activity is another important lifestyle factor in weight management. Physical activity and exercise

For successful weight management, some people find it helpful to limit their intake of foods high in fat and simple sugars. Foods made with fat and sugar substitutes are often promoted for weight loss. But just what are fat and sugar substitutes? And can they really contribute to weight management?

Fat Substitutes

A variety of substances are used to replace fats in processed foods and other products. Some contribute calories, protein, fiber, and/or other nutrients, while others do not. Fat replacers can be classified into three general categories:

- *Carbohydrate-based fat replacers* include starch, fibers, gums, cellulose, polydextrose, and fruit purees. They are the oldest and most widely used form of fat replacer and are found in dairy and meat products, baked goods, salad dressing, and many other prepared foods. Newer types such as Oatrim, Z-trim, and Nu-trim are made from types of dietary fiber that may actually lower cholesterol levels. Carbohydrate-based fat replacers contribute 0–4 calories per gram.

- *Protein-based fat replacers* are typically made from milk, egg whites, soy, or whey; trade names include Simplesse, Dairy-lo, and Supro. They are used in cheese, sour cream, mayonnaise, margarine spreads, frozen desserts, salad dressing, and baked goods. Protein-based fat replacers typically contribute 1–4 calories per gram.

- *Fat-based fat replacers* include glycerides, olestra, and other special types of fatty acids. Some of these compounds are not absorbed well by the body and so provide fewer calories per gram (5 calories compared with the standard 9 for fats); others are impossible for the body to digest and so contribute no calories at all. Olestra, marketed under the trade name Olean and used in fried snack foods, is an example of the latter type of compound. Concerns have been raised about the safety of olestra because it reduces the absorption of fat-soluble nutrients and certain antioxidants and because it causes gastrointestinal distress in some people.

Nonnutritive Sweeteners

Sugar substitutes are often referred to as nonnutritive sweeteners because they provide no calories or essential nutrients. By 2000, four types of nonnutritive sweeteners had been approved for use in the United States; acesulfame-K (Sunett, Sweet One), aspartame (NutraSweet, Equal, NatraTaste), saccharin (Sweet 'N Low), and sucralose (Splenda). They are used in beverages, desserts, baked goods, yogurt, chewing gum, and products such as toothpaste, mouthwash, and cough syrup. Other non-nutritive sweeteners currently under review include alitame, cyclamate, neotame, and stevia.

Fat and Sugar Substitutes in Weight Management

Whether fat and sugar substitutes help you achieve and maintain a healthy weight depends on your lifestyle—your overall eating and activity habits. The increase in the availability of fat-free and sugar-free foods in the United States has *not* been associated with a drop in calorie consumption. When evaluating foods containing fat and sugar substitutes, consider these issues:

- *Is the food lower in calories or just lower in fat?* Reduced-fat foods often contain extra sugar to improve the taste and texture lost when fat is removed, so such foods may be as high or even higher in total calories than their fattier counterparts. Limiting fat intake is an important goal for weight management, but so is controlling total calories.

- *Are you choosing foods with fat and/or sugar substitutes* instead of *foods you typically eat or* in addition to *foods you typically eat?* If you consume low-fat, no-sugar-added ice cream instead of regular ice cream, you may save calories. But if you add such ice cream to your daily diet simply because it is lower in fat and sugar, your overall calorie consumption—and your weight—may increase.

- *How many foods containing fat and sugar substitutes do you consume each day?* Although the FDA has given at least provisional approval to all the fat and sugar substitutes currently available, health concerns about some of these products linger. One way to limit any potential adverse effects is to read labels and monitor how much of each product you consume. Remember that fat and sugar substitutes are found in a wide variety of products.

- *Is an even healthier choice available?* Many of the foods containing fat and sugar substitutes are low-nutrient snack foods. Although substituting a lower-fat or lower-sugar version of the same food may be beneficial, fruits, vegetables, and whole grains are healthier snack choices.

burn calories and keep the metabolism geared to using food for energy instead of storing it as fat. Making significant cuts in food intake in order to lose weight is a difficult strategy to maintain; increasing your physical activity is a much better approach.

As described in Chapter 13, the first step in becoming more active is to incorporate more physical activity into your daily life. Accumulate 30 minutes or more of moderate-intensity physical activity—walking, gardening, housework, and so on—on most, or preferably all, days of the week. Take advantage of routine opportunities to be more active; in the long term, even a small increase in activity level can help maintain your current weight or help you lose a modest amount of weight. In fact, research suggests that fidgeting—stretching, squirming, standing up, and so on—may help prevent weight gain after overeating in some people. If you are overweight or obese and want to lose weight and keep it off, a greater amount of physical activity can help. Researchers have found that people who lose weight and don't regain it typ-

If you gaze into the mirror and wish you could change the way your body looks, consider getting some exercise—not to reshape your contours but to firm up your body image and enhance your self-esteem. In a recent study, 82 adults completed a 12-week aerobic exercise program and had 12 months of follow-up. Compared with the control group, these participants improved their fitness and also benefited psychologically in tests of mood, anxiety, and self-concept. These same physical and psychological benefits were still significant at the 1-year follow-up.

One reason for the findings may be that people who exercise regularly often gain a sense of mastery and competence that enhances their self-esteem and body image. In addition, exercise contributes to a more toned look, which many adults prefer. Research suggests that physically active people are more comfortable with their bodies and their image than sedentary people are. In one workplace study, 60 employees were asked to complete a 36-session stretching program whose main purpose was

to prevent muscle strains at work. At the end of the program, besides the significant increase by all participants in measurements of flexibility, their perceptions of their bodies improved and so did their overall sense of self-worth.

Similar results were obtained in a Norwegian study, in which 219 middle-aged people at risk for heart disease were randomly assigned to one of four groups: diet, diet plus exercise, exercise, and no intervention. The greater the participation of individuals in the exercise component of the program, the higher were their scores in perceived competence/self-esteem and coping.

SOURCES: DiLorenzo, T. M., et al. 1999. Long-term effects of aerobic exercise on psychological outcomes. *Preventive Medicine* 28(1): 75–85. Sorensen, M., et al. 1999. The effect of exercise and diet on mental health and quality of life in middle-aged individuals with elevated risk factors for cardiovascular disease. *Journal of Sports Science* 17(5): 369–377. Moore, T. M. 1998. A workplace stretching program. *AAOHN Journal* 46(12): 563–568.

ically burn about 2800 calories per week in physical activity—the equivalent of about 1 hour of brisk walking per day.

Once you become more active every day, consider beginning a formal exercise program that includes cardiorespiratory endurance exercise, resistance training, and stretching exercises. Moderate cardiorespiratory endurance exercise, sustained for 45 minutes to 1 hour, can help trim body fat permanently. Strength training helps increase fat-free mass, which results in more calorie burning even outside of exercise periods. See Chapter 13 for advice on creating a complete fitness program.

The message about exercise is that regular exercise, maintained throughout life, makes weight management easier and improves quality of life (see the box "Exercise, Body Image, and Self-Esteem"). The sooner you establish good habits, the better. The key to success is making exercise an integral part of the lifestyle you can enjoy now and will enjoy in the future. Chapter 13 contains many suggestions for becoming a more active, physically fit person.

Thinking and Emotions

What goes on in your head is another factor in a healthy lifestyle and successful weight management. The way you think about yourself and your world influences and is influenced by how you feel and how you act. Certain kinds of thinking produce negative emotions, which can undermine a healthy lifestyle.

Research on people who have a weight problem indicates that low self-esteem and the negative emotions that accompany it are significant problems. This often results

in part from mentally comparing the actual self to an internally held picture of the "ideal self." The greater the discrepancy, the larger the impact on self-esteem and the more likely the presence of negative emotions.

Often our internalized "ideal self" is the result of having adopted perfectionistic goals and beliefs about how we and others "should" be. Examples of such beliefs are "If I don't do things perfectly, I'm a failure" and "It's terrible if I'm not thin." These irrational beliefs may cause stress and emotional disturbance. The remedy is to challenge such beliefs and replace them with more realistic ones.

The beliefs and attitudes you hold give rise to self-talk, an internal dialogue you carry on with yourself about events that happen to and around you. Positive self-talk includes leading yourself through the steps of a job and then praising yourself when it's successfully completed. Negative self-talk takes the form of self-deprecating remarks, self-blame, and angry and guilt-producing comments. Negative self-talk can undermine efforts at self-control and lead to feelings of anxiety and depression (see Chapter 3).

Your beliefs and attitude influence how you interpret what happens to you and what you can expect in the future, as well as how you feel and react. A healthy lifestyle is supported by having realistic beliefs and goals and by engaging in positive self-talk and problem-solving efforts.

Coping Strategies

Adequate and appropriate coping strategies for dealing with the stresses and challenges of life are another lifestyle factor in weight management. One strategy that some people adopt for coping is eating. (Others use drugs, alcohol, smoking, spending, gambling, and so on to cope.) When boredom occurs, eating can provide entertainment. Food may be used to alleviate loneliness or as a pickup for fatigue. Eating provides distraction from difficult problems and is a means of punishing the self or others for real or imagined transgressions.

People with a healthy lifestyle have more effective ways to get their needs met. Having learned to communicate assertively and to manage interpersonal conflict effectively, they don't shrink from problems or overreact. The person with a healthy lifestyle knows how to create and maintain relationships with others and has a solid network of friends and loved ones. Food is used appropriately—to fuel life's activities and gain personal satisfaction, not to manage stress.

The healthy lifestyle that naturally and easily results in a reasonable body weight is one characterized by good nutrition, adequate exercise, positive thinking and emotions, and effective coping strategies and behavior patterns. You can make positive changes in your lifestyle to promote permanent weight control; see the box "Strategies for Successful Weight Management" for ideas.

COMMUNICATE! Some people overeat when they are angry or upset over misunderstandings or conflicts with people who are important to them. If this is the case for you, shape up your conflict-resolution skills instead of turning to food. To handle conflict effectively, remember to focus on the issue at hand, without dredging up old issues or expanding the discussion to unrelated problems; use "I" messages to say how you feel, when you feel that way, and why; take time out if your feelings are so strong they will get in the way of a productive conversation; edit out hurtful words; and try to think of solutions. Keep in mind that the purpose is to resolve the problem in the best interests of the relationship, not to win an argument.

APPROACHES TO OVERCOMING A WEIGHT PROBLEM

What should you do if you are overweight? There are several options available to you.

Doing It Yourself

Research indicates that people are far more successful than was previously thought at losing weight and keeping it off. One study found that about 64% of the subjects achieved long-term success without joining a formal program or getting special help. Supporting these findings, a U.S. Public Health Service survey indicated that nearly 50% of the general public succeed with long-term weight management.

Other researchers investigated the characteristics that distinguished those who lost at least 20% of their body weight and maintained this loss for 2 years or more. Although some had used diet alone to lose weight, some had used exercise alone, and others had used a combination of diet and exercise, virtually all maintained their success by making exercise a permanent part of their lifestyle. They also kept tabs on their weight and habits. In addition, they learned to develop their own diet, exercise, and maintenance plans, and they became more involved in and excited by activities other than eating—such as careers, projects, and special interests. Long-term success depends on maintaining the lifestyle changes that helped you lose the weight in the first place.

If you need to lose weight, focus on adopting the healthy lifestyle described throughout this book. The "right" weight for you will naturally evolve, and you won't have to diet. However, if you must diet, do so in combination with exercise, and avoid very-low-calorie diets. Don't try to lose more than 0.5–2 pounds per week. Realize that most low-calorie diets cause a rapid loss of body water at first. When this phase passes, weight loss declines. As a result, dieters are often misled into believing that their efforts are not working. They then give up, not realizing that smaller losses later in the diet are actually better than the initial big losses, because later loss is mostly fat loss, whereas initial loss was primarily fluid.

For more tips on losing weight on your own, refer to the Behavior Change Strategy at the end of the chapter.

Diet Books

Many people who try to lose weight by themselves fall prey to one or more of the dozens of diet books on the market. Although a very few of these do contain useful advice and tips for motivation, most make empty promises. Some guidelines for evaluating and choosing a diet book are as follows:

1. Reject books that advocate an unbalanced way of eating. These include books advocating a high-carbohydrate-only diet or those advocating low-carbohydrate, high-protein diets. Also reject books promoting a single food, such as cabbage or grapefruit.

2. Reject books that claim to be based on a "scientific breakthrough" or to have the "secret" to success.

3. Reject books that use gimmicks, like matching eating to blood type, hyping insulin resistance as the single cause of obesity, combining foods in special ways to achieve weight loss, rotating levels of calories, or purporting that a weight problem is due to food allergies, food sensitivities, yeast infections, or hormone imbalances.

Food Choices

- Follow the recommendations in the Food Guide Pyramid for eating a moderate, varied diet.

- Pay attention to the energy density and nutrient density of your food choices. Favor foods with a low energy density and a high nutrient density.

- Check food labels for serving sizes, calories, and nutrient levels.

- Watch for hidden calories. Reduced-fat foods often have as many calories as their full-fat versions. Fat-based condiments like butter, margarine, mayonnaise, and salad dressings provide about 100 calories per tablespoon; added sugars such as jams, jellies, and syrup are also packed with calories.

- Drink fewer calories. Many Americans consume high-calorie beverages such as soda, fruit drinks, sports drinks, alcohol, and specialty coffees and teas. (People who get extra calories from solid food tend to compensate by eating less later; those whose extra calories come in liquid form don't compensate and consume more calories overall.)

- For problem foods, try eating small amounts under controlled conditions. Go out for a scoop of ice cream, for example, rather than buying half a gallon for your freezer.

Planning and Serving

- Keep a log of what you eat. Before you begin your program, your log will provide a realistic picture of your current diet and what changes you can make. Once you start your program, a log will keep you focused on your food choices and portion sizes. Consider tracking the following:
  - food eaten
  - hunger level
  - circumstances (location, other activities)
  - outside influences (environment, other people)
  - thoughts and emotions

- Eat three meals a day, including breakfast. Replace impulse snacking with planned, healthy snacks. Keep low-calorie snacks on hand to combat the "munchies": baby carrots, popcorn, and fresh fruits and vegetables are good choices.

- When shopping for food, make a list and stick to it. Don't shop when you're hungry. Avoid aisles that contain problem foods.

- In a cafeteria, examine all the possible food choices before you begin making selections. This will help you avoid overloading your plate. Don't take dessert during your first trip through the line: What seems like an appropriate choice and portion size for dessert may look very different *after* you've eaten a meal.

- Pay special attention to portion sizes. Use measuring cups and spoons and a food scale to become more familiar with appropriate portion sizes.

- Serve meals on small plates and in small bowls to help you eat smaller portions without feeling deprived.

- Eat only in specifically designated spots. Remove food from other areas of your house or apartment.

- When you eat, just eat—don't do anything else, such as read or watch TV.

- Eat more slowly. It takes time for your brain to get the message that your stomach is full. Take small bites and chew food thoroughly. Pay attention to every bite, and enjoy your food. Between bites, try putting your fork or spoon down and taking sips of water or another beverage.

- When you're done eating, remove your plate. Cue yourself that the meal is over—drink a glass of water, suck on a mint, chew gum, or brush your teeth.

Special Occasions

- When you eat out, choose a restaurant where you can make healthy food choices. Ask the server not to put bread and butter on the table before the meal, and request that sauces and salad dressings be served on the side. If portion sizes are large, take half your food home for a meal later in the week.

- If you cook a large meal for friends, send leftovers home with your guests.

- If you're eating at a friend's, eat a little and leave the rest. Don't eat to be polite; if someone offers you food you don't want, thank the person and decline firmly: "No thank you, I've had enough" or "It's delicious, but I'm full."

- Take care during the winter holidays. Research indicates that people gain less than they think during the winter holidays (about a pound) but that the weight isn't lost during the rest of the year, leading to slow, steady weight gain.

Physical Activity and Stress Management

- Increase your level of daily physical activity. If you have been sedentary for a long time or are seriously overweight, increase your level of activity slowly. Start by walking 10 minutes at a time, and work toward 30 minutes or more of moderate physical activity per day.

- Begin a formal exercise program that includes cardiorespiratory endurance exercise, strength training, and stretching (see Chapter 13).

- Develop techniques for handling stress—go for a walk or use a relaxation technique. Practice positive self-talk.

- Develop strategies for coping with non-hunger cues to eat, such as boredom, sleepiness, or anxiety. Try calling a friend, taking a shower, or reading a magazine.

- Tell family members and friends that you're making some changes in your eating and exercise habits. Ask them to be supportive.

4. Reject books that promise quick weight loss or that limit the selection of foods.

5. Accept books that advocate a balanced approach to diet plus exercise and sound nutrition advice.

A recent crop of popular books has advocated diets high in protein, low in carbohydrate, and relatively high in fat. Weight loss on low-carbohydrate diets comes mainly from loss of water and protein, not fat, and weight is usually quickly regained when dieting ends. Low-carbohydrate diets may be high in unhealthy saturated fats, and they often limit or eliminate foods such as grains, fruits, and vegetables that are rich in nutrients and fiber. The American College of Sports Medicine, the American Dietetic Association, the Cooper Institute for Aerobics Research, and the Women's Sports Foundation released a joint statement saying that such diets are not a good weight-loss strategy, will not improve athletic performance, and can be harmful in some cases. The only reason such plans help some people lose weight is that the diets they advocate provide so few calories; but as with all such plans, they are difficult to maintain over any period of time. (See the January 1999 issue of *Environmental Nutrition* and the May 2000 issue of *Nutrition Action Healthletter* for reviews of many top-selling diet books; For More Information at the end of the chapter lists additional resources.)

Dietary Supplements and Diet Aids

The number of dietary supplements and other weight loss aids on the market has also increased in recent years. Promoted in advertisements, magazines, direct mail campaigns, infomercials, and Web sites, these products typically promise a quick and easy path to weight loss. Most of these products are marketed as dietary supplements and so are subject to fewer regulations than over-the-counter medications. If you are considering one of these products, use your critical thinking skills and the information in the box "Over-the-Counter Diet Pills and Diet Aids."

WW. Weight-Loss Programs

Weight-loss programs come in a variety of types, including noncommercial support organizations, commercial programs, Web sites, and medically supervised clinical programs.

Noncommercial Weight-Loss Programs Noncommercial programs such as TOPS (Take Off Pounds Sensibly) and Overeaters Anonymous (OA) mainly provide group support. They do not advocate any particular diet, but they do recommend seeking professional advice for creating an individualized diet and exercise plan. Like Alcoholics Anonymous, OA is a 12-step program with a spiritual orientation that promotes "abstinence" from compulsive overeating. These types of programs are generally free. Your physician or a registered dietitian can also provide information and support for weight loss.

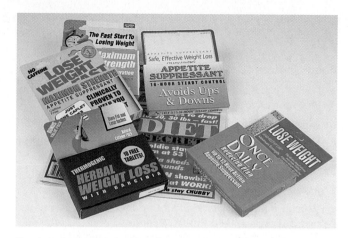

There are many plans and supplements promoted for weight loss, but few have any research supporting their effectiveness for long-term weight management. Developing lifelong healthy eating and exercise habits is the best approach for achieving and maintaining a healthy body composition.

Commercial Weight-Loss Programs Commercial programs such as Weight Watchers, Jenny Craig, Diet Workshop, and Richard Simmons Slimmons typically provide group support, nutrition education, physical activity recommendations, and behavior modification advice for changing habits. Some also make available packaged foods to assist in following dietary advice. Many commercial programs voluntarily belong to the Partnership for Healthy Weight Management established by the Federal Trade Commission in 1999. By doing so, they agree to provide clients with information on staff training and education, the risks associated with overweight and obesity, the risks associated with each program or product, the costs of the program, and the expected outcomes of the program, including rates of success.

Commercial programs can work, but only if you are motivated to decrease calorie intake and increase physical activity. A responsible and safe weight-loss program should have the following features:

1. The recommended diet should be safe and balanced, include all the food groups, and meet the DRIs for all nutrients. Physical activity and exercise should be strongly encouraged.

2. The program should promote slow, steady weight loss averaging ½–2 pounds per week. (There may be some rapid weight loss initially due to fluid loss.)

3. If a participant plans to lose more than 20 pounds, has any health problems, or is taking medication on a regular basis, physician evaluation and monitoring should be recommended. The staff of the program should include qualified counselors and health professionals.

4. The program should include plans for weight maintenance after the weight-loss phase is over.

Many over-the-counter (OTC) products are promoted for appetite control and fat loss, but few have evidence supporting their effectiveness. Testimonials and anecdotes are not good substitutes for scientific research findings. With herbs and other products marketed as dietary supplements, safety and cost are also a concern. In addition, use of OTC products doesn't help in the adoption of lifestyle behaviors that can help people achieve and maintain a healthy weight over the long term.

Formula Drinks and Food Bars

Canned diet drinks, powders used to make shakes, and diet food bars and snacks are designed to achieve weight loss by substituting for some or all of a person's daily food intake. However, most people find it difficult to use these products for long periods as a substitute for more satisfying "real" food, and serious health problems may result if they are used as the sole source of nutrition for extended periods of time. Use of such products can result in rapid weight loss for those who can stick with them, but such weight loss is accompanied by loss of muscle mass, and the weight is typically regained because users have not learned to change the eating and lifestyle behaviors that caused the weight problem in the first place.

Herbs and Herbal Products

Although many people believe that because herbs are "natural" they are safe, it is important to remember that herbs contain biologically active compounds that can be dangerous, especially if taken in large doses. As described in Chapter 12, herbs are marketed as dietary supplements, so there is little information about effectiveness, proper dosage, drug interactions, and side effects. In addition, labels may not accurately reflect the ingredients and dosages present, and safe manufacturing practices are not guaranteed. For example, the substitution of a toxic herb for another compound during the manufacture of a Chinese herbal weight-loss preparation caused more than 100 cases of kidney damage and cancer among users in Europe.

Ephedra, also known as ma huang or desert herb, is a popular herb found in weight-loss aids. Its active ingredient, ephedrine, is structurally similar to amphetamine. As a stimulant, ephedra may suppress appetite and increase body temperature and basal metabolic rate, causing calories to be burned at a faster rate. However, few studies have been done to identify safe and effective uses of ephedra, and long-term use is not recommended. In addition, many products containing ephedra also contain other stimulants—caffeine or herbal products that contain caffeine such as guarana seeds or kola nuts. There have been many reports of adverse effects from use of ephedra,

including elevated blood pressure, panic attacks, seizures, insomnia, headache, and nausea; it may also increase the risk of heart attack or stroke in some people, particularly if combined with another stimulant. The FDA is considering new regulations for ephedra, including dosage guidelines and warnings.

Herbal "dieter's teas" often contain a variety of strong botanical laxatives and diuretics such as senna, aloe, buckthorn, rhubarb root, cascara, and castor oil. These stimulate the colon and, if used in excess, can cause extreme diarrhea, nausea, vomiting, dehydration, fainting, and electrolyte imbalances that can lead to heart rhythm problems. If used regularly, the colon may become dependent on the laxative effect, resulting in chronic constipation. Any weight loss that occurs is due to fluid loss, not fat loss.

Other Dietary Supplements and Diet Aids

Supplements containing specific amino acids and proteins are also marketed for weight loss. Promoters claim that amino acids may ward off cravings and the impulse to binge-eat by affecting levels of neurotransmitters such as dopamine or hormones such as cholecystokinin (CCK) that are involved in appetite. However, there is little research to support these claims. In addition, even if such products do affect appetite, they may not be very helpful in weight management. Hunger is often not the reason that people consume high-calorie foods or overeat. The use of so-called "fat burners" or "fat inhibitors" such as carnitine, hydroxycitrate, chromium, or pyruvate is also not currently supported by research findings.

Fiber is another common ingredient in OTC diet aids. Manufacturers claim that fiber can swell in the stomach and control appetite by making people feel full. However, dietary fiber acts as a bulking agent in the large intestine, not in the stomach. The FDA has found no data to warrant classifying any type of fiber as an aid in weight control. In addition, most diet aids contain a mere 1–3 grams of fiber, which do not contribute much toward the recommended daily intake of 20–35 grams.

Until 2000, the synthetic compound phenylpropanolamine (PPA) was a common ingredient in OTC diet pills. Like ephedra, PPA acts as a mild stimulant and appetite suppressant. Although originally approved for short-term use, reports of increased risk for stroke led the FDA in 2000 to ask manufacturers to stop marketing products containing PPA.

The bottom line on nonprescription diet aids is *caveat emptor*—let the buyer beware. There is no quick and easy way to lose weight. The most effective approach is to develop healthy diet and exercise habits and make them a permanent part of your lifestyle.

---

5. The program should provide information on all fees and costs, including those of supplements and prepackaged foods, as well as data on risks and expected outcomes of participating in the program.

In addition, you should consider whether a program fits your lifestyle and whether you are truly ready to make a

commitment to it. A strong commitment and a plan for maintenance are especially important because studies indicate that only 10–15% of program participants maintain their weight loss—the rest gain back all or more than they had lost. One study of participants found that regular exercise was the best predictor of maintaining weight loss, whereas frequent television viewing was the best predictor of weight gain. This reinforces the idea that successful weight management requires long-term lifestyle changes.

Online Weight-Loss Programs A recent addition to the weight-loss program scene is the Internet-based program. Most such Web sites include a cross between self-help and group support through chat rooms, bulletin boards, and e-newsletters. Many sites offer online self-assessment for diet and physical activity habits as well as a meal plan; some provide access to a staff professional for individualized help. Many are free but some charge a small weekly or monthly fee. Preliminary research suggests that this type of program provides an alternative to in-person diet counseling and can lead to weight loss for some people. The criteria used to evaluate commercial programs can also be applied to Internet-based programs. In addition, check whether a program offers member-to-member support and access to staff professionals.

Clinical Weight-Loss Programs Medically supervised clinical programs are usually located in a hospital or other medical setting. Designed to help those who are severely obese, these programs typically involve a closely monitored very-low-calorie diet. The cost of a clinical program is usually high, but insurance will often cover part of the fee.

Prescription Drugs

The medications most often prescribed for weight loss are appetite suppressants that reduce feelings of hunger or increase feelings of fullness. Appetite suppressants usually work by increasing levels of catecholamine or serotonin, two brain chemicals that affect mood and appetite. All prescription weight-loss drugs have potential side effects. Those that affect catecholamine levels, including phentermine (Ionamin), diethylpropion (Tenuate), and mazindol (Sanorex), may cause sleeplessness, nervousness, and euphoria. Sibutramine (Meridia) acts on both the serotonin and catecholamine systems; it may trigger increases in blood pressure and heart rate. Other medications under study for weight loss include drugs that influence levels of leptin and cholecystokinin and certain antidepressants.

Most appetite suppressants are approved by the FDA only for short-term use. Sibutramine is the only such drug approved for longer-term use in significantly obese patients, but its safety and effectiveness have not been established beyond 1 year of use. Using weight-loss medications in combination or for long periods of time is considered "off-label" use, meaning that, although it is legal, the FDA has not approved such use.

A newer medication for obesity is orlistat (Xenical), which lowers calorie consumption by blocking fat absorption in the intestines; it prevents about 30% of the fat in food from being digested. Similar to the fat substitute olestra, orlistat reduces the absorption of fat-soluble vitamins and antioxidants. Side effects include diarrhea, cramping, and other gastrointestinal problems if users do not follow a low-fat diet.

Studies have generally found that appetite suppressants produce modest weight loss—about 5–22 pounds above the loss expected with nondrug obesity treatments. Individuals respond very differently, however, and some experience more weight loss than others. Unfortunately, weight loss tends to level off or reverse after 4 to 6 months on a medication, and many people regain the weight they've lost if they stop taking the drugs. Since most weight-loss medications are approved for only short-term use, regaining weight is a serious problem.

Side effects and risks are other concerns. In 1997, the FDA removed from the market two prescription weight-loss drugs, fenfluramine (Pondimin) and dexfenfluramine (Redux), after their use was linked to potentially life-threatening heart valve problems. (Fenfluramine was used most often in combination with phentermine, an off-label combination referred to as "fen/phen.") It appears that people who took these drugs over a long period or at high dosages are at greatest risk for problems, but the FDA recommends that anyone who has taken either of these drugs be examined by a physician.

Prescription weight-loss drugs are not for people who want to lose a few pounds to wear a smaller size of jeans. The latest federal guidelines advise people to try lifestyle modification for at least 6 months before trying drug therapy. Prescription drugs are recommended—in conjunction with lifestyle changes—only in certain cases: for people who have been unable to lose weight with nondrug options and who have a BMI over 30 (or over 27 if two or more additional risk factors such as diabetes and high blood pressure are present). For severely obese people who have been unable to lose weight by other methods, prescription drugs may provide a good option. Even modest weight loss provides significant health benefits for obese individuals.

Surgery

About 3% of Americans are severely obese, meaning they have a BMI of 40 or higher or are 100 pounds or more over recommended weight. For such people, obesity is a serious medical condition that is often complicated by other health problems such as diabetes, sleep disorders, heart disease, and arthritis. Surgical intervention may be necessary as a treatment of last resort for those who have not been successful in permanently reducing weight through other methods.

For surgery to treat extreme obesity, an expert panel from the National Institutes of Health has recommended a procedure called the *Roux-en-Y gastric bypass,* named after the Swiss surgeon who developed the technique. In this procedure, the stomach is divided in two with staples just below the esophagus to form a small (1-ounce) stomach pouch; a y-shaped intestinal junction is created by cutting the small intestine so that it connects to both the pouch and the bypassed portion of the stomach. Gastric bypass works primarily by restricting the amount of food that can be consumed at any one time, and it requires permanent lifestyle changes. If the patient eats or drinks too much, vomiting may result; some types of foods, including those high in sugar, may be difficult to digest. There is also no way to predict how much any individual will lose following surgery.

Another procedure, *liposuction,* has become popular for removing localized fat deposits. This cosmetic procedure is for body contouring, not weight loss; removing large amounts of fat is not recommended. In addition to being a medically serious operation, liposuction is associated with considerable pain and discomfort, bruising, swelling, discoloration, the risk of infection, and possible unexpected contour changes. Furthermore, it takes from 6 months to a year to see satisfactory results from a liposuction procedure, and the results are not always permanent.

Psychological Help

Many people can lose weight just by increasing their physical activity level and moderately restricting total calories, especially fat calories. When concern about body weight and shape have developed into an eating disorder, the help of a professional is recommended. In choosing a therapist, be sure to ask about credentials and experience (see Chapter 3). The therapist should have experience working with weight management, body image issues, eating disorders, addictions, and abuse issues. Your physician may be able to provide a referral.

Acceptance and Change

Most Americans, young and old, are unhappy with some aspect of their appearance and often their weight. The "can-do" attitude of Americans, together with the belief that there is a solution to this dissatisfaction, leads to even more problems with body image, as well as to dieting, disordered eating, and the desire for cosmetic surgery to "fix" perceived defects.

In fact, there are limits to the changes that can be made to body weight and body shape, both of which are influenced by heredity. The changes that can and should be made are lifestyle changes—engaging in regular physical activity, obtaining adequate nutrition, and maintaining healthy eating habits. With these changes, the body weight and shape that develop will be natural and appropriate for an individual's particular genetic makeup.

Knowing when the limits to healthy change have been reached—and learning to accept those limits—is crucial for overall wellness. Women in particular tend to measure

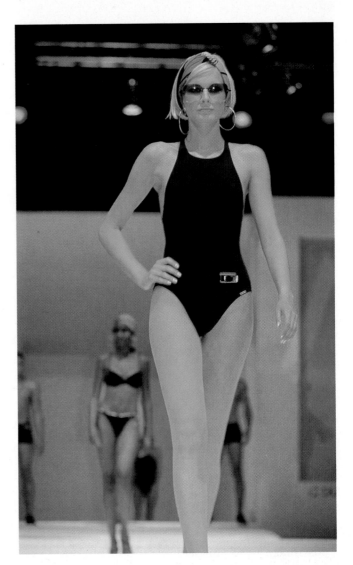

The image of the "ideal" female body promoted by the fashion and fitness industries doesn't reflect the wide range of body shapes and sizes that are associated with good health. An overconcern with body image can contribute to low self-esteem and the development of eating disorders.

self-worth in terms of their appearance; when they don't measure up to an unrealistic cultural ideal, they see themselves as defective and their self-esteem falls. The result can be negative body image, disordered eating, or even a full-blown eating disorder (see the box "Gender, Ethnicity, and Body Image").

Obesity is a serious health risk, but weight management needs to take place in a positive and realistic atmosphere. For an obese person, losing as few as 10 pounds can reduce blood pressure and improve mood. The hazards of excessive dieting and overconcern about body weight need to be countered by a change in attitude about what constitutes the perfect body and a reasonable body weight. A reasonable body weight must take into account a person's weight history, social circumstances, metabolic profile, and psychological well-being.

Body Image and Gender

Women are much more likely than men to be dissatisfied with their bodies, often wanting to be thinner than they are. In one study, only 30% of eighth-grade girls reported being content with their bodies, while 70% of their male classmates expressed satisfaction with their looks. Girls and women are much more likely than boys and men to diet, develop eating disorders, and be obese.

One reason that girls and women are dissatisfied with their bodies is that they are influenced by the media—particularly advertisements and women's fashion magazines. Most teen girls report that the media influence their idea of the perfect body and their decision to diet. In a study of adult women, viewing pictures of thin models in magazines had an immediate negative effect on their mood. Clearly, media images affect women's self-image and self-esteem. For American women of all ages, success is still too often equated with how we look rather than who we are.

It is important to note that the image of the "perfect" woman presented in the media is often unrealistic and even unhealthy. In a review of BMI data for Miss America pageant winners since 1922, researchers noted a significant decline in BMI over time, with an increasing number of recent winners having BMIs in the "underweight" category. The average fashion model is 4–7 inches taller and 20 pounds lighter than the average American woman.

Our culture may be promoting an unattainable masculine ideal as well. Researchers studying male action figures such as GI Joe from the past 40 years noted that they have become increasingly muscular. A recent Batman action figure, if projected onto a man of average height, would result in someone with a 30-inch waist, 57-inch chest, and 27-inch biceps. Such media messages can be demoralizing; and although not as commonly, boys and men also suffer from body image problems.

Body Image and Ethnicity

The thin, toned look as a feminine ideal is just a fashion, one that is not shared by all cultures. Although some groups espouse thinness as an "ideal" body type, others do not. In many traditional African societies, for example, full-figured women's bodies are seen as symbols of health, prosperity, and fertility. African American teenage girls have a much more positive body image than white girls; in one survey, two-thirds of them defined beauty as "the right attitude," whereas white girls were more preoccupied with weight and body shape. Nevertheless, recent evidence indicates that African American women are as likely to engage in disordered eating behavior, especially binge eating and vomiting, as their Latina, American Indian, and white counterparts. This finding underscores the complex nature of eating disorders and body image.

Avoiding Body Image Problems

To minimize your risk of developing a body image problem, keep the following strategies in mind:

- Focus on healthy habits and good physical health. Eat a moderate, balanced diet, and choose physical activities you enjoy. Avoid chronic or repetitive dieting.

- Focus on good psychological health and put concerns about physical appearance in perspective. Your worth as a human being is not dependent on how you look.

- Find things to appreciate in yourself besides an idealized body image. Men and women whose self-esteem is based primarily on standards of physical attractiveness can find it difficult to age gracefully. Those who can learn to value other aspects of themselves are more accepting of the physical changes that occur naturally with age.

- See the beauty and fitness industries for what they are. Realize that one of their goals is to prompt dissatisfaction with yourself so that you will buy their products.

WW. EATING DISORDERS

Problems with body weight and weight control are not limited to excessive body fat. A growing number of people, especially adolescent girls and young women, experience **eating disorders**, characterized by severe disturbances in eating patterns and eating-related behaviors. The major eating disorders are anorexia nervosa, bulimia nervosa, and binge-eating disorder. **Anorexia nervosa** is characterized by a refusal to maintain a minimally normal body weight. **Bulimia nervosa** is characterized by repeated episodes of binge eating followed by compensatory behaviors such as self-induced vomiting, the misuse of laxatives or diuretics, fasting, or excessive exercise. **Binge-eating disorder** is characterized by binge eating without regular use of compensatory behaviors. Eating disorders are associated with depression, anxiety, low self-esteem, and increased health risks, including, in some cases, increased risk of premature death.

Eating disorders are more prevalent in developed countries than in developing ones. At any given time, about 0.5–2.0% of Americans suffer from anorexia and 1.0–3.0% have bulimia. Binge-eating disorder may affect 2.0–5.0% of all adults and 8.0% of those who are obese. An even greater number of Americans exhibit disordered eating behavior but do not fully meet the criteria of one of the recognized eating disorders.

In the United States, anorexia and bulimia affect far more women than men: Of the 1 million Americans who develop anorexia or bulimia each year, 90% are female. Of those with binge-eating disorder, 60% are female. Eating disorders appear to be more prevalent among people of middle and upper-middle socioeconomic status. Preliminary research findings suggest that eating disorders are equally common among white females and Latinas, more common among Native American females, and less common among African American and Asian American females. Among minority groups, females most at risk for eating disorders are those who are younger, heavier, and better educated and who identify with middle-class values.

Factors in Developing an Eating Disorder

Many factors are probably involved in the development of an eating disorder. Although many widely different explanations have been proposed, they share one central feature: a dissatisfaction with body image and body weight. Such dissatisfaction is created by distorted thinking, including perfectionistic beliefs, unreasonable demands for self-control, and excessive self-criticism. Dissatisfaction with body weight leads to dysfunctional attitudes about eating, such as fear of fat and preoccupation with food, and problematic eating behaviors, including excessive dieting, constant calorie counting, and frequent weighing.

Heredity appears to play a role in the development of eating disorders, accounting for 30–50% of the risk. But as with other conditions, only the tendency to develop an eating disorder is explained by heredity; the expression of this tendency is affected by other factors. The home environment is one such factor: Families in which there is hostility, abuse, or lack of cohesion provide fertile ground for the development of an eating disorder; a rigid or overprotective parent can also increase risk. Cultural messages, as well as family, friends, and peers, shape attitudes toward the self and others. Comparing oneself negatively with others can damage self-esteem and increase vulnerability. Young people who see themselves as lacking control over their lives are also at high risk for eating disorders.

Certain turning points in life, such as beginning to date, leaving home for college, or the breakup of an important relationship, often trigger the onset of an eating disorder. How a person reacts to and copes with such stresses can influence risk, particularly in individuals who have few stress management skills. An eating disorder may become a means of coping: The abnormal eating behavior—starvation, **purging,** or binge eating—reduces anxiety by producing numbness and alleviating emotional pain. Restrictive dieting is another possible trigger for the development of eating disorders.

Anorexia Nervosa

A person suffering from anorexia nervosa does not eat enough food to maintain a reasonable body weight. Anorexia affects 1–3 million Americans, 95% of them female. Although it can occur later, anorexia typically develops between the ages of 12 and 18.

Characteristics of Anorexia Nervosa People suffering from anorexia have an intense fear of gaining weight or becoming fat. Their body image is distorted, so that even when emaciated, they think they are fat. (Distorted body image is also a hallmark of *muscle dysmorphia,* a disorder experienced by some body builders in which they see themselves as small and out of shape despite being very muscular.) People with anorexia may engage in compulsive behaviors or rituals that help keep them from eating, though some may also binge and purge. They commonly use vigorous and prolonged physical activity to reduce body weight as well. Although they may express a great interest in food, even taking over the cooking responsibilities for the rest of the family, their own diet becomes more and more extreme. People with anorexia often hide or hoard food without eating it.

Anorexic people are typically introverted, emotionally reserved, and socially insecure. They are often "model children" who rarely complain and are anxious to please others and win their approval. Although school performance is typically above average, they are often critical of themselves and not satisfied with their accomplishments. For people with anorexia nervosa, their entire sense of self-esteem may be tied up in their evaluation of their body shape and weight.

Health Risks of Anorexia Nervosa Because of extreme weight loss, females with anorexia often stop menstruating, become intolerant of cold, and develop low blood pressure and heart rate. They develop dry skin that is often covered by fine body hair like that of an infant. Their hands and feet may swell and take on a blue color.

Anorexia nervosa has been linked to a variety of medical complications, including disorders of the cardiovascular, gastrointestinal, and endocrine systems. When

eating disorder A serious disturbance in eating patterns or eating-related behavior, characterized by a negative body image and concerns about body weight or body fat.

Terms

anorexia nervosa An eating disorder characterized by a refusal to maintain body weight at a minimally healthy level and an intense fear of gaining weight or becoming fat; self-starvation.

bulimia nervosa An eating disorder characterized by recurrent episodes of binge eating and purging: overeating and then using compensatory behaviors such as vomiting, laxatives, and excessive exercise to prevent weight gain.

binge-eating disorder An eating disorder characterized by binge eating and a lack of control over eating behavior in general.

purging The use of vomiting, laxatives, excessive exercise, restrictive dieting, enemas, diuretics, or diet pills to compensate for food that has been eaten and that the person fears will produce weight gain.

body fat is virtually gone and muscles are severely wasted, the body turns to its own organs in a desperate search for protein. Death can occur from heart failure caused by electrolyte imbalances. As many as 16% of patients with anorexia nervosa die of complications related to the disorder. Depression is also a serious risk, and about half the fatalities relating to anorexia are suicides.

Bulimia Nervosa

A person suffering from bulimia nervosa engages in recurrent episodes of binge eating followed by purging. Bulimia is often difficult to recognize because sufferers conceal their eating habits and usually maintain a normal weight, although they may experience weight fluctuations of 10–15 pounds. Although bulimia usually begins in adolescence or young adulthood, it has recently begun to emerge at increasingly younger (11–12 years) and older (40–60 years) ages.

Characteristics of Bulimia Nervosa During a binge, a bulimic person may rapidly consume anywhere from 1,000 to 60,000 calories. This is followed by an attempt to get rid of the food by purging, usually by vomiting or using laxatives or diuretics. During a binge, bulimics feel as though they have lost control and cannot stop or limit how much they eat. Some binge and purge only occasionally, while others do so many times every day.

In public, people suffering from bulimia may appear to eat normally, but they are rarely comfortable around food. Binges usually occur in secret and can become nightmarish—ravaging the kitchen for food, going from one grocery store to another to buy food, or even stealing food. During the binge, all feelings are blocked out, and food acts as an anesthetic. Afterward, they feel physically drained and emotionally spent. They usually feel deeply ashamed and disgusted with both themselves and their behavior and terrified that they will gain weight from what they've eaten.

Major life changes such as leaving for college, getting married, having a baby, or losing a job can trigger a binge-purge cycle. At such times, stress is high and the person may have no good outlet for emotional conflict or tension. As with anorexia, bulimia sufferers are often insecure and depend on others for approval and self-esteem. They may hide difficult emotions such as anger and disappointment from themselves and others. Binge eating and purging becomes a way of dealing with feelings.

Health Risks of Bulimia Nervosa The binge-purge cycle of bulimia places a tremendous strain on the body and can have serious health effects. Contact with vomited stomach acids erodes tooth enamel. Bulimic people often develop tooth decay because they binge on foods that contain large amounts of simple sugars. Repeated vomiting or the use of laxatives, in combination with deficient calorie intake, can damage the liver and kidneys and cause cardiac arrhythmia. Chronic hoarseness and esophageal tearing with bleeding may also result from vomiting. More rarely, binge eating can lead to rupture of the stomach. Although many bulimic women maintain normal weight, even small amounts of weight loss to a lower-than-normal weight can cause menstrual problems. And although less often associated with suicide or premature death than anorexia, bulimia is associated with increased depression, excessive preoccupation with food and body image, and sometimes disturbances in cognitive functioning.

Binge-Eating Disorder

Binge-eating disorder is characterized by uncontrollable eating, usually followed by feelings of guilt and shame with weight gain. Common eating patterns are eating more rapidly than normal, eating until uncomfortably full, eating when not hungry, and preferring to eat alone. Binge eaters may eat large amounts of food throughout the day, with no planned mealtimes. Many people with binge-eating disorder mistakenly see rigid dieting as the only solution to their problem. However, rigid dieting usually causes feelings of deprivation and a return to overeating.

Compulsive overeaters rarely eat because of hunger. Instead, food is used as a means of coping with stress, conflict, and other difficult emotions or to provide solace and entertainment. People who do not have the resources to deal effectively with stress may be more vulnerable to binge-eating disorder. Inappropriate overeating often begins during childhood. In some families, eating may be used as an activity to fill otherwise empty time. Parents may reward children with food for good behavior or withhold food as a means of punishment, thereby creating distorted feelings about the use of food.

Binge eaters are almost always obese, so they face all the health risks associated with obesity. In addition, binge eaters may have higher rates of depression and anxiety. To overcome binge eating, a person must learn to put food and eating into proper perspective and develop other ways of coping with stress and painful emotions.

Treating Eating Disorders

The treatment of eating disorders must address both problematic eating behaviors and the misuse of food to manage stress and emotions. Anorexia nervosa treatment first involves averting a medical crisis by restoring adequate body weight; then the psychological aspects of the disorder can be addressed. The treatment of bulimia nervosa or binge-eating disorder involves first stabilizing the eating patterns and then identifying and changing the patterns of thinking that lead to disordered eating and improving coping skills. Concurrent problems, such as

- Educate yourself about eating disorders and their risks and about treatment resources in your community. (See the For More Information section at the end of this chapter for suggestions.)

- Write down specific ways the person's eating problem is affecting you or others in the household. Call a house meeting to talk about how others are affected by the problem and how to take action.

- Consider consulting a professional about the best way to approach the situation. Obtain information about how and where your friend can get help. Attend a local support group.

- Arrange to speak privately with the person, along with other friends or family members. Let one person lead the group and do most of the talking. Discuss specific incidents and the consequences of disordered eating.

- If you are going to speak with your friend, write down ahead of time what your concerns are and what you would like to say. Expect that the person you are concerned about will deny there is a problem, minimize it, or become angry

with you. Remain calm and nonjudgmental, and continue to express your concern.

- Avoid giving simplistic advice about eating habits. Gently encourage your friend to eat properly.

- Take time to listen to your friend, and express your support and understanding. Encourage honest communication. Emphasize your friend's good characteristics, and compliment all her or his successes.

- Help maintain the person's sense of dignity by encouraging personal responsibility and decision making. Be patient and realistic; recovery is a long process. Continue to love and support your friend.

- If the situation is an emergency—if the person has fainted or attempted suicide, for example—take immediate action. Call 911 for help.

- If you feel very upset about the situation, seek professional help. Remember, you are not to blame for another person's eating disorder.

---

depression or anxiety, must also be addressed. In 1996, the antidepressant Prozac became the first medication approved by the FDA for the treatment of bulimia.

Treatment of eating disorders usually involves a combination of psychotherapy and medical management. The therapy may be carried out individually or in a group; sessions involving the entire family may be recommended. A support or self-help group can be a useful adjunct to such treatment. Medical professionals, including physicians, dentists, gynecologists, and registered dietitians, can evaluate and manage the physical damage caused by the disorder. If a patient is severely depressed or emaciated, hospitalization may be necessary. Depending on the severity of the disorder, treatment may last from a few months to several years.

Friends and family members often want to know what they can do to help someone with an eating disorder. For suggestions, see the box "If Someone You Know Has an Eating Disorder. . . ."

Today's Challenge

Eating disorders can be seen as the logical extension of the concern with weight that pervades American society. Although most people don't succumb to irrational or distorted ideas about their bodies, many do become obsessed with dieting. The challenge facing Americans today is achieving a healthy body weight without excessive dieting—by adopting and maintaining sensible eating habits, an active lifestyle, realistic and positive attitudes and emotions, and creative ways of handling stress.

Tips for Today

Maintaining a healthy weight means balancing calories in with calories out. Many forces and factors in contemporary society work against a healthy balance, so it's imperative that individuals take active control of managing their weight. Many approaches work, but the simplest formula is moderate food intake coupled with regular exercise.

Right now you can

- Drink a glass of water instead of a soda.

- Throw away any high-calorie, low-nutrient snack foods in your kitchen and start a list of fruits and vegetables you can buy as snacks instead.

- Put a sign on your refrigerator reminding you of your weight-management goals.

- Go outside and walk or jog for 15 minutes or take a 15-minute bike ride.

- Review the information on portion sizes in Chapter 12 and consider whether the portions you usually take at meals are larger than they need to be.

SUMMARY

- Body composition is the relative amounts of fat-free mass and fat in the body. *Overweight* and *obesity* refer to body weight or the percentage of body fat that exceeds what is associated with good health.

The behavior management plan described in Chapter 1 provides an excellent framework for a weight-management program. Following are some suggestions about specific ways you can adapt that general plan to controlling your weight.

Motivation and Commitment

Make sure you are motivated and committed before you begin. Failure at weight loss is a frustrating experience that can make it more difficult to lose weight in the future. Think about the reasons you want to lose weight. Self-focused reasons, such as to feel good about yourself or to have a greater sense of well-being, are often associated with success. Trying to lose weight for others or out of concern for how others view you is a poor foundation for a weight-loss program. Make a list of your reasons for wanting to lose weight, and post it in a prominent place.

Setting Goals

Choose a reasonable weight you think you would like to reach over the long term, and be willing to renegotiate it as you get further along. Break your long-term weight and behavioral goals into a series of short-term goals. Develop a new way of behaving by designing small, manageable steps that will get you to where you want to go.

Creating a Negative Energy Balance

When your weight is constant, you are burning approximately the same number of calories as you are taking in. To tip the energy balance toward weight loss, you must either consume fewer calories or burn more calories through physical activity, or both. One pound of body fat represents 3500 calories. To lose weight at the recommended rate of 0.5–2.0 pounds per week, you must create a negative energy balance of 1750–7000 calories per week or 250–1000 calories per day. To generate your negative energy balance, it's usually best to begin by increasing your activity level rather than decreasing your calorie consumption.

Physical Activity

Consider how you can increase your energy output simply by increasing routine physical activity, such as walking or taking the stairs. (Figure 13-3, on p. 369, shows activities that use about 150 calories.) If you are not already involved in a regular exercise routine aimed at increasing endurance and building or maintaining muscle mass, seek help from someone who is competent to help you plan and start an appropriate exercise routine. If you are already doing regular physical exercise, evaluate your program according to the guidelines in Chapter 13.

Don't try to use exercise to "spot reduce." Leg lifts, for example, contribute to fat loss only to the extent that they burn calories; they don't burn fat just from your legs. You can make parts of your body appear more fit by exercising them, but the only way you can reduce fat in any specific part of your body is to create an overall negative energy balance.

Diet and Eating Habits

If you can't generate a large enough negative energy balance solely by increasing physical activity, you may want to supplement

---

- The key to weight management is maintaining a balance of calories in (food) and calories out (resting metabolism, food digestion, and physical activity).

- Standards for assessing body weight and body composition include body mass index (BMI) and percent body fat.

- Too much or too little body fat is linked to health problems; the distribution of body fat can also be a significant risk factor.

- An inaccurate or negative body image is common and can lead to psychological distress.

- Genetic factors help determine a person's weight, but the influence of heredity can be overcome with attention to lifestyle factors, especially diet and physical activity.

- Physiological factors involved in the regulation of body weight and body fat include metabolic rate, hormonal influences, and the size and number of fat cells.

- Nutritional guidelines for weight management include consuming a moderate number of calories; limiting portion sizes, energy density, and the intake of fat, simple sugars, refined carbohydrates, and

- protein to recommended levels; increasing the intake of complex carbohydrates; and developing an eating schedule and decision rules for food choices.

- Activity guidelines for weight management emphasize daily physical activity and regular sessions of cardiorespiratory endurance exercise and strength training.

- Weight management requires developing positive, realistic self-talk and self-esteem and a repertoire of appropriate techniques for handling stress and other emotional and physical challenges.

- People can be successful at long-term weight loss on their own, usually through a combination of diet and exercise.

- Diet books, OTC diet aids and supplements, and formal weight-loss programs should be assessed for safety and efficacy.

- Professional help is needed in cases of severe obesity; medical treatments include prescription drugs, surgery, and psychological therapy.

- Dissatisfaction with weight and shape are common to all eating disorders. Anorexia nervosa is charac-

exercise with modest cuts in your calorie intake. Don't think of this as "going on a diet"; your goal is to make small changes in your diet that you can maintain for a lifetime. Focus on cutting your fat intake and on eating a variety of nutritious foods in moderation. Don't try skipping meals, fasting, or going on a very-low-calorie diet or a diet that is unbalanced.

Making changes in eating habits is another important strategy for weight management. If your program centers on a conscious restriction of certain food items, you're likely to spend all your time thinking about the forbidden foods. Focus on *how* to eat rather than *what* to eat. Refer to the box "Strategies for Successful Weight Management" for suggestions.

Self-Monitoring

Keep a record of your weight and behavior change progress. Try keeping a record of everything you eat. Write down what you plan to eat, in what quantity, *before* you eat. You'll find that just having to record something that is "not OK" to eat is likely to stop you from eating it. If you also note what seems to be triggering your urges to eat (for example, you feel bored, someone offered you something), you'll become more aware of your weak spots and be better able to take corrective action. Also, keep track of your daily activities and your formal exercise program so you can monitor increases in physical activity.

Putting Your Plan into Action

- Examine the environmental cues that trigger poor eating and exercise habits, and devise strategies for dealing with them. For example, you may need to remove "problem" foods from your house temporarily or put a sign on the refrigerator reminding you to go for a walk instead of having a snack. Anticipate problem situations, and plan ways to handle them more effectively.

- Create new environmental cues that will support your new healthy behaviors. Put your walking shoes by the front door. Move fruits and vegetables to the front of the refrigerator.

- Get others to help. Talk to friends and family members about what they can do to support your efforts. Find a buddy to join you in your exercise program.

- Give yourself lots of praise and rewards. Think about your accomplishments and achievements and congratulate yourself. Plan special nonfood treats for yourself, such as a walk or a movie. Reward yourself often and for anything that counts toward success.

- If you do slip, tell yourself to get back on track immediately, and don't waste time on self-criticism. Think positively instead of getting into a cycle of guilt and self-blame. Don't demand too much of yourself.

- Don't get discouraged. Be aware that although weight loss is bound to slow down after the first loss of body fluid, the weight loss at this slower rate is more permanent than earlier, more dramatic losses.

- Remember that weight management is a lifelong project. You need to adopt reasonable goals and strategies that you can maintain over the long term.

---

terized by self-starvation, distorted body image, and an intense fear of gaining weight. Bulimia nervosa is characterized by recurrent episodes of uncontrolled binge eating and frequent purging. Binge-eating disorder involves binge eating without regular use of compensatory purging.

TAKE ACTION

1. Interview some people who have successfully lost weight and kept it off. What were their strategies and techniques? Do you think their approach would work for others?

2. Find out what percentage of your body weight is fat by taking one of the tests described in this chapter at your campus health clinic, sports medicine clinic, or health club. If you have too high or too low a proportion of body fat, consider taking steps to change it.

JOURNAL ENTRY

1. Monitor your diet for a week to see exactly how much fat and sugar you consume. If these amounts are excessive, make a list of specific steps you can take to reduce them.

2. Make a list of at least five things you could do each day to become more physically active. Your list might include things such as riding your bike to class instead of driving and walking up stairs instead of taking

the elevator. For each item on your list, describe the lifestyle adjustments you'd need to make—for example, leaving for class 10 minutes earlier to allow time to ride your bike rather than drive.

3. Critical Thinking Evaluate some of the weight-loss resources in your community. First, investigate a commercial weight-management program that operates in your community. Write an evaluation of it in terms of the criteria listed in the chapter. How does the program measure up? Next, look at the frozen diet dinners in your supermarket, such as Weight Watchers, Lean Cuisine, and Healthy Choice. How do they compare in terms of calories, fat content, and nutritional value?

FOR MORE INFORMATION

Books

Hensrud, D. D., ed. 2000. *Mayo Clinic on Healthy Weight.* New York: Kensington. *Presents basic information on determining and achieving a healthy body weight.*

Levenkorn, S. 2000. *Anatomy of Anorexia.* New York: Norton. *An up-to-date reference on the symptoms, diagnosis, and treatment of anorexia for patients, families, friends, and therapists.*

Milchovich, S. K., and B. Dunn-Long. 1999. *Diabetes Mellitus: A Practical Handbook,* 7th ed. Palo Alto, Calif.: Bull. *A user-friendly guide to diabetes.*

Nash, J. D. 1999. *Binge No More: Your Guide to Overcoming Disordered Eating.* Oakland, Calif.: New Harbinger. *Provides information and techniques for overcoming binge eating in the context of all types of disordered eating.*

Pope, H. G., K. A. Phillips, and R. Olivardia. 2000. *Adonis Complex: The Secret Crisis of Male Body Obsession.* New York: Free Press. *Provides a historical review of the changing fashions in male body type and information about male problems with body image.*

Rolls, B. J., and R. A. Barnett. 2001. *Volumetrics: Feel Full on Fewer Calories.* New York: HarperCollins. *Presents a research-based weight-management plan centering on the concept of energy density.*

Wilkins, F., and D. Wilkins. 2000. *DietMinder Personal Food and Fitness Journal.* Eugene, Ore.: Memory Minder. *An easy-to-use journal that helps track diet, physical activity, and the progress of a weight-loss program.*

WW. Organizations, Hotlines, and Web Sites

American Diabetes Association. Provides information, a free newsletter, and referrals to local support groups; the Web site includes and online diabetes risk assessment.

    800-342-2383

    http://www.diabetes.org

Ask the Dietitian/Overweight. Provides questions and answers on many topics related to weight control; is also linked to the Healthy Body Calculator™, which calculates BMI, waist-to-hip ratio, and daily nutrient and calorie goals.

    http://www.dietitian.com/overweig.html

Cyberdiet. Provides a variety of assessment and planning tools as well as practical tips for eating a healthy diet and being physically active.

    http://www.cyberdiet.com

National Heart, Lung, and Blood Institute (NHLBI): Aim for a Healthy Weight. Provides information and tips on diet and physical activity, as well as a BMI calculator.

    http://www.nhlbi.nih.gov/health/public/heart/obesity/lose_wt

National Institute of Diabetes and Digestive and Kidney Diseases (NIDDK). Health Information: Weight Loss and Control. Provides information and referrals for problems related to obesity, weight control, and nutritional disorders.

    877-946-4627

    http://www.niddk.nih.gov/health/nutrit/nutrit.htm

Partnership for Healthy Weight Management. Provides information on evaluating weight-loss programs and advertising claims.

    http://www.consumer.gov/weightloss

Phys: Weight Loss. A commercial site with resources for self-assessment, goal setting, dietary planning, and exercise; also includes the "diet debunker," which reviews popular diet books.

    http://www.phys.com/loseweight

Shape Up America! Provides materials about safe dietary and physical fitness strategies for successful weight management, including an online BMI calculator.

    http://shapeup.org

Thrive Online/Weight Control. Information and tools for weight management, including a BMI calculator, a weight-loss readiness quiz, and suggestions for diet and exercise.

    http://thriveonline.com/weight

U.S. Consumer Gateway: Health—Dieting and Weight Control. Provides links to government sites with advice on evaluating claims about weight-loss products and programs.

    http://www.consumer.gov/health.htm

There are also many resources for people concerned about eating disorders.

American Anorexia/Bulimia Association

    212-575-6200

    http://www.aabainc.org

Anorexia Nervosa and Related Eating Disorders (ANRED)

    http://www.anred.com

Eating Disorders Awareness and Prevention (EDAP)

    800-931-2237

    http://www.edap.org

National Association of Anorexia Nervosa and Associated Disorders (ANAD)

    847-831-3438 (referral line)

    http://www.anad.org

Something Fishy Website on Eating Disorders

    http://www.something-fishy.org

See also the listings in Chapters 12 and 13.

Allison, D. B., et al. 1999. Annual deaths attributable to obesity in the United States. *Journal of the American Medical Association* 282(16): 1530–1538.

American Institute for Cancer Research. 2000. *Fad Diets Versus Dietary Guidelines* (http://www.aicr.org/faddiets.htm; retrieved March 1, 2000).

Borzekowski, D. L., and T. N. Robinson. 2001. The 30-second effect: An experiment revealing the impact of television commercials on food preferences of preschoolers. *Journal of the American Dietetic Association* 101(1): 42–46.

Chemistry of fat substitutes: Can you stomach it? 2001. *Discover*, March.

Cohane, G. H., and H. G. Pope. 2001. Body image in boys: A review of the literature. *International Journal of Eating Disorders* 29(4): 373–379.

Crespo, C. J., et al. 2001. Television watching, energy intake, and obesity in U.S. children: Results from the third National Health and Nutrition Examination Survey, 1988–1994. *Archives of Pediatric and Adolescent Medicine* 155(3): 360–365.

Food and Drug Administration. 2001. FDA issues public health advisory on phenylpropanolamine in drug products. *FDA Consumer*, January/February.

Greeley, A. 2000. Planning to look flab-u-less? Know the facts about liposuction. *FDA Consumer*, November/December.

Guide to rating the weight-loss Websites. 2000. *Tufts University Health and Nutrition Letter*, July Special Supplement.

Haller, C. A., and N. L. Benowitz. 2000. Adverse cardiovascular and central nervous system events associated with dietary supplements containing ephedra alkaloids. *New England Journal of Medicine* 343(25): 1833–1838.

Harnack, L. J., R. W. Jeffery, and K. N. Boutelle. 2000. Temporal trends in energy intake in the United States: An ecologic perspective. *American Journal of Clinical Nutrition* 71: 1478–1484.

Hu, F. B., et al. 2001. Physical activity and risk for cardiovascular events in diabetic women. *Annals of Internal Medicine* 134: 96–106.

Jick, H. 2000. Heart valve disorders and appetite-suppressant drugs. *Journal of the American Medical Association* 283(13): 1738–1740.

Kernan, W. N., et al. 2000. Phenylpropanolamine and the risk of hemorrhagic stroke. *New England Journal of Medicine* 343(25): 1826–1832.

Khan, L. K., et al. 2001. Use of prescription weight loss pills among U.S. adults in 1996–1998. *Annals of Internal Medicine* 134(4): 282–286.

Leit, R. A., H. G. Pope, and J. J. Gray. 2001. Cultural expectations of muscularity in men: The evolution of playgirl centerfolds. *International Journal of Eating Disorders* 29(1): 90–93.

Levine, J., N. L. Eberhardt, and M. D. Jensen. 1999. Role of nonexercise activity thermogenesis in resistance to fat gain in humans. *Science* 283(5399): 212–214.

Liebman, B. 2000. Ten tips for staying lean. *Nutrition Action Healthletter* 26(6): 3–7.

Litt, A. S. 2000. *The College Student's Guide to Eating Well on Campus.* Bethesda, Md.: Tulip Hill Press.

Lotufo, P. A., et al. 2001. Diabetes and all-cause and coronary heart disease mortality among U.S. male physicians. *Archives of Internal Medicine* 161: 242–247.

Milligan, R. J., and G. Waller. 2000. Anger and bulimic psychopathology among nonclinical women. *International Journal of Eating Disorders* 28(4): 446–450.

Mokdad, A. H., et al. 2000. The continuing epidemic of obesity in the United States. *Journal of the American Medical Association* 284(13): 1650–1651.

Mokdad, A. H., et al. 2000. Diabetes trends in the U.S.: 1990–1998. *Diabetes Care* 23(9): 1278–1283.

National Center for Health Statistics. 2000. *Prevalence of Overweight and Obesity Among Adults: United States, 1999* (http://www.cdc.gov/nchs/products/pubs/pubd/hestats/obese/obse99.htm; retrieved December 15, 2000).

National Institute of Diabetes and Digestive and Kidney Disorders. 2001. *Prescription Medications for the Treatment of Obesity* (http://www.niddk.nih.gov/health/nutrit/pubs/presmeds.htm; retrieved April 19, 2001).

Oliver, G., J. Wardle, and E. L. Gibson. 2000. Stress and food choice. *Psychosomatic Medicine* 62(6): 853–865.

Pope, H. G., et al. 1999. Evolving ideals of male body image as seen through action toys. *International Journal of Eating Disorders* 26(1): 65–72.

Reseland, J. E., et al. 2001. Effect of long-term changes in diet and exercise on plasma leptin concentrations. *American Journal of Clinical Nutrition* 73(2): 240–245.

Rubinstein, S., and B. Caballero. 2000. Is Miss America an undernourished role model? *Journal of the American Medical Association* 283(12): 1569.

Schauer, P. R., et al. 2000. Outcomes after laparoscopic roux-en-Y gastric bypass for morbid obesity. *Annals of Surgery* 232(4): 515–529.

Seidell, J. C., et al. 2001. Report from a Centers for Disease Control and Prevention workshop on use of adult anthropometry for public health and primary health care. *American Journal of Clinical Nutrition* 73(1): 123–126.

Shalala, D. E. 2000. *Good Nutrition and Public Health: Remarks at the National Nutrition Summit, May 30, 2000* (http://www.hhs.gov/news/speeches/000530.html; retrieved November 3, 2000).

Steppan, C. M., et al. 2001. The hormone resistin links obesity to diabetes. *Nature* 409: 307–312.

Stevens, V. J., et al. 2001. Long-term weight loss and changes in blood pressure. *Annals of Internal Medicine* 134: 1–11.

Strober, M., et al. 2000. Controlled family study of anorexia nervosa and bulimia nervosa: Evidence of shared liability and transmission of partial syndromes. *American Journal of Psychiatry* 157(3): 393–401.

Tate, D. F., R. R. Wing, and R. A. Winett. 2001. Using Internet technology to deliver a behavioral weight loss program. *Journal of the American Medical Association* 285(9): 1172–1777.

Wagner, E. H., et al. 2001. Effect of improved glycemic control on health care costs and utilization. *Journal of the American Medical Association* 285(2): 182–189.

Westerterp, K. R. 2001. Pattern and intensity of physical activity. *Nature* 410(6828): 539.

Yanovski, J. A., et al. 2000. A prospective study of holiday weight gain. *New England Journal of Medicine* 342(12): 861–867.

Zipfel, S., et al. 2000. Long-term prognosis in anorexia nervosa: Lessons from a 21-year follow-up. *Lancet* 355(9205): 721–722.

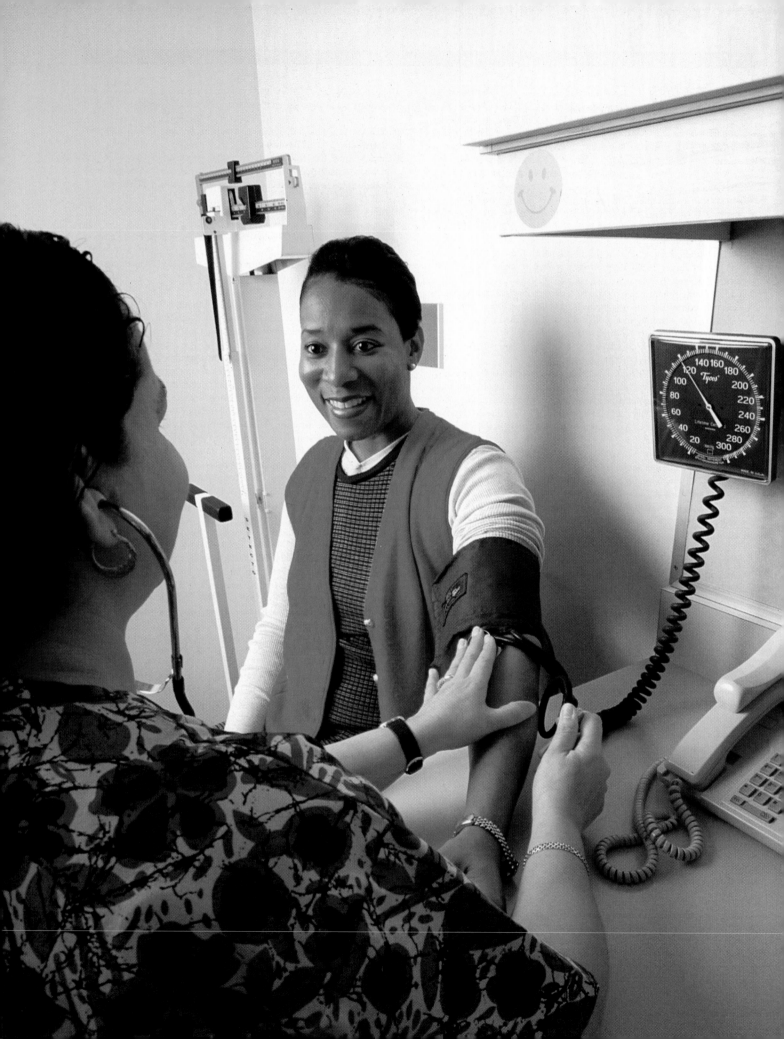

After reading this chapter, you should be able to

- List the major components of the cardiovascular system and describe how blood is pumped and circulated throughout the body

- Describe the controllable and uncontrollable risk factors associated with cardiovascular disease

- Discuss the major forms of cardiovascular disease and how they develop

- List the steps you can take to lower your personal risk of developing cardiovascular disease

Cardiovascular Health

15

TEST YOUR KNOWLEDGE

1. Reducing the amount of cholesterol you eat is the most important dietary change you can make to improve your blood cholesterol levels.
   True or false?

2. Women are about as likely to die of cardiovascular disease as they are to die of breast cancer.
   True or false?

3. How much earlier, on average, do people who do *not* exercise regularly develop heart disease compared with people who do exercise?
   a. 6 months
   b. 2 years
   c. 6 years

4. Which of the following is a possible sign of a heart attack?
   a. chest pain that spreads to the shoulders and arms
   b. uncomfortable pressure or fullness in the chest lasting more than a few minutes
   c. light-headedness and nausea

5. Which of the following foods would be a good choice for promoting heart health?
   a. tofu
   b. salmon
   c. bananas

ANSWERS

1. **FALSE.** Limiting your intake of saturated and trans fats, which promote the production of cholesterol by the liver, is the key dietary change for improving blood cholesterol levels; dietary cholesterol has much less of an effect on blood cholesterol.

2. **FALSE.** Cardiovascular disease kills far more. Among American women, about 1 in 2 deaths is due to cardiovascular disease and about 1 in 23 is due to breast cancer.

3. **C.** Both aerobic exercise and strength training significantly improve cardiovascular health.

4. **ALL THREE.** Quick recognition of symptoms and early treatment can greatly reduce the severity of a heart attack and increase the chances of survival.

5. **ALL THREE.** Soy protein (tofu), foods with omega-3 fatty acids (salmon), and foods high in potassium and low in sodium (bananas) all improve cardiovascular health.

ardiovascular disease (CVD) is the leading cause of death in the United States, claiming one life every 33 seconds. Nearly half of all Americans alive today will die from CVD. Though we typically think of CVD as primarily affecting men and older adults, heart attack is the number one killer of American women, and nearly a third of heart attacks occur in people under age 65. But not all the news is bad. In the past 50 years, lifestyle changes and medical advances have led to significant progress in the fight against CVD.

Much of the incidence of CVD is due to the American way of life. Too many Americans eat a high-fat diet, are overweight and sedentary, smoke, manage stress ineffectively, have uncontrolled high blood pressure or high cholesterol levels, and don't know the signs of CVD. Not all the risk factors for CVD are controllable—for example, the older you are, the greater your risk for CVD. But many factors can be changed, treated, or modified, and you have the power to significantly reduce your risk.

Exactly what is CVD, and how does it do its damage? More important, what steps can you take now to keep your heart healthy throughout your life? This chapter will provide some answers to these questions.

THE CARDIOVASCULAR SYSTEM

The cardiovascular system consists of the heart and blood vessels (veins, arteries, and capillaries); together, they pump and circulate blood throughout the body. A person weighing 150 pounds has about 5 quarts of blood, which is circulated about once every minute.

The heart is a four-chambered, fist-size muscle located just beneath the ribs under the left breast (Figure 15-1). Its role is to pump oxygen-poor blood to the lungs and oxygenated (oxygen-rich) blood to the rest of the body. Blood actually travels through two separate circulatory systems: The right side of the heart pumps blood to and from the lungs in what is called **pulmonary circulation,** and the left side pumps blood through the rest of the body in **systemic circulation.**

Used, oxygen-poor blood enters the right upper chamber, or **atrium,** of the heart through the **vena cava,** the largest vein in the body (Figure 15-2). Valves prevent the blood from flowing the wrong way. As the right atrium fills, it contracts and pumps blood into the right lower chamber, or **ventricle,** which, when it contracts, pumps blood through the pulmonary artery into the lungs. There, blood picks up oxygen and discards carbon dioxide. Cleaned, oxygenated blood then flows through the pulmonary veins into the left atrium. As this chamber fills, it contracts and pumps blood into the powerful left ventricle, which pumps it through the **aorta,** the body's largest artery, to be fed into the rest of the body's blood vessels. The period of the heart's contraction is called **systole;** the period of relaxation is called **diastole.**

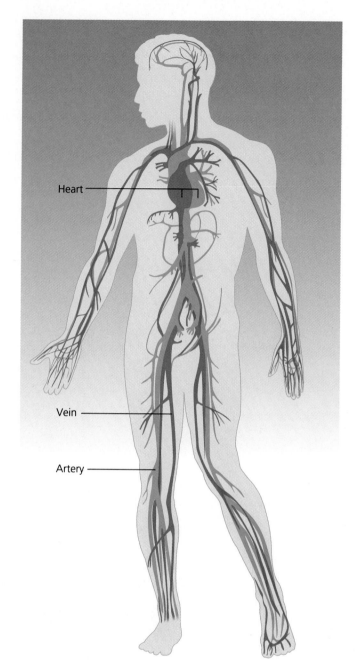

Figure 15-1   The cardiovascular system.

The heartbeat—the split-second sequence of contractions of the heart's four chambers—is controlled by electrical impulses. These signals originate in a bundle of specialized cells in the right atrium called the pacemaker. Unless the pace is speeded up or slowed down by the brain in response to such stimuli as danger or exhaustion, the heart produces electrical impulses at a steady rate.

Blood vessels are classified by size and function. **Veins** carry blood to the heart; **arteries** carry blood away from the heart. Veins have thin walls, but arteries have thick elastic walls that enable them to expand and relax with the volume of the blood being pumped through them. Af-

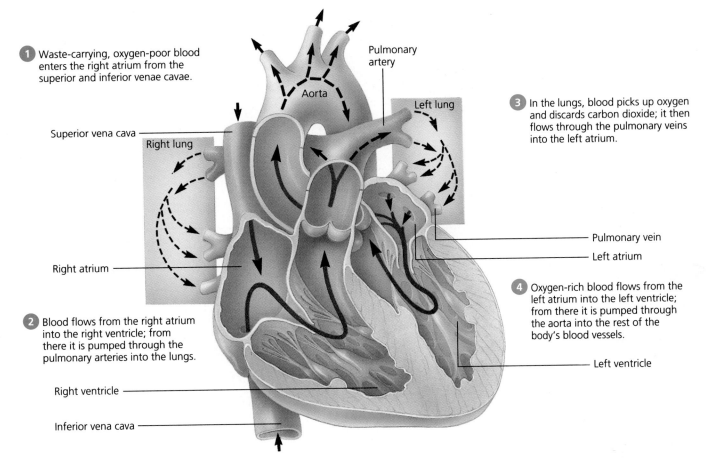

① Waste-carrying, oxygen-poor blood enters the right atrium from the superior and inferior venae cavae.

Aorta

Pulmonary artery

Superior vena cava

Right lung

Left lung

③ In the lungs, blood picks up oxygen and discards carbon dioxide; it then flows through the pulmonary veins into the left atrium.

Right atrium

Pulmonary vein

Left atrium

④ Oxygen-rich blood flows from the left atrium into the left ventricle; from there it is pumped through the aorta into the rest of the body's blood vessels.

② Blood flows from the right atrium into the right ventricle; from there it is pumped through the pulmonary arteries into the lungs.

Left ventricle

Right ventricle

Inferior vena cava

Figure 15-2   Circulation in the heart.

ter leaving the heart, the aorta branches into smaller and smaller vessels. Two vital arteries, called the **coronary arteries,** branch off the aorta to carry blood back to the heart tissues themselves (Figure 15-3).

The smallest arteries branch still further into **capillaries,** tiny vessels only one cell thick. The capillaries deliver oxygen and nutrient-rich blood to the tissues and receive oxygen-poor, waste-carrying blood. From the capillaries, this blood empties into small veins and then into larger veins that return it to the heart. From there the cycle is repeated.

▼ Ww. RISK FACTORS FOR CARDIOVASCULAR DISEASE

Researchers have identified a variety of factors associated with an increased risk of developing cardiovascular disease. They are grouped into two categories: major risk factors and contributing risk factors. Some major risk factors, such as diet, exercise habits, and use of tobacco, are linked to controllable aspects of lifestyle and can therefore be changed. Others, such as age, sex, and heredity, are beyond an individual's control.

Terms

cardiovascular disease (CVD) The collective term for various forms of diseases of the heart and blood vessels.

pulmonary circulation The part of the circulatory system governed by the right side of the heart; the circulation of blood between the heart and the lungs.

systemic circulation The part of the circulatory system governed by the left side of the heart; the circulation of blood between the heart and the rest of the body.

atria The two upper chambers of the heart in which blood collects before passing to the ventricles; also called *auricles*.

vena cava The large vein through which blood is returned to the right atrium of the heart.

ventricles The two lower chambers of the heart from which blood flows through arteries to the lungs and other parts of the body.

aorta The large artery that receives blood from the left ventricle and distributes it to the body.

systole Contraction of the heart.

diastole Relaxation of the heart.

veins Vessels that carry blood to the heart.

arteries Vessels that carry blood away from the heart.

coronary arteries Two arteries branching from the aorta that provide blood to the heart muscle.

capillaries Very small blood vessels that distribute blood to all parts of the body.

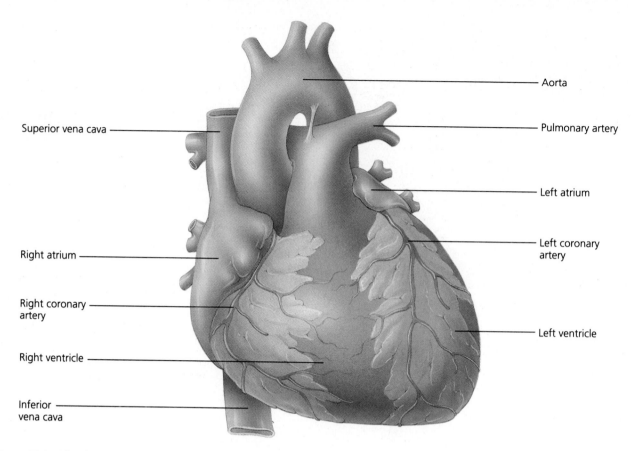

Figure 15-3 Blood supply to the heart.

Labels (clockwise from top):
- Aorta
- Pulmonary artery
- Left atrium
- Left coronary artery
- Left ventricle
- Inferior vena cava
- Right ventricle
- Right coronary artery
- Right atrium
- Superior vena cava

Major Risk Factors That Can Be Changed

The American Heart Association (AHA) has identified six major risk factors for CVD that can be changed: tobacco use, high blood pressure, unhealthy blood cholesterol levels, physical inactivity, obesity, and diabetes.

Tobacco Use   About 1 in 5 deaths from CVD is attributable to smoking. People who smoke a pack of cigarettes a day have twice the risk of heart attack that nonsmokers have; smoking two or more packs a day triples the risk. And when smokers do have heart attacks, they are two to four times more likely than nonsmokers to die from them. Women who smoke heavily and use oral contraceptives are up to 32 times more likely to have a heart attack and up to 20 times more likely to have a stroke than women who don't smoke and take the pill.

Smoking harms the cardiovascular system and raises risk for CVD in several ways. Nicotine, a central nervous system stimulant, increases blood pressure and heart rate; the carbon monoxide in cigarette smoke displaces oxygen in the blood, reducing the amount of oxygen available to the heart and other parts of the body. Smoking damages the linings of arteries, and it contributes to unhealthy blood fat levels by reducing levels of high-density lipo-

proteins (HDL), "good cholesterol," and raising levels of triglycerides and low-density lipoproteins (LDL), "bad cholesterol." It causes the **platelets** in blood to become sticky and cluster, promoting clotting. Smoking also permanently accelerates the rate at which fatty deposits are laid down in arteries.

You don't have to smoke to be affected. The risk of death from coronary heart disease increases up to 30% among those exposed to environmental tobacco smoke (ETS) at home or at work. Researchers estimate that 62,000 nonsmokers die from CVD each year as a result of exposure to ETS.

High Blood Pressure   High blood pressure, or **hypertension,** is a risk factor for many forms of CVD but is also considered a disease itself. High blood pressure occurs when too much force or pressure is exerted against the walls of the arteries. If your blood pressure is high, your heart has to work harder to push the blood forward. Over time, a strained heart weakens and tends to enlarge, which weakens it further. Increased blood pressure also scars and hardens arteries, making them less elastic. Heart attacks, strokes, **atherosclerosis,** and kidney failure can result.

Hypertension usually has no early warning signs, so it's important to have your blood pressure tested at least once

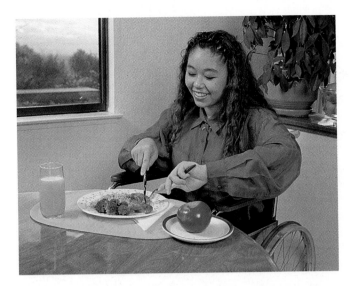

A diet high in fiber and low in saturated and trans fats can help lower levels of total cholesterol and LDL. This young woman is enjoying a healthy dinner of baked chicken, broccoli, rice, fruit, and juice.

every two years (more often if you have CVD risk factors). If yours is consistently high, your physician can help you lower it through diet, weight management, exercise, and, if necessary, medication. (High blood pressure and atherosclerosis are discussed later in the chapter.)

High Levels of Cholesterol   Cholesterol is a fatty, wax-like substance that circulates through the bloodstream and is an important component of cell membranes, sex hormones, vitamin D, the fluid that coats the lungs, and the protective sheaths around nerves. Adequate cholesterol is essential for the proper functioning of the body. However, excess cholesterol can clog arteries and increase the risk of cardiovascular disease. Our bodies obtain cholesterol in two ways: from the liver, which manufactures it, and from the foods we eat. Cholesterol levels vary depending on diet, age, sex, heredity, and other factors.

GOOD VERSUS BAD CHOLESTEROL   Cholesterol is carried in the blood in protein-lipid packages called lipoproteins. Lipoproteins can be thought of as shuttles that transport cholesterol to and from the liver through the circulatory system (Figure 15-4). **Low-density lipoproteins (LDLs)** shuttle cholesterol from the liver to the organs and tissues that require it. LDL is known as "bad" cholesterol because if there is more than the body can use, the excess is deposited in the blood vessels. LDL that accumulates and becomes trapped in artery walls may be oxidized by free radicals, speeding inflammation and damage to artery walls and increasing the likelihood of a blockage. If coronary arteries are blocked, the result may be a heart attack; if an artery carrying blood to the brain is blocked, a stroke may occur. **High-density lipoproteins (HDLs),** or "good" cholesterol, shuttle un-

used cholesterol back to the liver for recycling. By removing cholesterol from blood vessels, HDL helps protect against atherosclerosis.

RECOMMENDED BLOOD CHOLESTEROL LEVELS   The risk for cardiovascular disease increases with increasing blood cholesterol levels, especially LDL. The National Cholesterol Education Program (NCEP) recommends cholesterol testing at least once every 5 years for all adults, beginning at age 20. The recommended test is a lipoprotein profile that measures total cholesterol, LDL cholesterol, HDL cholesterol, and triglycerides (another blood fat). General cholesterol and triglyceride guidelines are given in Table 15-1. In general, high LDL levels and low HDL levels are associated with a high risk for CVD; low levels of LDL and high levels of HDL are associated with lower risk. HDL is important because a high HDL level seems to offer protection from CVD even in cases where total cholesterol is high

As shown in Table 15-1, LDL levels below 100 mg/dl (milligrams per deciliter) and total cholesterol levels below 200 mg/dl are desirable. An estimated 100 million American adults—over half the population—have total cholesterol levels of 200 mg/dl or higher. The CVD risk associated with elevated cholesterol levels also depends on other factors. For example, an above optimal level of LDL would be of more concern for an individual who also smoked and had high blood pressure than for an individual without these additional CVD risk factors.

BENEFITS OF CONTROLLING CHOLESTEROL   Experts calculate that people can cut their heart attack risk by 2% for every 1% that they reduce their total blood cholesterol levels. People who lower their total cholesterol from 250 to 200 mg/dl, for example, reduce their risk of heart attack by 40%. In addition, studies indicate that improving LDL and HDL levels not only reduces the likelihood that arteries will become clogged but can also

Terms

platelets Microscopic disk-shaped cell fragments in the blood that disintegrate on contact with foreign objects and release chemicals that are necessary for the formation of blood clots.

hypertension Sustained abnormally high blood pressure.

✓**atherosclerosis** A form of CVD in which the inner layers of artery walls are made thick and irregular by plaque deposits; arteries become narrow and blood supply is reduced.

low-density lipoproteins (LDL) Blood fat that transports cholesterol from the liver to organs and tissues; excess is deposited on artery walls, where it can eventually block the flow of blood to the heart and brain; "bad" cholesterol.

high-density lipoproteins (HDL) Blood fat that helps transport cholesterol out of the arteries and thus protects against heart diseases; "good" cholesterol.

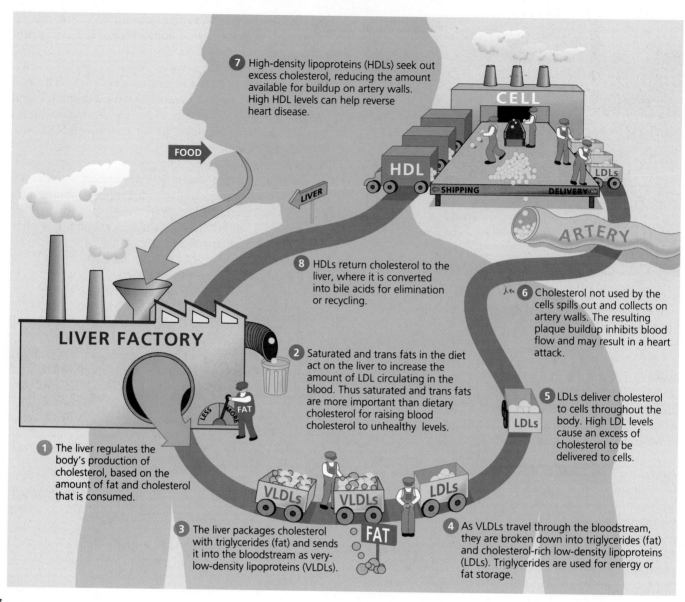

① The liver regulates the body's production of cholesterol, based on the amount of fat and cholesterol that is consumed.

② Saturated and trans fats in the diet act on the liver to increase the amount of LDL circulating in the blood. Thus saturated and trans fats are more important than dietary cholesterol for raising blood cholesterol to unhealthy levels.

③ The liver packages cholesterol with triglycerides (fat) and sends it into the bloodstream as very-low-density lipoproteins (VLDLs).

④ As VLDLs travel through the bloodstream, they are broken down into triglycerides (fat) and cholesterol-rich low-density lipoproteins (LDLs). Triglycerides are used for energy or fat storage.

⑤ LDLs deliver cholesterol to cells throughout the body. High LDL levels cause an excess of cholesterol to be delivered to cells.

⑥ Cholesterol not used by the cells spills out and collects on artery walls. The resulting plaque buildup inhibits blood flow and may result in a heart attack.

⑦ High-density lipoproteins (HDLs) seek out excess cholesterol, reducing the amount available for buildup on artery walls. High HDL levels can help reverse heart disease.

⑧ HDLs return cholesterol to the liver, where it is converted into bile acids for elimination or recycling.

Figure 15-4 Travels with cholesterol.

reverse deposits on artery walls, thereby actually helping clean out diseased arteries.

How can you improve your cholesterol levels? Your primary goal should be to reduce LDL to healthy levels. Important dietary changes for reducing LDL levels include substituting unsaturated for saturated and trans fats and increasing soluble fiber intake. Decreasing your intake of saturated and trans fats is particularly important because they promote the production and excretion of cholesterol by the liver. Exercising regularly and eating more fruits, vegetables, and whole grains also help. You can raise your HDL levels by exercising regularly, losing weight if you are overweight, quitting smoking, and altering the amount and type of fat you consume. These and other lifestyle changes promoting heart health are discussed in greater detail later in this chapter.

Physical Inactivity An estimated 35–50 million Americans are so sedentary that they are at high risk for developing CVD. Exercise is thought to be the closest thing we have to a "magic bullet" against heart disease. It lowers CVD risk by helping decrease blood pressure, increase HDL levels, maintain desirable weight, and prevent or control diabetes; exercise also improves the functioning of the endothelial cells that line coronary arteries. One recent study found that women who accumulated at least 3 hours of brisk walking each week cut their risk of heart attack and stroke by more than half. A minimum of 30 minutes per day of moderate physical activity is recommended; more intense or longer-duration exercise has even greater health benefits. Refer to Chapter 13 for more on the benefits of physical activity and guidelines for creating an exercise program.

Table 15-1	Cholesterol Guidelines

LDL cholesterol (mg/dl) *bad*

Less than 100	Optimal
100–129	Near optimal/above optimal
130–159	Borderline high
160–189	High
190 or more	Very high

Total cholesterol (mg/dl)

✓Less than 200	Desirable
200–239	Borderline high
240 or more	High

HDL cholesterol (mg/dl) *good*

Less than 40	Low
60 or more	High

Triglycerides (mg/dl)

Less than 150	Normal
150–199	Borderline high
200–499	High
500 or more	Very high

SOURCE: Expert Panel on Detection, Evaluation, and Treatment of High Blood Cholesterol in Adults. 2001. Executive Summary of the Third Report of the National Cholesterol Education Program (NCEP) Expert Panel on Detection, Evaluation, and Treatment of High Blood Cholesterol in Adults (Adult Treatment Panel III). *Journal of the American Medical Association* 285(19).

Obesity A person whose body weight is more than 30% above the recommended level is at higher risk for heart disease and stroke, even if no other risk factors are present. Excess weight increases the strain on the heart by contributing to high blood pressure and high cholesterol. It can also lead to diabetes, another CVD risk factor (see below). As discussed in Chapter 14, distribution of body fat is also significant: Fat that collects in the torso is more dangerous than fat that collects around the hips. A sensible diet and regular exercise are the best ways to achieve and maintain a healthy body weight. For someone who is overweight, even modest weight reduction can reduce CVD risk by lowering blood pressure, improving cholesterol levels, and reducing diabetes risk.

Diabetes As described in Chapter 14, diabetes is a disorder characterized by elevated blood glucose levels due to either insufficient supply or action of insulin. Having diabetes doubles the risk of CVD for men and triples the risk for women. Most people with diabetes die of CVD, and they usually die at younger ages than people without

diabetes. The reason for the increased CVD risk among people with diabetes is complex. Diabetics have higher rates of other CVD risk factors, including hypertension, obesity, and unhealthy blood lipid levels (typically, high triglyceride levels and low HDL levels). The elevated blood glucose levels that occur in diabetes can damage the lining of arteries, making them more vulnerable to atherosclerosis; diabetics also often have platelet and blood coagulation abnormalities that increase the risk of heart attacks and strokes.

Careful control of glucose levels is beneficial, but even people whose diabetes is under control face an increased risk of CVD. For that reason, careful control of other CVD risk factors is critical for people with diabetes.

Contributing Risk Factors That Can Be Changed

Various other factors that can be changed have been identified as contributing to CVD risk, including triglyceride levels and psychological and social factors.

High Triglyceride Levels Like cholesterol, triglycerides are blood fats that are obtained from food and manufactured by the body. High triglyceride levels are a reliable predictor of heart disease, especially if associated with other risk factors, such as low HDL levels, obesity, and diabetes. Factors contributing to elevated triglyceride levels include excess body fat, physical inactivity, cigarette smoking, excess alcohol intake, very high carbohydrate diets, and certain diseases and medications.

Much of the picture regarding triglycerides remains unclear, however. Studies have yet to show whether lowering triglyceride levels will actually decrease heart disease. Elevated triglyceride levels are most often seen in people with other lipid abnormalities; and the lifestyle modifications that help lower cholesterol also help decrease triglycerides, making it difficult to identify any potential independent benefit of lowering triglyceride levels.

A full lipid profile should include testing and evaluation of triglyceride levels (see Table 15-1). For people with borderline high triglyceride levels, increased physical activity and weight reduction can help bring levels down into the healthy range; for people with high triglycerides, drug therapy may be recommended. Being moderate in the use of alcohol and quitting smoking are also important.

Psychological and Social Factors Many of the psychological and social factors that influence other areas of wellness are also important risk factors for CVD.

- *Stress.* Excessive stress can strain the heart and blood vessels over time and contribute to CVD. A fullblown stress response causes blood pressure to rise; blood platelets become more likely to cluster, possibly enhancing the formation of artery-clogging clots. Stress can also trigger abnormal heart rhythms (arrhythmias),

Current research suggests that people with a quick temper, a persistently hostile outlook, and a cynical, mistrusting attitude toward life are more likely to develop heart disease than those with a calmer, more trusting attitude. People who are angry frequently, intensely, and for long periods experience the stress response—and its accompanying boosts in heart rate, blood pressure, and stress hormone levels—much more often than more relaxed individuals. Over the long term, these effects may damage arteries and promote CVD.

Are You Too Hostile?

To help answer that question, Duke University researcher Redford Williams, M.D., has devised a short self-test. It's not a scientific evaluation, but it does offer a rough measure of hostility. Are the following statements true or false for you?

1. I often get annoyed at checkout cashiers or the people in front of me when I'm waiting in line.
2. I usually keep an eye on the people I work or live with to make sure they do what they should.
3. I often wonder how homeless people can have so little respect for themselves.
4. I believe that most people will take advantage of you if you let them.
5. The habits of friends or family members often annoy me.
6. When I'm stuck in traffic, I often start breathing faster and my heart pounds.
7. When I'm annoyed with people, I really want to let them know it.
8. If someone does me wrong, I want to get even.
9. I'd like to have the last word in any argument.
10. At least once a week, I have the urge to yell at or even hit someone.

According to Williams, five or more "true" statements suggest that you're excessively hostile and should consider taking steps to mellow out.

Managing Your Anger

Begin by monitoring your angry responses and looking for triggers—people or situations that typically make you angry. Familiarize yourself with the patterns of thinking that lead to angry or hostile feelings, and then try to head them off before they develop into full-blown anger. If you feel your anger starting to build, try reasoning with yourself by asking the following questions:

1. *Is this really important enough to get angry about?* For example, is having to wait an extra 5 minutes for a late bus so important that you should stew about it for the entire 15-minute ride?
2. *Am I really justified in getting angry?* Is the person in front of you really driving slowly, or are you trying to speed?
3. *Is getting angry going to make a real and positive difference in this situation?* Will yelling and slamming the door really help your friend find the concert tickets he misplaced?

If you answer "yes" to all three questions, then calm but assertive communication may be an appropriate response. If your anger isn't reasonable, try distracting yourself or removing yourself from the situation. Exercise, humor, social support, and other stress-management techniques can also help (see Chapter 3 for additional anger-management tips). Your heart—and the people around you—will benefit from your calmer, more positive outlook.

SOURCES: Take it to heart: "Chill out." 2000. *Mind/Body Health Newsletter* 9(2): 1–2. Anger and heart-disease risk. 2000. *Harvard Heart Letter,* July. QUIZ SOURCE: Williams, Virginia and Williams, Redford, *Life Skills,* New York: Times Books. Reprinted by permission of the authors.

---

with potentially fatal consequences: Numerous studies have found an increase in CVD deaths following human-made and natural disasters such as wars and earthquakes. People sometimes also adopt unhealthy habits such as smoking or overeating as a means of dealing with severe stress.

- *Chronic hostility and anger.* Certain traits in the hard-driving "Type A" personality—hostility, cynicism, and anger—are associated with increased risk of heart disease. Men prone to anger have two to three times the heart attack risk of calmer men. In a 10-year study of young adults age 18–30 years, those with high hostility levels were more than twice as likely to develop coronary artery calcification (a marker of early atherosclerosis) as those with low hostility levels. See the box "Anger, Hostility, and Heart Disease" for more information.

- *Suppressing psychological distress.* Consistently suppressing anger and other negative emotions may also be hazardous to a healthy heart. People who hide psychological distress appear to have higher rates of heart disease than people who experience similar distress but share it with others. People with so-called Type D personalities tend to be pessimistic, negative, and unhappy and to suppress these feelings. Researchers are not yet certain why the Type D trait is dangerous. It may have physical effects, or it may lead to social isolation and poor communication with physicians.

- *Depression and anxiety.* Both mild and severe depression are linked to an increased risk of CVD, and researchers have also found a strong association between anxiety disorders and an increased risk of death from heart disease, particularly sudden death from heart at-

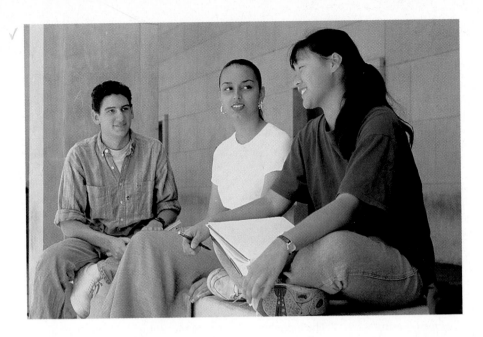

Stress and social isolation can increase risk of cardiovascular disease. A strong social support network improves both heart health and overall wellness.

tack. Both depression and anxiety have physical effects, including irregular heart rhythms, that have short- and long-term effects on the cardiovascular system.

• *Social isolation.* People with little social support are at higher risk for dying from CVD than people with close ties to others. A strong social support network is a major antidote to stress. Friends and family members can also promote and support a healthy lifestyle.

• *Low socioeconomic status.* Low socioeconomic status and low educational attainment also increase risk for CVD. These associations are probably due to a variety of factors, including lifestyle and access to health care.

COMMUNICATE! Does someone in your family have any major risk factors for cardiovascular disease that can be changed, such as smoking or physical inactivity? If so, practice how you might talk to the person about altering his or her behavior to reduce risk. Be prepared for some resistance; you may have to have more than one conversation about your concern. You might begin by saying, for instance, "Dad, I'm worried about what smoking might be doing to your heart. Can we talk about that for a minute?"

Major Risk Factors That Can't Be Changed

A number of major risk factors for CVD cannot be changed: heredity, aging, being male, and ethnicity.

Heredity The tendency to develop CVD seems to be inherited. If one of your parents has had heart or blood vessel disease, you have a greater risk of developing CVD yourself. High cholesterol levels, hypertension, abnormal blood-clotting problems, diabetes, and obesity are other CVD risk factors that have genetic links. But it's important to remember that people who inherit a tendency for CVD are not destined to develop it. They may, however, have to work harder than other people to prevent CVD.

Aging The risk of heart attack increases dramatically after age 65. About 70% of all heart attack victims are age 65 or older, and more than four out of five who suffer fatal heart attacks are over 65. For people over 55, the incidence of stroke more than doubles in each successive decade. However, many people in their thirties and forties, especially men, have heart attacks.

Being Male Although CVD is the leading killer of both men and women in the United States, men face a greater risk of heart attack than women, especially earlier in life. Until age 55, men also have a greater risk of hypertension than women. The incidence of stroke is about 19% higher for males than females. Estrogen production, which is highest during the childbearing years, may offer premenopausal women some protection against CVD (see the box "Women and CVD"). By age 75, the gender gap nearly disappears.

Ethnicity Death rates from heart disease vary among ethnic groups in the United States, with African Americans having much higher rates of hypertension, heart disease, and stroke than other groups (see the box "African Americans and CVD"). Puerto Rican Americans, Cuban Americans, and Mexican Americans are also more likely to suffer from high blood pressure and angina (a warning sign of heart disease) than non-Hispanic white Americans. These differences may be due in part to differences in education, income, and other socioeconomic factors. Asian Americans historically have had far lower rates of

Cardiovascular disease has traditionally been thought of as a "man's disease." It is true that men have a higher incidence of cardiovascular problems than women, especially before age 50. Until recently, this has been the justification for carrying out almost all CVD research on men. But heart disease is the leading cause of death among women, and more women actually die of CVD than men, though they tend to do so at older ages. On average, women live 10 to 15 more years free of coronary heart disease than men do. Polls indicate that women vastly underestimate their risk of dying of a heart attack and overestimate their risk of dying of breast cancer. In reality, nearly 1 in 2 women dies of CVD, while 1 in 23 dies of breast cancer.

Risk factors for CVD are generally similar for both sexes. But there are important gender differences in how and when CVD develops, is diagnosed, and is treated.

Estrogen: The Heart Protector

One important protective factor is unique to women—estrogen. It has long been observed that women seem to avoid heart disease until after menopause. The hormone estrogen, produced naturally by women's bodies until menopause or surgical removal of the ovaries, improves blood fat concentrations by increasing HDL levels and decreasing LDL levels. After menopause, when estrogen levels drop, rates of heart disease among women rapidly increase. Some women choose hormone replacement therapy (HRT) to keep estrogen levels high after menopause. Most studies have shown that HRT cuts CVD risk substantially. However, several recent studies have shown little cardiovascular benefit for HRT in women who already have heart disease. One study showed that women who already have heart disease might actually have more serious health problems during the first year of HRT than women with heart disease who are not on HRT. These findings are controversial, though, and do not apply to women with no history of CVD. Although more research is needed, many experts feel that for many postmenopausal women, the benefits of HRT outweigh the risks. (HRT is discussed further in Chapter 19.)

There is one special caution for premenopausal women: The combination of heavy smoking and using oral contraceptives makes a woman up to 32 times more likely to have a heart attack than a woman who doesn't both smoke and use birth control pills.

Postmenopausal Women: At Risk

Heart attack is the leading killer of women in the United States, and women are more likely than men to die within 2 years following a heart attack. Why are heart attacks more deadly for women? One answer is that women tend to develop heart disease at older ages, when they are more likely to have other health problems that complicate treatment. In addition, recent studies have shown that women tend to have more severe heart attacks than men. Because of physiological differences, some common diagnostic tests are less accurate for women (false positives on ECGs are common). Women also tend to have smaller hearts and arteries, possibly making surgery both more difficult and less successful.

The mortality difference cannot entirely be explained by age and anatomy, however. It also appears that medical personnel evaluate and treat women less aggressively than men. One study of emergency room treatment of heart attack patients found that women had to wait longer than men did—by about 23 minutes—before receiving clot-dissolving drugs. Women may complain less about their pain, or they may describe somewhat different symptoms than male heart attack victims. A recent study found that about one-third of all heart attack victims do not complain of chest pain and that women are more likely than men to have a heart attack without experiencing chest pain. Is physician bias an important factor in the differences in medical care for women and men with heart disease? This is an important question but one that is difficult to answer. There may also be unknown biological or psychosocial risk factors contributing to increased mortality among women.

Researchers are now focusing more attention on the health problems of women, and more accurate diagnostic techniques may soon be in use. In the meantime, women with chest pain or other symptoms should be persistent in seeking diagnosis and effective treatment.

CVD than white Americans. However, cholesterol levels among Asian Americans appear to be rising, presumably because of the adoption of a high-fat American diet.

Possible Risk Factors Currently Being Studied

In recent years, a number of other possible risk factors for cardiovascular disease have been identified. These include homocysteine, specific types of cholesterol, infectious agents, inflammation, and others.

Homocysteine   Elevated levels of homocysteine, an amino acid circulating in the blood, are associated with an increased risk of CVD. Researchers are not yet certain, however, whether it is a direct cause of CVD or simply a marker for some other risk factor. In laboratory studies, homocysteine appears to damage the lining of blood vessels, resulting in inflammation and the development of fatty deposits in artery walls. These changes can lead to the formation of clots and blockages in arteries, which in turn can cause heart attacks and strokes. Elevated homocysteine levels have also been associated with increased incidence of blood clots in veins.

Men generally have higher homocysteine levels than women, as do individuals with diets low in folic acid, vitamin B-12, and vitamin B-6. Many genes may cause elevated homocysteine levels, and some genes associated

Although cardiovascular disease is the leading cause of death for all Americans, African Americans are far more likely to suffer from CVD than whites in the United States. The CVD death rate is about 25% higher in black men and 33% higher in black women than in whites. The rate of hypertension among African Americans is among the highest in the world. Blacks tend to develop hypertension at an earlier age than whites, and their average blood pressures are much higher. As a result, the stroke rate among blacks is 1.5 times greater than that among whites. What accounts for these higher rates of CVD among African Americans? Contributing factors can be grouped into three areas: biological/genetic factors, low income and discrimination, and lifestyle factors.

Biological/Genetic Risk Factors

A number of genetic and biological factors may contribute to CVD in African Americans. Blacks appear to be more sensitive to dietary sodium, leading to greater blood pressure elevation in response to a given amount of sodium. African Americans may also experience less dilation of blood vessels in response to stress, an attribute that also raises blood pressure. Heredity also plays a large role in the tendency to develop diabetes, another important CVD risk factor that is more common in blacks than whites. A recent study of young children found that about 40% more black children than white children were relatively insensitive to insulin, increasing their risk for diabetes later in life. However, although the tendency to develop diabetes is largely hereditary, diet and lifestyle make a big difference in whether that tendency is actually expressed.

Low Income and Discrimination

Another factor in the high incidence of CVD among African Americans is low income. About 25% live below the official poverty line. Economic deprivation usually means reduced access to adequate health care and health insurance. Associated with low income are poorer educational opportunities, which often mean less information about preventive health measures, such as diet and stress management.

Discrimination may also play a role in CVD among blacks. Research has shown that many physicians and hospitals treat the medical problems of African Americans differently than those of whites. Discrimination, along with low income and other forms of deprivation, may also increase stress, which is linked with hypertension and CVD.

Lifestyle Factors

Lifestyle factors are important in explaining high CVD rates among African Americans. A recent large-scale study determined that birthplace, not ethnicity, is the key indicator of CVD risk among African Americans. The study found that among New Yorkers born in the Northeast, blacks and whites have nearly identical risk of CVD. But black New Yorkers who were born in the South have a sharply higher risk, and black New Yorkers born in the Caribbean have a significantly lower risk. Researchers speculate that some risk factors for CVD, including smoking and a high-fat diet, may be more common in the South. When combined with urban stress, these factors create a lifestyle that is far from heart-healthy. And people with low incomes, who are disproportionately African American, tend to smoke more, use more salt, and exercise less than those with higher incomes. In addition, half of black women and one-third of black men are significantly overweight.

All Americans are advised to have their blood pressure checked regularly, exercise, eat a healthy diet, manage stress, and avoid smoking. These general preventive strategies may be particularly critical for African Americans. In addition, recent research has indentified several specific dietary factors that may be of special importance for blacks. Studies have found that diets high in potassium and calcium improve blood pressure in African Americans. Fruits, vegetables, grains, and nuts are rich in potassium; dairy products are high in calcium.

---

with small-to-moderate elevations are quite common in the general population. The good news is that most people can lower homocysteine levels easily by adopting a healthy diet rich in fruits, vegetables, and grains and by taking supplements if needed. Studies are underway to determine if decreasing homocysteine levels will actually reduce CVD risk; at this point, testing for elevated homocysteine is usually recommended only for people with heart disease who have few of the traditional risk factors.

Lipoprotein(a)   A high level of a specific type of LDL called lipoprotein(a), or Lp(a), has been identified as a possible risk factor for coronary heart disease (CHD), es-

pecially when associated with high LDL or low HDL levels. Lp(a) levels have a strong genetic component and are difficult to treat. Research suggests that hormone replacement therapy in postmenopausal women, a diet rich in omega-3 fatty acids, and treatment for lowering elevated LDL levels may help reduce the associated risk.

LDL Particle Size   Recent research has shown that LDL particles differ in size and density and that the concentrations of different particles vary among individuals. LDL cholesterol profiles can be divided into three general types: people with pattern A have mostly large, buoyant LDL particles; people with pattern B have mostly small, dense LDL particles; and people with pattern C have a mixture of particle types. Small, dense LDL particles pose a greater CVD risk than larger particles; thus, people with LDL pattern B are at greater risk for CVD. At this time, testing to identify LDL particle size is expensive and not widely available, and further research is needed before routine screening and treatment for LDL pattern B can be recommended. Exercise, a low-fat diet, and certain lipid-lowering drugs may help lower CVD risk in people with LDL pattern B.

Infectious Agents   Several infectious agents have been identified as possible culprits in the development of CVD. *Chlamydia pneumoniae,* a common cause of flulike respiratory infections, has been found in sections of clogged, damaged arteries but not in sections of healthy arteries. In one study, evidence of infection with *C. pneumoniae* was found in 90% of patients who had recently had a heart attack but in only 25% of healthy control subjects. A few small studies indicate that antibiotic treatment of *C. pneumoniae* may be beneficial for some patients; however, further research is needed, and the role of antibiotics in the treatment of heart disease is still unclear.

Other infectious agents may also play a role in CVD. *Cytomegalovirus,* a common type of herpesvirus, is linked to the recurrence of blockages in patients who have been treated for CHD. The bacteria that cause gingivitis (gum disease) and *Helicobacter pylori,* the bacterium that causes the majority of peptic ulcers, have also been implicated as possible factors in the development of heart disease. Research findings have been mixed, however, and the jury is still out on whether infection is a significant trigger for atherosclerosis and CVD.

Inflammation and C-Reactive Protein   Recent research suggests that inflammation plays a key role in the development of CVD. When an artery is injured by smoking, cholesterol, infectious agents, or other factors, the body's response produces inflammation. A substance called C-reactive protein is released into the bloodstream during the inflammatory response, and studies suggest that high levels of C-reactive protein indicate a substantially elevated risk of heart attack and stroke. Aspirin, which reduces both clotting and inflammation, is often recommended for people at high risk for heart attacks and strokes.

Fibrinogen   Fibrinogen is a protein that is essential for the formation of blood clots. High levels of fibrinogen are linked to increased risk of coronary heart disease and stroke. Hormone replacement therapy and quitting smoking both help lower fibrinogen levels.

Blood Viscosity and Iron   High blood viscosity (thickness) may increase the risk of CVD; excess iron stores have also been linked to higher risk, especially for men

and postmenopausal women (iron stores are usually lower in younger women because of menstrual blood loss). Regular blood donation, which reduces iron stores and blood viscosity, is associated with lower CVD risk in men. Drinking five or more glasses of water a day may also reduce risk by reducing blood viscosity. On the flip side, high consumption of heme iron—found in meat, fish, and poultry—is associated with an increased risk of heart attack. Men and postmenopausal women should consult a physician before taking iron supplements.

Uric Acid   Recent research suggests a link between high blood levels of uric acid and CVD mortality, particularly among postmenopausal women and African Americans. Uric acid may raise CVD risk by increasing inflammation and platelet aggregation or by influencing the development of hypertension; high uric acid levels also cause gout (a type of arthritis), kidney stones, and certain forms of kidney disease. Medications to lower uric acid levels are available, but it is not yet known if they will be useful in preventing CVD.

Syndrome X   Researchers have found that certain CVD risk factors are often found in a cluster. As a group, these risk factors—abdominal obesity, high blood pressure, high triglycerides, low HDL, small LDL particles, and insulin resistance—are called syndrome X or metabolic syndrome. The underlying causes are not well understood, but syndrome X is thought to have a genetic basis. Because people with syndrome X have insulin resistance and often diabetes, some experts recommend a diet somewhat different from that recommended in the *Dietary Guidelines for Americans*—slightly higher in unsaturated fats and lower in carbohydrates—to help keep glucose and insulin levels under control (see the box "Dietary Fat: Eat More of the Right Type and Worry Less?"). The NCEP recommends weight control and physical activity to reduce all of the risk factors associated with syndrome X.

MAJOR FORMS OF CARDIOVASCULAR DISEASE

Collectively, the various forms of CVD kill more Americans than the next four leading causes of death combined (Figure 15-5). The financial burden of CVD, including the costs of medical treatments and lost productivity, exceeds $300 billion annually.

The main forms of CVD are hypertension, atherosclerosis, heart disease and heart attack, stroke, congestive heart failure, congenital heart disease, rheumatic heart disease, and heart valve problems. Many forms are interrelated and have elements in common; we treat them separately here for the sake of clarity.

IN THE NEWS   Dietary Fat: Eat More of the Right Type and Worry Less?

Is reducing the total amount of fat you eat always a good idea? Are you better off replacing saturated and trans fats with carbohydrates or with unsaturated fats? The answers to these hotly debated questions are not necessarily what you might think based on current dietary recommendations.

A diet with 30% or less of total calories from fat is advised by most major health organizations. However, some experts feel that the total amount of fat we consume is much less important than the type of fat we consume—and that we may benefit from eating more fat, as long as it's the right kind. Research has shown that people from Mediterranean countries whose diets are rich in olive oil (and thus monounsaturated fat) have low rates of CVD, even though their total fat intake is high. Since monounsaturated fats raise HDL levels, increasing the amount of these fats in our diets may be a good CVD prevention strategy, even if it raises total fat intake above 30% of daily calories. Omega-3 fatty acids from fish are also considered heart-healthy.

Most experts agree that reducing intake of saturated and trans fat is important for CVD prevention. There is less agreement, however, on whether it's best to replace saturated and trans fats with carbohydrates or with unsaturated fats. (For those trying to lose weight, the best strategy may be to simply cut back on saturated and trans fats without replacing them with anything else.) In some people, a diet high in carbohydrate and low in fat has a negative effect—lowering HDL levels and raising levels of triglycerides and glucose. These effects occur in part due to the high **glycemic index** of some carbohydrate-rich foods. Glycemic index refers to how quickly and how high a food causes blood glucose levels to rise. For example, white rice and potatoes have high glycemic indices and cause a dramatic rise in glucose and insulin levels a few hours after eating; legumes have a low index, and they break down more slowly and produce a more gradual rise in glucose and insulin levels. Eating lots of foods that rapidly raise glucose levels may con-

tribute to the development or worsening of diabetes and CVD in some people, including those with syndrome X. For this group, then, a diet relatively high in unsaturated and total fat might be a better choice than a diet high in carbohydrates.

It is important to note, however, that carbohydrate-rich foods typically have a lower calorie density than fat-rich foods, so substituting carbohydrates for fats can be helpful if it means consuming fewer total calories. If one chooses to substitute carbohydrates for fats, it's important to focus on healthy choices—fruits, vegetables, and whole grains—rather than low-fat or fat-free foods that are high in added sugars and calories and low in other nutrients. For people with insulin resistance or diabetes, choosing foods based on glycemic index may be a helpful strategy. Consuming high-fiber foods has also been shown to improve cholesterol and glucose levels.

The 2001 NCEP guidelines for people with elevated cholesterol allow total fat intake of up to 35% of total daily calories, with up to 10% of total calories from polyunsaturated fat, up to 20% from monounsaturated fat, and less than 7% as saturated fat. This slightly higher intake of total fat, primarily as unsaturated fat, can help raise HDL and lower triglycerides in people with syndrome X. However, simply adding unsaturated fats to the typical American diet is unlikely to yield all the benefits associated with the Mediterranean diet. In addition to being rich in olive oil, the Mediterranean diet is also low in saturated and trans fats, meats, and dairy products and rich in grains, fresh fruits and vegetables, and fish.

Ongoing research should help clarify the effects of different types and amounts of dietary fat. It may be that in the future, each of us will get individualized advice based on our particular risk profile—diets high in unsaturated fats for some people, diets high in healthy carbohydrates for others. Until that time, nearly all experts agree that eating fewer saturated and trans fats and more fruits, vegetables, and whole grains is a good idea.

Hypertension

Blood pressure, the force exerted by the blood on blood vessel walls, is created by the pumping action of the heart. When the heart contracts (systole), blood pressure increases; when the heart relaxes (diastole), pressure decreases. Many factors affect blood pressure; for example, excitement or exercise causes the heart to pump more blood into the arteries, resulting in a rise in blood pressure. Short periods of high blood pressure are normal, but blood pressure that is continually at an abnormally high level is known as hypertension.

Blood pressure is measured with a stethoscope and an instrument called a sphygmomanometer. It is expressed as two numbers—for example, 120 over 80—and measured in millimeters of mercury. The first and larger number is the systolic blood pressure; the second is the diastolic blood pressure. Average blood pressure readings for young adults in good physical condition are 110–120 systolic

over 70–80 diastolic. High blood pressure in adults is defined as equal to or greater than 140 over 90 (Table 15-2).

High blood pressure results from either an increased output of blood by the heart or, most often, increased resistance to blood flow in the arteries. The latter condition can be caused by atherosclerosis, discussed in the next section, or by constriction of smooth muscle surrounding the arteries. When a person has high blood pressure, the heart must work harder than normal to force blood through the narrowed arteries, thereby straining both the heart and arteries.

High blood pressure is often called a "silent killer," because it usually has no symptoms. A person may have high blood pressure for years without realizing it. But

glycemic index A measure of how the ingestion of a particular food affects blood glucose levels.

Terms

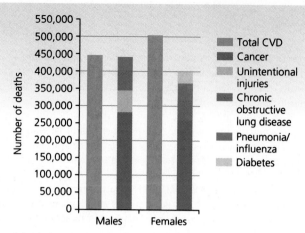

(a) Leading causes of death

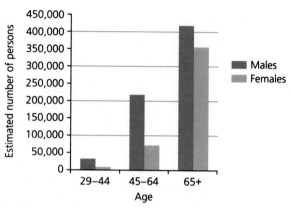

(b) Annual incidence of heart attack

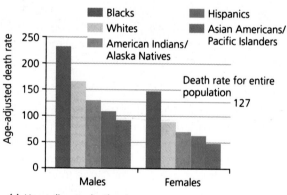

(c) Heart disease death rates

W. VITAL STATISTICS

Figure 15-5 A statistical look at cardiovascular disease in the United States. (a) The leading causes of death. CVD causes more deaths than the next four causes combined. (b) Estimated numbers of Americans who have a heart attack each year. Among heart attack victims under age 65, men significantly outnumber women; after age 65, women start to catch up. (c) Heart disease death rates by gender and ethnicity. SOURCES: American Heart Association. 2001. *2001 Heart and Stroke Facts Statistical Update.* Dallas, Tex.: American Heart Association. National Center for Health Statistics. 2000. *Health, United States, 2000.* Hyattsville, Md.: U.S. Public Health Service, DHHS Pub. No. (PHS) 00–1232.

Table 15-2	Blood Pressure Classification for Healthy Adults			
Category[a]	**Systolic (mm Hg)**		**Diastolic (mm Hg)**	
Optimal[b]	below 120	and	below 80	
Normal	below 130	and	below 85	
High-normal	130–139	or	85–89	
Hypertension[c]				
Stage 1	140–159	or	90–99	
Stage 2	160–179	or	100–109	
Stage 3	180 and above	or	110 and above	

[a]When systolic and diastolic pressure fall into different categories, the higher category should be used to classify blood pressure status.
[b]Optimal blood pressure with respect to cardiovascular risk is below 120/80 mm Hg; however, unusually low readings should be evaluated.
[c]Based on the average of two or more readings taken at different physician visits.

SOURCE: *The Sixth Report of the Joint National Committee on Prevention, Detection, Evaluation, and Treatment of High Blood Pressure.* 1997. Bethesda, Md.: National Heart, Lung, and Blood Institute. National Institutes of Health (NIH Publication No. 98-4080).

during that time, it damages vital organs and increases the risk of heart attack, congestive heart failure, stroke, kidney failure, and blindness. In about 90% of people with high blood pressure, the cause is unknown. So-called primary hypertension is probably due to a mixture of genetic and environmental factors, including obesity, stress, excessive alcohol intake, inactivity, and a high-fat, high-salt diet. In the remaining 10% of cases, the condition is caused by an underlying illness and is referred to as secondary hypertension.

Hypertension is common, occurring in about 1 in 4 adults. Its incidence rises dramatically with increasing age; however, it can occur among children and young adults, and women sometimes develop hypertension during pregnancy (blood pressure usually returns to normal after the baby is born).

Primary hypertension cannot be cured, but it can be controlled. The key to avoiding the complications of hypertension is to have your blood pressure checked regularly and to follow your physician's advice about lifestyle changes and medication. Unfortunately, of the estimated 50 million Americans with hypertension, only about 18% of them have it under control.

People with mild hypertension can frequently lower their blood pressure through lifestyle changes, including quitting smoking, exercising regularly, and improving diet. Controlling total calorie intake is important for achieving and maintaining a healthy body weight. Increasing intake of fruits, vegetables, and whole grains is

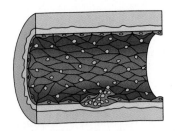

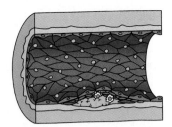

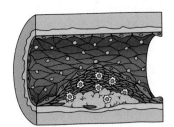

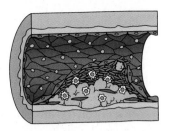

Plaque buildup begins when endothelial cells lining the arteries are damaged by smoking, high blood pressure, oxidized LDL, and other causes; excess cholesterol particles collect beneath these cells.

In response to the damage, platelets and other types of cells collect at the site; a fibrous cap forms, isolating the plaque within the artery wall. An early-stage plaque is called a fatty streak.

Chemicals released by cells in and around the plaque cause further inflammation and buildup; an advanced plaque contains LDL, white blood cells, connective tissue, smooth muscle cells, platelets, and other compounds.

The narrowed artery is vulnerable to blockage by clots. The risk of blockage and heart attack rises if the fibrous cap cracks (probably due to destructive enzymes released by white blood cells within the plaque).

Figure 15-6 Stages of plaque development.

recommended because these foods are rich in potassium and fiber, both of which may reduce blood pressure. Moderate sodium restriction can also be helpful. About half of all people with hypertension are "salt-sensitive," meaning that their blood pressure will decrease significantly when salt intake is restricted. Salt restriction has less impact on those who are not salt-sensitive, but it may still be beneficial. Most experts feel that restricting sodium intake to about 2400 mg per day is a good strategy for all people—whether they have hypertension or not. For people whose blood pressure isn't adequately controlled with lifestyle changes, medication is prescribed. There are many different types of antihypertensive drugs available, and it is usually possible to lower blood pressure effectively with a minimum of side effects.

Recent research has shed new light on the importance of lowering blood pressure to improving cardiovascular health. According to a recent large-scale study, death rates from coronary heart disease rise with increasing blood pressure even at pressures well below the traditional 140 over 90 cutoff for hypertension. According to this study, for example, if your blood pressure is 120 over 70, your risk for CVD would drop by about 25% if you lowered your blood pressure to 110 over 65. The bottom line is that lowering your blood pressure through healthy lifestyle changes is beneficial, even if your current blood pressure is already below 140 over 90.

Atherosclerosis

Atherosclerosis is a slow, progressive hardening and narrowing of the arteries that can begin in childhood. Arteries become narrowed by deposits of fat, cholesterol, and other substances. The process begins when the cells that line the arteries (endothelial cells) become damaged, most likely through a combination of factors such as smoking, high blood pressure, deposits of oxidized LDL particles, infection, and high homocysteine levels. The body's response to this damage results in inflammation and changes in the ar-

tery lining that create a sort of magnet for LDL, platelets, and other cells; these cells build up and cause a bulge in the wall of the artery. As these deposits, called **plaques,** accumulate on artery walls, the arteries lose their elasticity and their ability to expand and contract, restricting blood flow. Once narrowed by a plaque, an artery is vulnerable to blockage by blood clots (Figure 15-6). The risk of life-threatening clots and heart attacks increases if the fibrous cap covering a plaque ruptures.

If the heart, brain, and/or other organs are deprived of blood, and thus the vital oxygen it carries, the effects of atherosclerosis can be deadly. Coronary arteries, which supply the heart with blood, are particularly susceptible to plaque buildup, a condition called **coronary heart disease (CHD),** or *coronary artery disease.* The blockage of a coronary artery causes a heart attack. If a cerebral artery (leading to the brain) is blocked, the result is a stroke. If an artery in a limb becomes narrowed or blocked, it causes *peripheral vascular disease,* a condition that causes pain and sometimes loss of the affected limb.

The main risk factors for atherosclerosis are cigarette smoking, physical inactivity, high levels of blood cholesterol, high blood pressure, and diabetes.

Heart Disease and Heart Attacks

Every year, about 1.1 million Americans have a heart attack (see Figure 15-5). Although a **heart attack,** or myocardial infarction (MI), may come without warning, it is

Terms

plaque A deposit of fatty (and other) substances on the inner wall of the arteries.

coronary heart disease (CHD) Heart disease caused by atherosclerosis in the arteries that supply oxygen to the heart muscle; also called *coronary artery disease.*

heart attack Damage to, or death of, heart muscle, sometimes resulting in a failure of the heart to deliver enough blood to the body; also known as myocardial infarction (MI).

usually the end result of a long-term disease process. The most common form of heart disease is coronary artery disease caused by atherosclerosis. When one of the coronary arteries, the arteries that branch off the aorta and supply blood directly to the heart muscle, becomes blocked, a heart attack results. A heart attack caused by a clot is called a **coronary thrombosis.** During a heart attack, part of the heart muscle (myocardium) may die from lack of oxygen. If an MI is not fatal, the heart muscle may sometimes partially repair itself.

Symptoms of MI may include chest pain or pressure; arm, neck, or jaw pain; difficulty breathing; excessive sweating; nausea and vomiting; and loss of consciousness. Although chest pain occurs in the majority of MI victims, a recent study of over 750,000 MI patients revealed that about one-third of people having a heart attack do not experience chest pain. Women, ethnic minorities, older adults, and people with diabetes were the most likely groups to experience heart attack without chest pain.

Angina   Arteries narrowed by disease may still be open enough to deliver blood to the heart. At times, however—primarily during emotional excitement, stress, or physical exertion—the heart requires more oxygen than narrowed arteries can accommodate. When the need for oxygen exceeds the supply, chest pain, called **angina pectoris,** may occur. Angina pain is felt as an extreme tightness in the chest and heavy pressure behind the breastbone or in the shoulder, neck, arm, hand, or back. This pain, although not actually a heart attack, is a warning that the load on the heart must be reduced. Angina may be controlled in a number of ways (with drugs or surgical procedures), but its course is unpredictable. Over a period ranging from hours to years, the narrowing may go on to full blockage and a heart attack.

Arrhythmias and Sudden Cardiac Death   The pumping of the heart is controlled by electrical impulses that maintain a regular heartbeat of 60–100 beats per minute. If this electrical conduction system is disrupted, the heart may beat too quickly, too slowly, or in an irregular fashion, a condition known as **arrhythmia.** Arrhythmia can cause symptoms ranging from imperceptible to severe and even fatal.

Sudden cardiac death is most often caused by an arrhythmia called ventricular fibrillation, a kind of "quivering" of the ventricle that makes it ineffective in pumping blood. If ventricular fibrillation continues for more than a few minutes, it is fatal. Cardiac defibrillation, in which an electrical shock is delivered to the heart, can be effective in jolting the heart into a more efficient rhythm. Sudden cardiac death most often occurs in people with coronary heart disease, and serious arrhythmias frequently develop during or after a heart attack and are often the actual cause of death in cases of fatal MI.

Other potential causes of arrhythmia include congenital heart abnormalities, infections, drug use, chest trauma, and congestive heart failure. Some arrhythmias cause no problems and resolve without treatment; more serious arrhythmias are usually treated with medication or a surgically implanted pacemaker that delivers appropriate electrical stimulation to the heart to create a more normal rhythm.

Helping a Heart Attack Victim   Most people who die from a heart attack do so within 2 hours from the time they experience the first symptoms. Unfortunately, half of all heart attack victims wait more than 2 hours before getting help. If you or someone you are with has any of the warning signs of heart attack listed in the box "What to Do in Case of a Heart Attack or Stroke," take immediate action. Call your emergency medical service immediately or get to the nearest hospital emergency room or clinic that offers 24-hour emergency cardiac care. Get help even if the person denies there is something wrong. One additional step recommended by many experts is for the affected individual to chew and swallow one adult aspirin tablet (325 mg); aspirin has an immediate anticlotting effect.

If the person loses consciousness, emergency **cardiopulmonary resuscitation (CPR)** should be initiated by a qualified person. Damage to the heart muscle increases with time. If the victim receives emergency care quickly enough, a clot-dissolving agent can be injected to break up a clot in the coronary artery. These "clot-busting" drugs, such as streptokinase, urokinase, and tissue plasminogen activator (TPA), are being used successfully to treat not only heart attacks but

Terms

coronary thrombosis A clot in a coronary artery, often causing sudden death.

angina pectoris A condition in which the heart muscle does not receive enough blood, causing severe pain in the chest and often in the left arm and shoulder.

arrhythmia A change in the normal pattern of the heartbeat.

sudden cardiac death A nontraumatic, unexpected death from sudden cardiac arrest, most often due to arrhythmia; in most instances, victims have underlying heart disease.

cardiopulmonary resuscitation (CPR) A technique involving mouth-to-mouth breathing and chest compression to keep oxygen flowing to the brain.

electrocardiogram (ECG or EKG) A test to detect abnormalities by measuring the electrical activity in the heart.

magnetic resonance imaging (MRI) A computerized imaging technique that uses a strong magnetic field and radio frequency signals to examine a thin cross section of the body; also known as *nuclear magnetic resonance imaging* (NMR).

angiogram A picture of the arterial system taken after injecting a dye that is opaque to X rays; also called *arteriogram.*

balloon angioplasty A technique in which a catheter with a balloon on the tip is inserted into an artery; the balloon is then inflated at the point of obstruction in the artery, pressing the plaque against the artery wall to improve blood supply; also known as *percutaneous transluminal coronary angioplasty* (PTCA).

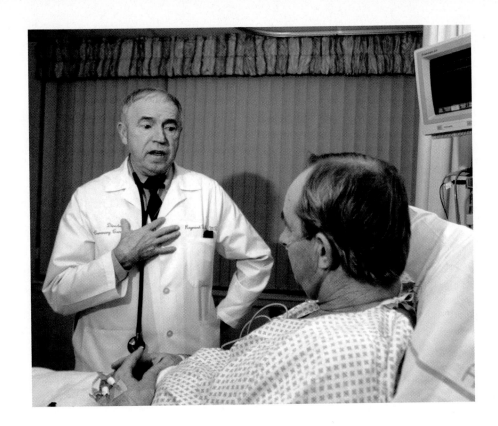

Many heart attack victims aren't sure they've had an attack and wait too long—2 hours or more—before getting help. Prompt medical attention greatly improves this man's chance of survival.

also some types of stroke. The sooner these drugs are used, the more effective they are.

Detecting and Treating Heart Disease Physicians have an expanding array of tools to evaluate the condition of the heart and arteries. Currently, the most common initial screening tool is the stress, or exercise, test, in which a patient runs or walks on a treadmill or pedals a stationary cycle while being monitored for abnormalities with an **electrocardiogram (ECG or EKG).** Certain characteristic changes in the heart's electrical activity while under stress can reveal particular heart problems, such as restricted blood flow. Exercise testing can also be performed in conjunction with techniques such as ultrasonography and X ray that provide further information about the heart and arteries.

Recently, several non-invasive tests for evaluating CVD have become available:

- Electron-beam computed tomography (EBCT) uses a sweeping electron beam to produce computerized cross-sectional images; it can detect calcium in the arteries, a marker for atherosclerosis.

- Echocardiographic equipment utilizes sound waves to examine the heart.

- **Magnetic resonance imaging** uses powerful magnets to look inside the body.

If symptoms of non-invasive tests suggest coronary artery disease, the next step is usually a coronary **an-giogram.** In this test, a catheter (small plastic tube) is threaded into an artery, usually in the groin, and a special dye is injected into the bloodstream. X rays are then used to trace the flow of blood through the coronary arteries and heart.

Various treatments, ranging from changes in diet to major surgery, are available if a problem is detected. Along with a low-fat diet, regular exercise, and smoking cessation, one frequent nonsurgical recommendation for people at high risk for CVD is to take half an aspirin tablet a day. Aspirin has an anticlotting effect, discouraging platelets in the blood from sticking to arterial plaques and forming clots; it also reduces inflammation. Prescription drugs can help control heart rate, dilate arteries, lower blood pressure, and reduce the strain on the heart—raising both quality and quantity of life in heart patients. In patients with coronary artery disease, a class of cholesterol-lowering drugs called statins has been effective in preventing heart attacks. Because statins are helpful even in people with normal cholesterol levels, experts suspect that they may also have beneficial anti-inflammatory effects.

A common surgical procedure for treating heart disease is **balloon angioplasty.** This technique involves threading a catheter with an inflatable balloon tip through the artery until it reaches the area of blockage. The balloon is then inflated, flattening the fatty plaque and widening the arterial opening. However, repeat clogging of the artery, known as *restenosis,* is common. To keep arteries open following angioplasty, many surgeons also

Heart Attack Warning Signs

The American Heart Association says these are the most common warning signs of a heart attack:

- Uncomfortable pressure, fullness, squeezing, or pain in the center of the chest lasting more than a few minutes
- Pain spreading to the shoulders, neck, or arms
- Chest discomfort with light-headedness, fainting, sweating, nausea, or shortness of breath

Less-common warning signs of a heart attack are . . .

- Atypical chest pain or stomach or abdominal pain
- Nausea or dizziness
- Shortness of breath and difficulty breathing
- Unexplained anxiety, weakness, or fatigue
- Palpitations, cold sweat, or paleness

Stroke Warning Signs

The American Stroke Association says these are the warning signs of a stroke:

- Sudden weakness or numbness of the face, arm, or leg, especially on one side of the body
- Sudden confusion or trouble speaking or understanding
- Sudden trouble seeing in one or both eyes
- Sudden trouble walking, dizziness, or loss of balance or coordination
- Sudden, severe headache with no known cause

Dial 9-1-1 Fast

Heart attack and stroke are life-and-death emergencies—every second counts. If you see or have any of these symptoms, immediately call 9-1-1. Not all these signs occur in every attack. Sometimes they go away and return. If some occur, get help fast! Treatment is more effective when given quickly.

---

permanently implant coronary stents—flexible, stainless steel mesh tubes that remain in place as a framework to prop the artery open and prevent restenosis.

Every year, **coronary bypass surgery** is performed on well over 300,000 men and women, about half of whom are under age 65. Surgeons remove a healthy blood vessel, usually a vein from one of the patient's legs, and graft it to one or more coronary arteries to bypass a blockage. A heart-lung machine maintains circulation during the surgery.

Terms

coronary bypass surgery Surgery in which a vein is grafted from a point above to a point below an obstruction in a coronary artery, improving the blood supply to the heart.

stroke An impeded blood supply to some part of the brain resulting in the destruction of brain cells; also called *cerebrovascular accident*.

ischemic stroke Impeded blood supply to the brain caused by the obstruction of a blood vessel by a clot.

hemorrhagic stroke Impeded blood supply to the brain caused by the rupture of a blood vessel.

thrombus A blood clot in a blood vessel that usually occurs at the point of its formation.

embolus A blood clot that breaks off from its place of origin in a blood vessel and travels through the bloodstream.

aneurysm A sac formed by a distention or dilation of the artery wall.

Whatever treatment is used, the person with heart disease is also advised to make behavior and lifestyle changes, such as changing the diet to improve blood cholesterol levels and quitting smoking. Otherwise, the arteries simply become clogged again, and the same problems recur a few years later.

> **COMMUNICATE!** An angry, hostile approach to life can increase your exposure to the stress response and can put you at risk for heart disease. Do your verbal and nonverbal communication patterns indicate underlying anger? For example, are you easily irritated by others? Do you fidget or tap your fingers while others are talking? Do you jump to conclusions or finish their sentences for them? Do you often interrupt? If you think you might have a problem with anger and hostility, look for solutions now, for your heart's sake. Try practicing relaxation techniques, investigating a spiritual path, reasoning with yourself as suggested in the box on anger in this chapter, or looking into some of the other approaches to stress and anger management described in Chapters 2 and 3.

Stroke

For brain cells to function as they should, they must have a continuous and ample supply of oxygen-rich blood. If brain cells are deprived of blood for more than a few min-

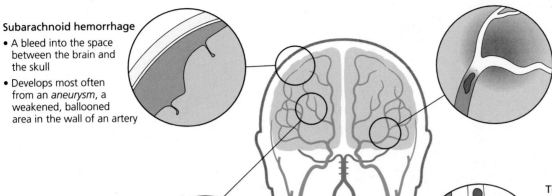

HEMORRHAGIC STROKE

- 20% of strokes
- Caused by ruptured blood vessels followed by blood leaking into tissue
- Usually more serious than ischemic stroke

Subarachnoid hemorrhage

- A bleed into the space between the brain and the skull
- Develops most often from an *aneurysm*, a weakened, ballooned area in the wall of an artery

Intracerebral hemorrhage

- A bleed from a blood vessel inside the brain
- Often caused by high blood pressure and the damage it does to arteries

ISCHEMIC STROKE

- 80% of strokes
- Caused by blockages in brain blood vessels; potentially treatable with clot-busting drugs
- Brain tissue dies when blood flow is blocked

Embolic stroke

- Caused by *emboli*, blood clots that travel from elsewhere in the body to the brain blood vessels
- 25% of embolic strokes are related to atrial fibrillation

Thrombotic stroke

- Caused by *thrombi*, blood clots that form where an artery has been narrowed by atherosclerosis
- Most often develops when part of a thrombus breaks away and causes a block-age in a "downstream" artery

 Figure 15-7 Types of stroke. SOURCE: Types of stroke. 2000. *Harvard Health Letter,* April. Copyright © 2000 by Harriet R. Greenfield. Used by permission.

utes, they die. A **stroke,** also called a *cerebrovascular accident (CVA),* occurs when the blood supply to the brain is cut off. Many experts now refer to strokes as "brain attacks" to emphasize their similarity to heart attacks and the importance of early treatment. In the past, not much could be done for stroke victims; today, however, prompt treatment of stroke can greatly decrease the risk of permanent disability. Everyone should know the warning signs for a stroke and seek immediate medical help, just as they would at the first sign of a heart attack.

Types of Strokes   There are two major types of strokes: **ischemic strokes,** which are caused by blockages in blood vessels, and **hemorrhagic strokes,** which are caused by rupture of blood vessels, leading to bleeding into the brain (Figure 15-7). One type of ischemic stroke, the *thrombotic stroke,* is caused by a **thrombus,** a blood clot that forms in a cerebral artery that has been narrowed or damaged by atherosclerosis. The second type of ischemic stroke, called an *embolic stroke,* is caused by an **embolus,** a wandering blood clot that is carried in the bloodstream and may become wedged in one of the cerebral arteries. Many embolic strokes are linked to a type of abnormal heart rhythm called atrial fibrillation; when this arrhythmia occurs, blood may pool in the atria and form clots. Ischemic strokes, which account for 80% of all strokes, are potentially treatable with clot-busting drugs,

so obtaining immediate medical help is critical to improve chances for recovery.

The other, less common but more severe, type of stroke is the hemorrhagic stroke. It occurs when a blood vessel in the brain bursts, spilling blood into the surrounding tissue. Cells normally nourished by the artery are deprived of blood and cannot function. In addition, accumulated blood from the burst vessel may put pressure on surrounding brain tissue, causing damage and even death. In a *subarachnoid hemorrhage,* a blood vessel on the brain's surface ruptures and bleeds into the space between the brain and the skull; a ruptured vessel within the brain causes an *intercerebral hemorrhage.* Hemorrhages can be caused by head injuries or the bursting of a malformed blood vessel or an **aneurysm,** a blood-filled pocket that bulges out from a weak spot in an artery wall. Aneurysms in the brain may remain stable and never break. But when they do, the result is a stroke. Aneurysms may be caused or worsened by high blood pressure.

The Effects of a Stroke   The interruption of the blood supply to any area of the brain prevents the nerve cells there from functioning—in some cases, causing death. Of the 600,000 Americans who have strokes each year, nearly one-third die within a year. Those who survive usually have some lasting disability. Which parts of the body are affected depends on the area of the brain that

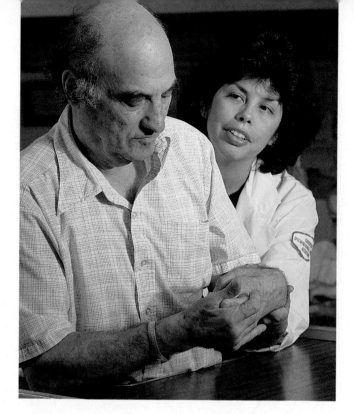

Rehabilitation after a stroke can be a long and arduous process. Complete recovery eludes many stroke victims.

has been damaged. Nerve cells control sensation and most of our body movements, and a stroke may cause paralysis, walking disability, speech impairment, memory loss, and changes in behavior. The severity of the stroke and its long-term effects depend on which brain cells have been injured, how widespread the damage is, how effectively the body can restore the blood supply, and how rapidly other areas of the brain can take over. Early treatment can significantly reduce the severity of disability resulting from a stroke.

Detecting and Treating Stroke Death rates from stroke have declined significantly over the past decades. In 1950, nearly 90% of victims died; today, about two-third of stroke victims survive. Effective treatment requires the prompt recognition of symptoms and correct diagnosis of the type of stroke that has occurred. Signals of a stroke are listed in the box "What to Do in Case of a Heart Attack or Stroke," on p. 442. Anyone who experiences one or more of these signs should obtain emergency medical help immediately.

Some stroke victims have a **transient ischemic attack (TIA),** or ministroke, days, weeks, or months before they have a full-blown stroke. A TIA produces temporary strokelike symptoms, such as weakness or numbness in an arm or a leg, speech difficulty, or dizziness, but these symptoms are brief, often lasting just a few minutes, and

do not cause permanent damage. However, TIAs should be taken as warning signs of a stroke, and anyone with a suspected TIA should get immediate medical help.

Strokes should be treated with the same urgency as heart attacks. A person with stroke symptoms should be rushed to the hospital. A **computed tomography (CT)** scan, which uses a computer to construct an image of the brain from X rays, can assess brain damage and determine the type of stroke. Newer diagnostic techniques using MRI and ultrasound are becoming increasingly available and should improve the speed and accuracy of stroke diagnosis.

If tests reveal that a stroke is caused by a blood clot— and if help is sought within a few hours of the onset of symptoms—the person can be treated with the same kind of clot-dissolving drugs that are used to treat coronary artery blockages. If the clot is dissolved quickly enough, brain damage is minimized and symptoms may disappear. (The longer the brain goes without oxygen, the greater the risk of permanent damage.) Drugs that help protect healthy brain cells from the effects of stroke are currently being tested. People who have had TIAs or who are at high risk for stroke due to narrowing of the carotid arteries may undergo a procedure called *carotid endarterectomy,* in which plaque is surgically removed.

If tests reveal that a stroke was caused by a cerebral hemorrhage, drugs may be prescribed to lower the blood pressure, which will usually be high. Careful diagnosis is crucial, because administering clot-dissolving drugs to a person suffering a hemorrhagic stroke would cause more bleeding and potentially more brain damage.

If detection and treatment of stroke come too late, rehabilitation is the only treatment. Although damaged or destroyed brain tissue does not normally regenerate, nerve cells in the brain can make new pathways, and some functions can be taken over by other parts of the brain. Some spontaneous recovery starts immediately after a stroke and continues for a few months.

Rehabilitation consists of various types of therapy: physical therapy, which helps strengthen muscles and improve balance and coordination; speech and language therapy, which helps those whose speech has been damaged; and occupational therapy, which helps improve hand-eye coordination and everyday living skills. Progress varies from person to person and can be unpredictable. Some people recover completely in a matter of days or weeks, but most stroke victims who survive must adapt to a lifelong disability.

Congestive Heart Failure

A number of conditions—high blood pressure, heart attack, atherosclerosis, rheumatic fever, birth defects—can damage the heart's pumping mechanism. When the heart cannot maintain its regular pumping rate and force, fluids begin to back up. When extra fluid seeps through capillary walls, edema (swelling) results, usually in the legs and ankles, but sometimes in other parts of the body as well. Fluid can collect in the lungs and interfere with breathing, particularly when a person is lying down. This condition is called **pulmonary edema,** and the entire process is known as **congestive heart failure.**

Congestive heart failure can be controlled. Treatment includes reducing the workload on the heart, modifying salt intake, and using drugs that help the body eliminate excess fluid. Drugs used to treat congestive heart failure include digitalis, which increases the pumping action of the heart, and diuretics, which help the body eliminate excess salt and water. Several other drugs have recently been shown to help prolong survival and improve the quality of life for people with congestive heart failure. This is an important area of research because the incidence of this disease is rising as our population ages.

Other Forms of Heart Disease

Other, less common, forms of heart disease include congenital heart disease, rheumatic heart disease, and heart valve disorders.

Congenital Heart Disease   About 40,000 children born each year in the United States have a defect or malformation of the heart or major blood vessels. These conditions are collectively referred to as **congenital heart disease,** and they cause about 5000 deaths a year. The most common congenital defects are holes in the wall that divides the chambers of the heart. With these defects the heart produces a distinctive sound, making diagnosis relatively simple. Another defect is *coarctation of the aorta,* a narrrowing, or constriction, of the aorta. Heart failure may result unless the constricted area is repaired by surgery.

Most of the common congenital defects can now be accurately diagnosed and treated with medication or surgery. Important in saving lives is early recognition that the newborn who has a bluish appearance or respiratory difficulty or who fails to thrive may be suffering from congenital heart disease.

Hypertrophic cardiomyopathy is the most common cause of sudden death among athletes younger than 35 years of age. It is an inherited condition that causes the heart muscle to become enlarged, primarily in the area between the two ventricles. Young children with this disorder usually have no obvious symptoms; the hypertrophy generally develops gradually between the ages of 5 and 15. People with hypertrophic cardiomyopathy are at high risk for sudden death, mainly due to serious arrhythmias. Possible treatments include medication and surgery to implant a pacemaker or internal defibrillator. Unfortunately, there is no cure for this disease, and the mortality rate is 2–4% per year. Individuals with hypertrophic cardiomyopathy should usually not participate in competitive sports because of the high risk of sudden death.

Rheumatic Heart Disease   Worldwide, a leading cause of heart trouble is **rheumatic fever,** a consequence of certain types of untreated streptococcal throat infections (group A beta-hemolytic). Rheumatic fever can permanently damage the heart muscle and heart valves, a condition called rheumatic heart disease (RHD). Many of the approximately 78,000 operations on heart valves performed annually are related to RHD, and about 5000 Americans die each year from RHD.

Symptoms of strep throat are the sudden onset of a sore throat, painful swallowing, fever, swollen glands, headache, nausea, and vomiting. Careful laboratory diagnosis is important because strep throat is treated with antibiotics, which are not useful in the treatment of far more common viral sore throats. Symptoms of rheumatic fever are generally vague, but in children they include weight loss or a failure to gain weight, fever, poor appetite, repeated nosebleeds, jerky body movements, fatigue, weakness, and pain in the arms, legs, or abdomen. Rheumatic fever can be prevented by treating strep throat, when it occurs, with antibiotics.

Heart Valve Disorders   Congenital defects and certain types of infections can cause abnormalities in the valves between the chambers of the heart. Heart valve problems generally fall into two categories—the valve fails to open fully or it fails to close completely. In either case, blood flow through the heart is impaired. Treatment for heart valve disorders depends on their location and severity; serious problems may be treated with surgery to repair or replace a valve. People with certain types of heart valve defects are advised to take antibiotics prior to some types of dental and surgical procedures in order to prevent bacteria, which may be dislodged into the bloodstream during the procedure, from infecting the defective valve.

transient ischemic attack (TIA) A small stroke; usually a temporary interruption of blood supply to the brain, causing numbness or difficulty with speech.

computed tomography (CT) The use of computerized X ray images to create a cross-sectional depiction (scan) of tissue density.

pulmonary edema The accumulation of fluid in the lungs.

congestive heart failure A condition resulting from the heart's inability to pump out all the blood that returns to it; blood backs up in the veins leading to the heart, causing an accumulation of fluid in various parts of the body.

congenital heart disease A defect or malformation of the heart or its major blood vessels, present at birth.

hypertrophic cardiomyopathy An inherited condition in which there is an enlargement of the heart muscle, especially between the two ventricles.

rheumatic fever A disease, mainly of children, characterized by fever, inflammation, and pain in the joints; often damages the heart muscle, a condition called rheumatic heart disease.

Terms

Do More

- Eat a diet rich in fruits, vegetables, whole grains, and low-fat or fat-free dairy products. Eat 5–9 servings of fruits and vegetables each day.
- Eat several servings of high-fiber foods each day.
- Eat 2 or more servings of fish per week; try a few servings of nuts and soy foods each week.
- Choose unsaturated fats rather than saturated and trans fats.
- Be physically active; do both aerobic exercise and strength training on a regular basis.
- Achieve and maintain a healthy weight.
- Develop effective strategies for handling stress and anger. Nurture old friendships and family ties, and make new friends; pay attention to your spiritual side.
- Obtain recommended screening tests and follow your physician's recommendations.

Do Less

- Don't use tobacco in any form: cigarettes, spit tobacco, cigars, pipes, bidis, or clove cigarettes.
- Avoid exposure to environmental tobacco smoke.
- Limit consumption of fats, especially trans fats and saturated fats.
- Limit consumption of cholesterol, added sugars, and refined carbohydrates.
- Avoid excessive alcohol consumption—no more than one drink per day for women and two drinks per day for men.
- Limit consumption of salt to no more than 2400 mg of sodium per day.
- Avoid excess stress, anger, and hostility.

Figure 15-8 Strategies for reducing your risk of cardiovascular disease.

The most common heart valve disorder is **mitral valve prolapse (MVP)**, which occurs in about 4% of the population. MVP is characterized by a "billowing" of the mitral valve, which separates the left ventricle and left atrium, during ventricular contraction; in some cases, blood leaks from the ventricle into the atrium. Most people with MVP have no symptoms; they have the same ability to exercise and live as long as people without MVP. The condition is often diagnosed during a routine medical exam when an extra heart sound (a click) or murmur is heard; the diagnosis can be confirmed with echocardiography. Treatment is usually unnecessary, although surgery may be needed in the rare cases where leakage through the faulty valve is severe. Experts disagree over whether patients with MVP should take antibiotics prior to dental procedures; most often, only those patients with significant blood leakage are advised to take antibiotics.

PROTECTING YOURSELF AGAINST CARDIOVASCULAR DISEASE

There are several important steps you can take now to lower your risk of developing CVD in the future (Figure 15-8). If you are a young adult, you may be wondering how CVD prevention advice applies to you, since most cases of CVD show up in people who are decades older. Evidence is mounting that the development of CVD begins very early in life. For example, young adults with relatively low cholesterol levels go on to live substantially longer than those with higher levels. Reducing CVD risk factors when you are young can pay off with many extra years of life and health (see the box "Are You at Risk for CVD?").

Eat Heart-Healthy

For most Americans, changing to a heart-healthy diet involves cutting total fat intake, substituting unsaturated fats for saturated and trans fats, and increasing fiber. Such changes can lower a person's blood levels of total cholesterol, LDL cholesterol, and triglycerides. A moderate amount of alcohol may also be beneficial for some people.

Decreased Fat and Cholesterol Intake The National Cholesterol Education Program (NCEP) recommends that all Americans over the age of 2 adopt a diet in which total fat consumption is no more than 30% of total daily calories, with no more than one-third of those fat calories (10% of total daily calories) coming from saturated fat. For people with heart disease or high LDL levels, the NCEP recommends a total fat intake of 25–35% of total daily calories and a saturated fat intake of less than 7% of total calories. (As described earlier, the higher total fat allowance is for people with syndrome X for whom high triglyceride and low HDL levels may also be a problem.)

Saturated fats are found in animal products; palm and coconut oil; and hydrogenated vegetables oils, which are also high in trans fats. Saturated and trans fats influence the

Terms

mitral valve prolapse (MVP) A condition in which the mitral valve "billows" out during ventricular contraction, possibly allowing leakage of blood from the left ventricle into the left atrium; often asymptomatic and usually only requiring treatment in cases of significant leakage.

Your chances of suffering an early heart attack or stroke depend on a variety of factors, many of which are under your control. The best time to identify your risk factors and change your behavior to lower your risk is when you are young. You can significantly affect your future health and quality of life if you adopt healthy behaviors. To help identify your risk factors, circle the response for each risk category that best describes you:

1. Gender and Age

- 0   Female age 55 or younger; male age 45 or younger
- 2   Female over age 55 or male over age 45

2. Heredity

- 0   Neither parent suffered a heart attack or stroke before age 60.
- 3   One parent suffered a heart attack or stroke before age 60.
- 7   Both parents suffered a heart attack or stroke before age 60.

3. Smoking

- 0   Never smoked
- 3   Quit more than 2 years ago and lifetime smoking is less than 5 pack-years*
- 6   Quit less than 2 years ago and/or lifetime smoking is greater than 5 pack-years*
- 8   Smoke less than ½ pack per day
- 13 Smoke more than ½ pack per day
- 15 Smoke more than 1 pack per day

4. Environmental Tobacco Smoke

- 0   Do not live or work with smokers
- 2   Exposed to ETS at work
- 3   Live with a smoker
- 4   Both live and work with smokers

5. Blood Pressure

The average of the last three readings:

- 0   130/80 or below
- 1   131/81–140/85
- 5   141/86–150/90
- 9   151/91–170/100
- 13 Above 170/100

6. Total Cholesterol

The average of the last three readings:

- 0   Lower than 190
- 1   190–210
- 2   Don't know
- 3   211–240
- 4   241–270
- 5   271–300
- 6   Over 300

7. HDL Cholesterol

The average of the last three readings:

- 0   Over 65 mg/dl
- 1   55–65
- 2   Don't know HDL
- 3   45–54
- 5   35–44
- 7   25–34
- 12 Lower than 25

8. Exercise

- 0   Exercise three times a week
- 1   Exercise once or twice a week
- 2   Occasional exercise less than once a week
- 7   Rarely exercise

9. Diabetes

- 0   No personal or family history
- 2   One parent with diabetes
- 6   Two parents with diabetes
- 9   Non–insulin-dependent diabetes
- 13 Insulin-dependent diabetes

10. Weight

- 0   Near ideal weight
- 1   6 pounds or less above ideal weight
- 3   7–19 pounds above ideal weight
- 5   20–40 pounds above ideal weight
- 7   More than 40 pounds above ideal weight

11. Stress

- 0   Relaxed most of the time
- 1   Occasional stress and anger
- 2   Frequently stressed and angry
- 3   Usually stressed and angry

Scoring

Total your risk factor points. Refer to the list below to get an approximate rating of your risk of suffering an early heart attack or stroke.

Score	Estimated Risk
Less than 20	Low risk
20–29	Moderate risk
30–45	High risk
Over 45	Extremely high risk

*Pack-years can be calculated by multiplying the number of packs you smoked per day by the number of years you smoked. For example, if you smoked a pack and a half a day for 5 years, you would have smoked the equivalent of $1.5 \times 5 = 7.5$ pack-years.

production and excretion of cholesterol by the liver, so decreasing saturated and trans fat intake is the most important dietary change you can make to achieve and maintain healthy cholesterol levels (see the Behavior Change Strategy at the end of the chapter). Choose unsaturated fats, especially monounsaturated fats, over saturated and trans fats.

Animal products contain cholesterol as well as saturated fat; vegetable products do not contain cholesterol. The NCEP recommends that most Americans limit dietary cholesterol intake to no more than 300 mg per day; for people with heart disease or high LDL levels, the suggested daily limit is 200 mg. The cholesterol content of packaged foods is provided on food labels, along with their total and saturated fat content. As described in Chapter 12, you can check for the presence of trans fats in a food by checking the list of ingredients for hydrogenated or partially hydrogenated vegetable oils.

Increased Fiber Intake Soluble fiber traps the bile acids the liver needs to manufacture cholesterol and carries them to the large intestine, where they are excreted. It also slows the production of proteins that promote blood clotting. Insoluble fiber may interfere with the absorption of dietary fat and may also help you cut total food intake because foods rich in insoluble fiber tend to be filling. Studies have shown that a high-fiber diet is associated with a 40–50% reduction in the risk of heart attack and stroke. To obtain the recommended 20–35 grams of dietary fiber per day, choose a diet rich in whole grains, fruits, and vegetables. Good sources of fiber include oatmeal, some breakfast cereals, barley, legumes, and most fruits and vegetables.

Alcohol The *Dietary Guidelines for Americans* state that moderate alcohol consumption may lower the risk of CHD among men over 45 and women over 55. (Moderate means no more than one drink per day for women and two drinks per day for men.) Moderate alcohol use may increase HDL cholesterol; it may also reduce stroke risk, possibly by dampening the inflammatory response or by affecting blood clotting. For most people under age 45, however, the risks of alcohol use probably outweigh any health benefit. Excessive alcohol consumption increases the risk of a variety of serious health problems, including hypertension, stroke, some cancers, liver disease, alcohol dependence, and injuries (see Chapter 10). If you do drink, do so moderately, with food, and at times when drinking will not put you or others at risk.

Other Dietary Factors Researchers have identified other dietary factors that may affect CVD risk:

- *Omega-3 fatty acids.* Found in fish, shellfish, and some plant foods (nuts and canola, soybean, and flaxseed oils), omega-3 fatty acids may reduce clotting and inflammation and have other heart-healthy effects. The American Heart Association recommends eating fish two or

more times a week; fish oil capsules may be appropriate for some people who won't eat fish, but they add fat and calories to the diet and may raise LDL levels.

- *Vitamin E.* The antioxidant vitamin E—found in nuts, vegetable oils, wheat germ, margarine, avocados, and leafy green vegetables—may help prevent CVD by inhibiting the buildup of fatty plaques on artery walls. Many experts now recommend that people increase their intake of foods high in vitamin E. Clinical trials have so far shown no consistent benefit to taking supplements.

- *Plant stanols and sterols.* Plant stanols and sterols, found in some new types of trans-free margarines and other products, reduce the absorption of cholesterol in the body and help lower LDL levels (see the box "Functional Foods and Dietary Supplements for Improving Cholesterol Levels"). For people with high LDL levels that do not respond to changes in fat intake, the NCEP suggests an intake of 2 grams per day of plant stanols or sterols.

- *Folic acid, vitamin B-6, and vitamin B-12.* These vitamins affect CVD risk by lowering homocysteine levels. See Chapter 12 for a list of foods rich in these vitamins and information on supplements.

- *Salt.* As described earlier, excessive salt consumption raises blood pressure in salt-sensitive people and is not recommended for anyone. Follow the *Dietary Guidelines'* recommendation of consuming no more than 2400 mg of sodium per day: limit your intake of processed and fast foods, choose low-sodium products, and eat plenty of naturally low-sodium foods such as fruits and vegetables.

- *Potassium and calcium.* Diets rich in potassium and calcium may help prevent and treat hypertension; they may also decrease the risk of stroke. The best way to ensure adequate intake of these minerals is to consume the recommended number of servings of fruits, vegetables, and low-fat or nonfat dairy products.

- *Soy protein.* Replacing some animal proteins with soy protein may lower LDL cholesterol. Soy-based foods include tofu and tempeh.

- *Total calories.* Some studies have found that reducing energy intake can improve cholesterol and triglyceride levels as much as reducing fat intake.

DASH A dietary plan that reflects many of the suggestions described here was released as part of a study called Dietary Approaches to Stop Hypertension, or DASH. The DASH study found that a diet low in fat and high in fruits, vegetables, and low-fat dairy products reduces blood pressure. (It also follows the recommendations for lowering one's risk of heart disease, cancer, and osteoporosis.) The DASH diet plan is as follows:

- 7–8 servings per day of grains and grain products
- 4–5 servings per day of vegetables
- 4–5 servings per day of fruits

Your local supermarket and health food store contain many products that claim to improve cholesterol levels. But do any of these products actually work? And are they worth the cost?

Perhaps the most widely advertised functional foods for improving cholesterol are margarine spreads that contain plant sterol or plant stanol esters. Studies show that if these spreads are used on a regular basis, they can help decrease LDL cholesterol by about 10%. In 2000, the FDA approved a health claim for these products, so their labels may now state that they can help lower the risk of heart disease. The 2001 NCEP guidelines recommend up to 2 grams per day of plant sterols for people with elevated cholesterol levels. However, because they are relatively high in calories, these spreads may be most beneficial for people who use them in place of margarine or butter, rather than for people who add them to their diets. These spreads also cost much more than standard butter or margarine.

Another popular product is a food bar that contains L-arginine, an amino acid typically found in protein-rich foods such as meat. The body uses L-arginine to make nitric oxide, a chemical that promotes dilation of blood vessels. A few small studies suggest that L-arginine may help improve blood flow in people with congestive heart failure or constricted arteries. However, the FDA has expressed concern that people who consume the food bar may discontinue their medication without first consulting a physician; in addition, the FDA is currently evaluating the advertising for this product to determine if it is misleading. For now, the safest approach may be to wait until further research clarifies the effects of L-arginine supplementation.

Garlic supplements have also received attention for their possible health benefits. Allacin, a component of garlic, may inhibit cholesterol production by the liver. Research findings on the effects of garlic supplements have been mixed, however, and it's likely that if there is a positive effect, it is minimal. A less expensive and more delicious strategy may be to enjoy garlic in healthy meals rather than to take garlic supplements.

Dietary supplements containing red rice yeast also claim to support healthy cholesterol levels. One of the substances in red rice yeast is chemically identical to lovastatin, the active ingredient in a prescription cholesterol-lowering medication. Various legal actions have been undertaken by the FDA relating to the marketing of these supplements and to their classification as supplements (rather than drugs).

In evaluating dietary supplements, it is important to remember the difference between a structure-function claim and a health claim (see Chapter 12). Most functional foods and dietary supplements carry structure-function claims that are not evaluated by the FDA; "promotes healthy cholesterol levels" is an example of a structure-function claim. However, there are a number of health claims relating to cardiovascular health that have been approved by the FDA and so can be considered based on solid science. As of 2001, these claims included the following:

- Foods low in saturated fat and cholesterol and reduced risk of coronary heart disease (CHD)
- Low-sodium foods and reduced risk of hypertension
- Soluble fiber and reduced risk of CHD
- Foods high in potassium and low in sodium and reduced risk of hypertension and stroke
- Soy protein and reduced risk of CHD
- Foods and supplements with plant sterol and plant stanol esters and reduced risk of CHD

For more strategies for evaluating supplements and functional foods, refer to Chapter 12 and visit the FDA web site listed in For Your Information at the end of the chapter.

- 2–3 servings per day of low-fat or nonfat dairy products
- 2 or fewer servings per day of meats, poultry, and fish
- 4–5 servings per *week* of nuts, seeds, and legumes
- 2–3 servings per day of added fats, oils, and salad dressings
- 5 servings per *week* of snacks and sweets

Before you act on new dietary advice, remember not to seize on one particular food as a cure-all for CVD. The fight against CVD will not be won by any single dietary change; success depends on the collective effects of your entire diet. Eat a varied, moderate diet rich in fruits, vegetables, and whole grains—the DASH diet provides a good model. And use your common sense. For example, substituting olive oil or canola oil for butter is a helpful change because it lowers saturated fat intake. But adding a new oil to your diet—without subtracting fat elsewhere—will add calories and fat and not be nearly as beneficial.

Exercise Regularly

You can significantly reduce your risk of CVD with a moderate amount of physical activity. Follow the guidelines for physical activity and exercise described in Chapter 13. Begin by accumulating at least 30 minutes of moderate-intensity physical activity each day. Activities like brisk walking, gardening, and stair climbing are appropriate. Increasing the duration or intensity of exercise can provide even greater health benefits. The next step, then, is to begin a formal exercise program that develops cardiorespiratory endurance and other components of fitness. The American Heart Association recently recommended strength training in addition to aerobic exercise for building and maintaining cardiovascular health. Strength training helps lower blood pressure, reduce body fat, and improve lipid levels and glucose metabolism.

Avoid Tobacco

Remember: The number one risk factor for CVD that you can control is smoking. If you smoke, quit. If you don't, don't start. The majority of people who start don't believe they will become hooked, but most do. If you live or work with people who smoke, encourage them to quit—for their sake and yours. Regular exposure to ETS in social settings, at home, or at work raises your risk of CVD. If you find yourself breathing in smoke, take steps to prevent or stop this exposure.

Until recently, many experts believed that 5 or more years after quitting smoking, a former smoker's CVD risk would drop to about that of a person who had never smoked. However, new research indicates that the rate of plaque formation in arteries is significantly greater in former smokers than in those who have never smoked. What seems to matter most for CVD risk is the total amount of smoking over a lifetime rather than whether a person is currently smoking. The same study also showed that people exposed to environmental tobacco smoke have a significantly higher rate of plaque formation than nonsmokers who are not exposed to ETS.

The bottom line? Quitting smoking is highly beneficial. But abstaining from cigarette smoking and avoiding ETS throughout your entire life is even better.

Know and Manage Your Blood Pressure

Currently, only about 18% of Americans with hypertension have their blood pressure under control; the *Healthy People 2010* report sets the goal of increasing this number to 50%. If you have no CVD risk factors, have your blood pressure measured by a trained professional at least once every 2 years; yearly tests are recommended if you have other risk factors. If your blood pressure is high, follow your physician's advice on how to lower it. For those with hypertension that is not readily controlled with lifestyle changes, a vast array of antihypertensive medications are available.

Know and Manage Your Cholesterol Levels

Everyone age 20 and over should have their cholesterol checked at least once every five years. The NCEP recommends a lipoprotein profile that measures total cholesterol, HDL, LDL, and triglyceride levels. Once you know your "numbers," you and your physician can develop an appropriate LDL goal and lifestyle plan. Your LDL goal depends in part on how many of the following major risk factors you have:

- Cigarette smoking
- High blood pressure
- Low HDL cholesterol (less than 40 mg/dl)
- A family history of heart disease
- Age (45 years and older for men, 55 years and older for women)

An HDL level of 60 mg/dl or higher is protective and counts as a "negative" risk factor, meaning it removes one risk factor from your total count of risk factors. Depending on your LDL level and other risk factors, your physician may recommend changes in lifestyle alone or lifestyle changes in combination with drug therapy. The lifestyle modifications recommended by the 2001 NCEP guidelines, known collectively as "Therapeutic Lifestyle Changes," or TLC, include the TLC diet, weight management, and increased physical activity. The TLC diet includes total fat intake of 25–35% of total daily calories, saturated fat intake less than 7% of total calories, and, for some people, 10–25 grams per day of soluble fiber and 2 grams per day of plant stanols and sterols.

- If you have two or fewer risk factors, the NCEP sets an LDL goal of less than 160 mg/dl. If your LDL is below that level, maintain a healthy lifestyle by eating a heart-healthy diet, getting regular exercise, maintaining a healthy body weight, and not smoking. If your LDL is 160 mg/dl or higher, you should begin TLC; if it is 190 mg/dl or higher, medication may also be needed to bring it into the healthy range.

- If you have two or more risk factors for heart disease, the NCEP sets an LDL goal of less than 130 mg/dl. If your LDL level is 130 or above, begin TLC; if your LDL level remains above the goal and your risk for CVD is fairly high, your physician may recommend medication.

- If you have heart disease or a condition such as diabetes that the NCEP considers the risk equivalent of heart disease, your goal for LDL is less than 100 mg/dl. TLC is recommended for all people in this risk category; a variety of medications are available to lower LDL and improve other blood fat levels. If you have syndrome X, your physician may suggest that you increase physical activity and, if needed, reduce your weight.

Develop Effective Ways to Handle Stress and Anger

To reduce the psychological and social risk factors for CVD, develop effective strategies for handling the stress in your life. Shore up your social support network, and try some of the techniques described in Chapter 2 for managing stress (see also the box "Religion and Wellness").

COMMUNICATE! Expressing chronic anger can put you at risk for heart disease, but suppressing and internalizing anger and resentment can also be dangerous. If someone is inconsiderate, rude, manipulative, or abusive toward you, you have the right to demand respect and fair treatment. Practice being assertive—defined as the ability to communicate your thoughts and feelings with confidence and skill—

In the past decade, numerous observational studies have shown a link between religious or spiritual factors and health. Regardless of why or how this relationship happens, the evidence clearly connects religion and wellness along several dimensions.

- *Reduced risk of disease and faster recovery.* Researchers have found that people who attend religious services regularly have especially low rates of heart disease, lung disease, cirrhosis of the liver, and some kinds of cancer. Older adults who attend religious services have healthier immune systems and recover from surgery more quickly.

- *Improved emotional health.* Religion also seems to aid in recovery from depression. Participating in religious activities, listening to religious programs on the radio, and watching religious programs on television are all associated with fewer symptoms of depression.

- *Longer life expectancy.* One study found that people who attend religious services one or more times a week live about 8 years longer than people who never attend services. How involved people are in their faith may be more important than was previously believed.

Although researchers are not sure why religion or spirituality seems to improve health, several explanations have been offered:

- *Social support.* Attending religious services helps people feel they are part of a community with similar values. It promotes social support and caring.

- *Healthy habits.* Religion may encourage healthy habits—such as eating less meat, drinking less alcohol, or eating a vegetarian diet—and also discourage behavior that is harmful to health, such as smoking and indiscriminate sex.

- *Positive attitude.* Having a sense of meaning and purpose in life results in a positive attitude. This outlook may help patients participate more in their own care.

- *Moments of relaxation.* Deep relaxation during prayer may invoke benefits by eliciting the relaxation response.

SOURCES: Strawbridge, W. J., et al. 2001. Religious attendance increases survival by improving and maintaining good health behaviors, mental health, and social relationships. Annals of Behavioral Medicine 23(1): 68–74. Hummer, R. A., et al. 1999. Religious involvement and U.S. adult mortality. *Demography* 36: 273–285. Can spirituality uplift your health? 1998. *Consumer Reports on Health,* June, 7–8. Hafen, B., et al. 1996. *Mind/Body Health: The Effects of Attitudes, Emotions, and Relationships.* Needham Heights, Mass.: Allyn & Bacon.

---

without being aggressive. Be specific about the behavior that bothers you, say how you feel about it, and specify how you would like it to change. For example, "I'm very upset that you forgot to tell me my brother called. This is the third time people have asked me why I haven't returned their calls. I feel as if you don't consider my calls important. In the future, can you please write it down when someone calls me and leave the message here by the phone?" Remember that suffering in silence is not good for your health *or* your relationship

Manage Other Risk Factors and Medical Conditions

Know your CVD risk factors and follow your physician's advice for testing, lifestyle modification, and any drug treatments. If you are a postmenopausal woman, discuss the health risks and benefits of hormone replacement therapy with your physician.

If you are at high risk for CVD, consult a physician about taking small doses of aspirin. As described earlier, aspirin reduces inflammation and the blood's tendency to clot, thereby reducing the risk of CVD for some people. The recommended prescription use of aspirin for treating CVD was recently updated by the FDA. Low doses (50–325 mg) are recommended for men and women to treat TIA, stroke, angina, heart attack, and certain other cardiovascular problems. Because of possible side effects, including gastrointestinal bleeding and increased risk of certain types of strokes, the FDA cautions people to consult with their physician before taking aspirin regularly.

Tips for Today

Risk factors for cardiovascular disease fall into two categories—those you can do something about, such as physical activity and levels of stress, and those you can't, such as age and ethnicity. Because cardiovascular disease is a long-term process that can begin when you're young, it's important to develop heart-healthy habits early in life.

Right now you can

- Plan to have fish for dinner two times this week.

- Practice time management by prioritizing your day's activities; work on accomplishing the most important tasks first.

- Resolve to address any nagging interpersonal issue that's been causing you stress.

- Go to the gym or fitness facility on your campus and get started on an aerobic exercise program.

The American Heart Association recommends that no more than 10% of the calories in your diet come from cholesterol-raising saturated and trans fats. Foods high in saturated fat include meat, poultry skin, full-fat dairy products, coconut and palm oils, and hydrogenated vegetable oils. Hydrogenated fats and products such as deep-fried fast food and snack foods that are made with them are high in trans fats.

Monitor Your Current Diet

To see how your diet measures up, keep track of everything you eat for 3 days in your health journal. Information about the calorie and saturated-fat content of foods is available on many food labels, in books, and on the Internet (see Chapter 12). Trans fat content may be more difficult to determine; the list below gives a few average values for foods that are rich sources of trans fats in the American diet.

	grams of trans fat/ serving		grams of trans fat/ serving
Pot pie	6	Danish pastry	3
French fries (large)	5	Vegetable shortening	3
Pound cake	5	Margarine (stick)	2
Fish sticks	5	Microwave popcorn	2
Doughnut	4	Sandwich cookies	2
Biscuit	4	Snack crackers	2
Fried, breaded chicken	3	Margarine (tub)	1

At the end of the monitoring period, write in the calories and grams of saturated and trans fat for as many as possible of the foods you've eaten. Determine the percentage of daily calories as fat that you consumed for each day: multiply grams of saturated and trans fat by 9 (fat has 9 calories per gram) and then divide by total calories. For example, if you consumed 30 grams of saturated and trans fat and 2100 calories on a particular day, then your saturated and trans fat consumption as a percentage of total calories would be 30 × 9 = 270 calories of fat ÷ 2100 total calories = 0.13, or 13%. If you have trouble obtaining all the data you need to do the calculations, you can still estimate whether your diet is high in saturated and trans fats by seeing how many servings of foods high in unhealthy fats you typically consume on a daily basis (see the table).

Making Heart-Healthy Changes

To reduce your intake of unhealthy fats, you may want to set a limit on the number of servings of foods high in saturated and trans fats that you consume each day. Or you may want to set a more precise goal and then continue to monitor your daily consumption. The 10% limit set by the American Heart Association corresponds to 18 grams of saturated and trans fat in a diet containing 1600 calories, 24 grams in a 2200-calorie diet, and 31 grams in a 2800-calorie diet. (If you have high cholesterol, you may want to follow the 7% limit set by the NCEP, which corresponds to 12 grams of saturated and trans fat in a 1600-calorie diet, 17 grams in a 2200-calorie diet, and 22 grams in a 2800-calorie diet.)

To plan healthy changes, take a close look at your food record. Do you choose many foods high in saturated and trans fat (see the table)? Do you limit your portion sizes to those recommended by the Food Guide Pyramid? Try making healthy substitutions. Do you have a salami and cheese sandwich for lunch? Try turkey for a change. Do you always order french fries when you eat out? Try a plain baked potato or a different vegetable next time. Do you snack on pastries, cookies, doughnuts, chips, or fatty crackers? Try fresh fruits and vegetables instead. If you frequently eat in fast-food restaurants or other places where the majority of the menu is heavy in saturated and trans fats, trying finding an appealing alternative—and recruit some friends to join you.

When you do choose foods that are rich in saturated and trans fats, *watch your portion sizes carefully.* Choose cuts of meat that have the least amount of visible fat, and trim off what you see. And try to balance your choices throughout the day: For example, if your lunch includes a hamburger and fries, choose broiled fish or poultry or a vegetarian pasta dish for dinner. There are plenty of delicious choices that are low in saturated and trans fats. Plan your diet around a variety of whole grains, vegetables, legumes, and fruits, which are nearly always low in fats and high in nutrients.

SUMMARY

- The cardiovascular system pumps and circulates blood throughout the body. The heart pumps blood to the lungs via the pulmonary artery and to the body via the aorta.

- The exchange of nutrients and waste products takes place between the capillaries and the tissues.

- The six major risk factors that can be changed are smoking, high blood pressure, unhealthy cholesterol levels, inactivity, obesity, and diabetes.

- Effects of smoking include lower HDL levels, increased blood pressure and heart rate, accelerated plaque formaton, and increased risk of blood clots.

- High LDL and low HDL cholesterol levels contribute to clogged arteries and increase the risk of CVD.

- Physical inactivity, obesity, and diabetes are interrelated and are associated with high blood pressure and unhealthy cholesterol levels.

- Contributing risk factors that can be changed include high triglyceride levels and psychological and social factors.

- Risk factors for CVD that can't be changed include being over 65, being male, being African American, and having a family history of CVD.

- Hypertension occurs when blood pressure exceeds normal limits most of the time. It weakens the heart, scars and hardens arteries, and can damage the eyes and kidneys.

Instead of . . .	Try . . .
Butter, stick margarine, vegetable shortening, coconut and palm oils	Vegetable oils, trans fat–free tub or squeeze margarines
Whole or 2% milk; regular cheese, mayonnaise, and sour cream	Fat-free or 1% milk, low-fat cheese, fat-free or low-fat sour cream, yogurt, or mayonnaise
Chips, cheese puffs, crackers, buttered popcorn	Fruits, vegetables, rice cakes, "light" popcorn, pretzels, fat-free chips, baked crackers
Cakes, cookies, pastries, doughnuts, cinnamon rolls, pie, regular ice cream	Fruit or a *small* serving of a low-fat sweet (angel food cake; fat-free ice cream, frozen yogurt, sherbet, or sorbet)
Biscuits, croissants, fried tortillas, regular granola, muffins, coffee cake	Whole-grain breads and rolls, baked tortillas, low-fat granola or cold cereal, English muffin or bagel
Creamy or cheesy sauces and soups	Tomato- and other vegetable-based sauces, clam sauce, clear soups
Ground beef, hamburger patty, meatloaf, ribs, T-bone or flank steak, prime grades of beef	Ground turkey, veggie burger, extra lean ground beef, round steak, sirloin, choice or select grades of beef
Pork chops, roast, or ribs; bone-end ham; lamb chops or ribs	Pork sirloin or tenderloin; boneless ham; veal chops and cutlets; leg of lamb
Bacon, sausage, lunch meats, hot dogs	Canadian bacon; turkey ham or pastrami, other low-fat lunch meats
Poultry with skin; fried chicken or fish	Skinless poultry, especially breast or drumstick; baked, broiled, grilled, or roasted poultry or fish; ground turkey
French fries, onion rings	Baked potato or other nonfried vegetable, rice
Pizza, pot pie, macaroni and cheese, and other high-fat convenience foods	Vegetarian or turkey chili, pasta with vegetables, grilled poultry and fish dishes

SOURCES: American Heart Association. 2000. *An Eating Plan for Healthy Americans: The New 2000 Food Guidelines.* Dallas, Tex.: American Heart Association. U.S. Department of Agriculture and U.S. Department of Health and Human Services. 2000. *Nutrition and Your Health: Dietary Guidelines for Americans,* 5th ed. Home and Garden Bulletin No. 232. Food and Drug Administration. 1999. *Questions and Answers on Trans Fat Proposed Rule* (http://vm.cfsan.fda.gov/~dms/qatrans.html). Center for Science in the Public Interest. 1997. The sat fat switch. *Nutrition Action Healthletter,* January/February.

- Atherosclerosis is a progressive hardening and narrowing of arteries that can lead to restricted blood flow and even complete blockage.
- Heart attacks are usually the result of a long-term disease process. Warning signs of a heart attack include chest discomfort, light-headedness, nausea, and sweating.
- A stroke occurs when the blood supply to the brain is cut off by a blood clot or hemorrhage. A transient ischemic attack (TIA) is a warning sign of stroke.
- Congestive heart failure occurs when the heart's pumping action becomes less efficient and fluid collects in the lungs or in other parts of the body.
- Dietary changes that can protect against CVD include decreasing your intake of fat, saturated fat, trans fat, and cholesterol; increasing your intake of fiber by eating more fruits, vegetables, and whole grains.
- CVD risk can also be reduced by engaging in regular exercise, not smoking cigarettes and avoiding environmental tobacco smoke, knowing and managing your blood pressure and cholesterol levels, developing effective ways of handling stress and anger, and managing other risk factors and medical conditions.

TAKE ACTION

1. The CPR courses given by the American Red Cross and other groups provide invaluable training that may help you save a life some day. Anyone can take these courses and become qualified to perform CPR. Investigate CPR courses in your community, and sign up to take one.

2. Do some research into your family medical history. Is there cardiovascular disease in your family, as indicated by premature deaths from heart attack, stroke, or congestive heart failure? Such a history is a risk factor for you. Keep that in mind as you consider whether you need to make lifestyle changes to avoid CVD.

1. If the quiz in the box "Anger, Hostility, and Heart Disease" indicates that you may have a quick temper, examine your thoughts and behavior more carefully. In your health journal, keep track of your cynical thoughts, angry feelings, and aggressive acts. For each entry, include the time, place, and cause of your cynical thoughts; what thoughts actually went through your head; the emotions you felt; and any actions you took. Review your journal at the end of a week to learn more about the frequency and kinds of situations that trigger these thoughts and behaviors.

2. *Critical Thinking* How much responsibility does an individual have for his or her health? Do people have an obligation to take care of themselves as best they can to help avoid becoming a burden on their family and on society? Do people have a right to choose whatever lifestyle they want—no matter how unhealthy? In your health journal, write an essay describing your opinion about individual responsibility for good health. Be sure to explain your reasoning.

FOR MORE INFORMATION

Books

American Heart Association and American Cancer Society. 1999. *Living Well, Staying Well: The Ultimate Guide to Help Prevent Heart Disease and Cancer.* New York: Times Books. *Provides practical, easy-to-follow guidelines to help you reduce your risk of developing CVD and cancer.*

Farquhar, J. W., and G. A. Spiller. 2001 *Diagnosis: Heart Disease.* New York: W. W. Norton. *Provides information about heart disease treatment and recovery for patients and their families.*

Gersh, B. J., ed. 2000. *The Mayo Clinic Heart Book.* New York: Morrow. *Covers risk factors, major forms of CVD, diagnosis, and treatment.*

Matthews, D. D., ed. 2000. *Healthy Heart Sourcebook for Women.* Detroit: Omnigraphics. *A guide to the causes, prevention, and treatment of CVD in women.*

Reaven, G. M. 2000. *Syndrome X: Overcoming the Silent Killer That Can Give You a Heart Attack.* New York: Simon & Schuster. *Provides information about syndrome X and insulin resistance, including lifestyle strategies for affected individuals.*

Williams, V., and R. Williams. 1999. *Lifeskills.* New York: Times Books. *An exploration of why relationships are essential for physical health, with practical tips for improving your interactions with others; written by the authors of* Anger Kills, *which focuses on why hostility is dangerous to heart health.*

W. Organizations, Hotlines, and Web Sites

American Heart Association. Provides information on hundreds of topics relating to the prevention and control of cardiovascular disease; sponsors a general Web site as well as several sites focusing on specific topics.
   800-AHA-USA1 (general information)
   888-MY-HEART (women's health information)
   888-4-STROKE (Stroke Connection)
   http://www.americanheart.org (general information)
   http://www.deliciousdecisions.org (dietary advice)
   http://www.justmove.org (fitness advice)
   http://women.americanheart.org (women and CVD)

Cardiology Compass. An index and links to cardiovascular information on the Internet.
   http://www.cardiologycompass.com

Dietary Approaches to Stop Hypertension (DASH). Provides information about the design, diets, and results of the DASH study, including tips on how to follow the DASH diet at home.
   http://dash.bwh.harvard.edu

Food and Drug Administration: Food Labeling. Provides information about food labels, including saturated and trans fat content and FDA-approved health claims relating to CVD.
   http://vm.cfsan.fda.gov/label.html

Franklin Institute Science Museum/The Heart: An On-Line Exploration. An online museum exhibit containing information on the structure and function of the heart, how to monitor your heart's health, and how to maintain a healthy heart.
   http://www.fi.edu/biosci/heart.html

Heart Disease Prevention System. Provides educational materials on improving lifestyle for heart health, including information on smoking cessation, low-fat diets, and exercise.
   http://www.fammed.wisc.edu/research/heart

HeartInfo—Heart Information Network. Provides information for heart patients and others interested in learning how to identify and reduce their risk factors for heart disease; includes links to many related sites.
   http://www.heartinfo.org

HeartPoint. Presents news, information, and tips relating to heart health.
   http://www.heartpoint.com

National Heart, Lung, and Blood Institute. Provides information on a variety of topics relating to cardiovascular health and disease, including cholesterol, smoking, obesity, and hypertension; Web site has special fact sheets covering women and heart disease.
   800-575-WELL
   http://www.nhlbi.nih.gov
   http://rover.nhlbi.nih.gov/chd

National Stroke Association. Provides information and referrals for stroke victims and their families; the Web site has a stroke risk assessment.
   800-STROKES
   http://www.stroke.org

See also the listings for Chapters 2, 3, and 12–14.

SELECTED BIBLIOGRAPHY

American Heart Association. 2000. *An Eating Plan for Healthy Americans: The New 2000 Food Guidelines.* Dallas, Tex.: American Heart Association.

American Heart Association. 2001. *Heart and Stroke Statistical Update, 2001.* Dallas, Tex.: American Heart Association.

American Heart Association Nutrition Committee. 2000. AHA Dietary Guidelines: Revision 2000. *Circulation* 102: 2296–2311.

Aranow, W., et al. 2000. Aiming for lower than 140/90 mm Hg. *Patient Care* 34(7): 60–176.

Ayanian, J. Z. 2001. Increased mortality among middle-aged women after myocardial infarction: Searching for mechanisms and solutions. *Annals of Internal Medicine* 134(3): 239–241.

Bersot, T. 2000. Strategies for raising HDL cholesterol levels. *Patient Care* 34(1): 151–157.

Bouknight, D., and R. O'Rourke. 2000. Current management of mitral valve prolapse. *American Family Physician* 61(11): 3343–3354.

Canto, J. 2000. Prevalence, clinical characteristics, and mortality among patients with myocardial infarction presenting without chest pain. *Journal of the American Medical Association* 283(24): 3223–3229.

Cardillo, C., et al. 2000. Racial differences in nitric oxide–mediated vasodilator responses to mental stress in the forearm circulation. *Hypertension* 31(6): 1235–1239.

Cooper, R. S., C. N. Rotimi, and R. Ward. 1999. The puzzle of hypertension in African-Americans. *Scientific American* 280(2): 56–63.

Fang, J., and M. Alderman. 2000. Serum uric acid and cardiovascular mortality: The NHANES I epidemiologic follow-up study, 1971–1992. *Journal of the American Medical Association* 283(18): 2404–2410.

Goldberg, I. J., et al. 2001. Wine and your heart: A science advisory for healthcare professionals from the Nutrition Committee, Council on Epidemiology and Prevention, and Council on Cardiovascular Nursing of the American Heart Association. *Circulation* 103: 472–475.

Goldstein, L. B., et al. 2001. Primary prevention of ischemic stroke: A statement for healthcare professionals from the Stroke Council of the American Heart Association. *Circulation* 103(1): 163–182.

Greenland, P. 2001. Beating high blood pressure with low-sodium DASH. *New England Journal of Medicine* 344(1): 53–55.

Ibarren, C., et al. 2000. Association of hostility with coronary artery calcification in young adults. *Journal of the American Medical Association* 283(19): 2546–2551.

Iso, H., et al. 2001. Intake of fish and omega-3 fatty acids and risk of stroke in women. *Journal of the American Medical Association* 285(3): 304–312.

Kiechl, S., et al. 2001. Chronic infections and the risk of carotid atherosclerosis. *Circulation* 103(8): 1064–1070

Lee, I-Min, et al. 2001. Physical activity and coronary heart disease in women. *Journal of the American Medical Association* 285(11): 1447–1454.

Lefkowitz, R. J., and J. T. Willerson. 2001. Prospects for cardiovascular research. *Journal of the American Medical Association* 285(5): 581–587.

Lewis, C. 2000. Health claims for foods that lower heart disease risk. *FDA Consumer,* November/December.

Liu, S., et al. 2000. Fruit and vegetable intake and risk of cardiovascular disease: The Women's Health Study. *American Journal of Clinical Nutrition* 72(4): 922–928.

Liu, S., et al. 2001. Dietary glycemic load assessed by food-frequency questionnaire in relation to plasma high-density-lipoprotein cholesterol and fasting plasma triacylglycerols in postmenopausal women. *American Journal of Clinical Nutrition* 733: 560–566.

Meagher, E. A., et al. 2001. Effects of vitamin E on lipid peroxidation in healthy persons. *Journal of the American Medical Association* 285(9): 1178–1182.

Ostir, G. V., et al. 2001. The association between emotional well-being and the incidence of stroke in older adults. *Psychosomatic Medicine* 63(2): 210–215.

Paterniti, S., et al. 2001. Sustained anxiety and 4-year progression of carotid atherosclerosis. *Arteriosclerosis, Thrombosis, and Vascular Biology* 21(1): 136–141.

Pinkowish, M. 2000. Diabetes and CVD risks in African American children: The role of insulin metabolism. *Patient Care* 34(9): 23–27.

Pollock, M. L., et al. 2000. AHA Science Advisory: Resistance exercise in individuals with and without cardiovascular disease. *Circulation* 101: 828–833.

Rader, D. J. 2000. Inflammatory markers of coronary risk. *New England Journal of Medicine* 343(16): 1179–1182.

Raeini-Sarjaz, M., et al. 2001. Comparison of the effect of dietary fat restriction with that of energy restriction on human lipid metabolism. *American Journal of Clinical Nutrition* 73: 262–267.

Rosenberg, L., et al. 2001. Low-dose oral contraceptive use and the risk of myocardial infarction. *Archives of Internal Medicine* 161(8): 1065–1070.

Rutledge, T., et al. 2001. Psychosocial variables are associated with atherosclerosis risk factors among women with chest pain. *Psychosomatic Medicine* 63(2): 282–288.

Sacks, F. M., et al. 2001. Effects on blood pressure of reduced dietary sodium and the Dietary Approaches to Stop Hypertension (DASH) diet. *New England Journal of Medicine* 344(1): 3–10.

Stamler, J., et al. 2000. Relationship of baseline serum cholesterol levels in 3 large cohorts of younger men to long-term coronary, cardiovascular, and all-cause mortality and to longevity. *New England Journal of Medicine* 284(3): 311–318.

Vaccarino, V., et al. 2001. Sex differences in 2-year mortality after hospital discharge for myocardial infarction. *Annals of Internal Medicine* 134(3): 173–181.

Vita, J., and J. Keaney. 2000. Exercise—Toning up the endothelium? *New England Journal of Medicine* 342(7): 503–505.

Vogel, R. 2000. The Mediterranean diet and endothelial function: Why some dietary fats may be healthy. *Cleveland Clinic Journal of Medicine* 67(4): 232–236.

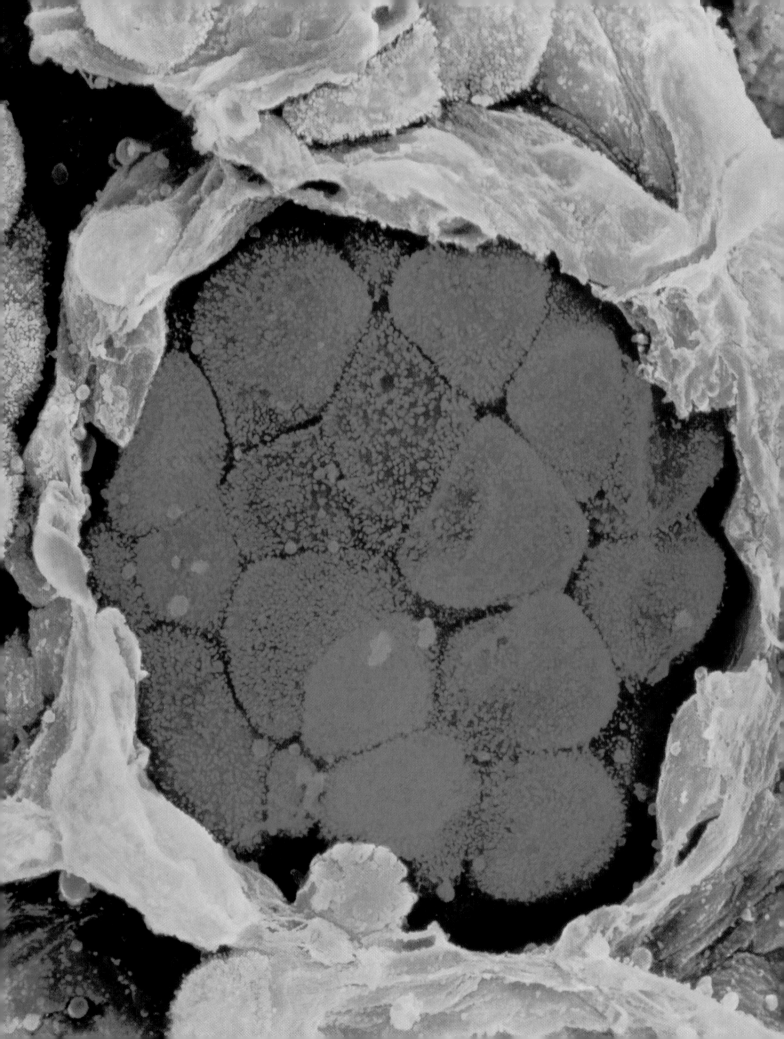

After reading this chapter, you should be able to

- Explain what cancer is and how it spreads

- List and describe common cancers—their risk factors, signs and symptoms, treatments, and approaches to prevention

- Discuss some of the causes of cancer and how they can be avoided or minimized

- Describe how cancer can be detected, diagnosed, and treated

- List specific actions you can take to lower your risk of cancer

Cancer

TEST YOUR KNOWLEDGE

1. Which type of cancer kills the most women each year?
   a. breast cancer
   b. lung cancer
   c. ovarian cancer

2. Testicular cancer is the most common cancer in men under age 30. True or false?

3. The use of condoms during sexual intercourse can prevent cancer in women. True or false?

4. Using a sunscreen with an SPF rating of 15 means that you
   a. can stay in the sun for 15 minutes without getting burned.
   b. can stay in the sun 15 times longer without getting burned than if you didn't use it.
   c. are protected against the full range of ultraviolet (UV) radiation.

5. Eating which of these foods may help prevent cancer?
   a. chili peppers
   b. broccoli
   c. oranges

ANSWERS

1. **B.** There are more cases of breast cancer each year, but lung cancer kills more women. Smoking is the primary risk factor for lung cancer.

2. **TRUE.** Although rare, testicular cancer is the most common cancer in men under age 30. Regular self-exams may aid in its detection.

3. **TRUE.** The primary cause of cervical cancer is infection with human papillomavirus (HPV), a sexually transmitted pathogen. The use of condoms helps prevent HPV infection.

4. **B.** Choose a sunscreen that has an SPF rating of 15 or higher and that protects against both UVA and UVB rays. Apply it generously; most people use less than half the recommended amount.

5. **ALL THREE.** These and many other fruits and vegetables are rich in phytochemicals, naturally occurring substances that may have anti-cancer effects.

Cancer is a word derived from the Greek for crab, *karkinos*. The early Greek physicians who first described cancerous tumors had no notion of their cause or true nature, but they were struck by the resemblance of some invasive tumors to crabs: a hard mass with clawlike extensions and an aggressive nature. Today, though we know a great deal about cancer, the old metaphor still has power; cancer has maintained its reputation as an alien presence in the body, capable of causing pain and great harm. Cancer causes more than 550,000 deaths in the United States each year, and it is the second most common cause of death, after heart disease.

While medical science struggles to find cures for the various cancers that plague us, evidence indicates that more than half of all cancers in the United States could be prevented by simple changes in lifestyle. Tobacco use is responsible for about one-third of all cancer deaths (Figure 16-1). Diet and exercise habits, including their effect on obesity, account for another large proportion of cancer deaths. Although cancer is primarily a disease of older adults, your behavior now will determine your cancer risk in the future. Experts estimate that through changes in lifestyle, most Americans can cut their lifetime cancer risk in half.

WHAT IS CANCER?

Cancer is the abnormal, uncontrolled growth of cells, which, if left untreated, can ultimately cause death.

Benign Versus Malignant Tumors

Most cancers take the form of tumors, although not all tumors are cancerous. A tumor is simply a mass of tissue that serves no physiological purpose. It can be benign, like a wart, or malignant, like most lung cancers. The term **malignant tumor** (or *neoplasm*) is synonymous with cancer.

Benign tumors are made up of cells similar to the surrounding normal cells and are enclosed in a membrane

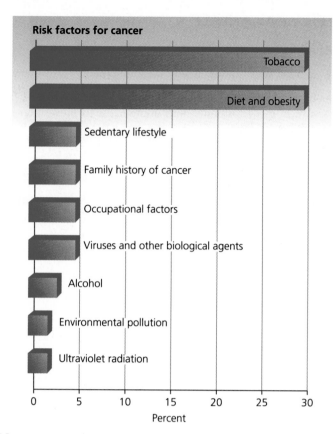

Risk factors for cancer

Tobacco

Diet and obesity

Sedentary lifestyle

Family history of cancer

Occupational factors

Viruses and other biological agents

Alcohol

Environmental pollution

Ultraviolet radiation

Percent

 VITAL STATISTICS

Figure 16-1   Percentage of all cancer deaths linked to risk factors. SOURCE: Harvard Center for Cancer Prevention. 1996. Harvard Report on Cancer Prevention. Vol. 1: Causes of Human Cancer. *Cancer Causes and Control* 7(Suppl).

that prevents them from penetrating neighboring tissues. They are dangerous only if their physical presence interferes with body functions. A benign brain tumor, for example, can cause death if it blocks the blood supply to the brain.

A malignant tumor, or cancer, is capable of invading surrounding structures, including blood vessels, the **lymphatic system,** and nerves. It can also spread to distant sites via the blood and lymphatic circulation, thereby producing invasive tumors in almost any part of the body. A few cancers, like leukemia, cancer of the blood, do not produce a mass and therefore are not properly called tumors. But since leukemia cells do have the fundamental property of rapid, uncontrolled growth, they are still malignant and therefore cancers.

Every case of cancer begins as a change in a cell that allows it to grow and divide when it should not. Normally (in adults), cells divide and grow at a rate just sufficient to replace dying cells. When you cut your finger, for example, the cells around the wound divide more rapidly to heal the wound. When the wound is healed, the rate of

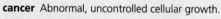

Terms

cancer Abnormal, uncontrolled cellular growth.

malignant tumor A tumor that is cancerous and capable of spreading.

benign tumor A tumor that is not cancerous.

lymphatic system A system of vessels that returns proteins, lipids, and other substances from fluid in the tissues to the circulatory system.

biopsy The removal and examination of a small piece of body tissue; a needle biopsy uses a needle to remove a small sample; some biopsies require surgery.

metastasis The spread of cancer cells from one part of the body to another.

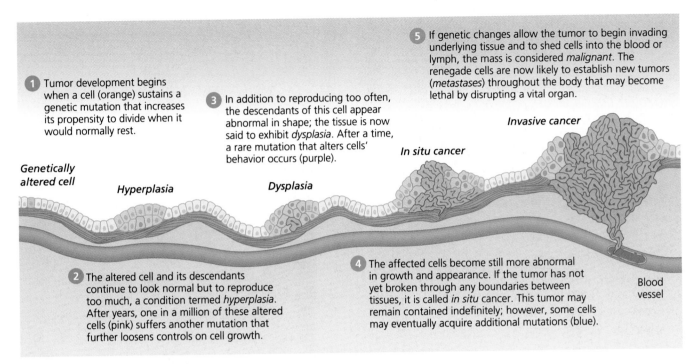

① Tumor development begins when a cell (orange) sustains a genetic mutation that increases its propensity to divide when it would normally rest.

③ In addition to reproducing too often, the descendants of this cell appear abnormal in shape; the tissue is now said to exhibit *dysplasia*. After a time, a rare mutation that alters cells' behavior occurs (purple).

⑤ If genetic changes allow the tumor to begin invading underlying tissue and to shed cells into the blood or lymph, the mass is considered *malignant*. The renegade cells are now likely to establish new tumors (*metastases*) throughout the body that may become lethal by disrupting a vital organ.

Invasive cancer

In situ cancer

Genetically altered cell

Hyperplasia

Dysplasia

② The altered cell and its descendants continue to look normal but to reproduce too much, a condition termed *hyperplasia*. After years, one in a million of these altered cells (pink) suffers another mutation that further loosens controls on cell growth.

④ The affected cells become still more abnormal in growth and appearance. If the tumor has not yet broken through any boundaries between tissues, it is called *in situ* cancer. This tumor may remain contained indefinitely; however, some cells may eventually acquire additional mutations (blue).

Blood vessel

Figure 16-2   Tumor development occurs in stages.   SOURCE: Weinberg, R. A. 1996. How cancer arises. *Scientific American,* September.

cell growth and division returns to normal. In contrast, a malignant cell divides without regard for normal control mechanisms and gradually produces a mass of abnormal cells, or a tumor. It takes about a billion cells to make a mass the size of a pea, so a single tumor cell must go through many divisions, often taking years, before the tumor grows to a noticeable size (Figure 16-2).

Eventually a tumor produces a sign or symptom that is determined by its location in the body. In the breast, for example, a tumor may be felt as a lump and diagnosed as cancer by an X ray or **biopsy.** In less accessible locations, like the lung, ovary, or intestine, a tumor may be noticed only after considerable growth has taken place and may then be detected only by an indirect symptom—for instance, a persistent cough or unexplained bleeding or pain. In the case of leukemia, there is no lump, but the changes in the blood will eventually be noticed as increasing fatigue, infection, or abnormal bleeding.

How Cancer Spreads: Metastasis

Metastasis, the spreading of cancer cells, occurs because cancer cells do not stick to each other as strongly as normal cells do and therefore may not remain at the site of the *primary tumor,* the original location. They break away and can pass through the lining of lymph or blood vessels to invade nearby tissue. They can also drift to distant parts of the body, where they establish new colonies of cancer cells. This traveling and seeding process is called

metastasizing, and the new tumors are called *secondary tumors,* or *metastases.*

Traveling cancer cells can follow two courses. They can produce secondary tumors in the lymph nodes and be carried through the lymph system to form secondary sites elsewhere, or they can invade blood vessels and circulate through the vessels to colonize other organs. This ability of cancer cells to metastasize makes early cancer detection critical. To control the cancer and prevent death, every cancerous cell must be removed. Once cancer cells enter either the lymphatic system or the bloodstream, it is extremely difficult to stop their spread to other organs of the body. In fact, counting the number of lymph nodes that contain cancer cells is one of the principal methods of predicting the outcome of the disease; the probability of a cure is much greater when the lymph nodes do not contain cancer cells.

Types of Cancer

The behavior of tumors arising in different body organs is characteristic of the tissue of origin. (Figure 16-3 shows the major cancer sites and the incidence of each type.) Because each cancer begins as a single (altered) cell with a specific function in the body, the cancer will retain some of the properties of the normal cell for a time. For instance, cancer of the thyroid gland may produce too much thyroid hormone and cause hyperthyroidism as well as cancer. Usually, however, cancer cells lose their

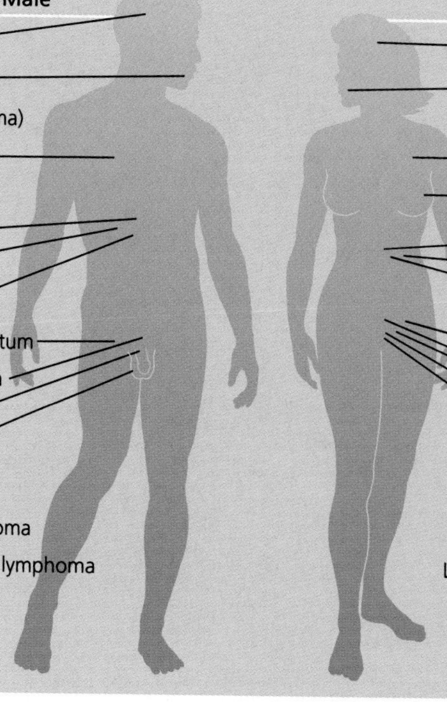

New cases	Deaths	Male	Female	New cases	Deaths
9,800	7,200	Brain	Brain	7,400	5,900
20,200	5,100	Oral	Oral	9,900	2,700
29,000	5,000	Skin (melanoma)	Skin (melanoma)	22,400	2,800
90,700	90,100	Lung	Lung	78,800	67,300
			Breast	192,200	40,200
13,400	7,400	Stomach	Stomach	8,300	5,400
10,700	8,900	Liver	Liver	5,500	5,200
14,200	14,100	Pancreas	Pancreas	15,000	14,800
67,300	27,700	Colon and rectum	Colon and rectum	68,100	29,000
59,400	16,100	Urinary system	Urinary system	28,100	8,900
198,100	31,500	Prostate	Ovary	23,400	13,900
7,200	400	Testes	Uterus	38,300	6,600
			Cervix	12,900	4,400
7,500	5,800	Multiple myeloma	Multiple myeloma	6,900	5,400
52,700	26,500	Leukemia and lymphoma	Leukemia and lymphoma	42,400	22,600
62,800	40,300	Other	Other	65,400	32,200
643,000	**286,100**	**Total**	**Total**	**625,000**	**267,300**

W. VITAL STATISTICS

Figure 16-3 Cancer cases and deaths by site and sex. The Incidence column indicates the number of cancers that occurred in each site; the Death column indicates the number of cancer deaths that were attributed to each type. SOURCE: American Cancer Society. 2000. *Cancer Facts and Figures, 2000.* Atlanta: American Cancer Society.

resemblance to normal tissue as they continue to divide, becoming groups of rogue cells with increasingly unpredictable behavior.

Malignant tumors are classified according to the types of cells that give rise to them:

- **Carcinomas** arise from **epithelia,** tissues that cover external body surfaces, line internal tubes and cavities, and form the secreting portion of glands. They are the most common type of cancers; major sites include the skin, breast, uterus, prostate, lungs, and gastrointestinal tract.

- **Sarcomas** arise from connective and fibrous tissues like muscle, bone, cartilage, and the membranes covering muscles and fat.

- **Lymphomas** are cancers of the lymph nodes, part of the body's infection-fighting system.

- **Leukemias** are cancers of the blood-forming cells, which reside chiefly in the **bone marrow.**

There is a great deal of variation in how easily different cancers can be detected and how well they respond to treatment. For example, certain types of skin cancer are easily detected, grow slowly, and are very easy to remove;

virtually all of the 1 million cases that occur each year in the United States are cured. Cancer of the pancreas, on the other hand, is very difficult to detect or treat, and very few patients survive the disease. In general, it is very difficult for an **oncologist** to predict how a specific tumor will behave because every tumor arises from a unique set of changes in a single cell.

The Incidence of Cancer

Each year, about 1.3 million people in the United States are diagnosed with cancer. More than half will be cured, but about 40% will eventually die as a result of their cancer. These grim statistics exclude more than 1 million cases of the curable types of skin cancer. At current U.S. rates, about 1 in 2 men and 1 in 3 women will develop cancer at some point in their lives.

Are cancer deaths increasing in the United States? Until 1991, the answer was yes, largely due to a wave of lethal lung cancers among men caused by smoking. In 1991, the death rate stopped increasing and began to fall slowly; it has dropped 3% since 1990. This is a very promising trend, as it suggests that efforts at prevention, early detection, and improved therapy are all bearing

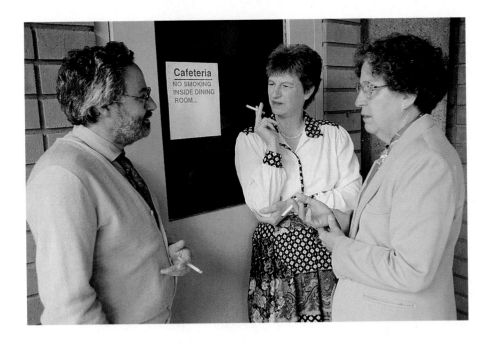

Smoking is responsible for about 30% of all cancer deaths. The benefits of quitting are substantial: Lung cancer risk decreases significantly after one smoke-free year and drops to half that of continuing smokers after 10 smoke-free years.

fruit. Experts estimate that if these trends continue, we may see a decline in death rates of as much as 15–50% over the next 20 years.

Could more people be saved from cancer? The American Cancer Society (ACS) estimates that 90% of skin cancer could be prevented by protecting the skin from the rays of the sun and 87% of lung cancer could be prevented by avoiding exposure to tobacco smoke. Thousands of cases of colon, breast, and uterine cancer could be prevented by improving the diet and controlling body weight. Regular screenings and self-examinations have the potential to save an additional 100,000 lives per year. Although cancer may seem like a mysterious disease, there are many concrete strategies you can adopt to reduce your risk.

WWW. COMMON CANCERS

A discussion of all types of cancer is beyond the scope of this book. In this section we look at some of the most common cancers and their causes, prevention, and treatment.

Lung Cancer

Lung cancer is the most common cause of cancer death in the United States; it is responsible for about 157,000 deaths each year. For over 40 years, breast cancer was the major cause of cancer death in women, but since 1987, lung cancer has surpassed breast cancer as a killer of women.

Risk Factors The chief risk factor for lung cancer is tobacco smoke, which accounts for 87% of cancers. (Other negative effects of tobacco smoke on the lungs were dis-

cussed in Chapter 11.) When smoking is combined with exposure to other **carcinogens,** such as asbestos particles, the risk of cancer can be multiplied by a factor of 10 or more. Elevated ozone levels tripled the risk of lung cancer for men in one 15-year study. (See Chapter 24 for more on asbestos, ozone, and other pollutants.)

The smoker is not the only one at risk. In 1993, the U.S. Environmental Protection Agency (EPA) classified environmental tobacco smoke (ETS) as a human carcinogen. Long-term exposure to ETS increases risk of lung cancer. Secondhand smoke, the smoke from the burning end of the cigarette, has significantly higher concentrations of the toxic and carcinogenic compounds found in mainstream smoke. It is estimated that ETS causes about 3000 lung cancer deaths each year.

Detection and Treatment Lung cancer is difficult to detect at an early stage and hard to cure even when detected early. Symptoms of lung cancer do not usually

---

carcinoma Cancer that originates in epithelial tissue (skin, glands, and lining of internal organs).

epithelial layer A layer of tissue that covers a surface or lines a tube or cavity of the body, enclosing and protecting other parts of the body.

sarcoma Cancer arising from bone, cartilage, or striated muscle.

lymphoma A tumor originating from lymphatic tissue.

leukemia Cancer of the blood or the blood-forming cells.

bone marrow Soft vascular tissue in the interior cavities of bones that produces blood cells.

oncologist A specialist in the study of tumors.

carcinogen Any substance that causes cancer.

Terms

appear until the disease has advanced to the invasive stage. Signals such as a persistent cough, chest pain, or recurring bronchitis may be the first indication of a tumor's presence. A recent study found that a relatively new option, spiral CT (computed tomography) scans, a computer-assisted body imaging technique, detected lung cancer significantly earlier than chest X rays did. This screening option is expensive and often not covered by insurance. In cases where it is not available, a diagnosis can usually be made by chest X ray or by studying the cells in sputum. Because almost all lung cancers arise from the cells that line the bronchi, tumors can sometimes be visualized by fiber-optic bronchoscopy, a test in which a flexible lighted tube is inserted into the windpipe and the surfaces of the lung passages are directly inspected.

Treatment for lung cancer depends on the type and stage of the cancer. If caught early, localized cancers can be treated with surgery. But because only about 15% of lung cancers are detected before they spread, radiation and **chemotherapy** are often used in addition to surgery. For cases detected early, 49% of patients are alive 5 years after diagnosis; but overall, the survival rate is only 14%. Phototherapy and gene therapy are being studied in the hope of improving these statistics. In addition, one form of lung cancer, known as small-cell lung cancer and accounting for about 20% of cases, can be treated fairly successfully with chemotherapy—alone or in combination with radiation. A large percentage of cases respond with **remission,** which in some cases lasts for years.

Colon and Rectal Cancer

Another common cancer in the United States is colon and rectal cancer (also called colorectal cancer). It is the second leading cause of cancer death.

Risk Factors Age is a key risk factor for colon and rectal cancer, with more than 90% of cases diagnosed in people age 50 and older. Heredity also plays a role: Many cancers arise from preexisting **polyps,** small growths on the wall of the colon that may gradually develop into malignancies. The tendency to form colon polyps appears to be determined by specific genes, and 15–30% of colon cancers may be due to inherited gene mutations. Chronic inflammation of the colon as a result of disorders such as ulcerative colitis also increases the risk of colon cancer.

Lifestyle is also a risk factor for colon and rectal cancer. Regular physical activity appears to reduce a person's risk, while obesity increases risk. A diet rich in red meat is thought to increase risk, although it is unclear whether fat or some other component of meat is the culprit. A diet rich in fruits, vegetables, and whole grains is associated with lower risk. However, recent findings have contradicted the long-standing view that dietary fiber prevents colon cancer. Further investigation of different types and sources of fiber and other properties of plant-based diets may help clarify the relationship between diet and colon cancer. Studies have suggested a protective role for folic acid and calcium; in contrast, high intake of simple sugars and smoked meats and fish may increase risk. A plant-based, high-fiber diet is still recommended because it is associated with a lower risk of cancer overall and also helps prevent heart disease, hypertension, and diabetes.

Other lifestyle factors that may increase the risk of colon and rectal cancer include excessive alcohol consumption and smoking. Use of oral contraceptives or hormone replacement therapy may reduce risk in women. In addition, research indicates that regular use of nonsteroidal anti-inflammatory drugs such as aspirin and ibuprofen decreases the risk of developing colon cancer and other cancers of the digestive tract.

Detection and Treatment If identified early, precancerous polyps and early-stage cancers can be removed before they become malignant or spread. Because polyps may bleed as they progress, the standard warning signs of colon cancer are bleeding from the rectum and a change in bowel habits. Regular screening tests are recommended beginning at age 50 (earlier for people with a family history of the disease). A stool blood test, which should be performed every year, can detect small amounts of blood in the stool long before obvious bleeding would be noticed. More involved screening tests are recommended at 5- or 10-year intervals. In sigmoidoscopy or colonoscopy, a flexible fiber-optic device is inserted through the rectum; part or all of the colon can be examined, and polyps can be biopsied or even removed without major surgery.

Surgery is the primary treatment for colon and rectal cancer. Radiation and chemotherapy may be used before surgery to shrink a tumor or after surgery to destroy any remaining cancerous cells. The survival rate is 90% for colon and rectal cancers detected early and 61% overall.

COMMUNICATE! Fear and embarrassment can sometimes prevent people from getting an early diagnosis of cancer, and this is especially true for colorectal cancer. If you have a family history of colorectal polyps or cancer, talk to your health care provider about what screening tests you should be having. For example, "My mother had colon cancer and I'm wondering if I should be screened earlier than usual." If you have a symptom that you're worried about—such as abdominal pain, rectal bleeding, or a change in bowel habits—bring it to your physician's attention right away. (Such symptoms can indicate conditions other than cancer, but if it is cancer, early detection can make an enormous difference in your prognosis.) Don't wait for your physician to ask; be assertive with your concerns. Direct and open communication with your health care provider is a key to continued good health.

Breast Cancer

Breast cancer is the most common cancer in women and causes almost as many deaths in women as lung cancer. In men, breast cancer occurs only rarely. In the United States, about one woman in nine will develop breast cancer during her lifetime. The incidence of breast cancer increased during the 1980s but now appears to have leveled off; each year, about 190,000 American women are diagnosed with breast cancer. Although mortality rates declined during the early 1990s, about 40,000 women die from breast cancer each year.

Less then 1% of breast cancer cases occur in women under age of 30, but a woman's risk doubles every 5 years between the ages of 30 and 45 and then increases more slowly, by 10–15% every 5 years after age 45. More than 75% of breast cancers are diagnosed in women over 50.

Risk Factors   There is a strong genetic factor in breast cancer. A woman who has two close relatives with breast cancer is four to six times more likely to develop the disease than a woman who has no close relatives with it. However, even though genetic factors are important, only about 15% of cancers occur in women with a family history of breast cancer. (Genetic factors in breast cancer are discussed later in the chapter.)

Other risk factors include early onset of menstruation, late onset of menopause, having no children or having a first child after age 30, current use of hormone replacement therapy, obesity, and alcohol use. The unifying factor for many of these risk factors may be the female sex hormone estrogen, which circulates in a woman's body in high concentrations between puberty and menopause. Fat cells also produce estrogen, and estrogen levels are higher in obese women. Alcohol can interfere with estrogen metabolism in the liver and increase estrogen levels in the blood. Estrogen promotes the growth of cells in responsive sites, including the breast and the uterus, so any factor that increases estrogen exposure may raise breast cancer risk. In addition, pregnancy and breastfeeding trigger changes in breast cells that make them less susceptible to cancerous changes.

Breast cancer has been called a "disease of civilization" because incidence is high in industrialized Western countries but remains low in developing non-Western countries. Differences in diet and exercise habits have been proposed to explain this pattern, but the connections are still being investigated. Recent studies indicate that a high-fat diet alone may not increase the risk of breast cancer but that the type of fat consumed may be important. Monounsaturated fats have been linked with reduced risk, while certain types of polyunsaturated fat may increase risk. Dietary fiber may also have a protective effects. Regular exercise is extremely important: A study of more than 25,000 women found that those who exercised regularly had a 37% lower risk of breast cancer than those who did not exercise. Vigorous exercise may reduce estrogen levels in the blood, and physical activity of all intensities helps control body weight. Both obesity and significant weight gain during adulthood are linked to increased risk of breast cancer.

Although some of the risk factors for breast cancer—such as heredity and some hormonal factors—cannot be changed, important lifestyle risk factors are under the control of the individual. Eating a low-fat, high-fiber diet, exercising regularly, limiting alcohol intake, and maintaining a healthy body weight can minimize the chance of developing breast cancer, even for women at risk from family history or other factors.

Early Detection   A cure is most likely if breast cancer is detected early, so regular screening is a good investment, even for younger women. The ACS advises a three-part personal program for the early detection of breast cancer:

1. Monthly breast self-examination (BSE) for all women over age 20 (see the box "Breast Self-Examination," on p. 464).

2. A clinical breast exam by a physician every 3 years for women between 20 and 39 and every year for women 40 and older.

3. **Mammograms** (low-dose breast X rays) every year for most women over 40. (Individual risk factors must be considered in determining the frequency of mammograms, and the value of mammograms for women in their forties is an area of debate.)

Treatment   If a lump is detected, it may be scanned by **ultrasonography** and biopsied to see if it is cancerous. The biopsy may be done either by needle in the physician's office or surgically. In 90% of cases, the lump is found to be a cyst or other harmless growth, and no further treatment is needed. If the lump does contain cancer cells, a variety of surgeries may be called for, ranging from a lumpectomy (removal of the lump and surrounding tissue) to a mastectomy (removal of the breast). To determine whether the cancer has spread, lymph nodes from

---

Terms

chemotherapy The treatment of cancer with chemicals that selectively destroy cancerous cells.

remission A period during the course of cancer in which there are no symptoms or other evidence of disease.

polyp A small, usually harmless mass of tissue that projects from the inner surface of the colon or rectum.

mammograms Low-dose X rays of the breasts used to check for early signs of breast cancer.

ultrasonography An imaging method in which sound waves are bounced off body structures to create an image on a TV monitor; also called *ultrasound*.

By regularly examining your own breasts, you are likely to notice any changes that occur. The best time for breast self-examination (BSE) is about a week after your period ends, when your breasts are not tender or swollen. If you are not having regular periods, do BSE on the same day every month.

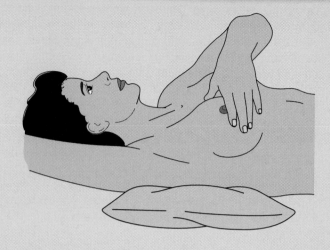

1. Lie down and put a pillow under your right shoulder. Place your right arm behind your head.

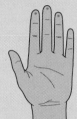

2. Use the finger pads of your three middle fingers on your left hand to feel for lumps or thickening in your right breast. Your finger pads are the top third of each finger.

3. Press firmly enough to know how your breast feels. If you're not sure how hard to press, ask your health care provider. Or try to copy the way your health care provider uses the finger pads during a breast exam. Learn what your breast feels like most of the time. A firm ridge in the lower curve of each breast is normal.

4. Move around the breast in a set way. You can choose either the circle (a), the up and down (b), or the wedge (c). Do it the same way every time. It will help you to make sure that you've gone over the entire breast area, and to remember how your breast feels.

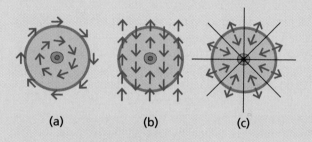

(a)   (b)   (c)

5. Now examine your left breast using right hand finger pads.

6. Repeat the examination of both breasts while standing, with one arm behind your head. The upright position makes it easier to check the upper and outer part of the breasts (toward your armpit). You may want to do the standing part of the BSE while you are in the shower. Some breast changes can be felt more easily when your skin is wet and soapy.

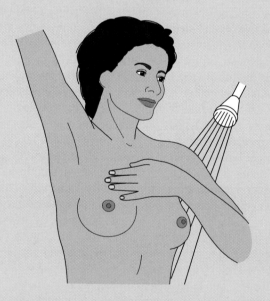

For added safety, you can also check your breasts for any dimpling of the skin, changes in the nipple, redness, or swelling while standing in front of a mirror right after your BSE each month.

If you find any changes, see your doctor right away.

SOURCE: *How to Do Breast Self-Examination.* © 2001 American Cancer Society, Inc. Reprinted by the permission of the American Cancer Society, Inc.

the armpit may be removed and examined. If cancer cells are found, tumor cells remaining in the body can often be slowed or killed by additional therapy, such as radiation, chemotherapy, or both.

The chance of survival in cases of breast cancer varies, depending both on the nature of the tumor and whether it has metastasized. If the tumor is discovered early, before it has spread to the adjacent lymph nodes, the patient has about a 97% chance of surviving more than 5 years. The survival rate for all stages is 85% at 5 years, 71% at 10 years, and 57% at 15 years.

New Strategies for Treatment and Prevention

A number of new drugs have recently been developed for the treatment or prevention of breast cancer. A family of drugs called selective estrogen-receptor modulators, or SERMs, act like estrogen in some tissues of the body but block estrogen's effects in others. One SERM, tamoxifen, has long been used in breast cancer treatment because it blocks the action of estrogen in breast tissue. In 1998, the FDA approved the use of tamoxifen to reduce the risk of breast cancer in healthy women who are at high risk for the disease. A large-scale study found that tamoxifen reduced the risk of breast cancer by 44% among high-risk women. However, the drug has serious potential side effects, including increased risk of blood clots and uterine cancer, and its long-term effects are unknown. Another SERM currently being tested as a potential preventive agent is raloxifene, a drug used to treat osteoporosis that has fewer side effects than tamoxifen. Although still controversial, the use of SERMs in the prevention of breast cancer is a major breakthrough.

A new therapy for advanced breast cancer is Herceptin (trastuzumab), a monoclonal antibody. Antibodies, discussed in Chapter 17, are proteins produced by the immune system that recognize and bind to foreign substances such as bacteria; monoclonal antibodies are a special type of antibody that are produced in the laboratory and designed to bind to a specific cancer-related target. About 30% of metastatic breast cancer tumors produce excess amounts of a growth-promoting protein called HER2. Herceptin binds to the excess HER2, thus blocking its action and slowing tumor growth. Herceptin is typically used alone or in combination with Taxol (paclitaxel), a drug that interferes with cell division.

Prostate Cancer

The prostate gland is situated at the base of the bladder in men. It produces seminal fluid; if enlarged, it can block the flow of urine. Prostate cancer is the most common cancer in men and, after lung cancer, the cause of the most deaths. More than 190,000 new cases are diagnosed each year, and about 32,000 American men die from the disease each year.

Risk Factors

Age is the strongest predictor of the risk, with about 75% of cases of prostate cancer diagnosed in men over age 65. Inherited genetic predisposition may be responsible for 5–10% of cases, and men with a family history of the disease should be particularly vigilant about screening. For reasons not well understood, African American men have the highest rate of prostate cancer of any group in the world; both genetic and lifestyle factors may be involved. Diets high in calories, dairy products, and animal fats and low in plant foods have also been implicated as possible culprits in the development of prostate cancer. Compounds in soy foods and cruciferous vegetables such as broccoli and cabbage are being investigated for their possible protective effects.

Detection

Warning signs of prostate cancer include changes in urinary frequency, weak or interrupted urine flow, painful urination, and blood in the urine. Screening tests for early detection are recommended annually for men age 50 and over—earlier for African Americans and those with a strong family history of the disease. Most cases of prostate cancer are first detected during a digital rectal exam. A physician can feel the prostate gland through the rectum and determine it is enlarged or if lumps are present.

The **PSA blood test,** which measures the amount of prostate-specific antigen (PSA) in the blood, can also be used to help diagnose prostate cancer. An elevated level or a rapid increase in PSA can signal trouble. A single measurement of PSA can help catch early prostate cancer, but it also registers benign conditions (more than half of men over 50 have benign prostate disease). Researchers are looking for ways to make the PSA test more sensitive. One strategy is to repeat the test over time to chart a rate of change. A newer approach involves measuring the percentage of PSA that is free-floating in the blood. PSA made by cancer cells is more likely to circulate bound to other proteins, while PSA from healthy prostate cells is more likely to be unbound. Thus, a low proportion of so-called free PSA indicates greater risk, while a high proportion of free PSA is associated with lower risk.

Ultrasound is used increasingly as a follow-up, to detect lumps too small to be felt and to determine their size, shape, and properties. A needle biopsy of suspicious lumps can be performed relatively painlessly, and whether the biopsied cells are malignant or benign can be determined by examining them under a microscope.

Treatment

Treatments vary based on the stage of the cancer and the age of the patient. A small, slow-growing tumor in an older man may be treated with "watchful waiting"

PSA blood test A diagnostic test for prostate cancer that measures blood levels of prostate-specific antigen (PSA).

Terms

because he is more likely to die from another cause before his cancer becomes life threatening. More aggressive treatment would be indicated for younger men or those with more advanced cancers. Treatment usually involves radical prostatectomy, in which the prostate is removed surgically. While radical surgery has an excellent cure rate, it is major surgery and often results in **incontinence** and **impotence.**

A less-invasive alternative involves surgical implantation of radioactive seeds. Radiation from the seeds destroys the tumor and much of the normal prostate tissue but leaves surrounding tissue relatively untouched. Although there is little risk of incontinence or impotence, this procedure is relatively new and its effectiveness for different stages of cancer is still being evaluated.

Alternative or additional treatments include external radiation, hormones, cryotherapy, and anti-cancer drugs. Survival rates for all stages of this cancer have improved steadily since 1940; the 5-year survival rate is currently about 93%.

Cancers of the Female Reproductive Tract

Because the uterus, cervix, and ovaries are subject to similar hormonal influences, the cancers of these organs can be discussed as a group.

Cervical Cancer Cervical cancer is at least in part a sexually transmitted disease. Probably more than 80% of cervical cancer stems from infection by the human papillomavirus (HPV), a large group of related viruses that cause both common warts and genital warts. When certain types of HPV are introduced into the cervix, usually by an infected sex partner, the virus infects cervical cells, causing the cells to divide and grow. If unchecked, this growth can develop into cervical cancer. Cervical cancer is associated with multiple sex partners and is extremely rare in women who have not had heterosexual intercourse. The regular use of condoms can reduce the risk of transmitting HPV.

Because only a very small percentage of HPV-infected women ever get cervical cancer, other factors must be involved. Two of the most important seem to be smoking and infection with genital herpes (discussed in Chapter 18

with other STDs). Both smoking and herpes infection can cause cancerous changes in cells in the laboratory and can speed and intensify the cancerous changes begun by HPV. Research also suggests that women with high levels of HPV 16, a specific form of HPV, are at particularly high risk for the infection to develop into cancer. Some studies show that past exposure to the bacterium that causes the STD chlamydia may also be a risk factor for cervical cancer that operates independently of HPV.

Screening for the changes in cervical cells that precede cancer is done chiefly by means of the **Pap test.** During a pelvic exam, loose cells are scraped from the cervix, spread on a slide, stained for easier viewing, and examined under a microscope to see whether they are normal in size and shape. If cells are abnormal, a condition commonly referred to as *cervical dysplasia,* the Pap test is repeated at intervals. Sometimes cervical cells spontaneously return to normal, but in about one-third of cases, the cellular changes progress toward malignancy. If this happens, the abnormal cells must be removed, either surgically or by destroying them with a cryoscopic (ultra-cold) probe or localized laser treatment. When the abnormal cells are in a precancerous state, the small patch of dangerous cells can be completely removed.

Without timely surgery, the malignant patch of cells goes on to invade the wall of the cervix and spreads to adjacent lymph nodes and to the uterus. At this stage, chemotherapy may be used with radiation to kill the fast-growing cancer cells, but chances for a complete cure are lower. Even when a cure can be achieved, it often means surgical removal of the uterus.

Because the Pap test is highly effective, all sexually active women and women between the ages of 18 and 65 should be tested annually. Unlike most cancers, which occur most often after the age of 60, cancer of the cervix occurs frequently in women in their thirties or even twenties. Although screening can clearly save lives, *Healthy People 2010* reports lower-than-average rates of Pap testing for certain groups, including women of low socioeconomic status and women with less than a high school education. Mortality rates for cervical cancer are twice as high for black women as for white women.

Uterine, or Endometrial, Cancer Cancer of the lining of the uterus, or **endometrium,** most often occurs after the age of 55. The risk factors are similar to those for breast cancer: prolonged exposure to estrogen, early onset of menstruation, late menopause, never having been pregnant, and other medical conditions, including obesity. The use of oral contraceptives, which combine estrogen and progestin, appears to provide protection.

Endometrial cancer is usually detectable by pelvic examination. It is treated surgically, commonly by hysterectomy, or removal of the uterus; radiation treatment and chemotherapy may be used in addition to surgery. When the tumor is detected at an early stage, about 96% of

Terms

incontinence The inability to control the flow of urine.

impotence The inability to have an erection or ejaculate; an inability to perform sexual intercourse.

Pap test A scraping of cells from the cervix for examination under a microscope to detect cancer.

endometrium The layers of tissue lining the uterus.

melanoma A malignant tumor of the skin that arises from pigmented cells, usually a mole.

ultraviolet (UV) radiation Light rays of a specific wavelength emitted by the sun; most UV rays are blocked by the ozone layer in the upper atmosphere.

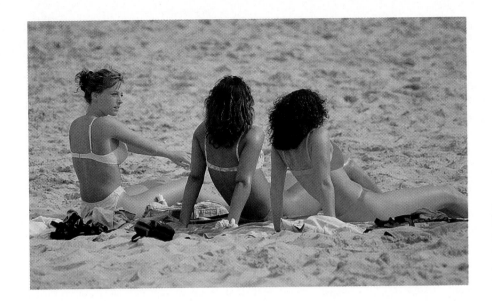

Cumulative exposure to sunlight, beginning in childhood, increases the risk of skin cancer later in life. Blistering sunburns are particularly dangerous, but tanning also poses a hazard. Sunscreens help protect the skin from the sun's radiation.

patients are alive and disease-free 5 years later. When the disease has spread beyond the uterus, the 5-year survival rate is less than 64%.

Ovarian Cancer   Although ovarian cancer is rare compared with cervical or uterine cancer, it causes more deaths than the other two combined. It cannot be detected by Pap tests or any other simple screening method and is often diagnosed only late in its development, when surgery and other therapies are unlikely to be successful. The risk factors are similar to those for breast and endometrial cancer: increasing age (most ovarian cancer occurs after age 60), never having been pregnant, a family history of breast or ovarian cancer, and specific genetic mutations. A high number of ovulations appears to increase the chance that a cancer-causing genetic mutation will occur, so anything that lowers the number of lifetime ovulation cycles—pregnancy, breastfeeding, or use of oral contraceptives—reduces a woman's risk of ovarian cancer.

There are often no warning signs of developing ovarian cancer. Therefore, women at high risk because of family history or because they harbor a mutant gene should have thorough pelvic exams at regular intervals, as recommended by their physician. Pelvic exams may include the use of ultrasound to view the ovaries. A blood test for a tumor marker called CA-125 may assist with diagnosis but is not yet recommended for routine screening.

Ovarian cancer is treated by surgical removal of both ovaries, the fallopian tubes, and the uterus. Radiation and chemotherapy are sometimes used in addition to surgery. When the tumor is localized to the ovary, the survival rate after 5 years is 95%. But for all stages, the survival rate is only 50%, reflecting the difficulty of early detection.

Other Female Reproductive Tract Cancers   From 1938 to 1971, millions of women were given a synthetic hormone called DES (diethylstilbestrol), which was thought to help prevent miscarriage. It was later discovered that daughters born to these women (DES daughters) have an increased risk, about 1 in 1000, of a vaginal or cervical cancer called clear cell cancer. This cancer is extremely rare in unexposed women. DES daughters may also have an anatomically abnormal reproductive tract and have problems with fertility or miscarriage. Though this is primarily a health threat for daughters, there is also some risk to DES sons, who may have an increased risk of abnormalities of the reproductive tract, including undescended testicles, a risk factor for testicular cancer.

If you suspect you may be a DES daughter or son, you should ask your mother if she took any medications while pregnant and, if possible, review her medical records for that time. A DES daughter should find a physician who is familiar with the problems of DES exposure; more frequent and more thorough pelvic exams are recommended. A recent animal study suggested the possibility of an increased third-generation cancer risk from DES, but further research is needed to determine if the finding applies to DES granddaughters.

WWW. Skin Cancer

Skin cancer is the most common cancer of all when cases of the highly curable forms are included in the count. (Usually these forms are not included, precisely because they are easily treated.) Of the more than 1 million cases of skin cancer diagnosed each year, 51,000 are of the most serious type, **melanoma**. Treatments are usually simple and successful when the cancers are caught early.

Risk Factors   Almost all cases of skin cancer can be traced to excessive exposure to **ultraviolet (UV) radiation** from the sun, including longer-wavelength ultraviolet A

Your risk of skin cancer from the ultraviolet radiation in sunlight depends on several factors. Take the quiz below to see how sensitive you are. The higher your UV-risk score, the greater your risk of skin cancer—and the greater your need to take precautions against too much sun.

Score 1 point for each true statement:

_____ 1. I have blond or red hair.

_____ 2. I have light-colored eyes (blue, gray, green).

_____ 3. I freckle easily.

_____ 4. I have many moles.

_____ 5. I had two or more blistering sunburns as a child.

_____ 6. I spent lots of time in a tropical climate as a child.

_____ 7. I have a family history of skin cancer.

_____ 8. I work outdoors.

_____ 9. I spend a lot of time in outdoor activities.

_____ 10. I like to spend as much time in the sun as I can.

_____ 11. I sometimes go to a tanning parlor or use a sunlamp.

_____ Total score

Score	Risk of skin cancer from UV radiation
0	Low
1–3	Moderate
4–7	High
8–11	Very high

SOURCE: Adapted from Shear, N. 1996. What's your UV-risk score? *Consumer Reports on Health*, June. Copyright © 1996 by Consumers Union of U.S., Inc., Yonkers, N.Y. 10703–1057. Reprinted by permission from *Consumer Reports on Health*. No photocopying or reproduction permitted. To order a subscription, call 1-800-234-1645.

(UVA) and shorter-wavelength ultraviolet B (UVB) radiation. UVB radiation causes sunburns and can damage the eyes and the immune system. UVA is less likely to cause an immediate sunburn, but by damaging connective tissue, it leads to premature aging of the skin, giving it a wrinkled, leathery appearance. (Tanning lamps and tanning-salon beds emit mostly UVA radiation.) Both UVA and UVB radiation have been linked to the development of skin cancer, and the National Toxicology Program has declared both solar and artificial sources of UV radiation to be known human carcinogens.

Both severe, acute sun reactions (sunburns) and chronic low-level sun reactions (suntans) can lead to skin cancer. People with fair skin have less natural protection against skin damage from the sun and a higher risk of developing skin cancer; people with naturally dark skin have a considerable degree of protection (see the box "What's Your UV Risk?"). Caucasians are about 20 times more likely than African Americans to develop melanoma. Severe sunburns in childhood have been linked to a greatly increased risk of skin cancer in later life, so children in particular should be protected. Because of damage to the ozone layer of the atmosphere (discussed in Chapter 24), there is a chance that we may all be exposed to increasing amounts of UV radiation in the future. Take time now to understand the risks of excessive sun exposure, because the precautions suggested here will become increasingly critical if the ozone shield continues to thin.

Other risk factors for skin cancer include having many moles, particularly large ones, spending time at high altitudes, and a family history of the disease. Skin cancer may also be caused by exposure to coal tar, pitch, creosote, arsenic, and radioactive materials; but compared to sunlight, these agents account for only a small proportion of cases.

Types of Skin Cancer   There are three main types of skin cancer, named for the types of skin cell from which they develop. **Basal cell** and **squamous cell carcinomas** together account for about 95% of the skin cancers diagnosed each year. They are usually found in chronically sun-exposed areas, such as the face, neck, hands, and arms. They usually appear as pale, waxlike, pearly nodules or red, scaly, sharply outlined patches. These cancers are often painless, although they may bleed, crust, and form an open sore on the skin.

Melanoma is by far the most dangerous skin cancer because it spreads so rapidly. Since 1973, the incidence of melanoma has increased by about 4% per year. It is the most common cancer among women age 25–29 years. It can occur anywhere on the body, but the most common sites are the back, chest, abdomen, and lower legs. A melanoma usually appears at the site of a preexisting mole. The mole may begin to enlarge, become mottled or varied in color (colors can include blue, pink, and white), or develop an irregular surface or irregular borders. Tissue invaded by melanoma may also itch, burn, or bleed easily.

Prevention   One of the major steps you can take to protect yourself against all forms of skin cancer is to avoid lifelong overexposure to sunlight. Blistering, peeling sun-

With proper clothing and the use of sunscreens, you can lead an active outdoor life *and* protect your skin against most sun-induced damage.

Clothing

- Wear long-sleeved shirts and long pants made of tightly woven fabric. Thin, white shirts or wet clothing will not protect you sufficiently.

- Wear a wide-brimmed hat to protect your ears and face.

- Wear UV-blocking sunglasses to protect your eyes. A dark color does not imply UV protection; check the label.

Sunscreen

- Use a sunscreen and lip balm with a sun protection factor (SPF) of 15 or higher. (An SPF rating refers to the amount of time you can stay out in the sun before you burn, compared to using no sunscreen; for example, a product with an SPF of 15 would allow you to remain in the sun without burning 15 times longer, on average, than if you didn't apply sunscreen.) If you're fair-skinned or will be outdoors for long hours, use a sunscreen with a high SPF (30+).

- Choose a "broad-spectrum" sunscreen that protects against both UVA and UVB radiation. The SPF rating of a sunscreen currently applies only to UVB, but a number of ingredients, including avobenzone (Parsol 1789), benzophenone, oxybenzone, titanium dioxide, and zinc oxide, are effective at blocking most UVA radiation. Use a water-resistant sunscreen if you swim or sweat quite a bit.

- Apply sunscreen 30 minutes before exposure to allow it time to penetrate the skin; shake it before applying.

- Reapply sunscreen frequently and generously to all sun-exposed areas (many people overlook their temples, ears, and sides and backs of their necks). Most people use less than half as much as they would need to attain the full SPF rating. One ounce of sunscreen—one-fourth of a 4-ounce container—is about enough to cover an average-size adult in a swimsuit.

- If you're taking medication, ask your physician or pharmacist about possible reactions to sunlight or interactions with sunscreens. Medications for acne (Retin-A), allergies, and diabetes are just a few of the products that can trigger reactions. If you're using sunscreen and an insect repellent containing DEET, use extra sunscreen (research has suggested that DEET may decrease sunscreen effectiveness).

- Don't let sunscreens give you a false sense of security. The effectiveness of sunscreens in preventing skin cancer has not been firmly established, so even if you wear sunscreen and don't burn, sun exposure may increase your cancer risk. For people at greatest risk—those with fair skin and the tendency to develop many moles—avoiding sun exposure may be the safest strategy.

Time of Day and Location

- Avoid sun exposure between 10 A.M. and 4 P.M., when the sun's rays are most intense. Clouds allow as much as 80% of UV rays to reach your skin. Stay in the shade when you can, and use an umbrella at the beach.

- Consult the day's UV Index, which predicts UV levels on a 0–10+ scale, to get a sense of the amount of sun protection you'll need; take special care on days with a rating of 5 or above. UV Index ratings are available in local newspapers, from the weather bureau, or from certain Web sites (see For More Information at the end of the chapter).

- UV rays can penetrate at least 3 feet in water, so swimmers should wear water-resistant sunscreen.

- Locations near the equator or at high altitudes have more intense sunlight, so stronger sunscreens should be used and applied often.

- Snow reflects the sun's rays, so don't forget to apply sunscreen before skiing and other snow activities. Sand and water also reflect the sun's rays, so you still need to apply a sunscreen if you are under a beach umbrella. Concrete and white-painted surfaces are also highly reflective.

---

burns from unprotected sun exposure are particularly dangerous, but suntans—whether from sunlight or tanning lamps—also increase your risk of developing skin cancer later in life. People of every age, including babies and children, need to be protected from the sun with **sunscreens** and protective clothing. For a closer look at sunlight and skin cancer, see the box "Protecting Your Skin from the Sun."

Detection and Treatment   The only sure way to avoid a serious outcome from skin cancer is to make sure it is recognized and diagnosed early. More than half of all melanomas are brought to a physician's attention by pa-

tients themselves. Make it a habit to examine your skin regularly. Most of the spots, freckles, moles, and blemishes on your body are normal; you were born with some of them, and others appear and disappear throughout

basal cell carcinoma Cancer of the deepest layers of the skin. Terms
squamous cell carcinoma Cancer of the surface layers of the skin.
sunscreen A substance used to protect the skin from UV rays; usually applied as an ointment or a cream.

your life. But if you notice an unusual growth, discoloration, sore that does not heal, or mole that undergoes a sudden or progressive change, see your physician or a dermatologist immediately.

The characteristics that may signal that a skin lesion is a melanoma—asymmetry, border irregularity, color change, and a diameter greater than ¼ inch—are illustrated in Figure 16-4. In addition, if someone in your family has had numerous skin cancers or melanomas, you may want to consult a dermatologist for a complete skin examination and discussion of your particular risk.

If you do have an unusual skin lesion, your physician will examine it and possibly perform a biopsy. If the lesion is cancerous, it is usually removed surgically, a procedure that can almost always be performed in the physician's office using a local anesthetic. Occasionally, other forms of treatment may be used. Even for melanoma, the outlook after removal in the early stages is good, with a 5-year survival rate of 96% if the tumor is localized but only 59% if the cancer has spread to adjacent lymph nodes. Since prevention requires a minimum of time and attention, it pays to be alert.

> **COMMUNICATE!** The media often portray beautiful people with a "healthy tan." Yet research studies as well as everyday experience confirm that the sun irreparably damages the skin and causes skin cancer. Both sunlight and tanning salons are human carcinogens. What messages are the media communicating with their images of tanned skin? Are you influenced by these messages? Can you look at the messages critically and counter them with scientific information and common sense?

Oral Cancer

Oral cancer—cancers of the lip, tongue, mouth, and throat—can be traced principally to cigarette, cigar, or pipe smoking, the use of spit tobacco, and the excess use of alcohol. These risk factors work together to multiply a person's risk of oral cancer. The incidence of oral cancer is twice as great in men as in women and most frequent in men over 40. Some prominent sufferers of oral cancer have included Sigmund Freud and Fidel Castro, both notorious cigar smokers. Sports figures who have cultivated a taste for spit tobacco are now also increasingly being diagnosed with oral cancer. Among long-term snuff users, the excess risk of cancers of the cheek, tongue, and gum is nearly fiftyfold (see Chapter 11 for more on cigars and spit tobacco).

Oral cancers do have the virtue of being fairly easy to detect, but they are often hard to cure. The primary methods of treatment are surgery and radiation. The 5-year survival rates vary from 91% for lip cancer to 26% for throat cancer; the overall survival rate is about 54%.

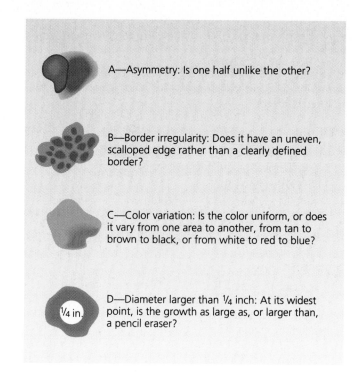

Figure 16-4 The ABCD test for melanoma.

Testicular Cancer

Testicular cancer is relatively rare, accounting for only 1% of cancer in men (about 7200 cases per year), but it is the most common cancer in men age 20–35. It is much more common among white Americans than Latinos, Asian Americans or African Americans and among men whose fathers had testicular cancer. Men with undescended testicles are at increased risk for testicular cancer, and for this reason the condition should be corrected in early childhood. Men whose mothers took DES during pregnancy have an increased risk of undescended testicles and other genital anomalies. For this reason, they may have a higher risk of testicular cancer.

Self-examination may help in the early detection of testicular cancer (see the box "Testicle Self-Examination"). Tumors are treated by surgical removal of the testicle and, if the tumor has spread, by chemotherapy. The 5-year survival rate for testicular cancer is 95%.

Other Cancers

Several other cancers affect a significant number of people each year. Some have identifiable risk factors, particularly smoking and obesity, that are controllable, while the causes of others are still under investigation.

Pancreatic Cancer   The pancreas, a gland found deep within the abdomen behind the stomach, produces both digestive enzymes and insulin. Because of the gland's hidden location, pancreatic cancer is usually well advanced

The best time to perform a testicular self-exam is after a warm shower or bath, when the scrotum is relaxed. First, stand in front of a mirror and look for any swelling of the scrotum. Then, examine each testicle with both hands. Place the index and middle fingers under the testicle and the thumbs on top; roll the testicle gently between the fingers and thumbs. Don't worry if one testicle seems slightly larger than the other—that's common. Also, expect to feel the epididymis, the soft, sperm-carrying tube at the rear of the testicle.

Perform the self-exam each month. If you find a lump, swelling, or nodule, consult a physician right away. The abnormality may not be cancer, but only a physician can make a diagnosis. Other possible signs of testicular cancer include a change in the way a testicle feels, a sudden collection of fluid in the scrotum, a dull ache in the lower abdomen or groin, a feeling of heaviness in the scrotum, or pain in a testicle or the scrotum.

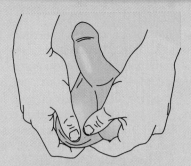

SOURCES: Testicular Cancer Resource Center. 2001. *How to Do a Testicular Self Examination* (http://www.acor.org/TCRC/tcexam.html; retrieved February 14, 2001). National Cancer Institute. 2000. *Questions and Answers About Testicular Cancer* (http://cis.nci.nih.gov/fact/6_34.htm; retrieved February 14, 2001).

before symptoms become noticeable. No effective cure is available, and it is the fifth leading cause of cancer death in the United States: In 2001, there were 29,000 new cases and about 29,000 deaths. About 3 out of 10 cases are linked to smoking. Other risk factors include being male, African American, or over age 60; having a family history of pancreatic cancer; having diabetes; and eating a diet high in fat and meat and low in vegetables.

Stomach Cancer   In many parts of the world, stomach cancer is the most common form of cancer. It is relatively unusual in the United States, with about 21,700 new cases and 12,800 deaths each year. It tends to occur after the age of 50 and is twice as common in men as in women. Risk factors include infection with the bacterium *Helicobacter pylori,* which has also been linked to the development of ulcers, and a diet high in smoked, salted, or pickled fish or meat. Bacteria, including *H. pylori,* can convert the nitrates in preserved foods into carcinogenic amines, and salt can break down the normal protective stomach coating, allowing these carcinogenic compounds access to the cells of the stomach wall. However, the great majority of people with *H. pylori* infection do not develop stomach cancer, particularly if they maintain a low-salt diet with adequate amounts of fruits, vegetables, and whole grains. There is no screening test for stomach cancer; it is usually recognized only after it has spread, and the 5-year survival rate is only 21% for all stages.

Bladder Cancer   This cancer is twice as common in men as in women, and smoking is the key risk factor. People living in urban areas and workers exposed to chemicals used in the dye, rubber, and leather industries are

also at increased risk. There is no screening test for it; the first symptoms are likely to be blood in the urine and/or increased frequency of urination. These symptoms can also signal a urinary infection but should trigger a visit to a physician, who can evaluate the possibility of cancer. With early detection, more than 90% of cases are curable. There are about 54,000 new cases and about 12,000 deaths each year.

Kidney Cancer   Although this cancer usually occurs in people over 50, anyone can develop it and there are few controllable risk factors. Smoking and obesity are mild risk factors, as is a family history of the disease. Symptoms may include fatigue, pain in the side, and blood in the urine. Kidney cancer has been difficult to treat, with a 5-year survival rate of only 61% for all stages. Recently, immune cell therapies have shown some promise in the disease's advanced stage. There are about 31,000 new cases each year and about 12,000 deaths.

Brain Cancer   Tumors can arise from most of the many types of cells that are found in the brain. The vast majority of brain cancers develop for no apparent reason; one of the few established risk factors is ionizing radiation, such as X rays. Before the risks were recognized, children with ringworm of the scalp (a fungal infection) often received low-dose radiation therapy, which substantially increased their risk of brain tumors later in life. Symptoms are often nonspecific and include headaches, fatigue, behavioral changes, and sometimes seizures. There has been a slight increase in the incidence of tumors over the past 20 years, but this may be due to improved methods of diagnosis. Some brain tumors are curable by surgery or by radiation and chemotherapy, but most are not. Survival time varies, depending on the type of the tumor, from 1 to 8 years. In 2001, there were about 17,200 new cases and 13,100 deaths.

Leukemia Leukemia, cancer of the white blood cells, can affect both children and adults. It starts in the bone marrow but can then spread to the lymph nodes, spleen, liver, other organs, and central nervous system. Like brain cancer, it is a complex disease with many different types and subtypes. Most people with leukemia have no known risk factors. About 20% of cases of adult leukemia are related to smoking; other possible risk factors include radiation and certain chemicals and infections. Most symptoms occur because leukemia cells crowd out the production of normal blood cells; the result can be fatigue, anemia, weight loss, and increased risk of infection. Treatment and survival rates vary, depending on the exact type and other factors. There were 31,500 new cases in 2001 and 21,500 deaths.

Lymphoma Arising from the lymph cells, lymphoma begins in the lymph nodes and then may spread to almost any part of the body. There are two types—Hodgkin's disease and non-Hodgkin's lymphoma (NHL). NHL is the more common and more deadly form of the disease. It is the fifth most common cancer in the United States, with about 56,000 people diagnosed annually; about half of all patients will eventually die from the disease. Risk factors for NHL are not well understood but may include genetic factors, radiation, and certain chemicals and infections. A new therapy based on the use of antibodies has shown promise in treating patients. Rates of Hodgkin's disease have fallen by more than 50% since the early 1970s, and there are now about 7400 cases and 1300 deaths each year.

Multiple Myeloma Normal plasma cells play an important role in the immune system, producing antibodies. Malignant plasma cells may produce tumors in several sites, particularly in the bone marrow; when they grow in multiple sites, they are referred to as multiple myeloma (MM). By crowding out normal bone marrow cells, MM can lead to anemia, excessive bleeding, and decreased resistance to infection. Age is the most significant risk fac-

tor: Only 2% of cases are diagnosed in people under 40, and the average age at diagnosis is about 70. Other risk factors are not well understood, although MM is about twice as common among African Americans as among whites. Although treated with chemotherapy and slow in its progression, the disease is usually fatal. There are about 14,400 new cases each year and 11,200 deaths.

W. THE CAUSES OF CANCER

Although scientists do not know everything about what causes cancer, they have identified genetic, environmental, and lifestyle factors. (For information on possible factors involved in cancer incidence, see the box "Can Poverty Cause Cancer?") There are usually several steps in the transformation of a normal cell into a cancer cell, and in many cases, different factors may work together in the development of cancer.

The Role of DNA

Almost daily, the mass media report on some new link between heredity and cancer. But how exactly do genes influence cancer? And what do these links mean for you and your risk of developing particular cancers?

DNA Basics The nucleus of each cell in your body contains 23 pairs of **chromosomes,** which are made up of tightly packed coils of **DNA** (deoxyribonucleic acid). As described in Chapter 1, DNA consists of two long strands wound around each other in a spiral structure, like a twisted ladder; scientists refer to this spiral as a double helix. The rungs of the ladder are made from four different nucleotide bases: adenine, thymine, cytosine, and guanine, or A, T, C, and G. The arrangement of nucleotide bases along the double helix constitutes the genetic code. You can think of this code as a set of instructions for building, operating, and repairing your body.

A **gene** is a smaller unit of DNA made up of a specific sequence of nucleotide bases. Each chromosome contains hundreds, and in some cases thousands, of genes; you have 30,000–40,000 genes in all. Each of your genes controls the production of a particular protein. The makeup of each protein—which amino acids it contains and in what sequence—is determined by its precise sequence of A, T, C, and G. Proteins build cells and make them work: They serve both as the structural material for your body and as the regulators of all chemical reactions and metabolic processes. By making different proteins at different times, genes can act as switches to alter the ways a cell works.

Except for sperm and egg cells, every cell in your body contains two copies of each gene, one on each of a pair of chromosomes. You inherit one copy of each gene from your mother and one from your father. Every cell contains a copy of the complete DNA sequence with all the genes.

Terms

chromosomes The threadlike bodies in a cell nucleus that contain molecules of DNA; most human cells contain 23 pairs of chromosomes.

DNA Deoxyribonucleic acid, a chemical substance that carries genetic information.

gene A section of a chromosome that contains the nucleotide base sequence for making a particular protein; the basic unit of heredity.

mutagen Any environmental factor that can cause mutation, such as radiation and atmospheric chemicals.

Americans with low incomes are more susceptible to cancer and are also more likely to die of it, even if their condition and treatment are similar to those of more affluent cancer victims. Why does cancer afflict the economically disadvantaged so disproportionately? A primary factor is lifestyle: People of low socioeconomic status are more likely to smoke, abuse alcohol, and eat high-fat foods—all of which have been associated with cancer. These unhealthy behaviors usually begin early: One study found that 63% of teenagers of parents with low incomes engage in two or more of five cancer-related behaviors: smoking, inactivity, an inadequate intake of fruits and vegetables, excessive fat consumption, and alcohol use. The rates of these behaviors among adolescents of more affluent parents are significantly lower.

Another reason is lack of knowledge and information. Studies have found that low-income people are less exposed to information about cancer, less aware of its early warning signs, and less likely to seek medical care when they have such symptoms. A third reason may be an inability to respond to health information and health needs. Many low-income people may not be able to afford nutritious foods and may not have transportation or access to health care facilities. A study comparing low-income Americans and Canadians found that Canadians in the poorest third of the population economically were about 35% more likely to survive cancer than similar Americans. The reason may be Canada's system of universal health care, which ensures access to treatment regardless of income. The difference in survival rates was even greater when Americans over 65 (who are eligible for government-funded Medicare) were removed from the study.

In fact, lifestyle differences account for only about 13% of the gap in death rates between Americans with high and low incomes. Many of the cancer-related threats that people with low incomes face are difficult or impossible to avoid. They may be forced to live and work in unsafe or unhealthy environments. They may have jobs, for example, in which they come into daily contact with carcinogenic chemicals, and they may not have been trained in handling them properly. They face similar risks in their homes and schools, where they may be exposed to asbestos or other carcinogens every day.

But even poor health habits and dangerous living and working conditions don't completely explain the high cancer mortality rates among the economically disadvantaged. One study of cancer patients found that chemotherapy was less effective on the tumors of the poorer patients. One possible explanation is the high levels of stress associated with poverty. Stress can impair the immune system, the body's first line of defense against cancer, and experiments with animals have shown that a stressful environment can enhance the growth of a variety of tumors. The link between poverty, stress, and cancer mortality in humans has not been proven, but studies have shown a link between stress and other illnesses.

What can be done about reducing the rate of cancer and cancer mortality in low-income populations? Educating people about prevention is clearly important, and elementary schools and high schools are places where people can be reached in time to encourage healthy habits and prevent bad habits before they begin. However, people from lower socioeconomic groups tend to have a high rate of school dropout. Furthermore, most people have a difficult time worrying about a disease they might get in 10 or 20 years when their immediate concern is survival.

For these reasons, some medical scientists look to policymakers for solutions. They maintain that living and working conditions in the inner cities must be improved and that access to quality health care must be assured for all Americans. Then, even without new miracle drugs or medical breakthroughs, the United States will see a real decrease in cancer rates in low-income populations.

SOURCES: Gorey, K. M., et al. 2000. An international comparison of cancer survival: Relatively poor areas of Toronto, Ontario and three U.S. metropolitan areas. *Journal of Public Health Medicine* 22(3): 343–348. Institute of Medicine. 1999. *The Unequal Burden of Cancer.* Washington, D.C.: National Academy Press. Lantz, P. M., et al. 1998. Socioeconomic factors, health behaviors, and mortality. *Journal of the American Medical Association* 279: 1703–1708. Grabmeier, J. 1992. Poverty can cause cancer. *USA Today,* July.

What makes the cells in your body different from one another in both structure and function—one a nerve cell and one a muscle cell, for example—is not which genes they contain, but which genes are "turned on," or expressed. Some genes are active and producing proteins all the time; others are expressed very seldomly.

Cells reproduce by dividing in two, and your body makes billions of new cells every day. When a cell divides, the DNA replicates itself so that each new cell has a complete set of chromosomes. Through the proteins for which they code, some genes are responsible for controlling the rate of cell division, and some types of cells divide much more rapidly than others. Genes that control the rate of cell division often play a critical role in the development of cancer.

DNA Mutations and Cancer   A mutation is any change in the normal sequence of nucleotide bases in a gene. Like a typographical error, it may involve a deletion or a substitution of a certain base—for example, CAA may become CA or CTA. Some mutations are inherited: If the egg or sperm cell that produces a child contains a mutation, so will every one of the child's 30 trillion cells. Environmental agents can also produce mutational damage; these **mutagens** include radiation, certain viruses, and chemical substances in the air we breathe. (When a mutagen also causes cancer, it is called a carcinogen.) Some mutations are the result of copying errors that occur when DNA replicates itself as part of cell division.

A mutated gene no longer contains the proper code for producing its protein. Since a cell has two copies of each gene, it can sometimes get by with only one functioning version. In this case, the mutation may have no effect on health. However, if both copies of a gene are damaged or if the cell needs two normal copies to function properly, then the cell will cease to behave normally.

It requires several mutational changes over a period of years before a normal cell takes on the properties of a cancer cell. Genes in which mutations are associated with the conversion of a normal cell into a cancer cell are known as **oncogenes**. In their undamaged form, many oncogenes play a role in controlling or restricting cell growth; they are called **tumor suppressor genes**. Mutational damage to these genes releases the brake on growth and leads to rapid and uncontrolled cell division—a precondition for the development of cancer.

A good example of how a series of mutational changes can produce cancer is provided by the p53 gene, located on chromosome 17. In its normal form, the protein that is coded for by this gene actually helps prevent cancer: If a cell's DNA is damaged, the p53 protein can either kill the cell outright or stop it from replicating until the damaged DNA is repaired. For example, if a skin cell's DNA is mutated by exposure to sunlight, the p53 protein activates the cell's "suicide" machinery. (The scientific term for this programmed cell death is **apoptosis**.) By thus preventing the replication of damaged DNA, the p53 protein keeps cells from progressing toward cancer. However, if the p53 gene itself undergoes a mutation, these controls are lost, and the cell can become cancerous. In fact, the damaged version of p53 can actually promote cell division and the spread of cancer.

A damaged p53 gene can be inherited, but carcinogenic damage or DNA copying errors are more common causes of p53 mutations. The carcinogen benzo(a)pyrene, found in tobacco smoke, causes a particular mutation in p53 that is linked to many cases of lung cancer. Other agents contribute to cancer by interfering with the p53 protein after it is produced. For example, human papillomavirus, the infectious agent linked to cervical cancer, neutralizes the p53 protein. Researchers believe that damage to the p53 gene and protein may be involved, directly and indirectly, in as many as 50–60% of all cancers.

Hereditary Cancer Risks As we've described, one way to obtain a mutated oncogene is to inherit it. For example, a form of inherited colon cancer is believed to account for one in six colon cancer cases; children who inherit the altered gene are thought to face a 70–80% chance of developing the disease. Using information from the Human Genome Project, scientists have been able to identify the genes responsible for the condition. Another example is BRCA1 (breast cancer gene 1): Women who inherit a damaged copy of this suppressor gene face a significantly increased risk of breast and ovarian cancer.

It is important to remember, however, that most cancers are not linked to heredity; mutational damage usually occurs after birth. For example, only about 5–10% of breast cancer cases can be traced to inherited copies of a damaged BRCA1 gene. In addition, lifestyle is important even for those who have inherited a damaged suppressor gene: Eating a high-fiber diet, exercising regularly, and maintaining a healthy body weight may protect against breast cancer.

Testing and identification of hereditary cancer risks can be helpful for some people, especially if it leads to increased attention to controllable risk factors and better medical screening. For more on hereditary cancer risks and the issues involved in genetic testing, see the box "Genetic Testing for Breast Cancer."

Cancer Promoters Substances known as cancer promoters make up another important piece of the cancer puzzle. Carcinogenic agents like UV radiation that cause mutational changes in the DNA of oncogenes are known as "initiators" of cancer. Cancer "promoters," on the other hand, don't directly produce DNA mutations. Instead, they accelerate the growth of cells without damaging or permanently altering their DNA. However, a faster growth rate means less time for a cell to repair DNA damage caused by initiators, so errors are more likely to be passed on. Estrogen, which stimulates cellular growth in the female reproductive organs, is an example of a cancer promoter.

Colon cancer provides a good example of how the combination of initiators and promoters contributes to the development of cancer. Colon cells may divide more rapidly if the diet is high in red meat. Under these circumstances of growth promotion, a cell with a preexisting mutation in an oncogene has an increased chance of progressing toward cancer. Increasing intake of fruits, vegetables, and calcium may reverse this effect and slow the growth of cells that line the colon, thereby decreasing the possibility of cancer developing.

Although much still needs to be learned about the role of genetics in cancer, it's clear that minimizing mutation

Terms

oncogene A gene involved in the transformation of a normal cell into a cancer cell.

tumor suppressor gene A type of oncogene that normally functions to restrain cellular growth.

apoptosis Genetically programmed cell death, in which the cell undergoes shrinkage, condensation of the nucleus, and fragmentation. Many cancer cells lose their ability to respond to the normal apoptosis triggers such as DNA damage.

Linda's mother, sister, and grandmother all developed breast cancer at around age 40. Now Linda is wondering if she should be tested for mutations in the so-called breast cancer gene, BRCA1. She is not alone. Recent discoveries of disease-related genes are opening up a host of issues related to genetic testing and associated legal, financial, and ethical concerns. Tests for hereditary mutations in breast cancer genes are now commercially available, but who should be tested?

Researchers identified BRCA1 in 1994. About 1 in 800 women in the general population carries a mutant copy of BRCA1, but in certain groups, most notably women of Ashkenazi (Eastern European) Jewish descent, as many as 1 in 100 may carry an altered gene. Defects in this gene cause breast cancer in as many as 50–60% of affected women; they also increase the risk of ovarian cancer and, in men, prostate cancer. Women with an altered BRCA1 gene tend to develop breast cancer at younger ages than other women, and the cancers that develop are more malignant. The situation is complex, however, because hundreds of different mutations of BRCA1 have been identified, and not all of them carry the same risks. Additional genes influencing risk have been identified—BRCA2 in 1995, TSG101 in 1997, BRAF35 in 2001—and others will no doubt be found in the future.

Genetic analysis of DNA from a blood sample can identify mutant copies of BRCA1. The tests can be expensive, however, ranging from $350 to more than $2000. (Searching for a mutation on a large gene is a bit like looking for a single typo in a novel.) Good news from a genetic test is reassuring, but it doesn't guarantee freedom from disease. Only 5–10% of all cases of breast cancer occur among women who inherit an altered version of BRCA1. And a woman with a family history of breast cancer must still be monitored closely, even if she carries a normal version of BRCA1; the cancer-causing genetic defect in her family could be located on another gene.

What about women who test positive for an altered copy of the gene? Options include close monitoring, drug treatment with a SERM such as tamoxifen, and surgical removal of currently healthy breasts or ovaries. None of these strategies completely eliminates risk, and they may expose a woman to a dangerous or drastic treatment that is actually unnecessary. And those who test positive can face problems in addition to an uncertain medical future. Some health insurers may use the results of a genetic test to justify canceling coverage. Although currently rare, such "genetic discrimination" could become a major problem as more and more disease-related genes are identified. Recent legislation has attempted to protect people from losing coverage due to the results of genetic tests.

In one study, 48% of women at risk for the BRCA1 mutation decided to take the test when it was offered. Women under the age of 50 and those with children were more likely to be tested. There is no simple answer to the question of who should undergo genetic testing for disease-related genes. If you think you are at high risk for a genetic abnormality because of your family or ethnic background, consider genetic counseling. A counselor can help you consider all the issues related to testing and can guide you into making the decision that is right for you.

---

damage to our DNA will lower our risk of many cancers. Unfortunately, a great many substances produce cancer-causing mutations, and we can't escape them all. By identifying the important carcinogens and understanding how they produce their effects, we can help keep our DNA intact and avoid activating "sleeping" oncogenes. The careful study of oncogenes should also lead to more precise methods of assessing cancer risk and to new methods of diagnosis and treatment.

W. Dietary Factors

Diet is one of the most important factors in cancer prevention, but it is also one of the most complex and controversial. Diets high in meat, fast food, refined carbohydrates, and simple surgars and low in fruits and vegetables are associated with a higher risk of cancer than are plant-based diets rich in whole grains, fruits, and vegetables. The picture becomes less clear, however, when researchers attempt to identify the particular constituents of foods that affect cancer risk. The foods you eat contain many biologically active compounds, and your food choices affect your cancer risk by both exposing you to potentially dangerous compounds and depriving you of potentially protective ones. For example, snacking on a doughnut instead of an apple means that you consume more fat and simple sugars *and* less fiber and fewer vitamins. Research into particular food components can help guide you in making dietary choices, but keep in mind that the overall quality of your diet is most important.

Let's take a look at some of the dietary factors that may affect cancer risk.

Dietary Fat and Meat   In general, diets high in fat and meat have been associated with higher rates of certain cancers, including those of the colon and prostate. Dietary fat may promote colon cancer by stimulating the production of bile acids, which are necessary to break down and digest material in the colon. Once produced, these bile acids remove layers of cells from the intestinal epithelium, which in turn are replaced by new cells. Newly formed and rapidly growing cells are particularly susceptible to carcinogens. Although the mechanism is unclear, diets high in animal fats and low in plant fats may also increase the risk of aggressive forms of prostate cancer, possibly by affecting hormone levels.

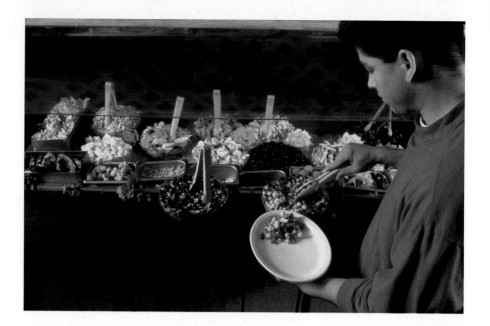

Your food choices significantly affect your risk of cancer. By consuming the recommended 5–9 servings of fruits and vegetables per day, this young man ensures that his diet is high in fiber and rich in cancer-fighting phytochemicals.

As is the case for heart disease, certain types of fats may be riskier than others. Some studies suggest that diets favoring omega-6 polyunsaturated fats over the omega-3 forms commonly found in fish may be associated with a higher risk of certain cancers, while monounsaturated fats may have a protective effect. Omega-3 fatty acids appear to slow the growth of colon cancer cells and may have protective factors against breast, prostate, and pancreatic cancers (see Chapter 12 for more on different types of fatty acids). Particular fatty acids found in meat as well as nonfat constituents of meat such as iron may also help explain the association between meat and cancer. In addition, curing, smoking, and grilling and other cooking methods utilizing a direct flame or high temperatures may produce carcinogenic compounds such as polycyclic aromatic hydrocarbons. (Grilling vegetables does not produce these compounds.)

Alcohol Alcohol is associated with an increased incidence of several cancers. An average alcohol intake of three drinks per day is associated with a doubling in the risk of breast cancer. Alcohol and tobacco interact as risk factors for oral cancer, and heavy users of both alcohol and tobacco have a risk of oral cancer up to 15 times greater than that of people who don't drink or smoke.

Fiber Determining the effects of fiber intake on cancer risk is complicated by the fact that fiber is found in foods that also contain many other potential anti-cancer agents—fruits, vegetables, and whole grains. Various potential cancer-fighting actions have been proposed for fiber, but none of these actions has been firmly established. Further study is needed to clarify the relationship between fiber intake and cancer risk, and experts still recommend a high-fiber diet for its overall positive effect on health.

Fruits and Vegetables A massive number of epidemiological studies provide evidence that high consumption of fruits and vegetables reduces the risk of many cancers. Exactly which constituents of fruits and vegetables are responsible for this reduction in risk is less certain. Researchers have identified many mechanisms by which food components may act against cancer: Some may prevent carcinogens from forming in the first place or block them from reaching or acting on target cells. Others boost enzymes that detoxify carcinogens and render them harmless. Still other anti-cancer agents act on cells that have already been exposed to carcinogens, slowing the development of cancer or starving cancer cells of oxygen and nutrients by cutting off their blood supply.

Some essential nutrients act as **anticarcinogens.** For example, vitamin C, vitamin E, selenium, and the **carotenoids** (vitamin A precursors) may help block the initiation of cancer by acting as **antioxidants.** As described in Chapter 12, antioxidants prevent **free radicals** from damaging DNA. Vitamin C may also block the conversion of nitrates (food preservatives) into cancer-causing agents. Folic acid may inhibit the transformation of normal cells into malignant cells and strengthen immune function. Calcium inhibits the growth of cells in the colon and may slow the spread of potentially cancerous cells.

Many other anti-cancer agents in the diet fall under the broader heading of **phytochemicals,** substances in plants that help protect against chronic diseases. One of the first to be identified was **sulforaphane,** a potent anticarcinogen found in broccoli. Sulforaphane induces the cells of the liver and kidney to produce higher levels of protective

Table 16-1   Choosing Foods with Phytochemicals

Food	Phytochemical and Its Potential Anti-Cancer Effects
Chili peppers (Note: hotter peppers contain more capsaicin)	Capsaicin: Neutralizes the effect of nitrosamines; may block carcinogens in cigarette smoke from acting on cells
Citrus fruits (oranges, lemons, limes), onions, apples, berries, eggplant	Flavonoids: Act as antioxidants; block access of carcinogens to cells; suppress malignant changes in cells; prevent cancer cells from multiplying
Citrus fruits, cherries	Monoterpenes: Help detoxify carcinogens; inhibit spread of cancer cells
Cruciferous vegetables (broccoli, cabbage, bok choy, cauliflower, kale, brussels sprouts, collards)	Isothiocyanates: Boost production of cancer-fighting enzymes; suppress tumor growth; block effects of estrogen on cell growth
Garlic, onions, leeks, shallots, chives	Allyl sulfides: Increase levels of enzymes that break down potential carcinogens; boost activity of cancer-fighting immune cells
Grapes, red wine, peanuts	Resveratrol: Acts as an antioxidant; suppresses tumor growth
Green, oolong, and black teas (Note: drinking tea that is burning hot may *increase* cancer risk)	Polyphenols: Increase antioxidant activity; prevent cancer cells from multiplying; help speed excretion of carcinogens from the body
Orange or deep yellow, red or pink, and dark-green vegetables and some fruits	Carotenoids: Act as anitoxidants; reduce levels of cancer-promoting enzymes; inhibit spread of cancer cells
Soy foods, whole grains, flax seeds, nuts	Phytoestrogens: Block effects of estrogen on cell growth; lower blood levels of estrogen; inhibit angiogenesis
Whole grains, legumes	Phytic acid: Binds iron, which may prevent it from creating cell-damaging free radicals

enzymes, which then neutralize dietary carcinogens. Most fruits and vegetables contain beneficial phytochemicals, and researchers are just beginning to identify them. Some of the most promising are listed in Table 16-1.

To increase your intake of these potential cancer fighters, eat a wide variety of fruits, vegetables, legumes, and grains. Don't try to rely on supplements. Many of these compounds are not yet available in supplement form, and optimal intakes have not been determined. Like many vitamins and minerals, isolated phytochemicals may be harmful if taken in high doses. Beta-carotene pills, for example, may increase smokers' risk of lung cancer. In addition, it is likely that the anti-cancer effects of many foods are the result of many chemical substances working in combination. Some practical suggestions for maximizing your intake of anti-cancer agents are included in the Behavior Change Strategy at the end of the chapter.

Inactivity and Obesity

Several common types of cancer are associated with an inactive lifestyle, and research has shown a relationship between increased physical activity and a reduction in cancer risk. There is good evidence that exercise reduces the risk of colon cancer, perhaps by speeding the movement of food through the digestive tract, strengthening immune function, and decreasing blood fat levels. When young girls get adequate exercise, they tend to gain weight more slowly, menstruation begins later, and their risk of breast and ovarian cancers is reduced.

In addition, exercise is important because it helps prevent obesity, an independent risk factor for cancer. A high percentage of body fat appears to increase the risk of cancers of the prostate, breast, female reproductive tract, and

anticarcinogen An agent that destroys or otherwise blocks the action of carcinogens.   Terms

carotenoid Any of a group of yellow-to-red plant pigments that can be converted to vitamin A by the liver; many act as antioxidants or have other anticancer effects. The carotenoids include beta-carotene, lutein, lycopene, and zeaxanthin.

antioxidant A substance that can lessen the breakdown of food or body constituents; actions include binding oxygen and donating electrons to free radicals.

free radicals Electron-seeking compounds that can react with fats, proteins, and DNA, damaging cell membranes and mutating genes in their search for electrons; produced through chemical reactions in the body and by exposure to environmental factors such as sunlight and tobacco smoke.

phytochemical A naturally occurring substance found in plant foods that may help prevent chronic diseases such as cancer and heart disease; *phyto* means plant.

sulforaphane A compound found in cruciferous vegetables that can turn on the body's detoxifying enzyme system.

kidney and possibly the colon and gallbladder. Obesity may affect hormone levels in the blood, slow the transit time of food through the colon, change the way the body metabolizes fat, and generally promote cell growth. All of these actions have the potential to increase cancer risk.

In the United States, about 170,000 cancer deaths per year appear to be due to a combination of dietary habits and a sedentary lifestyle. One expert estimates that if we were all to exercise for 20 minutes each day and make the dietary changes discussed in this chapter, about 40,000 cancer deaths could be prevented each year.

Microbes

It is estimated that about 15% of the world's cancers are caused by microbes, including viruses, bacteria, and parasites, although the percentage is much lower in developed countries like the United States. As discussed earlier, certain types of human papillomavirus cause many cases of cervical cancer, and the *Helicobacter pylori* bacterium has been definitely linked to stomach cancer.

Viruses seem to be the main cancer causers. The Epstein-Barr virus, best known for causing mononucleosis, is also suspected of contributing to Hodgkin's disease, cancer of the pharynx, and some stomach cancers. Human herpesvirus 8 has been linked to Kaposi's sarcoma and certain types of lymphoma. Hepatitis viruses B and C together cause as many as 80% of the world's liver cancers. Hepatitis B is spread mainly through sexual intercourse, though it can be passed through contact with any body fluid or with contaminated needles. Hepatitis C is most commonly acquired through blood transfusions or injection drug use, but it, too, can be spread sexually. Although most people who develop hepatitis recover, up to 10% of people with hepatitis B and 85% of people with hepatitis C become chronic carriers of the virus and are at high risk for liver cancer. A vaccine for hepatitis B is available; the best way to avoid contracting these viruses is to limit the number of sex partners you have, practice safer sex, and avoid sharing needles. (See Chapters 17 and 18 for more information on hepatitis.)

Carcinogens in the Environment

Some carcinogens occur naturally in the environment, like the sun's UV rays. Others are manufactured or synthetic substances that show up occasionally in the general environment but more often in the work environments of specific industries.

Ingested Chemicals The food industry uses preservatives and other additives to prevent food from becoming spoiled or stale (see Chapter 12). Some of these compounds are antioxidants and may actually decrease any cancer-causing properties the food might have. Other compounds, like the nitrates and nitrites found in processed meat, are potentially more dangerous.

Nitrates and nitrites are added to foods like beer and ale, ham, bacon, hot dogs, and lunch meats. The nitrates inhibit the growth of bacteria, which could otherwise cause food poisoning. They also preserve the pink color of the meat, which has no bearing on taste but looks more appetizing to many people. While nitrates and nitrites are not themselves carcinogenic, they can combine with dietary substances in the stomach and be converted to **nitrosamines**, which are highly potent carcinogens. Foods cured with nitrites, as well as those cured by salt or smoke, have been linked to esophageal and stomach cancer, and they should be eaten only in modest amounts.

Environmental and Industrial Pollution Pollutants in urban air have long been suspected of contributing to the incidence of lung cancer. Fossil fuels and their combustion products, such as complex hydrocarbons, have been of special concern, and most gas stations are now required to provide special nozzles to reduce the amount of gasoline vapor released when you fill your tank. The effect of air pollutants has been difficult to study because of the overwhelmingly greater influence of smoking on lung cancer rates. Urban air pollution appears to have a measurable but limited role in causing lung cancer. (Chapter 24 has more information on the health effects of air pollution.)

The best available data indicate that less than 2% of cancer deaths are caused by general environmental pollution, such as substances in our air and water. Exposure to carcinogenic materials in the workplace is a more serious problem. Occupational exposure to specific carcinogens may account for up to 5% of cancer deaths. For example, diesel exhaust may contribute to lung cancer in truck operators and railroad workers, soot may cause skin cancer in firefighters and bricklayers, and hair dyes have been linked to bladder cancer in hairdressers and barbers. With increasing industry and government regulations, we can anticipate that the industrial sources of cancer risk will continue to diminish, at least in the United States. By contrast, in the former Soviet Union and Eastern European countries, where environmental concerns were sacrificed to industrial productivity for decades, cancer rates from industrial pollution continue to climb.

Radiation All sources of radiation are potentially carcinogenic, including medical X rays, radioactive substances (radioisotopes), and UV rays from the sun. Striking examples of the effects of radiation can be seen in the survivors of the atomic bombings of Hiroshima and Nagasaki in 1945 and in residents of the area surrounding the Cher-

Terms   **nitrosamine** A carcinogen made in the stomach from nitrates and nitrites.

More than 100 million Americans now use mobile or cellular phones, some for security and many more simply to stay connected wherever they are. Media reports have sparked concerns over whether the radiation emitted by these phones as they are pressed against users' heads is causing brain tumors.

It is important to remember that the radiation from these phones is non-ionizing radiation, a different type of radiation from that used for medical X rays (see Chapter 24). At high intensity, non-ionizing radiation causes local heating, and it is used for this purpose in microwave ovens. Cell phones generate much lower levels of heating: Studies of cell phone use have found that the increase in temperature of nearby brain cells is within the normal fluctuations of the brain's temperature.

Researchers have not found conclusive evidence of a link between cell phone use and brain cancer. In one study, the use of cell phones was weakly linked to a higher-than-expected rate of one rare form of brain tumor; however, the increase may have occurred by chance, particularly because with increased hours of phone use, the cancer risk tended to decrease rather than increase, as one would expect. In another study, mobile phone users who developed brain tumors tended to report using the phone on the side of the head where the tumor developed. However, the patients' reports may have been biased because they already knew where the brain cancer had developed. The majority of studies have found no link between cell phone use and brain cancer; however, because cell phones have been in wide use for only a few years, more studies will be needed in the future to check for long-term effects.

It is predicted that there will be as many as 1.6 billion cell phone users worldwide by 2005. In some parts of the world, cell phones are the most reliable or the only phones available.

The need for further research into their health effects was underscored by the World Health Organization, which has undertaken a study in more than 10 countries to identify links, if any, between cell phone use and head and neck cancers. The study is to be completed in 2003.

In light of concerns about radiation, phone manufacturers have agreed to provide information on packaging about the phone's specific absorption rate (SAR). (The SAR measures the maximum quantity of radiation absorbed by a kilogram of tissue from a phone.) This information will allow consumers to compare radiation levels. The U.S. government already requires that phones meet radiation safety standards and that manufacturers report their phones' SAR levels to regulators before the phones are approved for sale.

There have been conflicting reports about whether the use of earpieces reduces the amount of radiation absorbed from a phone. While one study reported a 90% drop in absorption when a hands-free device was used, another study concluded that the amount of radiation reaching the brain increased threefold. If you are concerned about the effects of cell phone use, consider restricting your use to short calls and emergencies until more conclusive evidence is available.

SOURCES: U.S. Food and Drug Administration. 2000. Cell phones and cancer: No clear connection. *FDA Consumer Magazine,* November–December. Is hands-free safer? 2000. *CHOICE,* August. Niiler, Eric. 2000. Worrying about wireless. *Scientific American,* September. World Health Organization. 2000. *More Information Necessary to Establish Health Effects of Mobile Phones,* June 28 (http://www.who.int/peh-emf/publications/facts_press/press_release_mobilephone.htm; retrieved November 2, 2000).

nobyl nuclear reactor that blew up in 1986. In Japan, new cancers, especially leukemias, are still occurring over 50 years after the bombings. In Belarus, Russia, and Ukraine, the areas most affected by the radioactive debris from Chernobyl, rates of thyroid cancer in children are as much as 30 times higher than before the explosion. Researchers have also found that people living near Chernobyl suffered genetic damage that is being passed on to their children.

The continuing cancer cases in survivors of Hiroshima, Nagasaki, and Chernobyl are a warning to us that any unnecessary exposure to ionizing radiation should be avoided. Most physicians and dentists are quite aware of the risk of radiation, and successful efforts have been made to reduce the amount of radiation needed for mammograms, dental X rays, and other necessary medical X rays. (See the box "Cell Phones and Brain Cancer: Is There A Link?" for information on the non-ionizing radiation emitted by cell phones.)

Another source of environmental radiation is radon gas. Radon is a radioactive decomposition product of radium, which is found in small quantities in some rocks and soils. Because radon is inhaled with the air we breathe, it comes into intimate contact with the cells of the lungs, where its radiation can produce mutations. Radon and smoking together create a more-than-additive risk of lung cancer. Fortunately, in most of our homes and classrooms, radon is rapidly dissipated into the atmosphere, and very low levels of radon do not appear to increase cancer risk. But in certain kinds of enclosed spaces, such as mines, some basements, and airtight houses built of brick or stone, it can rise to dangerous levels (see Chapter 24).

Sunlight is a very important source of radiation, but because its rays penetrate only a millimeter or so into the skin, it could be considered a "surface" carcinogen. Most cases of skin cancer are the relatively benign and highly curable basal cell carcinomas, but a substantial minority are the potentially deadly malignant melanomas. As discussed earlier, all types of skin cancer are increased by early and excessive exposure to the sun, and severe sunburn early in childhood appears to carry with it an added risk of melanoma later in life.

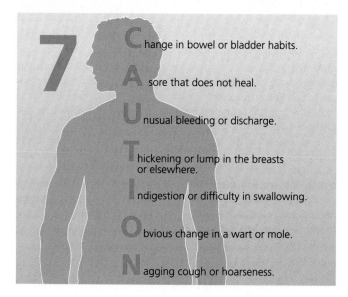

Figure 16-5   **The seven major warning signs of cancer.**

DETECTING, DIAGNOSING, AND TREATING CANCER

Early cancer detection often depends on our willingness to be aware of changes in our own body and to make sure we keep up with recommended diagnostic tests. Although treatment success varies with individual cancers, cure rates have increased—sometimes dramatically—in this century.

Detecting Cancer

Unlike those of some other diseases, early signs of cancer are usually not apparent to anyone but the person who has them. Even pain is not a reliable guide to early detection, because the initial stages of cancer may be painless. Self-monitoring is the first line of defense, and the American Cancer Society recommends that you watch for the seven major warning signs shown in Figure 16-5. Remember them by the acronym CAUTION.

Although none of the warning signs is a sure indication of cancer, the appearance of any one should send you to see your physician. By being aware yourself of the risk factors in your own life, including the cancer history of your immediate family and your own past history, you can often bring a problem to the attention of a physician long before it would have been detected at a routine physical.

In addition to self-monitoring, the ACS recommends routine cancer checkups, as well as specific screening tests for certain cancers (Table 16-2).

Diagnosing Cancer

Detection of a cancer by physical examination is only the beginning. Methods for determining the exact location, type, and degree of malignancy of a cancer continue to improve. Knowledge of the exact location and size of a tumor is necessary for precise and effective surgery or radiation therapy. This is especially true in cases where the tumor may be hard to reach, as in the brain.

A biopsy or exploratory surgery may be performed to identify a cancer's *stage*—a designation based on a tumor's size, location, and spread that helps determine appropriate treatment. New diagnostic imaging techniques have replaced exploratory surgery for some patients. In **magnetic resonance imaging (MRI)**, a huge electromagnet is used to detect hidden tumors by mapping, on a computer screen, the vibrations of different atoms in the body. **Computed tomography (CT)** scanning uses X rays to examine the brain and other parts of the body. The process allows the construction of cross sections, which show a tumor's shape and location more accurately than is possible with conventional X rays. For patients undergoing radiation therapy, CT scanning enables the therapist to pinpoint the tumor more precisely, thereby providing more accurate radiation dosage while sparing normal tissue.

Ultrasonography has also been used increasingly in the past few years to view tumors. It has several advantages: It can be used in the physician's office, it is less expensive than other imaging methods, and it is completely safe. Prostate ultrasound (a rectal probe using ultrasonic waves to produce an image of the prostate gland) is being investigated for its ability to detect small, hidden tumors that would be missed by a digital rectal exam.

Treating Cancer

The ideal cancer therapy would kill or remove all cancerous cells while leaving normal tissue untouched. Sometimes this is almost possible, as when a surgeon removes a small superficial tumor of the skin. Usually the tumor is less accessible, and some combination of surgery, radiation therapy, and chemotherapy must be applied instead. Some patients choose to combine conventional therapies with "alternative" treatments (see the box "Avoiding Cancer Quackery").

Table 16-2	Tests Recommended by the American Cancer Society for the Early Detection of Cancer in Asymptomatic People

Site	Recommendation
Cancer-related checkup	A cancer-related checkup is recommended every 3 years for people age 20–40 and every year for people age 40 or older. This exam should include health counseling and, depending on a person's age, might include examination for cancers of the thyroid, oral cavity, skin, lymph nodes, testes, and ovaries, as well as for some nonmalignant diseases.
Breast	Women age 20–39 should have a clinical breast exam (CBE) performed by a health care professional every 3 years and should perform monthly breast self-examination. Women 40 or older should have an annual mammogram, an annual CBE by a health care professional, and should perform monthly breast self-examination. The CBE should be conducted close to and preferably before the scheduled mammogram.
Colon and rectum	Beginning at age 50, men and women at average risk should follow one of these five examination schedules: (1) fecal occult blood test (FOBT) every year, (2) flexible sigmoidoscopy every 5 years, (3) FOBT every year and flexible sigmoidoscopy every 5 years, (4) double-contrast barium enema every 5 years, or (5) colonoscopy every 10 years. (Among the first three options, the ACS prefers option 3.) A digital rectal exam should be done at the same time as sigmoidoscopy, colonoscopy, or double-contrast barium enema. People who are at increased or high risk for colorectal cancer should talk with a physician about a different testing schedule.
Prostate	Beginning at age 50, the prostate-specific antigen (PSA) test and the digital rectal exam should be offered annually to men who have a life expectancy of at least 10 years. Men at high risk (African American men and men who have a first-degree relative who was diagnosed with prostate cancer at a young age) should begin testing at age 45.
Skin	All men and women should perform a monthly skin self-exam to look for early signs of skin cancer. A skin examination by a physician is recommended as part of a cancer-related checkup.
Testes	Men who choose to perform testicular self-exams should do so once a month.
Uterus	*Cervix:* All women who are or have been sexually active or who are 18 or older should have an annual Pap test and pelvic examination. After three or more consecutive satisfactory examinations with normal findings, the Pap test may be performed less frequently. Discuss the matter with your physician. *Endometrium:* Beginning at age 35, women with or at risk for hereditary non-polyposis colon cancer should be offered endometrial biopsy annually to screen for endometrial cancer.

SOURCES: American Cancer Society. 2001. *Cancer Facts and Figures, 2001.* Atlanta: American Cancer Society. Reprinted by permission of the American Cancer Society, Inc. American Cancer Society. 2000. *Testicular Cancer Detection and Symptoms* (http://www3.cancer.org/cancerinfo/load_cont. asp?st=ds&ct=41&language=english; retrieved April 20, 2001).

Surgery   For most cancers, surgery is the most useful therapy. In many cases, the organ containing the tumor is not essential for life and can be partially or completely removed. This is true especially for localized breast, prostate, or testicular cancer, where the surgical removal of one breast, the prostate gland, or one testicle may give a long-lasting cure. Surgery is less effective when the tumor involves cells of the immune system, which are widely distributed throughout the body, or when the cancer has already metastasized. In such cases, surgery must be combined with other techniques.

Chemotherapy   Chemotherapy, or the use of cell-killing drugs to destroy rapidly growing cancer cells, has been in use since the 1940s. Many of these drugs work by interfering with DNA synthesis and replication in rapidly dividing cells. Normal cells, which usually grow slowly, are not destroyed by these drugs. However, some normal tissues such as intestinal, hair, and blood-forming cells are always growing, and damage to these tissues produces the unpleasant side effects of chemotherapy, including nausea, vomiting, diarrhea, and hair loss.

Chemotherapy drugs are often used in combinations or with surgery. Recently, in a procedure called **induction chemotherapy,** physicians have begun to use chemotherapy before surgery, both to shrink the tumor and to kill any existing small metastases as soon as possible.

magnetic resonance imaging (MRI) A computerized imaging technique that uses a strong magnetic field and radio frequency signals to examine a thin cross section of the body; also known as *nuclear magnetic resonance imaging (NMR).*

computed tomography (CT) The use of computerized X ray images to create a cross-sectional depiction of tissue density.

induction chemotherapy The use of chemotherapy prior to surgery to shrink a cancerous tumor and prevent metastasis; sometimes eliminates the need for radical surgery.

Terms

Sometimes conventional treatments for cancer are simply not enough. A patient may be told that there is little conventional therapy can do, other than providing medication to ease pain. Even when therapy is available, it may be painful and even intolerable to some people. Not surprisingly, many cancer patients look for alternatives. These may be therapies within the bounds of legitimate medical practice that have not yet proven themselves in clinical trials. Or, at the other extreme, alternative therapies may be scientifically unsound and dangerous, as well as expensive.

The National Cancer Institute suggests that patients and their families consider the following questions when making decisions about cancer treatment:

- *Has the treatment been evaluated in clinical trials?* Advances in cancer treatment are made through carefully monitored clinical trials. If a patient wants to try a new therapy, participation in a clinical trial may be a treatment option. (See For More Information at the end of the chapter for more on clinical trials.)

- *Do the practitioners of an approach claim that the medical community is trying to keep their cure from the public?* No one genuinely committed to finding better ways to treat a disease would knowingly keep an effective treatment a secret or try to suppress such a treatment.

- *Does the treatment rely on nutritional or diet therapy as its main focus?* Although diet can be a key risk factor in the development of cancer, there is no evidence that diet alone can get rid of cancerous cells in the body.

- *Do those who endorse the treatment claim that it is harmless and painless and that it produces no unpleasant side effects?* Reputable researchers are working to develop less toxic cancer therapies, but because effective treatments for cancer must be very powerful, they frequently have unpleasant side effects.

- *Does the treatment have a "secret formula" that only a small group of practitioners can use?* Scientists who believe they have developed an effective treatment routinely publish their results in reputable journals so they can be evaluated by other researchers.

Some complementary approaches can benefit the patient without interfering with conventional treatments, such as art therapy, massage therapy, meditation, and yoga. It is always important that the patient inform the physician of any therapies being undertaken outside of the physician's care, so that any side effects or harmful interactions can be prevented.

SOURCES: American Cancer Society. 2000. *Complementary and Alternative Methods* (http://www.cancer.org/alt_therapy/index.html; retrieved November 2, 2000). Aulas, J. 1996. Alternative cancer treatments. *Scientific American*, September. National Cancer Institute. *Q and A About Complementary and Alternative Medicine in Cancer Treatment* (http://cancernet.nci.nih.gov; retrieved November 10, 2000).

Radiation   In cancer radiation therapy, a beam of X rays or gamma rays is directed at the tumor, and the tumor cells are killed. Occasionally, when an organ is small enough, radioactive seeds are surgically placed inside the cancerous organ to destroy the tumor and then removed later if necessary. Radiation destroys both normal and cancerous cells, but because it can be precisely directed at the tumor, it is usually less toxic for the patient than either surgery or chemotherapy, and it can often be performed on an outpatient basis. Radiation may be used as an exclusive treatment or in combination with surgery and/or chemotherapy.

New and Experimental Techniques   Many new and exciting possibilities for cancer therapy promise alternatives to the options of surgery, radiation, and chemotherapy. Although it is impossible to predict which of these new approaches will be most successful, researchers hope that cancer therapy overall will become increasingly safer and more effective.

- *Gene therapy.* Completion of the sequencing of the human genome in 2000 opened a treasure chest of new insights into cancer. Scientists have already discovered important new subtypes of tumors for breast cancer, melanoma, leukemia, and lymphomas based on patterns of gene expression. These patterns were revealed through the use of **gene chips,** which lay out thousands of specific DNA sequences on small glass chips for comparison with the sequences found in the tumor cells. Scientists can analyze which genes are present in the tumor, which have suffered mutations, and which are being expressed. Using this approach, researchers hope to develop a variety of powerful, targeted therapies for use in treatment of specific cancers, much as specific antibiotics are now used to treat specific bacterial diseases.

- *Bone marrow and stem cell transplants.* In cancers of the blood-forming cells or lymph cells, a patient's own bone marrow may have to be eliminated by radiation or chemotherapy to rid the body of cancer cells. Bone marrow can then be restored by transplanting healthy bone marrow cells from a compatible donor. Transplant incompatibility can be a problem, but progress on this front has been made recently through the use of **stem cells.** These unique, unspecialized cells can divide and produce more specialized cell types, including bone marrow cells. These stem cells can be identified, purified, and grown outside the body and then transplanted back into the cancer patient. This technique would allow

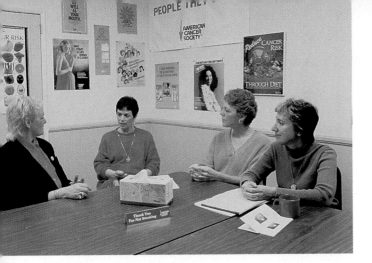

Social support can play a crucial role in cancer treatment for these patients. Studies indicate that support group participants have lower levels of anxiety and depression, manage pain more successfully, and possibly even live longer than cancer patients who are not in support groups.

for safe repopulation of bone marrow after radiation treatment.

- *Biological therapies.* Biological therapies are based on enhancing the immune system's reaction to a tumor. Techniques include cancer vaccines, genetic modification of the body's immune cells, and the use of genetically engineered **cytokines,** which enhance immune cell function. Melanomas seem particularly susceptible to these biological approaches.

- *Protease inhibitors.* To spread, cancer cells must activate a set of enzymes known as proteases, which enable them to dissolve the substances between cells and then migrate through normal tissues. **Protease inhibitors** are being developed to interfere with actions of specific proteases, thereby blocking cancer cells' ability to invade normal tissue and metastasize.

- *Anti-angiogenesis drugs.* To obtain nutrients, cancer cells signal the body to produce new blood vessels, a process called angiogenesis. Drugs that block angiogenesis could keep tumors from growing and spreading.

- *Telomerase inhibitors.* Normal human cells die after a limited number of divisions; cancer cells do not, in part because of the enzyme telomerase. Researchers hope to develop drugs to block the enzyme.

Living with Cancer

Earlier in this century, a diagnosis of cancer was almost equivalent to a death sentence. Gradually, however, survival has become the norm, and there are, in fact, 8.9 million cancer survivors in the United States today. However, for these people, the fear of cancer never completely disappears, and there is always the risk of a recurrence.

Cancer survivors may suffer economic prejudice from insurers, who can refuse to issue or renew health coverage. This sort of problem can be devastating to a cancer survivor who may be struggling both psychologically and financially to restore a normal existence. Several states have passed legislation to prevent this kind of discrimination, but it still exists.

Psychological support is an important factor during treatment for cancer (see the box "Coping with Cancer"). For some patients, family and friends plus a caring physician or nurse provide all the support that is necessary. But often, health care providers are busy or aloof, and family members and friends are just as fearful about the outcome as the patient. For many people, an organized support group can help provide needed social and psychological support. There is even some evidence that cancer patients may live longer when they become part of a professionally led support group (see the box "Support Groups and Cancer Survival"). The possibility that psychological health can enhance cancer survival is controversial, but no one doubts that support groups can promote emotional wellness in both patients and their families.

PREVENTING CANCER

Your lifestyle choices can radically lower your cancer risks, so you *can* take a very practical approach to cancer prevention (Figure 16-6).

Avoiding Tobacco

Smoking is responsible for 80–90% of all lung cancers and for about 30% of all cancer deaths. People who smoke two or more packs of cigarettes a day have lung cancer mortality rates 15–25 times greater than those of nonsmokers. The carcinogenic chemicals in smoke are transported throughout the body in the bloodstream, making smoking a carcinogen for many forms of cancer

gene chip Small glass chips on which tens of thousands of specific DNA sequences have been laid out in precise grids using a process similar to that used to make silicon chips.

stem cells Unspecialized cells that can divide and produce cells that differentiate into the many different types of specialized cells in the body (brain cells, muscle cells, skin cells, blood cells, and so on).

cytokine A chemical messenger produced by a variety of cell types that helps regulate many cell functions; immune system cells release cytokines that help amplify and coordinate the immune response.

protease inhibitor A drug that inhibits the action of any of the protein-splitting enzymes known as proteases. Because some proteases facilitate metastasis, protease inhibitors are being developed for cancer therapy.

Terms

Visiting a Cancer Patient

- Before you visit, call ahead to ask if it's a good time. Surprise visits are often not welcome. Don't overstay your welcome.

- Be a good listener. Allow the person to express all his or her feelings, and don't discount fears or minimize the seriousness of the situation. Let the patient decide whether the two of you talk about the illness. It's human to want to laugh and talk about other things sometimes.

- Ask "What can I get you?" or "How can I help?" instead of saying "Let me know if I can help." Make specific offers: to clean the bathroom, go grocery shopping, do laundry, or give caregivers a break.

- Refrain from offering advice. You may have heard about the latest treatment or hottest physician, but unless you are asked for suggestions, keep them to yourself.

- If you want to take food, ask about dietary restrictions ahead of time. Use a disposable container so the person doesn't have to worry about returning it.

- Don't be put off if your first visit gets a lukewarm reception. Many cancer victims are on an emotional roller coaster, and their feelings and needs will change over time.

If You Are the Patient

- Remember that cancer doesn't always mean death. Many cancers are curable or controllable for long periods, and survivors may return to a normal, healthy life. Hope and optimism can be important elements in cancer survival.

- Don't feel guilty if you can't keep a positive attitude all the time. Having cancer is difficult, and low moods will occur no matter how good you are at coping. But if they become frequent or severe, seek help.

- Use any strategies that have helped you solve problems and manage your emotions in the past. Some people respond to information gathering, talking with others, and prayer or meditation.

- Find a physician you trust and can communicate well with. Ask questions, and insist on being a partner in your treatment.

- Confide your worries to someone close to you. Don't bottle up your feelings to "spare" your loved ones. Ask someone you trust to accompany you on visits to your physician and treatment sessions.

- Explore groups that can help you get through this difficult time. There are many support groups for people who have cancer or who have survived it.

SOURCES: Life with cancer: How to provide support. 1996. *Women's Health Advocate.* September. Holland, J. C. 1996. Cancer's psychological challenges. *Scientific American,* September.

---

other than lung cancer. ETS is dangerous to nonsmokers. If you smoke, stop. If you don't smoke, avoid breathing the smoke from other people's cigarettes.

The use of spit tobacco, highly habit-forming because of its nicotine content, is also dangerous because it increases the risk of cancers of the mouth, larynx, throat, and esophagus. Refer to Chapter 11 for tips on breaking the tobacco habit.

Controlling Diet and Weight

Based on hundreds of studies, the National Cancer Institute estimates that about one-third of all cancers are in some way linked to what we eat. Choose a low-fat, plant-based diet containing a wide variety of fruits, vegetables, and whole grains rich in phytochemicals. See the specific suggestions in the Behavior Change Strategy at the end of this chapter.

Drink alcohol only in moderation, if at all. Oral cancer and cancers of the larynx, throat, esophagus, and liver occur more frequently among heavy drinkers of alcohol. The risk is even higher among heavy drinkers who smoke.

The risk of several cancers increases for obese people. Maintaining a healthy weight through a moderate diet and regular exercise lowers the risk. Chapters 12 and 14 provide strategies for improving your diet and maintaining a healthy body weight.

Regular Exercise

Regular exercise is linked to lower rates of colon and other cancers. It also helps control weight. Refer to Chapter 13 for advice on setting up a lifelong program of regular exercise.

Protecting Skin from the Sun

Almost all cases of nonmelanoma skin cancer are considered to be sun-related, and sun exposure is a major factor in the development of melanoma as well. Wear protective clothing when you're out in the sun, and use a sunscreen with an SPF rating of 15 or higher. Don't go to tanning salons; they do not provide "safe tans."

Avoiding Environmental and Occupational Carcinogens

Most medical X rays are adjusted to deliver the lowest dose of radiation possible without sacrificing image qual-

Stanford University psychiatrist Dr. David Spiegel and his colleagues carried out a 3-year study on women with advanced breast cancer to determine how participation in a support group would affect their psychological health. Women in the experimental group not only received standard medical care but also participated in weekly group therapy sessions. In the support group, women shared their fears, planned means of coping with the threat of death, grieved over the loss of group members, learned to control their pain with self-hypnosis, and looked for ways to live more fully in the time they had left.

At the conclusion of the study, researchers found that women in the study had, indeed, been helped by the support group. They were less anxious and depressed and were better able to control their pain than women in the control group, who received only standard medical treatment. The real surprise came several years later when Dr. Spiegel reexamined the data from this study. He found that the women who participated in the support group also lived on average more than twice as long from the start of the study than women in the control group.

How might support groups improve the survival as well as the psychological health of participants? Researchers have hypothesized several ways in which psychosocial support could be translated into changes in physical health:

- Social support may affect behavior, making patients in a support group more likely to engage in healthy behaviors such as eating well, exercising regularly, and getting plenty of sleep.

- Cancer patients who benefit from group support might interact more effectively with their physicians, eliciting more vigorous medical treatment.

- Support groups may buffer people against stress, cushioning the body from the effects of the stress response. Other studies have found that support groups are most beneficial for people who do not have a supportive spouse.

- Social support may be particularly helpful in reducing the negative effects of stress on the immune system: A strong immune system may enable the body to fight cancer more effectively.

Additional research should help clarify how support groups benefit cancer patients. In the meantime, this study can serve as a reminder of the powerful effects social support has on our physical and emotional well-being, whether we are coping with a life-threatening illness or the challenges of everyday life.

SOURCES: Helgeson, V. S., et al. 2000. Group support interventions for women with breast cancer: Who benefits from what? *Health Psychology* 19(2): 107–114. Spiegel, D., et al. 1998. Effects of psychosocial treatment in prolonging cancer survival may be mediated by neuroimmune pathways. *Annals of the New York Academy of Sciences* 840: 674–683. Spiegel, D. 1993. *Living Beyond Limits: New Hope and Help for Facing Life-Threatening Illness.* New York: Random House.

Do More

- Eat a varied, plant-based diet that is high in fiber-rich foods such as legumes and whole grains

- Eat 5–9 servings of fruits and vegetables every day, favoring foods from the following categories:
    Cruciferous vegetables
    Citrus fruits
    Berries
    Dark-green leafy vegetables
    Dark-yellow, orange, or red fruits and vegetables

- Be physically active

- Maintain a healthy weight

- Practice safer sex (to avoid HPV infection)

- Protect your skin from the sun with appropriate clothing and sunscreen

- Perform regular self-exams (breast self-exam, testicular self-exam, skin self-exam)

- Obtain recommended screening tests

Do Less

- Don't use tobacco in any form:
    Cigarettes
    Spit tobacco
    Cigars and pipes
    Bidis and clove cigarettes

- Avoid exposure to environmental tobacco smoke

- Limit consumption of fatty meats and other sources of saturated fat

- Avoid excessive alcohol consumption

- Limit consumption of salt

- Don't eat charred foods, and limit consumption of cured and smoked meats and meat and fish grilled in a direct flame

- Limit exposure to UV radiation from sunlight or tanning lamps or beds

- Avoid occupational exposure to carcinogens

Figure 16-6   Strategies for reducing your risk of cancer.

ity. Radiation from radon may pose a threat in some homes; remedial steps should be taken if tests indicate high levels of radon. A number of industrial agents that some people are exposed to on the job are associated with cancer, including nickel, chromate, asbestos, and vinyl chloride. Try to avoid occupational exposure to carcinogens, and don't smoke; the cancer risks of many of these agents increase greatly when combined with smoking.

Recommended Screening Tests

Your first line of defense against cancer involves the lifestyle changes described above that help you avoid cancer-causing agents. Your second line of defense involves having any cancers that do develop discovered as quickly as possible through regular self-exams and medical screening tests. Stay alert for the signs and symptoms that could indicate cancer (see Figure 16-5), and follow the American Cancer Society screening guidelines listed in Table 16-2. Both lifestyle changes and a program of early detection are important to your long-term health.

Tips for Today

Our knowledge about the causes of cancer has grown exponentially in the past few decades, and research in biology and genetics offers the hope of better cancer therapies in the future. A growing body of research also suggests that we can take an active role in preventing many cancers by adopting a wellness lifestyle. Exercise, diet, and awareness are three important keys to cancer prevention.

Right now you can

- Do a breast self-exam, if you are a woman, or a testicular self-exam, if you are a man.

- Plan to have two vegetables with dinner tonight, one of them broccoli, cauliflower, brussels sprouts, or kale.

- Put your sunscreen by the front door so you'll remember to apply it the next time you go out in the sun, or put a brimmed hat by the door or in the car.

- Memorize the seven major warning signs of cancer represented by the acronym CAUTION.

SUMMARY

- A malignant tumor can invade surrounding structures and spread to distant sites via the blood and lymphatic system, producing additional tumors.

- A malignant cell divides without regard for normal growth. As tumors grow, they produce signs or symptoms that are determined by their location in the body.

- One in two men and one in three women will develop cancer, but more than half will be cured.

- Lung cancer kills more people than any other type of cancer. Tobacco smoke is the primary cause.

- Colon and rectal cancer is linked to age, heredity, obesity, and a diet rich in red meat and low in fruits and vegetables. Most colon cancers arise from preexisting polyps.

- Breast cancer affects about one in nine women in the United States. Although there is a genetic component to breast cancer, diet and hormones are also risk factors.

- Prostate cancer is chiefly a disease of aging; diet and lifestyle probably are factors in its occurrence. Early detection is possible through rectal examinations, PSA blood tests, and sometimes ultrasound.

- Cancers of the female reproductive tract include cervical, uterine, and ovarian cancer. The Pap test is an effective screening test for cervical cancer.

- Abnormal cellular changes in the epidermis, often a result of exposure to the sun, cause skin cancer, as does chronic exposure to certain chemicals. Skin cancers occur as basal cell carcinoma, squamous cell carcinoma, and melanoma.

- Oral cancer is caused primarily by smoking, excess alcohol consumption, and use of spit tobacco. Oral cancers are easy to detect, but often hard to treat.

- Testicular cancer can be detected early through self-examination.

- Mutational damage to a cell's DNA can lead to rapid and uncontrolled growth of cells; mutagens include radiation, viral infection, and chemical substances in food and air.

- Cancer-promoting dietary factors include meat, certain types of fats, and alcohol.

- Diets high in fruits and vegetables are linked to a lower risk of cancer.

- Other possible causes of cancer include inactivity and obesity, certain types of infections and chemicals, and radiation.

- Self-monitoring and regular screening tests are essential to early cancer detection; early signs can be remembered by using the acronym CAUTION.

- Methods of cancer diagnosis include magnetic resonance imaging, computed tomography, and ultrasound.

- Treatment methods usually consist of some combination of surgery, chemotherapy, and radiation. Gene therapy, bone marrow and stem cell transplants, protease inhibitors, biological therapies, and drugs that inhibit angiogenesis or telomerase also hold promise as effective treatments.

When we think about the health benefits of fruits and vegetables, we usually focus on the fact that they are rich in carbohydrates, dietary fiber, and vitamins and low in fat. A benefit that we may overlook is that they contain specific cancer-fighting compounds, phytochemicals, that help slow, stop, or even reverse the process of cancer. The National Cancer Institute (NCI) reports that people who eat five or more servings a day of fruits and vegetables have half the risk of cancer of those who eat less than two; according to the NCI, five to nine servings per day is optimal. The NCI, along with industry groups, has developed a program to help more Americans increase their intake of fruits and vegetables to health-promoting levels—the "5 A Day for Better Health" program.

You don't have to make radical changes in your diet to increase the amount of fruits and vegetables you eat every day. Begin by monitoring your diet for 1–2 weeks to assess your current intake; then look for ways to incorporate these foods into your diet in easy and tasty ways. Here are some tips to get you started.

Breakfast

- Drink 100% juice every morning.
- Add raisins, berries, or sliced fruit to cereal, pancakes, or waffles. Top bagels with tomato slices.
- Try a fruit smoothie made from fresh or frozen fruit and orange juice or low-fat yogurt.

Lunch

- Choose vegetable soup or salad with your meal.
- Replace potato chips or french fries with cut-up vegetables.
- Add extra chunks of fruits or vegetables to salads.
- Try adding vegetables such as roasted peppers, cucumber slices, shredded carrots, avocado, or salsa to sandwiches.
- Drink tomato or vegetable juice instead of soda (watch for excess sodium).

Dinner

- Choose a vegetarian main course, such as stir-fry or vegetable stew. Have at least two servings of vegetables with every dinner.
- Microwave vegetables and sprinkle them with a little bit of Parmesan cheese.
- Substitute vegetables for meat in casseroles and pasta and chili recipes.

- At the salad bar, pile your plate with healthy vegetables and use low-fat or nonfat dressing.

Snacks and On the Go

- Keep "grab and eat" fruits and vegetables on hand (apples, plums, pears, and carrots).
- Keep small packages of dried fruit in the car (try dried apricots, peaches, and pears and raisins).
- Make ice cubes from 100% fruit juice and drop them into regular or sparkling water.
- Freeze grapes for a cool summer treat.

In the Grocery Store

- Stock up on canned, frozen, and dried fruits and vegetables when they go on sale. Buy fresh fruits and vegetables in season; they'll taste best and be less expensive.
- To save on preparation time, buy presliced vegetables and fruits and prepackaged salads.
- Try a new fresh fruit or vegetable every week.

The All-Stars

Different fruits and vegetables contribute different vitamins, phytochemicals, and other nutrients, so be sure to get a variety. The following types of produce are particularly rich in nutrients and phytochemicals:

- Cruciferous vegetables (broccoli, cauliflower, cabbage, bok choy, brussels sprouts, kohlrabi, turnips, etc.)
- Citrus fruits (oranges, lemons, limes, grapefruit, tangerines, etc.)
- Berries (strawberries, raspberries, blueberries, etc.)
- Dark-green leafy vegetables (spinach, chard, collards, beet greens, kale, mustard greens, romaine and other dark lettuces, etc.)
- Deep-yellow, orange, and red fruits and vegetables (carrots, pumpkin, sweet potatoes, winter squash, red and yellow bell peppers, apricots, cantaloupe, mangoes, papaya, etc.)

SOURCES: National Cancer Institute. 2000. *Eating 5 A Day: Steps to Sure Success* (http://www.5aday.gov/serving.html; retrieved November 2, 2000). The produce prescription. 2000. *Consumer Reports on Health,* December. Welland, D. 1999. Fruits and vegetables: Easy ways to five-a-day. *Environmental Nutrition,* June.

- Strategies for preventing cancer include avoiding tobacco; eating a varied, moderate diet and controlling weight; exercising regularly; protecting skin from the sun; avoiding exposure to environmental and occupational carcinogens; and getting recommended cancer screening tests.

1. Look through the foods listed in Table 16-1 and the Behavior Change Strategy and choose four or five that you don't typically eat. During the next week, make a point of trying each of the foods you've chosen.

2. Devise a plan for incorporating regular self-examinations for cancer (breast self-examination or testicle self-examination) into your life. What strategies will help you remember to do your monthly exam? How can you keep yourself motivated?

3. Interview your parents or grandparents about your family medical history. Are there any cases of cancer in your family, and has anyone died of cancer? Do you see any patterns?

JOURNAL ENTRY

1. In your health journal, list the positive behaviors that help you avoid cancer. How can you strengthen these behaviors? Also list the behaviors that tend to increase your risk, and plan ways to change them.

2. *Critical Thinking* Smoking is responsible for 85–90% of all lung cancers. Are tobacco companies in any way responsible for the high number of deaths from lung cancer each year? Or is each person entirely responsible for his or her own behavior and health? In your health journal, write a brief essay outlining your position on this issue. Then write a brief essay that supports the opposite viewpoint.

3. Make a list of risk factors for cancer over which you have no control, including heredity and personal history. Do these risk factors increase your risk for any cancers? If so, make a list of behaviors you can adopt that will lower your risk.

4. *Critical Thinking* Should people who inherit a genetic defect that increases their risk of cancer pay higher insurance premiums? Should companies be able to deny them employment or health, life, or disability insurance? Should people be held responsible for risk factors like heredity that they cannot control or only for risk factors they can control, such as smoking? What about risk factors like obesity that are due to a combination of heredity and lifestyle? Write an essay explaining your position.

FOR MORE INFORMATION

Books and Newsletters

American Cancer Society. 2000. *American Cancer Society's Guide to Complementary and Alternative Cancer Methods.* Atlanta, Ga.: American Cancer Society. *A scientific analysis of various complementary/alternative treatments for cancer.*

American Cancer Society and American Heart Association. 1999. *Living Well, Staying Well.* New York: Random House. *A practical guide to reducing cancer risk.*

American Institute for Cancer Research. 2000. *Stopping Cancer Before It Starts.* New York: Griffin. *Suggests research-based changes in diet and lifestyle to help prevent cancer.*

Cooper, G. M. 2001. *Elements of Human Cancer.* Sudbury, Mass.: Jones & Bartlett. *Provides a general overview of the biology and causes of cancer as well as information on specific types of cancers.*

Holland, J. C., and S. Lewis. 2000. *The Human Side of Cancer: Living with Hope, Coping with Uncertainty.* New York: HarperCollins. *A resource for dealing with the stresses and fears brought on by a serious illness.*

Prucha, E. J., ed. 2000. *Cancer Sourcebook.* Detroit: Omnigraphics. *Provides up-to-date information on the most common types of cancer.*

Organizations, Hotlines, and Web Sites

American Academy of Dermatology. Provides information on skin cancer prevention.

888-462-DERM
http://www.aad.org

American Cancer Society. Provides a wide range of free materials on the prevention and treatment of cancer.

800-ACS-2345
http://www.cancer.org

American Institute for Cancer Research. Provides information on lifestyle and cancer prevention, especially nutrition.

800-843-8114
http://www.aicr.org

Cancer Guide: Steve Dunn's Cancer Information Page. Links to many good cancer resources on the Internet and advice about how to make best use of information.

http://www.cancerguide.org

Cancer News. Provides links to news and information on many types of cancer.

http://www.cancernews.com

Clinical Trials. Information about clinical trials for new cancer treatments can be accessed at the following sites:

http://cancertrials.nci.nih.gov
http://www.centerwatch.com

Dole 5-A-Day/Nutrition Education. Provides resources for parents, children, and educators, including extensive nutrition information about fruits and vegetables.

http://www.dole5aday.com

EPA/UV Index. Information about the UV Index and the effects of sun exposure, with links to sites with daily UV Index ratings for cities in the United States and other countries.

http://www.epa.gov/ozone/uvindex/uvover.html

Food and Drug Administration, Center for Drug Evaluation and Research: Oncology Tools. Provides information about types of cancer, treatments, and clinical trials.

http://www.fda.gov/cder/cancer

Harvard Center for Cancer Prevention: Your Cancer Risk. Includes interactive risk assessments as well as tips for preventing common cancers.

http://www.yourcancerrisk.harvard.edu

National Cancer Institute. Provides information on treatment options, screening, and clinical trials and on the national "5 Day for Better Health Program" that promotes greater consumption of fruits and vegetables.

800-4-CANCER; 800-624-2511 (Cancer Fax)
http://www.nci.nih.gov
http://cancernet.nci.nih.gov
http://5aday.nci.nih.gov

New York Online Access to Health (NOAH)/Cancer. Provides information about cancer—causes, symptoms, types, treatments, clinical trials—and links to related sites.

http://www.noah-health.org/english/illness/cancer/cancer.html

Oncolink/The University of Pennsylvania Cancer Center Resources. Contains information on different types of cancer and answers to frequently asked questions.

http://www.oncolink.org

See also the listings in Chapters 10–14.

SELECTED BIBLIOGRAPHY

American Cancer Society. 2001. *Cancer Facts and Figures, 2001.* Atlanta: American Cancer Society.

American Institute for Cancer Research. 2000. *As Outdoor Grilling Season Begins, Cancer Experts Issue Yearly Warning,* May 17 (http://www.aicr.org/r051700.htm; retrieved November 3, 2000).

American Institute for Cancer Research. 2000. *New Survey: Older Americans Abandon Healthy Diets, Turn to Supplements for Lower Cancer Risk,* August 31 (http://www.aicr.org/r083100a.htm; retrieved November 13, 2000).

Anttila, T., et al. 2001. Serotypes of *Chlamydia trachomatis* and risk for development of cervical squamous cell carcinoma. *Journal of the American Medical Association* 285(1): 47–51.

Bonithon-Kopp, C., et al. 2000. Calcium and fibre supplementation in prevention of colorectal adenoma recurrence: A randomised intervention trial. *Lancet* 356(9238): 1300–1306.

Centers for Disease Control and Prevention. 2001. Trends in screening for colorectal cancer—United States, 1997 and 1999. *Morbidity and Mortality Weekly Report* 50(9): 162–165.

Cohen, J. H., A. R. Kristal, and J. L. Stanford. 2000. Fruit and vegetable intakes and prostate cancer risk. *Journal of the National Cancer Institute* 92(1): 61–68.

Fernandez, E., et al. 2001. Oral contraceptives and colorectal cancer risk: A meta-analysis. *British Journal of Cancer* 84(5): 722–727.

Food and Nutrition Science Alliance. 1999. *FANSA Statement on Diet and Cancer Prevention in the United States,* December (http://www.ift.org/resource/news/news_rel/FANSA/diet-cancer.shtml; retrieved November 13, 2000).

Garcia-Rodriguez, L. A., and C. Huerta-Alvarez. 2001. Reduced risk of colorectal cancer among long-term users of aspirin and nonaspirin nonsteroidal anti-inflammatory drugs. *Epidemiology* 12(1): 88–93.

Genetic testing for cancer: A complex decision. 2001. *Harvard Women's Health Watch,* February.

Hall, M. A. 2000. What are the positions and practices of insurance companies and HMOs when asked to pay or refer for genetic tests? *Looking Back at Five Years of Research: Conference on Cancer Genetics in the Ashkenazi Community to Examine Latest Findings in Areas of Frequency, Prevention, Treatment, Insurance and Genetic Testing,* September 25 (http://www.ajcongress.org/pages/RELS2000/SEP_2000/sep00_04.htm; retrieved November 13, 2000).

Han, S., and R. E. Peschel. 2000. Father-son testicular tumors: Evidence for genetic anticipation? A case report and review of the literature. *Cancer* 88(10): 2319–2325.

Johnston, C. 2000. Quantitative tests for human papillomavirus. *Lancet* 355(9222): 2179–2180.

Knekt, P., et al. 1999. Risk of colorectal and other gastro-intestinal cancers after exposure to nitrate, nitrite and N-nitroso compounds: A follow-up study. *International Journal of Cancer* 80(6): 852–856.

Lander, E. S., and R. A. Weinberg. 2000. Genomics: Journey to the center of biology. *Science* 287(5459): 1777–1782.

Marmorstein, L. Y., et al. 2001. A human BRCA2 complex containing a structural DNA binding component influences cell cycle progression. *Cell* 104(2): 247–257.

Meijers-Heijboer, E. J., et al. 2000. Presymptomatic DNA testing and prophylactic surgery in families with a BRCA1 or BRCA2 mutation. *Lancet* 355(9220): 2015–2020.

Murphy, M. E., et al. 2000. The effect of sunscreen on the efficacy of insect repellent: A clinical trial. *Journal of the American Academy of Dermatology* 43(2 Pt 1): 219–222.

National Human Genome Research Institute. 2000. *Hereditary Colon Cancer: Genetic Discoveries Offer Hope for Prevention* (http://www.nhgri.nih.gov/Policy_and_public_affairs/Communications/Publications/Maps_to_medicine/colon.html; retrieved May 10, 2000).

National Toxicology Program. 2000. *Ninth Report on Carcinogens.* Research Triangle Park, N.C.: U.S. Department of Health and Human Services.

Safe in the sun: How to enjoy the rays without getting burned. 2000. *Consumer Reports,* July.

Sano, T., and M. Sasako. 2001. Green tea and gastric cancer. *New England Journal of Medicine* 344(9): 675–676.

Screening for breast cancer. 2001. *Journal of the American Medical Association* 285(2): 246.

Slamon, D. J., et al. 2001. Use of chemotherapy plus a monoclonal antibody against HER2 for metastatic breast cancer that overexpresses HER2. *New England Journal of Medicine* 344(11): 783–792.

Strohsnitter, W. C., et al. 2001. Cancer risk in men exposed in utero to diethylstilbestrol. *Journal of the National Cancer Institute* 93(7): 545–551.

Verloop, J., M. A. Rookus, and F. E. van Leeuwen. 2000. Prevalence of gynecologic cancer in women exposed to diethylstilbestrol in utero. *New England Journal of Medicine* 342(24): 1838–1839.

Wohlfahrt J., and M. Melbye. 2001. Age at any birth is associated with breast cancer risk. *Epidemiology* 12(1): 68–73.

Ylitalo, N., et al. 2000. Consistent high viral load of human papillomavirus 16 and risk of cervical carcinoma in situ: A nested case-control study. *Lancet* 355(9222): 2194–2198.

Zenilman, J. M. 2001. Chlamydia and cervical cancer: A real association? *Journal of the American Medical Association* 285(1): 81–83.

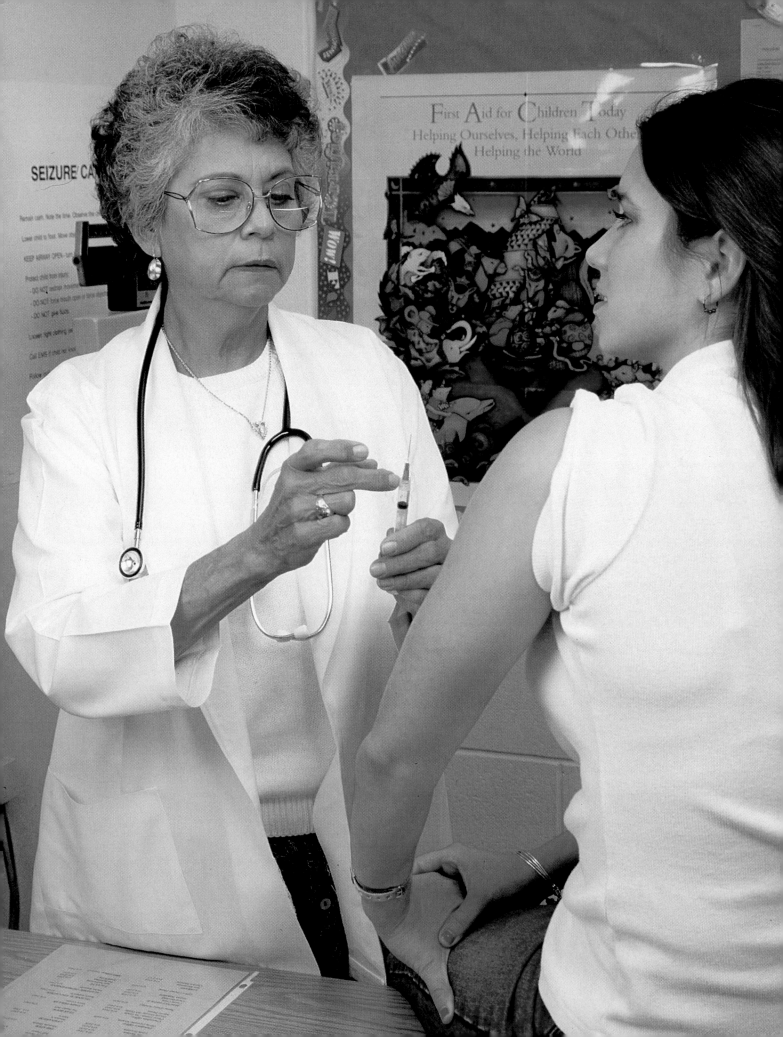

After reading this chapter, you should be able to

- Describe the step-by-step process by which infectious diseases are transmitted

- List the body's physical and chemical barriers to infection

- Explain how the immune system responds to an invading microorganism

- List the major types of pathogens and describe the common diseases they cause

- Discuss steps you can take to prevent infections and strengthen your immune system

Immunity and Infection

17

TEST YOUR KNOWLEDGE

1. A person with an infectious disease is not contagious unless he or she exhibits symptoms.
   True or false?

2. First-year college students, particularly those who live in dormitories or residence halls, are at moderately increased risk for contracting meningitis compared with others their age.
   True or false?

3. When taking a prescription antibiotic, you should stop taking the medicine as soon as your infection clears up.
   Ture or false?

4. Which of the following is most likely to increase your risk of catching a cold?
   a. Getting chilled or overheated
   b. Talking to someone who may have a cold
   c. Shaking hands with someone who may have a cold

5. Many stomach ulcers are caused by a bacterial infection.
   True or false?

6. You can lower your chances of getting sick by
   a. washing your hands frequently
   b. obtaining all recommended immunizations
   c. getting adequate sleep

ost of the time, we go about our daily lives thinking of the world as a place inhabited by beings more or less like ourselves. We seldom think of the countless, unseen microscopic organisms that live around, on, and in us. Although most microbes are beneficial, many of them can cause human disease. But the constant vigilance of our immune system keeps them at bay and our bodies intact and healthy.

Even without these "invaders," our bodies have a tendency to develop problems and diseases. The natural aging process of the human body is a prime example of the second law of thermodynamics: that all things have a tendency toward disorder or disintegration. The immune system works to keep the body from being overwhelmed not just by external invaders that cause **infections,** but also by internal changes, such as cancer.

Most people don't pay much attention to these internal skirmishes unless they become sick and find themselves deprived of their usual feelings of well-being. But many people today are more knowledgeable about the complexities of immunity because they have heard about, or had experience with, HIV infection, which directly attacks the immune system. This chapter provides information that will help you understand immunity, infection, and how to keep yourself well in a world of disease-causing microorganisms.

THE CHAIN OF INFECTION

Infectious diseases are transmitted from one person to another through a series of steps—a chain of infection (Figure 17-1). New infections can be prevented by interfering with any of the steps in this process.

Links in the Chain

The chain of infection has six major links: the pathogen, its reservoir, a portal of exit, a means of transmission, a portal of entry, and a new host.

Pathogen   The infectious disease cycle begins with a **pathogen,** a microorganism that causes disease. HIV, the virus that causes AIDS, and the tuberculosis bacterium

are examples of pathogens. Many pathogens cause illness because they produce **toxins** that harm human tissue; others do so by directly invading body cells.

Reservoir   The pathogen has a natural environment in which it typically resides. This so-called reservoir can be a person, an animal, or an environmental component like soil or water. A person who is the reservoir for a pathogen may be ill or may be an asymptomatic carrier who, although having no symptoms, is capable of spreading infection.

Portal of Exit   To transmit infection, the pathogen must leave the reservoir through some portal of exit. In the case of a human reservoir, portals of exit include saliva (for mumps, for example), the mucous membranes (for many sexually transmitted diseases), blood (for HIV and hepatitis), feces (for intestinal infections), and nose and throat discharges (for colds and influenza).

Means of Transmission   Transmission can occur directly or indirectly. In direct transmission, the pathogen is passed from one person to another without an intermediate component. Direct transmission usually requires fairly close association with an infected host, but not necessarily physical contact. For example, sneezing and coughing can discharge infectious particles into the air, where they can be inhaled by someone nearby. Most common respiratory infections are passed directly: A person with a cold blows her nose and gets some infectious droplets on her hands; she then shakes hands with someone, who later touches his nose and passes the pathogen into his own body. Many intestinal infections are also transmitted hand-to-hand; the initial contamination may result from a failure to wash hands after using the toilet or changing a diaper. Other means of direct transmission include sexual contact and contact with blood.

Transmission can also occur indirectly. Animals or insects such as rats, ticks, and mosquitoes can serve as **vectors,** carrying the pathogen from one host to another. Pathogens can also be transmitted via contaminated soil, food, or water or from inanimate objects, such as eating utensils, doorknobs, and handkerchiefs. Some pathogens float in the air for long periods, suspended on tiny particles of dust or droplets that can travel long distances before they are inhaled and cause infection.

Portal of Entry   To infect a new host, a pathogen must have a portal of entry into the body. Pathogens can enter in one of three general ways:

1. Penetration of the skin or direct contact.
2. Inhalation through the mouth or nose.
3. Ingestion of contaminated food or water.

Pathogens that enter the skin or mucous membranes can cause a local infection of the tissue, or they may penetrate into the bloodstream or **lymphatic system,** thereby

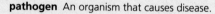

Terms

infection Invasion of the body by a microorganism.

pathogen An organism that causes disease.

toxin A poisonous substance produced by a microorganism.

vector An insect, rodent, or other organism that carries and transmits a pathogen from one host to another.

lymphatic system A system of vessels and organs that picks up excess fluid, proteins, lipids, and other substances from the tissues; filters out pathogens and other waste products; and returns the cleansed fluid to the general circulation.

systemic infection An infection spread by the blood or lymphatic system to large portions of the body.

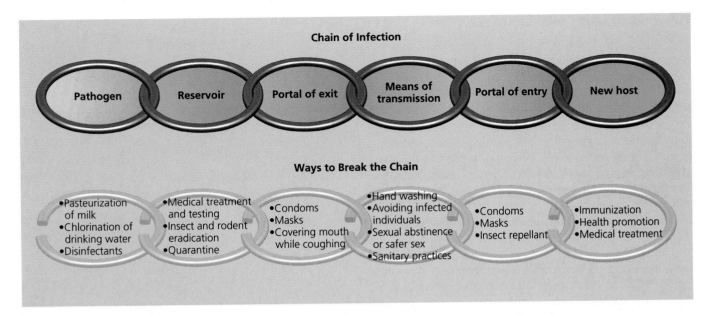

Figure 17-1 **The chain of infection.** Any break in the chain of infection can prevent disease.

causing a more extensive **systemic infection.** Agents that cause STDs usually enter the body through the mucous membranes lining the urethra (in males) or the cervix (in females). Organisms that are transmitted via respiratory secretions may cause upper respiratory infections or pneumonia, or they may enter the bloodstream and cause systemic infection. Foodborne and waterborne organisms enter the mouth and travel to the location that will best support their reproduction. They may attack the cells of the small intestine or the colon, causing diarrhea, or they may enter the bloodstream via the digestive system and travel to other parts of the body.

The New Host Once in the new host, a variety of factors determine whether the pathogen will be able to establish itself and cause infection. People with a strong immune system or resistance to a particular pathogen will be less likely to become ill than people with poor immunity (the concept of immunity will be discussed later in the chapter). The number of pathogens that enter the new host is also important; the body's defenses may be able to overcome a few bacteria, for example, but may be overwhelmed by thousands. If conditions are right, the pathogen will multiply and produce disease in the new host. In such a case, the new host may become a reservoir from which a new chain of infection can be started.

Breaking the Chain

Interruption of the chain of infection at any point can prevent disease. Strategies for breaking the chain include a mix of public health measures and individual action. For example, a pathogen's reservoir can be isolated or destroyed, as when a sick individual is placed under quar-

antine or when insects or animals carrying pathogens are killed. Public sanitation practices, such as sewage treatment and the chlorination of drinking water, can also kill pathogens. Transmission can be disrupted through strategies like hand washing and the use of facemasks. Immunization and the treatment of infected hosts can stop the pathogen from multiplying, producing a serious disease, and being passed on to a new host. Some methods of breaking the chain of infection are given in Figure 17-1.

> **COMMUNICATE!** People are sometimes reluctant to stay home from work when they have common communicable diseases, like a cold or the flu. However, it's legitimate and even advisable to stay home for a few days, until the infectious period has passed. Most employers are sympathetic, and you'll be doing your colleagues a favor. The next time you find yourself in this situation, think about calling in sick; for example, "I'm going to stay home today because I've caught a cold. If I can get some rest and avoid infecting the rest of the staff, I think it will be better for all of us in the long run."

THE BODY'S DEFENSE SYSTEM

Our bodies have very effective ways of protecting themselves against invasion by foreign organisms, especially pathogens. The body's first line of defense is a formidable array of physical and chemical barriers. When these barriers are breached, the body's immune system comes into play. Together, these defenses provide an effective response to nearly all the challenges and invasions our bodies will ever experience.

Physical and Chemical Barriers

The skin, the body's largest organ, prevents many microorganisms from entering the body. Although many bacterial and fungal organisms live on the surface of the skin, very few can penetrate it except through a cut or break. Wherever there is an opening in the body, or an area without skin, other barriers exist. The mouth, the main entry to the gastrointestinal system, is lined with mucous membranes, which contain cells designed to prevent the passage of unwanted organisms and particles. Body openings and the fluids that cover them (for example, tears, saliva, and vaginal secretions) are rich in antibodies (discussed in detail later in the chapter) and in enzymes that break down and destroy many microorganisms.

The respiratory tract is lined not only with mucous membranes but also with cells having hairlike protrusions called cilia. The cilia sweep foreign matter up and out of the respiratory tract. Particles that are not caught by this mechanism may be expelled from the system by a cough. If the ciliated cells are damaged or destroyed, as they are by smoking, a cough is the body's only way of ridding the airways of foreign particles. This is one reason smokers generally have a chronic cough—to compensate for damaged airways.

The Immune System

Once the body has been invaded by a foreign organism, an elaborate system of responses is activated. The immune system operates through a remarkable information network involving billions of cellular defenders who rush to protect the body when a threat arises. We discuss here two of the body's responses: the inflammatory response and the immune response. But before we cover these specific defenses, we'll briefly describe the defenders themselves and the mechanisms by which they work.

Immunological Defenders The immune response is carried out by different types of white blood cells, all of which are continuously being produced in the bone marrow. **Neutrophils,** one type of white blood cell, travel in the bloodstream to areas of invasion, attacking and ingesting pathogens. **Macrophages,** or "big eaters," take up stations in tissues and act as scavengers, devouring pathogens and worn-out cells. **Natural killer cells** directly destroy virus-infected cells and cells that have turned cancerous. **Lymphocytes,** of which there are several types, are white blood cells that travel in both the bloodstream and the lymphatic system. At various places in the lymphatic system there are lymph nodes (or glands), where macrophages congregate and filter bacteria and other substances from the lymph (Figure 17-2). When these nodes are actively involved in fighting an invasion of microorganisms, they fill with cells; physicians use the location of swollen lymph nodes as a clue to the location and cause of an infection.

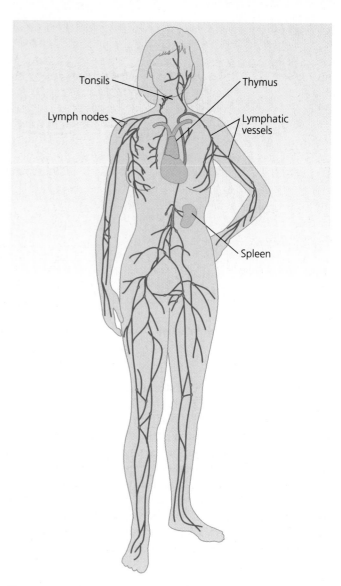

Figure 17-2 The lymphatic system. The lymphatic system consists of a network of vessels and organs, including the spleen, lymph nodes, thymus, and tonsils. The vessels pick up excess fluid and proteins, lipids, and other particles from body tissues. These pass through the lymph nodes, where lymphocytes and macrophages help clear the fluid (lymph) of debris and bacteria and other pathogens. The cleansed lymph is then returned to the bloodstream. The lymphatic organs are production centers for infection-fighting cells and sites for some immune responses.

The two main types of lymphocytes are known as **T cells** and **B cells.** T cells are further differentiated into **helper T cells, killer T cells,** and **suppressor T cells.** B cells are lymphocytes that produce **antibodies.** The first time T cells and B cells encounter a specific invader, some of them are reserved as **memory T and B cells,** enabling the body to mount a rapid response should the same invader appear again in the future. These cells and cell products—macrophages, natural killer cells, T cells, B cells and antibodies, and memory cells—are the primary players in the body's immune response.

The immune system is built on a remarkable feature of these defenders: the ability to distinguish foreign cells from the body's own cells. Because lymphocytes are capable of great destruction, it is essential that they not attack the body itself. When they do, they cause **autoimmune diseases,** such as lupus and rheumatoid arthritis.

How do lymphocytes know when they have encountered foreign substances? All the cells of an individual's body display markers on their surfaces—tiny molecular shapes—that identify them as "self" to lymphocytes that encounter them. Invading microorganisms also display markers on their surface; lymphocytes identify these as foreign, or "nonself." Nonself markers that trigger the immune response are known as **antigens.**

Antibodies have complementary surface markers that work with antigens like a lock and key. When an antigen appears in the body, it eventually encounters an antibody with a complementary pattern; the antibody locks onto the antigen, triggering a series of events designed to destroy the invading pathogen. The truly astonishing thing is that the body does not synthesize the appropriate antibody lock after it comes into contact with the antigen key. Rather, antibodies already exist for millions, if not billions, of possible antigens.

The Inflammatory Response

When the body has been injured or infected, one of the body's responses is the inflammatory response. Special cells in the area of invasion or injury release **histamine** and other substances that cause blood vessels to dilate and fluid to flow out of capillaries into the injured tissue. This produces increased heat, swelling, and redness in the affected area. White blood cells, including neutrophils and macrophages, are drawn to the area and attack the invaders—in many cases, destroying them. At the site of infection there may be pus, a collection of dead white blood cells and debris resulting from the encounter.

The Immune Response

The immune system can make two types of responses to invading pathogens: natural (innate) and acquired (adaptive). Neutrophils, macrophages, and natural killer cells are part of the natural response. They recognize pathogens as "foreign" but have no memory of past infections; they respond the same way no matter how many times a pathogen invades. These cells essentially "eat" the invaders, destroying them internally. Natural killer cells also destroy infected body cells, breaking the chain of reproduction of a pathogen and helping to stop an infection. T and B cells are part of the acquired response. They change after one contact with the pathogen, developing a memory for the antigen. If the body is invaded again, they recognize the pathogen and mount a much more potent response. Both natural and acquired responses occur each time the immune system is activated.

For convenience, we can think of the immune response as having four phases: (1) recognition of the invading pathogen, (2) amplification of defenses, (3) attack, and (4) slowdown (Figure 17-3). In each phase, crucial actions occur that are designed to destroy the invader and restore the body to health.

- *Phase 1.* Macrophages are drawn to the site of the injury and consume the foreign cells; they then provide information about the pathogen by displaying its antigen on their surfaces. Helper T cells "read" this information and rush to respond.

- *Phase 2.* Helper T cells multiply rapidly and trigger the production of killer T cells and B cells in the spleen and lymph nodes. **Cytokines,** chemical messengers secreted by lymphocytes, help regulate and coordinate the immune response; *interleukins* and *interferons* are two examples of cytokines. They stimulate increased production of T cells, B cells, and antibodies; promote the activities of natural killer cells; produce fever; and have special antipathogenic properties themselves.

Terms

neutrophil A type of white blood cell that engulfs foreign organisms and infected, damaged, or aged cells; particularly prevalent during the inflammatory response.

macrophage A large phagocytic (cell-eating) cell that devours foreign particles.

natural killer cell A type of white blood cell that directly destroys virus-infected cells and cancer cells.

lymphocytes A white blood cell continuously made in lymphoid tissue as well as in bone marrow.

T cell A lymphocyte that arises in bone marrow and matures in the thymus (thus its name).

B cell A lymphocyte that matures in the bone marrow and produces antibodies.

helper T cell A lymphocyte that helps activate other T cells and may help B cells produce antibodies.

killer T cell A lymphocyte that kills body cells that have been invaded by foreign organisms; also can kill cells that have turned cancerous.

suppressor T cell A lymphocyte that inhibits the growth of other lymphocytes.

antibody A specialized protein, produced by white blood cells, that can recognize and neutralize specific microbes.

memory T and B cells Lymphocytes generated during an initial infection that circulate in the body for years, "remembering" the specific antigens that caused the infection and quickly destroying them if they appear again.

autoimmune disease A disease in which the immune system attacks the person's own body.

antigen A marker on the surface of a foreign substance that immune system cells recognize as nonself and that triggers the immune response.

histamine A chemical responsible for the dilation and increased permeability of blood vessels in allergic reactions.

cytokine A chemical messenger produced by a variety of cell types that helps regulate many cell functions; immune system cells release cytokines that help amplify and coordinate the immune response.

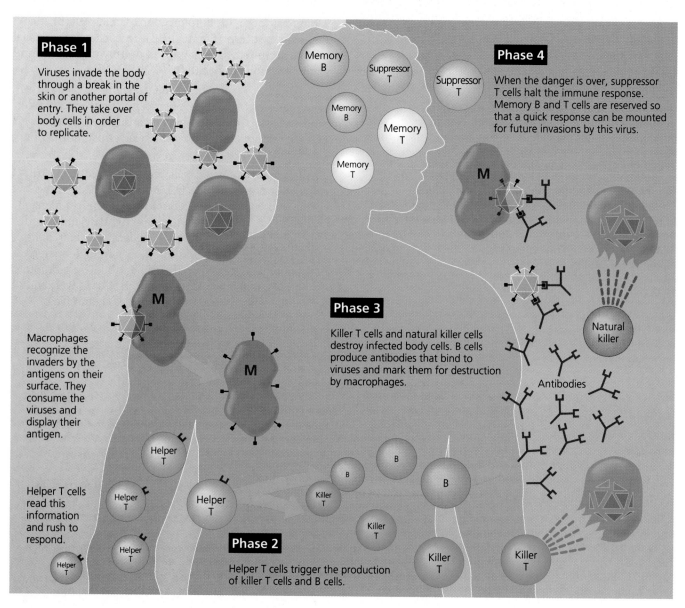

Phase 1

Viruses invade the body through a break in the skin or another portal of entry. They take over body cells in order to replicate.

Macrophages recognize the invaders by the antigens on their surface. They consume the viruses and display their antigen.

Helper T cells read this information and rush to respond.

Phase 2

Helper T cells trigger the production of killer T cells and B cells.

Phase 3

Killer T cells and natural killer cells destroy infected body cells. B cells produce antibodies that bind to viruses and mark them for destruction by macrophages.

Antibodies

Phase 4

When the danger is over, suppressor T cells halt the immune response. Memory B and T cells are reserved so that a quick response can be mounted for future invasions by this virus.

Figure 17-3   The immune response.   Once invaded by a pathogen, the body mounts a complex series of reactions to eliminate the invader. Pictured here are the principal elements of the immune response to a virus; not shown are the many types of cytokines that help coordinate the actions of different types of defenders.

• *Phase 3.* Killer T cells strike at foreign cells and body cells that have been invaded and infected, identifying them by the antigens displayed on the cell surfaces. Puncturing the cell membrane, they sacrifice body cells in order to destroy the foreign organism within. This type of action is known as a *cell-mediated immune response,* because the attack is carried out by cells. Killer T cells also trigger an amplified inflammatory response and recruit more macrophages to help clean up the site.

B cells work in a different way. Stimulated to multiply by helper T cells, they produce large quantities of antibody molecules, which are released in the blood-stream and tissues. Antibodies are Y-shaped protein molecules that bind to antigen-bearing targets and mark them for destruction by macrophages. This type of response is known as an *antibody-mediated immune response.* Antibodies work against bacteria and against viruses and other substances when they are in the body but outside cells. They do not work against infected body cells or viruses that are replicating inside cells.

• *Phase 4.* The last phase of the immune response is a slowdown of activity. When the danger is over, suppressor T cells halt the immune response and restore stability, or homeostasis. Dead cells, killed

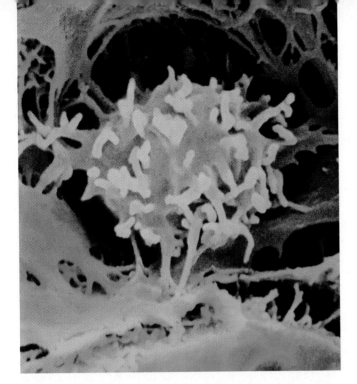

Macrophages are large, phagocytic (cell-eating) white blood cells that devour pathogens and worn-out body cells. The macrophage shown in this scanning electron micrograph is magnified 3350 times.

pathogens, and other debris that result from the immune response are scavenged by certain types of white blood cells; filtered out of circulation by the liver, spleen, and kidneys; and excreted from the body.

Immunity   In many infections, survival confers **immunity**; that is, an infected person will never get the same illness again. This is because some of the lymphocytes created during the amplification phase of the immune response are reserved as memory T and B cells. As part of the acquired immune response, they continue to circulate in the blood and lymphatic system for years or even for the rest of the person's life. If the same antigen enters the body again, the memory T and B cells recognize and destroy it before it can cause illness. This subsequent response takes only a day or two, whereas the original response lasted several days, during which time the individual suffered the symptoms of illness. The ability of memory lymphocytes to remember previous infections is known as **acquired immunity.**

Symptoms and Contagion   The immune system is operating at the cellular level within your body all the time, maintaining its vigilance when you're well and fighting invaders when you're sick. How does it all feel to you, the host for these activities? How do your symptoms relate to the course of the infection and the immune response?

During **incubation,** when viruses are multiplying in the body or when bacteria are actively multiplying before the immune system has gathered momentum, you may not have any symptoms of the illness, but you may be contagious. During the second and third phases of the immune response, you may still be unaware of the infection, or you may "feel a cold coming on." Symptoms first appear during the **prodromal period,** which follows incubation. If the infected host has prior immunity, the infection may be eradicated during the incubation period or prodromal period. In this case, although you may have felt you were coming down with a cold, for example, it does not develop into a full-blown illness.

Many of the symptoms of an illness are actually due to the immune response of the body rather than to the actions or products of the invading organism. For example, fever is thought to be caused by the release and activation of certain cytokines in macrophages and other cells during the immune response. Cytokines travel in the bloodstream to the brain, where they cause the body's thermostat to be "reset" to a higher level. The resulting elevated temperature is thought to help the body in its fight against pathogens by enhancing immune responses. (During an illness, it is necessary to lower a fever only if it is uncomfortably high [over 101.5°F] or if it occurs in an infant who is at risk for seizures from fever.)

Similarly, you get a runny nose when your lymphocytes destroy infected mucosal cells, leading to increased mucus production. You get a sore throat when your lymphocytes destroy infected throat cells, and the malaise and fatigue of the flu may be caused by interferons.

You are contagious when there are active microbes replicating in your body and they can gain access to another person. This may be before a vigorous immune response has occurred, so at times you may be contagious before experiencing any symptoms. This means that you can transmit an illness without knowing you're infected or catch an illness from someone who doesn't appear to be sick. On the other hand, your symptoms may continue after the pathogens have been mostly destroyed, when you are no longer infectious.

Terms

immunity Mechanisms that defend the body against infection; specific defenses against specific pathogens.

acquired immunity The body's ability to mobilize the cellular "memory" of an attack by a pathogen to throw off subsequent attacks; acquired through vaccination as well as the normal immune response.

incubation The period when bacteria or viruses are actively multiplying inside the body's cells; usually a period without symptoms of illness.

prodromal period The stage of an infection, following incubation, during which initial symptoms begin to appear but the host does not feel ill; a highly contagious period.

WWW. Immunization

The ability of the immune system to remember previously encountered organisms and retain its strength against them is the basis for immunization. When a person is immunized against a disease, the immune system is "primed" with an antigen similar to the pathogenic organism but not as dangerous. The body responds by producing antibodies to the organism, which prevent serious infection when and if the person is exposed to the disease itself. These preparations used to manipulate the immune system are known as **vaccines** (Table 17-1).

Vaccines can be made in several ways. In some cases, microbes are cultured in the laboratory in a way that weakens (attenuates) them. These "live, attenuated" organisms are used in vaccines against such diseases as measles, mumps, and rubella (German measles). In other cases, when it is not possible to breed attenuated organisms, vaccines are made from pathogens that have been killed in the laboratory but that still retain their ability to stimulate the production of antibodies. Vaccines composed of "killed" viruses are used against influenza viruses, among others.

Vaccines confer what is known as *active immunity*—that is, the vaccinated person produces his or her own antibodies to the microorganism. Another type of injection confers *passive immunity*. In this case, a person exposed to a disease is injected with the antibodies themselves, produced by other human beings or animals who have recovered from the disease. Injections of gamma globulin—a product made from the blood plasma of many individuals, containing all the antibodies they have ever made—are sometimes given to people exposed to a disease against which they have not been immunized. Such injections create a rapid but temporary immunity and are useful against certain viruses, such as hepatitis A. Gamma globulin is also sometimes used to treat antibody deficiency syndromes.

WWW. Allergy: The Body's Defense System Gone Haywire

Are you among the estimated 50 million Americans affected by **allergies**? Allergies result from a hypersensitive and overactive immune system. The immune system typically defends the body against only genuinely harmful pathogens such as viruses and bacteria. However, in someone with an allergy, the immune system also mounts a response to a harmless substance such as pollen or animal dander. The unpleasant and potentially serious symptoms of an allergy—stuffy nose, sneezing, wheezing, skin rashes, and so on—result primarily from the immune response rather than from the substances that provoke the response.

Allergens Substances that provoke allergies are known as **allergens;** they may cause a response if they are inhaled or swallowed or if they come in contact with the skin. Different people have allergic reactions to different substances. Common allergens include the following:

- *Pollen:* Referred to as hay fever or allergic rhinitis, pollen allergies are widespread; weeds, grasses, and trees are common producers of allergenic pollen.

- *Animal dander:* People with animal allergies are usually allergic not to fur but to dander (dead skin flakes), urine, or a protein found in saliva; allergies to mice, dogs, and/or cats are common.

- *Dust mites and cockroaches:* The droppings of microscopic dust mites can trigger allergies; mites live in carpets, upholstered furniture, and bedding. Cockroach droppings may also cause allergies.

- *Molds and mildew:* The small spores produced by these fungi can trigger allergy symptoms; molds and mildew thrive in damp areas of buildings.

- *Foods:* The most common food allergens in adults include peanuts, tree nuts, fish, and shellfish.

- *Insect stings:* The venom of insects such as yellow jackets, honeybees, hornets, paper wasps, and fire ants causes allergic reactions in some people.

People may also be allergic to certain medications, plants such as poison oak, metals such as nickel, latex, and compounds found in cosmetics.

The Allergic Response Most allergic reactions are due to the production of a special type of antibody known as immunoglobulin E (IgE). Initial exposure to a particular allergen may cause little response, but it sensitizes the immune system by causing the production of allergen-specific IgE, which binds to mast cells (Figure 17-4). When the body is subsequently exposed to the allergen, the allergen binds to IgE, causing the mast cells to release large amounts of histamine and other compounds into surrounding tissues.

Histamine has many effects, including increasing the inflammatory response and stimulating mucus production. The precise symptoms depend on what part of the body is affected. In the nose, histamine may cause congestion and sneezing; in the eyes, itchiness and tearing; in the skin, redness, swelling, and itching; in the intestines, bloating and cramping; and in the lungs, coughing, wheezing, and shortness of breath. In some people, an allergen can trigger an asthma attack (see the box "Asthma"). Symptoms often

---

Terms

vaccine A preparation of killed or weakened microorganisms, inactivated toxins, or components of microorganisms that is administered to stimulate an immune response; a vaccine protects against future infection by the pathogen.

allergy A disorder caused by the body's exaggerated response to foreign chemicals and proteins; also called hypersensitivity.

allergen A substance that triggers an allergic reaction.

anaphylaxis A severe systemic hypersensitive reaction to an allergen characterized by difficulty breathing, low blood pressure, heart arrhythmia, seizure, and sometimes death.

Table 17-1	Immunizations for Children and Adults

Vaccine	People for Whom Immunization Is Recommended
Diphtheria	All children; adults need boosters every 10 years
H. influenzae type b (Hib)	All children (protects against meningitis)
Hepatitis A	Children in selected states and regions; injection drug users, men who have sex with men, people with chronic hepatitis, and others at risk
Hepatitis B	All children and unvaccinated adolescents; adults at risk, including health care workers, household contacts and sex partners of infected people, injection drug users, and people with STDs
Influenza	Annual vaccination for adults age 50 and older; nursing home residents; anyone with heart, lung, or other chronic disorders (including asthma and diabetes) and others at high risk; women who will be in the second or third trimester of pregnancy during the influenza season; anyone over 6 months of age who wishes to reduce risk of influenza
Lyme disease	Adults over 15 with frequent or prolonged exposure to ticks in areas where Lyme disease is common
Measles and mumps	All children; unvaccinated adults born after 1956 who are not immune (those who received only one dose or were vaccinated between 1963 and 1967 may need revaccination)
Pertussis (whooping cough)	All children
Pneumococcal polysaccharide	Adults age 65 and older; anyone with chronic heart or lung disease or with no functional spleen; others at high risk, including Alaska Natives and certain American Indian groups
Pneumococcal conjugate	All children
Polio	All children; adults at risk, including certain laboratory and health care workers
Rabies	Anyone at risk from a bite, scratch, or mucous membrane exposure to a potentially rabid animal or from any direct contact with a bat (unless the person can be certain that exposure did not occur); people who work with animals may need preexposure immunization
Rubella (German measles)	All children; unvaccinated adults who are not immune, especially women
Tetanus (lockjaw)	All children; adults need boosters every 10 years (sooner if more than 5 years has elapsed since the previous booster and the individual has a contaminated wound)
Varicella (chicken pox)	Children over age 12 months; unvaccinated adolescents and adults who have not had varicella, especially health care workers and others at high risk for exposure

The CDC recommends that first-year college students who want to reduce their risk for meningococcal disease be vaccinated with the meningococcal polysaccharide vaccine. For international travelers, the CDC recommends that all standard childhood immunizations be up to date and that additional vaccines such as hepatitis A and influenza be considered. Travelers to areas where certain diseases are common may need others, including vaccines for yellow fever, typhoid fever, meningococcal meningitis, and Japanese or tickborne encephalitis; a one-time polio booster may also be given. Further information about immunization is available from the CDC's National Immunization Program (800-CDC-SHOT; http://www.cdc.gov/nip) and the CDC's Travel Information (877-394-8747; http://www.cdc.gov/travel).

SOURCES: Centers for Disease Control and Prevention. 2001. Recommended childhood immunization schedule. *Morbidity and Mortality Weekly Report* 50(1): 7–10. Centers for Disease Control and Prevention. 2000. Meningococcal disease and college students. *MMWR Recommendations and Reports* 49(RR-7). Centers for Disease Control and Prevention. 2000. *Summary of Adolescent/Adult Immunization Recommendations* (http:www.cdc.gov/nip/recs/adult-schedule.pdf; retrieved May 1, 2001). Centers for Disease Control and Prevention. 1999. Availability of Lyme disease vaccine. *Morbidity and Mortality Weekly Report* 48(2): 35–36, 43. Centers for Disease Control and Prevention. 1999. Human rabies prevention—Recommendations of the Advisory Committee on Immunization Practices. *MMWR Recommendations and Reports* 48(RR-1).

occur immediately, within minutes of exposure, but inflammatory reactions may take hours or days to develop and then may persist for several days.

The most serious, but rare, kind of allergic reaction is **anaphylaxis,** which results from a release of histamine throughout the body. Anaphylactic reactions can be life-threatening because symptoms may include swelling of the throat, extremely low blood pressure, fainting, heart arrhythmia, and seizures. Anaphylaxis is a medical emergency, and treatment requires immediate injection of epinephrine. People at risk for anaphylaxis should wear medical alert identification and keep self-administrable epinephrine readily available.

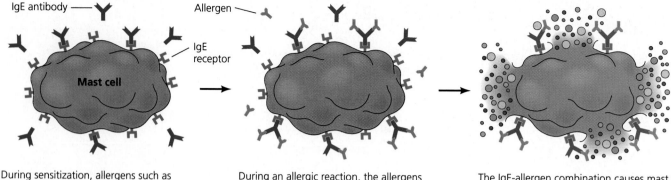

During sensitization, allergens such as pollen trigger the production of IgE antibodies, which bind to mast cells.

During an allergic reaction, the allergens enter the bloodstream and are recognized and bound by the IgE antibodies.

The IgE-allergen combination causes mast cells to release histamine and other compounds into surrounding tissue, producing allergy symptoms.

Figure 17-4   The allergic response.

Dealing with Allergies   If you suspect you might have an allergy, visit your physician or an allergy specialist. You may be asked to keep a diary to help identify allergens to which you are susceptible, or you may undergo allergy skin tests or blood tests. Your physician can help you put together a plan for your condition. There are three general strategies for dealing with allergies:

• *Avoidance:* You may be able to avoid or minimize exposure to allergens by making changes in your environment or behavior. For example, removing carpets from the bedroom and using special bedding can reduce dust mite contact. Pollen exposure can be limited by avoiding outdoor activities during peak pollination times and by showering and changing clothes following outdoor activities.

• *Medication:* A variety of medications are available for allergy sufferers. Many over-the-counter (OTC) antihistamines are effective at controlling symptoms, but the side effect of sedation may limit your daytime use of these medications; nonsedating antihistamines are available with a prescription. OTC decongestants may be useful for symptoms such as blocked nasal, sinus, or middle ear passages. Prescription corticosteroids markedly reduce allergy symptoms, but they have significant side effects, including reduced bone density, if used for long periods. Drug manufacturers have designed aerosol delivery systems for corticosteroids that help limit systemic absorption and side effects.

• *Immunotherapy:* Referred to as "allergy shots," immunotherapy desensitizes a person to a particular allergen through the administration of gradually increasing

doses of the allergen over a period of months or years. Allergy symptoms often diminish markedly during the period in which the person receives the injections and sometimes for years afterward.

> **COMMUNICATE!**   Do you have any life-threatening allergies—for example, to penicillin, bee stings, or shellfish? If so, make sure you've communicated the information to the appropriate parties. Inform your spouse or partner, your personal physician or health care professional, the medical or human relations department at work, the medical department of your school, and the person responsible for record keeping in any other organizations to which you belong. You might also want to carry a wallet card listing any such allergies.

THE TROUBLEMAKERS: PATHOGENS AND DISEASE

Now that we've discussed the intricate system that protects us from disease, let's consider some pathogens, the disease-producing organisms that live within us and around us. When they succeed in gaining entry to body tissue, they can cause illness and sometimes death to the unfortunate host. Worldwide, infectious diseases are responsible for more than 13 million deaths each year (Table 17-2).

Pathogens include bacteria, viruses, fungi, protozoa, parasitic worms, and prions (Figure 17-5). Infections can occur almost anywhere in or on the body; common types of infection include bronchitis, infection of the airways (bronchi); meningitis, infection of the tissue surrounding the brain and spinal cord; conjunctivitis, infection of the layer of cells surrounding the eyes; pharyngitis, or sore

Terms   **bacterium** (plural, **bacteria**) A microscopic single-celled organism; about 100 bacterial species can cause disease in humans.

More than 17 million Americans have asthma, including more than 5 million children and teenagers. The symptoms of asthma—wheezing, tightness in the chest, and shortness of breath—may be mild and occur only occasionally, or they may be severe and occur daily. Asthma can be disabling and even fatal if not controlled. Asthma is caused by both inflammation of the airways and a spasm of the muscles surrounding the airways. The spasm causes constriction, and the inflammation causes the airway linings to swell and secrete extra mucus, which further obstructs the passages. The inflammation can become chronic, making airways even more sensitive to triggers of attacks. The tendency to develop asthma may be hereditary.

An asthma attack begins when something sets off inflammation of the bronchial tubes. Usually it's an allergic reaction to an inhaled allergen, most commonly dust mites, mold, animal dander, or pollen. Anything that irritates or overtaxes the bronchial airways can also trigger spasms: exercise, cold air, environmental pollutants, tobacco smoke, infection, emotional stress, or even a hearty laugh. In female asthmatics, who make up about 60% of adults with asthma, hormonal changes that occur as menstruation starts may increase vulnerability to attacks.

Inhaling a muscle-relaxing medication from a bronchodilator can relieve an asthma attack immediately by opening the bronchial tubes. Inhaled anti-inflammatory drugs are designed to treat the underlying inflammation. Both types of treatments may be needed to get asthma under control. Other medications for asthma block the actions of molecules involved in the body's inflammatory response. Asthmatics can monitor their condition by self-testing their "peak air flow" several times a day (a drop in peak air flow can signal an upcoming attack). As with allergies, it's also a good idea to avoid allergens when possible.

The incidence of asthma is increasing throughout the world, for reasons not completely understood. Since 1980, the number of Americans with asthma has more than doubled, and despite better treatment options, the death rate has nearly tripled. Particularly affected are people over 65, children, African Americans, Latinos, and people living in inner cities. A combination of factors may well be responsible for this increased incidence, including greater exposure to indoor air pollutants and allergens due to poorer ventilation and more time spent indoors; higher levels of outdoor air pollution: and better diagnosis of asthma cases. Cockroach and mouse allergies have been shown to be an important cause of asthma-related illness among children in inner-city areas. The so-called hygiene hypothesis proposes that less exposure among children to dust, dirt, and certain childhood infections causes the immune system to become hypersensitive later in life.

throat; pneumonia, infection of the lung; gastroenteritis, infection of the gastrointestinal tract; cellulitis, infection of the soft tissues; osteomyelitis, infection of the bones; and so on, for every tissue and organ.

Bacteria

The most abundant living things on earth are **bacteria**, single-celled organisms that usually reproduce by splitting in two to create a pair of identical cells. Many species of bacteria feed on dead matter and play an important role in the recycling of nutrients for other organisms; other species of bacteria feed on living things and may cause disease. Bacteria are often classified according to their shape: they may be rod-shaped (bacilli), spherical (cocci), spiral-shaped (spirochete), or comma-shaped (vibrios).

We harbor both helpful and harmful bacteria on our skin and in our gastrointestinal and reproductive tracts. The human colon contains "friendly" bacteria that produce certain vitamins and help digest nutrients. (A large portion of human feces consists of bacteria). Friendly bacteria also keep harmful bacteria in check by competing for food and resources and secreting substances toxic to pathogenic bacteria. For example, *Lactobacillus acidophilus* resides in the vagina and produces chemicals that kill yeast and bacteria that cause vaginal infections.

VITAL STATISTICS

Table 17-2	Top Infectious Diseases Worldwide	
Disease		**Approximate Number of Deaths per Year**
Pneumonia		3,963,000
HIV/AIDS		2,673,000
Diarrheal diseases		2,213,000
Tuberculosis		1,669,000
Malaria		1,086,000
Measles		875,000
Tetanus		377,000
Pertussis (whooping cough)		295,000
Meningitis		171,000
Syphilis		153,000

In addition, many of the 589,000 deaths from liver cancer each year can be traced to viral hepatitis. Overall, infectious diseases kill more than 14 million people each year, representing nearly 25% of all deaths.

SOURCE: World Health Organization. 2000. *The World Health Report 2000: Health Systems: Improving Performance.* Geneva: World Health Organization.

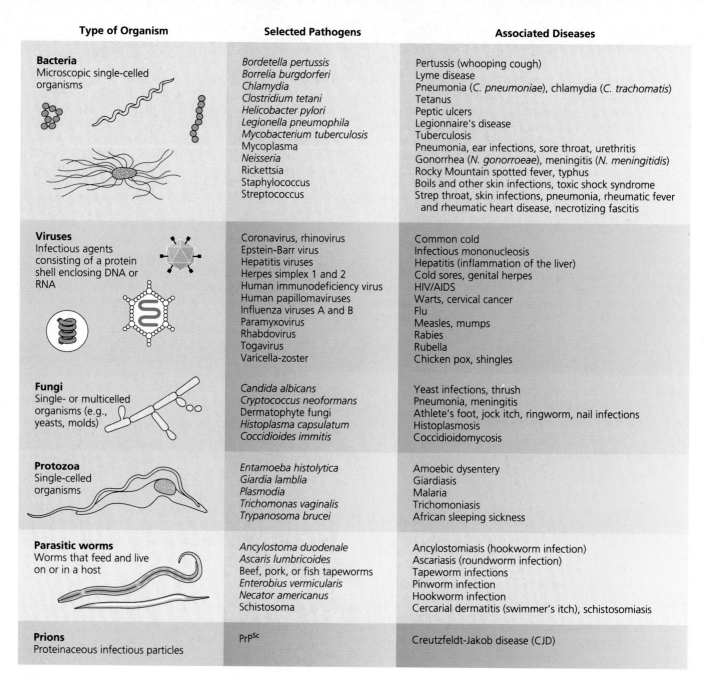

Type of Organism	Selected Pathogens	Associated Diseases
Bacteria Microscopic single-celled organisms	*Bordetella pertussis* *Borrelia burgdorferi* *Chlamydia* *Clostridium tetani* *Helicobacter pylori* *Legionella pneumophila* *Mycobacterium tuberculosis* Mycoplasma *Neisseria* Rickettsia Staphylococcus Streptococcus	Pertussis (whooping cough) Lyme disease Pneumonia (*C. pneumoniae*), chlamydia (*C. trachomatis*) Tetanus Peptic ulcers Legionnaire's disease Tuberculosis Pneumonia, ear infections, sore throat, urethritis Gonorrhea (*N. gonorroeae*), meningitis (*N. meningitidis*) Rocky Mountain spotted fever, typhus Boils and other skin infections, toxic shock syndrome Strep throat, skin infections, pneumonia, rheumatic fever and rheumatic heart disease, necrotizing fascitis
Viruses Infectious agents consisting of a protein shell enclosing DNA or RNA	Coronavirus, rhinovirus Epstein-Barr virus Hepatitis viruses Herpes simplex 1 and 2 Human immunodeficiency virus Human papillomaviruses Influenza viruses A and B Paramyxovirus Rhabdovirus Togavirus Varicella-zoster	Common cold Infectious mononucleosis Hepatitis (inflammation of the liver) Cold sores, genital herpes HIV/AIDS Warts, cervical cancer Flu Measles, mumps Rabies Rubella Chicken pox, shingles
Fungi Single- or multicelled organisms (e.g., yeasts, molds)	*Candida albicans* *Cryptococcus neoformans* Dermatophyte fungi *Histoplasma capsulatum* *Coccidioides immitis*	Yeast infections, thrush Pneumonia, meningitis Athlete's foot, jock itch, ringworm, nail infections Histoplasmosis Coccidioidomycosis
Protozoa Single-celled organisms	*Entamoeba histolytica* *Giardia lamblia* *Plasmodia* *Trichomonas vaginalis* *Trypanosoma brucei*	Amoebic dysentery Giardiasis Malaria Trichomoniasis African sleeping sickness
Parasitic worms Worms that feed and live on or in a host	*Ancylostoma duodenale* *Ascaris lumbricoides* Beef, pork, or fish tapeworms *Enterobius vermicularis* *Necator americanus* Schistosoma	Ancylostomiasis (hookworm infection) Ascariasis (roundworm infection) Tapeworm infections Pinworm infection Hookworm infection Cercarial dermatitis (swimmer's itch), schistosomiasis
Prions Proteinaceous infectious particles	Prp^{Sc}	Creutzfeldt-Jakob disease (CJD)

Figure 17-5 Pathogens and associated infectious diseases.

Not all bacteria found in the body are beneficial, however. If they gain access to the gastrointestinal tract via food or drink, unfriendly bacteria can disrupt the normal harmony in the intestines by invading cells or producing damaging toxins. Sexual activity can introduce pathogenic bacteria into the reproductive tract. Within the bloodstream, tissues, and organs, the human body is usually sterile—devoid of bacteria. If bacteria find their way into these areas, infection may result. It is here that the immune system keeps up its constant surveillance, seeking out and destroying any invaders. Some bacterial infections of concern are described below.

Pneumonia Inflammation of the lungs, called **pneumonia,** may be caused by infection with bacteria, viruses, or fungi or by contact with chemical toxins or irritants. Pneumonia can be serious if the alveoli (air sacs) become clogged with fluid, thus preventing oxygen from reaching the bloodstream. Pneumonia often follows another illness, such as a cold or the flu, but the symptoms are typically more severe—fever, chills, shortness of breath, increased mucus production, and cough. Pneumonia ranks sixth among the leading causes of death for Americans; people most at risk for severe infection include those under age 2 and over age 75 and those with chronic health problems such as heart disease, asthma, or HIV infection. Bacterial pneumonia can be treated with antibiotics.

Pneumococcus bacteria are the most common cause of bacterial pneumonia; a vaccine is available and recommended for all adults age 65 and older and others at risk. Other bacteria that may cause pneumonia include *Streptococcus pneumoniae, Chlamydia pneumoniae,* and **mycoplasmas.** Outbreaks of infection with mycoplasmas are relatively common among young adults, especially in crowded settings such as dormitories.

Legionnaires' disease is a severe form of pneumonia caused by the rod-shaped bacterium *Legionella pneumophila.* About 8,000–18,000 Americans get Legionnaires' disease each year, and the disease is fatal in 5–30% of cases. The disease usually occurs in single, isolated cases, but it was an outbreak at a 1976 American Legion convention that led to the bacterium's identification. Those most at risk include middle-aged and older persons, particularly those who smoke or have chronic health problems; younger, healthy individuals are more likely to contract a mild form of the infection known as Pontiac fever. *Legionella* flourish in moist environments like cooling towers, plumbing systems, and whirlpool spas.

Meningitis Infection of the *meninges,* the membranes covering the brain and spinal cord, is called **meningitis.** Viral meningitis is usually mild and goes away on its own; bacterial meningitis, however, can be life-threatening and requires immediate treatment with antibiotics. Symptoms of meningitis include fever, a severe headache, stiff neck, sensitivity to light, and confusion. Before the 1990s, *Haemophilus influenzae* type b (Hib) was the leading cause of bacterial meningitis, but routine vaccination of children has reduced the occurrence of Hib meningitis. Today, *Neisseria meningitidis* and *Streptococcus pneumoniae* are the leading causes of bacterial meningitis.

In the United States, approximately 2700 cases of meningitis are reported each year, although the actual number is probably higher. The disease is fatal in 10–15% of cases, and about 10% of people who recover have permanent hearing loss or other serious effects. Worldwide, about 170,000 people die from meningitis each year, particularly in the so-called meningitis belt in sub-Saharan Africa.

A vaccine is available, but it is not effective against all strains of meningitis-causing bacteria. First-year college students who live in dormitories have been found to be at a modestly increased risk for meningitis compared to other people their age. For this reason, the CDC recommended in 2000 that first-year college students be given information about meningitis and the benefits of vaccination and be offered the vaccine.

Strep Throat and Other Streptococcal Infections The **streptococcus** bacterium is spherical-shaped and often grows in chains. Streptococcal pharyngitis, or strep throat, is characterized by a red, sore throat with white patches on the tonsils, swollen lymph nodes, fever, and headache. It is typically spread through close contact with an infected person via respiratory droplets (sneezing or coughing). If left untreated, strep throat can develop into the more serious rheumatic fever (see Chapter 15 for more on rheumatic heart disease). Other streptococcal infections include scarlet fever (scarletina), characterized by a sore throat, fever, bright red tongue, and a rash over the upper body; impetigo, a superficial skin infection most common among children; and erysipelas, inflammation of skin and underlying tissues.

A particularly virulent type of streptococcus can invade the bloodstream, spread to other parts of the body, and produce dangerous systemic illness. It can also cause a serious but rare infection of the deeper layers of the skin, a condition called necrotizing fasciitis or "flesh-eating strep." This dangerous infection is characterized by tissue death and is treated with antibiotics and removal of the infected tissue or limb. Other species of streptococci are implicated in pneumonia, endocarditis (infection of the heart lining and valves), and serious infections in pregnant women and newborns.

Toxic Shock Syndrome and Other Staphylococcal Infections The spherical-shaped **staphylococcus** bacterium often appears in small clusters when viewed under a microscope. It is commonly found on the skin and in the nasal passages of healthy people. Occasionally, staphylococci enter the body and cause an infection, ranging from minor skin infections such as boils to very serious conditions such as blood infections or pneumonia.

A particular species of the bacteria, *Staphylococcus aureus,* is responsible for many cases of **toxic shock syndrome (TSS).** The bacteria produce a deadly toxin that causes

pneumonia Inflammation of the lungs, typically caused by infection or exposure to chemical toxins or irritants.

mycoplasma A small bacterium with an incomplete cell wall that may cause sore throats, ear infections, and pneumonia.

meningitis Infection of the membranes covering the brain and spinal cord (meninges).

streptococcus Any of a genus (*Streptococcus*) of spherical bacteria; streptococcal species can cause skin infections, strep throat, rheumatic fever, pneumonia, scarlet fever, and other diseases.

staphylococcus Any of a genus (*Staphylococcus*) of spherical, clustered bacteria commonly found on the skin or in the nasal passages; staphylococcal species may enter the body and cause such conditions as boils, pneumonia, and toxic shock syndrome.

toxic shock syndrome (TSS) Sudden onset of fever, aches, vomiting, and peeling rash, followed in some cases by shock and inflammation of multiple organs; often caused by a toxin produced by *Staphylococcus aureus.*

Terms

shock (potentially life-threatening low blood pressure), high fever, a peeling skin rash, and inflammation of several organ systems. TSS was first diagnosed in women using highly absorbent tampons, which appear to allow the growth of staphylococci; however, about half of all cases occur in men and in women not using tampons. The number of cases of TSS has dropped dramatically since a particular type of tampon was removed from the market, and there are now fewer than 10 cases per year of TSS occurring during menstruation.

Tuberculosis Caused by the rod-shaped bacterium *Mycobacterium tuberculosis*, **tuberculosis (TB)** is a chronic bacterial infection that usually affects the lungs. TB is spread via the respiratory route through prolonged contact with someone who has the disease in its active form. Symptoms include coughing, fatigue, night sweats, weight loss, and fever.

Ten to 15 million Americans have been infected with, and therefore continue to carry, *M. tuberculosis*. However, only about 10% of people with so-called latent TB infections actually develop an active case of the disease during their lifetime. Although their skin tests for TB antibodies register positive, the immune system prevents the disease from becoming active. In the United States, active TB is most common among people infected with HIV, recent immigrants from countries where TB is **endemic,** and those who live in the inner cities. Worldwide, about 2 billion people—one-third of the population—are infected with TB, and each year about 8 million develop active TB and more than 1.5 million die.

Many strains of tuberculosis respond to antibiotics, but only over a long course of treatment lasting 6–12 months. Failure to complete treatment can lead to relapse and the development of strains of antibiotic-resistant bacteria. The increase in recent years in the number of people with multidrug-resistant TB has alarmed public health officials and led to the development of new strategies to help ensure infected individuals receive and complete appropriate treatment.

Lyme Disease and Other Tickborne Infections As described earlier, one method of disease transmission is via insect vectors. Lyme disease is one such infection, and it accounts for more than 95% of all reported vector-borne illness in the United States—more than 15,000 cases per year. It is spread by the bite of a tick of the genus *Ixodes* that is infected with the spiral-shaped bacterium *Borrelia burgdorferi*. Ticks acquire the spirochete by ingesting the blood of an infected animal; they may then transmit the microbe to their next host. The deer tick is responsible for transmitting Lyme disease bacteria to humans in the northeastern and north-central United States; on the Pacific Coast, the culprit is the closely related western black-legged tick. Lyme disease has been reported in 48 states, but significant risk of infection is found in only about 100 counties in 10 states located in the northeastern and mid-Atlantic seaboard, the upper north-central region, and a few counties in northern California.

Symptoms of Lyme disease vary but typically occur in three stages. In the first stage, an expanding (bull's-eye-shaped) red rash develops from the area of the bite, usually about 2 weeks after the bite occurs. The second stage occurs weeks to months later in 10–20% of untreated patients; symptoms may involve the nervous and cardiovascular systems and can include impaired coordination, partial facial paralysis, and heart rhythm abnormalities. These symptoms usually disappear on their own within a few weeks. The third stage, which occurs in about half of untreated people, can develop months or years after the tick bite and usually consists of chronic or recurring arthritis. Lyme disease can also cause fetal damage or death at any stage of pregnancy.

Lyme disease is preventable by avoiding contact with ticks or by removing a tick before it has had the chance to transmit the infection (see the box "Protecting Yourself Against Tickborne Infections"). A vaccine is available for people age 15–70 years who are at high risk, but it is not 100% effective against the disease. Lyme disease is treatable at all stages, although arthritis symptoms may not completely resolve.

Rocky Mountain spotted fever and typhus are caused by **rickettsias** and are also transmitted via tick bites. Rocky Mountain spotted fever is characterized by sudden onset of fever, headache, and muscle pain, followed by development of a spotted rash. Prior to the development of antibiotics, as many as 30% of affected individuals died; the death rate has now dropped to 3–5%. Ehrlichiosis, another tickborne disease, typically causes less severe symptoms. As with Lyme disease, the risk of acquiring Rocky Mountain spotted fever and ehrlichiosis is greater in areas where specific bacteria-carrying tick species are common.

Ulcers About 25 million Americans suffer from ulcers, sores or holes in the lining of the stomach or the first part of the small intestine (duodenum). It used to be thought that spicy food and stress were major causes of ulcers, but it is now known that as many as 90% of ulcers are caused by infection with *Helicobacter pylori*. Ulcer symptoms include gnawing or burning pain in the abdomen, nausea, and loss of appetite. If tests show the presence of *H. pylori*, treatment with antibiotics often cures the infection and the ulcers.

Terms **tuberculosis (TB)** A chronic bacterial infection that usually affects the lungs.

endemic Persistent and relatively widespread in a given population.

rickettsia A bacterium that can reproduce only inside living cells, transmitted by ticks, fleas, and lice; causes Rocky Mountain spotted fever and typhus.

Avoid Tick Habitat

When possible, avoid areas that are likely to be infested with ticks, particularly in spring and summer, when the immature ticks, called nymphs, are most likely to feed. Ticks favor moist, shaded habitats, especially as provided by leaf litter and low-lying vegetation in wooded, brushy, or overgrown grassy habitats. State and local health departments, park personnel, and agricultural extension services can provide information on the distribution of ticks in your area.

Wear Protective Clothing and Apply Insect Repellent

Wear light-colored clothing so that ticks can be spotted more easily. Wear long-sleeved shirts and tuck pants into socks or the tops of boots to help keep ticks from reaching your skin. Ticks are usually located close to the ground, so wearing high boots may provide additional protection. Application of insect repellents containing DEET (n,n-diethyl-m-toluamide) to clothes and exposed skin, and permethrin to clothes, should also help reduce the risk of tick attachment. DEET can be used safely on adults and children, but it should be applied according to Environmental Protection Agency guidelines to reduce the possibility of toxicity.

Remove Attached Ticks

Transmission of an infectious agent is unlikely to occur until a tick has fed on you for several hours (36 hours in the case of Lyme disease), so daily checks for ticks and their prompt removal will help prevent infection. Search your entire body for ticks, using a handheld or full-length mirror; also check children and pets. Ticks are small; in the nymph phase, they may resemble poppy seeds (see figure).

To remove a tick, use fine-tipped tweezers and shield your fingers with rubber gloves or a paper towel. Grasp the tick as close to the skin surface as possible and pull upward (away from the skin) with steady, even pressure. Do not twist or jerk the tick, as this may cause the mouthparts to break off and remain in the skin. If this happens, remove the mouthparts with tweezers. Do not squeeze, crush, or puncture the body of the tick because its fluids may contain infectious organisms. After removing the tick, disinfect the bite site and wash your hands with soap and water. Save ticks for identification in case you become ill. Place the tick in a plastic bag in your freezer, and note the date of the bite.

Deer tick (actual size)

larva nymph female male

1   2

SOURCES: Centers for Disease Control and Prevention. 2000. *Lyme Disease: Prevention and Control* (http://www.cdc.gov/ncidod/dvbid/ lymeprevent.htm; retrieved December 5, 2000). Centers for Disease Control and Prevention. 2000. *Rocky Mountain Spotted Fever: Questions and Answers* (http://www.cdc.gov/ncidod/dvrd/rmsf/q&a.htm; retrieved November 30, 2000).

Other Bacterial Infections   The following are a few of the many other infections caused by bacteria:

• *Tetanus:* Also known as lockjaw, tetanus is caused by the bacterium *Clostridium tetani,* which thrives in deep puncture wounds and produces a deadly toxin. The toxin causes muscular stiffness and spasms, and infection is fatal in about 30% of cases. Due to widespread vaccination, tetanus is rare in the United States. Worldwide, however, nearly 400,000 deaths from tetanus occur each year, primarily among newborns who are infected through the unsterile cutting of the umbilical cord.

• *Pertussis:* Also known as whooping cough, pertussis is a respiratory illness most common among infants and young children; it is caused by a toxin produced by the bacterium *Bordetella pertussis.* Pertussis is characterized by bursts of rapid coughing, followed by a long attempt at inhalation that is often accompanied by a high-pitched "whoop"; symptoms may persist for 2–8 weeks. There are 3000–8000 cases each year in the United States.

• *Urinary tract infections (UTIs):* Infection of the bladder and urethra is most common among sexually active women but can occur in anyone. The bacterium *Escherichi coli* is the most common infectious agent, responsible for about 80% of all UTIs. Infection most often occurs when bacteria from the digestive tract that live on the skin around the anus get pushed toward the opening of the urethra during sexual intercourse; then, the bacteria travel up the urethra and into the bladder. (Women are more susceptible to UTIs than men because their urethra is much shorter, so it is easier for bacteria to reach the bladder.) Women who are particularly susceptible to UTIs may be given a supply of antibiotics to use after intercourse or at the first sign of infection; urinating before and after intercourse may also help prevent UTIs.

Bacteria responsible for foodborne illness were described in Chapter 12; Chapter 18 discusses sexually transmitted bacterial infections such as chlamydia, gonorrhea, and syphilis.

Antibiotic Treatments   The body's immune system can fight off many, if not most, bacterial infections. However, while the body musters its defenses, some bacteria can cause a great deal of damage: Inflammation, caused by the gathering of white blood cells, may lead to scarring and permanently damaged tissues. To help the body deal with these infections, science and medicine have made a considerable contribution: antibiotics.

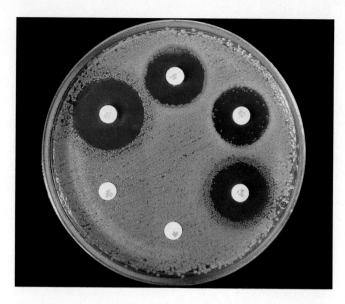

One of the dangers of antibiotic overuse is the development of bacteria resistant to drugs. Cultures of *E. coli* (a bacterium normally present in the human intestine) in this laboratory dish are sensitive to four different types of antibiotics, as indicated by the wide circles where no bacteria are growing, but they are resistant to two other types, which have no effect on their growth.

Antibiotics are both naturally occurring and synthetic substances having the ability to kill bacteria. Most antibiotics work in a similar fashion: They interrupt the production of new bacteria by damaging some part of their reproductive cycle or by causing faulty parts of new bacteria to be made. Penicillins inhibit the formation of the cell wall when bacteria divide to form new cells. Other antibiotics inhibit the production of certain necessary proteins by the bacteria, and still others interfere directly with the reading of genetic material (DNA) during the process of bacterial reproduction.

When antibiotics inhibit a specific bacterial strain's growth, these bacteria are said to be "sensitive." Unfortunately, antibiotic-resistant strains (types) of many common bacteria have developed, including strains of gonorrhea (an STD), salmonellosis (a foodborne illness), and tuberculosis. A bacterium can become resistant from a chance genetic mutation or through the transfer of genetic material from one bacterium to another. In any given population of bacteria, a few are always resistant. When exposed to antibiotics, these resistant bacteria can grow and flourish, while the antibiotic-sensitive bacteria die off. Eventually, an entire colony of bacteria can become resistant to one or more antibiotics. The more often bacteria encounter antibiotics, the more likely they are to develop resistance. Antibiotic resistance is a major factor contributing to the recent rise in problematic infectious diseases.

You can help prevent the development of antibiotic-resistant strains of bacteria by using antibiotics properly:

- Don't expect to take an antibiotic every time you get sick. They are mainly helpful for bacterial infections; against viruses, they are ineffective.
- Use antibiotics as directed, and finish the full course of medication even if you begin to feel better. This helps ensure that all targeted bacteria are killed off.
- Never take an antibiotic without a prescription. If you take an antibiotic for a viral infection, take the wrong one, or take an insufficient dose, your illness will not improve, and you'll give bacteria the opportunity to develop resistance.

Viruses

Visible only with an electron (high-magnification) microscope, **viruses** are on the borderline between living and nonliving matter. Viruses lack all the enzymes essential to energy production and protein synthesis in normal animal cells, and they cannot grow or reproduce by themselves. Viruses are **parasites;** they use what they need for growth and reproduction from the cells they invade. Once a virus is inside the host cell, it sheds its protein covering and its genetic material takes control of the cell and manufactures more viruses like itself (Figure 17-6). The normal functioning of the host cell is thereby disrupted. In order to fight viruses, the cellular immunity system produces substances such as interferon; unfortunately, these same substances are also responsible for most of the symptoms of a viral illness.

Illnesses caused by viruses are the most common forms of **contagious disease.** Different viruses affect different kinds of cells, and the seriousness of the disease they cause depends greatly on which kind of cell is affected. The viruses that cause colds, for example, attack upper respiratory tract cells, which are constantly cast off and replaced; the disease is therefore mild. Poliovirus, in contrast, attacks nerve cells that cannot be replaced, and the consequences, such as paralysis, are severe. HIV infection, a viral illness that destroys immune system cells, can destroy the body's ability to fight infectious diseases (see Chapter 18).

The Common Cold Although generally brief, lasting only 4–7 days, colds are nonetheless irritating and often interfere with one's normal activities. A cold may be caused by any of more than 200 different viruses that attack the lining of the nasal passages; rhinoviruses and coronaviruses cause a large percentage of all colds among adults. Cold viruses are almost always transmitted by hand-to-hand contact. To lessen your risk of contracting a cold, wash your hands frequently; if you touch someone else, avoid touching your face until after you've washed your hands. Colds are not caused by exposure to cold weather or by being chilled or overheated; more colds do occur in the fall and winter months, probably because of the opening of school season (children contract more colds than adults) and because people spend more time

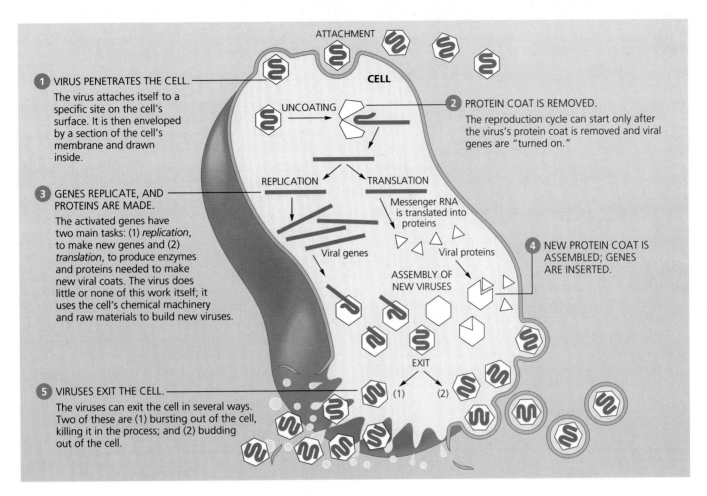

① VIRUS PENETRATES THE CELL.

The virus attaches itself to a specific site on the cell's surface. It is then enveloped by a section of the cell's membrane and drawn inside.

③ GENES REPLICATE, AND PROTEINS ARE MADE.

The activated genes have two main tasks: (1) *replication*, to make new genes and (2) *translation*, to produce enzymes and proteins needed to make new viral coats. The virus does little or none of this work itself; it uses the cell's chemical machinery and raw materials to build new viruses.

⑤ VIRUSES EXIT THE CELL.

The viruses can exit the cell in several ways. Two of these are (1) bursting out of the cell, killing it in the process; and (2) budding out of the cell.

ATTACHMENT

CELL

UNCOATING

② PROTEIN COAT IS REMOVED.

The reproduction cycle can start only after the virus's protein coat is removed and viral genes are "turned on."

REPLICATION   TRANSLATION

Messenger RNA is translated into proteins

Viral genes   Viral proteins

ASSEMBLY OF NEW VIRUSES

④ NEW PROTEIN COAT IS ASSEMBLED; GENES ARE INSERTED.

EXIT
(1)   (2)

Figure 17-6   Life cycle of a virus.

indoors in the fall and winter months, making person-to-person transmission of viruses more likely.

If you do catch a cold, over-the-counter cold remedies may help treat your symptoms but do not directly attack the viral cause (see the box "Preventing and Treating the Common Cold"). Sometimes it is difficult to determine whether your symptoms are due to a virus (as for colds, flu, and some sinus infections), a bacterium (as for other sinus infections), or an allergy, but this information is important for appropriate treatment (Table 17-3). For example, antibiotics will not help treat a cold but will help treat a bacterial sinus infection.

Influenza   Commonly called "the flu," **influenza** is an infection of the respiratory tract caused by the influenza virus. (Many people use the term "stomach flu" to describe gastrointestinal illnesses, but these infections are actually caused by organisms other than influenza viruses). Compared to the common cold, influenza is a more serious illness, usually including a fever and extreme fatigue. Most people who get the flu recover within 1–2 weeks, but some develop potentially life-threatening complications, such as pneumonia. Influenza is associated with more than 100,000 hospitalizations and 20,000

deaths each year, primarily among people over age 50 and those with chronic health problems. Influenza is highly contagious and is spread via respiratory droplets.

The two main types of influenza viruses are designated A and B; they are responsible for **epidemics** of respiratory illness that occur almost every winter. Influenza viruses undergo constant change, enabling them to evade the immune system and making people susceptible to influenza

virus A very small infectious agent composed of nucleic acid (DNA or RNA) surrounded by a protein coat; lacks an independent metabolism and reproduces only within a host cell.

parasite An organism that lives on or within a living host; the relationship benefits the parasite and harms the host.

contagious disease A disease that can be transmitted from one person to another; most are viral diseases, such as the common cold and flu.

influenza Infection of the respiratory tract by the influenza virus, which is highly infectious and adaptable; the form changes so easily that every year new strains arise, making treatment difficult; commonly known as the flu.

epidemic The occurrence in a particular community or region of more than the expected number of cases of a particular disease.

Terms

Unfortunately, there is no cure for the common cold. But there are some practical things you can do to avoid catching a cold and to relieve the symptoms of any colds you do catch.

Prevention

Colds are usually spread by hand-to-hand contact with another person or with objects such as doorknobs and telephones, which an infected person may have handled. The best way to avoid transmission is to wash your hands frequently with warm water and soap. Keeping your immune system strong is another good prevention strategy (see the guidelines provided later in the chapter).

Home Treatments

- Get some extra rest. It isn't usually necessary to stay home in bed, but you will need to slow down a little from your usual routine to give your body a chance to fight the infection.

- Drink plenty of liquids to prevent dehydration. Hot liquids such as herbal tea and clear chicken soup will soothe a sore throat and loosen secretions; gargling with a glass of slightly salty water may also help. Avoid alcoholic beverages when you have a cold.

- Hot showers or the use of a humidifier can help eliminate nasal stuffiness and soothe inflamed membranes.

Over-the-Counter Treatments

Avoid multisymptom cold remedies. Because these products include drugs to treat symptoms you may not even have, you risk suffering from side effects from medications you don't need. It's better to treat each symptom separately:

- *Analgesics*—aspirin, acetaminophen (Tylenol), ibuprofen (Advil or Motrin), and naproxen sodium (Aleve)—all help lower fever and relieve muscle aches. Use of aspirin is associated with an increased risk of a serious condition called Reye's syndrome in children and teenagers; for this reason, aspirin should be given only to adults.

- *Decongestants* shrink nasal blood vessels, relieving swelling and congestion. However, they may dry out mucous membranes in the throat and make a sore throat worse.

- *Cough medicines* may be helpful when your cough is nonproductive (not bringing up mucus) or if it disrupts your sleep or work. Expectorants make coughs more productive by increasing the volume of mucus and decreasing its thickness, thereby helping remove irritants from the respiratory airways. Suppressants (antitussives) reduce the frequency of coughing.

- *Antihistamines* decrease nasal secretions caused by the effects of histamine, so they are much more useful in treating allergies than colds. *Caution:* Many antihistamines can make you drowsy.

Antibiotics will not help a cold unless a bacterial infection such as strep throat is also present, and overuse of antibiotics leads to the development of drug resistance. The jury is still out on whether other remedies, including zinc gluconate lozenges, echinacea, and vitamin C, will relieve symptoms or shorten the duration of a cold. Researchers are also studying antiviral drugs that target the most common types of cold viruses.

Sometimes a cold leads to a more serious complication, such as bronchitis, pneumonia, or strep throat. If a fever of 102°F or higher persists, or if cold symptoms don't get better after 2 weeks, see your physician.

---

infection throughout life. A person who has been infected with influenza does develop antibodies, but as the virus changes, the antibodies no longer recognize the virus and reinfection can occur. Occasionally, an influenza type A virus undergoes a sudden, dramatic change. If this occurs, and the new virus spreads easily, a worldwide epidemic, called a **pandemic**, can occur because few people have any antibody protection against the virus. During the twentieth century, three influenza pandemics occurred, most dramatically in 1918–1919, when the so-called Spanish flu killed more than 500,000 Americans and 21 million people worldwide.

Terms
> **pandemic** A disease epidemic that is unusually severe or widespread; often used to refer to worldwide epidemics affecting a large proportion of the population.
>
> **herpesvirus** A family of viruses responsible for cold sores, mononucleosis, chicken pox, and the STD known as herpes; frequently cause latent infections.

The most effective way of preventing the flu is through annual vaccination. The influenza vaccine consists of killed virus and provides protection against the strains of the virus currently circulating; it is updated each year in response to changes in the virus. Vaccination is recommended for anyone age 6 months or older who is at increased risk for complications of influenza, who has close contact with people in high-risk groups, or who wants to reduce his or her risk of the flu. There are a number of medications that can treat influenza, but in most cases they can only shorten the duration of illness by about a day, and then only if treatment begins within 1–2 days after onset of symptoms. Several medications are also effective in reducing the risk of illness from influenza; however, they are less effective than the vaccine.

Measles, Mumps, and Rubella   Three childhood viral illnesses that have waned in the United States due to effective vaccines are measles, mumps, and rubella (German measles). Measles and rubella are generally charac-

Table 17-3   What's Causing My Symptoms?

Symptoms	Influenza	Common Cold	Allergy	Sinusitis
Headache	Usually	Occasionally	Occasionally	Usually
Muscle aches	Usually (severe)	Usually (mild)	Rarely	Rarely
Fatigue, weakness	Usually (severe; sudden onset; may last several weeks)	Usually (mild)	Rarely	Rarely
Fever	Usually (high, typically 102–104°F; sudden onset; lasts 3–4 days)	Occasionally (mild)	Never	Occasionally
Cough	Usually (often severe)	Occasionally	Occasionally	Usually
Runny, stuffy nose	Occasionally	Usually	Usually	Usually (stuffy)
Nasal discharge	Occasionally	Usually (thick, clear to yellowish green)	Usually (watery, clear)	Usually (thick, yellowish green)
Sneezing	Occasionally	Occasionally	Usually	Rarely
Sore throat	Occasionally	Usually	Occasionally	Rarely
Itchy eyes, nose, throat	Rarely	Rarely	Usually	Never

SOURCE: Is it the flu? 2000. *Consumer Reports,* November.

terized by rash and fever. Measles can occasionally cause more severe illness, including liver or brain infection or pneumonia; worldwide, nearly 900,000 people die each year from measles. Measles is a highly contagious disease, and prior to the introduction of vaccines, more than 90% of Americans contracted measles by age 15. Rubella, if it infects a pregnant woman, can be transmitted to a fetus, causing miscarriage, stillbirth, and severe birth defects, including deafness, eye and heart defects, and mental impairment. Mumps generally causes swelling of the parotid (salivary) glands, located just below and in front of the ears. This virus can also cause meningitis and, in males, inflammation of the testes.

Chicken Pox, Cold Sores, and Other Herpesvirus Infections

The **herpesviruses** are a large and important group of viruses. Once infected, the host is never free of the virus. The virus lies latent within certain cells and becomes active periodically, producing symptoms. Herpesviruses are particularly dangerous for people with a depressed immune system, as in the case of HIV infection. The family of herpesviruses includes the following:

• *Varicella-zoster virus,* which causes chicken pox and shingles. Chicken pox is a highly contagious childhood disease characterized by an itchy rash made up of small blisters; the infection is usually mild, although complications are more likely to occur in young infants and adults. After the rash resolves, the virus becomes latent, living in sensory nerves. Many years later, the virus may reactivate and cause shingles; symptoms of shingles include pain in the affected nerves and a rash on the skin that follows the pattern of the nerve pathways (often a band over the ribs on one side of the body). A vaccine is available to prevent chicken pox, and studies are ongoing to determine if the vaccine can be used later in life to prevent the recurrence of the virus as shingles.

• *Herpes simplex virus (HSV) types 1 and 2,* which cause cold sores and the STD herpes. Herpes infections are characterized by small, painful ulcers in the area around the mouth or genitals, at the site where a person first contacts the virus. Following the initial infection, HSV becomes latent and may reactivate again and again over time. Many infected people do not know they are infected, and the virus can be transmitted even when sores are not apparent. Heat and sunlight can trigger recurrences of lip ulcers, so using a lip balm with sunscreen may be a helpful strategy; antiviral medications are available to prevent recurrences of genital herpes. See Chapter 18 for more on sexually transmitted HSV infection.

• *Epstein-Barr virus (EBV),* which causes infectious mononucleosis. Mono, as it is commonly called, is characterized by fever, sore throat, swollen lymph nodes, and fatigue. It is usually spread by intimate contact with the saliva of an infected person—hence the name "kissing disease." Mono most often affects adolescents and young adults; by age 40, nearly 90% of Americans have become infected with EBV. Although EBV does reactivate throughout life, it generally does not cause any further symptoms. In a few people, especially those with HIV infection, EBV is associated with the development of cancers of the lymph system (see the box "Are All Diseases Infectious?").

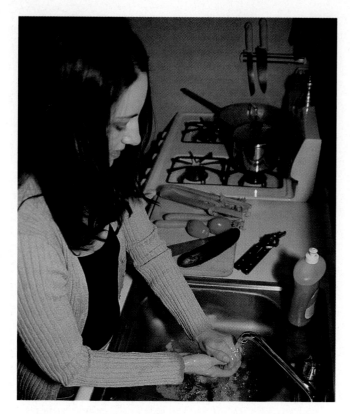

Hand washing is one of the best ways to prevent the spread of infectious diseases. Always wash your hands before, during, and after preparing food; before eating; and after using the bathroom. Wet your hands, apply soap, and rub vigorously for 10–20 seconds.

At one time, EBV was implicated as a cause of *chronic fatigue syndrome (CFS)*, a disorder characterized by severe chronic fatigue, impaired memory or concentration, and physical symptoms such as persistent sore throat or muscle pain. However, CFS has not been linked to any single infectious agent; other possible causes of CFS include abnormalities in immunity, hormone levels, and the regulation of blood pressure.

Two herpesviruses that can cause severe infections in people with a suppressed immune system are cytomegalovirus (CMV), which infects the lungs, brain, colon, and eyes, and human herpesvirus 8 (HHV-8), which has been linked to Kaposi's sarcoma.

Terms

encephalitis Inflammation of the brain; fever, headache, nausea, and lethargy are common initial symptoms, followed in some cases by memory loss, seizures, brain damage, and death.

hepatitis Inflammation of the liver, which can be caused by infection, drugs, or toxins.

jaundice Increased bile pigment levels in the blood, characterized by yellowing of the skin and the whites of the eyes.

poliomyelitis A disease of the nervous system, sometimes crippling; vaccines now prevent most cases of polio.

Viral Encephalitis HSV type 1 is a possible cause of viral **encephalitis**, inflammation of brain tissue due to a viral infection. Other possible causes include HIV and several mosquito-borne viruses, including Japanese encephalitis virus, equine encephalomyelitis virus, and West Nile virus. Mild cases of encephalitis may cause fever, headache, nausea, and lethargy; severe cases are characterized by memory loss, delirium, diminished speech function, and seizures, and they may result in permanent brain damage or death.

Viral Hepatitis Viral **hepatitis** is a term used to describe several different infections that cause inflammation of the liver. Hepatitis is usually caused by one of the three most common hepatitis viruses. Hepatitis A virus (HAV) causes the mildest form of the disease and is usually transmitted by food or water contaminated by sewage or an infected person. Hepatitis B virus (HBV) is usually transmitted sexually; it is discussed in detail in Chapter 18. Hepatitis C virus (HCV) can also be transmitted sexually, but it is much more commonly passed through direct contact with infected blood via injection drug use or, prior to the development of screening tests, blood transfusions. HBV and, to a lesser extent, HCV can also be passed from a pregnant woman to her child. Although there are effective vaccines for hepatitis A and B, there are up to 500,000 new cases of hepatitis in the United States each year.

Symptoms of acute hepatitis infection can include fatigue, **jaundice**, abdominal pain, loss of appetite, nausea, and diarrhea. Most people recover from hepatitis A within a month or so. However, 5–10% of people infected with HBV and 85–90% of people infected with HCV become chronic carriers of the virus, capable of infecting others for the rest of their lives. Some chronic carriers remain asymptomatic, while others slowly develop chronic liver disease, cirrhosis, or liver cancer. An estimated 5 million Americans and 500 million people worldwide may be chronic carriers of hepatitis. Each year in the United States, HBV and HCV are responsible for more than 15,000 deaths, and these numbers are expected to climb as more people infected in the 1970s and 1980s develop problems. HCV infection is already the most frequent reason for liver transplants among U.S. adults, and it is thought to be a major factor in the 70% increase in U.S. liver cancer rates since the 1970s.

The extent of HCV infection has only recently been recognized, and most infected people are unaware of their condition. To ensure proper treatment and prevention, testing for HCV may be recommended for people at risk, including people who have ever injected drugs (even once), who received a blood transfusion or a donated organ prior to July 1992, who have engaged in high-risk sexual behavior, or who have had body piercing, tattoos, or acupuncture involving unsterile equipment. Antiviral drugs are available to treat chronic hepatitis, but they are not completely effective and may have significant side effects.

Are all diseases infectious? Probably not, although researchers have recently been identifying infectious bases for more and more diseases—even diseases that have long been thought to be caused by other factors. Some scientists feel that the role of infectious agents in the major killers of today—cardiovascular disease, cancer, diabetes, and so on—has been greatly underestimated. The following are just a few examples.

- **Ulcers.** Although long believed to be caused by spicy food, stress, and smoking, most cases of ulcers are now known to be caused by infection with *Helicobacter pylori*.

- **Type 1 diabetes.** A viral infection is thought to trigger the immune system to destroy insulin-producing cells in the pancreas; when this occurs, the pancreas is no longer able to produce enough insulin to metabolize glucose.

- **Multiple sclerosis (MS).** Infection with a virus, possibly human herpesvirus 6, has been proposed as the precipitating cause of MS, a condition characterized by damage to nerve fiber coverings and progressive muscle weakness. Researchers have found MS to be more prevalent in some areas than others, and people who move from an area of low MS prevalence to an area of high MS prevalence before the age of 15 appear to increase their risk of getting MS.

- **Schizophrenia.** Some studies have found that people with schizophrenia are more likely than unaffected individuals to have elevated antibodies to the Borna virus. Researchers have proposed that the Borna virus may be one of several infectious agents that trigger changes in the brain leading to schizophrenia.

- **Childhood obsessive-compulsive disorder (OCD).** Some cases of OCD that begin in early childhood have been found to follow infection with streptococcus bacteria. It is thought that antibodies produced to fight the infection, rather than the infection itself, may cause OCD. Some affected children improve when they are given intravenous immunoglobulin or undergo plasma exchange to remove the antibodies from their blood.

- **Heart disease.** Several infectious agents have been implicated in the inflammatory processes underlying atherosclerosis, including *Chlamydia pneumoniae* and *Cytomegalovirus*. Research is underway to determine if antibiotics can lessen the risk of heart attack in infected individuals.

- **Cancer.** A number of infections have been linked to specific types of cancer: human papillomavirus and cervical cancer; Epstein-Barr virus and Burkitt's lymphoma, nasopharyngeal cancer, and some B-cell lymphomas; hepatitis B and C viruses and liver cancer; HTLV-1 and T-cell leukemia; *Helicobacter pylori* and stomach cancer; and human herpesvirus 8 and Kaposi's sarcoma.

Poliomyelitis   An infectious viral disease that affects the nervous system, **poliomyelitis** can cause irreversible paralysis and death in some affected individuals. As with other vaccine-preventable diseases, the incidence of polio declined dramatically in the United States following the introduction of the vaccine, and North and South America are now considered free of the disease. In 1998, the World Health Organization set the goal of eradicating polio from the world.

Rabies   Caused by a rhabdovirus, rabies is a potentially fatal infection of the central nervous system that is most often transmitted through an animal bite. U.S. rabies-related deaths among humans declined dramatically during the twentieth century due to the widespread vaccination of domestic animals and the development of a highly effective vaccine regimen that provides immunity following exposure ("post-exposure prophylaxis," or PEP). Although rabies is rare in the United States, most recent cases have been traced to bats. Unlike bites from larger animals that may carry rabies (raccoons, foxes, skunks, and so on), bat bites or scratches are likely to go unnoticed; thus, people may be unaware of their exposure and fail to seek treatment. The CDC recommends that PEP be considered for anyone who has had direct physical contact with a bat, including someone who has been in the same room as a bat and who might be unaware that contact has occurred (a sleeping child, for example). PEP consists of one dose of immune globulin and five doses of rabies vaccine over a 28-day period.

Warts   Infection by the human papillomavirus (HPV), which causes cell proliferation, can cause warts (noncancerous skin tumors). The more than 100 different types of HPV cause a variety of warts, including common warts on the hands, plantar warts on the soles of the feet, and genital warts around the genitalia. Depending on their location, warts may be removed using over-the-counter preparations or professional methods such as laser surgery or cryosurgery. Because HPV infection is chronic, warts can reappear despite treatment. Because of the link between HPV infection and cervical cancer, genital warts are of particular concern (see Chapter 18 for more information).

Treating Viral Illnesses   Although many viruses cannot be treated medically, researchers have recently begun to develop antiviral drugs. These typically work by interfering with some part of the viral life cycle; for example, they may prevent a virus from entering body cells or from successfully reproducing within cells. Antivirals are currently available to fight infections caused by HIV, influenza, herpes simplex, varicella-zoster, HBV, and HCV. Most other viral diseases must simply run their course.

> **COMMUNICATE!** A person who "feels a cold coming on" may be highly contagious, as may be the person sitting next to you in a meeting sneezing, blowing her nose, and leaving wadded-up tissues on the table. What can you do to protect yourself from being infected by another person? Offer information—"Did you know you're probably contagious even before you start sneezing?"—and assert your right to stay healthy—"Don't be offended, but I'm moving to the other side of the table. I can't afford to catch a cold right now."

Fungi

A **fungus** is a primitive plant. Fungi may be multicellular (like molds) or unicellular (like yeasts). Mushrooms and the molds that form on bread and cheese are all examples of fungi. Only about 50 fungi out of many thousands of species cause disease in humans, and these diseases are usually restricted to the skin, mucous membranes, and lungs. Some fungal diseases are extremely difficult to treat because some fungi form spores, an especially resistant dormant stage of the organism.

Candida albicans is a common fungus found naturally in the vagina of most women. In normal amounts, it causes no problems, but when excessive growth occurs, the result is itching and discomfort, commonly known as a yeast infection. Factors that increase the growth of *C. albicans* include the use of antibiotics, clothing that keeps the vaginal area excessively warm and moist, pregnancy, oral contraceptive use, and certain diseases, including diabetes and HIV infection. The most common symptom is usually a thick white or yellowish discharge. Treatment consists of OTC antifungal creams and suppos-

itories or prescription oral antifungal medication. Women should not self-treat unless they are certain from a past medical diagnosis that they have a yeast infection. (Misdiagnosis could mean that a different and more severe infection goes untreated.) *C. albicans* overgrowth can occur in other areas of the body, especially in the mouth in infants (a condition known as thrush).

Other common fungal conditions, including athlete's foot, jock itch, and ringworm, a disease of the scalp, affect the skin. These three mild conditions are usually easy to cure and rarely cause major problems.

Fungi can also cause systemic diseases that are severe, life-threatening, and extremely difficult to treat. Histoplasmosis causes pulmonary and sometimes systemic disease and is most common in the Mississippi and Ohio River Valleys. Coccidioidomycosis is also known as "valley fever" because it is most frequently seen in the San Joaquin Valley of California. Fungal infections can be especially deadly in people with an impaired immune system.

Protozoa

Another group of pathogens are single-celled organisms known as **protozoa**, microscopic single-celled animals. Many protozoal diseases are recurrent: The pathogen remains in the body, alternating between activity and inactivity. Hundreds of millions of people in developing countries suffer from protozoal infections.

Malaria, caused by a protozoan of the genus *Plasmodium,* is characterized by recurrent attacks of severe flu-like symptoms (chills, fever, headache, nausea, and vomiting). The protozoan is injected into the bloodstream via a mosquito bite; during its reproductive phase, it breaks down red blood cells and may cause anemia in severe cases. Although relatively rare in the United States, malaria is a major killer worldwide; each year, there are 300–500 million new cases of malaria and more than 1 million deaths, mostly among infants and children. Drugs are available to prevent and treat malaria.

Giardiasis is caused by *Giardia lamblia,* a single-celled parasite that lives in the intestines of humans and animals. Giardiasis is characterized by nausea, diarrhea, bloating, and abdominal cramps, and it is among the most common waterborne diseases in the United States. People may become infected with *Giardia* if they consume contaminated food or water or pick up the parasite from the contaminated surface of an object such as a bathroom fixture, diaper pail, or toy. People at risk include child care workers, children who attend day care, international travelers, and hikers and campers who drink untreated water. Giardiasis is rarely serious and can be treated with prescription medications.

Other protozoal infections include the following:

- *Trichomoniasis,* a common protozoal infection of the vagina. Although usually mild and treatable, "trich" may increase the risk of HIV transmission (see Chapter 18).

Terms

fungus A single-celled or multicelled organism that absorbs food from living or dead organic matter; examples include molds, mushrooms, and yeasts. Fungal diseases include yeast infections, athlete's foot, and ringworm.

protozoan A microscopic single-celled organism that often produces recurrent, cyclical attacks of disease.

malaria A severe, recurrent, mosquito-borne infection caused by the *Plasmodium* protozoan.

giardiasis An intestinal disease caused by the protozoan *Giardia lamblia.*

parasitic worm A pathogen that causes intestinal and other infections; includes tapeworms, hookworms, pinworms, and flukes.

prion Proteinaceous infectious particles thought to be responsible for a class of neurodegenerative diseases known as transmissible spongiform encephalopathies; Creutzfeldt-Jakob disease in humans and bovine spongiform encephalopathy ("mad cow disease") are examples of prion diseases.

- *Trypanosomiasis* (African sleeping sickness), which is transmitted through the bite of an infected tsetse fly and causes extreme fatigue, fever, rash, severe headache, central nervous system damage, and death.
- *Amoebic dysentery,* a severe form of amebiasis, infection of the intestines with the parasite *Entamoeba histolytica.* It is characterized by bloody diarrhea, stomach pain, and fever.

Parasitic Worms

The **parasitic worms** are the largest organisms that can enter the body to cause infection. The tapeworm, for example, can grow to a length of many feet. Worms, including such intestinal parasites as the tapeworm and hookworm, cause a great variety of relatively mild infections. Pinworm, the most common worm infection in the United States, primarily affects young children. Pinworms are white and about the size of a staple and live in the rectum of humans; they can cause itching and difficulty sleeping. Smaller worms known as flukes infect such organs as the liver and lungs and, in large numbers, can be deadly. Generally speaking, worm infections originate from contaminated food or drink and can be controlled by careful attention to hygiene.

Prions

In recent years, several fatal degenerative disorders of the central nervous system have been linked to "proteinaceous infectious particles," or **prions.** Unlike all other infectious agents, prions appear to lack DNA or RNA and to consist only of protein; their presence in the body does not trigger an immune response. Prions have an abnormal shape and form deposits in the brain. They may spread by triggering normal proteins to change their structure to the abnormal, damaging, form.

Prions are associated with a class of diseases known as *transmissible spongiform encephalopathies (TSEs),* which are characterized by spongelike holes in the brain; symptoms of TSEs include loss of coordination, weakness, dementia, and death. Known prion diseases include Creutzfeldt-Jakob disease (in humans), bovine spongiform encephalopathy ("mad cow disease" in cattle), and scrapie (in sheep). Some prion diseases are inherited or the result of spontaneous genetic mutations, while others are the result of eating infected tissue or being exposed to prions during medical procedures such as organ or tissue transplants. Ongoing research is exploring whether prions play a role in more common degenerative brain disorders such as Alzheimer's disease.

W. Emerging Infectious Diseases

The reduction in deaths from infectious diseases in the United States is one of the major public health achievements of the past century. Improvements in sanitation, hygiene, and water quality and the development of antibiotics all contributed to reduced death rates from tuberculosis, pneumonia, diarrhea, and other infections. However, after decades of decline, the U.S. death rate from infectious disease began to climb in 1981, largely due to the AIDS epidemic. Globally, infectious diseases remain a major killer.

Clearly, the battle has not been won, and new areas of concern have emerged in the past 20 years. Emerging infectious diseases are diseases of infectious origin whose incidence in humans has increased or threatens to increase in the near future. They include both known diseases that have experienced a resurgence, such as tuberculosis and cholera, and diseases that were previously unknown or confined to specific areas, such as Ebola or West Nile virus (see the box "Emerging Infections").

What's behind this rising tide of infectious diseases? Contributing factors are complex and interrelated. They include the following:

- *Drug resistance.* New or increasing drug resistance has been found in organisms that cause malaria, tuberculosis, gonorrhea, influenza, AIDS, and pneumococcal and staphylococcal infections. Infections caused by drug-resistant organisms prolong illness, and—if not treated in time with more expensive drugs—they can cause death. Some bacterial strains now appear to be resistant to all available antibiotics. The cost of drug resistance is increasing and exceeds $25 billion each year.

- *Poverty.* More than 1 billion people live in extreme poverty, and half the world's population has no regular access to essential drugs. Population growth, urbanization, overcrowding, and migration (including the movement of refugees) also contribute to the spread of infectious diseases.

- *The breakdown of public health measures.* A poor public health infrastructure is often associated with poverty and social upheaval, but problems such as contaminated water supplies can occur even in industrial countries. Inadequate vaccination has led to the reemergence of diseases such as diphtheria and pertussis.

- *Environmental changes.* Changes in land use—deforestation, the damming of rivers, the spread of ranching and farming—alter the distribution of disease vectors and bring people into contact with new pathogens. A shift in rainfall patterns caused by global warming may allow mosquito-borne diseases such as malaria and dengue fever to spread from the tropics into the temperate zones.

- *Travel and commerce.* More than 500 million travelers cross national borders each year, and international tourism and trade open the world to infectious agents. For example, the reintroduction of cholera into the Western Hemisphere is thought to have occurred through the discharge of bilge water from a Chinese freighter into the waters off Peru.

The appearance of West Nile virus in New York in 1999–2000 brought the issue of emerging infectious diseases back into the headlines. Although the chances of the average American contracting an exotic infection are very low, emerging infections are a concern to public health officials and represent a challenge to all nations in the future. Some of the emerging infections that concern scientists include the following:

- *West Nile virus.* A mini-outbreak of encephalitis in New York in 1999 led to identification of this virus, which had previously been restricted to Africa, the Middle East, and parts of Europe. Since that time, the virus has spread to more than 12 states and resulted in at least 8 deaths. Experts believe it arrived in this country in an infected bird or person from a country where the virus is common. West Nile virus is carried by birds and then passed to humans when mosquitoes bite first an infected bird and then a person. Most people who are bitten have few or no symptoms, but the virus can cause permanent brain damage or death in some cases.

- *Escherichia coli O157:H7.* This potentially deadly strain of *E. coli,* transmitted in contaminated food, can cause bloody diarrhea and kidney damage. The first major outbreak occurred in 1993, when over 600 people became ill and four children died after eating contaminated and undercooked fast-food hamburgers. Additional outbreaks have been linked to lettuce, alfalfa sprouts, unpasteurized juice, and contaminated public swimming pools. An estimated 70,000 cases and 6 deaths occur in the United States each year.

- *Hantavirus.* Since first being recognized in 1993, over 500 cases of hantavirus pulmonary syndrome (HPS) have been reported in the United States and South America. HPS is caused by the rodent-borne Sin Nombre virus (SNV) and is spread primarily through airborne viral particles from rodent urine, droppings, or saliva. It is characterized by a dangerous fluid buildup in the lungs and is fatal in about 45% of cases.

- *Necrotizing fascitis.* The "flesh-eating bacteria" that cause necrotizing fascitis are a virulent strain of streptococci that also cause scarlet fever, toxic shock syndrome, and the lethal type of pneumonia that killed Muppets creator Jim Henson in 1990. The bacteria break down tissue and damage blood vessels at the site of a wound, sometimes leading to gangrene, shock, and, in about 20% of cases, death. The disease is rare (500–1500 cases per year in the United States).

- *Mad cow disease.* By 2001, more than 90 cases of a new variant of a rare, incurable brain affliction called Creutzfeldt-Jakob disease (CJD) had been reported in the United Kingdom. The new variant of CJD has affected younger people, average age 29 years, and has several unique features. Researchers suspect that this new variant of CJD is caused by people eating beef contaminated with central nervous system tissue from cows infected with bovine spongiform encephalopathy (BSE), commonly called mad cow disease. No cases have been reported in the United States.

- *Ebola.* So far, outbreaks of the often fatal Ebola hemorrhagic fever (EHF) in humans have occurred only in Africa. The Ebola virus is transmitted by direct contact with infected blood or other body secretions, and many cases of EHF have been linked to unsanitary conditions in medical facilities. Because symptoms appear quickly and 75% of victims die, usually within a few days, the virus tends not to spread widely (unlike HIV or hepatitis, which can infect a person for years before any symptoms appear).

- *Influenza A(H5N1).* An outbreak in 1997–1998 of this unusual strain of influenza killed 6 people in Hong Kong. Local authorities contained the outbreak quickly by tracing its source to infected chickens. ducks, and geese and then ordering the slaughter of all domestic poultry. Although small, the outbreak raised the specter of the 1918–1919 influenza pandemic. A strain like A(H5N1) is so unique that few, if any, people have immunity from past exposure; had it mutated into a form that more easily infects humans, influenza A(H5N1) could conceivably have killed as many as 30% of the world's people.

- *Other infections.* A new strain of the bacterium that causes epidemic cholera, *Vibrio cholerae* O139, recently appeared in Asia and caused disease even in people who carry antibodies from previous exposure to other strains of the same organism. The recently discovered Nipah virus was linked to an outbreak of encephalitis in Malaysia in 1998–1999 that began in pigs and was then passed to humans; more than 30% of patients died. In 1999, Texas experienced the first outbreak of dengue fever in almost 20 years; the disease's reemergence in Central and South America has followed the deterioration of mosquito control programs and the spread of mosquitoes to urban areas. Finally, in 2000, three deaths from respiratory disease in California were traced to arenavirus, a rodent-borne virus that had almost never before infected humans in North America.

- *Mass food production and distribution.* Food now travels long distances to our table, and microbes are transmitted along with it. Mass production of food increases the likelihood that a chance contamination can lead to mass illness.

- *Human behaviors.* Changes in patterns of human behavior also have an impact on the spread of infectious diseases. The widespread use of injectable drugs rapidly transmits HIV infection and hepatitis. Changes in sexual behavior over the past 30 years have led to a proliferation of new and old STDs. The use of day-care facilities for children has led to increases in the incidence of several infections that cause diarrhea.

Public health officials are very much aware of the problem of emerging infections, and international efforts at monitoring, preventing, and controlling their spread are

Although the immune systems of men and women are essentially the same, women have much higher rates of many autoimmune diseases. The reason is somewhat of a mystery. One clue may come from pregnancy: In order to conceive and carry a baby to term, a woman's body must temporarily suppress its immune response so it doesn't attack the sperm or the fetus. Another factor seems to be related to estrogen. Estrogen receptors have been found on suppressor T cells, pointing to a possible link between the glands controlling immunity and those controlling sex hormones. Women also appear to have somewhat enhanced immunity compared to men, a factor that could be linked to both longer life spans and higher rates of autoimmune disorders.

Systemic lupus erythematosus is an autoimmune disease in which the immune system attacks the body's normal tissue, causing inflammation of the joints, blood vessels, heart, lungs, brain, and kidneys. Its symptoms include painful swollen joints, a rash on the nose and cheeks, sensitivity to sunlight, chest pain, fatigue, and dizziness. There are about 1.4–2 million Americans with lupus, 80% of them women; the disorder is especially common among Native American and African American women. Lupus usually begins before menopause and may flare up during pregnancy; for some women, symptoms also increase in severity during menstruation or with the use of oral contraceptives. A link between these exacerbating factors is increased levels of estrogen, but this connection is not well un-

derstood. Researchers have also identified genetic mutations that may be associated with lupus.

In rheumatoid arthritis, the body's immune system attacks the membranes lining the joints, causing pain and swelling. Among the estimated 1% of American adults with rheumatoid arthritis, women outnumber men 3 to 1. The causes of the disease are not well understood. Researchers have hypothesized that an as-yet-unidentified virus may stimulate the immune system and trigger the disease. When the disease is present in younger women, symptoms often improve during pregnancy, when estrogen levels are higher, the opposite of what is seen in the case of lupus. Therefore, although estrogen levels may play a role in these disorders, its effects appear to be influenced by many other factors.

Other autoimmune disorders more common among women than men include multiple sclerosis, a neurological disease caused by the destruction of the protective coating around nerves; scleroderma, a connective tissue disease characterized by thickening, hardening, and tightening of the skin; and Graves' disease, characterized by an increase in the production of thyroid hormone, which affects metabolism and many body systems. Continued scientific investigation will help pinpoint the causes and triggers of autoimmune disorders and explain their higher incidence among women.

---

underway. These efforts require worldwide coordination because microbes do not respect national borders. Only a global response can make the world a safer and healthier place for everyone.

Other Immune Disorders: Cancer and Autoimmune Diseases

The immune system has evolved to protect the body from invasion by foreign microorganisms. Sometimes, as in the case of cancer, the body comes under attack by its own cells. As explained in Chapter 16, cancer cells cease to cooperate normally with the rest of the body and multiply uncontrollably. The immune system can often detect cells that have recently become cancerous and then destroy them just as it would a foreign microorganism. But if the immune system breaks down, as it may when people get older, when they have certain immune disorders (including HIV infection), or when they are receiving chemotherapy for other diseases, the cancer cells may multiply out of control before the immune system recognizes the danger. By the time the immune system gears up to destroy the cancerous cells, it may be too late.

Another immune disorder occurs when the body confuses its own cells with foreign organisms. As described earlier, the immune system must recognize many thousands of antigens as foreign and then be able to recognize the same

antigens again and again. Our own tissue cells also are antigenic; that is, they would be recognized by another person's immune system as foreign. A delicate balance must be maintained to ensure that one's immune system recognizes only truly foreign antigens as enemies; erroneous recognition of one's own cells as foreign produces havoc.

This is exactly what happens in what are known as autoimmune diseases. In this type of malady, the immune system seems to be a bit too sensitive and begins to misapprehend itself as "nonself." Rheumatoid arthritis and systemic lupus erythematosus are examples of autoimmune diseases. For reasons not well understood, these conditions are much more common in women than men (see the box "Women and Autoimmune Diseases").

GIVING YOURSELF A FIGHTING CHANCE: HOW TO SUPPORT YOUR IMMUNE SYSTEM

Pathogens pose a formidable threat to wellness, but you can take many steps to prevent them from getting control of your body and compromising your health. Public health measures protect people from many diseases that are transmitted via water, food, or insects. A clean water supply and adequate sewage treatment help control typhoid fever and cholera, for example, and mosquito eradication programs control malaria and encephalitis. Proper food inspection

Many people believe that stress makes them more vulnerable to illness. Studies have shown that rates of illness are higher for weeks or even months in people who have experienced the severe emotional trauma of divorce or the death of a loved one. Can more commonplace anxieties and stresses also cause measurable changes in the immune system? And can common stress-management techniques actually boost the immune system? The answer to these questions appears to be yes. Consider the following research findings:

- Medical students taking final exams showed a much weaker immune response—as measured by levels of natural killer cells and other blood components—to a hepatitis vaccination than unstressed students. In other studies, stress was associated with lower T-cell responses and antibody levels following influenza vaccinations.

- Individuals who had higher levels of stress and who had a negative or pessimistic outlook developed more colds over the course of a yearlong study than individuals with lower levels of stress and a more positive outlook.

- Stressed caregivers of patients with Alzheimer's disease had higher blood levels of the stress hormone epinephrine and much lower levels of some types of T cells and cytokines than less-stressed caregivers. Stressed caregivers experienced more days of illness and slower wound healing.

- In a study of caregivers, relaxation sessions were associated with increased secretion of cytokines in minor wounds, thus speeding healing. Relaxation and imagery have also been shown to increase T-cell levels in some people.

In seeking to explain these effects, researchers are looking at the connections between stress, hormones, and immunity. Some hormones, such as cortisol, appear to impair the ability of immune cells to multiply and function. Others, such as prolactin, seem to give immune cells a boost. By matching stress levels and hormonal changes to the ups and downs of immune function, researchers hope to gain a better grasp of the shifting chemistry of mind and immunity.

SOURCES: Takkouche, B., et al. 2001. A cohort study of stress and the common cold. *Epidemiology* 12: 345–349. Bauer, M. E., et al. 2000. Chronic stress in caregivers of dementia patients is associated with reduced lymphocyte sensitivity to glucocorticoids. *Journal of Neuroimmunology* 103(1): 84–92. Cohen, S., W. J. Doyle, and D. P. Skoner. 1999. Psychological stress, cytokine production, and severity of upper respiratory illness. *Psychosomatic Medicine* 61(2): 175–180. Glaser, R., et al. 1999. Stress-induced immunomodulation: Implications for infectious diseases? *Journal of the American Medical Association* 281(41): 2268–2270. Mills, P. J., et al. 1999. Vulnerable caregivers of patients with Alzheimer's disease have deficit in circulation CD62L\-T lymphocytes. *Psychosomatic Medicine* 61(2): 168–174.

and preparation prevent illness caused by foodborne pathogens (see Chapter 12).

But what can you do as an individual to strengthen your immune system to help prevent infection? The most important thing you can do is to take good care of your body, with adequate nutrition, exercise, rest, and moderation in lifestyle. Medical science has not come up with anything that can improve upon the millions of years of evolution that have culminated in your immune system. Of course, once infection has begun, some diseases can be fought with the aid of antibiotics and antiviral drugs. But these medications are not helpful in *preventing* infection, except in circumstances where normal immunity is breached, such as in surgery.

Scientists have discovered, however, that even the strongest immune system (as measured by the number of helper T cells) fluctuates throughout a person's life. You are most susceptible to disease at the extremes of life—when first born, before you have developed active immunity against most pathogens, and in old age, when the immune system, like the rest of the body, starts to deteriorate. You can't avoid being young or old, but you can make sure you get appropriate vaccinations to help the immune system in case of invasion by specific pathogens (see Table 17-1).

One factor that is known to influence the immune response and that can also be affected by lifestyle and attitudes is stress. Research has shown that the actual number of helper T cells rises and falls inversely with stress; that is, the higher the stress, the lower the T-cell count

(see the box "Immunity and Stress"). As described in Chapter 2, stress encompasses many variables, ranging from emotional stressors, such as anger, anxiety, depression, and grief, to physical stressors, such as poor nutrition, sleep deprivation, overexertion, and substance abuse. Developing effective ways of coping with stress can improve many of the dimensions of wellness.

In addition to managing the stress in your life and getting all your immunizations, you can help your body defend itself against disease by following the guidelines in the box "How to Keep Yourself Well." As is the case with all your body systems, your immune system works best when you support it with a healthy lifestyle.

Tips for Today

The immune system is a remarkable information network; it operates continuously on the cellular level to keep you well. You can support your immune system by practicing a wellness lifestyle—getting enough sleep, managing stress, eating well, exercising, and protecting yourself against infectious agents.

Right now you can

- Go wash your hands, and count out 20 seconds while doing so; you can estimate 20 seconds by singing "Twinkle, Twinkle, Little Star" slowly or "Happy Birthday" twice.

- Eat a balanced diet, and maintain a healthy weight. Consume a variety of low-fat foods to obtain the recommended amount of nutrients every day (see Chapter 12).

- Get enough sleep, 6–8 hours every night. Sleep is extremely important in helping the body replenish itself. Adequate sleep allows the proper production and performance of all immune system cells and functions. Insufficient sleep predisposes you to a great number of illnesses and more severe infections.

- Exercise (but not while you're sick). Moderate endurance exercise is an excellent way to reduce stress and strengthen the body, thereby preventing infection. However, exercising vigorously while you are sick may actually decrease your immunity and can prolong the infection, probably by facilitating the replication of the viruses.

- Don't smoke, and drink alcohol only in moderation. Smoking decreases the levels of some immune cells, and heavy and long-term drinking interferes with the normal functioning of the immune system.

- Wash your hands frequently. Remove your rings, and rub all surfaces of your hands with lather for at least 10–20 seconds; rinse thoroughly. Antibacterial soaps may reduce the risk of infection, but some experts are concerned that widespread use of antibacterial products may contribute to the development of drug-resistant bacteria. The most important thing is to wash your hands well and often. (One study found that although 95% of adults claim they wash their hands after using a public restroom, only about 67% actually do.)

- Avoid contact with people who are contagious with infectious diseases transmitted via the respiratory route, such as influenza, chicken pox, and tuberculosis.

- Handle and prepare foods safely (see Chapter 12); don't drink water from streams or lakes, even in seemingly pristine wilderness areas.

- Avoid contact with mosquitoes and ticks. To help control mosquitoes, which breed in standing water, drain, remove, or turn over any outside objects that could hold water, such as roof gutters, discarded tires, and empty buckets. Wear thick, long-sleeved shirts and long pants, especially during the times of day when mosquitoes are most active—dawn, dusk, and evening (Refer to p.505 for tips on avoiding tick bites.)

- Avoid contact with rodents and other disease carriers. Don't touch or feed wild rodents or any wild animals. Air out unused cabins before occupying them, and avoid stirring up dust when cleaning rodent-infested areas by first wetting the areas with disinfectant.

- To protect yourself against diseases such as hepatitis and HIV infection, practice safer sex (see Chapter 18) and don't inject drugs.

- Get all appropriate immunizations, and use antibiotics appropriately.

- If you do become ill, allow yourself time to recover. Be courteous to others by washing your hands frequently and covering your nose and mouth when you sneeze or cough.

- Plan to move your bedtime up by 15 minutes, starting tonight.

- Put a small pack of tissues in your bag or coat pocket to use when you sneeze or cough, to avoid transmitting infection to others.

- Contribute a bar of soap or liquid hand soap to a public washroom you use frequently, such as in a common living area, in an academic building, or at work.

SUMMARY

- The step-by-step process by which infections are transmitted from one person to another includes the pathogen, its reservoir, a portal of exit, a means of transmission, a portal of entry, and a new host.

- Infection can be prevented by breaking the chain at any point. Strategies include public health measures such as treatment of drinking water and individual action such as hand washing.

- Physical and chemical barriers to microorganisms include skin, mucous membranes, and the cilia lining the respiratory tract.

- The immune response is carried out by white blood cells that are continuously produced in the bone marrow. These include neutrophils, macrophages, natural killer cells, and lymphocytes.

- The inflammatory response occurs when cells in the area of invasion or injury release histamines and other substances that cause blood vessels to dilate and fluid to flow out of capillaries.

- The immune response has four stages: recognition of the invading pathogen; rapid replication of killer T cells and B cells; attack by killer T cells and macrophages; suppression of the immune response.

- Immunization is based on the body's ability to remember previously encountered organisms and retain its strength against them.

- Allergic reactions occur when the immune system responds to harmless substances as if they were dangerous antigens.

- Bacteria are single-celled organisms; some cause disease in humans. Bacterial infections include pneumonia, meningitis, strep throat, toxic shock syndrome, tuberculosis, Lyme disease, and ulcers.

- Most antibiotics work by interrupting the production of new bacteria. Bacteria can become resistant to antibiotics, which do not work against viruses.
- Viruses cannot grow or reproduce themselves; different viruses cause the common cold, influenza, measles, mumps, rubella, chicken pox, cold sores, mononucleosis, encephalitis, hepatitis, polio, and warts.

- Other diseases are caused by certain types of fungi, protozoa, parasitic worms, and prions.
- Autoimmune diseases occur when the body identifies its own cells as foreign.
- The immune system needs little help other than adequate nutrition and rest, a moderate lifestyle, and protection from excessive stress. Vaccinations also help protect against disease.

TAKE ACTION

1. Find out from your parents or your health records which immunizations you have had, including when you last had a tetanus shot. Are your immunizations up to date? If they aren't, or if you're not sure, check with your school health center about what they recommend.

2. Go to your local pharmacy and examine the cold and cough remedies. Exactly which symptoms does each one claim to alleviate, and with what active ingredient? If possible, ask the pharmacist which ones he or she recommends for various symptoms.

Ww. JOURNAL ENTRY

1. In your health journal, list the positive behaviors that help you avoid or resist infection. Consider how you can strengthen those behaviors. Then list the behaviors that tend to block your positive behaviors and put you at risk for contracting an infection. Consider which of these you can change.

2. Monitor yourself the next time you feel a cold coming on. Write down the symptoms, how they felt, the time and date of their occurrence, what you were doing, how you were feeling emotionally, and what you did in response to the symptoms. Keep the record until the cold is gone, noting how long it takes to run its course. Is there an association between your emotional state and how you experienced the symptoms? Between your emotional state and the length of the cold? Does taking

medication (decongestant, cough syrup, etc.) make a difference in the symptoms or the duration of the cold?

3. *Critical Thinking* Does the government have the right to quarantine people who have serious infectious diseases such as tuberculosis or measles? Which should take precedence—concerns about public safety or the rights of individuals? Are there aspects of an illness, such as the seriousness of the illness or the mode of transmission, that should be considered in making this decision? Write an essay outlining your position on this issue; describe what circumstances, if any, you feel would warrant quarantining an infectious person.

FOR MORE INFORMATION

Books

Crawford, D. H. 2000. *The Invisible Enemy: A Natural History of Viruses.* New York: Oxford University Press. *Provides a comprehensive introduction to viruses.*

Garrett, L. 2000. *Betrayal of Trust: The Collapse of Global Public Health.* New York: Hyperion. *A look at the problems and challenges facing public health in today's climate of funding cuts, globalization, and superbugs.*

Karlen, A. 2000. *Biography of a Germ.* New York: Schocken Books. *An entertaining look at the natural history and life cycle of Borrelia burgdorferi, the bacterium that causes Lyme disease, from the microbe's point of view.*

Kolata, G. 2001. *Flu: The Story of the Great Influenza Pandemic of 1918 and the Search for the Virus That Caused It.* New York: Touchstone Books. *A fascinating look at the 1918 flu pandemic.*

Postgate, J. R. 2000. *Microbes and Man,* 4th ed. New York: Cambridge University Press. *An updated introduction to microbes and how they affect people's everyday lives.*

Sompayrac, L. M. 1999. *How the Immune System Works.* Malden, Mass.: Blackwell Science. *A highly readable overview of basic concepts of immunity.*

Ww. Organizations, Hotlines, and Web Sites

Alliance for the Prudent Use of Antibiotics. Provides information on antibiotics and their proper usage as well as tips for avoiding infections.

http://www.healthsci.tufts.edu/apua/apua.html

American Academy of Allergy, Asthma, and Immunology. Provides information and publications; pollen counts are available from the hotline and Web site.

800-822-2762; 800-9-POLLEN

http://www.aaaai.org

American Autoimmune-Related Diseases Association. Provides background information, coping tips, and an online knowledge quiz about autoimmune diseases.

http://www.aarda.org

American College of Allergy, Asthma, and Immunology. Provides information for patients and physicians; Web site includes an extensive glossary of terms related to allergies and asthma.

http://allergy.mcg.edu

American Society for Microbiology. Resources geared toward the public include a library of images and an introduction to microbes.

http://www.asmusa.org

http://www.microbeworld.org/mlc (Microbe World online)

http://www.washup.org (Clean Hands Campaign)

Bugs in the News! Provides information about microbiology—allergies, antibodies, antibiotics, mad cow disease, and more—in easy-to-understand language.

http://falcon.cc.ukans.edu/~jbrown/bugs.html

CDC National Center for Infectious Diseases. Provides extensive information on a wide variety of infectious diseases, including emerging infections.

888-CDC-FAXX

http://www.cdc.gov/ncidod

CDC National Immunization Program. Information and answers to frequently asked questions about immunizations.

800-CDC-SHOT

http://www.cdc.gov/nip

877-FYI-TRIP (international travel information)

http://www.cdc.gov/travel

Cells Alive! Includes micrographs of immune cells and pathogens at work.

http://www.cellsalive.com

Lung Facts/National Jewish Medical and Research Center. Provides information about allergies, asthma, chronic bronchitis, and other lung-related problems.

800-552-LUNG

http://www.NationalJewish.org

Lyme Disease Foundation. Provides strategies for the prevention and treatment of Lyme disease and other tickborne infections.

800-886-LYME (24-hour recorded information)

http://www.lyme.org

National Foundation for Infectious Diseases. Provides information about a variety of diseases and disease issues.

http://www.nfid.org

National Institute of Allergy and Infectious Diseases. Includes fact sheets about many topics relating to allergies and infectious diseases, including tuberculosis and STDs.

http://www.niaid.nih.gov

World Health Organization: Infectious Diseases. Provides fact sheets about many emerging and tropical diseases as well as information about current outbreaks.

http://www.who.int/health-topics/idindex.htm

See also the listings in Chapter 12 (food safety), Chapter 18, and Appendix B.

SELECTED BIBLIOGRAPHY

American Academy of Pediatrics Committee on Infectious Diseases. 2000. Meningococcal disease prevention and control strategies for practice-based physicians (Addendum: Recommendations for college students). *Pediatrics* 106(6): 1500–1504.

American Society for Microbiology. 2000. *Don't Get Caught Dirty Handed.* Washington, D.C.: American Society for Microbiology.

Arvin, A. M. 2001. Varicella vaccine: The first six years. *New England Journal of Medicine* 344(13): 1007–1009.

Bren, L. 2001. Fighting the flu. *FDA Consumer,* January/February.

Bren, L. 2001. Trying to keep "mad cow disease" out of U.S. herds. *FDA Consumer,* March–April.

Cassell, G. H., and J. Mekalanos. 2001. Development of antimicrobial agents in the era of new and reemerging infectious diseases and increasing antibiotic resistance. *Journal of the American Medical Association* 285(5): 601–605.

Centers for Disease Control and Prevention. 2000. *Influenza: General Information* (http://www.cdc.gov/ncidod/diseases/flu/fluinfo.htm; retrieved December 1, 2000).

Centers for Disease Control and Prevention. 2000. Meningococcal disease and college students. *MMWR Recommendations and Reports* 49(RR07): 11–20.

Centers for Disease Control and Prevention. 2001. Lyme disease—United States, 1999. *Morbidity and Mortality Weekly Report.* 50(10): 181–184.

Centers for Disease Control and Prevention. 2001. Serosurveys for West Nile Virus infection. *Morbidity and Mortality Weekly Report* 50(3): 37–39.

Centers for Disease Control and Prevention, Division of Bacterial and Mycotic Diseases. 2000. *Legionellosis: Legionnaire's Disease and Pontiac Fever* (http://www.cdc.gov/ncidod/dbmd/diseaseinfo/legionellosis_g.htm; retrieved November 30, 2000).

Centers for Disease Control and Prevention, National Immunization Program. 2000. *Epidemiology and Prevention of Vaccine-Preventable Diseases,* 6th ed. Washington, D.C.: Public Health Foundation.

Delves, P. J., and I. M. Roitt. 2000. The immune system. *New England Journal of Medicine* 343(1): 37–49.

El-Serag, H. B., and A. C. Mason. 2000. Risk factors for the rising rates of primary liver cancer in the United States. *Archives of Internal Medicine* 160(21): 3227–3230.

Enserink, M. 2000. New arenavirus blamed for recent deaths in California. *Science* 289(5481): 842–843.

Flu vaccine: Preparing for battle. 2001. *Scientific American,* February.

Gonzales, R., et al. 2001. Principles of appropriate antibiotic use for treatment of acute respiratory tract infections in adults: Background, specific aims, and methods. *Annals of Internal Medicine* 1344(6): 479–486.

Marsland, A. L., et al. 2001. Associations between stress, trait negative affect, acute immune reactivity, and antibody response to hepatitis B injection in healthy young adults. *Health Psychology* 20(1): 4–11.

Meadows, M. 2000. Tampon safety: TSS now rare, but women still should take care. *FDA Consumer,* March–April.

Moore, P. S. 2000. The emergence of Kaposi's sarcoma–associated herpesvirus (human herpesvirus 8). *New England Journal of Medicine* 343(19): 1411–1413.

National Institute of Allergy and Infectious Diseases. 2000. *Fact Sheet: Group A Streptococcal Infections* (http://www.niaid.nih.gov/factsheets/strep.htm; retrieved July 24, 2000).

Sparrer, H. E., et al. 2000. Evidence for the prion hypothesis. *Science* 289(5479): 595–599.

Subramanian, C., M. A. Cotter, and E. S. Robertson. 2001. Epstein-Barr virus nuclear protein EBNA-3C interacts with the human metastatic suppressor Nm23-H1: A molecular link to cancer metastasis. *Nature Medicine* 7(3): 350–355.

Super-germ alert: How to avoid antibiotic misuse and overuse. 2001. *Consumer Reports,* January.

World Health Organization. 2000. *Fact Sheet: Variant Creutzfeldt-Jakob Disease* (http://www.who.int/inf-fs/en/fact180.html; retrieved December 4, 2000).

World Health Organization. 2000. *Global Polio Eradication Initiative: The Disease and Virus* (http://www.polioeradication.org/virus.html; retrieved December 4, 2000).

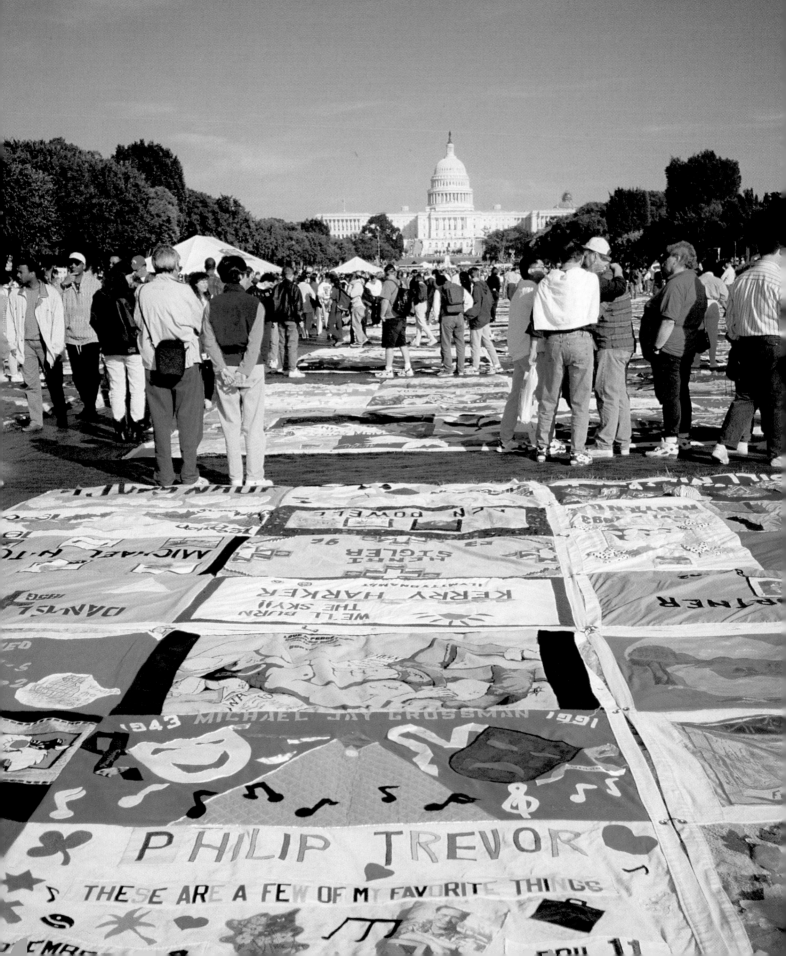

Sexually Transmitted Diseases

18

TEST YOUR KNOWLEDGE

1. If you have a sexually transmitted disease (STD), you will know it.
   True or false?

2. STDs can cause infertility in women.
   True or false?

3. About _____ Americans are infected with HIV, the virus that causes AIDS; and about _____ Americans are infected with HSV-2, the virus that causes most cases of genital herpes.
   a. 1 in 30,000 (HIV); 1 in 20 (HSV-2)
   b. 1 in 3000 (HIV); 1 in 10 (HSV-2)
   c. 1 in 300 (HIV); 1 in 5 (HSV-2)

4. A man with an STD is more likely to transmit the infection to a female partner than vice versa.
   True or false?

5. After you have had an STD once, you become immune to that disease and cannot get it again.
   True or false?

6. Douching after intercourse helps decrease the risk of STDs.
   True or false?

ANSWERS

1. **FALSE.** Many people with STDs have no symptoms and do not know they are infected; however, they can still pass an infection to their partners.

2. **TRUE.** Untreated STDs, especially gonorrhea and chlamydia, are the leading cause of infertility in young women.

3. **C.** Worldwide, about 1 in 100 people is infected with HIV. Most of the approximately 22% of Americans infected with HSV-2 are asymptomatic and unaware they are infected.

4. **TRUE.** For many STDs, infected men are at least twice as likely as infected women to transmit an STD to their partner. And many STDs are more physically damaging to women than to men.

5. **FALSE.** Reinfection with STDs is very common. For example, if you are treated and cured of chlamydia and then you have sex with your untreated partner, the chances are very good that you will be infected again.

6. **FALSE.** Douching can actually increase a woman's chance of getting pelvic inflammatory disease.

Acquired immunodeficiency syndrome (AIDS) is a leading cause of death in many parts of the world. Most of the more than 36 million people around the world who are infected with **human immunodeficiency virus (HIV),** the virus that causes AIDS, will likely die within the next 10 years. Although the death rate from AIDS in the United States began to decline in 1996, more than 430,000 of the 750,000 Americans who had been diagnosed with AIDS by 2000 had died from the disease, and it remains a major killer of Americans.

Although recent public education campaigns have focused primarily on HIV infection, all the **sexually transmitted diseases (STDs)**—gonorrhea, genital warts, chlamydia, herpes, syphilis, and others—continue to have a high incidence among Americans. The United States has the highest rate of STDs of any developed nation. Worldwide, nearly 300 million people are affected by STDs each year.

STDs are a particularly insidious group of diseases because a person can be infected and be able to transmit the disease to others, yet not look or feel sick. The cost of unprotected sex may not become apparent for many years. Then a person may find that an undiagnosed STD has led to infertility, contributed to the development of cancer, or caused a birth defect in a child. In the case of HIV infection, the immune system becomes weakened and can no longer provide protection from disease.

It is important that everyone have a clear understanding of what STDs are, how they are transmitted, and—most important—how they can be prevented. The crucial message is that they *can* be prevented. And many can also be cured if they are treated early and properly. This chapter is designed to provide information about healthy, safer sexual behavior and to help you understand what you can do to reduce the further spread of these diseases.

WWW. THE MAJOR STDS

In general, seven different STDs pose major health threats: HIV/AIDS, hepatitis, syphilis, chlamydia, gonorrhea, herpes, and genital warts. These diseases are considered major because they are serious in themselves, cause serious complications if left untreated, and/or pose risks to a fetus or newborn. In addition, pelvic inflammatory disease (PID) is a common complication of gonorrhea and chlamydia and merits discussion as a separate disease. The pathogens responsible for these and other STDs are listed in Table 18-1.

The bacterial STDs, including chlamydia, gonorrhea, and syphilis, are curable with antibiotics. Unfortunately, previous infection does not confer immunity, so a person can be reinfected despite treatment. The viral STDs—herpes, genital warts, hepatitis, and HIV infection—are not curable with current therapies. Although antiviral drugs and other medications can help target the effects of these STDs, the virus remains in the body and may cause chronic or recurrent infection. A further risk of all STDs is that they can substantially contribute to the spread of HIV. The sores and inflammation caused by STDs allow HIV to pass more easily from one person to another.

HIV Infection and AIDS

HIV infection is one of the most serious and challenging problems facing the United States and the world today. Worldwide, it is estimated that more than 57 million people have been infected since the epidemic began—nearly 1% of the world's population—and that more than 21 million have died (see the box "HIV Infection Around the World"). About 10 people are infected every minute, and half of these new infections are in people age 15–24. By 2000, an estimated 650,000–1,000,000 Americans were believed to be living with HIV—about 1 in 160 males and 1 in 800 females over age 12. Although the death rate from AIDS among Americans has declined, new infections are holding steady at about 40,000 per year, meaning the number of Americans living with HIV infection is growing.

HIV is a relatively new disease for humans. Experts believe that the virus initially spread from chimpanzees to people during the 1930s as a result of the trapping, butchering, or eating of infected chimps. In the middle part of the twentieth century, HIV infection was relatively rare, but the disease began to spread rapidly in the 1970s and 1980s. Despite the best efforts of health professionals all around the world, HIV infection continues to spread, and a cure is yet to be found.

What Is HIV Infection? **HIV infection** is a chronic disease that progressively damages the body's immune system, making an otherwise healthy person less able to

Terms

acquired immunodeficiency syndrome (AIDS) A generally fatal, incurable, sexually transmitted viral disease.

human immunodeficiency virus (HIV) The virus that causes HIV infection and AIDS.

sexually transmitted disease (STD) A disease that can be transmitted by sexual contact; some STDs can also be transmitted by other means.

HIV infection A chronic, progressive disease that damages the immune system.

CD4 T cell A type of white blood cell that helps coordinate the activity of the immune system; the primary target for HIV infection. A decrease in the number of these cells correlates with the risk and severity of HIV-related illness.

opportunistic infection An infection caused when organisms take the opportunity presented by a primary (initial) infection to multiply and cause a secondary infection.

asymptomatic Showing no signs or symptoms of a disease.

| Table 18–1 | Sexually Transmitted Pathogens and Associated Diseases |

Bacteria[a]

Chlamydia trachomatis	Chlamydia, pelvic inflammatory disease, epididymitis, urethritis
Gardnerella vaginalis[b]	Bacterial vaginosis
Haemophilus ducreyi	Chancroid
Neisseria gonorrhoeae	Gonorrhea, pelvic inflammatory disease, epididymitis, urethritis
Treponema pallidum	Syphilis

Viruses[c]

Hepatitis B virus (HBV)	Hepatitis, cirrhosis, liver cancer
Herpes simplex viruses (HSV)	Genital herpes, oral-labial herpes (cold sores)
Human immunodeficiency virus (HIV)	HIV infection/AIDS
Human papillomavirus (HPV)	Genital warts, cervical cancer

Protozoa[a]

Trichomonas vaginalis	Trichomoniasis

Ectoparasites[a]

Phthirus pubis	Pubic lice
Sarcoptes scabiei	Scabies

[a]Treatable with antibiotics or topical medications.
[b]Other organisms associated with bacterial vaginosis include *Mycoplasma hominis*, *Bacteroides*, and *Mobiluncus*.
[c]Incurable with current treatment methods, although medications may reduce symptoms and limit the damage from infection; viral STDs are usually chronic/recurrent.

resist a variety of infections and disorders. Under normal conditions, when a virus or other pathogen enters the body, it is targeted and destroyed by the immune system. But the human immunodeficiency virus (HIV) attacks the immune system itself, invading and taking over **CD4 T cells**, monocytes, and macrophages, which are essential elements of the body's defense system. HIV enters a human cell and converts its own genetic material, RNA, into DNA. It then inserts this DNA into the chromosomes of the host cell. The viral DNA takes over the CD4 cell, causing it to produce new copies of HIV; it also makes the CD4 cell incapable of performing its immune functions. HIV primarily affects the T-cell part of the immune system (see Chapter 17).

Immediately following infection with HIV, billions of infectious particles are produced every day. For a time, the immune system keeps pace, also producing billions of new cells. Unlike the virus, however, the immune system cannot make new cells indefinitely; as long as the virus keeps replicating, it wins in the end. The destruction of the immune system is signaled by the loss of CD4 T cells (Figure 18-1). As the number of CD4 cells declines, an infected person may begin to experience mild to moderately severe symptoms. A person is diagnosed with full-blown AIDS when he or she develops one of the conditions defined as a marker for AIDS or when the

number of CD4 cells in the blood drops below a certain level (200/μl). People with AIDS are vulnerable to a number of serious, often fatal, secondary, or **opportunistic, infections.** The infections that most often prove deadly for people with HIV are seldom serious in people with a healthy immune system. In fact, opportunistic infections are usually caused by organisms that are very common in the environment and generally do not cause illness in healthy people.

Shortly after being infected with HIV, about 50% of people develop flulike symptoms that disappear after a few days or weeks. Once the initial symptoms resolve, most people feel generally well. This **asymptomatic** (symptom-free) period of HIV infection can last from 2 to 20 years, with an average of 11 years in untreated adults. During this time the virus is progressively infecting and destroying the cells of the immune system. People infected with HIV can pass the virus to others—even if they have no symptoms and even if they do not know they have been infected. In the early days and weeks of infection, the most commonly used test for HIV remains negative. An infected individual may feel fine, but viral levels are often high at this stage. These asymptomatic individuals, unaware that they are infected but with high viral levels, are responsible for much of the spread of HIV.

Although first detected among heterosexuals in Africa, AIDS captured world attention in the early 1980s as a disease occuring primarily among homosexual men in the United States and Europe. Since then, AIDS has spread around the world. Nearly 60 million people worldwide have been infected with HIV since the epidemic began, and more than 21 million have died.

The vast majority of cases—95%—have occurred in developing countries, where heterosexual contact is the primary means of transmission, responsible for 75–85% of all adult infections. In the developed world, HIV is increasingly becoming a disease that disproportionately affects the poor and ethnic minorities, especially women, youth, and children. Worldwide, women are the fastest-growing group of newly infected people, and nearly half the new cases of HIV infection in 2000 occurred in women. In addition, an estimated 1.4 million children are living with HIV infection and about 13.2 million children are AIDS orphans. It is estimated that the number of AIDS orphans will reach 40 million by 2010.

Currently, more than 25 million of those infected with HIV are in Africa, where AIDS has become the leading cause of death. Sub-Saharan Africa remains the hardest hit of all areas of the world; in some countries, 20–35% of adults carry the virus, and overall life expectancy has begun to decline dramatically. However, because the epidemic started about 10 years later in Asia than in Africa, experts expect an explosion of new cases in Asia, where already nearly 6 million people are infected. And because Asia accounts for more than 50% of the world's population, the pool of people at risk is much larger than in Africa. HIV is also spreading rapidly in Eastern Europe, where injection drug use and commercial sex are increasing.

Efforts to combat AIDS are complicated by political, economic, and cultural barriers in many parts of the world. Education and prevention programs are often hampered by resistance from social and religious institutions and by the taboo on openly discussing sexual issues. Condoms are unfamiliar in many countries, and women in many societies do not have sufficient control over their lives to demand that men use condoms during sex. Prevention approaches that have had success include STD treatment and education, public education campaigns about safer sex, and syringe exchange programs for injection drug users. In countries where there is a substantial imbalance in the social power of men and women, focusing prevention efforts on men is an essential step. International efforts are underway to make condoms more available by lowering their price and to develop effective antiviral creams that women can use without the knowledge of their partners. In countries such as Thailand and Uganda, where governments have worked hard to prevent the spread of HIV through education and other public health measures, rates of new infection have declined substantially.

In developed nations such as the United States, new drugs are reversing AIDS symptoms and lowering viral levels dramatically for some patients. But these drugs are almost entirely unavailable in the developing world. Ultimately what is needed are effective vaccines. But until vaccines or a low-cost cure is developed, efforts must continue to focus on widespread educational campaigns and prevention through behavior change.

SOURCES: Joint United Nations Programme on HIV/AIDS (UNAIDS). 2000. *AIDS Epidemic Update: December 2000*. Geneva: UNAIDS/WHO. Centers for Disease Control and Prevention. 2000. World AIDS Day—December 1, 2000. *Morbidity and Mortality Weekly Report* 49(47): 1061.

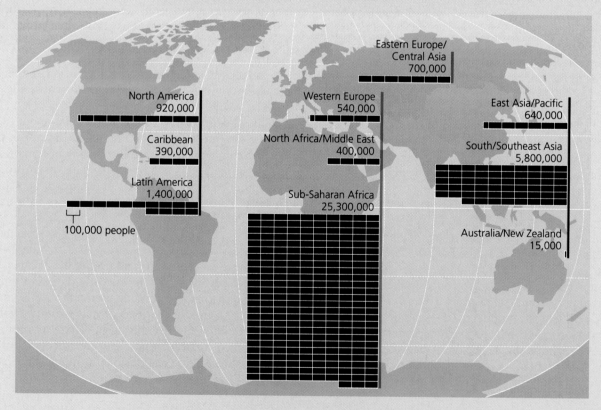

Approximate number of people with HIV/AIDS at the beginning of 2001.

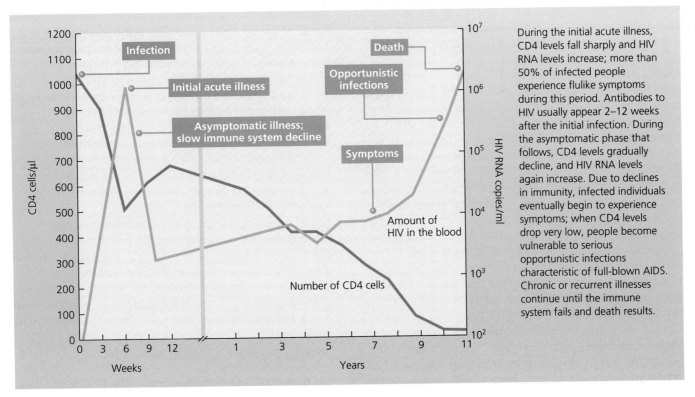

During the initial acute illness, CD4 levels fall sharply and HIV RNA levels increase; more than 50% of infected people experience flulike symptoms during this period. Antibodies to HIV usually appear 2–12 weeks after the initial infection. During the asymptomatic phase that follows, CD4 levels gradually decline, and HIV RNA levels again increase. Due to declines in immunity, infected individuals eventually begin to experience symptoms; when CD4 levels drop very low, people become vulnerable to serious opportunistic infections characteristic of full-blown AIDS. Chronic or recurrent illnesses continue until the immune system fails and death results.

Figure 18-1   The general pattern of untreated HIV infection.   The purple line represents the number of CD4 cells in the blood, a marker for the status of the immune system. The orange line shows the amount of HIV RNA in the blood.   SOURCE: Adapted from Fauci, A. S., et al. 1996. Immunopathogenic mechanisms of HIV infection. *Annals of Internal Medicine* 124: 654–663. Reprinted with permission of the publisher.

Transmitting the Virus   HIV lives only within cells and body fluids, not outside the body. It is transmitted by blood and blood products, semen, vaginal and cervical secretions, and breast milk. It cannot live in air, in water, or on objects or surfaces such as toilet seats, eating utensils, or telephones. The three main routes of HIV transmission are (1) from specific kinds of sexual contact, (2) from direct exposure to infected blood, and (3) from an HIV-infected woman to her fetus during pregnancy or childbirth or to her infant during breastfeeding.

SEXUAL CONTACT   Of the different types of sexual contact, HIV is more likely to be transmitted by unprotected anal or vaginal intercourse than by other sexual activities. Being the receptive partner during unprotected anal intercourse is the riskiest of all sexual activities. Oral-genital contact carries some risk of transmission, although less than anal or vaginal intercourse. Oral sex is responsible for a small but significant number of cases of HIV transmission; a recent study of newly HIV-infected gay men found that up to 8% of infections were transmitted through unprotected oral sex. HIV can be transmitted through tiny tears in the fragile lining of the vagina, cervix, penis, anus, and mouth and through direct infection of cells in some of these areas.

The presence of lesions, blisters, or inflammation from other STDs in the genital, anal, or oral areas makes it two to nine times easier for the virus to be passed. In addition, any trauma or irritation of tissues, such as might occur from rough or unwanted intercourse or the use of enemas prior to anal intercourse, increases the risk. Spermicides may also cause irritation and increase the risk of HIV transmission. A recent large-scale study of female sex workers in Africa and Thailand found a higher rate of HIV transmission among women who used nonoxynol-9, a widely used spermicide.

The risk of HIV transmission during oral sex increases if a person has poor oral hygiene, has oral sores, or has brushed or flossed just before or after oral sex. During vaginal intercourse, male-to-female transmission is more likely to occur than female-to-male transmission. HIV has been found in preejaculatory fluid, so transmission can occur before ejaculation.

Studies in developing nations with high rates of HIV infection have found that circumcised males have a lower risk of HIV infection than uncircumcised males. Studies are ongoing to determine the magnitude of protection offered by circumcision, but most experts doubt whether circumcision, which is uncommon in most parts of the world, would ever be a practical preventive measure. In the United States, where circumcision is common and HIV infection rates are much lower, circumcision does not appear to offer any significant protection against HIV.

DIRECT CONTACT WITH INFECTED BLOOD   Direct contact with the blood of an infected person is the second major route of HIV transmission. Needles used to inject drugs (including heroin, cocaine, and anabolic steroids) are routinely contaminated by the blood of the user. If needles are shared, small amounts of one person's blood are directly injected into another person's bloodstream. HIV may be transmitted through subcutaneous and intramuscular injection as well, from needles or blades used in acupuncture, tattooing, ritual scarring, and piercing of the earlobes, nose, lip, nipple, navel, or other body part.

Nearly half of all new cases of HIV in the United States are caused, directly or indirectly, by sharing drug injection equipment contaminated with HIV. Drug users, their sex partners, and their children are all at extremely high risk for HIV infection. Most experts agree that syringe exchange programs combined with increased substance abuse treatment and prevention could significantly reduce the spread of HIV. However, syringe exchange programs are controversial and not available in many communities (see Chapter 9 for more information).

HIV has been transmitted in blood and blood products used in the medical treatment of injuries, serious illnesses, and **hemophilia,** resulting in about 14,000 cases of AIDS in the United States. The blood supply in all licensed blood banks and plasma centers in the United States is now screened for HIV. The odds are less than 1 in 650,000 that a unit of HIV-infected donated blood will fail to be detected with today's testing methods, and new genetic tests may further reduce the risk. Unfortunately, the blood supply is much less safe in the rest of the world. In the developing world in particular, blood is not adequately tested and blood donors are not appropriately screened. In these countries, the risk of contracting HIV or another serious infection from a blood transfusion is very high. The World Health Organization (WHO) estimates that 5–10% of all cases of HIV infection worldwide have resulted from the transfusion of infected blood and blood products.

A small number of health care workers have acquired HIV on the job; most of these cases involve needle sticks, in which a health care worker is accidentally stuck with a needle used on an infected patient. The only reported cases of possible transmission *to* patients are those of six patients of a Florida dentist, one patient of a nurse in France, and one patient of a French orthopedic surgeon. A method of transmission was never determined with cer-

tainty in the first two cases; in the third, an injury to the hand of the surgeon during an operation may have exposed the patient to infected blood. Intensive investigations of over 22,000 patients of 63 HIV-infected health care workers showed no other cases of HIV transmission from health care workers to patients in the United States. The likelihood of a patient acquiring HIV infection from a health care worker is almost negligible; the risk to health care workers from infected patients is much greater.

What about contact with other body fluids? Trace amounts of HIV have been found in the saliva and tears of some infected people. However, researchers believe that these fluids do not carry enough of the virus to infect another person. (In the rare cases of HIV infection linked to deep kissing or biting, the virus is thought to have been transmitted in blood from oral sores rather than in saliva.) HIV has been found in urine and feces, and contact with the urine or feces of an infected person may carry some risk. Contact with an infected person's sweat is not believed to carry any risk. There is absolutely no evidence that the virus can be spread by insects such as mosquitoes.

MOTHER-TO-CHILD TRANSMISSION   The final major route of HIV transmission is mother-to-child, also called *vertical, or perinatal, transmission,* which can occur during pregnancy, childbirth, or breastfeeding. About 25–30% of infants born to untreated HIV-infected mothers are also infected with the virus; treatment, discussed later in the chapter, can dramatically lower this infection rate. Worldwide, about two-thirds of vertical transmission occurs during pregnancy and childbirth and one-third through breastfeeding. An estimated 600,000 infants are infected with HIV each year, 90% of them in developing countries. Primarily because of voluntary HIV testing and treatment of pregnant women, the number of new cases of AIDS diagnosed each year among U.S. children has declined more than 80% since 1992. However, by 2000, over 8000 cases of AIDS in children infected by vertical transmission had been reported in the United States.

NOT THROUGH CASUAL CONTACT   A person is not at risk of getting HIV infection by being in the same classroom, dining room, or even household with someone who is infected. Before this was generally known, many people with HIV infection, including children, were the targets of ostracism, hysteria, and outright violence. Today, it is an acknowledged responsibility of everyone to treat people with HIV infection with respect and compassion, regardless of their age or how they became infected.

Populations of Special Concern for HIV Infection
Among Americans with AIDS, the most common means of exposure to HIV has been sexual activity between men; injection drug use (IDU) and heterosexual contact are the next most common (Figure 18-2). Changes in the sexual

Terms   **hemophilia** A hereditary blood disease in which blood fails to clot and abnormal bleeding occurs, requiring transfusions of blood products with a specific factor to aid coagulation.

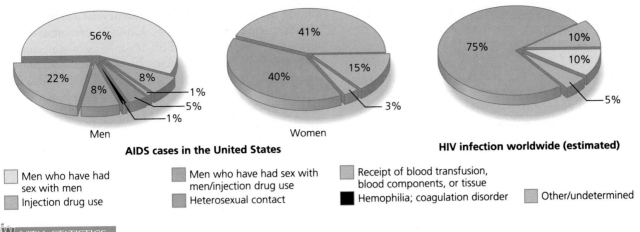

Men	Women	HIV infection worldwide (estimated)
56%	41%	75%
22%	40%	10%
8%	15%	10%
8%	3%	5%
1%		
5%		
1%		

AIDS cases in the United States | **HIV infection worldwide (estimated)**

☐ Men who have had sex with men   ☐ Men who have had sex with men/injection drug use   ☐ Receipt of blood transfusion, blood components, or tissue

☐ Injection drug use   ☐ Heterosexual contact   ■ Hemophilia; coagulation disorder   ☐ Other/undetermined

VITAL STATISTICS

Figure 18-2   **Routes of HIV transmission among adults.**   SOURCES: Centers for Disease Control and Prevention. 2000. *HIV/AIDS Surveillance Report* 12(1). Joint United Nations Programme on HIV/AIDS (UNAIDS). 2000. *AIDS Epidemic Update: December 2000.* Geneva: UNAIDS/WHO.

behavior of homosexual men and the screening of all donated blood have slowed the rate of infection from these sources, and HIV in the United States is increasingly becoming a disease that disproportionately affects minorities, women, children, and the poor.

The rate of HIV infection is eight times higher in African Americans than it is in whites, and the rate among Hispanics is twice that of whites. African American and Hispanic women account for nearly 80% of new HIV cases among women in the United States. In 2000, about 85% of children reported with AIDS were African American or Hispanic. While a large majority of HIV infection among whites in the United States is due to sexual contact between men, among minorities, IDU contributes to about half of cases. Of young women with AIDS, more than half were infected through heterosexual contact, often with an injection drug user.

AIDS incidence and deaths have declined since 1996 among all groups of Americans, but these declines have been smaller among women and minorities compared to other groups. Between 1985 and 2000, the proportion of new U.S. AIDS cases reported each year in women increased from 7% to 24%. Women with HIV infection or AIDS often face tremendous challenges when they are ill because they may be caring for family members—children and spouses—who are also infected and ill. Many women are also dealing with substance-abuse problems in themselves or in family members. In addition, there is some evidence that women may actually become sicker at lower viral loads compared to men.

More than 90% of all cases of HIV infection in children are the result of transmission from infected mothers. HIV-infected children rarely appear ill at birth, but they begin to develop health problems over the first months and years of life. About 20% of infected children become very

ill and progress to AIDS or death by age 4; the remaining 80% develop problems more slowly. In the United States, new treatments to reduce vertical transmission are in use, and the number of new cases of HIV infection in children has declined significantly. The situation worldwide is bleak, however: By 2000, fewer than 1 in 20 children born to HIV-positive women in the United States became infected with HIV; in developing countries, the average was about 1 in 3. The major reasons for this disparity are the lack of HIV testing and treatment in developing countries and breastfeeding practices. In developing countries, infants often acquire HIV through breastfeeding, whereas in the United States, HIV-infected mothers generally do not breastfeed their infants.

Also of concern are younger homosexual men. Although the overall transmission rates of HIV infection have dropped substantially among gay men in general, the reductions are not as great for men under 30. Surveys indicate that younger gay and bisexual men are much more likely to engage in unsafe sexual activity, especially unprotected receptive anal intercourse, than older men.

These patterns of HIV infection reflect complex social, economic, and behavioral factors. Reducing the rates of HIV transmission and AIDS death in minorities, women, and other groups at risk will require dealing with the difficult problems of drug abuse, poverty, and discrimination. HIV prevention programs must be tailored to meet the special needs of minority communities.

Symptoms of HIV Infection   Within a few days or weeks of infection with HIV, about half of people will develop symptoms of acute HIV infection. These can include fever, fatigue, rashes, headache, swollen lymph nodes, body aches, night sweats, sore throat, nausea, and diarrhea. Because the symptoms of acute HIV infection are similar to those of many common viral illnesses, the condition often goes undiagnosed, even if an infected individual sees a physician.

Diagnosis of HIV at this very early stage of infection, although uncommon, is extremely beneficial. Immediate treatment may help preserve immune function, slow the progress of the disease, and reduce transmission of HIV to others. For these reasons, it is critical for people who have engaged in behavior that places them at risk for HIV infection and who then experience symptoms of acute HIV infection to immediately inform their physician of their risk status. Standard tests for HIV will usually be negative in the very early stages of infection, so specialized tests such as the **HIV RNA assay,** which directly measures the amount of virus in the body, must be used.

Other than the initial flulike symptoms associated with acute HIV infection, most people in the first months or years of HIV infection have few if any symptoms. As the immune system weakens, however, a variety of symptoms can develop—persistent swollen lymph nodes; lumps, rashes, sores, or other growths on or under the skin or on the mucous membranes of the eyes, mouth, anus, or nasal passages; persistent yeast infections; unexplained weight loss; fever and drenching night sweats; dry cough and shortness of breath; persistent diarrhea; easy bruising and unexplained bleeding; profound fatigue; memory loss; difficulty with balance; tremors or seizures; changes in vision, hearing, taste, or smell; difficulty in swallowing; changes in mood and other psychological symptoms; and persistent or recurrent pain. Obviously, many of these symptoms can also occur with a variety of other illnesses.

Because the immune system is weakened, people with HIV infection are highly susceptible to infections, both common and uncommon. The infection most often seen among people with HIV is ***Pneumocystis carinii* pneumonia,** a protozoal infection. **Kaposi's sarcoma,** a rare form of cancer, is common in HIV-infected men. Women with HIV infection often have frequent and difficult-to-treat vaginal yeast infections. Cases of tuberculosis (TB) are also increasingly being reported in people with HIV, and the Centers for Disease Control and Prevention recommends TB testing for anyone with HIV infection. In Africa, drug-resistant strains of TB are now the most deadly infection among people with AIDS.

Diagnosing HIV Infection Early diagnosis of HIV infection is important to minimize the impact of the disease. The most common tests for HIV check for the presence of antibodies to the virus. As described earlier, HIV infection primarily disrupts T-cell immunity; B cells are still able to produce antibodies to HIV, which will show up in tests. Unfortunately, these antibodies do not protect against the spread of the virus. For most other diseases, the presence of an antibody to a particular pathogen may indicate protective immunity. In the case of HIV, however, the presence of the antibody indicates an active case of the disease. **HIV antibody tests** are used for screening because they are accurate and relatively inexpensive. An initial test, called an **ELISA,** is performed; if it is positive, a second test called a **Western blot** is done to confirm the results (see the box "Getting an HIV Test").

Not everyone with HIV infection will test positive on antibody tests, however. Antibodies may not appear in the blood for weeks or months after infection, so people who are newly infected are likely to have a negative antibody test. The infection can be detected with a more expensive test that directly measures the presence of the virus, such as an HIV RNA test. The reverse situation is seen in babies born to HIV-infected mothers: They may carry HIV antibodies, passed from their mother, without being infected with HIV. Antibodies can pass through the placenta to a fetus, but in the majority of cases, even without treatment, an infant does not acquire HIV. Thus, an infant may test positive on an HIV antibody test but actually be uninfected. Further tests such as the HIV RNA assay must be done to determine if an infant is actually infected.

If a person is diagnosed as **HIV-positive,** the next step is to determine the current severity of the disease in order to plan appropriate treatment. The status of the immune system can be gauged by taking CD4 T-cell measurements every few months. The infection itself can be monitored by tracking the amount of virus in the body (the "viral load") through HIV RNA assay. Keeping track of viral load changes helps physicians evaluate the effects of treatment and can also help predict the likelihood of long-term survival in a person infected with HIV.

Although rates vary from state to state, surveys indicate that about 40% of adults in the United States have been tested for HIV. About 20% of those tested had the test for personal or health reasons. The majority were tested to

Terms

HIV RNA assay A test used to determine the amount of HIV in the blood (the "viral load").

***Pneumocystis carinii* pneumonia** A protozoal infection that is common in people infected with HIV.

Kaposi's sarcoma A form of cancer characterized by purple or brownish lesions that are generally painless and occur anywhere on the skin; usually appears in men infected with HIV.

HIV antibody test A blood test to determine whether a person has been infected by HIV; becomes positive within weeks or months of exposure.

ELISA (enzyme-linked immunosorbent assay) A blood test that detects the presence of antibodies to HIV.

Western blot A blood test that detects the presence of HIV antibodies; a more accurate and more expensive test, and used to confirm positive results from an ELISA test.

HIV-positive A diagnosis resulting from the presence of HIV in the bloodstream; also referred to as *seropositive.*

seroconversion The appearance of antibodies to HIV in the blood of an infected person; usually occurs 1–6 months after infection.

Getting an early diagnosis of HIV infection is more important than ever, but many people with HIV do not know they are infected. Anyone who has engaged in any of the following activities is potentially at risk and should consider being tested

- You have had unprotected sex (vaginal, anal, or oral) with more than one partner or with a partner who was not in a mutually monogamous relationship with you.

- You have used or shared needles, syringes, or other paraphernalia for injecting drugs (including steroids).

- You received a transfusion of blood or blood products prior to 1985.

- You have been diagnosed with an STD.

Testing Options

If you decide to get an HIV test, either you can visit a physician or health clinic or you can take a home test. A big advantage to having the test performed by a physician or clinician is that you will get one-on-one counseling about the test, your results, and ways to avoid future infection or spreading the disease. If you have good reason to think you may test positive, it is probably best to be tested by a physician or clinic, where follow-up counseling and medical care will be intensive. The home test is a good alternative for people at low risk who just want to be sure. The advantages of the home test are that it can be done privately and anonymously, and it may be attractive to people who would not otherwise get tested.

Physician or Clinic Testing

Your physician, student health clinic, Planned Parenthood, public health department, or local AIDS association can arrange your HIV test. It usually costs $50–$100, but public clinics often charge little or nothing. The test itself is fairly simple. The procedure will be explained to you, and then a sample of blood will be drawn and sent to a laboratory for analysis for the presence of antibodies to HIV. If the first stage of testing, the ELISA test, proves positive, it is followed by a confirmatory test, the Western blot. You'll be asked to phone or come in personally to get your results, which should include appropriate counseling. (Some clinics now also offer "rapid tests" that yield results within 10–30 minutes; positive results must still be confirmed with the standard antibody tests and may require an additional week or two.) If you test negative, you need to know how to stay uninfected. If you test positive, you'll need to know what your medical options are; what the psychological, social, and financial repercussions might be; and how to avoid spreading the disease.

Alternative tests may be used in some circumstances. The Orasure test uses oral fluid, which is collected by placing a treated cotton pad in the mouth for several minutes. Urine tests are also available. Oral fluid and urine tests may be helpful for people who avoid blood tests because of fear of needles. If you are ill and have reason to think your symptoms could be due to acute (very recent) HIV infection, see your physician and request an HIV RNA test. Remember, HIV antibody tests are generally negative in the earliest stage of infection, so it is important to have the more expensive HIV RNA test.

Before you get an HIV test, be sure you understand what will be done with the results. Results from confidential tests may still become part of your medical record and/or reported (with your name or some other identifier) to state and federal public health agencies. If you decide you want to be tested anonymously—in which case the results will not be reported to anyone but yourself—check with your physician or counselor about how to obtain an anonymous test or use a home test.

Home Testing

Home test kits for HIV are now available; they cost about $40. (Take care to avoid testing kits that are not FDA-approved; many such unapproved kits are being sold over the Internet.) To use a home test, you prick a finger with a supplied lancet, blot a few drops of blood onto blotting paper, and mail it to the company's laboratory. There the sample is tested for HIV by the same methods used for samples collected by physicians. In about a week, you call a toll-free number to find out your results. Anyone testing positive is routed to a trained counselor, who can provide emotional and medical support.

The results of home test kits are completely anonymous. Your blood sample is assigned an identification number, and you never give your name or address. Even if you test positive and receive counseling, your conversation will be anonymous.

Understanding the Results

A negative test result means that no antibodies were found in your sample. However, it usually takes at least a month (and possibly as long as 6 months in some people) after exposure to HIV for antibodies to appear, a process called **seroconversion.** Therefore, an infected person may get a false-negative result. If you think you've been exposed to HIV, get a test immediately; if it's negative but your risk of infection is high, ask about obtaining an HIV RNA assay, which allows very early diagnosis.

A positive result means that you are infected. It is important to seek medical care and counseling immediately. Rapid progress is being made in treating HIV, and treatments are potentially much more successful when begun early.

---

obtain insurance or enter the military or for reasons related to employment.

Diagnosing AIDS   As mentioned earlier, AIDS is the most severe form of HIV infection. The CDC's criteria for

a diagnosis of AIDS reflect the stage of HIV infection at which a person's immune system becomes dangerously compromised. Since January 1993, a diagnosis of AIDS has been made if a person is HIV-positive and either has developed an infection defined as an AIDS indicator or has a severely damaged immune system (as measured by CD4 T-cell counts).

Reporting   All diagnosed cases of AIDS must be reported to public health authorities. Before effective treatments for HIV infection were available, officials could use AIDS statistics to track the epidemic because nearly everyone with HIV eventually developed AIDS within a fairly predictable time frame. However, the advent of more effective treatments has lengthened the time between infection and the onset of full-blown AIDS for many patients, making it more difficult to track the U.S. epidemic based on AIDS statistics alone. For this reason, the CDC recommended in 1999 that states require reporting of both HIV infection and full-blown AIDS. These data may be available by 2002.

Despite efforts to safeguard confidentiality and prohibit discrimination, mandatory reporting of HIV infection remains a controversial issue. If people believe they are risking their jobs, friends, or social acceptability, they may be less likely to be tested. At the same time, it is essential that enough information be disclosed through reporting to monitor the epidemic. The CDC recommends that states continue to provide opportunities for people to be tested anonymously; home HIV tests also allow anonymous testing.

Treatment   Although there is no known cure for HIV infection, medications can significantly alter the course of the disease and extend life. The drop in the number of U.S. AIDS deaths that has occurred since 1996 is in large part due to the increasing use of combinations of new drugs. Researchers hope that HIV infection will become a chronic disease that can be managed with medication.

ANTIVIRAL DRUGS   Antiviral drugs in current use to combat HIV fall into two major categories. The first type is **reverse transcriptase inhibitors,** which include the widely used drug zidovudine (AZT). These drugs work by inhibiting the enzyme reverse transcriptase, which is used by HIV to integrate its genetic material into human cells (Figure 18-3). The second class of antivirals is the **protease inhibitors;** these target the enzyme HIV protease, which is used by the virus to create a protein coat for each new copy of the virus. Treatment with combinations of drugs, referred to as highly active antiretroviral therapy,

or HAART, can reduce HIV in the blood to undetectable levels in some people. However, research indicates that latent virus is still present in the body and that HIV-infected men on HAART carry potentially transmissible HIV in their semen.

A new medication under study is hydroxyurea, which blocks the function of an enzyme that is necessary for both HIV and human cells to multiply. When combined with other antivirals, hydroxyurea may slow the development of drug resistance and allow antiviral drugs to work better for longer periods. Researchers are also pairing antivirals with drugs such as interleukin-2 that stimulate the immune system.

Another new approach to HIV treatment is the use of *structured intermittent therapy,* in which HAART is used for a period of time, then discontinued completely, and then restarted again in a planned, cyclical fashion. Researchers hope that drug-free intervals will help stimulate the patient's own immune response against HIV. This approach, if successful, could greatly reduce the side effects and cost of HIV treatment. So far, only a few patients have tried structured intermittent therapy, and researchers do not yet know how effective it will be and who will be most likely to benefit. Experts urge people with HIV not to try intermittent therapy on their own because stopping drug therapy could increase drug resistance and even be life-threatening if done inappropriately.

Researchers are hoping to develop new antiviral drugs that will attack HIV at different parts of its life cycle. For example, human CD4 cells contain several receptors that interact in a complex manner with HIV, allowing the virus to enter the cell. One of these receptors is called CCR-5, and researchers have found that people who have a particular genetic mutation in one copy of the CCR-5 gene have half the normal number of CCR-5 receptors. Because of this, these individuals are much less likely than average to become infected with HIV, and if they do become infected, they tend to stay healthy much longer. People with mutations in both CCR-5 genes are even more resistant to HIV infection. Researchers hope to develop drugs that mimic the effects of the CCR-5 mutation, but further studies of safety and effectiveness are needed; for example, it appears that people with the CCR-5 mutation are *more* susceptible to hepatitis C.

For more on treatment, refer to the resources listed in For More Information at the end of the chapter.

POST-EXPOSURE PROPHYLAXIS   Antiviral medications are being used in some cases in an attempt to prevent infection in people who have been exposed to the virus. The CDC currently recommends that health care workers who have significant exposure to HIV-infected blood or body fluids via a needle stick or other mishap consider starting antiviral medication as soon as possible (preferably within a few hours of exposure) to decrease the risk of infection. Some experts feel that in certain situations

Terms

reverse transcriptase inhibitor An antiviral drug used to treat HIV infection that works by inhibiting reverse transcriptase, the enzyme that converts viral RNA to DNA.

protease inhibitor A drug that inhibits the action of any of the protein-splitting enzymes known as proteases. Protease inhibitors have been developed to block the action of HIV protease and thus prevent the replication of HIV.

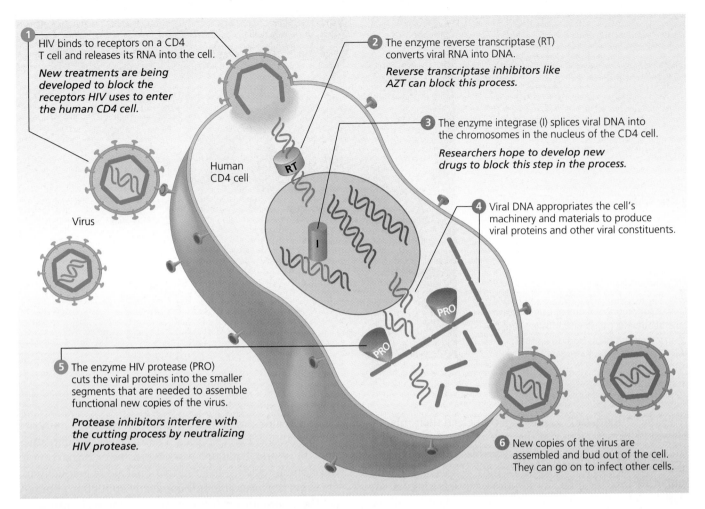

Figure 18-3 The life cycle of HIV: How antiviral drugs work. Different classes of drugs block the replication of HIV at different points in the virus's life cycle. SOURCES: Dickinson, G., et al. 1998. The latest recommendations for antiretroviral therapy. *Patient Care*, 15 August. Disrupting the assembly line. 1996. *Newsweek*, 2 December.

The labeled text within the figure reads:

1. HIV binds to receptors on a CD4 T cell and releases its RNA into the cell.
   New treatments are being developed to block the receptors HIV uses to enter the human CD4 cell.

2. The enzyme reverse transcriptase (RT) converts viral RNA into DNA.
   Reverse transcriptase inhibitors like AZT can block this process.

3. The enzyme integrase (I) splices viral DNA into the chromosomes in the nucleus of the CD4 cell.
   Researchers hope to develop new drugs to block this step in the process.

4. Viral DNA appropriates the cell's machinery and materials to produce viral proteins and other viral constituents.

5. The enzyme HIV protease (PRO) cuts the viral proteins into the smaller segments that are needed to assemble functional new copies of the virus.
   Protease inhibitors interfere with the cutting process by neutralizing HIV protease.

6. New copies of the virus are assembled and bud out of the cell. They can go on to infect other cells.

Human CD4 cell

Virus

people who have had nonoccupational exposure to HIV—such as unprotected high-risk sex or needle sharing with an HIV-positive individual—should also have the option of this type of post-exposure treatment. This approach is controversial for many reasons, and its effectiveness is unknown; it is not currently recommended in most cases.

TREATMENTS FOR OPPORTUNISTIC INFECTIONS In addition to antiviral drugs, most patients with low CD4 T-cell counts also take a variety of antibiotics to help prevent opportunistic infections such as *Pneumocystis carinii* pneumonia and tuberculosis. A person with advanced HIV infection may need to take 20 or more pills every day. All these medications have potential side effects, which can become severe when so many drugs are used in combination.

HIV AND PREGNANCY Early-stage HIV infection does not appear to significantly affect a woman's chance of becoming pregnant. Without treatment, 25–30% of infants born to HIV-infected women are themselves infected with the virus. But treatment with antiviral drugs during pregnancy, labor, and early infancy has been shown to decrease a child's chance of contracting HIV by as much as 90%. Cesarean delivery can lower the risk of infection in women who have high blood levels of HIV; women who have undergone antiviral treatment and have very low levels of HIV can usually deliver vaginally. Because treatment can make such a dramatic difference in the health of the baby, HIV testing is strongly recommended for all pregnant women.

HIV-infected women are usually advised not to breastfeed, because this has been shown to transmit HIV. In developed countries, women infected with HIV generally

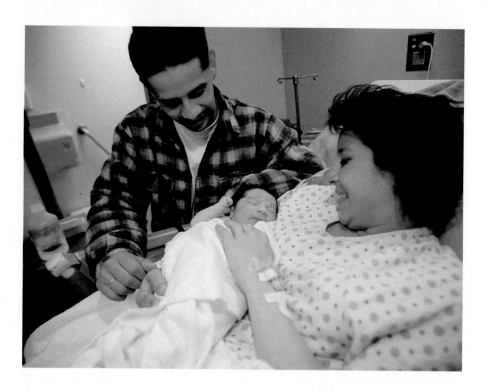

Early diagnosis and treatment of HIV infection are important for everyone, but particularly so for pregnant women. Currently available treatments can significantly increase the chance that this baby, born to an HIV-infected mother, will be free of the virus.

have the support and resources to bottlefeed their infants. However, this is often not the case in developing countries: Infant formula is often unavailable and/or unaffordable, and many regions lack a supply of safe water with which to mix formula. In addition, bottlefeeding is socially unacceptable in some cultures and may be seen as a sign that the mother has AIDS. Many infants in Africa whose mothers do receive treatment during pregnancy and delivery are born uninfected but then acquire the infection later, through breastfeeding.

Testing and the use of antiviral drugs by pregnant HIV-positive women has had a dramatic effect in the United States: The number of new cases of HIV infection in children has declined by more than 80% since 1992. Unfortunately, long-term combination antiviral therapy is very expensive and is out of reach for most of the world's HIV-positive women. Recent studies indicate that very short courses of antiviral drugs given around the time of birth can also reduce vertical transmission, and health authorities are working with drug companies to provide less expensive treatment regimens that will meet the needs of women in developing nations.

TREATMENT CHALLENGES The cost of treatment for HIV continues to be an area of major concern. A recent study revealed an average cost of over $18,000 per year to treat an HIV-infected person in the United States. These costs are tremendous even for relatively wealthy countries. But 95% of people with HIV infection live in developing countries, where these treatments are unlikely to be available to anyone except the wealthiest few. The average per-

person health expenditure in many developing countries is only about $10 per year. Pharmaceutical companies and the World Bank are working to lower drug costs in developing regions, and international aid is gradually increasing; however, it is still not nearly enough to counteract the devastating impact of AIDS on these countries.

Toxicity of antiretroviral drugs is another concern. Long-term use of HAART can cause a number of serious effects, including bone loss and dangerously high levels of cholesterol. For this reason, the National Institutes of Health issued new HIV treatment guidelines in 2001 that recommend that asymptomatic patients hold off on treatment until they are at a more advanced stage of the disease. However, immediate treatment is still recommended for anyone who has acute (very recent) infection or who is experiencing symptoms.

Even for those who have access to the drugs and can tolerate the side effects, treatment is difficult. The drug combinations require people to take dozens of pills every day at precise times. If the drugs are not taken on schedule, their effectiveness is reduced and the virus is much more likely to develop drug resistance. Some people cannot tolerate the toxic side effects of these powerful drugs. In addition, the drugs are much more effective for some people than others. Currently available antiviral drugs do not appear able to completely eliminate the virus from the body, even if viral levels in the blood become undetectable. The optimal duration of drug therapy is not currently known, although many scientists feel that lifelong drug therapy will probably be necessary. It is also unclear to what degree a damaged immune system can rebound

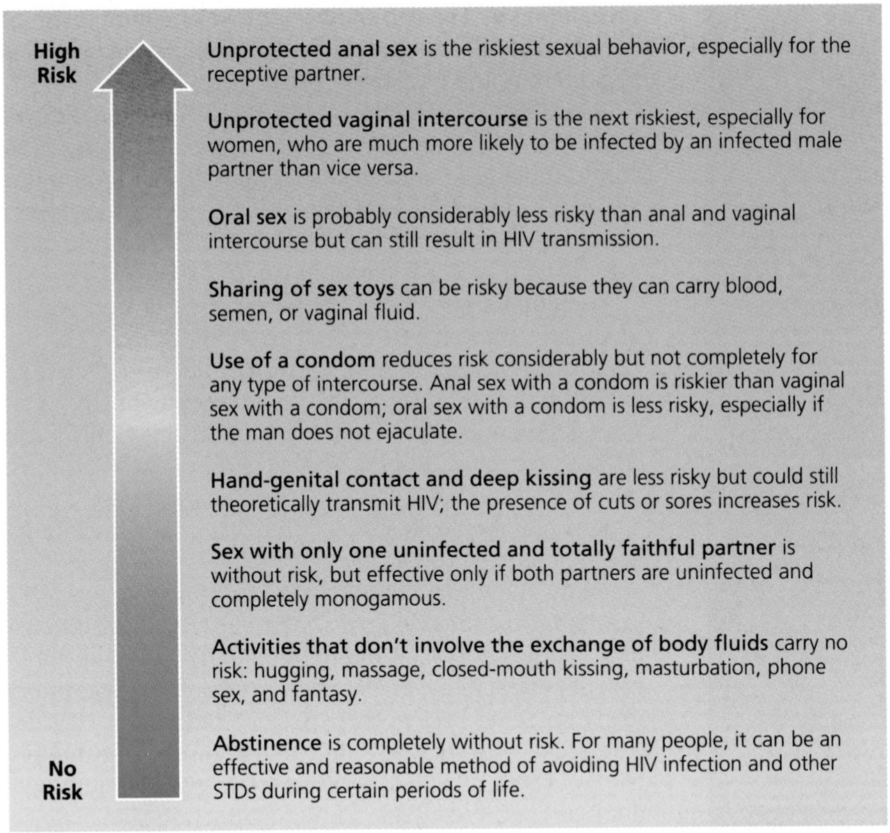

High Risk

Unprotected anal sex is the riskiest sexual behavior, especially for the receptive partner.

Unprotected vaginal intercourse is the next riskiest, especially for women, who are much more likely to be infected by an infected male partner than vice versa.

Oral sex is probably considerably less risky than anal and vaginal intercourse but can still result in HIV transmission.

Sharing of sex toys can be risky because they can carry blood, semen, or vaginal fluid.

Use of a condom reduces risk considerably but not completely for any type of intercourse. Anal sex with a condom is riskier than vaginal sex with a condom; oral sex with a condom is less risky, especially if the man does not ejaculate.

Hand-genital contact and deep kissing are less risky but could still theoretically transmit HIV; the presence of cuts or sores increases risk.

Sex with only one uninfected and totally faithful partner is without risk, but effective only if both partners are uninfected and completely monogamous.

Activities that don't involve the exchange of body fluids carry no risk: hugging, massage, closed-mouth kissing, masturbation, phone sex, and fantasy.

Abstinence is completely without risk. For many people, it can be an effective and reasonable method of avoiding HIV infection and other STDs during certain periods of life.

No Risk

Figure 18-4 What's risky and what's not: The approximate relative risk of HIV transmission of various sexual activities. Safer sex strategies that reduce the risk of HIV infection will also help protect you against other STDs. The main point to re-member is that any activity that involves con-tact with blood, semen, or vaginal fluid can transmit HIV.

from the effects of long-term HIV infection even if the virus is brought under control with antiviral medication.

What About a Vaccine? The best hope for preventing the spread of HIV worldwide rests with the development of a safe, effective, and inexpensive vaccine. Many different approaches to the development of an AIDS vac-cine are currently under investigation, and human trials have begun on several vaccines. It is likely that numerous vaccines will be needed because of the variety of HIV sub-types found around the world and the virus's ability to mutate. No vaccine is likely to be ready for widespread use within the next 5 years.

Vaccines are also being tested as therapy for people al-ready infected with HIV. Clinical trials have found that some patients improve in response to HIV vaccines, which may stimulate the immune system to attack HIV. In addition to vaccines, researchers are also working to de-velop effective **microbicides** as a prevention strategy against HIV. A cream or gel that kills HIV on contact and could be applied topically, similar to a spermicide, would be especially valuable for women in developing countries.

Prevention Although AIDS is currently incurable, it is preventable. You can protect yourself by avoiding behav-iors that may bring you into contact with HIV. This means making careful choices about sexual activity and not shar-ing needles if you inject drugs.

MAKE CAREFUL CHOICES ABOUT SEXUAL ACTIVITY In a sexual relationship, the current and past behaviors of you and your partner determine the amount of risk involved. If you are uninfected and in a mutually monogamous re-lationship with another uninfected person, you are not at risk for HIV. Of course, it is often hard to know for sure whether your partner is completely faithful and is truly uninfected. Having a series of monogamous relationships is not a safe prevention strategy.

For anyone not involved in a long-term, mutually monogamous relationship, abstinence from any sexual activity that involves the exchange of body fluids is the only sure way to prevent HIV infection (Figure 18-4). Safer sex includes many activities that carry virtually no risk of HIV infection, like hugging, massaging, closed-lip kissing, rubbing clothed bodies together, kissing your partner's skin, and mutual masturbation.

Anal and vaginal intercourse are the sexual activities asso-ciated with the highest risk of HIV infection. If you have in-tercourse, always use a latex condom. Condoms are not per-fect, and they do not provide risk-free sex; however, used properly, a latex condom provides a high level of protection

microbicide An agent that destroys microorganisms; also known as an antiseptic.

Terms

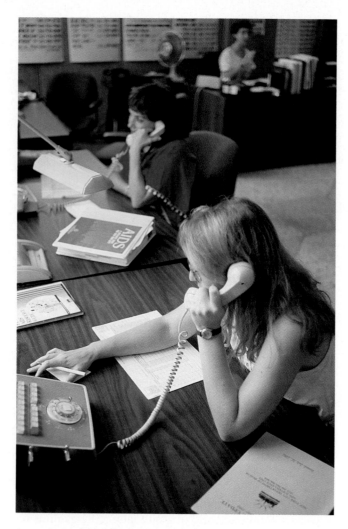

Accurate, confidential answers to personal questions are available from local and national STD hotlines. Separate AIDS hotlines, such as the one shown here, provide referrals, information, and updates on the success of the latest treatments for HIV infection and AIDS.

against HIV. One study of 124 couples in which one partner was infected showed that with consistent condom use, none of the uninfected partners acquired the virus during the 20-month study period. Condoms should also be worn during oral sex. Some experts also suggest the use of latex squares and dental dams, rubber devices that can be used as barriers during oral-genital or oral-anal sexual contact.

Limiting the number of partners you have—particularly those who have engaged in risky sexual behaviors in the past—can also lower your risk of exposure to HIV. Take the time to talk with a potential new partner about HIV and safer sex. Talking about sex may seem embarrassing and uncomfortable, but good communication is critical for your health. Asking a partner about past sexual experiences can also be helpful, but you cannot always depend on that information. Recent surveys of HIV-positive people found that 40–50% failed to reveal their HIV status to sexual partners; of these, nearly two-thirds failed to always use a condom. Take precautions with every partner. Don't agree to have intercourse or give up

precautions as a way to show your love or commitment to a relationship. Your specific sexual practices can be just as important as the number of partners you have.

Removing alcohol and other drugs from sexual activity is another crucial component of safer sex. The use of alcohol and mood-altering drugs may lower inhibitions and affect judgment, making you more likely to engage in unsafe sex. The use of drugs is also associated with sexual activity with multiple partners.

Remember, you can't tell if someone is infected by looking at him or her. Researchers believe that HIV has been in the United States since the mid- to late 1970s; anyone who has engaged in an unsafe behavior since that time is potentially at risk for HIV infection. Consider in advance what you will say and do in particular situations. Be assertive, and negotiate for safer sex practices.

Surveys of college students indicate that the majority of students are not engaging in safer sex. Although most students know that condom use can protect against HIV infection, this knowledge is often not translated into action. Many students also report a willingness to lie about past sexual activity in order to obtain sex. In addition, many students believe their risk of contracting HIV depends on "who they are" rather than on their sexual behavior. These attitudes and behaviors place college students at continued high risk for contracting HIV.

If you are sexually active, take responsibility for undergoing testing for HIV and other STDs at least once a year—more often if you have a new sexual partner or multiple partners. Remember that having any other STD makes you much more likely to acquire HIV infection. Prompt detection and treatment of other STDs can help decrease your risk of HIV infection.

DON'T SHARE DRUG NEEDLES People who inject drugs should avoid sharing needles, syringes, or anything that might have blood on it. Any injectable drug, legal or illegal, can be associated with HIV transmission. Needles can be decontaminated with a solution of bleach and water, but it is not a foolproof procedure and HIV can survive in a syringe for a month or longer. (Boiling needles and syringes does not necessarily destroy HIV either.) If you are an injection drug user, your best protection against HIV is to obtain treatment and refrain from using drugs. (See Chapter 9 for more information about drug abuse.)

PARTICIPATE IN AN HIV EDUCATION PROGRAM Many schools and colleges have peer education programs about preventing the transmission of HIV. These programs give you a chance to practice communicating with potential sex partners and negotiating safer sex, to engage in role playing to build self-confidence, and to learn how to use condoms. Studies show that educational programs in which students learn from their peers and then try out what they've learned through role playing are more likely to result in real behavior change.

Many young people still believe that they are invulnerable to most kinds of harm and persist in thinking of

For those who don't have a long-term monogamous relationship with an uninfected partner, abstinence is the only truly safe option. Individuals should remember that it's OK to say no to sex and drugs.

Safer sexual activities that allow close person-to-person contact with almost no risk of contracting STDs or HIV include fantasy, hugging, massage, rubbing clothed bodies together, self-stimulation by both partners, and kissing with lips closed.

If you choose to be sexually active, talk with potential partners about HIV, safer sex, and the use of condoms before you begin a sexual relationship. The following behaviors will help lower your risk of exposure to HIV during sexual activities:

- Limit the number of partners. Avoid sexual contact with people who have HIV or an STD or who have engaged in risky behaviors in the past, including unprotected sex and injection drug use.

- Use latex condoms during every act of intercourse and oral sex. Even if your partner claims to have been tested for HIV and STDs, there is no guarantee that he or she is uninfected. Many STDs are not easy to diagnose in their asymptomatic stage, which can last for years; and asymptomatic individuals can still infect others. No matter what your partner says, you have no guarantee that you will not contract an STD during any sexual encounter. If you choose to have intercourse, your best protection is to *always* use a condom. They do not provide perfect protection, but they greatly reduce your risk of contracting an infection.

- Use condoms properly to obtain maximum protection (refer to the instructions for condom use in Chapter 6). Use a water-based lubricant; don't use oil-based lubricants such as petroleum jelly or baby oil or any vaginal product containing mineral or vegetable oil. Unroll condoms gently to avoid tearing them, and smooth out any air bubbles.

- Avoid sexual contact that could cause cuts or tears in the skin or tissue. Using extra lubricant (water-based) can help prevent damage to delicate tissues.

- Get periodic screening tests for STDs and HIV. Young women need yearly pelvic exams and Pap tests.

- Get vaccinated for hepatitis B. Take advantage of this safe and effective vaccine.

- Get prompt treatment for any STDs you contract.

- Don't drink or use drugs in sexual situations. Mood-altering drugs can affect your judgment and make you more likely to engage in risky behaviors. Having sex when intoxicated is associated with a significantly increased risk of STDs.

If you inject drugs of any kind, don't share needles, syringes, or anything that might have blood on it. If your community has a syringe exchange program, use it. Seek treatment; stop using injectable drugs.

If you are at risk for HIV infection, don't donate blood, sperm, or body organs. Don't have unprotected sex or share needles or syringes. Get tested for HIV soon, and get treated. HIV-infected people who get early treatment generally feel better and live longer than those who delay.

---

themselves as not being at risk for HIV. The attitude of "It won't happen to me" is pervasive among high school and college students and is a major stumbling block to HIV/AIDS prevention. Until there is an effective vaccine and a cure, HIV infection will remain one of the biggest challenges of this generation. Education and individual responsibility can lead the way to controlling this devastating epidemic (see the box "Preventing HIV Infection and Other STDs").

> **COMMUNICATE!** If you've decided that abstinence is your best protection against STDs, remember that you have a right to say no to sexual relations with a partner. To make the conversation easier for both of you, don't wait until you are in an intimate setting to let your partner know how you feel. Choose a quiet time alone together to discuss your decision, your reasons for it, and sexual activities such as hugging and massage that you might be ready for. Practice ways of expressing yourself on the subject of abstinence until you can do so confidently.

Chlamydia

Chlamydia trachomatis causes **chlamydia,** the most prevalent bacterial STD in the United States. About 3 million new cases occur each year, down from a high of about 4 million; the drop is likely due to increased screening and treatment. An estimated 5–10% of all sexually active American women are infected with chlamydia; rates among men are similar. The highest rates of infection occur in single people between ages 18 and 24 (see the box "College Students and STDs"). Twenty to 40% of people who are diagnosed with gonorrhea also have chlamydia. *C. trachomatis* can be transmitted by oral sex as well as by other forms of sexual intercourse.

Both men and women are susceptible to chlamydia, but, as with most STDs, women bear the greater burden

> **chlamydia** An STD transmitted by the pathogenic bacterium *Chlamydia trachomatis.*

Terms

How many college students have STDs?

- By age 21, 25% of all people will have had an STD. More than half the people who contract STDs are under age 25.

- Among sexually active college students, 5–20% test positive for chlamydia and nearly half are infected with HPV. Although incidence varies at different campuses, about 1 in 500 college students carries HIV.

Why do college students have high rates of STDs?

- Risky sexual behavior is common. One study of college students found that fewer than half used condoms consistently and one-third had had ten or more sex partners. Another study found that 19% of male students and 33% of female students had consented to sexual intercourse simply because they felt awkward refusing.

- College students underestimate their risk of STDs and HIV. Although students may have considerable knowledge about STDs, they often feel the risks do not apply to them—a dangerous assumption. One study of students with a history of STDs showed that more than half had unprotected sex while they were infected, and 25% of them continued to have sex without ever informing their partner(s).

- Young women are more vulnerable to STDs than older women because the less-mature cervix is more easily infected. As a woman ages, the type of cells at the opening of the cervix gradually changes so that the tissue becomes tougher and more resistant to infection. If an 18-year-old woman and a 30-year-old woman are exposed to the same pathogen, the younger woman is far more likely to develop a serious STD.

What effect does alcohol or drug use have on my likelihood of getting an STD?

- Between one-third and one-half of college students report participating in sexual activity as a direct result of being intoxicated. All too often, sexual activity while intoxicated leads to unprotected intercourse.

- Students who binge-drink are more likely to have multiple partners, use condoms inconsistently, and delay seeking treatment for STDs than students who drink little or no alcohol. Sexual assaults occur more frequently when either the perpetrator or the victim has been drinking.

What can students do to protect themselves against STDs?

- Limit the number of sex partners. Even people who are always in a monogamous relationship can end up with extensive potential exposure to STDs if, over the years, they have numerous relationships.

- Use condoms consistently, and don't assume it's safe to stop after you've been with a partner for several months. HIV infection, HPV infection, herpes, and chlamydia can be asymptomatic for months or years and can be transmitted at any time. If you haven't been using condoms with your current partner, start now.

- Think about how you use alcohol or other drugs. If alcohol or drug use is causing problems in your life, get help.

- Enjoy sexuality on your own terms. Don't let the expectations of friends and partners cause you to ignore your own feelings. Let your own wellness be your first priority. If you choose to be sexually active, learn about safer sex practices.

- Get to know your partner, and talk to him or her before becoming intimate. Be honest about yourself, and encourage your partner to do the same. Unfortunately, studies show that many people lie about their sexual past. So listen to your intuition, and practice safer sex no matter what.

---

because of possible complications and consequences of the disease. In most women, chlamydia produces no early symptoms. If left untreated, it can lead to pelvic inflammatory disease (PID), a serious infection involving the oviducts (fallopian tubes) and uterus. PID, discussed later in this chapter, is a leading cause of infertility, and even an infection that produces no symptoms can cause significant scarring of the oviducts. Chlamydia also greatly increases a woman's risk for ectopic (tubal) pregnancy. Because rates of infection are high and most women with chlamydia have no symptoms, many physicians screen sexually active women at the time of their routine pelvic exam; for young sexually active women, some experts recommend screening every 6 months.

Chlamydia can also lead to infertility in men, although not as often as in women. In men under age 35, chlamydia is the most common cause of **epididymitis,** inflammation of the sperm-carrying ducts. And up to half of all cases of **urethritis,** inflammation of the urethra, in men are caused by chlamydia. Despite these statistics, many infected men have no symptoms. And although equally likely to be infected, men are much less likely than women to be screened routinely for chlamydia.

Infants of infected mothers can acquire the infection through contact with the pathogen in the birth canal during delivery. Every year, over 150,000 newborns suffer from eye infections and pneumonia as a result of untreated maternal chlamydial infections.

Symptoms In men, chlamydia symptoms include painful urination, a slight watery discharge from the penis, and sometimes pain around the testicles. Although most women with chlamydia are asymptomatic, some notice increased vaginal discharge, burning with urination, pain or bleeding with intercourse, and lower abdominal pain. Less common symptoms in both men and women include arthritis, conjunctivitis, and rectal inflammation and pain (in people who become infected during receptive anal intercourse). Symptoms in both men and women can begin within 5 days of infection. However, most people experience few or no symptoms, increasing the likelihood that they will inadvertently spread the infection to their partners.

Diagnosis Chlamydia is typically diagnosed through laboratory tests. Specimens are usually obtained by collecting a urine sample or a small amount of fluid from the urethra or cervix with a swab. The lab test may involve growing the organism in culture, special dyes to detect bacterial proteins, or a process that quickly copies and detects genetic material from the bacteria. Testing pregnant women and treating those with chlamydia is a highly effective way to prevent infection of newborns. A home test currently being studied could help increase the diagnosis and treatment of chlamydia.

Treatment Once chlamydia has been diagnosed, the infected person and his or her partner(s) are given antibiotics—usually doxycycline, erythromycin, or a newer drug, azithromycin, which can cure infection in one dose. Treatment of partners is important because people who have been treated for chlamydia are susceptible to getting the disease again if they have sexual contact with an infected person. Chlamydia is an expensive disease, wih costs running higher than $2 billion annually in the United States. And for an individual, the physical and emotional costs—damaged reproductive organs, infertility, or an infected infant—can be devastating.

Gonorrhea

In the United States, an estimated 700,000 new cases of **gonorrhea** are diagnosed every year. The highest incidence is among 15–24-year-olds. Like chlamydia, untreated gonorrhea can cause PID in women and urethritis and epididymitis in men. It can also cause arthritis, rashes, and eye infections, and it occasionally involves internal organs. A woman who is infected during pregnancy is at risk for preterm delivery and for having a baby with life-threatening gonorrheal infection of the blood or joints. An infant passing through the birth canal of an infected mother may contract **gonococcal conjunctivitis,** an infection in the eyes that can cause blindness if not treated. In most states, all newborn babies are routinely treated with antimicrobial eyedrops to prevent eye infection.

Gonorrhea is caused by the bacterium *Neisseria gonor-rhoeae,* which flourishes in mucous membranes, including the moist linings of the mouth, throat, vagina, cervix, urethra, and anal canal. The microbe cannot thrive outside the warm, moist environment of the human body and dies within moments of exposure to light and air. Consequently, gonorrhea cannot be contracted from toilet seats, towels, or other objects.

Symptoms In males, the incubation period for gonorrhea is brief, generally 2–7 days. The first symptoms are due to urethritis, which causes urinary discomfort and a thick, yellowish white or yellowish green discharge from the penis. The lips of the urethral opening may become inflamed and swollen. In some cases, the lymph glands in the groin become enlarged and swollen. Up to half of males have very minor symptoms or none at all.

Most females with gonorrhea are asymptomatic. Those who do have symptoms often experience pain with urination, increased vaginal discharge, and severe menstrual cramps. Up to 40% of women with untreated gonorrhea develop PID. Women may also develop painful abscesses in the Bartholin's glands, a pair of glands located on either side of the opening of the vagina.

Gonorrhea can also infect the throat or rectum of people who engage in oral or anal sex. Gonorrhea symptoms in the throat may be a sore throat or pus on the tonsils, and those in the rectum may be pus or blood in the feces or rectal pain and itching.

Diagnosis Several tests—gram stain, detection of bacterial genes or DNA, or culture—may be performed; depending on the test, samples of urine or cervical, urethral, throat, or rectal fluids may be collected.

Treatment A variety of new and relatively expensive antibiotics are usually effective in curing gonorrhea. Older, less expensive antibiotics such as penicillin and tetracycline are not currently recommended for treating gonorrhea because of widespread drug resistance. People with gonorrhea often also have chlamydia, so additional antibiotics are typically given to treat chlamydia. Follow-up tests are sometimes performed to make sure the infection has been eradicated. If you have had gonorrhea and have been treated, you can still get the disease again if you have sexual contact with an infected partner.

epididymitis An inflammation of the small body of ducts that rests on the testes. **Terms**

urethritis Inflammation of the tube that carries urine from the bladder to the outside opening.

gonorrhea A sexually transmitted bacterial infection that usually affects mucous membranes.

gonococcal conjunctivitis An inflammation of the mucous membrane lining of the eyelids, caused by the gonococcus bacterium.

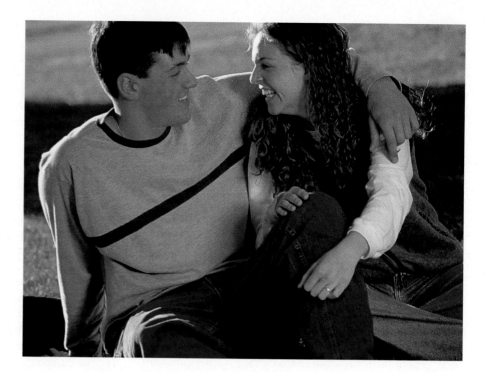

By taking a responsible attitude toward STDs, people show respect and concern for themselves and their partners. This couple's plans for the future could be seriously disrupted if one of them contracted an STD like gonorrhea or chlamydia. Either of these diseases, if untreated, could result in PID, the leading cause of infertility in young women.

Pelvic Inflammatory Disease

A major complication in 10–40% of women who have been infected with either gonorrhea or chlamydia and have not received adequate treatment is **pelvic inflammatory disease (PID)**. PID occurs when the initial infection with gonorrhea and/or chlamydia travels upward, often along with other bacteria, beyond the cervix into the uterus, oviducts, ovaries, and pelvic cavity. PID is often serious enough to require hospitalization and sometimes surgery. Even if the disease is treated successfully, about 25% of affected women will have long-term problems such as a continuing susceptibility to infection, ectopic pregnancy, infertility, and chronic pelvic pain.

PID is the leading cause of infertility in young women, often undetected until later, when the inability to become pregnant leads to further evaluation. Infertility occurs in 8% of women after one episode of PID, 20% after two episodes, and 40% after three episodes. The risk of ectopic pregnancy increases significantly in women who have had PID.

Young women under age 25 are much more likely to develop PID than older women. As with all STDs, the more sex partners a woman has had, the greater her risk of PID. Smokers have twice the risk of PID as nonsmokers. Using IUDs for contraception and vaginal douching also increases the risk of PID. In general, women should avoid douching because this practice may actually force bacteria up through the cervix and into the uterus and oviducts. Research into whether the use of other contraceptives protects against PID has yielded mixed results; OC use may reduce the severity of PID symptoms.

Symptoms Symptoms of PID vary greatly. Some women, especially those with PID from chlamydia, may be asymptomatic; others may feel very ill with abdominal pain, fever, chills, nausea, and vomiting. Early symptoms are essentially the same as those described earlier for chlamydia and gonorrhea. Symptoms often begin or worsen during or soon after a woman's menstrual period. Many women have abnormal vaginal bleeding—either bleeding between periods or heavy and painful menstrual bleeding.

Diagnosis Diagnosis of PID is made on the basis of symptoms, physical examination, ultrasound, and laboratory tests. Laparoscopy may be used to confirm the diagnosis and obtain material for cultures. Cultures from the rectum or cervix may also be taken to help identify the specific organism. The symptoms of PID, ectopic pregnancy, and appendicitis can be quite similar, so careful evaluation is required to make the correct diagnosis.

Treatment Starting treatment of PID as quickly as possible is important in order to minimize damage to the reproductive organs. Antibiotics are usually started immediately; in severe cases, the woman may be hospitalized and antibiotics given intravenously. It is especially important that an infected woman's partners be treated. As many as 60% of the male contacts of women with PID are infected but asymptomatic.

Genital Warts

Genital warts, also known as condyloma, are caused by infection with **human papillomavirus (HPV).** The CDC estimates that more than 20 million people in the United States have this persistent viral infection, and another 5.5 million people are infected each year. Approximately 15% of Americans age 15–49 years have HPV infection and are contagious. The vast majority of these people have no visible warts and have no idea that they are infected with HPV. Rates are even higher among college students. Condyloma is the most common STD for which diagnosis and treatment are sought in student health services. The disease appears to be most prevalent in young people age 16–25.

HPV infection presents a challenge to the medical community because of its known relationship to cervical cancer. A precancerous condition known as cervical dysplasia often occurs among women with genital HPV infection (see Chapter 16). If untreated, women with this condition sometimes develop cervical cancer. (Other factors that increase a woman's chance of getting cervical cancer include smoking, sexual activity at a young age, and multiple sex partners.) Recent evidence suggests that HPV infection also speeds the progression of HIV/AIDS.

Human papillomaviruses cause many types of human warts. There are more than 100 different strains of HPV, and different strains infect specific locations. More than 20 types are likely to cause genital infections, and 5 of these are often implicated in cervical cancer; other strains are linked to anal, penile, and other genital cancers. The HPV strains that cause most visible genital warts are less likely to cause cancer than some of the other HPV strains. A person can be infected with several different strains of HPV.

Genital HPV infection is quite contagious. Condoms and other barrier methods can help prevent the transmission of HPV, but HPV infection frequently occurs in areas where condoms are not fully protective. These areas are the labia in women, the base of the penis and the scrotum 'n men, and around the anus in both men and women.

Controlling the current genital HPV epidemic is difficult for several reasons. First, many people who carry HPV have no visible warts or symptoms (see the box "STDs: The Stealth Diseases"). And although people with visible genital warts may be more likely to transmit the disease, asymptomatic people can also infect others. Second, although current treatments can often (but not always) eliminate visible warts, HPV continues to infect healthy tissue nearby. So even after treatment, a person can still transmit HPV to someone else. Third, as mentioned above, condoms do not provide complete protection against the transmission of HPV.

Symptoms   Genital warts can look like warts that are seen on other parts of the body. They are often dry, painless growths, rough in texture and gray or pink in color. They can be flat or raised, and they vary in size. Early on, genital warts look like small, barely noticeable bumps. Untreated warts can grow together to form a cauliflower-like mass. In males, they appear on the penis and often involve the urethra, appearing first at the opening and then spreading inside. The growths may cause irritation and bleeding, leading to painful urination and a urethral discharge. Warts may also appear around the anus or within the rectum.

In women, warts may appear on the labia or vulva and may spread to the perineum, the area between the vagina and the rectum. They may also appear on the cervix. If warts occur only on the cervix, the woman will generally have no symptoms or awareness that she has HPV.

The incubation period ranges from 1 month to 2 years from the time of contact. People can be infected with the virus and be capable of transmitting it to their sex partners without having any symptoms at all. The vast majority of people with HPV infection have no visible warts or symptoms of any kind.

Genital warts sometimes grow very large during pregnancy and can occasionally be large enough to make vaginal delivery difficult. However, most pregnant women with HPV infection can deliver vaginally. HPV infection is infrequently transmitted to an infant during delivery but can occasionally cause warts to form on the infant's vocal cords.

Diagnosis   Genital warts are usually diagnosed based on the appearance of the lesions. Sometimes examination with a special magnifying instrument or biopsy is done to evaluate suspicious lesions. Frequently, HPV infection of the cervix is detected on routine Pap tests. Special tests are now available to detect the presence of HPV infection and to distinguish among the more common strains of HPV, including those that cause most cases of cervical cancer. These tests are not yet widely used, but they may prove useful in the future to help decide how aggressively to treat women with abnormal Pap tests.

Treatment   Treatment of genital warts focuses on reducing the number and size of warts. The currently available treatments do not eradicate HPV infection. Warts may be removed by cryosurgery (freezing), electrocautery (burning), or laser surgery. Direct applications of podophyllin or other cytotoxic acids may be used. Two treatments may be applied by patients at home: imiquimod, an immune system enhancer, and podofilox, a drug that destroys warts. The success rates of methods vary, and warts often recur despite initial improvement.

Terms

pelvic inflammatory disease (PID) An infection that progresses from the vagina and cervix to the uterus, oviducts, and pelvic cavity.

genital warts A sexually transmitted viral infection characterized by growths on the genitals; also called *genital HPV infection.*

human papillomavirus (HPV) The pathogen that causes human warts, including genital warts.

According to data released at the 2000 National STD Prevention Conference, the annual incidence of STDs in the United States—the number of new cases each year—exceeds 15 million (see the table). HPV infection, trichomoniasis, and chlamydia top the list, each with an annual incidence of 3 million or more cases. However, the statistics for prevalence, the number of currently infected people capable of transmitting a disease, are even more striking. Because the viral STDs are typically persistent and incurable, the prevalence of these diseases greatly exceeds the number of new cases each year. This means there is a large pool of people capable of infecting others. For example, studies suggest that more than 1 in 5 American adults are infected with the virus that causes genital herpes—and the vast majority don't know it.

HIV/AIDS and many of the other major STDs have become widespread in large part because people carry pathogens and infect others without realizing it. If a person becomes obviously ill shortly after acquiring an infection, he or she will be much less likely to infect others. However, the most common major STDs in the United States, HPV infection, herpes, and chlamydia, and the most deadly, HIV infection, often infect people for long periods without causing symptoms. The high number of disease carriers who are unaware of their infection makes these diseases extremely difficult to control.

Some of the recent news on the incidence of STDs has been good. Chlamydia rates in the United States have begun to drop, probably because screening tests are widely used. Many physicians and clinics now routinely test all young, sexually active women for chlamydia, even if they have no symptoms. Chlamydia is also easily and effectively treated, so diagnosis can be quickly followed by a cure. Syphilis rates have also continued to decline in recent years, following efforts to target affected groups in high-risk areas. Declining infection rates among adults have led to a dramatic decrease in the number of infants affected by syphilis: The rate of congenital syphilis dropped by 50% between 1997 and 1999.

For other STDs, however, the news is not so encouraging. In 2000, the CDC announced the first increase in gonorrhea rates in nearly two decades. Although tests and effective treatments for gonorrhea are available, the recent rise in the number of cases is worrisome because gonorrhea can have serious consequences, including ectopic pregnancy, PID and infertility, and increased risk of HIV transmission.

Herpes and HPV infection are particularly challenging. Screening tests for these STDs have been unavailable or underutilized. And even when infections are diagnosed, there is no cure. The rates of these diseases will likely remain extremely high until easy screening and effective treatment of these viruses become possible. Many experts believe that the best hope for controlling diseases such as herpes, HPV, and HIV/AIDS is the development and widespread use of effective vaccines. Research is ongoing, but hepatitis B is the only STD for which a vaccine is currently available and widely used. The effects of the HBV vaccine have been dramatic: In the years since its introduction, the rate of new cases of hepatitis B has dropped by more than 50%, and further declines are expected.

Until STDs are controllable with vaccines or effective screening and treatment, the only way to reduce your risk is to limit the number of sexual partners and to use condoms consistently. For those who choose abstinence or a mutually monogamous relationship with one uninfected partner, there is no risk of STDs.

Estimated Incidence and Prevalence of STDs in the United States

	Estimated Annual Incidence	Estimated Prevalence[a]
HPV infection	5,500,000	20,000,000
Trichomoniasis	5,000,000	n/a
Chlamydia	3,000,000	2,000,000
Genital herpes	1,000,000	45,000,000
Gonorrhea	700,000	n/a
Hepatitis B[b]	130,000	1,250,000
Syphilis (all stages)[c]	70,000	n/a
HIV infection[b]	40,000	900,000

n/a = not available.

[a]Because the viral STDs are persistent and incurable, the number of currently infected people capable of transmitting the infection (prevalence) greatly exceeds the annual number of new cases (incidence) of the viral STDs. Chlamydia prevalence remains high because most cases are asymptomatic and undiagnosed.

[b]Hepatitis B and HIV infection can be transmitted in a variety of ways; about half of all cases of HIV and 30–60% of cases of hepatitis B are transmitted sexually.

[c]Total includes about 8,000 cases of primary- and secondary-stage syphilis, the stages of the disease during which it can be easily transmitted to others.

SOURCES: Centers for Disease Control and Prevention. 2000. *Tracking the Hidden Epidemics: Trends in STDs in the United States.* Atlanta, Ga.: Centers for Disease Control and Prevention. Centers for Disease Control and Prevention. 2000. Gonorrhea—United States, 1998. *Morbidity and Mortality Weekly Report* 49(24): 538–542. Kaiser Family Foundation. 1998. *Sexually Transmitted Diseases in America: How Many Cases and at What Cost?* (http://www.kff.org/archive/repro/policy/std/std_rep.html; retrieved December 16, 1998).

Recent research indicates that HPV infection often resolves on its own after a number of months, although this is unpredictable. Even after treatment and the disappearance of visible warts, the individual may continue to carry HPV in healthy-looking tissue and can probably still infect others. Anyone who has ever had HPV should inform all partners. Condoms should be used, even though they do not provide total protection. Because of the relationship between HPV and cervical cancer, women who have had genital warts should have Pap tests at least every 12 months.

Genital Herpes

Genital herpes affects about 45 million people in the United States and is also very common worldwide. It plays a significant role in HIV infection because the sores associated with genital herpes facilitate the transmission of HIV. Two types of herpes simplex viruses, HSV-1 and HSV-2, cause genital herpes and oral-labial herpes (cold sores). Genital herpes is usually caused by HSV-2, and oral-labial herpes is usually caused by HSV-1, although both virus types can cause either genital or oral-labial lesions. HSV can also cause rectal lesions, usually transmitted through anal sex. (Other types of herpesviruses cause different illnesses; see Chapter 17.) Infection with HSV is generally lifelong; after infection, the virus lies dormant in nerve cells and can reactivate at any time.

HSV-1 infection is so common that 50–80% of U.S. adults have antibodies to HSV-1 (indicating previous exposure to the virus); most were exposed to HSV-1 during childhood. HSV-2 infection usually occurs during adolescence and early adulthood, often between ages 18 and 25. Approximately 22% of adults—nearly one in four—have antibodies to HSV-2; about a million are infected each year.

HSV-2 is almost always sexually transmitted. It is theoretically possible, but much less common, to become infected through contaminated clothing, towels, or other objects. The infection is more easily transmitted when people have active sores, but HSV-2 can be transmitted to a sex partner even when no lesions are present. Because HSV is asymptomatic in 80–90% of people, the infection is often acquired from a person who has no awareness that he or she is infected. This makes controlling the spread of genital herpes very difficult. If you have ever had an outbreak of genital herpes, you must always consider yourself contagious and inform your partners. Avoid intimate contact when any sores are present, and use condoms during all sexual contact.

Newborns can occasionally be infected with HSV, usually during passage through the birth canal of an infected mother or due to HSV infection acquired by the mother during the third trimester of pregnancy. Without treatment, 65% of newborns with HSV will die, and most who survive will have some degree of brain damage. The risk of mother-to-child HSV transmission during pregnancy and delivery is low (less than 1%) in women with long-standing herpes infection. However, a woman who acquires the infection during pregnancy, especially in the third trimester, has a much higher risk of transmitting the infection to her infant. Some experts believe that the use of new herpes blood tests to screen pregnant women and their sexual partners could substantially reduce the number of neonatal herpes infections. If an uninfected pregnant woman's partner carries HSV, abstinence or the use of condoms could prevent infection during pregnancy.

Pregnant women who have been exposed to genital herpes should inform their physician so that appropriate precautions can be taken to protect the baby from infection. These precautions sometimes include cesarean section if active lesions are present at the time of delivery. Fortunately, most babies born to mothers with a history of genital herpes do not acquire the infection, and most women are able to have normal vaginal deliveries.

Symptoms　Up to 90% of people who are infected with HSV have no symptoms. Those that do develop symptoms often first notice them within 2–20 days of having sex with an infected partner. (However, it is not unusual for the first outbreak to occur months or even years after initial exposure.) The first episode of genital herpes frequently causes flulike symptoms in addition to genital lesions. The lesions usually heal within 3 weeks, but the virus remains alive in an inactive state within nerve cells. A new outbreak of herpes can occur at any time. On average, newly diagnosed people will experience 5–8 outbreaks per year, with a decrease in the frequency of outbreaks over time. Recurrent episodes are usually less severe than the initial one, with fewer and less painful sores that heal more quickly. Outbreaks can be triggered by stress, illness, fatigue, sun exposure, sexual intercourse, and menstruation (see the box "Stress and Genital Herpes").

Diagnosis　Genital herpes is often diagnosed on the basis of symptoms; a sample of fluid from the lesions may also be sent to a laboratory for evaluation. A new blood test that can determine if a person is infected with HSV-1 or HSV-2 is now available and may potentially alert many asymptomatic people to the fact that they are infected. This knowledge may help prevent transmission of HSV in couples where one partner is infected and the other is not (particularly important for uninfected women who are pregnant). However, the new test is likely to cause both personal and medical dilemmas for many individuals who are currently unaware that they have genital herpes.

Treatment　There is no cure for herpes. Once infected, a person carries the virus for life. Antiviral drugs such as acyclovir can be taken at the beginning of an outbreak to shorten the severity and duration of symptoms. People who have frequent outbreaks, more than six per year, can take acyclovir or other similar drugs on a daily basis to

genital herpes A sexually transmitted infection caused by the herpes simplex virus.

Terms

For decades, patients and health care workers alike have suspected that stress and genital herpes outbreaks are related. Research studies that have investigated this potential link have yielded mixed results. There is no doubt that having genital herpes is a considerable stress to many people, but does stress itself make a person with herpes infection more likely to have an outbreak? A recent study of women with genital herpes found that persistent stressors (those lasting more than a week) and persistent high levels of anxiety were associated with increased genital herpes outbreaks. Short-term stress, mood changes, and brief negative life experiences did not influence the rate of herpes outbreaks.

Why should persistent stress make a person with genital herpes have more frequent outbreaks? No one knows for sure, but experts suspect that stress has a negative impact on the immune system. Studies have shown that cell-mediated immune function and antibody levels may drop in response to psychological stress. Perhaps herpesviruses that are usually dormant in nervous system tissue become activated when immune function declines due to stress.

The next logical step is to investigate whether stress-reduction techniques such as meditation or exercise result in reduced rates of herpes outbreaks. Until such research becomes available, it makes sense for people who suffer recurrent genital herpes outbreaks to do what they can to reduce stress, especially long-term stress and anxiety (see Chapter 2). If you have herpes, joining a support group may help reduce your stress and improve your ability to cope with this chronic disease (see For More Information at the end of the chapter). If you have more than six outbreaks a year, consider taking an antiviral medication. Keep in mind that regardless of stress level, genital herpes outbreaks naturally tend to become less and less frequent over time. Knowing that your outbreaks are likely to diminish can, in and of itself, help reduce your feelings of stress.

SOURCE: Rein, M. 2000. Stress and genital herpes recurrences in women: Commentary. *Journal of the American Medical Association* 283(11): 1394.

suppress outbreaks. Support groups are available to help people learn to cope with herpes (see For More Information at the end of the chapter). Researchers are working on a vaccine for HSV-2, but it is not expected to be available for some time.

> **COMMUNICATE!**   How can you find out whether your partner could expose you to a sexually transmitted disease? The simplest and most direct way is to ask. You can say something like, "It seems as if we're getting to a point in our relationship where we should talk about STDs and safer sex." If your partner is agreeable, you might continue, "I'm wondering whether you've had other partners, and if you have, whether any of them ever had an STD, or if you've ever had an STD." Remember that your partner has a right to know your health status as well, so be prepared to answer his or her questions.

Hepatitis B

Hepatitis (inflammation of the liver) can cause serious and sometimes permanent damage to the liver, which can result in death in severe cases. One of the many types of hepatitis is caused by hepatitis B virus (HBV). HBV is somewhat similar to HIV; it is found in most body fluids, and it can be transmitted sexually, by injection drug use, and during pregnancy and delivery. However, HBV is much more contagious than HIV, and it can also be spread through nonsexual close contact. Health care workers who are exposed to blood are frequently infected, as are people who live in close contact with each other, such as prisoners and residents of mental health care facilities. In the Far East and in developing countries, hepatitis B is extremely common, and the virus is primarily transmitted from the mother to child during pregnancy or delivery.

Hepatitis B is a potentially fatal disease with no cure, but fortunately there is an effective vaccine. The number of cases of acute hepatitis B in the United States has dropped by more than 50% in the past decade, primarily as a result of the vaccine. In addition, mother-to-child transmission has been greatly reduced because of routine HBV screening of pregnant women. Vaccination is recommended for everyone under age 19 and for all adults at increased risk for hepatitis B.

Transmission   HBV is found in all body fluids, including blood and blood products, semen, saliva, urine, and vaginal secretions. It is easily transmitted through any sexual activity that involves the exchange of body fluids, the use of contaminated needles, and any blood-to-blood contact, including the use of contaminated razor blades, toothbrushes, and eating utensils. The primary risk factors for acquiring HBV are sexual exposure and injection drug use; having multiple partners greatly increases risk. As mentioned, a pregnant woman can transmit HBV to her unborn child.

Symptoms   Many people infected with HBV never develop symptoms; they have what are known as "silent" infections. The normal incubation period is 30–180 days.

Mild cases of hepatitis cause flulike symptoms such as fever, body aches, chills, and loss of appetite. As the illness progresses, there may be nausea, vomiting, dark-colored urine, abdominal pain, and jaundice. Some people with hepatitis also develop a skin rash and joint pain or arthritis. Acute hepatitis B can sometimes be severe, resulting in prolonged illness or even death.

People with hepatitis B sometimes recover completely, but they can also become chronic carriers of the virus, capable of infecting others for the rest of their lives. Some chronic carriers remain asymptomatic, while others develop chronic liver disease. Chronic hepatitis can cause cirrhosis of the liver, liver failure, and a deadly form of liver cancer. Hepatitis kills some 6000 Americans each year; worldwide, the annual death toll exceeds 700,000.

Diagnosis and Treatment Blood tests can be used to diagnose hepatitis through analysis of liver function and detection of the specific organism causing the infection. There is no cure for hepatitis B and no specific treatment for acute infections; antiviral drugs may be used for cases of chronic HBV infection. For people exposed to HBV, treatment with hepatitis B immunoglobulin can provide protection against the virus.

Prevention Preventive measures for hepatitis B are similar to those for HIV infection: Avoid sexual contact that involves sharing body fluids, including saliva; use condoms during sexual intercourse; and don't share needles. If you choose to have tattooing or body piercing done, make sure all needles and equipment are sterile. The vaccine for hepatitis B is safe and highly effective.

Syphilis

Syphilis, a disease that once caused death and disability for millions, can now be effectively treated with antibiotics. Each year, there are about 7000–10,000 new cases of early syphilis in the United States, and about 70,000 people are diagnosed at all stages of the disease. The number of new cases hit an all-time low in 1999, and most were clustered in a few counties in the South and Northeast. Some experts feel that aggressive public health measures could eliminate syphilis in the United States. Syphilis is unfortunately still very common in the developing world, and aside from the suffering and death caused directly by the disease, it also is a major cofactor in the transmission of HIV. The open sores associated with syphilis dramatically increase the risk of acquiring HIV or transmitting it to someone else.

Syphilis is caused by a spirochete called *Treponema pallidum,* a thin, corkscrew-shaped bacterium. The disease is usually acquired through sexual contact, although infected pregnant women can transmit it to the fetus. The pathogen passes through any break or open-

ing in the skin or mucous membranes and can be transmitted by kissing, vaginal or anal intercourse, or oral-genital contact. Although easy to treat, syphilis can be difficult to recognize, and if left untreated, the disease can cause devastating damage to almost any system of the body.

Symptoms Syphilis progresses through several stages. *Primary syphilis* is characterized by an ulcer called a **chancre** that appears within 10–90 days after exposure. The chancre is usually found at the site where the organism entered the body, such as the genital area, but it may also appear in other sites such as the mouth, breasts, or fingers. Chancres contain large numbers of bacteria and make the disease highly contagious when present; they are often painless and typically heal on their own within a few weeks. If the disease is not treated during the primary stage, about a third of infected individuals progress to chronic stages of infections.

Secondary syphilis is usually marked by mild, flulike symptoms and a skin rash that appears 3–6 weeks after the chancre. The rash may cover the entire body or only a few areas, but the palms of the hands and soles of the feet are usually involved. Areas of skin affected by the rash are highly contagious but usually heal within several weeks or months.

If the disease remains untreated, the symptoms of secondary syphilis may recur over a period of several years; affected individuals may then lapse into an asymptomatic latent stage in which they experience no further consequences of infection. However, in about a third of cases of untreated secondary syphilis, the individual develops *late,* or *tertiary, syphilis.* Late syphilis can damage many organs of the body, possibly causing severe dementia, cardiovascular damage, blindness, and death.

In infected pregnant women, the syphilis bacterium can cross the placenta. If the mother is not treated, the probable result is stillbirth, prematurity, or congenital deformity. In many cases, the infant is also born infected (*congenital syphilis*) and requires treatment.

Diagnosis and Treatment Syphilis is diagnosed by examination of infected tissues and with blood tests. All stages can be treated with antibiotics, but damage from late syphilis can be permanent.

Terms

hepatitis Inflammation of the liver, which can be caused by infection, drugs, or toxins; some forms of infectious hepatitis can be transmitted sexually.

syphilis A sexually transmitted bacterial infection caused by the spirochete *Treponema pallidum.*

chancre The sore produced by syphilis in its earliest stage.

OTHER STDS

Although less serious than the diseases already described, a few other diseases are transmitted sexually or linked to sexual activity. They include trichomoniasis, bacterial vaginosis, chancroid, pubic lice, and scabies.

Trichomoniasis, often called "trich," is a common STD, with about 5 million new cases per year. The single-celled organism that causes trich, *Trichomonas vaginalis,* thrives in warm, moist conditions, making women particularly susceptible to these infections in the vagina. This protozoan can remain alive on external objects for as long as 60–90 minutes, in urine for 3 hours, and in seminal fluid for 6 hours. Thus it is possible, although rare, to contract trich by nonsexual means.

Women who become symptomatic with trich develop a greenish, foul-smelling vaginal discharge 5–28 days after the time of contact with the organism. The discharge can cause severe itching and irritation of the vagina and vulva, causing redness and pain. Although most males do not have any symptoms, some may experience slight itching, clear discharge, and sometimes painful urination.

Diagnosis of trich can be done through microscopic examination of the discharge. The drug of choice is metronidazole (Flagyl). Partners should also be treated, to prevent the "Ping-Pong" effect that occurs when partners pass infection back and forth. Treatment is important because studies suggest that trich may increase the risk of HIV transmission. *Trichomonas* infection may also increase a pregnant woman's risk of premature delivery.

Bacterial vaginosis (BV) is the most common cause of abnormal vaginal discharge in women of reproductive age. BV involves a shift in the makeup of the bacteria that normally inhabit the vagina: Instead of *Lactobacillus* being most numerous, there is an overgrowth of anaerobic microorganisms and bacteria such as *Gardnerella vaginalis.* BV is clearly associated with sexual activity, often occurring after a change in partners. However, research on the degree to which BV is sexually transmitted is ongoing. Recent research suggests that a sexually transmitted virus that infects and kills *Lactobacillus* may be the under-lying cause of BV. Topical and oral antibiotics are used to treat BV, but BV often recurs after treatment.

Symptoms of BV include a vaginal discharge with a fishlike odor and, in some cases, vaginal irritation; many women with BV have no symptoms. Some studies have shown an association between BV and increased risk of PID, HIV transmission, infection following childbirth or gynecological surgery (including abortion), and in pregnant women, premature delivery. The CDC recommends that any pregnant woman who has symptoms of BV or who is at risk for premature delivery be screened and, if necessary, treated for BV. The recognition that BV may contribute to more serious conditions has led to an increase in screening and treatment.

Chancroid is a sexually transmitted bacterial infection caused by *Haemophilus ducreyi.* Prevalent in some parts of the world, chancroid is relatively uncommon in the United States, although there are periodic outbreaks. The infection is characterized by painful open sores in the genital area that may resemble the sores associated with herpes or syphilis; other symptoms may include painful urination and vaginal discharge. As with any STD that causes genital sores, chancroid can increase the risk of HIV transmission. Chancroid is treated with antibiotics.

Pubic lice, commonly known as "crabs," are highly contagious, both sexually and nonsexually. They are often difficult to see but are the color and size of small freckles until they have fed, and then they become dark brown in color. Like mosquitoes, lice feed on human blood. Although usually found attached to pubic hair, they have been known to attach themselves to hair on the head, eyelashes, underarm hair, and even mustaches and beards. (Head lice belong to a different species than pubic lice.) Separated from their human hosts, lice can survive for about 24 hours.

Easily passed from person to person, lice can also be transmitted via infested bedding, towels, clothing, sleeping bags, and even toilet seats. Intense itching is the usual symptom, and with careful examination, both the parasite and its eggs, or nits, can be seen. Treatment is generally easy, although the infestation can require repeated applications of nonprescription medications. These preparations are in lotion or shampoo form and include a fine comb for removing any remaining lice or nits from body hair. Carefully washing clothing and linen is also essential for preventing reinfestation. If the infestation persists, other medications are available by prescription.

Scabies is another fairly common infestation. A burrowing parasite, the scabies mite deposits eggs beneath the skin, especially in the creases of the body. The eggs hatch in a few days, and the new mites congregate around hair follicles. This burrowing parasite produces intense itching, especially at night. The usual sites of infestation are between the fingers, on wrists, in armpits, underneath the breasts, along the inner surfaces of the thighs, on penis and scrotum, and occasionally on the female genitals.

Terms

trichomoniasis A protozoal infection caused by *Trichomonas vaginalis,* transmitted sexually and externally.

bacterial vaginosis (BV) A condition linked to sexual activity; caused by an overgrowth of certain bacteria inhabiting the vagina.

chancroid A sexually transmitted bacterial infection caused by *Haemophilus ducreyi.*

pubic lice Parasites that infest the hair of the pubic region, commonly called crabs.

scabies A contagious skin disease caused by a type of parasitic mite.

All sexually transmitted diseases are preventable. You have control over the behaviors and attitudes that place you at risk for contracting STDs and for increasing their negative effects on your health. To identify your risk factors, read the following list of statements and identify whether they're true or false for you.

T or F

_____ 1. I have never been sexually active. (If false, continue. If true, you are not at risk; respond to the remaining statements based on how you realistically believe you would act.)

_____ 2. I am in a mutually monogamous relationship with an uninfected partner or am not currently sexually active. (If false, continue. If true, you are at minimal risk now; respond to the remaining statements according to your attitudes and past behaviors.)

_____ 3. I have only one sex partner.

_____ 4. I always use a latex condom for each act of intercourse, even if I am fairly certain my partner has no infections.

_____ 5. I do not use oil-based lubricants or other products with condoms.

_____ 6. I discuss STDs and prevention with new partners before having sex.

_____ 7. I do not use alcohol or another mood-altering drug in sexual situations.

_____ 8. I would tell my partner if I thought I had been exposed to an STD.

_____ 9. I am familiar with the signs and symptoms of STDs.

_____ 10. I regularly perform genital self-examination.

_____ 11. When I notice any sign or symptom of any STD or if I engage in risky sexual behavior, I consult my physician immediately.

_____ 12. I obtain screening for HIV and STDs regularly. In addition (if female), I obtain yearly pelvic exams and Pap tests.

_____ 13. When diagnosed with an STD, I inform all recent partners.

_____ 14. When I have a sign or symptom of an STD that goes away on its own, I still consult my physician.

_____ 15. I do not use drugs prescribed for friends or partners or left over from other illnesses to treat STDs.

_____ 16. I do not share syringes or needles to inject drugs.

False answers indicate attitudes and behaviors that may put you at risk for contracting STDs or for suffering serious medical consequences from them.

Scabies is easily spread from person to person, not only through sexual contact but also through any direct or close contact. Diagnosis is made by actual identification of the mite, the eggs, or the larvae in scrapings taken from the burrows in the skin of the human host. Scabies is generally treated with prescription permethrin cream. Clothing and bedding must be washed to prevent reinfestation with the scabies mite.

WHAT YOU CAN DO

You can take responsibility for your health and contribute to a general reduction in the incidence of STDs in three major areas: education, diagnosis and treatment, and prevention. To assess your current level of responsibility about STD prevention, complete the quiz in the box "Do Your Attitudes and Behaviors Put You at Risk for STDs?"

Education

Since the AIDS epidemic began, public and private agencies have grown more serious about educating the public and increasing their awareness of all STDs. This campaign may already be paying off in changing attitudes and sexual behaviors, at least among certain segments of the population. Recent surveys indicate that condom use is increasing, and the number of new cases of HIV infection in the gay population has been smaller in recent years. On the other hand, surveys also reveal that many younger gay men are participating in very high risk behaviors, and a "second wave" of the AIDS epidemic among homosexual men can be expected if younger men fail to use preventive measures. Also discouraging is the fact that the number of cases of HIV infection among harder-to-reach groups, such as injection drug users and their partners and children, is still increasing.

Education efforts targeted at increasing public awareness about AIDS through the media have included public service announcements, dramatic presentations, and support from well-known public figures. Colleges offer courses in human sexuality. Free pamphlets and other literature are available from public health departments, health clinics, physicians' offices, student health centers, and Planned Parenthood; and easy-to-understand books are available in libraries and bookstores. Several national hotlines have been set up to

You can't take back an unwise sexual choice, but quickly owning up to the fact that you are at risk for infection and taking action right away can make a big difference. Treating STDs like chlamydia and gonorrhea within a few days of infection is very likely to prevent complications such as PID and infertility. You will also be much less likely to pass the infection on to anyone else. If you have had a recent risky sexual encounter, visit your physician, student health center, or local STD clinic and ask for testing. Don't wait for symptoms to develop—you may never have any. Permanent damage from STDs, including infertility, can occur even if you have no symptoms.

If you feel a recent sexual encounter puts you at high risk for HIV, ask for an HIV RNA test in addition to standard STD tests. (HIV antibody tests may not register early HIV infection.) Flulike illness within a few days or weeks of risky sexual or drug-taking behavior is an emergency. If HIV treatment is begun within the first weeks of the infection, there is a good chance that damage to the immune system can be reduced or even prevented. Many physicians will not think of acute HIV infection when you describe flulike symptoms, so be sure to speak up about your recent risky activities and your concerns about HIV.

If tests come back positive for a particular STD, you need to be tested for others, including HIV infection. Infection with any STD means that you are at higher risk for all others. Women should also have a pelvic exam and a Pap test, which can often detect asymptomatic HPV infection long before cervical cancer has a chance to develop. If you are given medication to treat an STD, take all of it as directed. Incomplete treatment can result in an incomplete cure, thereby contributing to the development of drug-resistant organisms. Do not share your medication with a partner; he or she should see a physician for testing and treatment.

Do not have sexual intercourse until your treatment—and your partner's treatment—is complete. If your partner still carries the infection, you are likely to be reinfected when you resume sexual activity. If you have an incurable STD such as herpes or HPV infection, always use a condom and make sure your partner is fully informed of the potential risks of being intimate with you, even if you are using condoms.

Avoiding risky sexual encounters is by far the best course of action. But if you do make a mistake, improve your odds of staying healthy by getting tested and treated as soon as possible. And think seriously about what steps you can take to protect yourself in the future.

provide free, confidential information and referral services to callers anywhere in the country (see the For More Information section at the end of the chapter).

Although information about STDs is widely disseminated, learning about STDs is still up to every person individually. You must assume responsibility for learning about the causes and nature of STDs and their potential effects on you, the children you may have, and others with whom you have sexual relationships. Once you know about STDs—their symptoms, how they're transmitted, how they can be prevented—you are in a position to educate others. Providing information to your friends and partners, whether in casual conversation or in more serious decision-making discussions, is an important way that you can make a difference in your own wellness and that of others.

Diagnosis and Treatment

Early diagnosis and treatment of STDs can help you and your sex partner(s) avoid unnecessary complications and help prevent the spread of STDs.

Be Alert for Symptoms   If you are sexually active, be alert for any sign or symptom of disease, such as a rash, a discharge, sores, or unusual pain, and don't hesitate to have a professional examination if you notice such a symptom. Although only a physician can make a proper diagnosis of an STD, you can perform *genital self-examination* between checkups to look for early warning signs of infection. Women should examine the entire genital area, including the area covered by pubic hair, the outer and inner lips of the vagina, the clitoris, and the area around the urinary and vaginal openings. Men should look at the entire head, shaft, and base of the penis and the scrotum. (A mirror may be helpful for checking difficult-to-see areas.) Throughout the exam, look for bumps, sores, blisters, or warts on the skin. Bumps or blisters may be red or light colored; they may look like pimples or they may develop into open sores. Genital warts may appear as very small bumpy spots or they may have a fleshy, cauliflower-like appearance. Also stay alert for other signs of STDs, including pain or burning upon urination, itchiness in the genital area, abnormal discharge from the vagina or penis, pelvic pain, and, in women, bleeding between menstrual periods. Be alert for these signs or symptoms in your partner too, and don't hesitate to question him or her if you notice something unusual.

Get Tested   Remember that almost all STDs—including HIV infection—can be completely asymptomatic for long periods of time. If you are sexually active, be sure to get periodic STD and HIV checks, even if you have no symptoms; if you have a risky sexual encounter, see a physician as soon as possible (see the box "Don't Wait— Early Treatment of STDs Really Matters"). Sexually active young women should have pelvic exams and Pap tests at least once a year, with chlamydia and gonorrhea screening in most cases. Sexually active men, especially if they have had more than one partner, should receive periodic STD and HIV screening.

Testing for STDs is done through private physicians, public health clinics, community health agencies, and most student health services. If you are diagnosed as having an STD, you should begin treatment as quickly as possible. Inform your partner(s), and avoid any sexual activity until your treatment is complete and testing indicates that you are cured. If your partner tells you that he or she has contracted an STD, get tested immediately, even if you don't have any symptoms. Asymptomatic partners are often treated to ensure that an infection will not spread or recur.

Inform Your Partners   Telling a partner that you have exposed him or her to an STD isn't easy. You may be afraid your partner will be angry or resentful, or you may worry that your partner will think less of you or reject you. At the same time, you may be feeling afraid, ashamed, embarrassed, or angry yourself. Despite the awkwardness and difficulty, it is crucial that your sex partner or partners be informed and urged to seek testing and/or treatment as quickly as possible.

You can get help telling your partner if you need it. Public health departments will notify sex partners of their possible exposure while maintaining your confidentiality and anonymity. Peer counseling and student health programs often help students with practice in role playing in these circumstances, and concerned health care personnel can provide assistance.

As emphasized throughout this chapter, undetected and untreated STDs can lead to serious medical complications and even death. In asymptomatic cases, the only way infected people can find out they have a disease is by being told they need to be tested. Uninformed partners can go on to spread the disease, contributing to anguish for others as well as spiraling public health problems. The responsibility of informing partners is an ethical task too important to shirk.

Get Treated   With the exception of AIDS treatments, treatments for STDs are safe and generally inexpensive. If you are being treated, follow instructions carefully and complete all the medication as prescribed. Don't stop taking the medication just because you feel better or your symptoms have disappeared. Above all, don't give any of your medication to your partner or to anyone else. Doing so will only make your treatment incomplete and reinfection more likely. Being cured of an STD does not mean that you will not get it again, and exposure does not confer lasting immunity, nor does it prevent you from getting any other STD—all the more reason to be informed, to inform your partners, and to practice safer sex.

COMMUNICATE!   Talking with your health care provider is a critical step in protecting yourself from STDs and their potentially lasting effects. Don't wait for your provider to bring up the topic; if you have concerns or questions, it's important to ask, even if you feel embarrassed or uncomfortable. For example, "My girlfriend thinks she may have genital warts. I'd like to be examined for warts and other STDs," or "I have a new sexual partner who thinks he may have been exposed to herpes in the past. Should I be checked for herpes?" Make sure you understand what your provider tells you about your health status and any treatments prescribed for you. If there are medical terms you don't understand, ask for clarification; you have the right to fully understand issues related to your health.

WW. Prevention

STDs *are* preventable. As discussed earlier, the only sure way to avoid exposure to STDs is to abstain from sexual activity. But if you do choose to be sexually active, the key is to think about prevention *before* you have a sexual encounter or find yourself in the "heat of the moment." Find out what your partner thinks before you become sexually involved. Remember, you can become infected with an STD from just one unprotected encounter.

All your good intentions are likely to fly out the window if you enter into a sexual situation when you are intoxicated. If you or your partner (or both of you) is drunk, you are likely to be less cautious about sex than you would be if you were sober. Many people use alcohol and drugs as a way to deal with their anxiety in social and sexual situations. However, being intoxicated leaves you vulnerable to sexual assault and greatly increases your risk of acquiring a serious STD.

Most people don't want to think, talk, or ask questions about STDs for a variety of reasons. They may think it detracts from the appeal and excitement of the moment, that it takes away from the spontaneity of the experience, or that it will be perceived as a personal insult. For others, simply not knowing how to talk about STDs and safer sex may prevent them from bringing up the issue with a partner. (For advice on communicating with potential sex partners, see the box "Talking About Condoms and Safer Sex.")

Plan ahead for safer sex. Know what sexual behaviors are risky. Find out about your partner's sexual history and practices. Be honest, and ask your partner to do the same, but don't stake your health and life on assumptions about your partner's honesty. Even if your partner's past seems low-risk, still insist on using a condom every time you have sex. Many honest people are simply unaware that they have an STD.

You may find that your partner is just as concerned as you are. By thinking and talking about responsible sexual

The only sure way to prevent STDs, including HIV infection, is to abstain from sexual activity. If you choose to be sexually active, you should do everything possible to protect yourself from STDs. This includes good communication with your sex partner(s).

The time to talk about safer sex is before you begin a sexual relationship. However, even if you've been having unprotected sex with your partner, it is still worth it to start practicing safer sex now. If you're nervous about initiating a conversation about safer sex, rehearse what you will say first. Practice in front of a mirror or with a friend.

There are many ways to bring up the subject of safer sex and condom use with your partner. Be honest about your concerns and stress that protection against STDs means that you care about yourself and your partner. Here are a few suggestions:

- "I heard on the news that more and more people are buying and using condoms. I think it shows that people are being more responsible about sex. What do you think?"

- "I'm worried about the diseases we can get from having sex because so many don't have symptoms. I want to protect both of us by using condoms whenever we have sex."

- "I've been thinking about making love with you. But first we need to talk about how to have safer sex and be protected."

You may find that your partner shares your concerns and also wants to use condoms. He or she may be happy and relieved that you have brought up the subject of safer sex. However, if he or she resists the idea of using condoms, you may need to negotiate. Stress that you both deserve to be protected and that sex will be more enjoyable when you aren't worrying about STDs (see the suggestions to the right). If you and your partner haven't used condoms before, buy some and familiarize yourselves with how to use them. Once you feel more comfortable handling condoms, you'll be able to use them correctly and incorporate them into your sexual activity in fun ways.

If your partner still won't agree to use condoms, think carefully about whether you want to have a sexual relationship with him or her. Safer sex is part of a responsible, caring sexual relationship, and it's smart to say "no" to a partner who won't use a condom. It's up to you to protect yourself.

If your partner says . . .	Try saying . . .
"They're not romantic."	"Worrying about AIDS isn't romantic, and with condoms we won't have to worry." OR "If we put one on together, a condom could be fun."
"You don't trust me."	"I do trust you, but how can I trust your former partners or mine?" OR "It's important to me that we're both protected."
"I don't have any diseases. I've been tested."	"I'm glad you've been tested, but tests aren't foolproof for all diseases. To be safe, I always use condoms."
"I forgot to bring a condom. But it's OK to skip it just this once."	"I'd really like to make love with you, but I never have sex without a condom. Let's go get some."
"I don't like the way they feel."	"They might feel different, but let's try." OR "Sex won't feel good if we're worrying about diseases."
"I don't use condoms."	"I use condoms every time." OR "I don't have sex without condoms."
"But I love you."	"Being in love can't protect us from diseases." OR "I love you, too. We still need to use condoms."
"But we've been having sex without condoms."	"I want to start using condoms now so we won't be at any more risk." OR "We can still prevent infection or reinfection."

SOURCES: Dialogue from San Francisco AIDS Foundation. 1988. *Condoms for Couples*. (IMPACT AIDS, 3692 18th Street, San Francisco, CA 94110). Copyright © 1998 San Francisco AIDS Foundation. All rights reserved. Used with permission.

behavior, you are expressing a sense of caring for yourself, your potential partner, and your future children. Taking STDs seriously is practical, courageous, and loving; it means giving yourself the respect you deserve.

Everyone can reduce the risk of infection by behaving responsibly. Aside from abstinence, the next most effective approach to preventing STDs is having sex only with one mutually monogamous uninfected partner. If you are sexually active, use a condom during every act of intercourse to reduce your risk of contracting a disease. Although not foolproof, a properly used condom provides an effective barrier against pathogens, including HIV. A disease can be transmitted if there is contact with an infected area that isn't protected by the condom, however. The use of a barrier over the cervix (diaphragm or cervical cap) in addition to a condom may provide women with some additional protection against the organisms that cause gonorrhea, genital warts, and chlamydia (see Chapter 6).

Approaches to STD prevention that do not work include urinating or douching after intercourse, engaging in oral sex, and genital play without full penetration. Birth

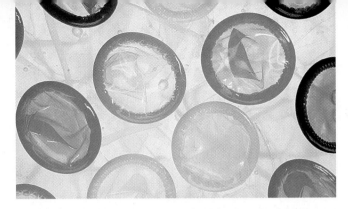

The use of condoms declined as more advanced methods of contraception, such as birth control pills and IUDs, became available. But condoms are once again gaining in popularity because of the protection they provide against STDs.

control pills and sterilization protect you against conception and unwanted pregnancy but not against STDs.

The decision to have a sexual relationship is accompanied by uncertainties and risks, both physical and emotional. It also carries the responsibility of safeguarding your own health and that of others. You and your partner must have mutual respect and honesty in order to make good decisions together. Caring about yourself and your partner means asking questions and being aware of signs and symptoms. It may be a bit awkward, but the temporary embarrassment of asking intimate questions is a small price to pay to avoid contracting or spreading disease. If your partner thinks less of you for being concerned, you may want to reconsider the relationship in terms of your personal values. Concern about STDs is part of a sexual relationship, not an intrusion into it, just as sexuality is part of life, not separate from it.

Tips for Today

STDs are among the most common infections you can contract—and some are among the most dangerous. Because they can have serious, long-term effects, it's important to be vigilant about exposure, treatment, and, most critically, prevention.

Right now you can

- Perform a genital self-examination, following the instructions on p. 546, if there is any possibility that you might have been exposed to an STD.

- Call to make an appointment with your health care provider if you need or want to see someone about possible STD infection.

- Inform a friend or roommate that people can have an STD and not have any symptoms.

- Resolve to discuss condom use with your partner if you are sexually active and are not already using condoms.

SUMMARY

- HIV affects the immune system, making an otherwise healthy person less able to resist a variety of infections.

- HIV is carried in blood and blood products, semen, vaginal and cervical secretions, and breast milk. HIV is transmitted through the exchange of these fluids.

- There is currently no cure or vaccine for HIV infection. Drugs have been developed to slow the course of the disease and to prevent or treat certain secondary infections.

- HIV infection can be prevented by making careful choices about sexual activity, not sharing drug needles, and learning about how to protect oneself from contracting HIV.

- Chlamydia causes epididymitis and urethritis in men; in women, it can lead to PID and infertility if untreated.

- Untreated, gonorrhea can cause PID in women and epididymitis in men, leading to infertility. In infants, untreated gonorrhea can cause blindness.

- Pelvic inflammatory disease (PID), a complication of untreated gonorrhea or chlamydia, is an infection of the uterus and oviducts that may extend to the ovaries and pelvic cavity. It can lead to infertility, ectopic pregnancy, and chronic pelvic pain.

- Genital warts, caused by the human papillomavirus (HPV), are associated with cervical cancer. Treatment does not eradicate the virus, which can be passed on even by asymptomatic people.

- Genital herpes is a common incurable infection that can be fatal to newborns. After an initial infection, outbreaks may recur at any time.

- Hepatitis B is a viral infection of the liver transmitted through sexual and nonsexual contact. Following an initial infection, most people recover; but some become chronic carriers of the virus who may develop serious, potentially fatal, complications.

- Syphilis is a highly contagious bacterial infection that can be treated with antibiotics. If left untreated, it can lead to deterioration of the central nervous system and death.

- Less serious diseases that can be transmitted sexually or are linked to sexual activity include trichomoniasis, bacterial vaginosis, chancroid, pubic lice, and scabies. Any STD that causes sores or inflammation can increase risk of HIV transmission.

- Successful diagnosis and treatment of STDs involves being alert for symptoms, getting tested, informing partners, and following treatment instructions carefully.

- All STDs are preventable; the key is practicing responsible sexual behaviors. Those who are sexually active are safest with one mutually monogamous uninfected partner. Using a condom properly with every act of sexual intercourse helps protect against STDs.

1. Go to a drugstore and examine the OTC contraceptives. Which ones provide protection against STDs? If you are sexually active, make sure you use the best protection available.

2. More and more communities have treatment and support programs for people with HIV infection. Look in the yellow pages or contact local health agencies to find out what services are available where you live. If any of these agencies use volunteers, consider donating some of your time to help.

3. If you have ever engaged in unprotected sex or another behavior that puts you at risk for STDs, talk with your health care provider about being screened for common STDs. What tests are available and useful for your situation?

JOURNAL ENTRY

1. In your health journal, list the positive behaviors that help you avoid exposure to sexually transmitted diseases. Consider what additions you can make to this list or how you can strengthen your existing behaviors. Then list the behaviors that may block your positive behaviors or put you at risk for contracting an STD. Consider which ones you can change and how you can begin doing so.

2. In your health journal, write a brief script for four different ways you could bring up the subject of STDs and safer sex with a potential sex partner. Then write out a response you could use if a potential partner brought up the subject of safer sex.

3. **Critical Thinking** What responsibility do you think the federal government has for funding programs for the prevention and treatment of HIV infection? Do you think the government should pay for national prevention programs or increase financial aid to cities bearing the medical costs of caring for people with HIV? Or should these costs be borne by individuals, families, communities, or private insurance companies? Should the new, more effective (and expensive) drugs be available only to people who can afford them or who have private insurance? Write an essay describing what role, if any, you think the government should play; explain your reasoning.

FOR MORE INFORMATION

Books

Bayer, R., and G. Oppenheimer. 2000. *AIDS Doctors: Voices from the Epidemic.* New York: Oxford University Press. *The AIDS epidemic as seen through the eyes of 74 physicians on the front lines.*

Ebel, C. 1998. *Managing Herpes: How to Live and Love with a Chronic STD.* Durham, N.C.: American Social Health Association. *Helpful advice and support.*

Hatcher, R. A. 1999. *Safely Sexual.* New York: Ardent Media. *Provides practical advice for STD prevention.*

Marr, L. 1999. *Sexually Transmitted Disease: A Physician Tells You What You Need to Know.* Baltimore, Md.: Johns Hopkins University Press. *Provides practical information about protecting oneself against infection and obtaining appropriate medical care.*

Matthews, D. D., ed. 2000. *Sexually Transmitted Diseases Sourcebook.* Detroit, Mich.: Omnigraphics. *Includes consumer-oriented information on a wide variety of topics.*

Smith, R. A., ed. 2001. Encyclopedia of AIDS. New York: Penguin. *An overview of the scientific, medical, and social aspects of HIV/AIDS.*

Organizations, Hotlines, and Web Sites

American College Health Association. Offers free brochures on STDs, alcohol use, acquaintance rape, and other college health issues.

410-859-1500
http://www.acha.org

American Social Health Association (ASHA). Provides written information and referrals on STDs; sponsors support groups for people with herpes and HPV.

800-230-6039
http://www.ashastd.org

ASHA/CDC STD and AIDS Hotlines. ASHA operates several hotlines related to STDs, including those sponsored by the CDC; callers can obtain information, counseling, and referrals for testing and treatment. The general hotline offers information on more than 20 STDs and includes Spanish and TTY service. Specific hotlines for herpes and HPV infection are also available.

800-342-AIDS or 800-227-8922
800-344-SIDA (Spanish)
800-243-7889 (TTY, deaf access)
919-361-8488 (herpes)
919-361-4848 (HPV infection)

The Body/A Multimedia AIDS and HIV Information Resource. Provides basic information about HIV—prevention, testing, treatment—and links to related sites.

http://www.thebody.com

CDC National Prevention Information Network. Provides extensive information and links on HIV/AIDS and other STDs.

800-458–5231

http://www.cdcnpin.org

HIV InSite: Gateway to AIDS Knowledge. Provides information about prevention, education, treatment, statistics, clinical trials, and new developments.

http://hivinsite.ucsf.edu

Joint United Nations Programme on HIV/AIDS (UNAIDS). Provides statistics and information on the international HIV/AIDS situation.

http://www.unaids.org

Journal of the American Medical Association Information Centers. Provides daily news summaries, patient information, expert advice, and glossaries.

http://www.ama-assn.org/special/hiv (HIV/AIDS Center)

http://www.ama-assn.org/special/std (STDs Center)

Latex Love. Sponsored by the makers of Trojan condoms, this site includes directions for condom use and sample dialogues for overcoming excuses for not using condoms.

http://www.trojancondoms.com/quizzes/safer_sex

The NAMES Project Foundation AIDS Memorial Quilt. Includes the story behind the quilt, images of quilt panels, and information and links relating to HIV infection.

http://www.aidsquilt.org

National Institute of Allergies and Infectious Disease/STDs Information. Provides up-to-date fact sheets and brochures.

http://www.niaid.nih.gov/publications/stds.htm

Planned Parenthood Federation of America. Provides information on STDs, family planning, and contraception.

http://www.plannedparenthood.org

Safer Sex Page. Provides information on a variety of topics related to safer sex and STD prevention; includes audio of sample dialogues for talking about safer sex and condom use with partners. (Information is geared to people of all sexual orientations, and some is explicit.)

http://www.safersex.org/safer.sex

See also the listings for Chapters 6 and 17.

SELECTED BIBLIOGRAPHY

Anderson, J. E., et al. 1999. Condom use and HIV risk behaviors among U.S. adults: Data from a national survey. *Family Planning Perspectives* 31(1): 24–28.

Barroso, P. F., et al. 2000. Effect of antiretroviral therapy on HIV shedding in semen. *Annals of Internal Medicine* 133(4): 280–284.

Blankson, J., and R. Siliciano. 2000. Interleukin 2 treatment for HIV infection. *Journal of the American Medical Association* 284(2): 236–238.

Bozzette, S. A., et al. 2001. Expenditures for the care of HIV-infected patients in the era of highly active antiretroviral therapy. *New England Journal of Medicine* 344(11): 817–823.

Burstein, G. R., et al. 2001. Predictors of repeat *Chlamydia trachomatis* infections diagnosed by DNA amplification testing among inner city females. *Sexually Transmitted Infections* 77(1): 26–32.

Centers for Disease Control and Prevention. 1998. 1998 guidelines for treatment of sexually transmitted diseases. *MMWR Recommendations and Reports* 47(RR-1).

Centers for Disease Control and Prevention. 2000. CDC statement on study results of product containing nonoxynol-9. *Morbidity and Mortality Weekly Report* 49(31): 717–718.

Centers for Disease Control and Prevention. 2001. Primary and secondary syphilis—United States, 1999. *Morbidity and Mortality Weekly Report* 50(7): 113–117.

Centers for Disease Control and Prevention, Division of Viral and Rickettsial Diseases. 2000. *Hepatitis Surveillance Report*, No. 57. Atlanta: Centers for Disease Control and Prevention.

Centers for Disease Control and Prevention. 2001. Prevalence of risk behaviors for HIV infection among adults—United States, 1997. *Morbidity and Mortality Weekly Report* 50(14): 262–265.

Corey, L., and H. Handsfield. 2000. Genital herpes and public health: Addressing a global problem. *Journal of the American Medical Association* 283(6): 791–794.

Daar, E. S., et al. 2001. Diagnosis of primary HIV-1 infection. *Annals of Internal Medicine* 134(1): 25–29.

Deeks, S. G., et al. 2001. Virologic and immunologic consequences of discontinuing combination antiretroviral-drug therapy in HIV-infected patients with detectable viremia. *New England Journal of Medicine* 344(7): 472–480.

Dorenbaum, A. 2001. *Report of the Results of PACTG 316: An International Phase III Trial of Standard Antiretroviral (ARV) Prophylaxis plus Nevirapine (NVP) for Prevention of Perinatal HIV Transmission.* Presented at the 8th Conference on Retroviruses and Opportunistic Infections (http://www.retroconference.org/2001/abstracts/abstracts/abstracts/LB7.htm; retrieved March 7, 2001).

Folks, T. 2000. Chimpanzees as original source for HIV. *Journal of the American Medical Association* 283(3): 310.

Friedrich, M. 2000. HAART stopping news: Experts examine structured therapy interrruption for HIV. *Journal of the American Medical Association* 283(2): 2917–2918.

Gage, J. R., et al. 2000. Effects of human papillomavirus–associated cells on human immunodeficiency virus gene expression. *Obstetrics and Gynecology* 96(6): 879–885.

Goujon, C. P., et al. 2000. Phylogenetic analyses indicate an atypical nurse-to-patient transmission of human immunodeficiency virus type 1. *Journal of Virology* 74(6): 2525–2532.

Hader, S. L., et al. 2001. HIV infection in women in the United States. *Journal of the American Medical Association* 285(9): 1186–1192.

Joint United Nations Programme on HIV/AIDS (UNAIDS). 2000. *AIDS Epidemic Update: December 2000.* Geneva: UNAIDS/WHO.

Kirchner, J., and D. Emmert. 2000. Sexually transmitted diseases in women: *Chlamydia trachomatis* and herpes simplex infection. *Postgraduate Medicine* 107(1): 55–65.

Lee, L. M., et al. 2001. Survival after AIDS diagnosis in adolescents and adults during the treatment era, United States, 1984–1997. *Journal of the American Medical Association* 285(10): 1308–1315.

Levy, J. A. 2001. What can be achieved with an HIV vaccine? *Lancet* 357(9251): 223–224.

Miller, K., and J. Graves. 2000. Update on the prevention and treatment of sexually transmitted diseases. *American Family Physician* 61(2): 379–386.

Ness, R. B., et al. 2001. Douching and endometritis: Results from the PID evaluation and clinical health (PEACH) study. *Sexually Transmitted Diseases* 28(4): 240–245.

Richwald, G., and P. Langley. 1999. Management of external genital warts: Diagnosis and clinical management. *Family Practice Recertification* 21(9): 5–12.

Screening and prevention of sexually transmitted diseases. 2001. *Journal of the American Medical Association* 285(1): 118.

Siegal, H. A., et al. 1999. Under the influence: Risky sexual behavior and substance abuse among DUI offenders. *Sexually Transmitted Diseases* 26(2): 87–92.

Stephenson, J. 2000. HIV risk from oral sex higher than many realize. *Journal of the American Medical Association* 283(10): 1279.

U.S. Department of Health and Human Services and the Henry J. Kaiser Family Foundation. 2001. *Guidelines for the Use of Antiretroviral Agents in HIV-Infected Adults and Adolescents* (http://www.hivatis.org/trtgdlns.html; retrieved February 10, 2001).

Wald, A., et al. 2000. Reactivation of genital herpes simplex virus type 2 infection in asymptomatic seropositive persons. *New England Journal of Medicine* 342(12): 844–850.

Woitas, R. P., et al. 2001. *CCR5-D32 Mutation—Protective Against HIV, but Bad for Hepatitis C Virus?* Presented at the 8th Conference on Retroviruses and Opportunistic Infections (http://www.retroconference.org/2001/abstracts/abstracts/abstracts/499.htm; retrieved March 7, 2001).

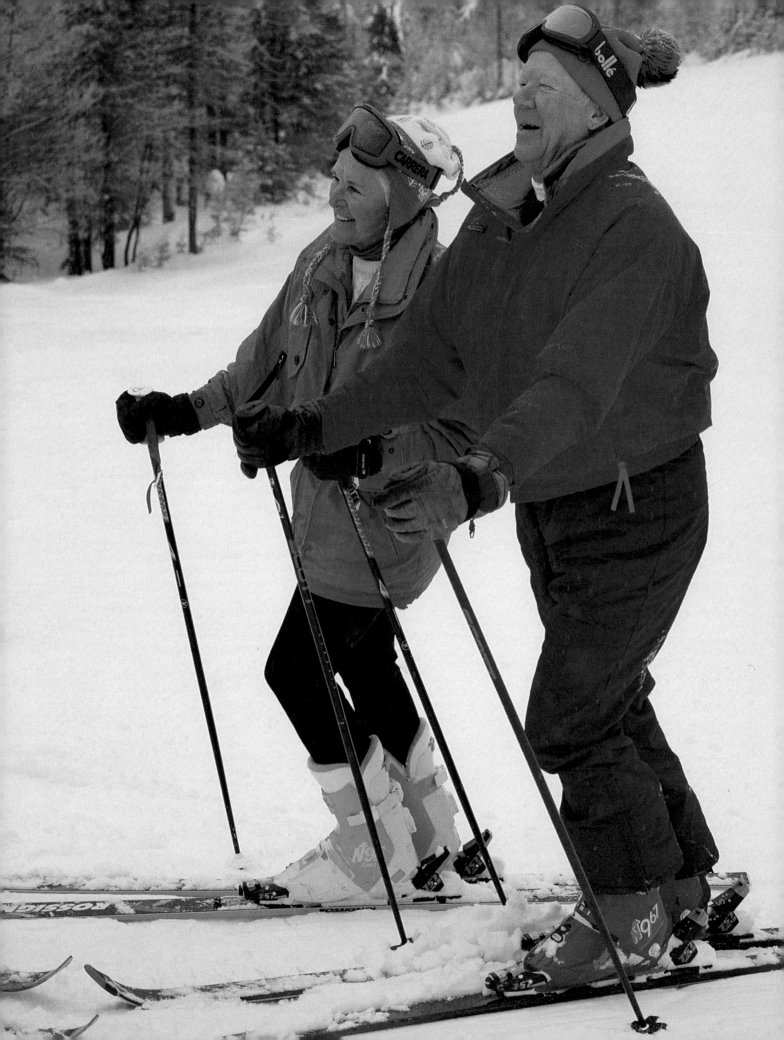

After reading this chapter, you should be able to

- List strategies for healthful aging

- Explain the physical, social, and mental changes that may accompany aging and discuss how people can best confront these changes

- Compare different theories on the causes of aging

- Describe practical considerations of older adults, including housing, finances, health care, and transportation

Aging: A Vital Process

19

TEST YOUR KNOWLEDGE

1. Women do not need to take preventive measures against osteoporosis until after menopause.
   True or false?

2. Medicare and private insurers pay for what percentage of nursing home costs overall?
   a. 3%
   b. 33%
   c. 66%

3. On average, a woman will spend more time caring for an aging relative than raising children.
   True or false?

4. Exercise is beneficial for older people because it
   a. protects against osteoporosis.
   b. maintains alertness and intelligence.
   c. prevents falls.

5. Alcohol abuse is rare among older adults.
   True or false?

ANSWERS

1. **FALSE.** Women need to pay attention to diet and exercise in younger years in order to build bone mass.

2. **A.** Medicare pays less than 2% of costs, and private insurers pay less than 1% for the more than 1 million older Americans currently living in nursing homes.

3. **TRUE.** The average woman will spend 17 years raising children and 18 years caring for an aging relative.

4. **ALL THREE.** Even for people over 80, exercise can improve physical functioning and balance and reduce falls and injuries.

5. **FALSE.** Alcohol abuse affects about 10% of elderly people. It often goes undetected because its symptoms may mimic those of other conditions, such as Alzheimer's disease.

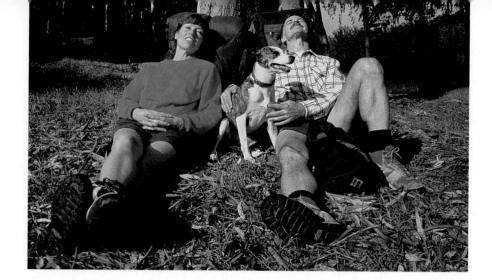

Middle age is a time of reassessment and readjustment in preparation for the second half of life. Many people in their forties and fifties who have cultivated healthy lifestyles will continue to lead vigorous lives well into old age.

Many people would like to live for a long time and never grow old. When we see that old age has taken us in its grip, we're stunned. We regard old age as something foreign: Can I become a different person while I still remain myself? Yes. And no. Life is like a river. The flow is continuous, and you can never step in the same place twice.

Aging does not begin on the sixty-fifth birthday, and there is no precise age at which a person becomes "old." Rather, aging is a normal process of development that occurs over the entire lifetime. It happens to everyone, but at different rates for different people. Some people are "old" at 25, and others are still "young" at 75.

Although youth is not entirely a state of mind, your attitude toward life and your attention to your health significantly influence the satisfaction you will derive from life, especially when new physical, mental, and social challenges occur in later years. If you optimize wellness during young adulthood, you can exert great control over the physical and mental aspects of aging, and you can better handle your response to events that might be out of your control. With foresight and energy you can shape a creative, graceful, and even triumphant old age.

GENERATING VITALITY AS YOU AGE

As we age, we experience both gains and losses. Physical and mental changes occur gradually, over a lifetime. Biological aging includes all the normal, progressive, irreversible changes to one's body that begin at birth and continue until death. Psychological and social aging usually involve more abrupt changes in circumstance and emotion: relocating, changing homes, losing a spouse and friends, retiring, having a lower income, and changing roles and social status. These changes represent opportunities for growth throughout life.

Not all of them happen to everybody, and their timing varies, partly depending on how we have prepared for our later days. Some people never have to leave their homes and appear to be in good health until the day they die. Others have tremendous adjustments to make—to entirely new surroundings with fewer financial resources, to new acquaintances, to the changing physical condition of their bodies and new health problems, and possibly to loneliness and loss of self-esteem.

Successful aging requires preparation. People need to establish good health habits in their teens and twenties. During their twenties and thirties, they usually develop important relationships and settle into a particular lifestyle. By their mid-forties, they generally know how much money they need to support the lifestyle they've chosen. At this point, they must assess their financial status and perhaps adjust their savings in order to continue enjoying that lifestyle after retirement. In their mid-fifties, they need to reevaluate their health insurance plans and may want to think about retirement housing. In their seventies, eighties, and nineties, they need to consider ways of sharing their legacy with the next generation. Throughout life, people should cultivate interests and hobbies they enjoy, both alone and with others, so they can continue to live an active and rewarding life in their later years.

What Happens As You Age?

Many of the characteristics associated with aging are not due to aging at all. Rather, they are the result of neglect and abuse of our bodies and minds. These assaults lay the foundation for later psychological problems and chronic conditions like arthritis, heart disease, diabetes, hearing loss, and hypertension. We sacrifice our optimal health by smoking, having poor nutrition, overeating, abusing alcohol and drugs, bombarding our ears with excessive noise, and exposing our bodies to too much ultraviolet radiation from the sun. We also jeopardize our bodies through inactivity, encouraging our muscles and even our bones to wither and deteriorate. And we endure abuse from the toxic chemicals in our environment.

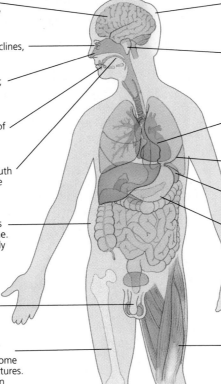

Blood flow to the brain decreases and nerve cells atrophy. Neuron loss does not necessarily mean a decline in mental ability.

The ability to focus on objects close to you declines, and night driving may become more difficult.

Many of the sensory receptors in the nose die; long-term exposure to smoke also lessens the ability to smell.

Teeth can last a lifetime; however, a buildup of plaque can lead to tooth loss if brushing and flossing are neglected.

About two-thirds of the taste buds in the mouth die by age 70; some medications can interfere with taste.

Body fat increases and muscle mass decreases as activity levels drop and calorie needs decline. Regular exercise helps maintain a healthy body composition

Men take longer to attain an erection and it may not be as firm or as large as when they were younger. Enlargement of the prostate gland is common. In women, menopause occurs and estrogen levels drop.

Women in particular are prone to bone loss, especially after menopause, when bones become weaker, more porous, and more likely to fractures. Calcium intake and weight-bearing exercise in younger years can slow bone loss later.

Cells at the base of hair follicles produce progressively less pigment and eventually die, causing hair to turn gray and some men to go bald. Hair also becomes finer.

Ability to hear high-pitched and sibilant (hissing) sounds such as s, z, sh, and ch declines. Some losses may be due to damage from loud music or machinery.

The heart pumps less blood with each beat; this is particularly noticeable during exercise. A healthy diet and regular exercise can often counteract potential cardiovascular problems.

Lung capacity stays steady or even increases with regular exercise. Colds are fewer and less severe due to a buildup in immunity.

Kidneys filter waste more slowly, affecting drug clearance and increasing frequency of urination.

Decreases in acid production and digestive enzymes make digestion take longer; constipation may become more common unless fiber intake increases.

Long-term sun exposure produces wrinkles and spotty pigmentation ("age spots"). Skin gets looser, stretches more easily, and is less resilient.

Muscle fibers atrophy and lose their ability to contract as more protein is broken down and less is synthesized. Regular exercise can slow this process. Muscles are also less flexible and more susceptible to injury.

Figure 19-1 Age-related changes in the body. The body changes in predictable ways as we age. Many of these changes can be slowed by choices we make throughout our lives.

But even with the healthiest behavior and environment, aging inevitably occurs. It results from biochemical processes we don't yet fully understand. The physiological changes in organ systems are caused by a combination of gradual aging and impairment from disease. Because of redundancy in most organ systems, the body's ability to function is not affected until damage is fairly extensive. Studies of healthy people indicate that functioning remains essentially constant until after age 70. Figure 19-1 shows some of the changes that are a part of aging. Some diseases are associated with aging, but the precise risk factors that make a person susceptible to them are still unclear (for example, see the box "Parkinson's Disease").

Life-Enhancing Measures: Age-Proofing

You can prevent, delay, lessen, or even reverse some of the changes associated with aging through good habits. Simple things you can do daily will make a vast difference to your appearance, level of energy, and vitality—your overall wellness. The following suggestions have been mentioned throughout this text. But because they are profoundly related to health in later life, we highlight them here.

Challenge Your Mind Creativity and intelligence remain stable in healthy individuals. Develop interests and hobbies you can enjoy throughout your life. Staying involved in learning as a lifelong process can help you remain alert and keep your mental abilities.

Develop Physical Fitness Exercise enhances both psychological and physical health. We cannot say enough about the positive effects of appropriate exercise throughout your life, particularly when weighed against the physical and mental deterioration of older people who have not kept their minds and bodies fit. The benefits include:

- Lower blood pressure and healthier cholesterol levels
- Better protection against heart attacks and an increased chance of survival should one occur
- Sustained capacity of the lungs and respiratory reserves
- Weight control through less accumulation of fat
- Maintenance of strength, flexibility, and balance
- Protection against osteoporosis and Type 2 diabetes
- Increased effectiveness of the immune system
- Maintenance of mental agility and flexibility, response time, memory, and hand-eye coordination

The news that television actor Michael J. Fox has **Parkinson's disease** brought increased attention to a disease that is usually associated with older adults. Parkinson's is a degenerative illness caused by a decrease in the production of dopamine, a chemical in the brain crucial for muscle control and movement.

The early signs and symptoms of Parkinson's usually develop on one side of the body. They include shaking or trembling; changes in handwriting (which becomes smaller or more cramped, for example); problems with movement, such as hands, arms, or legs not moving as smoothly as they have in the past; and diminished facial expression. A person with these symptoms should see a physician for evaluation. As the disease progresses, other symptoms appear. The most common include the following:

- Rigidity of muscles: contraction and tension causing stiffness and resistance to movement

- Tremor: involuntary shaking, trembling, or movement of parts of the body such as fingers, hands, jaw, or head, usually appearing when the person is at rest

- Postural instability: inability to hold a body position, with problems of balance and coordination

- Bradykinesia: a slowing down of movement and loss of the ability to move automatically and spontaneously

The main risk factor for developing Parkinson's disease is age. Although 15% of patients are diagnosed before age 50, it is more common among older adults, affecting 1 out of every 100 persons over the age of 60. It is estimated that up to 1.5 million Americans have the disease. A recent study suggests that men may be at higher risk for developing the disease than women. The reasons for this are not clear, although estrogen may be a protective factor for women. Other than age, risk factors for the disease are unclear. Exposure to pesticides or other environmental hazards has been investigated as a cause, but results have been inconclusive. There is no evidence that the disease is hereditary, although some research has indicated that there may be genes that make a person more susceptible to the disease if combined with an as yet unknown environmental factor.

As researchers continue to search for a cure, Parkinson's can be treated and managed with medication. The most common drug used is levodopa (called L-dopa for short), which can mask symptoms of the disease for several years. L-dopa is closely related to dopamine; when taken orally by a patient, it is absorbed by the brain cells that normally release dopamine. They convert L-dopa into dopamine and release it as needed to allow the body to move normally. This regained mobility comes at the price of side effects that can include hallucinations and agitation caused by overstimulation of other brain cells by the dopamine and, after prolonged use, dyskinesias, or wild involuntary movements. Other drugs may be used to postpone the effects of L-dopa.

Patients may turn to surgery as their drug regimen becomes more problematic. Treatments that have had some success include destroying a small mass of cells within the brain to calm tremors and implanting an electrode to stimulate targeted parts of the brain. A controversial area of research, but one that has held out some promise, is fetal-cell implantation, in which dopamine-producing fetal cells are implanted in the brain.

SOURCES: Parkinson disease. 2000. *Journal of the American Medical Association* 284(5). The National Parkinson Foundation. 2000. What the patient should know (http://www.parkinson.org/pdedu.htm; retrieved December 21; 2000). Perry, P. 2000. Understanding Parkinson's disease, *Saturday Evening Post* 272(6). Baldereschi, M., et al. 2000. Parkinson's disease and Parkinsonism in a longitudinal study: Two-fold higher incidence in men. ILSA Working Group. Italian Longitudinal Study on Aging. *Neurology* 55(9): 1358–1363.

The stimulus that exercise provides also seems to protect against the loss of **fluid intelligence,** the ability to find solutions when confronted with a new problem. Fluid intelligence depends on rapidity of responsiveness, memory, and alertness. Individuals who exercise regularly have also been found to be less susceptible to depression than those whose level of physical activity has declined.

Find a variety of activities that you enjoy and can do regularly. Accumulate at least 30 minutes of moderate-intensity physical activity every day, and begin a formal exercise program to develop cardiorespiratory endurance, muscular strength and endurance, and flexibility (see Chapter 13). Older individuals who have been sedentary should be encouraged to become more active. Studies have shown that it's never too late to start exercising. Even in people over 80, endurance and strength training can improve balance, flexibility, and physical functioning and reduce the potential for dangerous falls.

Eat Wisely   Good health at any age is enhanced by eating a varied diet, paying special attention to lower fat and calorie intake. A new version of the Food Guide Pyramid (see Chapter 12) has been developed to address the changing dietary concerns of older individuals. The pyramid for people age 70 and older differs from the original pyramid in several ways:

- The new pyramid contains the same food groups and range of recommended servings as in the original pyramid, but because of decreased energy levels, most individuals only need the number of servings at the low end of the range.

- A new base includes eight 8-ounce glasses a day of water or any other nonalcoholic or caffeine-free beverages. Decreased sensitivity to thirst and changes in fluid needs from medications and kidney function make it important to monitor fluid intake.

- Recommended choices within groups emphasize foods that are high in nutrient density and fiber. (Fiber is important for preventing constipation and diverticulitis, and it is associated with lower levels of cholesterol and reduced incidence of cardiovascular disease and cancer.)
- Fiber-rich whole fruits and vegetables are recommended instead of juices, especially a variety of fruits and vegetables for vitamin C, beta-carotene, and folate content and cruciferous vegetables (such as cabbage, cauliflower, and broccoli) for the phytochemicals they contain.
- Three key supplements are mentioned: calcium, vitamin D, and vitamin B-12, which are the nutrients most often lacking in seniors' diets.

Maintain a Healthy Weight   Weight management is especially difficult if you have been overweight most of your life. A sensible program of expending more calories through exercise, cutting calorie intake, or a combination of both will work for most people who want to lose weight, but there is no magic formula. Obesity is not physically healthy, and it leads to premature aging (see Chapter 14).

Control Drinking and Overdependence on Medications   Alcohol abuse ranks with depression as a common hidden mental health problem, affecting about 10% of older adults. (The ability to metabolize alcohol decreases with age.) The problem is often not identified because the effects of alcohol or drug dependence can mimic disease, such as Alzheimer's disease. Signs of potential alcohol or drug dependence include unexplained falls or frequent injuries, forgetfulness, depression, and malnutrition. Older people who retire or lose a spouse are especially at risk. Problems can be avoided by not using alcohol to relieve anxiety or emotional pain and not taking medication when safer forms of treatment are available. Women taking hormone replacements should use alcohol cautiously because it appears to raise blood levels of estrogen to more than three times the intended dose.

Don't Smoke   The average pack-a-day smoker can expect to live about 12 years less than a nonsmoker. Furthermore, smokers suffer more illnesses that last longer, and they are subject to respiratory disabilities that limit their total vigor for many years before their death. Premature balding, skin wrinkling, and osteoporosis have been linked to cigarette smoking. Smokers at age 50 often have wrinkles resembling those of a person of 60.

Schedule Physical Examinations to Detect Treatable Diseases   When detected early, many diseases, including hypertension, diabetes, and many types of cancer, can be successfully controlled by medication and lifestyle

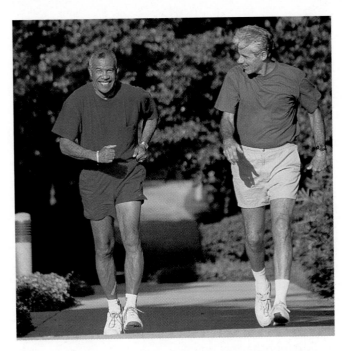

Regular exercise throughout life is an important key to successful aging. By keeping fit, these men have maintained a high level of physical functioning. Regular exercise also helps prevent depression, boredom, and losses in fluid intelligence typically associated with aging.

changes (see Chapter 21 for medical testing guidelines). Regular testing for **glaucoma** after age 40 can prevent blindness from this eye disease. Recommended immunizations, including those for influenza and pneumococcus, can protect you from preventable infectious diseases (see Chapter 17).

Recognize and Reduce Stress   Stress-induced physiological changes increase wear and tear on your body. Cut down on the stresses in your life. Don't wear yourself out through lack of sleep, substance abuse or misuse, or overwork. Practice relaxation, using the techniques described in Chapter 2. If you contract a disease, consider it your body's attempt to interrupt your life pattern; reevaluate your lifestyle, and perhaps slow down.

Parkinson's disease A neurological disorder caused by a deficiency of the neurotransmitter dopamine; symptoms include muscle rigidity, tremors, and difficulty walking.

fluid intelligence The ability to develop a solution when confronted with a new problem.

glaucoma A disease in which fluid inside the eye is under abnormally high pressure; can lead to the loss of peripheral vision and blindness.

Terms

The health behaviors you practice *now* are more influential in determining how long and how well you will live than your behaviors at a later age. Retiring from your life's occupation with a physically healthy body will allow far more options for enjoying yourself than will retiring with frail health or disabilities. Poor health that could have been prevented drains finances, emotions, and energy and contributes to poor psychological health. By enhancing your wellness today, you're buying some insurance for the future.

CONFRONTING THE CHANGES OF AGING

The changes that occur with aging have repercussions that must be grappled with and resolved. Just as you can act now to prevent or limit the physical changes of aging, you can also begin preparing yourself psychologically, socially, and financially for changes that may occur later in life. If you have aging parents, grandparents, and friends, the following information may give you insight into their lives and encourage you to begin cultivating appropriate and useful behaviors now.

WW. Planning for Social Changes

Retirement marks a major change in the second half of life. As the longevity of Americans has increased, people spend a larger proportion of their lives in retirement: 17 years or more. This has implications for reestablishing important relationships, developing satisfying interests outside work, and saving for an adequate retirement income. People who have well-developed leisure pursuits adjust better to retirement than those with few interests outside work.

Changing Roles and Relationships Changes in social roles are a major feature of middle age. Children become young adults and leave home, putting an end to daily parenting. Parents experiencing this "empty nest syndrome" must adapt to changes in their customary responsibilities and personal identities. And while retirement may be a desirable milestone for most people, it may also be viewed as a threat to prestige, purpose, and self-respect—the loss of a valued or customary role—and will probably require a period of adjustment.

Retirement and the end of child rearing also bring about changes in the relationship between marriage partners. The amount of time a couple spend together will increase and activities will change. Couples may need a period of adjustment, in which they get to know each other as individuals again. Discussing what types of activities each partner enjoys can help couples set up a mutually satisfying routine of shared and independent activities.

Terms   **arthritis** Inflammation of a joint or joints, causing pain and swelling.

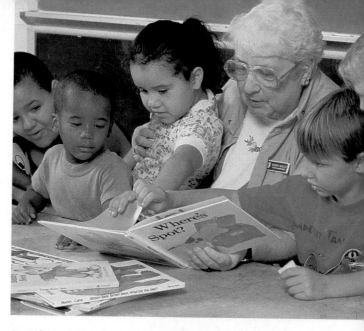

One of the challenges of aging is finding satisfying activities that provide meaningful connections with others. This retired woman reads to a group of children as part of a foster grandparent program.

Increased Leisure Time Planning ahead for retirement is crucial. What kinds of things do you enjoy doing? How will you spend your days? Although retirement confers the advantages of leisure time and freedom from deadlines, competition, and stress, many people do not know how to enjoy their free time. If you have developed diverse interests, retirement can be a joyful and fulfilling period of your life. It can provide opportunities for expanding your horizons by giving you the chance to try new activities, take classes, and meet new people. Volunteering in your community can enhance self-esteem and allow you to be a contributing member of society (see the box "Help Yourself by Helping Others").

The Economics of Retirement Retirement is usually accompanied by a new economic situation. It may mean a severely restricted budget or possibly even financial disaster if you don't take stock of your finances and plan ahead. Financial planning for retirement should begin early in life. People in their twenties and thirties should estimate how much money they need to support their standard of living, calculate their projected income, and begin a savings program. The earlier such a program is begun, the more money they will have at retirement.

Financial planning for retirement is especially critical for women. American women are much less likely than men to be covered by pension plans, reflecting the fact that many women have lower-paying jobs or work part-time during their childbearing years. They tend to have less money vested in other types of retirement plans as well. Although the gap is narrowing, women currently outlive men by about 7 years, and they are more likely to

Choosing to help others—whether as a volunteer for a community organization or through spontaneous acts of kindness—can enhance emotional, social, spiritual, and physical wellness. Surveys and studies indicate that the sense of purpose and service, and the feelings of generosity and kindness, that go with helping others may be as important a consideration for wellness as good nutrition and regular exercise. For example, a recent study of 1211 older adults found that about 35 percent of them did some volunteer work. Those who spent up to 40 hours a year helping others were less likely to die during the 7½-year length of the study than those who didn't volunteer at all.

In a national survey of volunteers from all fields, helpers reported the following benefits:

- "Helper's high"—physical and emotional sensations such as sudden warmth, a surge of energy, and a feeling of euphoria that occur immediately after helping

- Feelings of increased self-worth, calm, and relaxation

- A perception of greater physical health

- Fewer colds and headaches, improved eating and sleeping habits, and some relief from the pain of chronic diseases such as asthma and arthritis

Just how might helping benefit the health of the helper? By helping others, we may relieve our own distress and guilt over their problems. We focus on things other than our own problems, and we get a special kind of attention from the people we help. Helping others can be effective at banishing a bad mood or a case of the blues. Helping may block physical pain because we can pay attention to only a limited number of things at a given time. Helping others can also expand our perspective and enhance our appreciation for our own lives. Helping may benefit physical health by providing a temporary boost to the immune system and by combating stress and hostile feelings linked to the development of chronic diseases.

Helping others doesn't require a huge time commitment or a change of career. To get the most out of helping, keep the following guidelines in mind:

- *Make contact.* Choose an activity that involves personal contact.

- *Help as often as possible.* If your schedule allows, volunteer at least once a week. But, as with many parts of a wellness lifestyle, any amount of time helping is better than none.

- *Make helping voluntary.* Voluntary helping has positive results, whereas obligatory helping situations can actually increase stress.

- *Volunteer with others.* Working with a group enables you to form bonds with other helpers who can support your interests and efforts. Studies have found that the health benefits of volunteering are strongest for people who otherwise have low levels of social interaction.

- *Focus on the process, not the outcome.* We can't always measure or know the results of our actions.

- *Practice random acts of kindness.* Smile, let people go ahead of you in line, pick up litter, and so on.

- *Adopt a pet.* Several studies suggest that pet owners enjoy better health, perhaps by feeling needed or by having a source of unconditional love and affection.

- *Avoid burnout.* Recognize your own limits, pace yourself, and try not to feel guilty or discouraged. Take pride in being a volunteer or caregiver.

You can experience the "helper's high" and the other personal rewards of volunteering as soon as you begin helping others. In addition to the benefits for you, volunteering has the added bonus of having a positive impact on the wellness of others. It fosters a sense of community and can provide some practical help for many of the problems facing our society today.

SOURCES: Musick, M. A., A. R. Herzog, and J. S. House. 1999. Volunteering and mortality among older adults: Findings from a national sample. *Journal of Gerontology: Social Sciences* 54B(3): 5173. Adapted with permission from Sobel, D. S., M.D., and R. Ornstein, Ph.D. 1996. *The Healthy Mind, Healthy Body Handbook* (Los Altos, Calif.: DRx).

develop chronic conditions that impair their daily activities later in life. The net result of these factors is that older women are almost twice as likely as older men to live in poverty. Women should investigate their retirement plans and take charge of their finances to be sure they will be provided for as they get older.

Adapting to Physical Changes

As described earlier in the chapter, there are many things a person can do to avoid or minimize the impact of the physical changes associated with aging. However, some changes in physical functioning are inevitable, and successful aging involves anticipating and accommodating these changes.

Decreased energy and changes in health mean that older people have to develop priorities for how to use their energy. Rather than curtailing activities to conserve energy, they need to learn how to generate energy. This usually involves saying "yes" to enjoyable activities and paying close attention to the need for rest and sleep.

Adapting, rather than giving up, favorite activities may be the best strategy for dealing with physical limitations. For example, if **arthritis** interferes with piano playing, a person can continue to enjoy music by attending concerts or checking out music from the local library.

Hearing Loss   The loss of hearing is a common physical disability that can have a particularly strong effect on the lives of older adults. Hearing loss affects a person's ability to interact with others and can lead to a sense of isolation and depression. If someone you know complains that words are difficult to understand, that another person's speech sounds slurred or mumbled, or that people are not speaking loudly enough, that person may have suffered some hearing loss. You may also notice that the person sets the volume of a radio or TV very high.

Hearing loss should be assessed and treated by a health care professional; in some cases, hearing can be completely restored by dealing with the underlying cause of hearing loss. In other cases, hearing aids may be prescribed.

COMMUNICATE! How can you ease communication with a person suffering hearing loss? First, don't leave the person out of the conversation; practice can improve his or her ability to communicate. Speak more slowly and at a slightly louder level, and lower the pitch of your voice. Talking too loudly raises your pitch (hearing loss usually involves high-pitched sounds) and distorts your speech, making it more difficult for the other person to follow visual cues. Stand about 3 to 6 feet away from the person, in good light that allows your lip movements, facial expressions, and gestures to be seen clearly. Reduce background noise as much as possible. Finally, if the person does not understand you, rephrase your message in shorter, simpler sentences.

Vision Changes   Vision usually declines with age. For some individuals this can be traced to conditions such as glaucoma or **age-related macular degeneration (AMD)** that can be treated medically. For others, the effects of a decline in vision can be managed using strategies to make the most of remaining vision.

Glaucoma is caused by increased pressure within the eye due to built-up fluid. The optic nerve can be damaged by this increased pressure, resulting in a loss of side vision and, if untreated, blindness. Medication can relieve the pressure by decreasing the amount of fluid produced or by helping it drain more efficiently. Laser and conventional surgery are other options. Of the 3 million Americans with glaucoma, only half know that they have it; others lose the

opportunity to control the condition and preserve their sight. People over 60, African Americans over 40, and anyone with a family history of glaucoma are at risk.

AMD is a slow disintegration of the macula, the tissue at the center of the retina where fine, straight-ahead detail is distinguished. Losing this vision makes it difficult to read, drive, or perform other close-up activities. It is not known what causes the 90% of AMD cases known as "dry," in which usually one eye is gradually affected. About 10% of AMD cases are the more serious "wet" type, in which new blood vessels in the eye grow toward the macula and leak fluid, quickly causing serious damage. Risk factors for AMD are age, gender (women may be at higher risk than men), smoking, elevated cholesterol levels, and family history. Although dry AMD cannot be treated, it progresses so gradually that many people can adjust to it. Some cases of wet AMD can be treated with laser surgery. Both glaucoma and AMD can be detected with regular screening.

Vision can also be affected by conditions that are products of aging. By the time they reach their forties, many people have developed **presbyopia**, a gradual decline in the ability to focus on objects close to them. This occurs because the lens of the eye no longer expands and contracts as readily. **Cataracts,** a clouding of the lens caused by lifelong oxidation damage (a by-product of normal body chemistry) may dim vision by the sixties.

Whether vision is affected by disease or simply as a function of aging, there are many strategies to deal with reduced vision. Older people may need about a 30% increase in light in order to work more effectively; increasing light sources and painting rooms in a lighter color can help. Improving the light in dark areas such as stairwells can reduce falls from the slower light-to-dark accommodation that occurs with age. Wearing a hat and sunglasses outside helps reduce glare. If visual losses are more severe, large-print books, talking clocks, magnifying mirrors, large numbers on telephone keypads, and a variety of electronic devices are available to help. Not every person with low vision needs assistance, and steps can be taken to preserve independence. For example, when walking with a person with vision problems, ask if she needs help. If she does, offer your arm (don't take her arm unasked) and walk a half step in front of her. Warn quietly as you approach steps, ramps, curbs, and corridors. Every state has an association for the blind or visually impaired.

Arthritis   Half of all people over the age of 65 have some form of arthritis. This degenerative disease causes joint inflammation leading to chronic pain, swelling, and loss of mobility. Its warning signs include swelling, pain, redness, warmth, tenderness, changes in joint mobility, early morning stiffness, and unexplained weight loss, fever, or weakness in combination with joint pain.

There are more than 100 different types of arthritis; osteoarthritis (OA) is by far the most common. (Rheuma-

---

Terms

age-related macular degeneration (AMD) A deterioration of the macula (the central area of the retina) leading to blurred vision and sensitivity to glare; some cases can lead to blindness.

presbyopia The inability of the eyes to focus sharply on nearby objects, caused by a loss of elasticity of the lens that occurs with advancing age.

cataracts Opacity of the lens of the eye that impairs vision and can cause blindness.

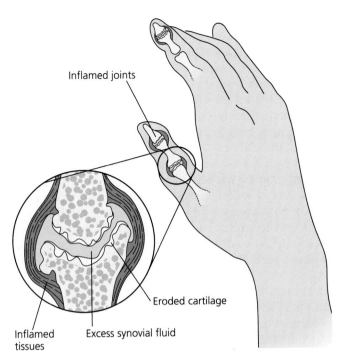

Figure 19-2 Osteoarthritis. When cartilage wears aways within a joint, sharp spurs form and the amount of fluid increases, causing pain and swelling. SOURCE: Clayman, C., ed. 1995. *The Human Body: An Illustrated Guide to Its Structure, Function, and Disorders.* New York: DK.

Labels in figure: Inflamed joints; Eroded cartilage; Excess synovial fluid; Inflamed tissues

toid arthritis and lupus, both autoimmune disorders that affect the joints, are described in Chapter 17.) In a person with OA, the cartilage that caps the bones in joints wears away, forming sharp spurs (Figure 19-2). It most often affects the hands and weight-bearing joints of the body—knees, ankles, and hips. OA is second only to heart disease in disabling people so that they cannot work; 74% of those it affects are women.

Strategies for reducing the risk of arthritis and, for those who already have OA, for managing it include exercise, weight management, and avoidance of heavy or repetitive muscle use. Exercise lubricates joints and strengthens the muscles around them, protecting them from further damage. Swimming, walking, and t'ai chi are good low-impact exercises; knitting and crocheting are excellent ways to exercise the hands. Maintaining an appropriate weight is important to avoid placing stress on the hips, knees, and ankles. Assistive devices such as kitchen utensils and repair tools with large handles can help people with arthritis maintain independence.

It is also important to visit a physician as soon as arthritis symptoms occur so appropriate treatment can be started to reduce pain and swelling, keep joints moving safely, and prevent further joint damage. Many people with OA take nonsteroidal anti-inflammatory drugs (NSAIDs). NSAIDs block the action of the enzyme cyclooxygenase (COX), which is involved in the production of a family of hormones called prostaglandins. Traditional

NSAIDs such as aspirin and ibuprofen block both COX-1 enzymes, which produce "good" prostaglandins that protect the lining of the stomach, and COX-2 enzymes, which make "bad" prostaglandins that cause pain and inflammation. For this reason, traditional NSAIDs can produce stomach irritation and even gastric ulcers and bleeding. A new type of NSAID known as COX-2 inhibitors has been effective in blocking only the inflammatory COX-2 prostaglandins; COX-1 is unaffected, so the drugs may cause less stomach irritation. Acetaminophen (Tylenol) also reduces pain without upsetting the stomach, although exceeding the recommended dosage, especially if combined with alcohol use, can cause liver damage.

Recent studies seem to indicate that two dietary supplements, glucosamine and chondroitin sulfate, do have a mild anti-inflammatory effect that eases some of the symptoms of OA. It is not clear if the two compounds need to be taken together to be effective or even exactly how they work. Glucosamine is extracted from crustacean shells and thus should not be taken by people with shellfish allergies; neither supplement should be taken in combination with blood-thinning medications. A health care provider should be consulted before either compound is taken.

Another treatment designed to ease OA is the injection of a synthetic version of hyaluronic acid, a component of joint lubricating fluid, into affected joints. If joints are severely damaged and activity is limited, surgery to repair or replace joints may be considered.

Menopause A special concern for women is menopause and the changes accompanying it. During their forties or fifties, women's ovaries gradually stop functioning and menstruation ceases. About 85% of women experience symptoms related to menopause, such as hot flashes, vaginal dryness, and emotional changes (see Chapter 5). Health care providers agree that menopause is not an illness but a natural part of a woman's life cycle, a time that provides the opportunity for new energy, self-discovery, and growth.

One important decision that women need to make after menopause is whether to start hormone replacement therapy (HRT). The advantages of HRT include a reduction in hot flashes and vaginal dryness, improvement in short-term memory, reduced stress incontinence, and lowered risk of osteoporosis. HRT's effect on heart disease is less clear; as described in Chapter 15, recent studies have shown that it may reduce cholesterol levels but may not slow the progression of heart disease. There are drawbacks to HRT: an increase in breast density and cancer risk (especially for long-time users) and the possibility of rapid weight gain, depression, increased need for some vitamins and minerals, breast tenderness, and headache. Women should carefully review their personal risk factors with their physician before deciding whether to begin HRT.

As described in earlier chapters, drugs called selective estrogen-receptor modulators (SERMs) mimic estrogen's effects on some body tissues while blocking its effects on others. Researchers hope to develop SERMs that provide all estrogen's beneficial effects without the risks currently associated with HRT. Raloxifene (Evista), for example, protects bone density and has beneficial effects on cholesterol levels. Unlike estrogen, it does not increase the risks of breast and uterine cancer. However, it does increase the occurrence of hot flashes, one of the main reasons that women start HRT. Some dietary supplements are also being investigated for their potential in easing the effects of menopause. Phytoestrogens, plant-based substances similar to estrogen, are found as isoflavones in soy protein and as lignans in whole grains and some fruits and vegetables. They may provide the protective effects of estrogen without some of its drawbacks. Black cohosh and a combination of ginseng and vitamin E are also being studied.

Osteoporosis As described in Chapter 12, **osteoporosis** is a condition in which bones become dangerously thin and fragile over time. Fractures are the most serious consequence of osteoporosis; up to 25% of all people who suffer a hip fracture die within a year. Other problems associated with osteoporosis are loss of height and a stooped posture due to vertebral fractures, severe back and hip pain, and breathing problems caused by changes in the shape of the skeleton.

Women are at greater risk than men for osteoporosis because they have 10–25% less bone in their skeleton. As they lose bone mass with age, women's bones become dangerously thin sooner than men's bones (although more men will probably develop osteoporosis in the future as they live into their eighties and nineties). Bone loss accelerates in women during the first 5–10 years after the onset of menopause because of the drop in estrogen production. (Estrogen improves calcium absorption and reduces the amount of calcium the body excretes.) Black women have higher bone density and fewer fractures than white or Asian women. Other risk factors include a family history of osteoporosis, early menopause (before age 45), abnormal or irregular menstruation, a history of anorexia, and a thin, small frame. Thyroid medication and corticosteroid drugs for arthritis or asthma can also have a negative impact on bone mass.

Terms   **osteoporosis** The loss of bone density, causing bones to become weak, porous, and more prone to fractures.

dementia Deterioration of mental functioning (including memory, concentration, and judgment) resulting from a brain disorder; often accompanied by emotional disturbances and personality changes.

Alzheimer's disease A disease characterized by a progressive loss of mental functioning (dementia), caused by a degeneration of brain cells.

Preventing osteoporosis requires building as much bone as possible during your young years and then maintaining it as you age. Diet and exercise play key roles in this process; see Chapter 12 for recommendations for calcium, vitamin D, and vitamin K intake. Weight-bearing aerobic activities must be performed regularly throughout life to have lasting effects. Strength training improves bone density, muscle mass, strength, and balance, protecting against both bone loss and falls, a major cause of fractures. Even for women in their seventies, low-intensity strength training has been shown to improve bone density.

Two other lifelong strategies for reducing the effects of osteoporosis are avoiding tobacco use and managing depression and stress. Smoking reduces the body's estrogen levels and is linked to earlier menopause and more rapid postmenopausal bone loss. Some women with depression experience significant bone loss. Researchers have not identified the reason, but it may be linked to increases in the stress hormone cortisol.

Bone mineral density testing can be used to gauge an individual's risk of fracture and help determine if any treatment is needed. It is recommended for all women over age 65 and for younger postmenopausal women who have a fracture or one or more risk factors. In addition to HRT, drug treatments that are effective in treating and preventing osteoporosis include alendronate (Fosamax) and calcitonin (Miacalcin), which slow the resorption of bone by the body, and fluoride, which helps build bone. Risedronate (Actonel) is a new drug related to alendronate that significantly reduced the risk of fractures in a study of postmenopausal women with osteoporosis. Research continues into injections of parathyroid hormone, which regulates calcium in the body, and cholesterol-lowering drugs that may have bone benefits.

Handling Psychological and Mental Changes

Many people associate old age with forgetfulness, and slowly losing one's memory was once considered an inevitable part of growing old. However, we now know that most older adults in good health remain mentally alert and retain their full capacity to learn and remember new information. Slight confusion and occasional forgetfulness may indicate only a temporary information overload, or fatigue. Many people become smarter as they become older and more experienced.

Dementia Severe and significant brain deterioration in elderly individuals, termed **dementia**, affects about 7% of people under age 80 (the incidence rises sharply for people in their eighties and nineties). Early symptoms include slight disturbances in a person's ability to grasp the situation he or she is in. As dementia progresses, memory failure becomes apparent, and the person may forget conversations, the events of the day, or how to perform simple tasks. It is important to have any symptoms evaluated by a

Alzheimer's disease (AD) is a fatal brain disorder that causes physical and chemical changes in the brain. As the brain's nerve cells are destroyed, the system that produces the neurotransmitter acetylcholine breaks down, and communication among parts of the brain deteriorates. Autopsies reveal that the interiors of the affected neurons are filled with clusters of proteins known as tangles; the spaces between the neurons are filled with protein deposits called amyloid plaques. More than 4 million Americans have Alzheimer's disease, and that number is expected to quadruple in the next 50 years, as more people live into their eighties and nineties. AD usually occurs in people over 60 but can occur in people as young as 40.

Symptoms

The first symptoms of AD are forgetfulness and inability to concentrate. A person may have difficulty performing familiar tasks at home and work and have problems with abstract thinking. As the disease progresses, people experience severe memory loss, especially for recent events. They may vividly remember events from their childhood but be unable to remember the time of day or their location. Depression and anxiety are also common. In the later stages, people with AD are disoriented and may even hallucinate; some experience personality changes—becoming very aggressive or very docile. Eventually, they lose control of physical functioning and are completely dependent on caregivers. On average, a person will survive 8 years after the development of the first symptoms.

Causes

Scientists do not yet know what causes Alzheimer's disease. Age is the main risk factor, although about 10% of cases seem tied to inherited gene mutations. Inherited familial AD generally strikes people before age 65, while the more common late-onset AD occurs in people 65 and older. Other possible clues are provided by substances that appear to delay the onset or progression of the disease. People who regularly take nonsteroidal anti-inflammatory drugs (NSAIDS) like ibuprofen (often to control arthritis) and people who regularly consume fish rich in omega-3 fatty acids appear to have lower rates of AD, indicating a possible protective effect of substances that reduce inflammation. Some studies indicate that vitamin E and other antioxidants may reduce risk for AD or slow the progress of the disease, suggesting that oxidative stress caused by free radicals may play a role. (As described in Chapter 12, antioxidants block damage by free radicals.) Other possible risk factors include a high-fat diet, high blood levels of homocysteine, a history of head injuries, brain damage from small strokes, and a sedentary lifestyle.

Diagnosis and Treatment

Currently, the only certain way to diagnose AD is to examine brain tissue during an autopsy. In most cases, physicians use physical, psychological, and neurological tests. A recent study that combined a positron emission tomography (PET) scan of the brain with a blood test for a genetic disposition for AD diagnosed the disease in people without symptoms. Often a 7-minute pencil-and-paper test is given to evaluate whether memory and related mental functions are appropriate for a person of a particular age. A behavior diary can also aid in diagnosis.

For people with mild to moderate AD, there are several drugs that provide modest improvements in memory. Several medications help maintain cognitive function by inhibiting the breakdown of the neurotransmitter acetylcholine but do not alter the course of the disease. They include donepezil, rivastigmine, physostigmine, and metrifonate. People with AD may also be prescribed antidepressant or antianxiety medications. Many new treatments are under study, including selegiline, a drug used to treat Parkinson's disease; high doses of the antioxidant vitamin E; and the herbal compound ginkgo biloba, which may improve blood flow to the brain and act as an antioxidant. As scientists gain more insight into Alzheimer's disease, they hope to develop more effective treatments that will ease the burden of AD for both families and society.

---

health care professional because some of the over 50 known causes of dementia are treatable (for example, depression, dehydration, malnutrition, vitamin B-12 deficiency, alcoholism, misuse of medications, and thyroid gland problems). The two most common forms of dementia among older people—**Alzheimer's disease** and multi-infarct dementia—are irreversible. Alzheimer's disease is characterized by changes in brain nerve cells. Multi-infarct dementia results from a series of small strokes or changes in the brain's blood supply that destroy brain tissue. Even for the incurable forms of dementia, however, appropriate treatment may greatly improve an affected person's quality of life (see the box "Alzheimer's Disease").

Repeatedly telling stories about the past—something older people often do—doesn't necessarily indicate dementia. Reminiscence is a normal part of development and allows an older person to integrate life by making past events meaningful in the present. Reminiscing can be of great significance to members of the younger generations because it is a rich source of social, cultural, and family history.

Grief Another psychological and emotional challenge of aging is dealing with grief and mourning. Aging is associated with loss—the loss of friends, peers, physical appearance, possessions, and health. Grief is the process of getting through the pain of loss, and it can be one of the loneliest and most intense times in a person's life. It can take a year or two or more to completely come to terms with the loss of a loved one. (See Chapter 20 for more information about responses to loss and how to support a grieving person.)

Unresolved grief can have serious physical and psychological or emotional health consequences and may

One group of Americans is more than twice as likely to commit suicide than any other. From mass media accounts, you might imagine this group to be adolescents; however, suicide is much more common among the elderly—especially white males over the age of 65. Women and minorities of all ages have much lower rates of suicide than white men.

Why is this so? One explanation is that because white men generally have greater power and status in our society, aging and retirement represent a relatively greater loss for them. Women, more accustomed to "secondary" status, are not as threatened by the loss of economic and social power. Another theory is that white men tend to have weaker social ties than women or than men from other cultural groups, and as they retire, their increasing social isolation leads to depression and suicide. Indeed, depression is probably the single most significant factor associated with suicidal behavior in older adults.

Why are rates for other groups lower? In general, women are more likely than men to attempt suicide, but men are more likely to succeed, due in large part to their choice of more lethal methods. Some cultural groups, particularly Latinos and Native Americans, afford greater respect and status to older people, who are valued for their wisdom and experience. Cultural groups that emphasize family and social ties also seem to have lower rates of suicide.

The high rate of suicide among the elderly often fails to receive much attention. As a society, we are less disturbed about the deaths of older Americans from any cause than the deaths of younger people. What does it say about our society if, after a lifetime of contributions, an older person finds himself or herself in a position where suicide seems to be the best option?

---

require professional help. Signs of unresolved grief include hostility toward people connected with the death (physicians or nurses, for example), talking about the death as if it occurred yesterday, and unrealistic or harmful behavior (such as giving away all of one's own belongings). Many people become depressed after the loss of a loved one or when confronted with retirement or a chronic illness. But after a period of grieving, people are generally able to resume their lives.

Depression   Unresolved grief can lead to depression, a common problem in older adults (see Chapter 3). If you notice the signs of depression in yourself or someone you know, consult a mental health professional. A marked loss of interest in usually pleasurable activities, decreased appetite, insomnia, fatigue, and feelings of worthlessness are signs of depression. Listen carefully when an older friend or relative complains about being depressed; it may be a request for help. Suicide rates are relatively high among the elderly, and depression should be taken seriously (see the box "Suicide Among Older Men").

It is a mistake to think that a depressed person will "snap out of it" or that people are too old to be helped. Both professional treatment and support groups can help people deal successfully with major life changes, such as retirement, moving, health problems, or loss of a spouse. If someone refuses help, be reassuring and emphasize that treatment helps make people feel better; in some cases, a mental health professional can make a home visit.

One of the most important ways of dealing with the changes associated with aging is to adopt a flexible attitude toward whatever life brings you. Self-acceptance can help make the later years more meaningful and enjoyable. Accepting limitations, having an optimistic outlook, and having a sense of humor are tools that can help you cope with all of life's changes.

COMMUNICATE!   Communicating with a person who suffers from dementia requires patience and compassion. Here are some tips that may help: Approach the person from the front, and wait to make eye contact before talking. Turn off the television or radio to reduce distraction. Communicate in a calm, clear, and supportive way. Speak slowly to give the person more time to process information, and simplify your message. If you can't understand what the person is saying, listen for the feeling, tone, or basic meaning behind the person's communication. If the person talks about an event that happened long ago as if it were happening now, accept that perception of reality. Ask the person to tell you more. Don't make corrections; the person can't help making mistakes in memory or cognition, and you will not be able to "talk sense" into him or her. Reassure and support the person if he or she feels confused, lost, abandoned, or disoriented.

AGING AND LIFE EXPECTANCY

Life expectancy is the average length of time we can expect to live. It is calculated by averaging mortality statistics, the ages of death of a group of people over a certain period of time. A female born in the United States in 2000 has a longer life expectancy (79.4 years) than her male counterpart (73.6 years). Individuals who reach their sixty-fifth birthday can expect to live even longer—17 more years or longer—because they have already survived hazards to life in the younger years (Table 19-1).

Factors Influencing Life Expectancy

The reason for the gender gap in life expectancy is not known, but estrogen production and other factors during a woman's fertile years appear to protect her from heart

Table 19-1	Life Expectancy	

Year	Men	Women
At birth:		
1900	47.9	50.7
1950	65.5	71.0
2000	73.6	79.4
2050 (projected)	79.7	84.3
At age 65:		
1900	11.5	12.2
1950	12.7	15.0
2000	15.9	19.2
2050 (projected)	20.3	22.4

SOURCES: Federal Interagency Forum on Aging-Related Statistics. 2000. *Older Americans 2000: Key Indicators of Well-Being.* Hyattsville, Md.: National Center for Health Statistics. Administration on Aging. 1997. *Life Expectancy: 1995 and 2050* (http://www.aoa.dhhs.gov/aoa/stats/aging21/table17.html; retrieved March 7, 2001).

disease. Her risks increase after menopause. Increased male mortality can also be traced to smoking (lung cancer, heart and respiratory disease), more injuries, and more alcoholism. Where these factors are not operative, men live as long as women, as with the Amish, a religious sect that has strict rules against smoking and drinking. Life expectancy also varies among ethnic groups; reasons for these differences include socioeconomic, genetic, and lifestyle factors.

Life expectancy in the United States has increased dramatically in this century, as described in Chapter 1. This does not mean that every American now lives longer than in 1900; rather, far fewer people die young now, because childhood and infectious diseases are better controlled and diet and sanitation are much improved. Only 30% of people born in 1900 would live to age 70; of those born in 2000, closer to 70% can expect to live that long.

How long can humans expect to live in the best of circumstances? It now seems possible that our maximum potential **life span** is 100–120 years. (A man in Japan reached the age of 120 years, 237 days, in 1986.) Failure to achieve that span in good health results to some degree from destructive environmental and behavioral factors—factors over which we can exert considerable control. Long life does not necessarily mean a longer period of disability, either. People often live longer because they have been well longer. A healthy, productive old age is very often an extension of a healthy, productive middle age. However, behavior changes cannot extend the maximum human life span, which seems to be built into our genes.

Theories on Aging

Throughout history, people have searched in vain for ways to preserve youth. Now scientists are studying the aging process and looking for ways to help people to live longer and maintain much of their youthful vigor. What causes the eventual breakdown of the body? No existing theory on aging accommodates all the facts. Perhaps aging is caused by a variety of different processes and affected by a multitude of factors, both environmental and biological.

A cellular theory of aging based on the genetic makeup of cells suggests that a cell contains "aging" genes that specify the exact number of times the cell can duplicate itself. The limiting number varies from species to species. This is why the maximum life span for fruit flies is about 100 days, for dogs 25–30 years, for humans about 110 years, and for giant tortoises about 180 years.

Another cellular theory is that the body generates free radicals, which undermine the integrity of cell membranes, damage DNA, and inactivate many enzymes and proteins required for normal cellular functioning. Environmental pollution also promotes free radical activity, but a diet rich in antioxidants can reduce it (see Chapter 12). As scientists map the human genome, a number of genes are being identified as playing a role in the aging process.

A theory of aging involving the immune system suggests that the body begins to make errors in protein synthesis, producing proteins that the immune system cannot recognize. The immune system then attacks them as it would any foreign substance, destroying cells and impairing body functions (see Chapter 17). Also, the immune system itself may weaken as we age, producing fewer antibodies to fight disease. Researchers are testing drugs that would reinforce faltering immune systems.

A theory of aging that focuses on metabolic function helps explain the immobility seen in old age. Connective tissue all over the body is given structural support by fibers of a class of proteins called collagen. Collagen becomes stiffer and chemically immobilized with age. This is because by-products of metabolism, called cross-links, form between parallel collagen fibers, making it impossible for the two fibers to slip past each other or stretch. Lowering the metabolic rate by not overeating has been shown to reduce age-related diseases like diabetes.

life expectancy The average length of time a person is expected to live.

life span A theoretically projected length of life based on the maximum potential of the human body in the best environment.

Terms

As life expectancy increases, a larger proportion of the population will be in their later years. This change will necessitate new government policies and changes in our general attitudes toward older adults.

America's Aging Minority

People over 65 are a large minority in the American population—over 35 million people, about 13% of the total population in 2000 (Figure 19-3). As birth rates drop, the percentage increases dramatically. Many older people are happy, healthy, and self-sufficient. Changes that come with age, including negative ones, normally occur so gradually that most people adapt, some even gracefully.

Today the status of older adults is improving more than ever before. The enormous increase in the over-55 population is markedly affecting our stereotypes of what it means to grow old. The misfortunes associated with aging—frailty, forgetfulness, poor health, isolation—occur in fewer people in their sixties and seventies and are shifting instead to burden the very old, those over 85.

The "younger" elderly who are in good physical and psychological health are gaining status in our society; politicians are listening to them, and advertisers have targeted them as a valuable market. In general, today's older adults are better off than they have ever been in the past. They have more money than they did 20 years ago. The poverty rate of the elderly has dropped from 28.5% to 11% since the 1960s, largely from the effects of Social Security payments and health care benefits from Medicare.

About 78% of older Americans own their homes. Their living expenses are lower after retirement because they no longer support children and have fewer work-related expenses; they consume and buy less food. They are more likely to continue practicing their expertise for years after retirement: Thousands of retired consultants, teachers, technicians, and craftspeople work until their middle and late seventies. They receive greater amounts of assistance, such as Medicare, pay proportionately lower taxes, and have greater net worth from lifetime savings.

As the aging population increases proportionately, however, the number of older people who are ill and dependent rises. Health care remains the largest expense for older adults. On average, they visit a physician 10–12 times a year and are hospitalized more frequently and require twice as many prescription drugs as the general population. Tens of thousands of older Americans live in poverty, particularly minorities and women living alone. These other elderly—poverty-stricken, isolated, lonely—are just as ignored as they ever were, and their numbers are increasing.

Retirement finds many older people with their incomes reduced to subsistence levels. This is especially true of the very old. The majority of older Americans live with fixed sources of income, such as pensions, that are

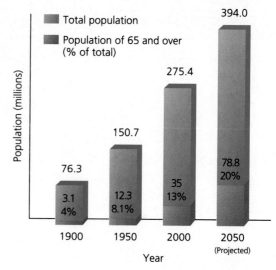

(a) Population growth over age 65 as a proportion of the total population.

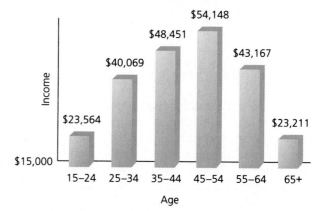

(b) Average household income by age of the household head.

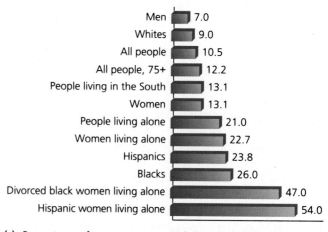

(c) Percentages of groups over age 65 below the poverty level.

WW. VITAL STATISTICS

Figure 19-3 A statistical look at older Americans. SOURCE: U.S. Bureau of the Census. U.S. Administration on Aging.

At some point in their lives, many people will be called on to care for an older family member. People who have mental impairments due to dementia, Alzheimer's disease, stroke, head injury, or other brain disorders can become confused or disoriented and have memory and behavioral problems. These tips can help make caregiving more effective and satisfying and can help keep the older adult safe from harm.

Keep Your Loved One Safe

- Supervise or limit the use of potentially hazardous equipment or appliances such as stoves, knives, scissors, and blenders.

- Supervise and record the taking of medication.

- Supervise eating and alcohol use.

- Help with bathing; monitor the water temperature.

- Restrict consumption of caffeine if the person has difficulty sleeping or is overly agitated.

- Have the person wear a bracelet with name, address, and telephone number.

Create a Safe Environment

- Make sure entries, landings, stairways, and bathrooms are well lit.

- Use childproof locks and doorknobs.

- Install grab bars and nonskid decals in bathtub and shower areas.

- Remove locks from doors that cannot be unlocked from the outside.

Help with Daily Tasks

- Establish a routine and stay with it as much as possible.

- Go one step at a time and move slowly.

- Use a structured approach for completing routine tasks; for example, lay clothes out in sequence to help with dressing.

- Perform for the person only those tasks that he or she is no longer able to do without assistance.

Remember to keep yourself healthy by arranging regular breaks from caregiving. You might also want to consider joining a support group for caregivers.

SOURCE: Caring for loved ones who are mentally impaired. 2000. *Journal of the American Medical Association* 284(1).

---

eroded by inflation. Expenses tend to increase more rapidly, especially those due to circumstances over which people have little or no control, such as deteriorating health. Many Americans rely on Social Security payments as their only source of income; they are not covered by other types of retirement plans. **Social Security** was intended to serve as a supplement to personal savings and private pensions, not as a sole source of income. It is vital that people plan early for an adequate retirement income.

Family and Community Resources for Older Adults

With help from friends, family members, and community services, people in their later years can remain active and independent. About 66% of noninstitutionalized older Americans live with a spouse or other family member; the other 34% live alone or with a nonrelative. Only 4% live in nursing homes or other institutional settings at any point in time.

Family Involvement in Caregiving   Most families do not abandon their aging relatives when they need help. Studies show that in about three out of four cases, a grown daughter or daughter-in-law assumes a caregiving role for elderly relatives. This may mean bringing them into the home, helping them remain in their own homes, or arranging for alternative housing. With more parents living into their eighties and with fewer children per fam-

ily, many people, especially women, will face the choice of how to care for an aging relative. Recent surveys indicate that the average woman will spend about 17 years raising children and 18 years caring for an aging relative.

Caregiving can be rewarding, but it is also hard work. If the experience is stressful and long-term, family members may become emotionally exhausted. Caregivers should use available community services and consider their own needs for relaxation and relief from caregiving duties. Corporations are increasingly responsive to the needs of their employees who are family caregivers by providing such services as referrals, flexible schedules and leaves, and on-site adult care. Professional health care advice is another critical part of successful home care. An aging relative who is mentally impaired by Alzheimer's disease or another form of dementia poses special challenges for caregivers (see the box "Caring for a Person with Dementia or Alzheimer's Disease").

The best thing a family can do to prepare for the task of caring for aging parents is to talk frankly about the future. What does everyone expect will happen? What living and

Social Security A government program that provides financial assistance to people who are unemployed, disabled, or retired (and over a certain age); financed through taxes on business and workers.

Terms

Later in life many older people need help with everyday activities like shopping, cooking, walking, or bathing. Help from family and friends may be all some people need to stay active and healthy in their own homes, while others may choose to move to a place that offers more services. A variety of options are available:

- *Retirement communities* allow maximum independence with very little supervision. They may offer transportation, activities, and other services but do not routinely offer assistance with basic needs.

- *Residential care homes* are licensed to provide services to three or more residents in a smaller environment, typically in a private home. They may provide assistance with medications, bathing, dressing, transportation, daily laundry, daily housekeeping, and meals.

- *Assisted living facilities* allow independence with supervision and are licensed by the state. They provide some meals, housekeeping and laundry, transportation, and activities.

- *Nursing homes* provide 24-hour medical care and rehabilitation for residents, who are mostly very frail or suffer from the later stages of dementia.

Some providers offer all levels of care at one site. These continuing-care communities allow people to move from one level to another as their needs change.

Finding the right place to live takes some investigation. Because the best homes often have a waiting list, plan ahead, and don't wait until your family member is too sick to function. Once you have an initial list of facilities in your area start visiting the homes, keeping the following evaluation points in mind:

- Ask questions about specific facilities. Doctors, friends, relatives, local hospital discharge planners, social workers, and religious organizations can help. The ombudsperson at your state's office of long-term care can let you know if there have been problems in a particular nursing home. Residential care homes and assisted living facilities do not follow the same licensing requirements as nursing homes. Talk to people in the community to find out about these options.

- Contact the places that interest you. Ask basic questions about vacancies, number of residents, cost, and any services of interest to you, such as transportation and meals.

- Visit several places. Talk to the staff, residents, and, if possible, family members of residents. Set up an appointment, but also go unannounced and at different times of the day. Make sure residents are clean, well groomed, involved in activities, and treated with respect.

- Evaluate the facility's financial agreements. Have a lawyer look them over before you sign. Nursing homes may accept Medicare or Medicaid, but most other facilities are private-pay only. Costs can range from $1500 per month to $5500 per month or more.

- Moving is a big change that affects the whole family. Talk about how you feel. Once a family member has moved to a new home, visit often and pay attention to the quality of care. Say something nice when care is good, and speak up when care is poor. If you have trouble resolving a complaint, your local ombudsperson or citizen advocacy groups may be able to help.

caring options are available, and which ones do family members prefer? What community resources are available? Planning ahead can reduce the stress on everyone involved and help ease difficult transitions.

Other Living and Care Options

If living together is not possible for aging parents and adult children, other living and care options are available. There are agencies that specialize in recruiting and matching like-minded individuals for shared living situations. Homesharing, as this is called, offers older adults who are in fairly good health the opportunity for new relationships, either with peers or with a younger family. Intergenerational homesharing may relieve elders of transportation problems and demanding physical tasks, which can be taken care of by younger household members. Conversely, elders in good health can help busy, working families with child care and household chores.

Retirement communities are an option for individuals in good health, with a good income, who want to maintain home ownership. Other types of facilities are available for people who need more assistance with daily living (see the box "Choosing a Place to Live").

Community Resources

Different kinds of community resources are available to help older adults remain active and in their own homes. The key to success is matching services with the needs of the individual person. Typical services include the following:

- *Senior citizens' centers or adult day-care centers,* which may provide meals, social activities, and health care services for those unable to be alone during the day

- *Homemaker services,* which may include light housekeeping, cooking, running errands, doing shopping, and providing escort service

- *Visiting nurses,* who provide some basic health care services

- *Household services,* which may include basic household repairs and seasonal work

- *Friendly visitor or daily telephone reassurance services,* which provide daily contacts for older people who live alone and may feel isolated

- *Home food delivery services,* which provide daily meals to homebound people

- *Adult day hospital care,* which provides day care plus physical therapy and treatment for chronic illnesses

- *Low-cost legal aid,* which can help in managing finances and health care
- *Transportation,* which includes buses with special senior rates for visits to doctors' offices, hospitals, or grocery stores
- *Case management,* which helps seniors navigate through complex and confusing health care services

Services can usually be located by looking in the phone book under local government agencies or in the yellow pages under Senior Citizens' Services.

Transportation Older drivers usually have safe driving records compared with young adults because they tend to be more cautious; however, crashes in the older age group are more likely to be fatal. Many states require special driver's testing for people over age 70 and may restrict some drivers as to the time, area, and distances they may drive. Because of changes in vision or other health problems, some older drivers may be required to give up their license before they feel ready. Elderly people report that the loss of a driver's license, and the loss of independence that it brings, is one of the most severe hardships they face.

Whatever their circumstances, older adults have the same needs as people at any other stage of life, including the need to feel that their lives have meaning. Becoming dependent on others for daily care and transportation is difficult for many people to accept. Most caregivers are motivated by love and responsibility and want to do the best they can for their aging friend or relative. However, some situations can lead to abuse, physical or economic. Assistance is available, including respite care for caregivers and legal and protective services for abused elders.

COMMUNICATE! As your parents age, you may find, as many people do, that you want to resolve long-standing tensions and let go of old hurts and grudges. If your parents are open to it, you may be able to discuss incidents or situations from the past with them. Try to set up a structured dialogue in which you give your perspective without interruption for a certain period of time (say, five minutes), your parents recap what you've said, and you confirm or correct the recap. Then, in the same way, you listen to your parents' version of the event, you provide a recap, and they confirm or correct your understanding. Continue the dialogue until you feel your parents have heard your point of view and you have heard theirs. With each step, you should come closer to mutual understanding and to the resolution of hurt feelings.

Government Aid and Policies

The federal government helps older Americans through several programs, such as food stamps, housing subsidies,

Social Security, Medicare, and Medicaid. Social Security, the life insurance and old-age pension plan, has saved many from destitution, although it is intended not as a sole source of income but as a supplement to other income. Social Security funds have been used to cover other government financial deficits, so the future solvency of the program is uncertain.

Medicare is a major health insurance program for the elderly and the disabled. It has two parts: Part A is financed by part of the payroll (FICA) tax that also pays for Social Security; Part B is financed by monthly premiums paid by people who choose to enroll. Part A helps pay for inpatient hospital care, some inpatient care in a skilled nursing facility, and some types of home and hospice care. Medicare Part B helps pay for physicians' services and other services not covered by Part A.

Medicare pays about 30% of the medical costs of older Americans. It provides basic health care coverage for acute episodes of illness that require skilled professional care; it does not pay for custodial or preventive care, including most expenses for routine checkups, dental care and dentures, immunizations, and prescription drugs. Over 1 million older people currently live in nursing homes, but Medicare pays less than 2% of nursing home costs, and private insurers pay less than 1%, creating a tremendous financial burden for nursing home residents and their families. Because of these gaps in coverage, many older people are joining managed health care plans to get more care for their money. See Chapter 22 for more information on insurance options.

When their financial resources are exhausted, people may apply for Medicaid. A 1965 amendment to the Social Security Act, Medicaid provides medical insurance to low-income people of any age. Funded by state and federal contributions, the services vary from state to state but typically include hospital, nursing home and home health care, physician services, and some medical supplies and services. The portion of federal Medicaid spending attributed to the elderly has declined since 1980 from about 37% to about 30%.

A crucial question regarding aid for the elderly is, Who will pay for it? The government picks up many of the health care expenses, primarily through Medicare and Medicaid. Total health care expenditures are about 14.3% of the U.S. gross national product; about one-third of these expenditures go to care for older Americans.

Health care policy planners hope that rising medical costs for older adults will dwindle dramatically through education and prevention. Health care professionals, including **gerontologists** and **geriatricians,** are beginning

gerontologist One who studies the biological, psychological, and social phenomena associated with aging and old age.

geriatrician A physician specializing in the diseases, disabilities, and care of older adults.

Terms

The following is excerpted from an article written by Dr. Robert Coles, a professor of psychiatry and medical humanities at Harvard Medical School.

Why are so many Americans afraid of growing old? This question occurred to me often during the three years my wife and I lived in New Mexico and Arizona. Not a day went by when we weren't reminded of how much Native American and Hispanic families value old age. These are cultures that grant dignity and authority to their elders.

One young Hispanic woman described to us her relationship with her parents, both in their seventies, in this way: "When I am wondering what to do about a problem, I turn to my mother or my father. Even if they are not here, I still turn to them. I picture them in my mind and I hear them saying words that make good sense." One day, this woman's father made a show of his humorous and practical good sense before his young grandson. "You know what my son said to me that night when he was going to bed?" the woman asked. "He told me he wished he could be old like his grandpapa!"

To be old is to "last" oneself—to go through ups and downs, to survive bad luck and avoid all sorts of hazards. To be old is to be blessed by fate, by chance and circumstance. Pueblo Indians know that. One Hopi child drew me a picture of an old woman shaking hands with the moon. Then she explained, "When you're old, you're a full moon; you make the night a little less dark." For Hopi children, an older person is a source of encouragement, instruction, inspiration, a part of nature's awesome presence.

For many young people living in other parts of America, old age is regarded not as a major achievement but rather as a last, sad, brief way station. One boy in Boston commented, "It's no fun to be old; it's the worst thing in the world, except to die." To many of us, old age means abandonment, rejection, loneliness, a loss of respect from others, and subsequently a loss of self-respect. This is not the case, though, in Hispanic and Native American cultures. The elders we met in New Mexico and Arizona showed a great deal of self-confidence, and in general they seemed contented with their lives. In their contentment and harmony with nature lies a lesson for all of us.

SOURCE: Adapted from Coles, R. 1989. Full-moon wisdom. *New Choices for the Best Years*, September. Reprinted with permission of Robert Coles, James Agee Professor of Social Ethics, Harvard University.

to practice preventive medicine, just as pediatricians do. They advise older people about how to avoid and, if necessary, how to manage disabilities. They try to instill an ethic of physical and psychological maintenance that will prevent chronic disease and enable older people to live long, healthy, vigorous lives.

Changing the Public's Idea of Aging

Aging people may be one of our least used and least appreciated resources. (For another view, see the box "Multicultural Wisdom About Aging.") How can we use the knowledge and productivity of our growing numbers of older citizens, particularly those now leaving the work force through mandatory early retirement?

First, we must change our thinking about what aging means. We must learn to judge productivity rather than age. Capacity to function should replace age as a criterion for usefulness. Instead of singling out 65 as a magic number, we could consider ages 50–75 as the third quarter of life. Changes occur around 50 that signal a new era: Children are usually grown and gone; a person has often achieved a level in career, earnings, and accomplishments that meets his or her ambitions. The upper end of the quarter is determined by the fact that most people today are vigorous, in good health, mentally alert, and capable of making a productive contribution until they are at least in their seventies.

However we define old age, the costs of losing what these people can contribute to our national productivity and quality of life are too high. Through their early retirement we forfeit substantial income tax and Social Security tax revenues on their earnings. Those who retire at 62 start using their Social Security benefits earlier than otherwise.

A far better arrangement would be to make available full-time and part-time volunteer and paid employment. We would benefit by providing retraining programs for both occupational and leisure time activities. Volunteer opportunities, such as preparing recordings for the blind, helping with activities for the disabled, and performing necessary tasks in hospitals, could be expanded. At the same time, we could possibly change both public and private pension programs to make partial retirement possible. In such cases we could allow people to borrow against their Social Security benefits to finance retraining or enrollment in new educational programs.

There can be benefits to aging, but they don't come automatically. They require planning and wise choices earlier in life. One octogenarian, Russell Lee, founder of a medical clinic in California, perceived the advantages of aging as growth: "The limitations imposed by time are compensated by the improved taste, sharper discretion, sounder mental and esthetic judgment, increased sensitivity and compassion, clearer focus—which all contribute to a more certain direction in living. . . . The later years can be the best of life for which the earlier ones were preparation."

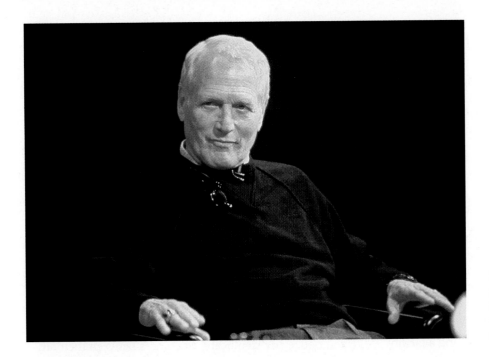

Some extraordinary individuals defy all preconceived ideas about old age. Actor and philanthropist Paul Newman, now in his seventies, continues to live an intensely vigorous and creative life.

SUMMARY

- People who take charge of their health during their youth have greater control over the physical and mental aspects of aging.

- Biological aging takes place over a lifetime, but some of the other changes associated with aging are more abrupt.

- A lifetime of interests and hobbies helps maintain creativity and intelligence.

- Exercise throughout life enhances physical and psychological health.

- A low-fat, high-carbohydrate diet that includes a variety of foods promotes health at every age. Obesity leads to premature aging.

- Alcohol abuse is a common but often hidden problem, as is overdependence on medications. Tobacco use not only shortens life but also may cause severe health impairment for many years.

- Regular physical examinations help detect conditions that can shorten life and make old age less healthy.

- Stress increases wear and tear on the body; getting enough sleep, avoiding drugs, and practicing relaxation help reduce stress.

- Retirement can be a fulfilling and enjoyable time of life for those who adjust to their new roles, enjoy participating in a variety of activities, and have planned ahead for financial stability.

- Successful aging involves anticipating and accommodating physical changes and limitations.

- Slight confusion and forgetfulness are not signs of a serious illness; however, severe symptoms may indicate Alzheimer's disease or another from of dementia.

- Resolving grief and mourning and dealing with depression are important tasks for older adults.

- Life expectancy, which has risen dramatically since the 1900s, is generally longer for women.

- Theories on aging examine the influences of cellular changes, free radicals, inappropriate immune responses, and changes in metabolism.

- Older adults can be role models for the successful integration of life's experiences and the ability to adapt to challenges.
- People over 65 form a large minority in the United States, and their status is improving.
- Those who are ill and dependent—often those who were already poor—experience major social and economic problems.

- About 66% of all noninstitutionalized older people are cared for by their spouse or by family members, usually daughters and daughters-in-law.
- Community resources can help older adults stay active and independent.
- Government aid to the elderly includes food stamps, housing subsidies, Social Security, Medicare, and Medicaid.

TAKE ACTION

1. Interview your parents or grandparents to find out how they want to spend their later years. Do they want to live at home, in a retirement community, with a relative? Do they plan to live on a pension, retirement account, Social Security? Have they made any concrete plans, or have they not yet confronted those decisions?

2. Develop a project that benefits you and a facility for the elderly in your community. For example, teach an older adult how to send an e-mail. Have an older adult teach you how to repair an old faucet or make bread.

3. Interview several people from different cultural backgrounds about their attitudes toward aging and older people. How do they view the aging process? How are elderly people treated or viewed in their culture? Do you notice any significant differences between their attitudes and yours?

WW. JOURNAL ENTRY

1. Imagine that you are very old and are looking back on your life. What will have given you satisfaction—a successful career, parenthood, happiness, travel, self-knowledge? Make a list in your health journal of your life goals and priorities. What actions can you take now to work toward your goals? Choose one goal, and take an action this week that moves you toward it.

2. *Critical Thinking* Assuming that government funding for medical care is limited, should more money be allocated for children's services or for medical care for older adults? Write a brief essay making a case for each side of the debate. Provide evidence to support each position.

FOR MORE INFORMATION

Books
Cassel, C. K., and G. A. Vallasi. 2001. *The Practical Guide to Aging: What Everyone Needs to Know.* New York: New York University Press. A practical, comprehensive reference to many aspects of aging.

Cohen, D., and C. Eisdorfer. 2001. *The Loss of Self: A Family Resource for the Care of Alzheimer's Disease and Related Disorders.* Rev. ed. New York: W. W. Norton. A resource for caregivers of people with dementia that addresses biological, emotional, medical, and social issues.

Cohen, H. J. 2000. *Taking Care After 50: A Self-Care Guide for Seniors.* New York: Three Rivers Press. *Addresses a variety of issues for older adults, including nutrition, mental health, safety, and sexuality.*

Gillick, M. R., M.D. 2000. *Lifelines: Living Longer, Growing Frail, Taking Heart.* New York: Norton. *Examines some common health problems associated with aging. Follows people who have faced these difficulties and looks at various solutions.*

Perls, T. T., M. H. Silver, and J. F. Lauerman. 2000. *Living to 100: Lessons in Living to Your Maximum Potential at Any Age.* New York: Basic Books. *Looks at the lifestyles of people who have lived to 100 and offers advice on how to stay healthy throughout the later years.*

WW. Organizations and Web Sites
AARP. Provides information on all aspects of aging, including health promotion, health care, and retirement planning.
800-424-2277
http://www.aarp.org

Access America for Seniors. A gateway to government resources on the Internet for older Americans.
http://www.seniors.gov

Aging Well. A practical resource for seniors that includes information on diet, exercise, safety, and medical care.
http://agingwell.state.ny.us

Alzheimer's Association. Offers tips for caregivers and patients, as well as information on research into the causes and treatment of Alzheimer's disease.

800-272-3900

http://www.alz.org

American Association of Homes and Services for the Aging (AAHSA). Provides information about living and care arrangements available for older adults.

202-783-2242

http://www.aahsa.org

Arthritis Foundation. Provides information about arthritis, including free brochures, referrals to local services, and research updates.

800-283-7800

http://www.arthritis.org

ElderWeb. A gateway to aging resources on the Internet, with information about health, housing, and financial issues.

http://www.elderweb.com

Exercise: A Guide from the National Institute on Aging. Provides practical advice on fitness for seniors; includes animated instructions for specific exercises.

http://www.nih.gov/nia/health/pubs/nasa-exercise

Health Care Financing Administration (HCFA). Provides information about Medicare.

http://www.hcfa.gov http://Medicare.gov

National Council on Aging. Promotes the well-being of older persons through research and advocacy; Web site provides helpful information on retirement planning, health promotion, and lifelong learning.

http://www.ncoa.org

National Institute on Aging. Provides fact sheets and brochures on aging-related topics.

http://www.nih.gov/nia

National Institutes of Health Osteoporosis and Related Bone Diseases—National Resource Center. Provides information about osteoporosis prevention and treatment; includes a special section on men and osteoporosis.

http://www.osteo.org/

National Osteoporosis Foundation. Provides information on the causes, prevention, detection, and treatment of osteoporosis.

http://www.nof.org

U.S. Administration on Aging. Provides fact sheets, statistical information, and Internet links to other resources on aging.

202-619-7501

http://www.aoa.gov

SELECTED BIBLIOGRAPHY

Angerer, P., et al. 2001. Effect of oral postmenopausal hormone replacement on progression of atherosclerosis: A randomized, controlled trial. *Arteriosclerosis, Thrombosis, and Vascular Biology* 21(2): 262–268.

Centers for Disease Control and Prevention. 2000. Health-related quality of life among adults with arthritis. *Morbidity and Mortality Weekly Report* 49(17): 366–369.

Charles, S. T., C. A. Reynolds, and M. Gatz. 2001. Age-related differences and change in positive and negative affect over 23 years. *Journal of Personality and Social Psychology* 80(1): 136–151.

Farrer, L. A. 2001. Intercontinental epidemiology of Alzheimer disease. *Journal of the American Medical Association* 285(6): 796–798.

Felson, D. T., et al. 2000. Osteoarthritis: New insights Part 1: The disease and its risk factors. *Annals of Internal Medicine* 133(8): 635–646.

Friedland, R. P., et al. Patients with Alzheimer's disease have reduced activities in midlife compared with healthy control-group members. *Proceedings of the National Academy of Sciences* 98(6): 3440–3445.

Hartman, C. A., et al. 2000. Effects of t'ai chi training on function and quality of life indicators in older adults with osteoarthritis. *Journal of the American Geriatrics Society* 48(12): 1553–1559.

Kritz-Silverstein, D., E. Barrett-Connor, and C. Corbeau. 2001. Cross-sectional and prospective study of exercise and depressed mood in the elderly. *American Journal of Epidemiology* 153(6): 596–603.

Laurin, D., et al. 2001. Physical activity and risk of cognitive impairment and dementia in elderly persons. *Archives of Neurology* 58(3): 498–504.

Leranth, C., et al. 2001. Estrogen is essential for maintaining nigrostriatal dopamine neurons in primates: Implications for Parkinson's disease and memory. *Journal of Neuroscience* 20(23): 8604–8609.

Lewis, C. 2000. Arthritis: Timely treatments for an ageless disease. *FDA Consumer Magazine*, May–June.

McClung, M. R., et al. 2001. Effect of risedronate on the risk of hip fracture in elderly women. *New England Journal of Medicine* 344(5): 333–340.

Michael, Y. L., et al. 2001. Living arrangements, social integration, and change in functional health status. *American Journal of Epidemiology* 153(2): 123–131.

Mulnard, R. A., et al. 2000. Estrogen replacement therapy for treatment of mild to moderate Alzheimer disease: A randomized controlled trial.

Alzheimer's Disease Cooperative Study. *Journal of the American Medical Association* 283(8): 1007–1015.

National Eye Institute. 2000. *Age-Related Macular Degeneration* (http://www.nei.nih.gov/publications /armd-p.htm; retrieved November 15, 2000).

National Eye Institute. 2000. *Glaucoma* (http://www.nei.nih.gov/publications/glau-pat.htm; retrieved November 15, 2000).

Nicodemus, K. K., A. R. Folsom, and K. E. Anderson. 2001. Menstrual history and risk of hip fractures in postmenopausal women in the Iowa Women's Health Study. *American Journal of Epidemiology* 153(3): 251–255.

NIH Consensus Development Panel on Osteoporosis Prevention, Diagnosis, and Therapy. 2001. Osteoporosis prevention, diagnosis, and therapy. *Journal of the American Medical Association* 285(6): 785–795.

Ostir, G. V., et al. 2000. Emotional well-being predicts subsequent functional independence and survival. *Journal of the American Geriatrics Society* 48(5): 473–478.

Plassman, B. L., et al. 2000. Documented head injury in early adulthood and risk of Alzheimer's disease and other dementias. *Neurology* 55(8): 1158–1166.

Psychiatric illness in older adults. 2000. *Journal of the American Medical Association* 283(21): 2886.

Reginster, J. Y., et al. 2001. Long-term effects of glucosamine sulphate on osteoarthritis progression: A randomised, placebo-controlled clinical trial. *Lancet* 357(9252): 251–256.

Russell, R. M., H. Rassmussen, and A. Lichenstein. 1999. Modified food guide pyramid for people over seventy years of age. *Journal of Nutrition* 129: 751–753.

Rutter, C. M., et al. 2001. Changes in breast density associated with initiation, discontinuation, and continuing use of hormone replacement therapy. *Journal of the American Medical Association* 285(2): 171–176.

Small, G. W., et al. 2000. Cerebral metabolic and cognitive decline in persons at genetic risk for Alzheimer's disease. *Proceedings of the National Academy of Sciences of the United States* 97(11): 6037–6042.

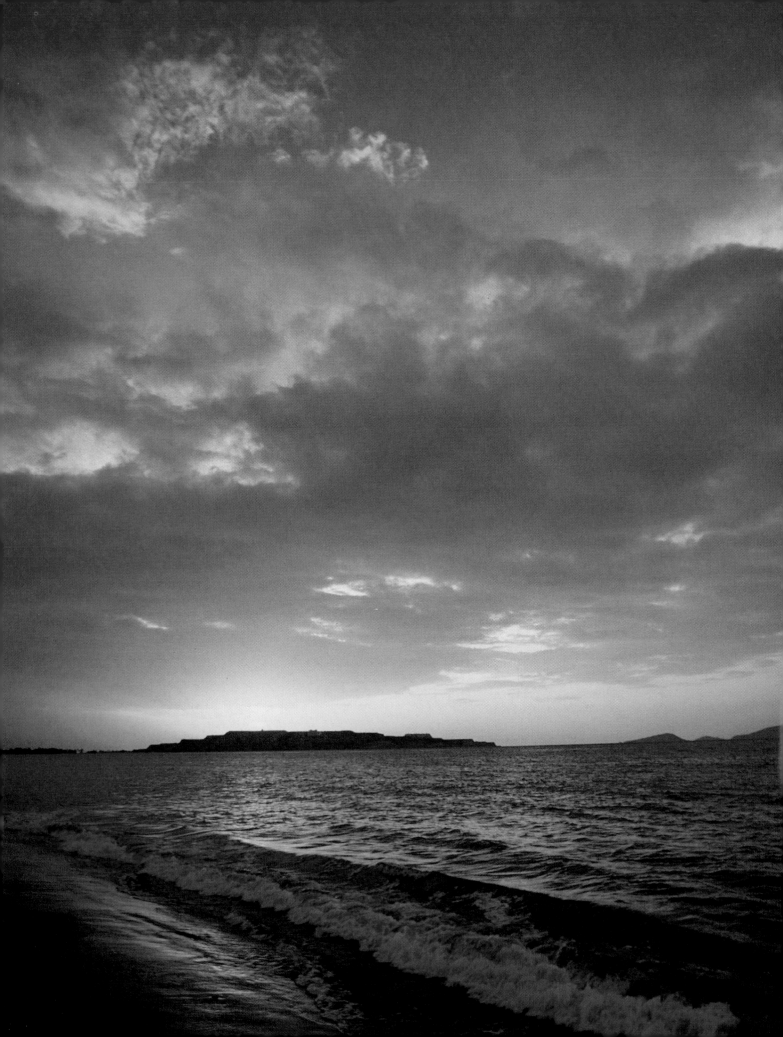

After reading this chapter, you should be able to

- Identify the physical, mental, social, behavioral, and spiritual dimensions of dying and death

- Describe various ways of defining death and the components of a mature concept of death

- Understand personal considerations in preparing for death, including making a will, assessing choices for end-of-life care, and making arrangements for a funeral or memorial service

- Describe the experience of living with a life-threatening illness and list ways to support a person who is dying

- Explain the grieving process and how support can be offered to adults and children who have experienced a loss

Dying and Death

20

TEST YOUR KNOWLEDGE

1. If you die in a car crash, your organs will automatically be donated to people waiting for transplants.
   True or false?

2. How many Americans die without leaving a will?
   a. 1 in 10
   b. 4 in 10
   c. 7 in 10

3. Historically, death has been ascertained by
   a. breathing and heartbeat
   b. consciousness
   c. brain waves

4. Physician-assisted suicide is considered murder and is illegal in all 50 states.
   True or false?

5. The best way to help a friend who is grieving is to distract her or him from the loss by talking about sports, gossip, or other lighthearted topics.
   True or false?

ANSWERS

1. **FALSE.** For your organs to be donated, you must have authorized it prior to your death (such as by completing an organ donor card), or the donation must be authorized by relatives at the time of your death.

2. **C.** In such cases, the estate is distributed according to state law, which may not reflect what the individual would have wanted.

3. **A.** The conventional signs of death, cessation of breathing and heartbeat, have been supplemented more recently by medical criteria for establishing brain death when a person's breathing and heartbeat are sustained by life-support systems.

4. **FALSE.** Physician-assisted suicide is legal in Oregon, where the Death with Dignity Act was approved in 1997. By 2001, 70 terminally ill people participating in PAS had died from lethal doses of prescription medication.

5. **FALSE.** Most people who are grieving need to talk about their loss, and a friend who will let them talk freely is very valuable. The best strategy is simply to be a good listener.

A man hiking a high mountain trail suddenly lost his footing and found himself hurtling toward certain death. As he plummeted past a small bush growing out of the sheer rock wall, he caught a berry in his hand and ate it. It was the most delicious berry he had ever eaten.

Each of us is that man, hurtling toward certain death. Yet we tend to avoid thinking about our mortality. Death represents losing everything and everyone dear to us. The death of a best friend, parent, mate, or child evokes confusion and pain. The prospect of our own death is emotionally devastating. If you suddenly discovered that you had a terminal illness, how would you want to spend your last year or months? What kind of final ceremony would you want held to mark your passing? How would you want to dispose of your possessions? Have you discussed issues of this kind with your family? The manner in which we choose to confront death can greatly influence how we live our lives.

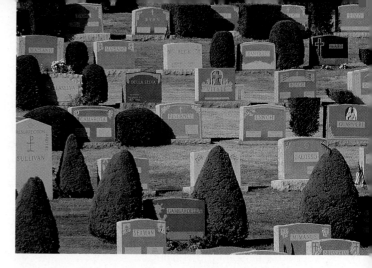

Death awaits all of us at the end of our lives, and accepting and dealing with death are difficult but important tasks. Some people have found that facing the prospect of death makes them more aware of the preciousness of life.

WHY IS THERE DEATH?

Ultimately, no answer to the question of why death exists is completely satisfying. When we look at the big picture, we see that death promotes variety through the evolution of species. The average human life span is long enough to allow us to reproduce ourselves and ensure that the lineage of our species continues. Yet it is brief enough to allow for new genetic combinations, thereby providing a means of adaptation to changing conditions in the environment. From the perspective of species survival, the cycle of life and death makes sense.

From a personal point of view, however, death challenges our emotional and intellectual security. We may acknowledge the fact that all living things eventually die, that this is nature's way of renewal, but this recognition offers little comfort when death touches our own lives. Questions about the meaning of death and what happens when we die are central concerns of the great religions and philosophies. Some promise a better life after death. Others teach that everyone is evolving toward perfection or divinity, a goal reached after successive rounds of death and rebirth. There are also those who suggest that it is not possible to know what happens—if anything—after death, that any judgment about whether life is worth living must be made on the basis of satisfactions or rewards that we create for ourselves in this life.

It is worth noting that, even in modern secular societies, religion plays a major role in shaping our attitudes and behaviors toward death. Religion offers solace to the extent that it suggests some meaning in dying. The mourning ceremonies associated with various religious practices ease the pangs of grief for many people. Dying and death are more than biological events; they have social and spiritual dimensions. Our beliefs—religious or philosophical—can be a key to how we relate to the prospect of our own death, as well as the deaths of others.

UNDERSTANDING DEATH AND DYING

Death forces us to puzzle out an understanding of its meaning in our lives. We may choose not to think about some issues, such as the possibility of an afterlife, but we cannot keep from facing the reality of dying and death. Regardless of our explanations or efforts to minimize its effects, death is painful—both to the person who is dying and to those left behind.

Defining Death

Traditionally, death has been defined as cessation of the flow of vital bodily fluids. This occurs when the heart stops beating and breathing ceases. These traditional signs are adequate for determining death in most cases. However, the use of respirators and other **life-support systems** in modern medicine allows some body functions to be artificially sustained. To make a determination of death in such cases requires investigating the presence or absence of a physical response other than heartbeat or breathing. The concept of **brain death** has been developed to determine whether a person is alive or dead when the traditional signs are inadequate because of supportive medical technology.

According to the standards published in 1968 by a Harvard Medical School committee, brain death involves the following four characteristics: (1) lack of receptivity and response to external stimuli, (2) absence of spontaneous muscular movement and spontaneous breathing, (3) absence of observable reflexes, and (4) absence of brain activity, as signified by a flat **electroencephalogram (EEG)**. The Harvard criteria require a second set of tests to be performed after 24 hours have elapsed, and they exclude cases of hypothermia (body temperature below 90°F), as well as situations involving central nervous system depressants, such as barbiturates.

In contrast to **clinical death**, which is determined by either the cessation of heartbeat and breathing or the criteria for establishing brain death, **cellular death** refers to a gradual process that occurs when heartbeat, respiration, and brain activity have stopped. It encompasses the breakdown of metabolic processes and results in complete nonfunctionality at the cellular level. In a biological sense, therefore, death can be defined as the cessation of life due to irreversible changes in cell metabolism.

The way in which death is defined has potential legal and social consequences in a variety of areas, including criminal prosecution, inheritance, taxation, treatment of the corpse, even mourning. It also affects the practice of organ transplantation because some organs—hearts, most obviously—must be harvested from a human being who is legally determined to be dead. Timing is critical in removing a heart from someone who has been declared dead and transplanting it into a person whose life can thereby be saved. Safeguards are necessary to ensure that the determination of death occurs without regard to any plans for subsequent transplantation of the deceased's organs.

Learning About Death

Our understanding of death changes as we grow and mature, as do our attitudes toward it. Very young children view death as an interruption and an absence, but their lack of a mature time perspective means that they do not understand death as final and irreversible. A child's understanding of death evolves greatly from about age 5 to age 9. During this period, most children come to understand that death is final, universal, and inevitable. A child who consciously recognizes these facts is said to possess a **mature understanding of death.** This understanding of death is further refined during the years of adolescence and young adulthood by considering the impact of death on close relationships and contemplating the value of religious or philosophical answers to the enigma of death.

Based on work done by Mark Speece and Sandor Brent, a formal statement of the empirical, or observable, facts about death includes four components:

1. *Universality*. All living things eventually die. Death is all-inclusive, inevitable, and unavoidable (although unpredictable with respect to its exact timing).

2. *Irreversibility*. Organisms that die cannot be made alive again.

3. *Nonfunctionality*. Death involves the cessation of all physiological functioning, or signs of life.

4. *Causality*. There are biological reasons for the occurrence of death.

It is important to add, however, that individuals who possess a mature understanding of death commonly hold nonempirical ideas about it as well. Such nonempirical ideas—that is, ideas not subject to scientific proof—deal mainly with the notion that human beings survive in some form beyond the death of the physical body. What happens to an individual's "personality" after he or she dies? Does the self or soul continue to exist after the death of the physical body? If so, what is the nature of this "afterlife"? Developing personally satisfying answers to such questions, which involve what Speece and Brent term **noncorporeal continuity,** is also part of the process of acquiring a mature understanding of death.

Denying Versus Welcoming Death

Understanding death in a mature fashion does not imply that we never experience anxiety about the deaths of those we love or about the prospect of our own death. The news of a friend's or loved one's serious illness can shock us into an encounter with mortality that creates a need to cope not only with the painful reality of our friend's or loved one's illness, but also with our own eventual death. Our ability to find meaning and comfort in the face of mortality depends not only on our having an understanding of the facts of death, but also on our attitudes toward it.

Many people seek to avoid any thought or mention of death. The sick and old are often isolated in hospitals and nursing homes. Relatively few Americans have been present at the death of a loved one. Where the reality of death is concerned, "out of sight, out of mind" often appears to be the rule of the day. Instead of facing death directly, we tend to amuse ourselves with unrealistic portrayals on television and movie screens. The fictitious deaths of characters we barely know do not cause us to confront the

---

Terms

life-support systems Medical technologies, such as the respirator, that allow vital body functions to be artificially sustained.

brain death A medical determination of death as the cessation of brain activity indicated by various diagnostic criteria, including a flat EEG reading.

electroencephalogram (EEG) A record of the electrical activity of the brain (brain waves).

clinical death A determination of death made according to accepted medical criteria.

cellular death The breakdown of metabolic processes at the level of the cell.

mature understanding of death The recognition that death is universal and irreversible, that it involves the cessation of all physiological functioning, and that there are biological reasons for its occurrence.

noncorporeal continuity The notion that human beings survive in some form after the death of the physical body.

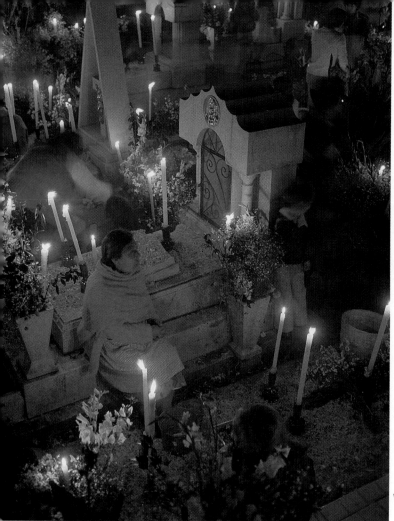

Día de los Muertos in Mexico is characterized by a mixture of reverent remembrance of the departed, festivity to make them happy upon their return, and irony and mockery to defy the fear of death itself. After cleaning the graves and decorating them with candles and flowers, these families will spend the night in the graveyard—eating, singing, praying, and talking with the departed.

reality of death as it is experienced in real life. Moreover, such faked death is often presented as reversible. Children watch a daily fare of superhuman heroes, invincible to bullets and other weapons. In their games, they reenact these false ideas about death—falling down "dead" and jumping up again unharmed. Cartoons and video games present death in a two-dimensional world where one can "die" and then be "reborn" to play another day.

Although some commentators characterize the predominant attitude toward death in the United States as "death denying," others are reluctant to paint society as a whole with such a broad brush. Individuals often maintain conflicting or ambivalent attitudes toward death. Those who come to view death as a relief or release from insufferable pain may have at least a partial sense of welcoming death. Few people wholly avoid or

wholly welcome death. Problems can arise, however, when avoidance or denial fosters the notion that death happens to others, but not to you or me. (For another perspective, see the box "Día de los Muertos: The Day of the Dead.")

PLANNING FOR DEATH

Acknowledging the inevitability of death allows us to plan for it. Adequate planning can help ensure that a sudden, unexpected death is not made even more difficult for survivors. Even when sudden death is not the issue, individuals with a debilitating illness may become unable to make decisions that could have been made before the onset of crisis. Although some decisions cannot be made until one is actually in a particular situation, many decisions relating to dying and death can be anticipated, considered, and discussed with close relatives and friends.

Basic tasks in planning for death include making a will, anticipating medical care needs and expressing preferences for end-of-life care, considering whether to become an organ donor, and helping our survivors plan tasks that will be carried out after we die. It is reasonable to begin such planning and decision making during the college years and to periodically review and revise one's choices throughout life.

WW. Making a Will

Statistics indicate that seven out of ten Americans die without leaving a will. Perhaps the failure to plan ahead for death by making a will is attributable to the discomfort people feel about their own mortality. Whatever the reason, dying without having made a will can lead to unnecessary hardships for survivors, even when an estate is modest in size. If an estate is substantial, the complications can be formidable.

A **will** is a legal instrument expressing a person's intentions and wishes for the disposition of his or her property after death. It is a declaration of how one's **estate**—that is, money, property, and other possessions—will be distributed after death. During the life of the **testator** (the person making the will), a will can be changed, replaced, or revoked. Upon the testator's death, it becomes a legal instrument governing the distribution of the testator's estate.

When a person dies **intestate**—that is, without having left a valid will—property is distributed according to rules set up by the state. The failure to execute a will may result in a distribution of property that is not compatible with a person's wishes nor best suited to the interests and needs of heirs. In making a will, it is generally advisable to involve close family members to prevent problems that can arise when actions are taken without the knowledge of those who will be affected.

In contrast to the solemn attitude toward death so prevalent in the United States, a familiar and even ironic attitude is more common among Mexicans and Mexican Americans. In the Mexican worldview, death is another phase of life, and those who have passed into it remain accessible. Ancestors are not forever lost, nor is the past dead. This sense of continuity has its roots in the culture of the Aztecs, for whom regeneration was a central theme. When the Spanish came to Mexico in the sixteenth century, their beliefs about death, along with such symbols as skulls and skeletons, were absorbed into the native culture.

Mexican artists and writers confront death with humor and even sarcasm, depicting it as the inevitable fate that all—even the wealthiest—must face. At no time is this attitude toward death livelier than at the beginning of each November on the holiday known as Día de los Muertos, "the Day of the Dead." This holiday coincides with All Souls' Day, the Catholic commemoration of the dead, and represents a unique blending of indigenous ritual and religious dogma.

Festive and gay, the celebration in honor of the dead typically spans two days—one day devoted to dead children, one to adults. It reflects the belief that the dead return to Earth in spirit once a year to rejoin their families and partake of holiday foods prepared especially for them. The fiesta usually begins at midday on October 31, with flowers and food—candies, cookies, honey, milk—set out on altars in each house for the family's dead. The next day, family groups stream to the graveyards, where they have cleaned and decorated the graves of their loved ones, to celebrate and commune with the dead. They bring games, music, and special food—chicken with *mole* sauce, enchiladas, tamales, and *pan de muertos,* the "bread of the dead," sweet rolls in the shape of bones. People sit on the graves, eat, sing, and talk with the departed ones. Tears may be shed as the dead are remembered, but mourning is tempered by the festive mood of the occasion.

During the season of the dead, graveyards and family altars are decorated with yellow candles and yellow marigolds—the "flower of death." In some Mexican villages, yellow flower petals are strewn along the ground, connecting the graveyard with all the houses visited by death during the year.

As families cherish memories of their loved ones on this holiday, the larger society satirizes death itself—and political and public figures. The impulse to laugh at death finds expression in what are called *calaveras,* a word meaning "skeletons" or "skulls" but also referring to humorous newsletters that appear during this season. The *calaveras* contain biting, often bawdy, verses caricaturing well-known public figures, often with particular reference to their deaths. Comic skeletal figures march or dance across these pages, portraying the wealthy and influential as they will eventually become.

Wherever Mexican Americans have settled in the United States, Día de los Muertos celebrations keep the traditions alive, and the cultural practices associated with the Day of the Dead have found their way into the nation's culture. Books and museum exhibitions have brought to the public the "art of the dead," with its striking blend of skeletons and flowers, bones and candles. Even the schools in some areas celebrate the holiday. Students create paintings and sculptures depicting skeletons and skulls with the help of local artists.

Does this more familiar attitude toward death help people accept death and come to terms with it? Keeping death in the forefront of consciousness may provide solace to the living, reminding them of their loved ones and assuring them that they themselves will not be forgotten when they die. Yearly celebrations and remembrances may help people keep in touch with their past, their ancestry, and their roots. The festive atmosphere may help dispel the fear of death, allowing people to look at it more directly. Although it is possible to deny the reality of death even when surrounded by images of it, such practices as Día de los Muertos may help people face death with more equanimity.

SOURCES: Adapted from DeSpelder, L., and A. Strickland. 2002. *The Last Dance,* 6th ed. New York: McGraw-Hill. Puente, T. 1991. Día de los Muertos. *Hispanic,* October. Milne, J. 1965. *Fiesta Time in Latin America.* Los Angeles: Ward Ritche Press. Azcentral. 2000. *Día de los Muertos* (http://www.azcentral.com/rep/dead; retrieved March 8, 2001).

COMMUNICATE! Many experts suggest that people make their wills quite early in life, often at the time of marriage, the birth of a child, or the purchase of a home. Think about what you would put in your own will, including the disposition of your property, and practice ways to discuss these ideas with your friends and family. For example, "I expect to live a long time, but I also want to make sure I don't leave you with any problems when I do die. Here's what I've been thinking about writing into my will." Follow up this conversation by actually writing a valid will and putting it in a safe but accessible place. It's also helpful to keep a written record of the location of important documents, such as insurance policies, pensions, bank accounts, mortgages, property deeds, and Social Security records.

Considering Options for End-of-Life Care

If you were facing the prospect of dying soon, would you prefer to spend your last days or weeks at home, cared for by relatives and friends? Or would you rather have access to the sophisticated medical technologies available in the hospital? An appropriate balance in end-of-life care may

Terms

will A legal instrument expressing a person's intentions and wishes for the disposition of his or her property after death.

estate The money, property, and other possessions belonging to a person.

testator The person who makes a will.

intestate Referring to the situation in which a person dies without having made a legal will.

involve a combination of home care, hospital stays, and hospice or palliative care. By becoming aware of our options, we and our families are empowered to make informed, meaningful choices.

Home Care   Many people express a preference to be cared for at home during the end stage of a terminal illness. An obvious advantage of home care is the fact that the dying person is in a familiar setting, ideally in the company of family and friends. For home care to be an option, however, support generally must be provided not only by family and friends, but also by skilled, professional caregivers.

Home care is a full-time job, and it is not always possible to provide a sufficient level of care in the home. Success depends on adequate preparation and commitment. When a patient requires sophisticated medical procedures, does not have access to qualified caregivers, or intends to be an organ donor, institutional care may be more appropriate. When suitable, however, home care is arguably the most satisfying option for care as a person's life comes to a close.

Hospital-Based Palliative Care   Although hospitals are primarily organized to provide short-term intensive treatment for acute injury and illness, they are also adopting the principles of **palliative care** for patients who require comprehensive care at the end of life. Unlike acute care, which involves taking active measures to sustain life, palliative care focuses on controlling pain and relieving suffering by caring for the physical, psychological, spiritual, and existential needs of the patient. Although the emphasis is generally placed on comfort care, palliative therapies can be combined with cure-oriented treatment approaches in some cases. In all cases, the goal of palliative care is to achieve the best possible quality of life for patients and their families.

Hospice Programs   As a comprehensive program of care offering a set of services designed to support terminally ill patients and their families, **hospice** is a well-known form of palliative care. Although the term *hospice* sometimes refers to a freestanding medical facility to which terminally ill patients are admitted, most hospice care takes place in patients' homes with family members as primary caregivers. "Entering hospice care" usually means affiliating with a hospice program—that is, arranging to receive the services of a local hospice. Such hospices are generally community-based organizations that coordinate a range of palliative care services that may be provided in nursing homes and hospitals, as well as in patients' homes. (For more on the history and development of hospice, see the box "Hospice: Comfort and Care for the Dying.") Qualifying for hospice care usually requires a doctor's certification that a patient's life expectancy is 6 months or less, and both patient and physician agree to forgo treatment aimed at prolonging life.

Hospice (and palliative care generally) involves a team-oriented approach to care that typically includes physicians, nurses, social workers, home health aides, pharmacists, chaplains, physical and occupational therapists, and trained volunteers. This team-oriented approach seeks to provide state-of-the-art care to prevent or relieve pain and other distressing symptoms, as well as to offer emotional and spiritual support to both patient and family. The notion that hospice is appropriate only when there is no hope is a myth. Much can be done even when recovery or cure is not a realistic possibility.

The primary aim of hospice and palliative care is to help people live as fully as possible until the end of their lives. In addition to its goal of helping patients achieve a "good" or "peaceful" death, an important gift of such care is the potential to help patients and families discover how much can be shared at the end of life through personal and spiritual connections that might not have been possible otherwise.

Deciding to Prolong Life or Hasten Death

If you were given a prognosis of only a very short time to live and told that any further treatment toward a cure was useless, would you want aggressive treatment to keep you alive, even if it meant that your vital bodily functions were maintained on life-support systems? The decision to limit treatment, to stop "doing everything that can be done," is often a difficult one for patients and their families. Many people owe their lives to the advanced medical technologies now available. Yet a medical stance that strives to keep people alive by all means and at any cost is increasingly questioned.

Modern medicine can keep the human organism alive despite the cessation of normal heart, brain, respiratory, or kidney function. But should a patient without any hope of recovery be kept alive by means of artificial life support? At what point does such treatment become futile? What if a patient has fallen into a **persistent vegetative state**, a state of profound unconsciousness, lacking any sign of normal reflexes and unresponsive to external stimuli, with no reasonable hope of improvement?

Ethical questions about the "right to die" have become prominent since the landmark case of Karen Ann Quinlan in 1975. At age 22, she was admitted in a comatose state

Hospice is a special kind of care for people in the final phase of a terminal illness. Instead of being in a hospital, where the emphasis is on curing disease, most hospice patients stay in their home or another homelike setting surrounded by family and friends. The goals of hospice care include the following:

- To make every terminally ill patient as pain-free as possible

- To support the patient and family as a unit

- To respect the feelings and beliefs about death held by patients and their families

- To involve patients in decision making regarding their care

- To help patients and family members deal with feelings of loneliness and fears of abandonment

- To counsel family members after a patient's death

Although institutions dedicated to the care of the dying have existed throughout history, the modern hospice movement began in 1967, when Dr. Cicely Saunders founded St. Christopher's Hospice near London. The first hospice program in the United States began in 1974. Today there are more than 3000 such programs, serving an estimated 700,000 terminally ill patients and their families each year. Once a patient can no longer benefit from medical treatment based on curing disease, the primary physician may refer the patient to hospice. Referrals can also be made by family members, friends, clergy, or health professionals.

Most patients receive care at home, with the primary caregiver often a partner or family member. Providing medical care and other types of support to the patient, family, and caregivers is a team of trained professionals—physicians, nurses, counselors, therapists, social workers, home health aides, and volunteers. The emphasis of care is on enhancing the quality of life rather than extending its length. Most hospice patients have a life expectancy of 6 months or less at the time they enter hospice, and about two-thirds of them are over 65 years old.

Hospice care is often less expensive than conventional care—high-cost technology is much less likely to be used, and family, friends, and volunteers provide much of the day-to-day patient care at home. Because a principle of hospice is to offer services based on need rather than the ability to pay, many hospices rely on grants, donations, and a large volunteer staff. At the same time, hospice has grown into a more formal, regulated industry. Hospice care is a covered benefit under most private insurance plans, Medicare, and, in many states, Medicaid. Medicare-certified hospice programs meet quality standards set by the federal government, including 24-hour access to professional care.

Some experts believe hospice could serve many more patients than it does. There are several stumbling blocks, however. Physicians may be reluctant to stop treatment and tell patients and their families that nothing further can be done to effect a cure. Establishing a specific timeline for a patient's expected death is difficult. Patients and family members may be reluctant to face an imminent death.

In addition, under Medicare rules, a physician must certify that the patient will likely die in 6 months or less. Although the rules do provide for extensions, many hospices feel pressured to accept only patients near death, turning away those who may linger beyond the half-year cutoff. The Health Care Financing Administration, which manages Medicare, has recently emphasized that the 6-month rule is based on life expectancy at the time of the physician's certification, not an absolute deadline by which the patient must die. Nevertheless, some hospices have been subjected to audits that have left them feeling bitter and suspicious about how Medicare benefits are administered. A proposal currently being discussed would let hospices obtain preauthorization for cases in which prognosis is difficult. Whether or not this solves the problem, nearly everyone agrees that there is a need for eligibility criteria that are not time-dependent, so that hospice services can be extended to more patients and their families.

SOURCES: National Hospice and Palliative Care Organization. 2000. *Facts and Figures on Hospice Care in America* (http://www.nhpco.org; retrieved October 2, 2000). Lagnado, L. 2000. Medicare head tackles criticism on hospice care. *Wall Street Journal,* September 15. Hospice care. 1997. *Mayo Clinic Health Letter,* July.

to an intensive care unit, where her breathing was sustained by a respirator. When she remained unresponsive in a persistent vegetative state, her parents asked that the respirator be disconnected, but the medical staff responsible for Karen's care denied their request. The request to withdraw treatment eventually reached the New Jersey Supreme Court, which ruled that artificial respiration could be discontinued.

Since then, courts have ruled on removing other types of life-sustaining treatment, including artificial feeding mechanisms that provide nutrition and hydration to permanently comatose patients who are able to breathe on their own. Most notable was the case of Nancy Beth Cruzan, heard before the United States Supreme Court in 1990. As a result of injuries she received in 1983, Cruzan was in a persistent vegetative state. To provide nourishment, Nancy's physicians implanted a feeding tube, the only form of life support she was receiving. When Nancy's parents requested that the feeding tube be taken out, hospital personnel refused, arguing that the state had an inherent interest in preserving life.

In the Cruzan case, the U.S. Supreme Court ruled that the right to refuse unwanted treatment, even if it is life-sustaining, is constitutionally protected. However, the court said that states are justified in requiring that only the patient can decide to withdraw treatment. Because

Nancy apparently had not provided a clear expression of her wishes prior to her injury, the state of Missouri was not bound to honor her parents' request. A few months later, however, in light of new testimony from several of Nancy's friends that she had expressed a wish "not to live like a vegetable," a state court ruled that the legal standard of "clear and convincing" evidence of Nancy's wishes had been met, and therefore permission was granted for removal of the feeding tube. This case emphasized the importance of expressing one's preferences about life-sustaining treatment—preferably in writing—before the need arises.

Withholding or Withdrawing Treatment   The right of a competent patient to refuse unwanted treatment is now generally established in both law and medical practice. The consensus is that there is no medical or ethical distinction between withholding (not starting) a treatment and withdrawing (stopping) a treatment once it has been started. The choice to forgo life-sustaining treatment involves refusing treatments that would be expected to extend life. The right to refuse treatment remains constitutionally protected even when a patient is unable to communicate. Although specific requirements vary, all of the states authorize some type of written advance directive to honor the decisions of individuals unable to speak for themselves, but who have previously recorded their wishes in an appropriate legal document. (Advance directives are discussed later in this chapter.)

The practice of withholding or withdrawing a treatment that could potentially sustain life is sometimes termed **passive euthanasia,** although many people consider this term a misnomer because it tends to confuse the widely accepted practice of withholding or withdrawing treatment with the generally unacceptable and unlawful practice of taking active steps to cause death. It can be argued that "passive euthanasia" is not euthanasia at all, but rather letting nature take its course. This distinction is sometimes phrased as the difference between "killing" and "allowing to die."

Assisted Suicide and Active Euthanasia   In contrast to withdrawing or withholding treatment, assisted suicide and active euthanasia refer to practices that intentionally hasten the death of a person. Although some ethicists argue that the constitutional basis for the right to refuse treatment provides the same basis for a right to active euthanasia, this argument has not been accepted by the Supreme Court or by the majority of health care practitioners.

Assisted suicide refers to providing someone with the means to commit suicide, knowing that the recipient intends to use them to end his or her life. In **physician-assisted suicide (PAS),** a physician provides lethal drugs or other interventions—at the patient's explicit request—with the understanding that the patient plans to use them to end his or her life. The patient, not the doctor, administers the fatal dose.

In 1997, the Supreme Court reviewed two cases relating to physician-assisted suicide. The decisions in these cases (*Washington v. Glucksberg* and *Vacco v. Quill*) are important for several reasons. First, the Court upheld the distinction between, on the one hand, withholding or withdrawing treatment, and, on the other hand, physician-assisted suicide. In doing so, the Court clarified its ruling in the Cruzan case, noting that the right to *refuse treatment* is based on the right to maintain one's bodily integrity, not on a right to *hasten death.* When treatment is withheld or withdrawn, the Court said, the intent is to honor the patient's wishes, not cause death, unlike with PAS, where the patient is "killed" by the lethal medication. Second, the Court affirmed the rights of states to craft policy concerning physician-assisted suicide, prohibiting it, as most states now do, or permitting it under some regulatory system, as is now happening in Oregon.

Oregon is currently the only state where PAS is permitted. The Death with Dignity Act, a ballot initiative, was passed by Oregon voters in 1994 and, after surviving judicial challenges, was reaffirmed in 1997. During its first three years of implementation, 70 people were reported

Terms

passive euthanasia The practice of withholding (not starting) or withdrawing (stopping) treatment that could potentially sustain a person's life, with the recognition that, without such treatment, death is likely to occur.

physician-assisted suicide (PAS) The practice of a physician intentionally providing, at the patient's request, lethal drugs or other means for a patient to hasten death with the understanding that the patient plans to use them to end his or her life.

double effect A situation in which a harmful effect occurs as an unintended side effect of a beneficial action, such as when medication intended to control a patient's pain has the unintended result of causing the patient's death.

active euthanasia A deliberate act intended to end another person's life; voluntary active euthanasia involves the practice of a physician administering—at the request of a patient—medication or other intervention that causes death.

advance directive Any statement made by a competent person about his or her choices for medical treatment should he or she become unable to make such decisions or communicate them in the future.

living will A type of advance directive that allows individuals to provide instructions about the kind of medical care they wish to receive if they become unable to participate in treatment decisions.

health care proxy A type of advance directive that allows an individual to appoint another person as an agent in making health care decisions in the event he or she becomes unable to participate in treatment decisions; also known as a durable power of attorney for health care.

surrogate The agent or substitute decision maker appointed by a person to act on his or her behalf by means of a health care proxy.

to have legally committed suicide with the assistance of their physicians. These patients exhibited strong beliefs in personal autonomy and determination to control the end of their lives. The decision to request a prescription for lethal medication was associated mainly with concerns about loss of autonomy and control. Specific quality-of-life concerns included decreasing ability to participate in activities that make life enjoyable, losing control of bodily functions, and physical suffering.

A third finding of importance in the Supreme Court's 1997 rulings about PAS relates to the concept of **double effect** in the medical management of pain. The doctrine of double effect states that a harmful effect of treatment, even if it results in death, is permissible if the harm is not intended and occurs as a side effect of a beneficial action. Sometimes the dosages of medication needed to relieve a patient's pain (especially those in the end stage of some diseases) must be increased to levels that can cause respiratory depression, resulting in the patient's death. Thus, the relief of suffering (the intended good effect) may have a potential bad effect, which is foreseen but not the primary intention. The Court said that such medication for pain, even if it hastens death, is not physician-assisted suicide if the intent is to relieve pain.

Unlike physician-assisted suicide, **active euthanasia** involves a deliberate act to end another person's life. Generally, it is understood as the intentional act of killing someone who would otherwise suffer from an incurable and painful disease. It is important, however, to recognize that active euthanasia can be involuntary, nonvoluntary, or voluntary. Involuntary euthanasia (or involuntary active euthanasia) refers to the ending of a patient's life by a medical practitioner *without* the patient's consent. The most notorious example of this is the medical killing programs of the Nazi regime. Nonvoluntary euthanasia occurs when a surrogate decision maker (not the patient) asks a physician for assistance to end another person's life.

Voluntary euthanasia (also known as voluntary active euthanasia, or VAE) is the intentional termination of life at the patient's request by someone other than the patient. In practice, this generally means that a competent patient requests direct assistance to die, and he or she receives assistance from a qualified medical practitioner.

At present, active euthanasia has found greatest acceptance in the Netherlands, where physicians are permitted to give lethal injections to patients who request death. The guidelines for VAE in the Netherlands include the presence of a terminal diagnosis, the patient's unwavering desire to die, the presence of suffering that the patient finds unbearable, and a second medical opinion. Voluntary active euthanasia is currently unlawful in the United States, and it is for this practice that Michigan physician Dr. Jack Kevorkian was convicted of second-degree murder in 1999. Taking active steps to end someone's life is a crime—even if the motive for doing so results from good intentions as an act of mercy.

Many people believe that the emphasis on a "right to die," along with the movement to legalize physician-assisted suicide and active euthanasia, results from inattention to the needs of the dying by the health care system. Inadequate pain management has been called "the shame of American medicine." The advocates of hospice and palliative care have highlighted the need for adequate pain management, not only for patients with terminal illness, but for all patients with untreated or undertreated pain and suffering. Increasingly, pain is being viewed as a "fifth vital sign," one that should be added to the four vital signs—temperature, pulse, respiration, and blood pressure—now recorded and assessed as a standard part of patient care. Unfortunately, there is tremendous variation among health care providers with respect to assessing and managing pain adequately.

Completing an Advance Directive

To make our preferences known about medical treatment to health care providers and others who should be aware of them, it is important to document them through a written **advance directive.** In a general sense, an advance directive is any statement made by a competent person about choices for medical treatment should he or she become unable to make such decisions or communicate them at some time in the future.

Two forms of advance directives are legally important. First is the **living will,** which enables individuals to provide instructions about the kind of medical care they wish to receive if they become incapacitated or otherwise unable to participate in treatment decisions (Figure 20-1). Many people believe that living wills are appropriate only for stating a desire to forgo life-sustaining procedures or to avoid medical heroics when death is imminent; and, indeed, most "standard" forms for completing a living will reflect this purpose. In fact, however, a living will can be drafted to express very different ideas about the kinds of treatment a person would or would not want, and they can be written to cover various contingencies.

The second important form of advance directive is the **health care proxy,** which is also known as a durable power of attorney for health care. This document makes it possible to appoint another person to make decisions about medical treatment if you become unable to do so. This decision maker, also known as a **surrogate,** may be a family member, close friend, or attorney with whom you have discussed your treatment preferences. The proxy is expected to act in accordance with your wishes as stated in an advance directive or as otherwise made known.

For advance directives to be of value, you must do more than merely complete the paperwork. Discuss your wishes ahead of time with caregivers and family members as well as with your physician. If you have completed an advance directive in one state and subsequently move

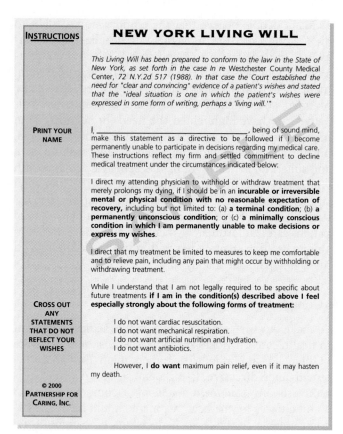

Figure 20-1   Sample living will.   Because of differences in state law, each state has its own format for advance directives.   SOURCE: Partnership for Caring, 1035 30th St., Washington, DC 20007 (800-989-9455; http://www.partnershipforcaring.org).

elsewhere, find out if you need to complete a new one. Indeed, it is a good idea to revisit the issue occasionally to be sure the preferences expressed in the directive continue to match your wishes.

Becoming an Organ Donor

A human body is a valuable resource. Of all the advances in medical techniques for helping patients who were formerly beyond recovery, perhaps the best known is the transplantation of human organs. Yet the demand for organs continues to drastically outpace the number of organ donations. Each day about 60 people receive an organ transplant while another 18 people on the waiting list die because not enough organs are available (Figure 20-2).

If you decide to become a donor, the first step is to indicate your wish by completing a **Uniform Donor Card** (Figure 20-3); alternatively, you can indicate your wish on your driver's license. (In 2001, federal officials announced plans for a national organ donor card that would carry more weight than the current unofficial cards or driver's license notifications.) Because relatives are called upon to make decisions about organ and tissue donation at the time of a loved one's death, your second step is to

discuss your decision with your family. Decisions about whether to become an organ donor are often based on both personal and cultural values (see the box "Organ Donation and Transplantation in Japan").

Planning a Funeral or Memorial Service

Just as people gather to commemorate other major transitions in a person's life, such as birth and marriage, funerals and memorial services are rites of passage that commemorate a person's life in a community and acknowledge his or her passing from that community. Funerals and memorial services provide a framework that allows survivors to support one another as they cope with the fact of their loss and express their grief. The presence of death rites in every human culture suggests that they serve innate human needs.

Disposition of the Body   When a death occurs, one of the immediate concerns of survivors is the disposition of the corpse. Although corpses must be disposed of for sanitary reasons, the disposition of a body is surrounded by a web of social, cultural, religious, psychological, and interpersonal considerations that influence how this basic human task is accomplished.

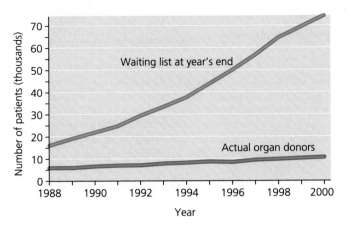

Figure 20-2   The need for organ donors.   As organ transplants have become an option for more and more patients, the number of people waiting for transplants has increased. The number of actual donations has not grown nearly so significantly.   SOURCE: United Network for Organ Sharing (http://www.unos.org).

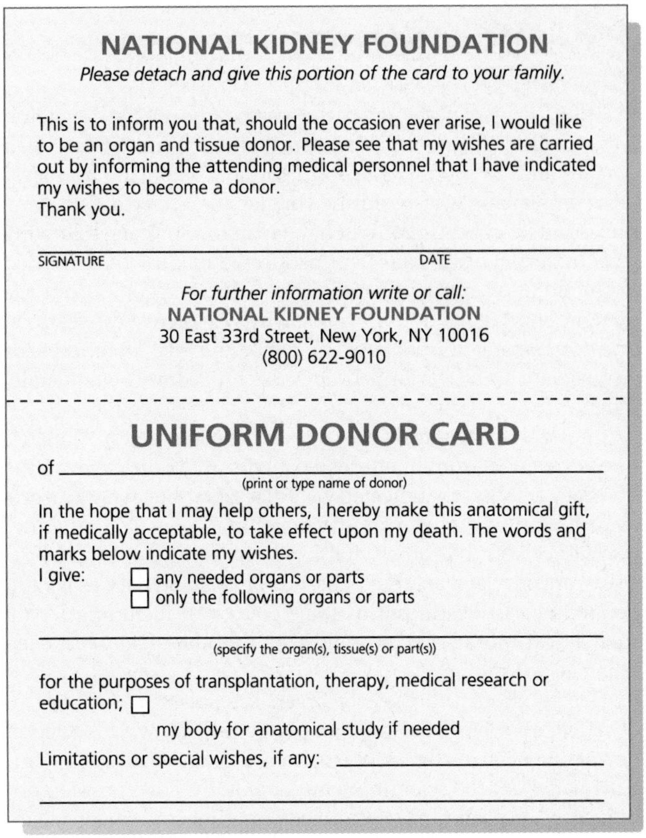

People generally have a preference about the final disposition of their body. For must Americans, the choice is either burial or cremation. *Burial* usually involves a grave dug into the soil or entombment in a mausoleum. *Cremation* involves subjecting a body to intense heat, thereby reducing its organic components to a mineralized skeleton. The remaining bone fragments are then usually put through a "cremulator," which reduces them to a granular state, often referred to as "ashes" (which actually resemble coarse coral sands). Cremated remains can be buried, placed in a columbarium niche, put into an urn kept by the family or interred in an urn garden, or scattered at sea or on land. A body destined for burial or cremation may or may not be embalmed. If the body is to be viewed during a wake or will be present at the funeral, **embalming** is generally done.

Arranging a Service   In commemorating a person's life and death, the choice of "last rites" may involve a traditional funeral ceremony or a simple memorial service. Whereas the casketed body is typically present at a funeral, it is not at a memorial service. In some cases, both a funeral and a memorial service are held, the former occurring within a few days after death and the latter being held sometime later (perhaps in a different town where the deceased had a large social network). Although it is becoming more common for individuals and families to express a preference for no services, bereaved relatives and friends can derive important benefits from having an opportunity to honor the deceased and express their grief through ceremony.

Decisions about one's own last rites are ideally made with a view to the needs and wishes of one's survivors. It can be worthwhile to consider such decisions early in life,

NATIONAL KIDNEY FOUNDATION
Please detach and give this portion of the card to your family.

This is to inform you that, should the occasion ever arise, I would like to be an organ and tissue donor. Please see that my wishes are carried out by informing the attending medical personnel that I have indicated my wishes to become a donor.
Thank you.

SIGNATURE _____ DATE _____

For further information write or call:
NATIONAL KIDNEY FOUNDATION
30 East 33rd Street, New York, NY 10016
(800) 622-9010

- -

UNIFORM DONOR CARD

of _____
(print or type name of donor)

In the hope that I may help others, I hereby make this anatomical gift, if medically acceptable, to take effect upon my death. The words and marks below indicate my wishes.

I give: ☐ any needed organs or parts
         ☐ only the following organs or parts

_____
(specify the organ(s), tissue(s) or part(s))

for the purposes of transplantation, therapy, medical research or education; ☐
         my body for anatomical study if needed

Limitations or special wishes, if any: _____
_____

Figure 20-3   A sample organ donor card.   SOURCE: Uniform Donor Card. Copyright © 1996 the National Kidney Foundation, Inc. Reprinted with permission.

while it's possible to gather information about options and to discuss plans with family members (see the box "A Consumer Guide to Funerals"). Religious and cultural or ethnic traditions play a major role in shaping the way people honor their dead. The diversity of life and death in the United States calls for a diversity of rites. A meaningful funeral or memorial service can be designed in many different ways.

Costs also may influence the choices people make for last rites. According to the latest available figures, the average cost of a funeral, not including cemetery costs, is $5800. About $2200 of this cost goes toward purchase of a casket, which people usually feel is the centerpiece of a funeral due to its symbolic and emotional significance in honoring the deceased. Less expensive options for disposal

Uniform Donor Card A consent form authorizing the use of the signer's body parts for transplantation or medical research upon his or her death.

embalming The process of removing blood and other fluids and replacing them with chemicals to disinfect and temporarily retard deterioration of a corpse.

Terms

In 1997 the Japanese legislature passed the Organ Donation Law, a bill legalizing organ transplantation from a brain-dead person; and 18 months later, in February 1999, the first legal heart transplant was performed in Japan. Prior to this date, transplants had been prohibited in Japan for 30 years, following a controversial heart transplant performed in 1968 that resulted in the filing of murder charges against the surgeon. Given the extreme shortage of donor organs, why was there a 30-year ban on heart transplants in Japan, and why did it take 18 months for a transplant to be performed after the procedure was officially sanctioned?

Central to this issue is how a society defines death. Donated hearts are taken from brain-dead patients, individuals who have no brain activity, as indicated by a flat EEG, but whose hearts are still beating and who are still breathing—that is, brain function has ceased, but other vital functions continue. Most Western countries have accepted absence of brain activity as a valid determinant of death, but in some countries, including Japan, such a definition is so culturally alien that the society has been reluctant to embrace it.

Debate about the issue of organ transplantation began in 1968, when a Japanese surgeon performed the world's second heart transplant using an organ from a brain-dead donor. Initially hailed for the scientific achievement, the surgeon was subsequently accused of illegal human experimentation and disregard for the rights of both donor and recipient. The concept of brain death was quite new at the time, and no public consensus existed in Japan concerning this new definition of death. The case left a legacy of mistrust about brain death and transplantation in Japan.

Among technologically advanced countries, Japan is unique in its reliance on living donors. Recent statistics indicate that, in Japan, about 70% of transplanted kidneys and 80% of liver segments are taken from live donors. This is almost the opposite of the situation in the United States, where, in 1999, 64% of transplanted kidneys—about 8000 kidneys—and 98% of transplanted livers—about 4700 livers—as well as about 2200 hearts—were from brain-dead donors. Although many scientific and technological advances have been eagerly adopted in Japan, persistent questions about brain death have resulted in a reluctance to actively pursue organ transplantation.

The Japanese attitude toward organ transplantation from brain-dead donors is influenced by many cultural factors, including religious beliefs. Many Japanese believe that body and soul remain together after death and arise together in the next life, a belief supported by both Buddhist and Shinto teachings. Buddhism teaches further that personal identity is found in the whole person, not in the brain or any other single physical organ. Brain dysfunction does not necessarily mean that a person is dead; the notion of brain death is inconsistent with the Japanese idea of death of the whole person.

According to Shinto teachings, life is still present as long as the body is warm. Shinto claims that death occurs when the soul leaves the body, but when this occurs cannot be known with certainty. Shinto customs also require a waiting period before a person is declared dead, because there is a possibility that the soul will return to the body.

The Japanese also have distinctive cultural views on bodily integrity. Many Japanese are concerned about keeping the body intact, not only during life—the body is viewed as a gift from one's ancestors—but also after death, when body and soul remain together. Related to the concern with bodily integrity is Japan's long history of concerns about impurity. Procedures involved in organ donation and transplantation may be construed as defiling the body.

Traditional practices involving gift giving are involved as well. In Japan, receiving a gift incurs an obligation to return the favor. When an organ is donated, there is no way of repaying such a valuable gift, even to the family of the donor. Moreover, the absence of a social relationship between donor and receiver tends to taint organ donation with an aura of commercialism.

Another factor is the traditional relationship between physicians and patients in Japan. Until fairly recently, most Japanese physicians practiced a kind of "closed door" medicine in which patients were neither given information about their health nor permitted to criticize their physicians. To many Japanese, such paternalistic conduct is worrisome in the context of transplantation procedures. They fear that physicians might apply the criteria for brain death too readily or even be influenced by the market demand for organs, especially in the absence of family involvement.

Given all these cultural factors, it is not surprising that heart transplants are not widely accepted in Japan, despite the fact that, according to surveys, nearly half of Japanese people accept brain death as a valid definition of death. Currently, only 50% of the institutions authorized by the 1997 Organ Donation Law to perform organ transplants are prepared to do so. Japanese surgeons have urged the government to clarify some of the issues related to brain death and organ transplants, including legal responsibilities, costs, diagnosis, and education of the public. At the same time, it is clear that the issue is not just about medicine and technology, nor should resistance to transplantation be viewed simply as an obstacle to overcome. The approach developed by Japan or any society must take into account the complex historical, religious, and cultural factors that make up its unique identity.

SOURCES: Wicks, M. N. 2000. *Brain Death and Transplantation: The Japanese* (http://www.medscape.com/medscape/transplantation/journal/2000/v01.no2/mt0425.wick/html; retrieved November 15, 2000). United Network for Organ Sharing. 2001. UNOS Transplant Patient Data Source (http://www.unos.org; retrieved March 8, 2001). Brannigan, M., and J. A. Boss. 2000. *Healthcare Ethics in a Diverse Society* (Mountain View, Calif.: Mayfield). Kimura, R. 1998. Organ transplantation and brain-death in Japan: Cultural, legal, and bioethical background. *Annals of Transplantation* 3: 55–58.

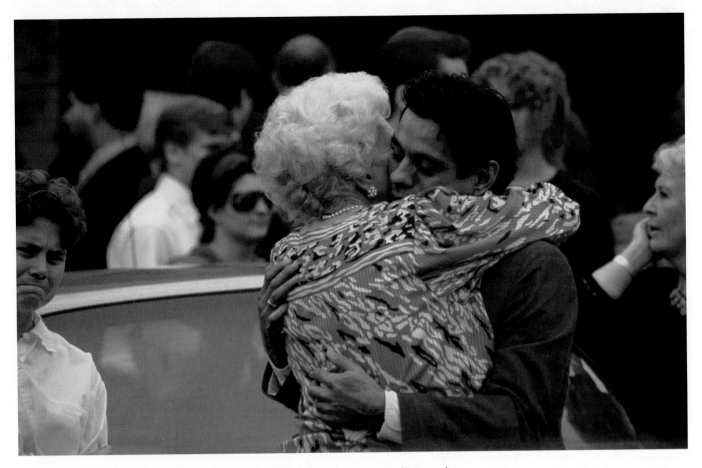

Funeral or memorial services give friends and relatives of the deceased the opportunity to mark their grief through ritual and ceremony.

of the body include direct cremation or immediate burial, both of which involve no viewing and no funeral ceremony. Although both of these options are generally available from mortuaries that also offer traditional funeral services, people who prefer a no-frills approach may have the option of arranging economic burial or cremation through a non-profit **memorial society.** Veterans are eligible for burial in a national cemetery, an option that can also reduce costs.

The bottom line is that a wide range of options is available to meet consumers' diverse needs and wishes. Making at least some plans ahead of time and discussing the options with family members can help reduce the burden on survivors who find themselves facing a number of tasks and decisions once death occurs (see the box "Tasks for Survivors").

COPING WITH DYING

There is no one right way to live with or die of a life-threatening illness. Every disease has its own set of problems and challenges, and each person copes with these problems and challenges in his or her own way. It is said that doctors treat *disease;* people suffer from *illness.* Much of the suffering experienced by people with a life-threatening illness comes from overwhelming feelings of loss on all levels. Besides the emotional havoc accompanying news of a potentially life-ending disease, there are usually concerns about costly medical care, loss of income, repeated and perhaps lengthy hospitalization, and physical pain. How a person copes with such an experience is likely to reflect his or her personality and life history, as well as the nature of family relationships and patterns of interaction in the person's wider social environment.

Awareness of Dying

Living with an illness that is life-threatening and incurable can be described as a "living-dying" experience. From the time discomforting symptoms are first noticed and one's worst fears confirmed by a diagnosis, through the ups and downs of treatment, and on to the final days or hours of life, hope and honesty are often delicately

memorial society A nonprofit membership group that provides simple and economical burial or cremation.

Terms

Funerals are a consumer product. They are also among the most expensive purchases many consumers will ever make. A traditional funeral costs about $5500, and many funerals run to $10,000 or more. When no preplanning has been done, as often occurs, family members have to make decisions under time pressure and in the grip of strong feelings. As a result, they may make poor decisions and spend more than they need to.

To avoid these problems, millions of consumers are now making funeral arrangements in advance, comparing prices and services so they can make well-informed purchasing decisions. Many people see funeral planning as an extension of will and estate planning. It is also possible to prepay some or all of the expenses involved.

A federal law called the Funeral Rule, enforced by the Federal Trade Commission, regulates the funeral provider business. It includes many requirements designed to protect consumers from unprofessional business practices. To ensure that you make the best possible decisions, follow these guidelines:

- Plan ahead. Think about what type of funeral you want—simple or elaborate, public or private, religious or secular. Do you want your funeral to be held in a house of worship, a funeral home, or a private setting? Also think about the disposition of the body—do you want your remains to be buried or cremated?

- Shop around. Look for a funeral home that belongs to the National Funeral Directors Association (NFDA), and compare prices from at least two funeral homes. You are not legally required to use a funeral home, but many people find it makes arrangements easier.

- Ask for a price list. The Funeral Rule requires funeral directors to give you an itemized price list when you ask either in person or over the telephone. Many funeral homes offer package funerals that cost less than individual items, but you may not need or want everything included in the package.

- Decide on the goods and services you want. Basic services include planning the funeral and coordinating arrangements with the cemetery or crematory. Embalming is not necessary or legally required if the body is buried or cremated shortly after death. The casket is usually the single most expensive item; an average casket costs about $2000, but some caskets sell for as much as $10,000. You do not have to buy the casket from the funeral home you use. The Funeral Rule prohibits funeral directors from claiming that some caskets can preserve a body indefinitely; they can't.

- Resist pressure to buy goods and services you don't really want or need. Funeral directors are required to inform you that you need buy only those goods and services you want.

- In choosing a cemetery, take into consideration its location; its religious affiliation, if any; the types of monuments allowed; and cost. Visit the cemetery ahead of time to make sure it's suitable.

- Once you have made decisions, put them in writing, give copies to family members, and keep a copy accessible. It's a good idea to review your decisions every few years and revise them if necessary.

- Know the facts, including which goods and services are required by law in your state and which are optional. Many organizations provide information about making funeral arrangements; see the For More Information section at the end of the chapter.

- If you need help dealing with a funeral home, contact consumer protection agencies listed in the telephone book, the Funeral Consumer's Alliance (800-458-5563 or http://www.funerals.org), or the Funeral Service Consumer Assistance Program (800-662-7666). To file a complaint about a funeral home, contact the Federal Trade Commission at 877-FTC-HELP or http://www.ftc.gov.

SOURCES: Federal Trade Commission. 2000. *Funerals: A Consumer Guide* (http://www.ftc.gov/bcp/conline/pubs/services/funeral.htm; retrieved July 14, 2000). National Funeral Directors Association. 2000. *Ensure Wise Decision-Making: Know the Facts* (http://www.nfda.org/resources/ensure.html; retrieved July 14, 2000).

balanced—honesty to face reality as it is, hope for a positive outcome. The object of hope changes. The early hope that the symptoms are not really serious gives way to hope that a cure is possible. When the illness is deemed incurable, there is hope for more time. As time begins to run out, one hopes for a pain-free death, a good death.

Psychiatrist Avery Weisman described this process of coping as involving **middle knowledge,** with patients and their families seeking a balance between sustaining hope and acknowledging the reality. Maintaining a sense of self-worth, setting goals and striving to reach them, engaging in fruitful interactions with one's environment—all of these reflect a coping strength that sustains the will to live fully despite a bleak prognosis.

The Tasks of Coping

In her 1969 book *On Death and Dying* Elisabeth Kübler-Ross suggested that the response to an awareness of imminent death involves five psychological stages: denial, anger, bargaining, depression, and acceptance. The notion that these "five stages" occur in a linear progression has since become a kind of modern myth of how people *ought* to cope with dying. Unfortunately, this can lead to the idea that it is a person's "task" to move sequentially through these stages, one after another; and, if this is not

Some of the following tasks must be attended to soon after a death occurs, others take weeks or months to complete. Many of these tasks, especially those that need to be dealt with in the first hours and days following the death, can be taken care of by friends and relatives of the immediate survivors.

- Prepare a list of relatives, close friends, and business colleagues, and arrange to telephone them about the death as soon as possible. Friends can help with the notification process.

- Find out whether the deceased left instructions or made plans for disposition of the body or for a funeral or memorial service.

- If no prior plan exists, contact a mortuary or memorial society for help in making arrangements. Clergy, friends, and other family members can be asked to help decide what is most appropriate.

- If flowers are to be omitted from the funeral or memorial service, choose an appropriate charity or other memorial to which gifts can be made.

- Write the obituary. Include the deceased's age, place of birth, cause of death, occupation, academic degrees, memberships, military service record, accomplishments, names and relationships of nearest survivors, and an announcement of the time and place of the funeral or memorial service.

- Arrange for family members or close friends to take turns welcoming those who come to express their condolences in person and responding to those who telephone their condolences.

- Ask friends to help coordinate the supplying of meals for the first few days following the death, as well as the management of other household tasks and child care, if necessary.

- Arrange hospitality for relatives and friends who are visiting from out of town.

- If a funeral ceremony is planned, choose the individuals who are to be pallbearers, and notify them that you would like their participation.

- Notify the lawyer, accountant, and other personal representatives who will be helping to settle the deceased's estate.

- Send handwritten or printed notes of acknowledgment to the people who have provided assistance or who have sent flowers, contributions, or their condolences.

- With the help of a lawyer or an accountant, review all insurance policies as well as other sources of potential death benefits, such as Social Security, military service, fraternal organizations, and unions.

- Review all debts, mortgages, and installment payments. Some may carry clauses that cancel debt in the event of death. If payments must be delayed, contact creditors to arrange for a grace period.

---

accomplished, the person has somehow failed. In fact, however, Kübler-Ross said that individuals go back and forth among the stages during the course of an illness and different stages can occur simultaneously.

The stage-based model devised by Kübler-Ross more than three decades ago has been a stimulus toward a better understanding of how people cope with dying. The notion of sequential stages, however, has been deemphasized in favor of highlighting the *tasks* that deserve attention in coping with a life-threatening illness. Charles Corr, for example, distinguishes four primary dimensions in coping with dying:

1. *Physical:* Satisfying bodily needs and minimizing physical distress

2. *Psychological:* Maximizing a sense of security, self-worth, autonomy, and richness in living

3. *Social:* Sustaining significant relationships and addressing the social implications of dying

4. *Spiritual:* Identifying, developing, or reaffirming sources of meaning and fostering hope

Contemplating these dimensions gives us a framework for considering the specific tasks that need to be addressed in coping with dying. In addition to an *acute* phase initiated by the diagnosis, a *chronic* phase of living with the disease, and a *terminal* phase that involves coping with impending death, there are sometimes two other phases. First, a *prediagnostic* phase, during which a person suspects the illness and may seek medical attention; and, second, a *recovery* phase following a cure or remission of a previously life-threatening disease. Even as the threat of dying recedes into the background, however, there can be a need to cope with the fact that one has had a potentially terminal illness.

To avoid mistaking the map for the territory, we must remember that a person's death is as unique as his or her life. Thus, although models can help us gain understanding, they need to be balanced by paying attention to the dying person's own unfolding *life* story. Each person's

middle knowledge A state of knowing when a person both acknowledges the reality of a threatening situation and maintains hope for a positive outcome.

Terms

What does it mean to die a "good death"? Participants in a recent study were asked to discuss the deaths of family members, friends, or patients and reflect on what made those deaths good or bad. From these discussions and interviews, six major themes emerged as components of a good death.

The first component was pain and symptom management. Many people fear dying in pain, and portrayals of bad deaths usually included inadequate pain management. Every health care provider in the study told regret-filled stories of patients who died in pain. Patients were concerned with both current and future pain control; when reassured that pain could be managed with drugs, they were less anxious.

The second major component of a good death was clear decision making. Both providers and families feared entering a medical crisis without knowledge of patient preferences. Patients and families who had good communication with health care providers and had discussed treatment decisions ahead of time felt empowered, and providers felt they were giving good care. Researchers noted that although all uncertainty about end-of-life decisions cannot be eliminated, tolerance for uncertainty may increase if values and preferences are clarified.

The third component was preparation for death. Patients expressed satisfaction when they had adequate time to prepare their wills and help plan the events that would follow their death, such as funeral arrangements. Many times, providers avoided end-of-life discussions to prevent their patients from losing hope, thus depriving them of the opportunity to plan ahead. Patients and families also wanted to know what to expect during the course of the illness and what physical and psychosocial changes would take place as death approached. It was important for providers and families to have reached some personal comfort with death so they felt prepared when death occurred.

The fourth element was completion, the opportunity to review one's life, to resolve conflicts, to spend time with loved ones, and to say good-bye. Participants confirmed the deep importance of spirituality or meaningfulness at the end of life. Many times, patients were able to view their experience of dying as part of a broader life trajectory and thus continue to grow emotionally and spiritually in their last days. Issues of faith were often mentioned as important to healing, but participants emphasized that the cues about the particular expression of faith must be taken from the patient.

The fifth component was contributing to others. Patients wanted to know that they still had something to offer to others, whether it was making someone laugh or lightening the load of someone closer to death. Many patients found that as they reflected on their lives, what they valued most was their personal relationships with family and friends, and they were anxious to impart this wisdom to others.

The last component of a good death was affirmation of the whole person. Patients appreciated empathic health care providers, and family members were comforted by those who treated their loved ones as unique and whole people, rather than as a "disease." The quality of dying is related to the acknowledgment that people die "in character," that is, as an extension of who they have been in their lives. Health care providers also focused on their personal relationships with patients and family members as important to a satisfying death.

The study affirmed that most people think of death as a natural part of life, not as a "failure of technology." Although the biomedical aspects of end-of-life care are crucial, they merely provide a point of departure toward a good death. When pain is properly managed and the practical aspects of dying are taken care of, patients and their families have the opportunity to address the important emotional, psychological, and spiritual issues that all human beings face at the end of life.

SOURCE: Steinhauser, K. S., et al. 2000. In search of a good death: Observations of patients, families, and providers. *Annals of Internal Medicine* 132(10): 825–832.

pathway through life-threatening illness is determined by such factors as the specific disease and its course, his or her personality, and the available supportive resources (see the box "In Search of a Good Death").

Terms

defense mechanisms Unconscious mental processes that alter a person's internal psychological states in reaction to a threat without affecting the external problem.

coping strategies Conscious, purposeful efforts employed with the intention of controlling a threatening or stressful situation or problem.

trajectory of dying The duration and nature of a person's experience in approaching death as influenced by the underlying cause of dying.

Patterns of Coping

When confronted by a stressful situation, our first response is to evaluate it. Whether or not we are fully aware of this process, we consider the significance of the threatening situation and assess our resources for coping with it. Our evaluation influences the way we subsequently cope.

The threat of a potentially fatal illness evokes a variety of responses to make the threat somehow manageable. These responses can be divided into two main categories: defense mechanisms and coping strategies. **Defense mechanisms** occur unintentionally and without conscious effort or awareness; they function to change a person's internal psychological states, not the external reality. **Coping strategies** involve conscious, purposeful effort; they are employed with the intention of solving a problem. Although coping strategies are generally viewed more positively than defense mechanisms, both involve psychological processes that can help ease a distressful situation. The defense mechanism *denial,* for example, is sometimes adaptive and sometimes not, depending on the person and the situation. In the short term, denial can give a person "breathing room" in living with a distressing situation; over the long term, however, such defenses may hinder a positive outcome because they prevent a person from mobilizing needed resources and taking appropriate action.

The main aim of the mental processes and behaviors involved in coping is to establish control over a stressful situation. Achieving this typically requires different coping strategies at different times. One way of distinguishing different strategies is to examine their purpose and focus. *Emotion-focused coping,* for example, helps regulate the level of distress. It allows a person to escape the impact of the stressful situation by reframing it or distancing the self from it. Reframing a situation to put it in a positive light can reduce the sense of threat. Another strategy, *problem-focused coping,* deals with managing the problem that is causing distress. A cancer patient who seeks out information about her disease and takes an active role in determining her options is engaging in problem-focused coping. A hallmark of this style of coping is the person's pursuit of personally meaningful goals. Recalling that the main aim of coping is to establish a sense of control, it is worth mentioning that a greater sense of control is associated with problem-focused coping, whereas less control is associated with emotion-focused coping. Even so, each of these strategies has a role in coping.

A third strategy, *meaning-based coping,* is employed to maintain a person's sense of positive well-being. Examples include giving up goals that are no longer achievable and formulating new ones, making some sense of what is happening, and, where possible, finding benefit in the distressing situation. In this search for meaning, people often turn to spiritual beliefs for insight in making the best of a bad situation. Finding some redeeming value in loss can make the burden easier to bear.

People vary their styles of coping depending on the opportunities for problem solving in a situation, the intensity of their emotional responses and their ability to regulate them, and the changes in their environment as the distressing situation unfolds. Thus, the various coping strategies are dynamic rather than static, with the overall pattern of coping resembling a more-or-less-continual flow or rhythm among the various styles. It is a mistake to pit one style against another, because they are interdependent and work together, each supplementing the others.

People who apparently cope best with life-threatening illness often exhibit a "fighting spirit" that views the illness not only as a threat, but also as a challenge. These people strive to inform themselves about their illness and take an active part in treatment decisions. They are optimistic and have a capacity to discover positive meaning in ordinary events. Holding to a positive outlook despite distressing circumstances involves creating a sense of meaning that is bigger than the threat. In the context of life-threatening illness, this encompasses a person's ability to comprehend the implications an illness has for the future, as well as for his or her ability to accomplish goals, maintain relationships, and sustain a sense of personal vitality, competence, and power. Although life-threatening illness disrupts virtually all aspects of a person's life, there is a vital link between finding meaning and achieving a sense of mastery.

COMMUNICATE! If someone you know tells you that he or she is facing a life-threatening illness, you may not be sure what to say. Give the person the opportunity to express his or her concerns and needs, and respond with questions, such as "Can you tell me more?" Practice active, empathic listening, avoiding statements such as "Everything will be OK" or "You should see another doctor." Stay present with the person, and offer practical assistance if you feel comfortable doing so ("Do you need anything right now?"). Keep in mind that you don't have to have answers or make things better; all you need to offer is your caring presence.

The Trajectory of Dying

Our expectations about dying may be quite different from what most people actually experience. The concept of a **trajectory of dying** is useful for understanding patients' experiences as they near death. Although sudden death from an unexpected cause—a massive heart attack or an accident, for example—is one type of dying trajectory, our focus here is on deaths that occur when there is forewarning. Among these, some trajectories involve a steady and fairly predictable decline. This is the case with many cancers, which tend to follow the course of a progressive disease with a terminal phase. Other kinds of advanced, chronic illness involve a long period of slow decline marked by episodes of crisis, the last of which proves to be "suddenly" fatal.

We can also distinguish between different stages in a dying trajectory; namely, a period when a person is known to be terminally ill but is living with a life expectancy of perhaps weeks or months, possibly years; and a later period when dying is imminent and the person is described as "actively dying." The way in which such trajectories are estimated—their duration and expected course—can affect both patients and caregivers and influence their actions. Deaths that occur "out of time" (too quickly or too slowly) may pose special difficulties.

When a person is actively dying, his or her death is expected to occur within hours or, at most, a few days. During the last phase of a fatal illness, a dying person may

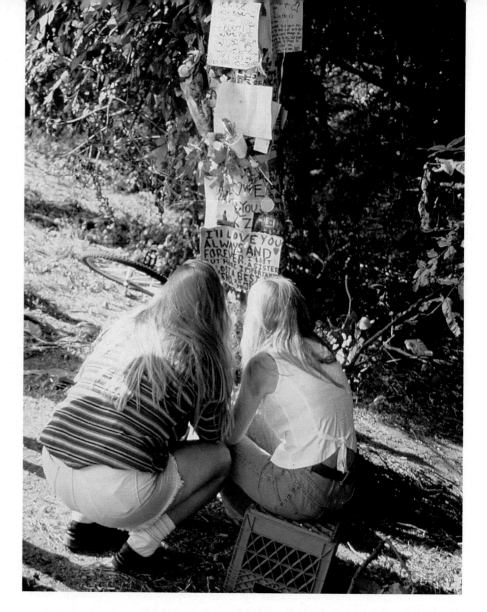

Death can challenge our sense of emotional and intellectual security, particularly the sudden death of a young person. This roadside marker was placed in memory of people killed in an automobile crash at this site.

exhibit irregular breathing or shortness of breath, decreased appetite and thirst, nausea and vomiting, incontinence, restlessness and agitation, disorientation and confusion, and diminished consciousness. These symptoms usually can be managed by skilled palliative care. Pain, if it is present, should be treated aggressively as part of a comprehensive approach to comfort care. Since most patients are more comfortable without eating or drinking at the end of life, forcing food or liquids is usually not beneficial. The stopping of eating and drinking has always been part of the last phase of a terminal condition. Near the time of death, relaxation of the throat muscles or secretions in the throat may cause the person's breathing to become noisy, resulting in a sound called the "death rattle." Most dying patients are not aware of this noisy breathing. If it unnerves family or caregivers, giving medication or repositioning the person can help. Just before death, the person may take a breath and sigh or shudder.

When a family member or close friend is dying, people often feel that they should be at the bedside at the very moment of death. This is not always possible, however, because the exact timing of death is difficult to predict. Sometimes people keep a deathwatch for days. Then, when they step out briefly for a break, the person dies. Perhaps this phenomenon is just a matter of chance, or perhaps it is the case that the dying person was "waiting" for a moment to be "on her own" before letting go.

Supporting a Dying Person

People often feel uncomfortable in the presence of a person who is close to dying. What can we say? How should we act? It may seem that any attempt to be comforting could only result in words that are little more than stale platitudes. Yet we want to express concern and establish meaningful contact with the person who is facing the major loss of his or her life. In such circumstances, the most important gift we can bring is the gift of listening. Offering the person opportunities to speak openly and honestly about his or her experience can be crucial, even when such conversation is initially painful.

We tend to place dying persons in a special category, but the reality is that their needs are not fundamentally different from anyone else's, although their situation is perhaps more urgent. Dying people need to know that they are valued, that they are not alone, that they are not being unfairly judged, and that those closest to them are also striving to come to terms with a difficult situation. As with any relationship, there are opportunities for growth on both sides.

Besides friends and family, the dying person may need other supportive resources. These may include counselors and clergy. Many hospitals, hospices, and other health care providers sponsor programs for dying patients and their families, offering opportunities for them to share their concerns in a supportive and validating atmosphere. Programs of this kind can be located by asking hospital staff or other medical personnel. Local chapters of support groups affiliated with organizations such as the American Cancer Society and Make Today Count also can be found in many cities.

In supporting someone who is facing the prospect of dying from a terminal illness, the most important thing is simply to be there for the person and his or her family. Listen more than talk. At the same time, remember to take care of yourself. Especially if you are a member of the caregiving team, be sure to make time for yourself. To accomplish this, it may be necessary to find others to help you. It can be important to strengthen your own support system even as you offer support.

COPING WITH LOSS

Even if we have not experienced the death of someone close, we are all survivors of losses that occur in our lives because of changes and endings. The loss of a job, the ending of a relationship, transitions from one school or neighborhood to another—these are examples of the kinds of losses that occur in all our lives. Such losses are sometimes called "little deaths," and, in varying degrees, they all involve grief.

Experiencing Grief

Grief is the reaction to loss. It encompasses thoughts and feelings, as well as physical and behavioral responses. Mental distress may involve disbelief, confusion, anxiety, disorganization, and depression. The emotions that can be present in normal grief include not only sorrow and sadness, but also relief, anger, and self-pity, among others. Bereaved people experience a range of feelings, even conflicting

ones. Recognizing that grief can involve many different feelings—not just sadness—makes us more able to cope with it. Common behaviors associated with grief include crying, "searching" for the deceased, and talking incessantly about the deceased and the circumstances of the death. Bereaved people may be restless, as if not knowing what to do with themselves. Physically, grief may involve frequent sighing, insomnia, and loss of appetite. Grief may also evoke a reexamination of religious or spiritual beliefs as a person struggles to make meaning of the loss. All such manifestations of grief can be present as part of one's total response to **bereavement**—that is, the event of loss.

Mourning is closely related to grief and is often used as a synonym for it. However, mourning refers not so much to the *reaction* to loss, but to the *process* by which a bereaved person adjusts to loss and incorporates it into his or her life. How this process is managed is determined, at least partly, by cultural norms for the expression of grief. Considered jointly, grief and mourning are the means to healing the pain of loss.

Tasks of Mourning Experiencing grief is part of the process by which a bereaved person integrates a significant loss into his or her life. Psychologist William Worden has identified four tasks that must be attended to:

1. *Accepting the reality* of the loss
2. *Working through the pain* of grief
3. *Adjusting to a changed environment* in which the deceased is absent
4. *Emotionally relocating the deceased and moving on with life*

Accomplishing the fourth task does not mean dishonoring the deceased's memory or denying normal feelings of connection that persist beyond death. Finding healthy ways to maintain bonds with the deceased is a testimony to the enduring strength of love. When this task is managed successfully, however, the bereaved is not "stuck" in the past. Making the journey of grief and attending to the various tasks along the way, we come to a place where we learn how to keep a special place for the deceased in our heart and memory while moving forward with our lives.

The Course of Grief Grieving, like dying, is highly individual. In the first hours or days following a death, a bereaved person is likely to experience overwhelming shock and numbness, as well as a sense of disbelief. There is often a period of denial—"No! This can't be true!"—

grief A person's reaction to loss as manifested physically, emotionally, mentally, and behaviorally.

bereavement The objective event of loss.

mourning The process whereby a person actively copes with grief in adjusting to a loss and integrating it into his or her life.

Terms

- Recognize and acknowledge the loss.
- React to grief by accepting and expressing it.
- Take time for nature's process of healing.
- Know that powerful, overwhelming feelings will change with time.
- Review and remember the relationship with the deceased.
- Share your pain by accepting support from others.
- Surround yourself with life: plants, animals, friends.
- Make use of mementos to promote your mourning, not to live in the past.

- Avoid major decisions, if possible, and give yourself time to readjust.
- Adapt to a new world without forgetting the old.
- Prepare for change, new interests, new friends, creativity, and growth.
- Reinvest in life.

SOURCES: The Centre for Living with Dying (554 Mansion Park Dr., Santa Clara, CA 95054; 408-980-9801). Rando, T. A. 1993. *The Treatment of Complicated Mourning.* Champaign, Ill.: Research Press.

especially if the death was unexpected. Consider the ways in which people die: the aged grandmother, dying quietly in her sleep; the young child pronounced DOA after a bicycle crash; the despondent executive who commits suicide; the chronically ill person who dies a "lingering death." The cause or mode of death—natural, accidental, homicide, or suicide—has an impact on how grief is experienced. Even when a death is anticipated, grief is not necessarily diminished when the loss becomes real.

The sense of disorganization experienced by survivors during the early period of grief is set against the need to attend to decisions and actions surrounding the disposition of the deceased's body. As family and friends gather to offer mutual support, funeral ceremonies are held. Engaging in such activities promotes accepting the reality of the death and moving beyond the initial shock and numbness.

In its middle phase, the course of grief is characterized by anxiety, apathy, and pining for the deceased. The "pangs of grief" are felt as the bereaved person deeply experiences the pain of separation. There is often a sense of despair as a person repeatedly goes over the events surrounding the loss, perhaps fantasizing that somehow everything could be undone and be as it was before. During this period, the bereaved also begins looking toward the future and taking the first steps toward building a life without the deceased.

This can be a difficult time in grieving. Yet the bereaved often find themselves without the social support of the relatives and friends who were present during the initial period. Grief always occurs within a particular social or cultural context, and individual grievers differ in their particular styles of grieving. This leads to the recognition that there is no "standard" way of coping with loss. Colin Murray Parkes points to three main influences on a person's course of grieving:

1. The urge to look back, cry, and search for what is lost

2. The urge to look forward, explore the world that emerges out of the loss, and discover what can be carried forward from the past into the future

3. The social and cultural pressures that influence how the first two urges are inhibited or expressed

As these influences interact in various ways, at times the bereaved tries to avoid the pain of grief and at other times confronts it. The goal is to achieve a balance between avoidance and confrontation that facilitates coming to terms with the loss. Attaining this goal can be seen as an oscillation between what Margaret Stroebe and Henk Schut call "loss-oriented" and "restoration-oriented" mourning. From this perspective, looking at old photographs and yearning for the deceased are examples of loss-oriented coping, whereas doing what is needed to reorganize life in the wake of the loss—for example, learning to do tasks that the deceased had always managed, such as finances or cooking—is part of restoration-oriented coping.

There is no predetermined timetable for completing this mourning process. In moving toward the restoration of one's well-being, however, the last phase of "active" grief involves coming to a sense of resolution. The acute pain and emotional turmoil of grief subsides. Physical and mental balance is reestablished. The bereaved becomes increasingly reintegrated into his or her social world. Sadness doesn't go away completely, but it recedes into the background. Although reminders of the loss stimulate active grieving from time to time, the main focus is the present, not the past. Adjusting to loss may sometimes feel like a betrayal of our deceased loved one, but it is healthy to engage again in our ongoing lives and our future (see the box "Coping with Grief").

Coming to terms with loss doesn't mean forgetting our loved one or minimizing the significance of the lost relationship. Rather, making the journey of grief allows us to incorporate the loss into our lives. We learn to maintain connections with deceased loved ones through memories and other means that sustain relationships beyond the grave. The "course of grief" has no absolute end point as long as the deceased is kept alive in our memory.

Supporting a Grieving Person

In experiencing a significant loss, a person initially may feel and behave much like a frightened, helpless child. He or she may respond best to the kind of loving support that is given by a parent. A hug may be more comforting than any words. Also, because talking about a loss is an important way that survivors cope with the changed reality, simply listening can be very helpful. The key to being a good listener is to refrain from making judgments about whether the feelings expressed by a survivor are "right" or "wrong," "good" or "bad." The emotions, thoughts, and behaviors evoked by loss may not be the ones we expect, but they can nonetheless be valid and appropriate within a survivor's experience of loss.

Talking and crying, even yelling in rage, are among the ways of coping with intense feelings of grief. Bereaved persons should not be urged to hold back their feelings or be "strong" and "brave." Expressions of grief are healing. On the other hand, if strong emotions aren't expressed, the bereaved need not pretend to grieve or exaggerate his or her feelings to satisfy others' expectations. Funerals and other leave-taking ceremonies generally help survivors gain a sense of closure and begin to integrate a loss into their lives. For some, funerals are occasions of weeping and wailing; for others, stoic and subdued emotions are the rule. Different styles of mourning behavior can be equally valid and appropriate.

Social support is as critical during the later course of grief as it is during the first days after a loss. Bereaved people need the reliable support of those they trust. In offering support, we can reassure them that grief is normal and confirm that it is permissible and appropriate to express grief. They may also need permission to occasionally give themselves a break from grieving. As they move forward in life, the bereaved may need encouragement from others to face the world confidently. An extended need for support often continues through the first year or two of mourning. The first anniversary following a significant loss can be a time of renewed grieving when the support of others is important and appreciated. Knowing that others remember and acknowledge the loss and that they take time to "touch base" is usually perceived as very helpful.

Besides the support from individuals who are part of their social network, bereaved people may want to share their stories and concerns through organized support groups, such as those intended for widowed persons. Many support groups are organized around a focus for some specific type of bereavement. Compassionate Friends, for example, is a nationwide organization composed of parents who have experienced a child's death. Referrals to support groups for bereaved people are available through community service organizations.

> **COMMUNICATE!** Few of us know just what to say to a friend who has lost a loved one. Some things to *avoid* are making references to the deceased person's advanced age, declaring that the death was "for the best," asking the widow or widower to let you introduce him or her to new people, suggesting the adoption of a pet, saying "I know how you feel," and expecting the person to be consoled by the presence of his or her remaining family. Very often, the most appreciated expression of sympathy is just "I'm so sorry."

Helping Children Cope with Loss

Children tend to cope with loss in a healthier fashion when they are included as part of their family's experience of grief and mourning. Although adults may be uncomfortable about sharing potentially disturbing or painful news with children, a child's natural curiosity usually negates the option of withholding information. Sudden changes in family communication patterns without any explanation can alarm a child and create anxiety. When children are asked about their experiences of family crises involving death, many say that the most difficult times occurred when they did not know what was happening. Thus, the question is, How should we offer our help to a child who is bereaved?

In talking about death with children, the most important guideline is to be honest. Set the explanation you are offering at the child's level of understanding. Children generalize from familiar concepts to make new experiences fit. We don't want to overwhelm a child with excessive detail, but we must beware of talking down to the child as if he or she were incapable of any comprehension. In general, it's advisable to keep the explanation simple, stick to basics, and verify what the child has understood from your explanation. A child's readiness for more details can usually be assessed by paying attention to his or her questions.

COMING TO TERMS WITH DEATH

We may wish we could keep death out of view and not make a place for it in our lives. But this wish cannot be fulfilled. With the death of a beloved friend or relative, we are confronted with emotions and thoughts that relate not only to the immediate loss but also to our own mortality.

Our encounters with dying and death teach us that relationships are more important than things and that life offers no guarantees. In discovering the meaning of death in our own lives, we find that life is both precious and precarious.

Allowing ourselves to make room for death, we discover that it touches not only the dying or bereaved person and his or her family and friends, but also the wider community of which we are all part. We recognize that dying and death offer opportunities for extraordinary growth in the midst of loss. Denying death, it turns out, results in denying life.

Tips for Today

Death is inevitable for all living things. When we contemplate the meaning of death in our own lives, we see that loss is profoundly woven into the fabric of human life. Facing death clear-sightedly, despite our fears and discomfort, can deepen our appreciation of life.

Right now you can

- Think about how you want your body to be disposed of when you die.

- Think about how you would want your worldly goods to be distributed if you were to die now.

- Think about whether you want to be an organ donor; if you do, look into filling out a donor card (see Take Action at the end of the chapter).

- Consider asking your parents or grandparents what their wishes are for end-of-life care and for funeral arrangements, if you don't already know.

SUMMARY

- Although death makes rational sense in terms of species survival and evolution, there may be no completely satisfying answer to the question of why death exists from a personal point of view.

- Dying and death are more than biological events; they have social and spiritual dimensions.

- The traditional criteria for determining death focus on vital signs such as breathing and heartbeat. Brain death is characterized by a lack of physical responses other than breathing and heartbeat.

- Between ages 5 and 9, most children develop a mature understanding of death; that is, they come to understand death as final, universal, and inevitable.

- A mature understanding of death can include ideas about the survival of the human personality after death.

- Problems arise when avoidance or denial of death fosters the notion that it happens only to others.

- Many basic tasks in preparing for death can and should be accomplished while one is young.

- A will is a legal instrument that governs the distribution of a person's estate after death.

- End-of-life care may involve a combination of home care, hospital stays, and hospice or palliative care.

- Palliative care is devoted to making dying patients comfortable by controlling pain and relieving suffering.

- Hospice programs apply a team-oriented approach to caring for dying patients and their families with the goal of helping people live as fully as possible until the end of their lives.

- Exercising choices about end-of-life care can involve making decisions about prolonging life or hastening death.

- The practice of withholding or withdrawing potentially life-sustaining treatment is sometimes termed passive euthanasia.

- Physician-assisted suicide occurs when a physician provides lethal drugs or other interventions, at a patient's request, with the understanding that the patient plans to use them to end his or her life. Voluntary active euthanasia refers to the intentional ending of a patient's life, at his or her request, by someone other than the patient.

- Advance directives, such as living wills and health care proxies, are used to express one's wishes about the use of life-sustaining treatment.

- People can donate their bodies or specific organs for transplantation and other medical uses after death.

- For Americans, the decision about what to do with the body after death usually involves either burial or cremation.

- Bereaved people usually benefit from participating in a funeral or memorial service to commemorate a loved one's death.

- Coping with dying involves physical, psychological, social, and spiritual dimensions.

- A variety of defense mechanisms and coping strategies may be appropriate as a person confronts the need to deal with tasks related to life-threatening illness.

- It is useful for patients and caregivers to understand the trajectory, or course, of dying.

- In offering support to a dying person, the gift of listening can be especially important.

- Grief encompasses thoughts and feelings, as well as physical and behavioral responses.

- Mourning, the process by which a person integrates a loss into his or her life, is determined partly by social and cultural norms for expressing grief.

- Children tend to cope with death in a healthier fashion when they are included in their family's experience of grief and mourning.

- Dying and death offer opportunities for growth in the midst of loss.

1. In most states, the Department of Motor Vehicles provides organ donor forms. You can also request a donor form or download one from the National Kidney Foundation (800-622-9010; http://www.kidney.org), the Coalition on Donation (800-355-7427; http://www.shareyourlife.org), or the Department of Health and Human Services (http://www.organdonor.gov). When you receive your donor form, consider the advantages and disadvantages of becoming a donor. If you decide to be a donor, fill out the card and keep it with your driver's license. Discuss your decision with members of your family.

2. Obtain sample copies of advance directives that are appropriate for the state you live in. Check with your local hospital or health services organization for these forms, or request them from Partnership for Caring (800-989-9455; http://www.partnershipforcaring.org).

Review the forms and consider the advantages and disadvantages of using them. If you decide to execute a living will or health care proxy, discuss your decision with members of your family and anyone else who might become involved in your health care.

3. Talk with your parents, grandparents, spouse, or other family members about their wishes for care at the end of their lives. Ask if they have made wills or completed advance directives. If they do not wish to discuss these matters, let them know that you are open to such a discussion in the future.

4. Investigate the services in your community that provide care for the dying, including hospitals, hospices, and counseling resources. Visit one or more of them, and evaluate their services.

JOURNAL ENTRY

1. What do you believe happens after death—heaven or hell, eternal sleep, nothingness, return to life in another form, union with a higher consciousness, something mysterious and unknowable? Write a brief essay explaining your concept or belief. Where did it come from? Is it what you wish would happen after death?

2. **Critical Thinking** Research the issue of physician-assisted suicide. Write a brief essay that presents the main arguments on both sides of the issue, and conclude with a statement of your own opinion. Be sure to explain your reasoning. What are the most important factors in your decision? Why do you think you have the opinion you do?

FOR MORE INFORMATION

Books

Brannigan, M. C., and J. A. Boss. 2000. *Healthcare Ethics in a Diverse Society.* Mountain View, Calif.: Mayfield. *A comprehensive overview of U.S. health care ethics that introduces a cross-cultural perspective on many issues.*

Byock, I. 1998. *Dying Well: Peace and Possibilities at the End of Life.* New York: Riverhead. *An eminent hospice physician offers a blueprint for care at the end of life.*

DeSpelder, L. A., and A. L. Strickland. 2002. *The Last Dance: Encountering Death and Dying,* 6th ed. New York: McGraw-Hill. *A comprehensive and readable text highlighting a broad range of topics related to dying and death.*

Doka, K. J. 1998. *Living with Life-Threatening Illness: A Guide for Patients, Their Families, and Caregivers.* San Francisco: Jossey-Bass. *Sheds light on coping with life-threatening illness, from diagnosis through treatment to eventual recovery or impending death.*

Kessler, D. 2000. *The Needs of the Dying: A Guide for Bringing Hope, Comfort, and Love to Life's Final Chapter.* New York: HarperCollins. *A compassionate and honest guide for people facing life-threatening illness and those caring for them.*

MacPherson, M. 1999. *She Came to Live Out Loud: An Inspiring Family Journey Through Illness, Loss, and Grief.* New York: Simon & Schuster. *The journey of a woman with breast cancer, from diagnosis to death, with attention to both its unique and universal aspects.*

Mitford, J. 2000. *The American Way of Death Revisited.* Reprint Edition. New York: Vintage. *A scathing, witty exposé of the funeral industry, updated from the 1963 classic.*

Silverman, P. R. 2000. *Never Too Young to Know: Death in Children's Lives.* New York: Oxford University Press. *A compassionate book that challenges mistaken beliefs about how children cope with grief and loss.*

Organizations and Web Sites

Association for Death Education and Counseling (ADEC). Provides resources for education, bereavement counseling, and care of the dying.
860-586-7503
http://www.adec.org

Caregiver Survival Resources. Designed to help people cope with the demands of caregiving.
http://www.caregiver911.com

The Dougy Center. Offers education about childhood bereavement and support groups for bereaved children.

503-775-5683

http://www.dougy.org

Dying Well. A Web site focused on wellness through the end of life.

http://www.dyingwell.com

GriefNet. A site where you can communicate with others via e-mail support groups in the areas of death, grief, and major loss.

http://www.griefnet.org

Growth House. Offers an extensive directory of Internet resources relating to life-threatening illness and end-of-life care.

http://www.growthhouse.org

Hospice Foundation of America. Promotes the hospice concept of care through education and leadership.

202-638-5419

http://www.hospicefoundation.org

Longwood College Library: Doctor Assisted Suicide—A Guide to Web Sites and the Literature. Information on physician-assisted suicide and links to related sites.

http://web.lwc.edu/administrative/library/suic.htm

National Funeral Directors Association (NFDA). Provides resources related to funerals and funeral costs, body disposition, and bereavement support.

800-228-6332; 262-789-1880

http://www.nfda.org

National Hospice and Palliative Care Organization (NHPCO). Provides information about hospice care and supplies an online national directory of hospices listed by state and city.

703-243-5900

http://www.nhpco.org

National Public Radio: The End of Life—Exploring Death in America. Download transcripts of this 1998 NPR series on end-of-life issues, as well as resources, a bibliography, and readings.

http://www.npr.org/programs/death

Nolo Press: Wills and Estate Planning. Provides answers to questions about planning for death, from writing a basic will to organ donation.

http://www.nolo.com

On Our Own Terms: Public Broadcasting System. A companion Web site to the Bill Moyers PBS series on improving end-of-life care.

http://www.pbs.org/wnet/onourownterms

Oregon Health Division, Center for Health Statistics and Vital Records. Provides information about Oregon's Death with Dignity Act.

http://www.ohd.hr.state.or.us/chs/pas/pas.htm

Partnership for Caring. Provides information about right-to-die issues and supplies advance directives that meet specific state requirements.

800-989-9455

http://www.partnershipforcaring.org

Soros Foundation: Project on Death in America. A Web site focusing on different approaches to achieving a good death.

http://www.soros.org/death/index.htm

The following organizations provide information about organ donation and donor cards.

National Kidney Foundation

212-889-2210

http://www.kidney.org

U.S. Department of Health and Human Services

http://www.organdonor.gov

SELECTED BIBLIOGRAPHY

Attig, T. 1996. *How We Grieve: Relearning the World.* New York: Oxford University Press.

Byock, I. 2000. Palliative care. In *On Our Own Terms: Moyers on Dying,* ed. Public Affairs Television, 10–11. New York: WNET.

Callanan, M., and P. Kelley. 1997. *Final Gifts: Understanding the Special Awareness, Needs, and Communications of the Dying.* New York: Bantam.

Cantor, N. L., and G. C. Thomas. 2000. The legal bounds of physician conduct hastening death. *Buffalo Law Review* 48: 83–173.

Capron, A. M. 2001. Brain death—well settled yet still unresolved. *New England Journal of Medicine* 344(16): 1244–1246.

Choice in Dying. 1999. *Issue: Background on the Right to Die* (http://www.choices.org/issues.htm; retrieved September 9, 2000).

Corr, C. A. 1998. Enhancing the concept of disenfranchised grief. *Omega: Journal of Death and Dying* 38: 1–20.

Corr, C. A., K. J. Doka, and R. Kastenbaum. 1999. Dying and its interpreters: A review of selected literature and some comments on the state of the field. *Omega: Journal of Death and Dying* 39: 239–259.

Cramer, P. 2000. Defense mechanisms in psychology today: Further processes for adaptation. *American Psychologist* 55: 637–646.

DeSpelder, L. A., and A. L. Strickland. 1995. Using life experiences as a way of helping children understand death." In *Beyond the Innocence of Childhood: Factors Influencing Children's and Adolescents' Perceptions and Attitudes Toward Death,* ed. D. W. Adams and E. J. Deveau, 45–54. Amityville, N.Y.: Baywood.

Ditto, P. H., et al. 2001. Advance directives as acts of communication: A randomized controlled trial. *Archives of Internal Medicine* 161(3): 421–430.

Doka, K. J. 1996. Coping with life-threatening illness: A task model. *Omega: Journal of Death and Dying* 32: 111–122.

Folkman, S., and S. Greer. 2000. Promoting psychological well-being in the face of serious illness: When theory, research and practice inform each other. *Psycho-Oncology* 9: 11–19.

Folkman, S., and J. T. Moskowitz. 2000. Positive affect and the other side of coping. *American Psychologist* 55: 647–654.

Golin, C. E., et al. 2000. A prospective study of patient-physician communication about resuscitation. *Journal of the American Geriatrics Society* 48: S52–S60.

Health Resources and Services Administration. 2000. *Organ Donation* (http://www.organdonor.gov; retrieved September 9, 2000).

Hospice care. 2001. *Journal of the American Medical Association* 285(7): 970.

Kendall, C. E. 2000. A double dose of double effect. *Journal of Medical Ethics* 26: 204–205.

Kübler-Ross, E. 1997. *On Death and Dying.* Reprint Edition. New York: Simon & Schuster.

Lynn, J. 2001. Serving patients who may die soon and their families. The role of hospice and other services. *Journal of the American Medical Association* 285(7): 925–932.

Lynn, J., and J. Harrold. 1999. *Handbook for Mortals: Guidance for People Facing Serious Illness.* New York: Oxford University Press.

Merboth, M. K., and S. Barnason. 2000. Managing pain: The fifth vital sign. *Nursing Clinics of North America* 35: 375–383.

Naierman, N. 2000. *Debunking the Myths of Hospice* (http://www.choices.org/newsf98.htm; retrieved September 9, 2000).

National Funeral Directors Association. 1999. *Funeral Price Information* (http://www.nfda.org/resources/99gpl.html; retrieved September 9, 2000).

O'Brien, C. N., G. A. Madek, and G. R. Ferrera. 2000. Oregon's guidelines for physician-assisted suicide: A legal and ethical analysis. *University of Pittsburgh Law Review* 61: 329–365.

Oregon Health Division. 2001. *Oregon's Death with Dignity Act: Three Years of Legalized Phyusician-Assisted Suicide* (http://www.ohd.hr.state.or.us/chs/pas/ar-smmry.htm; retrieved May 2, 2001).

Parkes, C. M. 1998. Bereavement in adult life. *British Medical Journal* 316: 856–859.

Saunders, C. 2000. The evolution of palliative care. *Patient Education and Counseling* 41: 7–13.

Silveira, M. J., et al. 2000. Patients' knowledge of options at the end of life. *Journal of the American Medical Association* 284(19): 2483–2488.

Speece, M. W., and S. B. Brent. 1996. The development of children's understanding of death. In *Handbook of Childhood Death and Bereavement*, ed. C. A. Corr and D. M. Corr. New York: Springer.

Strickland, A. L., and L. A. DeSpelder. 1995. Communicating about death and dying. In *A Challenge for Living: Dying, Death, and Bereavement*, ed. I. B. Corless, B. B. Germino, and M. A. Pittman, 37–51. Boston: Jones & Bartlett.

Stroebe, M., and H. Schut. 1995. *The Dual Process Model of Coping with Bereavement.* Paper presented at the meeting of the International Work Group on Death, Dying, and Bereavement, Oxford, England, June 29, 1995.

The SUPPORT Principal Investigators. 1995. A controlled trial to improve care for seriously ill hospitalized patients: The study to understand prognoses and preferences for outcomes and risks of treatment. *Journal of the American Medical Association* 274: 1591–1598.

Tierney, W. M., et al. 2001. The effect of discussions about advance directives on patients' satisfaction with primary care. *Journal of General Internal Medicine* 16(1): 32–40.

United Network for Organ Sharing. 2000. *The Critical Organ Shortage* (retrieved September 9, 2000; http://www.unos.org/about/numone_main.htm).

Weisman, A. D. 1984. *The Coping Capacity: On the Nature of Being Mortal.* New York: Human Sciences Press.

Weithman, P. J. 1999. Of assisted suicide and "the philosophers' brief." *Ethics* 109: 548–578.

Windler, D., and N. Dickert. 2001. The consent process for cadaveric organ procurement. How does it work? How can it be improved? *Journal of the American Medical Association* 285(3): 329–333.

Worden, J. W. 1991. *Grief Counseling and Grief Therapy: A Handbook for the Mental Health Practitioner,* 2nd ed. New York: Springer.

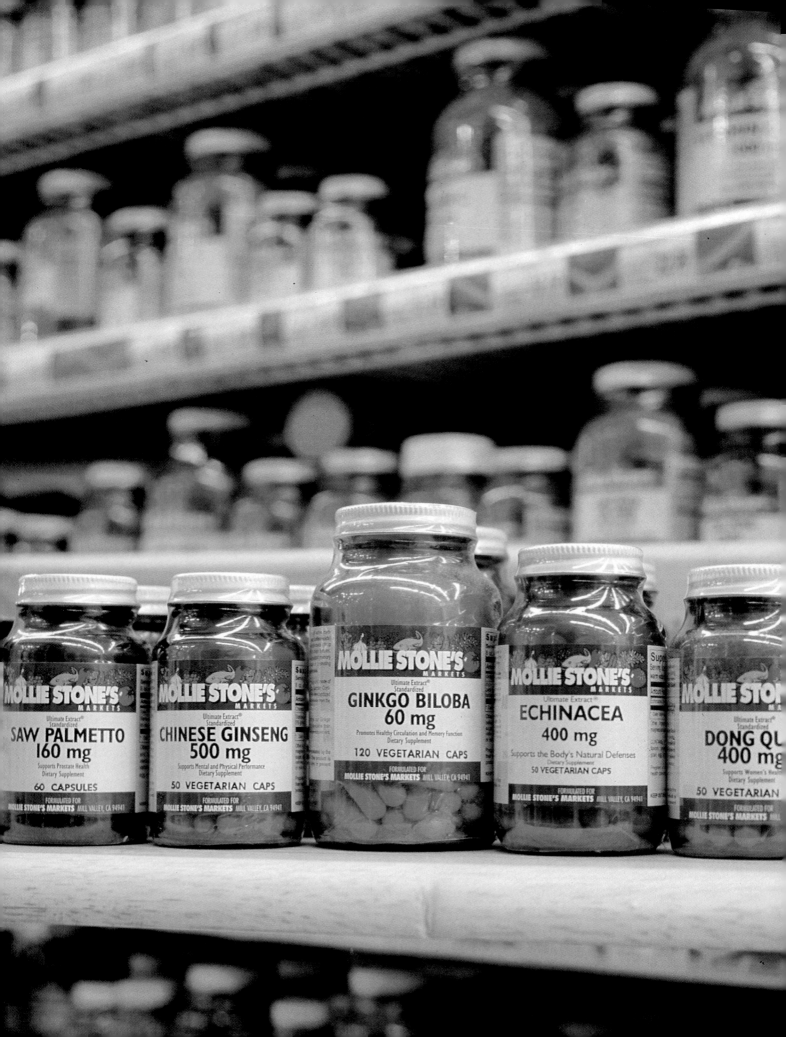

After reading this chapter, you should be able to

- Describe the basic premises of conventional medicine, and list the different types of conventional health care providers

- Explain how to choose and evaluate a primary care physician

- Describe the different types of complementary and alternative medicine, and explain their basic philosophies and treatments

- Explain how to choose and evaluate a practitioner of a complementary or alternative form of treatment

- Discuss both the safety issues associated with the use of complementary and alternative medicine and possible reasons for its appeal

Health Care: Conventional and Complementary Medicine

21

TEST YOUR KNOWLEDGE

1. The people most likely to use complementary and alternative medicine are those without a regular primary care physician.
   True or false?

2. Which practice or interest is shared by both conventional Western medicine and complementary and alternative medicine?
   a. careful observation of symptoms
   b. treatment with remedies derived from plants
   c. concern with the patient-physician relationship

3. Herbal remedies and dietary supplements like ginkgo and St. John's wort must meet FDA standards for safety and effectiveness before they can be put on the market.
   True or false?

4. About what percentage of Americans use some form of complementary and alternative medicine?
   a. 5%
   b. 25%
   c. 50%

5. Herbal remedies are from natural plant sources and are therefore safer than pharmaceutical drugs.
   True or false?

ANSWERS

1. **FALSE.** The more often a person visits a primary care physician, the more likely he or she is to use complementary and alternative medicine.

2. **ALL THREE.** Although there are profound philosophical differences between the approaches, they share many characteristics.

3. **FALSE.** Manufacturers are responsible for the safety of the dietary supplements they sell; the FDA has the power to restrict a product if it is found to pose a health risk after it is on the market. Manufacturers do not have to prove that their products are effective.

4. **B.** The most commonly used therapies are acupuncture, chiropractic, massage, and dietary supplements.

5. **FALSE.** Herbal remedies may contain substances that are toxic or that are not listed on the label, may have more or less of the active ingredient than claimed, may be contaminated, and may interact dangerously with prescription and over-the-counter drugs; they are not subject to the same strict controls as pharmaceutical drugs.

Have you ever visited a chiropractor, had acupuncture or a massage, or taken echinacea for a cold? If so, you are one of millions of Americans who have used **complementary and alternative medicine (CAM)**, defined as those therapies or practices that do not form part of conventional, or "mainstream," health care and medical practice as taught in most U.S. medical schools and offered in most U.S. hospitals. Consumer surveys and industry reports show that more and more people in the United States are using various forms of CAM (Table 21-1).

Consumers turn to CAM for a large variety of purposes related to health and well-being, such as boosting their immune system, lowering their cholesterol levels, losing weight, quitting smoking, or enhancing their memory. There are indications that people with chronic conditions, including cancer, asthma, autoimmune diseases, and HIV infection, are particularly likely to try CAM therapies. It has been estimated, for example, that up to 80% of patients suffering from arthritis, an autoimmune disorder, have tried various CAM approaches.

Despite their growing popularity, many CAM practices remain controversial, and individuals need to be critically aware of safety issues. In this chapter we examine the principles and providers of both conventional medicine and CAM, with particular attention to consumer issues.

Table 21-1   Use of Complementary and Alternative Therapies in the United States

	Percent Who Used Therapy at Least Once in Past 12 Months
Relaxation techniques	16.3
Herbal medicine	12.1
Massage	11.1
Chiropractic	11.0
Spiritual healing (by others)	7.0
Megavitamins	5.5
Self-help group	4.8
Imagery	4.5
Commercial diet	4.4
Folk remedies	4.2
Lifestyle diet	4.0
Energy healing	3.8
Homeopathy	3.4
Hypnosis	1.2
Biofeedback	1.0
Acupuncture	1.0
Any therapy	42.1

SOURCE: Eisenberg, D. M., et al. 1998. Trends in alternative medicine use in the United States, 1990–1997: Results of a follow-up national survey. *Journal of the American Medical Association* 280: 1569–1575.

Ww. THE RISE OF COMPLEMENTARY MEDICINE IN THE UNITED STATES

Over the past several millennia, every great culture has developed an extensive medical system—that is, a system for the diagnosis, treatment, and prevention of disease. The medical system you are likely to be most familiar with is **conventional medicine**, also called standard Western medicine or biomedicine. This is the dominant medical system in the United States, Europe, and other countries whose culture developed out of the Greek and Roman traditions.

Conventional medicine has historically viewed health as an absence of disease. It looks for the cause of illness in physical factors such as pathogens and biochemical imbalances, and it treats disease by destroying or otherwise acting on the identified or suspected cause. Scientific methods are used in diagnosis, and drugs, surgery, and radiation are the primary means of treatment. Areas of specialization include dentistry, dermatology, neurology, obstetrics and gynecology, ophthalmology, pediatrics, and many others.

Although conventional medicine is also taught and practiced in non-Western countries, many cultures have developed and continue to use medical systems based on philosophies and concepts very different from those of Western medicine. Today, many forms of medicine from Asia, as well as from indigenous systems of healing that developed in societies around the world, are being prac-

ticed in the United States and are becoming increasingly popular. These systems are referred to as **traditional medicine,** or, in the context of conventional Western medicine, complementary and alternative medicine.

These traditional systems and practices tend to view health more holistically, as a balance of body systems—mental, emotional, and spiritual, as well as physical. All aspects of the person are thought to be interrelated, forming an integrated system—a principle called **holism.** An imbalance or disharmony in any aspect can stress the body and lead to illness; the goal of traditional medicine is to strengthen the body's defenses and restore harmony. Examples of alternative therapies include acupuncture, massage, chiropractic, herbal therapies, homeopathy, and many others.

With the objective of encouraging scientific research on some of the more promising alternative therapies, the National Institutes of Health created the Office of Alternative Medicine in 1992. It was soon recognized that many people were using such "alternative" approaches in addition to conventional medical treatments, rather than in their place. In other words, they wanted to complement, not replace, conventional medical practices. Thus, the term "complementary and alternative" has become accepted to describe therapies that are not currently considered mainstream health care practices in the United States. Accordingly, the Office of Alternative Medicine has been renamed the National Center for Complementary and Alternative Medicine (NCCAM).

Currently, many Americans use some form of CAM; the most commonly used therapies are relaxation techniques, herbal medicine, massage, and chiropractic. Users of CAM tend to have higher-than-average incomes and levels of education; they typically have conditions not easily treated by conventional medicine, such as chronic pain, HIV infection, cancer, or mental health problems like depression or anxiety. People often use CAM therapies in addition to their conventional medical treatments, but they may be reluctant to tell their physicians about it.

Some of the treatments that are regarded as outside mainstream U.S. medical practices, such as acupuncture, already form part of standard medical care in several other Western countries. In many of these countries, a variety of other CAM approaches, such as acupressure, botanical remedies, homeopathy, and mind-body therapies, are also more widely accepted as part of conventional medical treatment than they are in the United States. It can be expected that, as scientific evidence proves certain CAM practices to be safe and effective, they will eventually cease to be considered "complementary or alternative." Instead, they will be integrated into a comprehensive approach to treating patients.

It is also worth noting that for large portions of the world population, CAM is neither complementary nor alternative. The World Health Organization estimates that 80% of the world population lives in developing countries and that 80% of those people either have no access to or choose not to use standard Western medicine. Instead, they turn to traditional medicine for their primary health care. One of the reasons U.S. government agencies and the World Health Organization actively encourage research on CAM therapies is the hope that some of them might offer effective and fairly inexpensive ways of treating people in developing countries. For example, the millions of AIDS patients in sub-Saharan Africa, most of whom do not have access to Western AIDS drugs, might be able to obtain some benefit from CAM treatments.

Before we consider the various types of CAM, let's take a closer look at the practice of conventional medicine in the United States, including a brief look at its underlying philosophy and assumptions.

CONVENTIONAL MEDICINE

Referring to conventional medicine as "standard Western medicine" draws attention to the fact that it differs from the various medical systems that have developed in China, Japan, India, and other parts of the world. Calling it "bio-medicine" reflects the concept that conventional medicine is based on the findings of a variety of biological sciences.

Premises and Assumptions of Conventional Medicine

One of the important characteristics of Western medicine is the belief that disease is caused by identifiable physical factors. This belief can be traced back to Hippocrates, the Greek physician of the fourth century B.C. who is credited with placing the practice of medicine on a scientific footing. Hippocrates attacked the idea that disease was caused by spirits or gods and suggested instead that it could be caused by such internal and external factors as climate and diet. He advocated a reliance on careful observation of symptoms, experimentation, and attention to cause and effect. The form of medicine invented by Hippocrates and other Greek physicians was referred to as "rational medicine" because of its focus on facts and observable phenomena.

In Hippocrates' time, the causes of disease were thought to include the interplay of various forces and elements; today, Western medicine identifies the causes of disease as pathogens, such as bacteria and viruses, genetic factors, and unhealthy lifestyles that result in changes at the molecular and cellular levels. In most cases, however, the focus is primarily on the physical causes of the illness rather than mental or spiritual imbalance.

Another feature that distinguishes Western biomedicine from other medical systems is the concept that every disease is defined by a certain set of symptoms and that these symptoms are similar in most patients suffering from this disease. Western medicine tends to treat illness as an isolated biological disturbance that can occur in any human being, rather than as integral in some way to the individual with the illness.

Related to the idea of illness as the result of invasion by outside factors is the strong orientation toward methods of

complementary and alternative medicine (CAM) Therapies or practices that are not part of conventional or mainstream health care and medical practice as taught in most U.S. medical schools and available at most U.S. health care facilities; examples of CAM practices include acupuncture, herbal remedies, and homeopathy.

conventional medicine A system of medicine based on the application of the scientific method; diseases are thought to be caused by identifiable physical factors and characterized by a representative set of symptoms; also called biomedicine or standard Western medicine.

traditional medicine Medical systems that have developed in many non-Western cultures; also referred to as complementary and alternative medicine.

holism The principle that all aspects of a person are interrelated and form an integrated system.

Terms

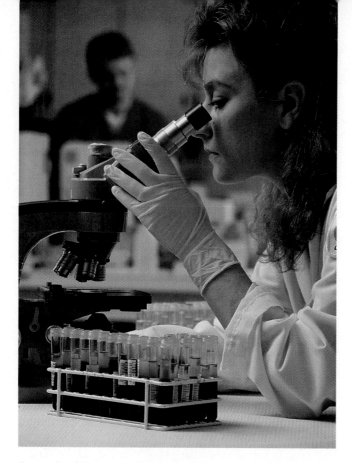

Conventional Western medicine is firmly grounded in scientific explanations resulting from the application of the scientific method to a question or problem. The identification of viruses, bacteria, and other microorganisms as a key cause of disease led to many public health measures and treatments that reduced deaths from infectious diseases in the United States.

Finally, Western medicine is based on scientific ways of obtaining knowledge and explaining phenomena. Scientific explanations result from the application of the scientific method to a question or problem; they have a blend of characteristics that set them apart from other types of explanation, such as those based on common sense, faith, belief, or authority. Scientific explanations are

- *Empirical*—they are based on the evidence of the senses and on objective and systematic observation, often carried out under carefully controlled conditions; they must be capable of verification by others.
- *Rational*—they follow the rules of logic and are consistent with known facts.
- *Testable*—either they are verifiable through direct observation or they lead to predictions about what should occur under conditions not yet observed.
- *Parsimonious*—they explain phenomena with the fewest number of assumptions.
- *General*—they have broad explanatory power.
- *Rigorously evaluated*—they are constantly evaluated for consistency with the evidence and known principles, for parsimony, and for generality.
- *Tentative*—scientists are willing to entertain the possibility that their explanations are faulty.

The scientific method is both a way of acquiring knowledge and a way of thinking, of approaching a problem by carefully defining its parameters, seeking out relevant information, and subjecting proposed solutions to rigorous testing.

Western medicine translates the scientific method into practice through the research process, a highly refined and well-established approach to exploring the causes of disease and ensuring the safety and efficacy of treatments. Research studies range from case studies—descriptions of a single patient's illness and treatment—to clinical trials conducted on large populations and carried out under carefully controlled conditions over a period of many years. The process of drug development is equally rigorous. Drugs are developed and tested through an elaborate course that begins with preliminary research in the lab and continues through trials with human participants, review and approval by the FDA, and monitoring of the drug's effects after it is on the market (Figure 21-1). The process may take 12 years or more, and only about 20% of drugs for which applications are filed are eventually approved.

When results of research studies are published in medical journals, a community of scientists, physicians, researchers, and scholars have the opportunity to share the findings and enter a dialogue about the subject. Publication of research often prompts further research designed to replicate and confirm the findings, challenge the conclusions, or pursue a related line of thought or experiment. (For guidelines on how to interpret research when

destroying pathogens or preventing them from causing serious infection. The public health measures of the nineteenth and twentieth centuries—chlorination of drinking water, sewage disposal, food safety regulations, vaccination programs, education about hygiene, and so on—are an outgrowth of this kind of orientation. (As described in Chapter 1, these public health measures are largely responsible for the 25-year increase in life expectancy that Americans have experienced in the twentieth century.)

The implementation of public health measures is one way to control pathogens; another is the use of drugs. The discovery and development of sulfa drugs, antibiotics, and steroids in the twentieth century, along with advances in chemistry that made it possible to identify the active ingredients in common herbal remedies, paved the way for the current close identification of Western medicine with **pharmaceuticals** (medical drugs, both prescription and over-the-counter). Western medicine also relies heavily on surgery and on advanced medical technology to discover the physical causes of disease and to remove or destroy them.

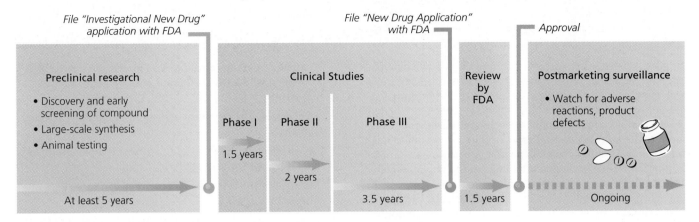

Figure 21-1 Timeline for drug development. Once preclinical research indicates that a drug is both safe and effective, it can be tested in humans. In Phase I trials, a small group of healthy human volunteers is given the treatment to screen it for safety and to establish a maximum safe dose. In Phase II trials, a small group of patients with the condition the drug is supposed to improve is given the treatment to help screen for adverse effects and to determine appropriate dosages. In Phase III trials, a larger group of patients is given the treatment to determine if it is effective and what the common side effects are. Researchers and the FDA have made efforts to shorten the process, but thorough drug testing takes many years. SOURCE: Timeline for drug development. 2000. *Scientific American*, April.

it is reported in the popular press, see the box "Evaluating Health News.")

The assumptions of conventional medicine are so basic to Western culture that we may not even recognize them as ideas or premises. They become clearer when we examine some of the very different assumptions of alternative and complementary practices.

The Providers of Conventional Medicine

Conventional medicine is practiced by a wide range of health care professionals in the United States. Several kinds of professionals are permitted to practice medicine independently; these include medical doctors, osteopaths, podiatrists, optometrists, and dentists.

• **Medical doctors** are practitioners who hold a doctor of medicine (M.D.) degree from an accredited medical school. In the United States, an education in medicine has several stages: four years of premedical education in a college or university, with an emphasis on the sciences; four years of medical school, which teaches basic medical skills and awards the M.D. degree; graduate medical study, called a residency and lasting from three to eight years, during which a specialty is chosen and studied and a medical license is obtained; and continuing medical education to keep abreast of advances in medical science. Twenty-three medical specialties are currently approved by the American Board of Medical Specialties, each with its own rule-making and certifying body. The larger specialties are further divided into subspecialties; for example, internal medicine includes such subspecialties as cardiology and gastroenterology

(see the box "Selected Medical Specialties"). Becoming a subspecialist generally requires several more years of formal training after the completion of a residency.

• **Doctors of osteopathic medicine** (D.O.) receive a medical education similar to that of medical doctors, but their training places special emphasis on musculoskeletal problems and manipulative therapy. M.D.s and D.O.s are the two types of "complete" physicians in the United States, meaning they are fully trained and licensed to perform surgery and prescribe medication. D.O.s are graduates of osteopathic medical schools, which emphasize training students to be primary care physicians and to practice a "whole person" approach to medicine.

• **Podiatrists** are practitioners who specialize in the medical and surgical care of the feet. They hold a doctor of podiatric medicine (D.P.M.) degree; the length of training is similar to that of M.D.s. They can prescribe drugs and perform surgery on the feet.

Health-related research is now described in popular newspapers and magazines rather than just medical journals, meaning that more and more people have access to the information. Greater access is certainly a plus, but news reports of research studies may oversimplify both the results and what those results mean to the average person. Researchers do not set out to mislead people, but they must often strike a balance between reporting promising preliminary findings to the public, thereby allowing people to act on them, and waiting 10–20 years until long-term studies confirm (or disprove) a particular theory.

All this can leave you in a difficult position. You cannot become an expert on all subjects, capable of effectively evaluating all the available health news. However, the following questions can help you better assess the health advice that appears in the popular media:

1.   *Is the report based on research or on an anecdote?* Information or advice based on one or more carefully designed research studies has more validity than one person's experiences.

2.   *What is the source of the information?* A study published in a respected peer-reviewed journal has been examined by editors and other researchers in the field, people who are in a position to evaluate the merits of a study and its results. Research presented at medical meetings should be considered very preliminary because the results have not yet undergone a thorough pre-publication review. It is also wise to ask who funded a study to determine whether there is any potential for bias. Information from government agencies and national research organizations is usually considered fairly reliable.

3.   *How big was the study?* A study that involves many subjects is more likely to yield reliable results than a study involving only a few people. Another important indication that a finding is meaningful is if several different studies yield the same results.

4.   *Who were the participants involved in the study?* Research findings are more likely to apply to you if you share important characteristics with the participants of the study. For example, the results of a study on men over age 50 who smoke may not be particularly meaningful for a 30-year-old nonsmoking woman. Even less applicable are studies done in test tubes or on animals. Such research should be considered very preliminary in terms of its applicability to humans. Promising results from laboratory or animal research frequently cannot be replicated in human study subjects.

5.   *What kind of study was it?* Epidemiological studies involve observation or interviews in order to trace the relationship among lifestyle, physical characteristics, and diseases. While epidemiological studies can suggest links, they cannot establish cause-and-effect relationships. Clinical or interventional studies or trials involve testing the effects of different treatments on groups of people who have similar lifestyles and characteristics. They are more likely to provide conclusive evidence of a cause-and-effect relationship. The best interventional studies share the following characteristics:

- *Controlled.* A group of people who receive the treatment is compared with a matched group who do not receive the treatment.

- *Randomized.* The treatment and control groups are selected randomly.

- *Double-blind.* Researchers and participants are unaware of who is receiving the treatment.

- *Multicenter.* The experiment is performed at more than one institution.

A third type of study, meta-analysis, involves combining the results of individual studies to get an overall view of the effectiveness of a treatment.

6.   *What do the statistics really say?* First, are the results described as "statistically significant"? If a study is large and well designed, its results can be deemed statistically significant, meaning there is less than a 5% chance that the findings resulted from chance. Second, are the results stated in terms of relative or absolute risk? Many findings are reported in terms of relative risk—how a particular treatment or condition affects a person's disease risk. Consider the following examples of relative risk:

- According to some estimates, taking estrogen without progesterone can increase a postmenopausal woman's risk of dying from endometrial cancer by 233%.

- Giving AZT to HIV-infected pregnant women reduces prenatal transmission of HIV by about 90%.

The first of these two findings seems far more dramatic than the second—until one also considers absolute risk, the actual risk of the illness in the population being considered. The absolute risk of endometrial cancer is 0.3%; a 233% increase based on the effects of estrogen raises it to 1%, a change of 0.7%. Without treatment, about 25% of infants born to HIV-infected women will be infected with HIV; with treatment, the absolute risk drops to about 2%, a change of 23%. Because the absolute risk of an HIV-infected mother passing the virus to her infant is so much greater than a woman's risk of developing endometrial cancer (25% compared with 0.3%), a smaller change in relative risk translates into a much greater change in absolute risk.

7.   *Is new health advice being offered?* If the media report new guidelines for health behavior or medical treatment, examine the source. Government agencies and national research foundations usually consider a great deal of evidence before offering health advice. Above all, use common sense, and check with your physician before making a major change in your health habits based on news reports.

SOURCES: Medical research: Finding the best information. 2000. *Journal of the American Medical Association* 284(10): 1336. Medicine and the media. 1999. *Harvard Women's Health Watch,* February. Medical hype: How to read between the lines. 1998. *Consumer Reports on Health,* October. Making sense of health research. 1998. *Healthline,* May.

The following are some of the approved general specialties recognized by the American Board of Medical Specialties.

Allergy and immunology   Evaluation and management of disorders involving the immune system, including asthma, adverse food and drug reactions, and immune deficiency diseases.

Anesthesiology   Pain relief and maintenance of a stable condition during and immediately following an operation or other medical procedure.

Dermatology   Diagnosis and treatment of benign and malignant disorders of the skin, mouth, external genitalia, hair, and nails, as well as a number of STDs.

Emergency medicine   Immediate initial recognition, evaluation, and treatment of patients in response to acute illness and injury.

Family practice   Prevention, diagnosis, and treatment of a wide variety of conditions in patients of all ages, with special emphasis on caring for families on a continuing basis.

Internal medicine   Long-term, comprehensive care of both common illnesses and complex problems of adolescents, adults, and the elderly; subspecialties of internal medicine include cardiology, endocrinology (care of glandular and metabolic disorders), gastroenterology (care of problems of the digestive tract), geriatric medicine, hematology (focusing on diseases of the blood, spleen, and lymph glands), and sports medicine.

Neurology   Diagnosis and treatment of disease or impaired function of the brain, spinal cord, peripheral nerves, muscles, and autonomic nervous system.

Obstetrics and gynecology   Medical and surgical care of the female reproductive system and associated disorders.

Ophthalmology   Diagnosis and medical or surgical treatment of all problems affecting the eyes and visual pathways.

Pathology   Diagnosis and monitoring of disease by means of information gathered from microscopic examination of tissue specimens, cells, and body fluids and from clinical laboratory tests.

Pediatrics   Care of the physical, emotional, and social health of children from birth to young adulthood; services range from preventive care to the diagnosis and treatment of acute and chronic diseases.

Plastic surgery   Repair, reconstruction, or replacements of physical defects of form or function involving the skin, musculoskeletal system, face and head, hands, breast, trunk, extremities, and external genitalia.

Psychiatry   Prevention, diagnosis, and treatment of mental, addictive, and emotional disorders.

Radiology   Diagnosis and treatment of disease using radiologic methods such as X ray, ultrasonography, and computed tomography.

Surgery (general)   Diagnosis and surgical care for conditions affecting almost any area of the body.

Urology   Medical and surgical care of benign and malignant disorders of the adrenal gland and reproductive and urinary systems.

Information on physicians, including their training and board certification, is available from a variety of sources, including the American Medical Association, the American Board of Medical Specialties, and the American Osteopathic Association (see For More Information at the end of the chapter).

SOURCE: American Board of Medical Specialties. 2000. *Approved ABMS Specialty Boards and Certificate Categories* (http://www.abms.org/certs1.html; retrieved July 20, 2000).

• **Optometrists** are practitioners trained to examine the eyes, detect eye diseases, and treat vision problems. They hold a doctor of optometry (O.D.) degree. All states permit optometrists to use drugs for diagnostic purposes, and most permit them to use drugs to treat minor eye problems. (Ophthamologists are M.D. eye specialists who care for all types of eye problems and can perform eye surgery.)

• **Dentists** specialize in the care of the teeth and mouth. They are graduates of four-year dental schools and hold the doctor of dental surgery (D.D.S.) or doctor of medical dentistry (D.M.D.) degree. Those who wish to become specialists receive additional education. Dentists can perform surgery and prescribe drugs within the scope of their training. (Care of the teeth and mouth is an area where individual effort makes a huge difference; see the box "Caring for Your Teeth and Gums.")

In addition to these practitioners, there are millions of other trained health care professionals, known as **allied health care providers,** working in the United States. Some of them are licensed to work independently; others are permitted to work under medical supervision or medical referral. They include registered nurses (R.N.),

optometrist A practitioner who holds a doctor of optometry degree and is trained to examine the eyes, detect eye diseases, and prescribe corrective lenses.

dentist A practitioner who holds a doctor of medical dentistry or doctor of dental surgery degree and who specializes in the prevention and treatment of diseases and injuries of the teeth, mouth, and jaws.

allied health care providers Health care professionals who typically provide services under the supervision or control of independent practitioners.

Terms

The health of your teeth and gums has a major impact on your quality of life. Good dental health requires teamwork between you and your dentist. Regular dental visits are not likely to result in healthy teeth and gums if you don't care for your own teeth on a daily basis. Likewise, even if you are diligent about keeping your teeth clean, you still need regular visits to the dentist, preferably twice each year. Here are some tips on how to do your part in keeping your teeth and gums in top condition.

Brushing

Brush your teeth at least twice a day, in the morning and before bed; if possible, also brush after each meal and snack. Choose a soft-bristled brush of a size and shape that allows you to reach all areas of your mouth easily. Use a toothpaste that contains fluoride, a mineral that helps protect your teeth from decay.

- Place the toothbrush at a 45-degree angle where your gums meet your teeth. Press gently and move the brush back and forth in short (tooth-wide) strokes.

- Brush all the surfaces—inner, outer, and chewing—of each tooth. Brush for at least three minutes.

- Hold the brush vertically and use the "toe" of the brush to clean the inner surfaces of the front teeth, using a gentle up-and-down stroke.

- Brush your tongue to remove bacteria and freshen breath, and then rinse your mouth with water.

Flossing

Because there are many areas of your teeth that a toothbrush can't reach, flossing is a critical step for preventing gum disease. Use a piece of floss about 18 inches long, and hold it tightly between your thumbs and forefingers; take up used, dirty floss by winding it around one of your middle fingers.

- Guide the floss between your teeth using a gentle motion; never snap floss into the gums. Run the floss up and down both sides of each tooth.

- When the floss reaches the gum line, curve it into a C shape against one tooth, and gently slide it into the space between the gum and the tooth. Hold the floss tightly against the tooth, and gently rub the side of the tooth with up and down motions.

- Repeat this process on each tooth, remembering the back side of your last tooth.

Flossing is a learned skill that gets easier with practice. If you have difficulty handling dental floss, you may be able to use another kind of interdental cleaner such as a pick or a special brush. If you use one of these cleaners, ask your dentist about how to do it properly to avoid injuring your gums.

---

licensed vocational nurses (L.V.N.), physical therapists, social workers, registered dietitians (R.D.), physician assistants (P.A.), nurse practitioners, and certified nurse midwives.

WWW. Choosing a Primary Care Physician

Most experts believe it is best to have a primary care physician, someone who gets to know you, who coordinates your medical care, and who refers you to specialists when you need them. Primary care physicians include those certified in family practice, internal medicine, pediatrics, and obstetrics-gynecology. These physicians are able to diagnose and treat the vast majority of common health problems; they also provide many preventive health services. The best time to look for a physician is before you are sick.

To select a physician, begin by making a list of possible choices. If your insurance limits the health care providers you can see, check the plan's list first. Ask for recommendations from family, friends, coworkers, local medical societies, and the physician referral service at a local clinic or hospital. Some clinics provide brief biographies of physicians on staff who are taking new patients. If you have a particular health problem, you may want to identify physicians who are board-certified in appropriate spe-

cialties. Once you have a list of possible physicians, find out if a consumer or other independent group has rated doctors in your area; this will help you check on the quality of care they provide.

Once you have the names of a few physicians you might want to try, call their offices to find out information such as the following:

- Is the physician covered by your health plan and accepting new patients?

- What are the office hours, and when is the physician or office staff available? What do patients do if they need urgent care or have an emergency?

- Which hospitals does the physician use?

- How many other physicians are available to "cover" when he or she isn't available, and who are they?

- How long does it usually take to get a routine appointment?

- Does the office send reminders about preventive tests such as Pap tests?

- Does the physician (or a nurse or physician assistant) give advice over the phone for common medical problems?

Finally, schedule a visit with the physician you think you would most like to use. During that first visit, you'll get a sense of how well matched you are and how well he or she might meet your medical needs. After the visit, consider the following:

- Do you feel you were listened to, and did you have a chance to ask questions?
- Do you feel you were treated with respect and made to feel comfortable?
- Do you understand what the physician told you, and did he or she spend enough time with you?
- Do you feel that the physician addressed your health problems or concerns, and do you feel comfortable with the recommended course of action?

Although you may want to give the relationship some time to develop, you should trust your own reactions when deciding whether a particular health care provider is the right one for you.

Choosing a Medical Facility

Choosing a medical facility depends on the type and urgency of the problem as well as health insurance coverage and other financial considerations. For college students, the best choice is usually the student health center. Individuals in managed-care programs usually receive care at their physician's private medical office or clinic. Most communities have urgent care or ambulatory care centers where patients can get medical attention when their regular physician's office or clinic is closed. For serious emergencies, a hospital emergency room is the best choice (see Chapter 22 for guidelines on when to go to the emergency room).

Not all hospitals are alike. Many specialize in the care of patients with specific types of medical problems. For example, some hospitals have trauma centers where surgeons and other specialists are always available to treat individuals with very severe injuries; other hospitals may have burn units, units that specialize in organ transplantation, or nurseries that can care for very premature infants. Large hospitals, especially those that are affiliated with a medical school, often have multiple special services for patients with more complex medical problems.

COMMUNICATE! Drug manufacturers try to sell their products directly to the public through their advertising, whether for over-the-counter medications, prescription drugs, or dietary supplements. Critically examine and evaluate an ad in a magazine or on TV for a health-related product or service. What is the manufacturer communicating about the product and about health in general? What underlying premises can you discern in the way the product is presented and the promises the manufacturer makes? Does the ad contain any hidden messages? Are there any aspects of the ad you feel are misleading? Do you find it easy or difficult to resist the appeal of the ad and the product?

W. COMPLEMENTARY AND ALTERNATIVE MEDICINE

Where conventional Western medicine tends to focus on the body, on the physical causes of disease, and on ways to eradicate pathogens in order to restore health, traditional medicine tends to focus on an integration of mind, body, and spirit and to seek ways to restore the whole person to harmony so that he or she can regain health. Where conventional medicine is based on science, traditional medicine tends to be based on accumulated experience.

Many alternative medical systems with long-standing traditions have concepts and theories of medicine that are very different from those making up current Western medical thought. Some people consider all of CAM "quackery" and tell you that you can recognize a quack by his or her use of "pseudoscientific" language. However, the use of phrases like "bringing into harmony with nature" or "enhancing the flow of vital energy" does not necessarily mean that a practitioner is a quack; rather, it may reflect this practitioner's different concept of health and healing.

You might have heard that there are only anecdotal reports and testimonials to support the value of many forms of CAM and that because such reports do not constitute scientific proof of effectiveness, they are therefore meaningless. Although it is correct that anecdotes and testimonials cannot be considered scientifically reliable evidence, that does not mean that they are meaningless. What is called "anecdotal evidence" can actually be a form of case report, a valuable and standard form of study in which a researcher describes a single patient, his or her medical history, the treatments administered, and the outcome of the case. Still, case reports alone are not sufficient to scientifically prove the effectiveness of a medical treatment. Caution is in order when choosing any mode of treatment that has not been scientifically evaluated for safety and effectiveness (see the box "Avoiding Health Fraud and Quackery").

NCCAM groups CAM practices into five domains: alternative medical systems, mind-body interventions, biological-based therapies, manipulative and body-based methods, and energy therapies (Figure 21-2). It is impossible to discuss all of these forms fully in a single chapter. Instead, what follows is a general introduction to the types of CAM available and a brief description of some of the more widely used ones. To learn more about any of these approaches, consult the For More Information section at the end of the chapter.

Alternative Medical Systems

Many cultures elaborated complete systems of medical philosophy, theory, and practice long before the current biomedical approach was developed. The complete systems that are best known in the United States are probably traditional Chinese medicine (TCM), also known as

According to the Federal Trade Commission, consumers waste billions of dollars on unproven, fraudulently marketed, and sometimes useless health care products and treatments. In addition, those with serious medical problems may waste valuable time before seeking proper treatment. Worse yet, some of the products they're buying may cause serious harm. Health fraud is a business that sells false hope. It preys on people who are victims of diseases that have no medical cure and on people who want shortcuts to weight loss or improvements to personal appearance.

The first rule of thumb for evaluating any health claim is that if it sounds too good to be true, it probably is. Also, be on the lookout for the typical phrases and marketing techniques fraudulent promoters use to deceive consumers:

- The product is advertised as a quick and effective cure-all for a wide range of ailments.

- The promoters use words like *scientific breakthrough, miraculous cure, exclusive product, secret ingredient,* or *ancient remedy.* Also remember that just because a product is described as "natural" or unprocessed does not necessarily mean it's safe.

- The text is written in "medicalese"—impressive-sounding terminology to disguise a lack of good science.

- The promoter claims the government, the medical profession, or research scientists have conspired to suppress the product.

- The advertisement includes undocumented case histories claiming amazing results.

- The product is advertised as available from only one source, and payment is required in advance.

- The promoter promises a no-risk "money-back guarantee." Be aware that many fly-by-night operators are not around to respond to your request for a refund.

To check out a particular product, talk to a physician or another health care professional and to family members and friends. Be wary of treatments offered by people who tell you to avoid talking to others. Check with the Better Business Bureau or local attorney general's office to see whether other consumers have lodged complaints about the product or the product's marketer. You can also check with the appropriate health professional group. For example, check with the American Diabetes Association or the National Arthritis Foundation if the products are promoted for diabetes or arthritis.

If you think you have been a victim of health fraud or if you have an adverse reaction that you think is related to a particular supplement, you can report it to the appropriate agency:

- *False advertising claims:* Contact the FTC by phone (877-FTC-HELP); by mail (Consumer Response Center, Federal Trade Commission, Washington, DC 20580); or online (http://www.ftc.gov; click on Complaint form). You can also contact your state attorney general's office, your state department of health, or the local consumer protection agency (check your local telephone directory).

- *False labeling on a product:* Contact the FDA district office consumer complaint coordinator for your geographic area. (The FDA regulates safety, manufacturing, and product labeling.)

- *Adverse reaction to a supplement:* Call a doctor or other health care provider immediately. You may also report your adverse reaction to FDA MedWatch by calling 800-FDA-1088 or by visiting the MedWatch Web site (http://www.fda.gov/medwatch/report/hcp.htm)

SOURCES: Federal Trade Commission. 1999. *Fraudulent Health Claims: Don't Be Fooled.* Washington, D.C.: Federal Trade Commission. Kurtzweil, P. 1999. How to spot health fraud. *FDA Consumer,* November/December. Food and Drug Administration. 1999. *How to Report Adverse Reactions and Other Problems with Products Regulated by FDA* (http://www.fda.gov/opacom/backgrounders/problem.html; retrieved July 19, 2000).

traditional Oriental medicine, and homeopathy. Traditional medical systems have also been developed in many other regions of the world, including North, Central, and South America; the Middle East; India; Tibet; and Australia. In many countries, these medical approaches continue to be used today—frequently alongside Western medicine and quite often by physicians trained in Western medicine.

Alternative medical systems tend to have concepts in common, perhaps because of contact between the Mediterranean area, the Middle East, India, and China in ancient times. For example, the concept of life force or energy exists in many cultures. In traditional Chinese medicine, the life force contained in all living things is called *qi* (sometimes spelled chi). Qi resembles the *vis vitalis* (Latin for "life force") of Greek, Roman, and European medical systems, and *prana* of Ayurveda, the traditional medical system of India.

Most traditional medical systems think of disease as a disturbance or imbalance not just of physical processes but also of forces and energies within the body, the mind, and the spirit. Treatment aims at reestablishing equilibrium, balance, and harmony. In traditional Chinese medicine, for example, the principle of balance is expressed as yin and yang, which are opposites yet complement each other. Disease is a disturbance of qi reflecting an imbalance between yin and yang; treatment aims at restoring equilibrium.

Because the whole patient, rather than an isolated set of symptoms, is treated in most comprehensive alternative medical systems, it is rare that only a single treatment approach is used. Most commonly, multiple techniques

Domain	Characteristics	Examples
Alternative Medical Systems	Involve complete systems of theory and practice that have evolved independently of and often long before the conventional biomedical approach	Traditional Chinese medicine; Kampo; Ayurveda (India); Native American, Aboriginal, African, Middle-Eastern, Tibetan, Central and South American medical systems; homeopathy; naturopathy
Mind-Body Interventions	Employ a variety of techniques designed to make it possible for the mind to affect bodily function and symptoms	Meditation, certain uses of hypnosis, prayer, mental healing
Biological-Based Therapies	Include natural and biologically based practices, interventions, and products, many of which overlap with conventional medicine's use of dietary supplements	Herbal, special dietary, orthomolecular,* and individual biological therapies
Manipulative and Body-Based Methods	Include methods that are based on manipulation and/or movement of the body	Chiropractic, osteopathy, massage therapy
Energy Therapies	Focus on energy fields within the body (biofields) or from other sources (electromagnetic fields)	Qi gong, Reiki, therapeutic touch, bioelectromagnetic-based therapies

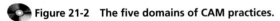

*Orthomolecular therapies are treatments of diseases with varying, but usually high, concentrations of chemicals, including minerals (e.g., magnesium), hormones (e.g., melatonin), or vitamins.

Figure 21-2   The five domains of CAM practices.

and methods are employed and are continually adjusted according to the changes in the patient's health status that occur naturally or are brought about by the treatment. For example, in traditional Chinese medicine, a patient might be treated with acupuncture, herbal medicine, massage, and qigong, a type of energy therapy.

Traditional Chinese Medicine (TCM)   **Traditional Chinese medicine (TCM)** is based on highly abstract concepts; a sophisticated set of techniques and methods; and individualized diagnosis, treatment, and prevention. No identical diseases exist in TCM. Two patients with the same diagnosis in Western medicine will get different diagnoses in TCM and will be given different treatments.

In TCM, the free and harmonious flow of qi produces health—a positive feeling of well-being and vitality in body, mind, and spirit. Illness occurs when the flow of qi is blocked or disturbed. TCM works to restore and balance the flow of blocked qi; the goal is not only to treat illnesses but also to increase energy, prevent disease, and support the immune system.

Two of the primary treatment methods in TCM are herbal remedies and **acupuncture.** Chinese herbal remedies number about 5,800 and include plant products, animal parts, and minerals. Herbal remedies, like everything else, have yin and yang properties. When a disease is perceived to be due to a yin deficiency, remedies with more

yin characteristics might be used for treatment. Since yin and yang are interconnected, an overbalance in the opposite direction needs to be avoided. Therefore, small amounts of herbs with yang characteristics are likely to also be added. The use of a single medicinal botanical is rare in Chinese herbal medicine; rather, several different plants are combined in very precise proportions, often to make a tea or soup. For example, a remedy might include a primary herb that targets the main symptom, a second herb that enhances the effects of the primary herb, a third that lessens side effects, and a fourth that helps deliver ingredients to a particular body site.

Acupuncture works to correct disturbances in the flow of qi through the insertion of long, thin needles at appropriate points in the skin. Qi is believed to flow through the body along several meridians, or pathways, and there are approximately 360 acupuncture points located along these meridians. Acupuncturists use a variety of diagnostic

traditional Chinese medicine (TCM) The traditional medical system of China, which views illness as the result of a disturbance in the flow of qi, the life force; therapies include acupuncture, herbal medicine, and massage.

acupuncture Insertion of long, thin needles into the skin at points along meridians, pathways through which qi is believed to flow; needles correct imbalances in qi; a practice common in traditional Chinese medicine.

Terms

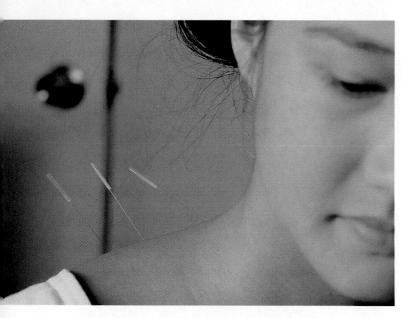

Acupuncture is one of the key treatment methods in traditional Chinese medicine. It involves the insertion of long, thin needles at appropriate points in the skin to restore balance to the flow of qi.

techniques to identify the nature of the imbalance in a patient and to choose the points at which acupuncture needs to be applied. The traditional method consists of inserting the needle and then manipulating it manually, but other means of manipulation, such as heat, pressure, friction, suction, or electric stimulation, can also be used.

In addition to treating internal problems, needles can also work on external injuries. Needles inserted near the area of a pulled tendon or overstrained muscle will increase qi flow to relieve pain and quicken the healing process. The points chosen for acupuncture are highly individualized for each patient, and they change over the course of treatment as the patient's health status changes.

The World Health Organization has compiled a list of over 40 conditions in which acupuncture may be beneficial. At a conference called by the National Institutes of Health (NIH), a panel of experts recently analyzed the available information on the scientific evidence for the efficacy of acupuncture in many of these conditions. Their conclusions were published as an NIH consensus statement, "consensus" meaning an agreement reached by experts in a given field. These experts found evidence that acupuncture was effective in relieving nausea and vomiting after chemotherapy and pain after surgery, including dental surgery. They added, however, that there is not yet enough evidence to show that acupuncture is effective for

headaches, menstrual cramps, tennis elbow, back pain, carpal tunnel syndrome, asthma, or other conditions. Western researchers typically use a different framework for understanding the effects of acupuncture. For example, they might explain pain relief not in terms of qi but in terms of stimulation of the central nervous system and release of hormones and neurotransmitters.

Although more than 1 million Americans receive acupuncture each year, there have been few adverse events (negative effects) associated with it in the United States. Nonetheless, problems can occur from the improper insertion and manipulation of needles and from the use of unsterile needles. The FDA regulates acupuncture needles like other standard medical devices and requires that they be sterile. Most acupuncture practitioners follow these regulations, but, if you consider acupuncture, you should ask your practitioner about the relative risks of the procedure and the safety practices he or she observes. A majority of states require some form of licensing or credentialing for practitioners of acupuncture, but the requirements for licensure vary widely.

Homeopathy　An alternative medical system of Western origin, **homeopathy** was developed about 200 years ago by the German physician Samuel Hahnemann (1755–1843) and is based on two main principles: "like cures like," and remedies become more effective with greater dilution. "Like cures like" summarizes the concept that a substance that produces the symptoms of an illness or disease in a healthy person can cure the illness when given in very minute quantities. Remedies containing very small quantities of a particular substance are obtained by repeatedly diluting the original solution. The extent of dilution varies, but the final extract is often so dilute that few, if any, of the original molecules are left in it. According to homeopathic thinking, such highly diluted extracts not only retain some form of biological activity but actually become more potent.

Over 1000 different substances (plant and animal parts, minerals, and chemicals) can be used to prepare homeopathic remedies, and each of these substances is thought to have different effects at different dilutions. That means a homeopath must not only choose the correct remedy for a particular patient but also decide on the specific dilution of that remedy in order to achieve the desired effect.

Like other traditional systems of medicine, homeopathy constitutes a highly individualized form of therapy; that is, the treatment of each patient is determined by the overall condition of the patient rather than by specific symptoms. In order to assess a patient's condition, homeopaths generally spend quite a bit of time talking with a patient and assessing his or her physical, psychological, and emotional health before deciding on the correct remedy at the proper dilution. This intensive interaction between the practitioner and the patient might play an im-

Terms

homeopathy An alternative medical system of Western origin in which illnesses are treated by giving very small doses of drugs that in larger doses in a healthy person would produce symptoms like those of the illness.

A placebo is a chemically inactive substance or ineffective procedure that a patient believes is an effective medical therapy for his or her condition. Researchers frequently give placebos to the control group in an experiment testing the efficacy of a particular treatment. By comparing the effects of the actual treatment with the effects of the placebo, researchers can judge whether or not the treatment is effective. The so-called placebo effect occurs when a patient improves after receiving a placebo. In such cases, the effect of the placebo on the patient cannot be attributed to the specific actions or properties of the drug or procedure. Placebos are most often used in trials of new drugs but can also be used in studies of medical treatments such as surgery. For example, in a placebo-controlled trial of fetal tissue transplants in Parkinson's disease patients, half the study participants underwent a sham surgery in which holes were drilled in their skulls but no cells were implanted.

Researchers have consistently found that 30–40% of all patients given a placebo show improvement. This result has been observed for a wide variety of conditions or symptoms, including coughing, seasickness, depression, migraines, and angina. For some conditions, placebos have been effective in up to 70% of patients. In some cases, people given a placebo even report having the side effects associated with an actual drug. Placebos are particularly effective when they are administered by a physician whom the patient trusts.

A clear demonstration of the placebo effect occurred in a recent study that examined the effectiveness of a drug used to treat benign enlargement of the prostate. The men who participated in the study were randomly assigned to one of two groups: One group received the medication; the other received a placebo, a look-alike dummy pill. More than half the men who got the placebo pills reported significant relief from their symptoms, including faster urine flow. This despite the fact that men on the placebo actually experienced an *increase* in the size of their prostates. Many placebo recipients also reported side effects of the "medication," ranging from fatigue and nausea to impotence. How did the men in the study experience fewer symptoms despite no improvement in their condition (prostate enlargement)? Researchers hypothesize that the patients' positive expectations of the medication's effects may have resulted in decreased nerve activity and muscle relaxation affecting the bladder, prostate, and urethra.

The placebo effect can be exploited by unscrupulous people who sell worthless medical treatments to the scientifically unsophisticated public. But placebo power can also be harnessed for its beneficial effects. When a skilled and compassionate medical practitioner provides a patient with a sense of confidence and hope, the positive aspects of placebo power can boost the benefits of standard medical treatment. Getting well, like getting sick, is a complex process. Anatomy, physiology, mind, emotions, and the environment are all inextricably entwined. But the placebo effect does show that belief can have both psychological and physical effects.

SOURCES: Nordenberg, T. 2000. The healing power of placebos. *FDA Consumer*, January/February. The powerful placebo: An effect without a cause. 2000. *Harvard Men's Health Watch*, June. Brown, W. A. 1998. The placebo effect. *Scientific American* 278(1): 90–95.

portant role in the success of the therapy. Indeed, critics of homeopathy often attribute its reported effectiveness to this nonspecific "placebo effect" (see the box "The Power of Belief: The Placebo Effect").

However, when the results of 185 homeopathic trials were analyzed recently, it was concluded that the clinical effects of homeopathy could not be completely explained by the placebo effect. At the same time, homeopathy was not found to be effective for any single clinical condition. Homeopathy remains one of the most controversial forms of CAM.

Because of the extremely dilute nature of homeopathic remedies, it is generally assumed that they are safe. To date, the FDA has not found any serious adverse events associated with the use of homeopathy, with the possible exception of situations in which a patient might have been successfully treated with standard medical approaches but chose to rely solely on homeopathy. The FDA regulates homeopathic remedies, but they are subject to many fewer restrictions than prescription or over-the-counter drugs. Remedies designed to treat self-limiting conditions such as colds and headaches can be sold over the counter; products that claim to treat serious conditions such as heart disease can be sold only by prescription. A few states require practitioners to have special licenses, but most providers practice homeopathy as a specialty under another medical license, such as medical doctor or nurse practitioner.

COMMUNICATE! If you are interested in exploring an alternative or complementary therapy, talk with the practitioner over the phone or during your first appointment. You can ask about the underlying philosophy of the therapy, how it claims to improve your condition, how diagnoses are made, what treatments consist of, and whether the practitioner has any written material about the therapy that you can read. You can also ask about the practitioner's training, credentials, and certification. For example, "My aunt got chiropractic treatments for back pain, and she said it helped. I'm interested in trying it for my stiff neck, but I don't know much about it. Can you tell me what a treatment would consist of and explain to me how it's supposed to work?"

Mind-Body Interventions

Mind-body interventions make use of the integral connection between mind and body and the effect each can have on the other. They include many of the stress-management techniques discussed in Chapter 2, including meditation, yoga, visualization, t'ai chi ch'uan, and biofeedback. Psychotherapy, support groups, prayer, and music, art, and dance therapy can also be thought of as mind-body interventions. Obviously, there is no clear line between these forms of CAM and conventional medicine. The placebo effect is one of the most widely known examples of mind-body interdependence.

Some forms of **hypnosis** are considered to be CAM therapies, although the use of hypnotherapy for certain conditions was accepted more than 40 years ago by the American Medical Association. Hypnosis involves the induction of a state of deep relaxation during which the patient is more suggestible (more easily influenced). While the patient is in such a hypnotic trance, the practitioner tries to help him or her change unwanted behavior or deal with pain and other symptoms. An NIH-sponsored report found strong evidence for the effectiveness of relaxation techniques and hypnosis in reducing chronic pain stemming from a variety of medical conditions, although subsequent studies have cast some doubt on this conclusion. Hypnosis is sometimes used in smoking cessation programs and as a nondrug approach to anxiety disorders such as phobias and chronic conditions such as irritable bowel syndrome.

Hypnosis can be used by medical professionals (M.D.s, D.O.s, D.D.S.s) but is also offered by hypnotherapists. Physicians are certified by their own associations; many states require hypnotherapists to be licensed, but the requirements for licensing vary substantially. There is little regulation of practitioners of other relaxation techniques, but it is very rare that adverse events result from such techniques. Many studies have shown that support groups, friendships, strong family relationships, and prayer can all have a positive impact on health.

Biological-Based Therapies

Biological-based therapies consist primarily of herbal therapies or remedies, botanicals, and dietary supplements. Herbal therapies are sometimes referred to as *materia medica,* Latin for "medical matter," a term that can include a much larger variety of compounds than just "herbs" (which are plants that die down at the end of a growing season and do not produce woody tissue). Some herbal remedies are not technically herbs, such as the leaves of the ginkgo biloba tree, and some are not even from plants, such as shark cartilage and bear gallbladder. Other items that constitute *materia medica* are algae, bacteria, fungi, and minerals. For traditional remedies that are of plant origin, many scientists prefer to use the term *botanicals.* Nonetheless, because even official government definitions use the word *herbs* to designate substances from the categories of herbs, botanicals, and other *materia medica,* the terms are used somewhat interchangeably in this chapter.

Herbal remedies are a major component of all indigenous forms of medicine; prior to the development of pharmaceuticals at the end of the nineteenth century, people everywhere in the world relied on materials from nature for pain relief, wound healing, and treatment of a variety of ailments. Herbal remedies are also a common element in most systems of traditional medicine. For example, many popular botanicals are derived from plants that were used by American Indians for the very purposes for which they are touted today. Much of the **pharmacopoeia** of modern scientific medicine originated in the folk medicine of native peoples, and many drugs used today are derived from plants.

A majority of botanical products are sold as dietary supplements, that is, in the form of tablets, pills, capsules, liquid extracts, or teas. Like foods, dietary supplements must carry ingredient labels (see Chapter 12 for more about dietary supplement labeling). As with food products, it is the responsibility of the manufacturers to ensure that their dietary supplements are safe and properly labeled prior to marketing. The FDA is responsible for monitoring the labeling and accompanying literature of dietary supplements and for overseeing their safety once they are on the market.

Well-designed clinical studies have been conducted on only a small number of botanicals. Among the most thoroughly tested plant extracts are St. John's wort (*Hypericum perforatum*), ginkgo (*Ginkgo biloba*), and the different coneflowers (*Echinacea purpurea, Echinacea angustifolia,* and *Echinacea pallida*). These and other commonly used botanicals, their uses, and the evidence supporting their efficacy are presented in Table 21-2. Participants in clinical trials with St. John's wort, ginkgo, and echinacea experienced only minor adverse events. However, most clinical trials of this type last only for a few weeks, so the tests did not indicate whether it is safe to take these botanicals for longer periods of time. They also didn't indicate whether higher or lower dosages would be more or less effective or cause more or fewer adverse events.

For the vast majority of other botanicals, there are almost no reliable research findings on efficacy or safety. That is extremely worrisome since, of all the CAM approaches, the consumption of botanical supplements has the greatest potential to result in serious and even life-

Table 21-2

Commonly Used Botanicals, Their Uses, Evidence for Their Effectiveness, and Contraindications

Botanical	Use	Evidence	Contraindications
Echinacea (*Echinacea purpurea, E. angustifolia, E. pallida*)	Stimulation of immune functions; to prevent colds and flulike diseases; to lessen symptoms of colds and flus	Some trials showed that it prevents colds and flus and helps patients recover from colds faster, but others found it ineffective	Might cause liver damage if taken over long periods of time (more than 8 weeks); since it is an immune stimulant, it is not advisable to take it with immune suppressants (e.g., corticosteroids)
Evening primrose oil* (*Oenothera biennis L.*)	Reduction of inflammation	Long-term supplementation effective in reducing symptoms of rheumatoid arthritis	None known
Feverfew (*Tanacetum parthenium*)	Prevention of headaches and migraines	The majority of trials indicate that it is more effective than placebo, but the evidence is not yet conclusive	Should not be used by people allergic to other members of the aster family; has the potential to increase the effects of warfarin and other anticoagulants
Ginkgo (*Ginkgo biloba*)	Improvement of circulation and memory	Improves cerebral insufficiency and slows progression of Alzheimer's disease and other types of senile dementia in some patients	Could increase bleeding time; should not be taken with nonsteroidal anti-inflammatory drugs or anticoagulants
Ginseng** (*Panax ginseng*)	Improvement of physical performance, memory, immune function, and glycemic control in diabetes; treatment of herpes simplex 2	No conclusive evidence exists for any of these uses	Interacts with warfarin and alcohol in mice and rats; hence should probably not be used with these drugs
Kava kava (*Piper methysticum*)	Treatment of depression and anxiety	Is significantly better than placebo and about equal to some standard antidepressants	May cause sedation, boost the effects of alcohol, and interact with antidepressants and other drugs
St. John's wort (*Hypericum perforatum*)	Treatment of depression	There is strong evidence that it is significantly more effective than placebo, is as effective as some standard antidepressants for mild to moderate depression, and causes fewer adverse effects	Known to interact with a variety of pharmaceuticals and should not be taken together with digoxin, theophylline, cyclosporine, indinavir, and serotonin-reuptake inhibitors
Saw palmetto (*Serenoa repens*)	Improvement of prostate health	Appears to be moderately effective, but the evidence is not yet considered conclusive	Has no known interactions with drugs, but should probably not be taken with hormonal therapies
Valerian (*Valeriana officinalis*)	Treatment of insomnia	Appears to help with sleep disorders, but further trials are needed	Interacts with thiopental and pentobarbital and should not be used with these drugs

* Similar results have been obtained with borage oil (*Borago officinalis L.*).
** There are two other species of ginseng, namely *Panax quinquefolium* (American ginseng) and *Eleutherococcus senticosus* (Siberian ginseng), but in clinical trials for cerebral insufficiency and dementia only *Panax ginseng* has been tested.

threatening consequences. For more on concerns associated with botanicals, see the box "Herbal Remedies: Are They Safe?"

Manipulative and Body-Based Methods

Touch and body manipulation are long-standing forms of health care. Manual healing techniques are based on the idea that misalignment or dysfunction in one part of the body can cause pain or dysfunction in another part; correcting these misalignments can bring the body back to optimal health.

Manual healing methods are an integral part of osteopathic medicine, now considered a form of conventional medicine. Other physical healing methods include massage, acupressure, Feldenkrais, Rolfing, and numerous other techniques. The most commonly accepted of the

In February 2000, the FDA issued a Public Health Advisory warning of drug interactions between St. John's wort (*Hypericum perforatum*) and drugs used to treat HIV infection, heart disease, and several other conditions. St. John's wort was found to substantially reduce blood levels of indinavir, an HIV-fighting protease inhibitor; it was expected that the herb would have the same effect on other HIV antiretroviral drugs, as well as several other drugs that are metabolized via the same chemical pathway. These include oral contraceptives; digitalis, warfarin, and other drugs used to treat CVD; cyclosporine and other antirejection drugs used with organ transplants; and some medications used to treat infections, depression, seizure disorders, cancer, asthma, and other conditions. Because St. John's wort uses the same metabolic pathway as these drugs, it reduces their concentration in the blood and thus their effectiveness.

In May of the same year, the FDA issued a warning about botanical products that contain aristolochic acid, a powerful carcinogen and nephrotoxin (a substance that causes kidney damage). In 1990–1992, Chinese herbs containing aristolochic acid had caused severe kidney damage, renal failure, and bladder cancer in patients at a weight-loss clinic in Belgium; due to a manufacturing error, aristolochia had been inadvertently substituted for another ingredient in weight-loss pills. Several European countries have banned the use of herbal products containing aristolochic acid, but such products are still obtainable in the United States, as are products believed to be contaminated with aristolochic acid.

These FDA warnings reflect growing safety concerns about herbal remedies, botanicals, and dietary supplements, which now represent a more than $15-billion-a-year industry in the United States. Some problems result from lack of regulation, standardization, and quality control, in both the United States and other countries, and other problems result from attempts to apply Western manufacturing methods to traditional herbal remedies. Safety concerns include drug interactions, lack of standardization, contamination, and toxicity.

Drug Interactions

As in the case of St. John's wort, the chemicals in botanical supplements can interact dangerously with prescription and over-the-counter drugs. HIV-infected patients were taking St. John's wort (for depression) and thereby reduced the concentration of indinavir to ineffective levels. In other cases, heart and kidney transplant patients who were taking St. John's wort had lower than expected plasma concentrations of cyclosporine and experienced symptoms of acute transplant rejection. These patients' lives were probably saved because they told their physicians that they were taking St. John's wort. Alarmingly, a high percentage of patients fail to tell their physicians about their use of herbal substances. Botanicals may decrease the effects of drugs, making them ineffective, or increase their effects, in some instances making them toxic. Botanicals can also interact with alcohol, usually heightening alcohol's effects.

There are also complex interactions among the constituents of a single herbal preparation. Certain constituents might cause more or less digestion or absorption of one of the other constituents, and even otherwise inert (inactive) constituents may stabilize active ingredients. This is one of the reasons that herbal remedies in traditional Chinese medicine commonly contain at least three or four and occasionally up to twelve different herbs. Although there is little research on the interactions in Chinese herbal preparations, the precise combination of herbs is based on observations of patient reactions gathered over a period of more than 2000 years. In the United States, many manufacturers are offering new combinations of botanical preparations without empirical or scientific information about the interactions of the individual ingredients.

Lack of Standardization

A related problem is the lack of standardization in the manufacturing of herbal products in the United States. The Dietary Supplement Health and Education Act of 1994 requires that dietary supplement labels list the name and quantity of each ingredient; if a product contains botanical ingredients, the label must also specify the part of the plant from which the ingredient is derived.

In listing the names of ingredients, manufacturers can use either common names or Latin names. Latin names are the same throughout the world, but common names differ. Sometimes different plant species have the same common name, as in the

CAM manual healing methods is **chiropractic**, a method that focuses on the relationship between structure, primarily of joints and muscles, and function, primarily of the nervous system, to maintain or restore health. An important therapeutic procedure is the manipulation of joints, particularly those of the spinal column. However, chiropractors also use a variety of other techniques, including physical therapy, exercise programs, patient education and lifestyle modification, and orthotics (mechanical supports and braces) to treat patients. They do not use drugs or surgery.

Chiropractors, or doctors of chiropractic, are trained for a minimum of four full-time academic years at accredited chiropractic colleges and can go on to postgraduate training in many countries. Although specifically listed by NCCAM as one of the manipulative and body-based

Terms

chiropractic A system of manual healing most frequently used to treat musculoskeletal problems; the primary treatment is manipulation of the spine and other joints. Practitioners hold a doctor of chiropractic degree and are licensed.

energy therapies Forms of CAM treatment that use energy fields originating either within the body or from outside sources to promote healing.

case of ginseng, which may be Chinese ginseng (*Panax ginseng*), American ginseng (*Panax quinquefolium*), or Siberian ginseng (*Eleutherococcus senticosus*). Even Latin names may refer to different species, as in the case of the coneflower, Echinacea. At least three different species of Echinacea are found in commercial preparations: *Echinacea purpurea, Echinacea angustifolia,* and *Echinacea pallida.* Although these plants look similar, they have quite distinct chemical compositions and, as a result, different biological activities.

The content of herbal preparations is also variable. A *Consumer Reports* study found that the amount of the active ingredient in ten widely sold ginseng products varied widely, with some pills containing twenty times as much as others. Even those with the same labeled milligram dosage had tenfold differences in concentration.

Part of the reason for such variation is the difficulty of isolating individual ingredients. Manufacturers are trying to standardize the process of preparing plant extracts so that every pill, tablet, capsule, or bottle of liquid contains the same amount of the active ingredient. First, though, they have to determine which of the hundreds of chemicals in a plant extract are responsible for its medicinal effects. This is a difficult task; scientists are far from having a complete list of all the chemical constituents of even a single plant. The types and amounts of chemicals present in an extract are also affected by the growing, harvesting, processing, and storage conditions of plants.

Contamination, Adulteration, and Toxicity

A variety of traditional Chinese and Ayurvedic remedies contain heavy metals, such as lead, mercury, and arsenic, as part of the formula, all of which can be highly toxic and can cause irreversible damage. Some Chinese herbal remedies have been found to contain pharmaceutical drugs, including tranquilizers and steroids. Others contain herbs not listed on the label, sometimes substitute herbs that have toxic effects, as in the case of the weight-loss pills used in the Belgian clinic.

Furthermore, many plants are poisonous. Most medical systems with extensive knowledge of herbal remedies use poisonous plants because of their beneficial effects in very low dosages. (Even conventional medicine uses such drugs—for example, digitalis, derived from the foxglove plant, for heart disease.) Adverse events can occur if the safe dosage is exceeded; the problem is that for many botanicals, the safe dosage is not known. Most manufacturers provide ranges of intakes on the label of a botanical dietary supplement that they deem to be safe.

Some botanicals are not poisonous but can cause damage to the liver or kidney if taken over long periods of time; for many others it is not known if their regular long-term use is safe. Experts have also advised against taking supplements that contain raw animal parts, particularly central nervous system tissue, out of concern that disease may be transmissible this way.

The Role of Government in Safety Issues

Some European governments assume greater responsibility in regulating botanicals than the U.S. government. In Germany, herbal medicine has a long history, but herbs are considered medicines rather than supplements; they are prescribed by physicians, although preparations with lower concentrations of herbs are available over the counter. Manufacturing is standardized so that content, quantity, quality, and purity are guaranteed. Botanicals do not have to be proven effective to be marketed, but they do have to be proven safe.

In the United States, because herbs are considered supplements rather than food or drug products, they do not have to meet FDA food and drug standards for safety or effectiveness, nor do they currently have to meet any manufacturing standards. The manufacturer is responsible for ensuring that a supplement is safe before it is marketed; the FDA has the power to restrict a substance if it is found to pose a health risk after it is on the market, usually on the basis of voluntary reporting of adverse events by the manufacturer. Under U.S. law, if a supplement is suspected of causing harm, the burden of proof lies with the FDA. Because U.S. manufacturers can put almost anything into an herbal supplement, American consumers are at risk for buying and using products that may be not just useless but harmful as well. Part of the reasoning behind this situation is that "natural" products are considered safer than conventional medicines. As the incidents with St. John's wort and aristolochic acid demonstrate, this is not always the case.

methods of CAM, chiropractic is accepted by many health care and health insurance providers to a far greater extent than the other types of CAM therapies. Based on research showing the efficacy of chiropractic management in acute low-back pain, spinal manipulation has been included in the federal guidelines for the treatment of this condition. Promising results have also been reported with the use of chiropractic techniques in neck pain and headaches. However, there are no well-controlled studies to support manipulation for asthma, gastrointestinal problems, infectious diseases, or other nonmechanical problems.

A caution is in order regarding chiropractic: Spinal manipulation performed by a person without proper chiropractic training can be extremely dangerous. There are several organizations, in particular the American Chiropractic Association, that can help you locate a licensed chiropractor near you.

Energy Therapies

Energy therapies are forms of treatment that use energy fields originating either within the body (biofields) or from other sources (electromagnetic fields). Biofield therapies are based on the idea that energy fields surround and penetrate the body and can be influenced by movement, touch, pressure, or the placement of hands in or

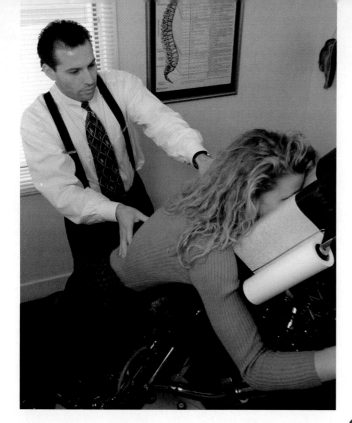

The primary treatment used by chiropractors is spinal manipulation. Properly applied, manipulation can benefit people with some types of musculoskeletal disorders.

through the fields. **Qigong,** a component of traditional Chinese medicine, combines movement, meditation, and regulation of breathing to enhance the flow of qi, improve blood circulation, and enhance immune function. **Therapeutic touch** is derived from the ancient technique of "laying-on of hands"; it is based on the premise that healers can identify and correct energy imbalances by passing their hands over the patient's body. **Reiki** is one form of therapeutic touch; it is intended to correct disturbances in the flow of life energy (ki is the Japanese form of the Chinese qi) and enhance the body's healing powers through the use of thirteen specific hand positions on the patient.

Terms

qigong A component of traditional Chinese medicine that combines movement, meditation, and regulation of breathing to enhance the flow of qi, improve blood circulation, and enhance immune function.

therapeutic touch A CAM practice based on the premise that healers can identify and correct energy imbalances by passing their hands over the patient's body.

Reiki A CAM practice intended to correct disturbances in the flow of life energy and enhance the body's healing powers through the use of thirteen hand positions on the patient.

bioelectromagnetic-based therapies CAM therapies based on the notion that electromagnetic fields can be used to promote healing and manage pain.

Bioelectromagnetics is the study of the interaction between living organisms and electromagnetic fields, both those produced by the organism itself (endogenous) and those produced by outside (exogenous) sources. The recognition that the body produces electromagnetic fields has led to the development of many diagnostic procedures in Western medicine, including electroencephalography (EEG), electrocardiography (ECG), and nuclear magnetic resonance (NMR) scans. **Bioelectromagnetic-based therapies** involve the use of electromagnetic fields, such as pulsed fields, magnetic fields, or alternating current or direct current fields, to manage pain and to treat conditions such as asthma. There are some indications that the use of electromagnetic fields might be useful in the areas of bone repair, wound healing, nerve stimulation, immune system stimulation, and modulation of the neuroendocrine (nerve and hormonal) system. Although promising, the available research is still very limited and does not allow firm conclusions about the efficacy of these therapies. Most scientists believe that consumer products containing small magnets have no significant effect on the human body.

Evaluating Complementary and Alternative Therapies

Because there is less information available about complementary and alternative therapies, as well as less regulation of associated products and providers, it is important for consumers to take an active role when they are thinking about using them.

Working with Your Physician If you are considering a CAM therapy, your first source of information should be your physician or primary health care provider. The NCCAM advises consumers not to seek complementary therapies without first visiting a conventional health care provider for an evaluation and diagnosis of their symptoms. It's usually best to discuss and try conventional treatments that have been shown to be beneficial for your condition. If you are thinking of trying any alternative therapies, it is critically important to tell your physician in order to avoid any dangerous interactions with conventional treatments you are receiving. Areas to discuss with your physician include the following:

- *Safety:* Is there something unsafe about the treatment in general or for you specifically? Are there safety issues you should be aware of, such as the use of disposable needles in acupuncture?

- *Effectiveness:* Is there any research about the use of the therapy for your condition?

- *Timing:* Is the immediate use of a conventional treatment indicated?

- *Cost:* Is the therapy likely to be very expensive, especially in light of the potential benefit?

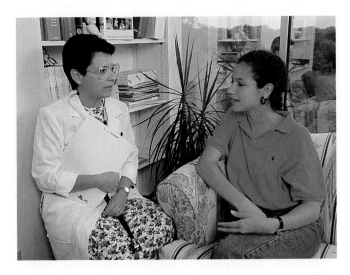

Good communication between consumers and health care providers is important in both conventional and complementary medicine. It is important for consumers who choose to use CAM to discuss their choice with their physician to prevent any dangerous interactions with conventional treatments.

If you are not comfortable discussing complementary and alternative therapies with your physician, ask yourself why. Are you embarrassed about it? Do you think your doctor will think less of you? Do you think he or she doesn't know enough about the therapy you are considering? You have the right to expect your physician to take you and your concerns seriously, to respect your interest in a CAM therapy, to be informed about CAM approaches or at least make an effort to find out about them, and to be willing to discuss the evidence for and against them with you.

If appropriate, schedule a follow-up visit with your physician to assess your condition and your progress after a certain amount of time using a complementary therapy. Keep a symptom diary to more accurately track your symptoms and gauge your progress. (Symptoms such as pain and fatigue are very difficult to recall with accuracy, so an ongoing symptom diary is an important tool.) If you plan to pursue a therapy against your physician's advice, you need to tell him or her.

For dietary supplements, particularly botanicals, pharmacists can also be an excellent source of information, especially if they are familiar with other medications you are taking.

Questioning the CAM Practitioner   You can also get information from individual practitioners and from schools, professional organizations, and state licensing boards. Ask about education, training, licensing, and certification. If appropriate, check with local or state regulatory agencies or the consumer affairs department to determine if any complaints have been lodged against the practitioner. Some guidelines for talking with a CAM practitioner include the following:

- Ask the practitioner why he or she thinks the therapy will be beneficial for your condition. Ask for a full description of the therapy and any potential side effects.
- Describe in detail any conventional treatments you are receiving.
- Ask how long the therapy should continue before it can be determined if it is beneficial.
- Ask about the expected cost of the treatment. Does it seem reasonable? Will your health insurance pay some or all of the costs?

If anything an alternative practitioner says or recommends directly conflicts with advice from your physician, discuss it with your physician before making any major changes in any current treatment regimen or in your lifestyle.

Doing Your Own Research   You can investigate CAM therapies on your own by going to the library or doing research online, although caution is in order when using Web sites for the various forms of CAM. A good place to start is the Web sites of government agencies like the FDA or NCCAM and of universities and similar organizations that conduct government-sponsored research on CAM approaches (see For More Information at the end of the chapter).

If possible, also talk to people with the same condition you have who have received the same treatment. Remember, though, that patient testimonials shouldn't be used as the sole criterion for choosing a therapy or assessing its safety and efficacy. Controlled scientific trials usually provide the best information and should be consulted whenever possible. The absence of documented danger is not the same thing as proof of safety. Quite often, people working in health food stores are only too willing to give advice and make recommendations, particularly about botanical supplements. Many of these people are not qualified to give this kind of advice. Ask about qualifications (training or education) before accepting recommendations from anyone. Perhaps more so than for any other consumer products and services, the use of complementary and alternative medicine calls for consumer skills, critical thinking, and caution.

COMMUNICATE!   It makes sense to talk with your physician if you are thinking about trying a complementary therapy, such as acupuncture or chiropractic, and it is critically important to talk with him or her about any dietary supplements you are taking or thinking about taking. As mentioned in the text, you have a right to expect your physician to be able to discuss complementary and alternative therapies with you. To get started, you might say something like, "A friend of mine tried acupuncture for tendinitis and he said it helped. What do you think about my trying it for my elbow?" or "I've read that St. John's wort can help with mild depression. Do you think I should try it? Is there any reason I shouldn't?"

WHY DO CONSUMERS USE COMPLEMENTARY MEDICINE?

Why are American consumers attracted to complementary and alternative medicine? Numerous reasons have been proposed. CAM often offers hope to people who have been disappointed by conventional medical therapies or who have chronic conditions that are incurable with conventional medical treatments. People with cancer, AIDS, and arthritis are among the heaviest users of CAM. Those most likely to use CAM are elderly people, approximately 80% of whom have at least one chronic health problem, and teenagers, who are concerned about their appearance and respond to a variety of appeals. Both these groups may be particularly susceptible to fraudulent claims for products promising new, quick, or easy ways to stay thin, strong, or attractive. A major source of CAM's appeal is that CAM practitioners often spend much more time listening and touching their patients than conventional physicians. Patients may find CAM practitioners to be warmer, more empathetic, and less rushed than their conventional counterparts.

Some experts speculate that the persuasive appeal of complementary and alternative medicine may be related to the power of its underlying beliefs and cultural assumptions, which offer patients an experience they are missing in conventional medicine. According to this view, the appeal of CAM may be found in four "themes."

One such theme is a belief in the benevolent power of "nature," which is viewed as pure, whole, and simple. People using CAM feel they are connecting with a more natural, organic version of both self and society. Conventional medicine suffers in comparison because of its association with sophisticated technology; it may be viewed as artificial, synthetic, or toxic.

A second theme is a connection to vital energy or life-supporting cosmic forces, such as qi. As these healing energies are mobilized, the patient is empowered to influence his or her own condition. An optimistic perspective pervades this approach, despite the usually overlooked implication that such self-determinism might also include personal fault for the disease in the first place.

A third theme is "science," though not in the Western sense. Many CAM disciplines involve years of study of complex knowledge systems and have long intellectual traditions. They use the label "science" (as in "chiropractic science") as a source of legitimacy, power, moral au-

thority, and self-definition. The CAM version of science is more holistic, unified, and person-centered than Western science. When illness threatens a person's sense of self and understanding of the world, CAM validates his or her subjective experience.

The fourth theme is that the quest for health takes on a sacred dimension; patients often find meaning, purpose, and connection with the universe in CAM therapies. Regimens of exercise, diet, meditation, and other practices become daily activities of affirmation and commitment. The focus on mind, body, and spirit nurtures the spiritual side of the person as well as the physical.

According to this view, then, CAM is attractive because of what it offers people when their sense of intactness and connection with the world is threatened by illness: empowerment, participation, authenticity, connection to nature and the universe, a renewed sense of purpose and meaning, and a new set of behavioral options. The assumptions of CAM can redefine the experience of illness in ways that inspire, empower, and transform the individual.

It is worth noting that the differences between conventional medicine and CAM are to some extent a matter of degree, according to this view. Western medicine is based on a set of core values that include respect for patients, a compelling interest in the truth, and service to humanity. Physicians often rely on the "power of nature" for healing and cures. "Nonscientific" phenomena and forces can be found in the biomedical world in the form of the placebo effect and the patient-physician relationship. A major difference, however, is that conventional medicine has a more rigorous and self-critical scientific method.

THE FUTURE: CONFLICT, CONVERGENCE, OR COLLABORATION?

Despite many profound and irreconcilable philosophical differences between conventional medicine and CAM, there are abundant opportunities for learning, collaborating, and providing parallel care. Conventional medicine has already adopted many principles prevalent in complementary and alternative disciplines, including the ideas of health promotion, of personal responsibility for health, and of wellness as a multidimensional ideal. Western medicine is looking at the soaring use of CAM to discover what patients are missing in conventional care—perhaps more information, interest, or time from their physicians. At the same time, practitioners of CAM are looking to Western methods to modernize and optimize some of their practices, such as the preparation and standardization of herbal remedies. Within each is an enormous amount of time-tested information that has its own logic and use. In the future, greater understanding and collaboration across boundaries will certainly benefit the patient-consumer.

Conventional Western medicine is responsible for many of the health practices that benefit us today, including vaccination, trauma care, surgery, public health measures, and the use of drugs to control infectious diseases. At the same time, alternative and complementary medicine offers practices that support health as a balance among the many dimensions of mind, body, and spirit. Both can be used to work toward wellness.

Right now you can

- Consider whether you are satisfied with your primary care physician; if not, think about what steps you can take to improve the situation, either by resolving problems with your existing physician or by looking for a new one.

- Research any alternative or complementary practice or product you are using, either at the library or online, to find out if it is considered safe.

- Sit back in your chair and practice relaxation through breathing: Inhale slowly and deeply, imagining warm air flowing to all parts of your body; exhale from your abdomen, imagining tension flowing out of your body; continue for five or ten minutes or until you feel relaxed.

SUMMARY

- Complementary and alternative medicine (CAM) is defined as those therapies and practices that do not form part of conventional or "mainstream" health care and medical practice as taught in most U.S. medical schools and offered in most U.S. hospitals.

- Conventional medicine is characterized by a focus on the external, physical causes of disease; the identification of a set of symptoms for different diseases; the development of public health measures to prevent disease and drugs and surgery to treat them; the use of rational, scientific thinking to understand and explain phenomena; and a well-established research methodology.

- Conventional practitioners include medical doctors, doctors of osteopathic medicine, podiatrists, optometrists, and dentists, as well as allied health care providers.

- CAM is characterized by a view of health as a balance and integration of body, mind, and spirit; a focus on ways to restore the individual to harmony so that he or she can fight disease and regain health; and a body of knowledge based on accumulated experience and observations of patient reactions.

- Alternative medical systems are complete systems of medical philosophy, theory, and practice. Traditional Chinese medicine makes use of many treatment methods, including herbal remedies and acupuncture, to restore the free flow of qi, or life energy. Homeopathy is based on the principles that like cures like and that remedies become more effective with greater dilution.

- Mind-body interventions include meditation, yoga, breathwork, group support, hypnosis, and prayer.

- Biological-based therapies consist of herbal remedies, botanicals, and dietary supplements.

- Manipulative and body-based methods include massage and other physical healing techniques; the most commonly accepted is chiropractic.

- Energy therapies are designed to influence the flow of energy in and around the body; they include qigong, therapeutic touch therapies, and Reiki.

- Because there is less information available about CAM and less regulation of its practices and providers, consumers must be proactive in researching and choosing treatments, using critical thinking skills and exercising caution.

- In general, CAM may be attractive to consumers because it allows people to redefine the experience of illness in ways that empower the individual.

TAKE ACTION

1. Visit the student health center on your campus or another health care facility. and evaluate the services available. Consider such things as hours, waiting time, health literature available, the scope of services, the availability of specialists, and so on. Would you make any recommendations for improvement? Pass your ideas along to the director of your health center.

2. Take an informal survey of your friends and family members about their use of CAM. How many have used alternative therapies? What types of therapies were most common? Why did people choose a particular CAM therapy? Did they use the therapy in addition to or instead of conventional treatments? What were the results?

3. Visit a local drugstore and compare different brands of the same herbal remedy or dietary supplement. How similar are the supplements in terms of ingredients, recommended dosages, and price? What aspect of health do the supplements claim to benefit, and how do they make the claim? Research any unfamiliar ingredients using the resources listed in Chapter 12 and For More Information at the end of this chapter.

1. Interactions among over-the-counter and prescription drugs and herbal remedies are potentially serious. Make a list of every drug and herbal remedy you've used in the past three months. How many did you use? Do you know for certain that you haven't risked a dangerous interaction? Check the labels on all the products you used for warnings; if you are unsure about any interactions, take your list to your pharmacist or health care practitioner for advice.

2. *Critical Thinking* Examine a news report on a research study. From the report, try to determine key facts about the research (see the box on p. 606 in the chapter): source of the information, size and type of the study, characteristics of the participants, findings, and conclusions. How much information is actually included in the media report? Is there enough information for you to critically evaluate the findings? If possible, compare the media report to the actual study findings. (Abstracts of most medical studies can be found on the Library of Medicine's PubMed Web site: http://www.ncbi.nlm.nih.gov/entrez.) Write a short essay about your findings.

3. *Critical Thinking* In your health journal, describe the criteria you use or would use to evaluate a CAM therapy and decide on its use. Under what circumstances do you think you would use it? What would you want to know about the therapy and where would you obtain information? What assumptions do you have about the safety and efficacy of the therapy? Where do you think your ideas come from? How do they compare with your ideas about conventional medical treatment of the same condition?

FOR MORE INFORMATION

Books and Articles

Alvord, L. A., and E. C. Van Pelt. 1999. *The Scalpel and the Silver Bear: The First Navajo Woman Surgeon Combines Western Medicine and Traditional Medicine.* New York: Bantam. *A personal account of a physician who combines advanced conventional medical care (surgery) with traditional Navajo healing practices.*

Brody, H. 2000. *The Placebo Response.* New York: Cliff Street Books. *Describes the placebo effect and how it may be used to benefit health.*

Consumer Reports magazine frequently publishes articles that help consumers make informed decisions about health care, including the following: Alternative medicine (May 2000); Herbal remedies for prostate problems (September 2000); Dietary supplements for improving mood (December 2000).

Howard Hughes Medical Institute, ed. 2000. *Exploring the Biomedical Revolution.* Baltimore: Johns Hopkins University Press. *Explores biomedical research and its impact on the fight against human disease.*

Micozzi, M. S. 2001. *Fundamentals of Complementary and Alternative Medicine.* 2nd ed. St. Louis: Mosby. *Provides information on the development and key ideas and approaches of alternative and complementary systems and therapies.*

W. Organizations, Hotlines, and Web Sites

Agency for Healthcare Research and Quality (AHRQ). Provides practical, evidence-based information on health care treatments and outcomes for consumers and practitioners.
888-358-9295
http://www.ahrq.gov

American Academy of Medical Acupuncture (AAMA). Provides information about acupuncture and a searchable directory of medical doctors who have been certified by the American Board of Medical Acupuncture.
323-937-5514
http://www.medicalacupuncture.org

American Board of Medical Specialties. Provides information on board certification, including information on specific physicians.
866-275-2267
http://www.abms.org

American Chiropractic Association. Provides information on chiropractic care, consumer tips, and a searchable directory of certified chiropractors.
http://www.amerchiro.org

American Medical Association (AMA). Provides information about physicians, including their training, licensure, and board certification.
http://www.ama-assn.org

American Osteopathic Association. Provides information on osteopathic physicians, including board certification.
800-621-1773
http://www.aoa-net.org

ConsumerLab.com. Provides information on the results of tests of dietary supplements, including information on actual ingredients and concentrations.
http://www.consumerlab.com

Food and Drug Administration: Information for Consumers. Provides materials on dietary supplements, foods, prescription and OTC drugs, and other FDA-regulated products.
888-INFO-FDA
http://www.fda.gov/opacom/morecons.html

National Center for Complementary and Alternative Medicine (NCCAM). Provides general information packets, answers to frequently asked questions about CAM, consumer advice for safer use of CAM, research abstracts, and bibliographies.
888-644-6226
http://nccam.nih.gov

National Center for Homeopathy. Provides information about homeopathy and a directory of member practitioners.

http://www.homeopathic.org

National Certification Commission for Acupuncture and Oriental Medicine (NCCAOM). Promotes nationally recognized standards of competency and safety in acupuncture, Chinese herbology, and Oriental bodywork therapy; includes a searchable directory of certified practitioners.

703-548-9004

http://www.nccaom.org

National Council Against Health Fraud. Provides news and information about health fraud and quackery and links to related sites.

http://www.ncahf.org

Quackwatch. Provides information on health fraud, quackery, and health decision making.

http://www.quackwatch.com

See also the listings for Chapters 2, 12, and 22; the section on dietary supplements in Chapter 12 (pp. 341–343) suggests books and Web sites with more information on supplements.

SELECTED BIBLIOGRAPHY

Avants, S. K., et al. 2000. A randomized controlled trial of auricular acupuncture for cocaine dependence. *Archives of Internal Medicine* 160 (15): 2305–2312.

Bauer, B. A. 2000. Herbal therapy: What a clinician needs to know to counsel patients effectively. *Mayo Clinic Proceedings* 75(8): 835–841.

Berman, B. M., et al. 2000. The evidence for acupuncture as a treatment for rheumatologic conditions. *Rheumatic Disease Clinics of North America* 26 (1): 103–115.

Borchers, A. T., et al. 2000. Inflammation and Native American medicine: The role of botanicals. *American Journal of Clinical Nutrition* 72(2): 339–347.

Bordens, K. S., and B. B. Abbott. 2002. *Research Design and Methods: A Process Approach*. 5th ed. New York: McGraw-Hill.

Cauffield, J. S. 2000. The psychosocial aspects of complementary and alternative medicine. *Pharmacotherapy* 20(11): 1289–1294.

DiBlasi, Z., et al. 2001. Influence of context effects on health outcomes. *Lancet* 357(9258): 757–762.

Eisenberg, D. M. 1997. Advising patients who seek alternative medical therapies. *Annals of Internal Medicine* 127: 61–69.

Eisenberg, D. M., et al. 1998. Trends in alternative medicine use in the United States, 1990–1997: Results of a follow-up national survey. *Journal of the American Medical Association* 280(18): 1569–1575.

Ernst, E. 2001. A primer of complementary and alternative medicine commonly used by cancer patients. *Medical Journal of Australia* 174(2): 88–92.

Foster, D. F., et al. 2000. Alternative medicine use in older Americans. *Journal of the American Geriatric Society* 48(12): 1560–1565.

Gardiner, P., and W. Wornham. 2000. Recent review of complementary and alternative medicine used by adolescents. *Current Opinion in Pediatrics* 12(4): 298–302.

Kaptchuk, T. J., and D. M. Eisenberg. 1998. The persuasive appeal of alternative medicine. *Annals of Internal Medicine* 129(12): 1061–1065.

LaFrance, W. C., Jr., et al. 2000. The use of herbal alternative medicines in neuropsychiatry: A report of the ANPA Committee on Research. *Journal of Neuropsychiatry and Clinical Neuroscience* 12(2): 177–192.

Linde, K., et al. 1998. Are the clinical effects of homeopathy placebo effects? A meta-analysis of placebo-controlled trials. *Lancet* 350(9081): 834–843.

Miller, L. G., et al. 2000. White paper on herbal products; American College of Clinical Pharmacy. *Pharmacotherapy* 20(7): 877–891.

Murphy, D. R. 2000. Chiropractic rehabilitation of the cervical spine. *Journal of Manipulative and Physiological Therapeutics* 23(6): 404–408.

National Center for Complementary and Alternative Medicine. 2000. Major domains of complementary and alternative medicine. (http://nccam.nih.gov/nccam/fcp/classify; retrieved December 20, 2000).

National Center for Complementary and Alternative Medicine. 2001. *Considering Complementary and Alternative Therapies?* (http://nccam.nih.gov/nccam/fcp/faq/cconsidercam.html; retrieved May 2, 2001).

National Institutes of Health. 1997. *Acupuncture: NIH Consensus Statement* (http://odp.od.nih.gov/consensus/cons/107/107statement.htm; retrieved December 29, 2000).

Nortier, J. L., et al. 2000. Urothelial carcinoma associated with the use of a Chinese herb (*Aristolochia fangchi*). *The New England Journal of Medicine* 342(23): 1686–1692.

Participating in medical research studies. 2001. *Journal of the American Medical Association* 285(5): 686.

Piscitelli, S. C., et al. 2000. Indinavir concentrations and St. John's wort. *Lancet* 355(9203): 547–548.

Ruschitzka, R., et al. 2000. Acute heart transplant rejection due to Saint John's wort. *Lancet* 355(9203): 548–549.

Sollner, W., et al. 2000. Use of complementary and alternative medicine by cancer patients is not associated with perceived distress or poor compliance with standard treatment but with active coping behavior: A survey. *Cancer* 89(4): 873–880.

Soon, S. L., and R. I. Crawford. 2001. Recurrent erythema nodosum associated with Echinacea herbal therapy. *Journal of the American Academy of Dermatology* 44(2): 298–299.

Taylor, M. A., et al. 2000. Randomised controlled trial of homoeopathy versus placebo in perennial allergic rhinitis with overview of four trial series. *British Medical Association* 321(7259): 471–476.

Tomlinson, B., et al. 2000. Toxicity of complementary therapies: An Eastern perspective. *Journal of Clinical Pharmacology* 40(5): 451–456.

Veeramah, E. K., and S. Holmes. 2000. Complementary therapy: Complement or threat to modern medicine? *Journal of the Royal Society of Health* 120(1): 42–46.

Yoon, S. J., and C. H. Horne. 2001. Herbal products and conventional medicines used by community-residing older women. *Journal of Advanced Nursing* 33(1): 51–59.

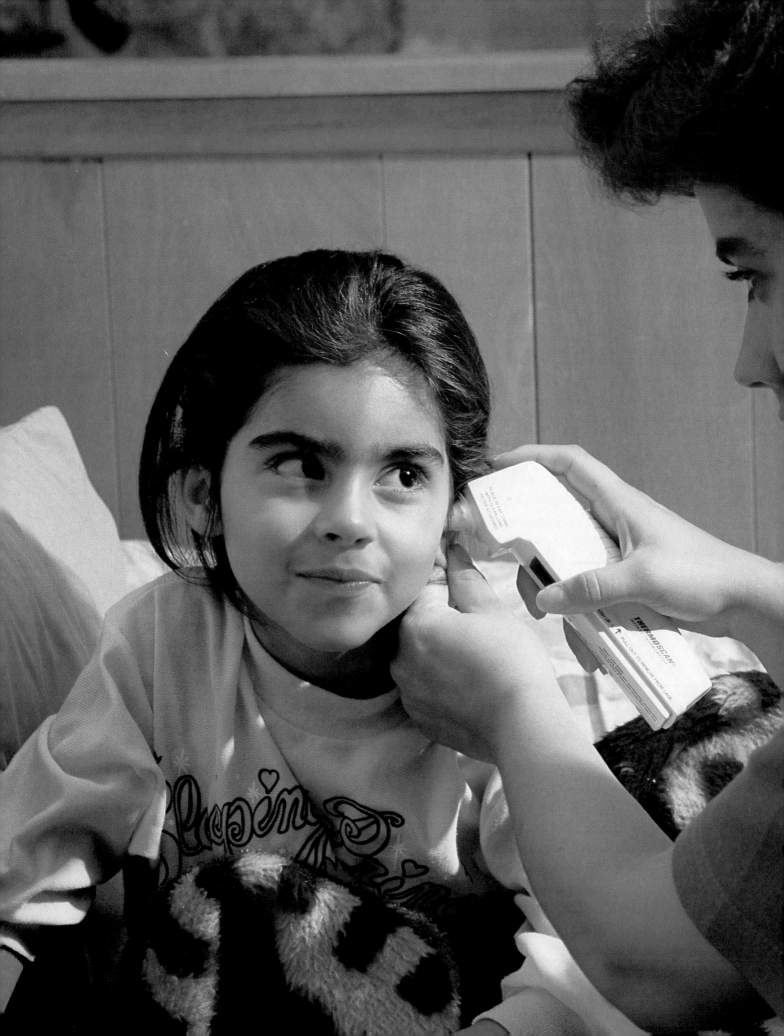

After reading this chapter, you should be able to

- Explain the self-care decision-making process, including how to decide whether to see a physician

- Discuss options for self-treatment

- Explain the physician-patient partnership, including how to communicate effectively with a health care professional

- Describe how medical problems are diagnosed, tested, and treated and list ways that patients can participate fully in each step

- Discuss different types of health insurance plans

Self-Care: Skills for the Health Care Consumer

TEST YOUR KNOWLEDGE

1. About what percentage of medical symptoms are self-diagnosed and self-treated?
   a. 40%
   b. 60%
   c. 80%

2. Generic drugs are generally less effective than brand-name drugs.
   True or false?

3. Physician fees are the fastest-growing component of health care costs in the United States.
   True or false?

4. What proportion of Americans do not have health insurance?
   a. 1 in 6
   b. 1 in 10
   c. 1 in 20

5. Including payments made by individuals, insurance companies, and the government, about how much is spent on health care for each American?
   a. $600 per year
   b. $2600 per year
   c. $4600 per year

ANSWERS

1. **C.** The health care system would be overwhelmed if people started visiting their physicians for even a small proportion of the symptoms they now treat themselves.

2. **FALSE.** Price is often the only difference. The generic version of a drug has the same active ingredient as the brand-name drug, but it may have different inactive ingredients.

3. **FALSE.** Drug expenditures are the fastest-growing component. High drug costs are of particular concern to older Americans because they typically take more medications and because Medicare does not cover outpatient drugs.

4. **A.** More than 48 million Americans currently have no health insurance, a figure that could grow to more than 60 million by 2009.

5. **C.** Costs are expected to increase to about $8700 per person by 2010.

When you think of the health care system, do you envision physicians, nurses, clinics, hospitals, and medical laboratories? This is an accurate picture as far as it goes, but don't forget your own role in the health care system—as a self-care provider. Even with today's dazzling medical technology, highly effective medications, and wide variety of skilled practitioners, the individual plays a crucial role in the health care system. In fact, the professional medical care system depends on the functioning of nonprofessional care. If people were to stop practicing self-care and seek professional care for even a small percentage of the complaints they usually manage themselves—colds, backaches, stomachaches, headaches, fatigue, and so on—the professional health care system would be overwhelmed. The average person has about four new medical symptoms each *month* yet consults a physician only four times a *year*. At least 80% of medical symptoms are self-diagnosed and self-treated.

Today, people are becoming more confident of their own ability to solve personal health problems. With increased knowledge of when and how to self-treat and when to seek professional care, they can become even more competent in self-care. And even a small increase in appropriate self-care could result in billions of health care dollars saved. People who manage their own health care gather information and learn skills from physicians, friends, classes, books, magazines, Web sites, or self-help groups; solicit opinions and advice; make decisions; and take action. They recognize that everyday choices about diet, exercise, and other habits are critical determinants of health. They participate in every phase of their health care and accept personal responsibility for it. They realize that the choices are theirs.

Health promotion and a healthy lifestyle include being an informed partner in medical care and practicing safe, effective self-care. How can you develop this self-care attitude and take a more active role in your health care? The first step is to learn the skills you need to identify and manage medical problems. The second step is to learn how to make the health care system work effectively for you. This chapter provides information that will help you become competent in both these areas.

SELF-CARE: MANAGING MEDICAL PROBLEMS

Effectively managing medical problems involves developing several skills. First, you need to learn how to be a good observer of your own body and assess your symptoms. You also must be able to decide when to seek professional advice and when you can safely deal with the problem on your own. You need to know how to safely and effectively self-treat common medical problems. Finally, you need to know how to develop a partnership with physicians and other care providers and how to carry out treatment plans.

Self-Assessment

Self-care begins with careful observation of your own body, scanning for unusual sensations, aches, or pains. Symptoms are signals from our bodies. They alert us that something may be wrong.

Observing Symptoms   Symptoms are often an expression of the body's attempt to heal itself. For example, the pain and swelling that occur after an ankle injury immobilize the injured joint to allow healing to take place. A fever may be an attempt to make the body less hospitable to infectious agents. A cough can help clear the airways and protect the lungs. Understanding what a symptom means and what is going on in your body helps reduce anxiety about symptoms and enables you to practice safe self-care that supports your body's own healing mechanisms.

Carefully observing symptoms also lets you identify those signals that suggest you need professional assistance. You should begin by noting when the symptom began, how often and when it occurs, what makes it worse, what makes it better, and whether you have any associated symptoms. You can also monitor your body's vital signs, such as temperature and heart rate. These signs may give important clues to how your body is managing an illness.

Medical Self-Tests   Not too long ago, the thermometer was the only tool available for evaluating medical problems at home. Now new medical self-tests are available: home blood pressure machines; home blood sugar tests for diabetics; pregnancy tests; self-tests for urinary tract infections, hepatitis C, and HIV infection; and over a dozen other do-it-yourself kits and devices. All these tools are designed to help you make a more informed decision about when to seek medical help and when to self-treat (see the box "Choosing and Using Medical Self-Tests").

Decision Making: Knowing When to See a Physician

When confronted with a symptom, you must ask a series of questions: "What's going on in my body?" "Is this dangerous?" "Have I or anyone else I know had something like this before?" Some of the answers you give to these questions are conscious and rational; others are more unconscious, emotional responses.

Evaluating Symptoms   Your decision to seek professional assistance for a symptom is generally guided by

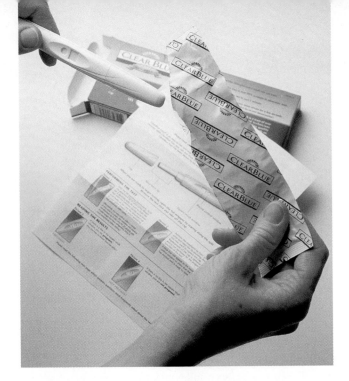

Home pregnancy test kits are just one type of self-test that can be obtained without a prescription in a pharmacy or even your supermarket. Using one of these kits, a woman can determine whether she is pregnant within a week of having missed her period.

your history of medical problems and the nature of the symptom you are experiencing. In general, you should check with a physician for symptoms that are described as follows:

1. *Severe.* If the symptom is very severe or intense, medical assistance is advised. Examples include severe pains, major injuries, and other emergencies.

2. *Unusual.* If the symptom is peculiar and unfamiliar, it is wise to check it out with your physician. Examples include unexplained lumps, changes in a mole, problems with vision, difficulty swallowing, numbness, weakness, unexplained weight loss, and blood in sputum, urine, or stool.

3. *Persistent.* If the symptom lasts longer than expected, seek medical advice. Examples in adults include fever for more than 5 days, a cough lasting longer than 2 weeks, a sore that doesn't heal within a month, and hoarseness lasting longer than 3 weeks.

4. *Recurrent.* If a symptom tends to return again and again, medical evaluation is advised. Examples include recurrent headaches, stomach pains, and backache.

Sometimes a single symptom is not a cause for concern, but when the symptom is accompanied by other symptoms, the combination suggests a more serious problem. For example, a fever with a stiff neck suggests meningitis.

Getting Professional Assistance If you evaluate your symptoms and think that you need professional help, you must decide how urgent the problem is. If it is a true emergency, you should go (or call someone to take you) to the nearest emergency room (ER). Emergencies would include:

- Major trauma or injury, such as head injury, suspected broken bone, deep wound, severe burn, eye injury, or animal bite
- Uncontrollable bleeding or internal bleeding, as indicated by blood in the sputum, vomit, or stool
- Intolerable and uncontrollable pain or severe chest pain
- Severe shortness of breath
- Persistent abdominal pain, especially if associated with nausea and vomiting
- Poisoning or drug overdose
- Loss of consciousness or seizure
- Stupor, drowsiness, or disorientation that cannot be explained
- Severe or worsening reaction to an insect bite or sting or to a medication, especially if breathing is difficult

If your problem is not an emergency but still requires medical attention, call your physician's office. Often you can be given medical advice over the phone without the inconvenience of a visit. You will also be advised if you do need to schedule an appointment.

To help you make wise medical decisions, a Self-Care Guide for Common Medical Problems is provided in Appendix B. This guide includes some specific suggestions on when to call a physician for certain medical problems and on when and how to self-treat. Of course, you should also see a health care professional for help with preventive care, including lifestyle counseling, immunizations, and screening tests.

W. Self-Treatment: Many Options

When confronted with a new symptom, many people try to find some pill or potion that will relieve or cure it. However, other self-treatment options are available.

Watchful Waiting In most cases, your body can itself relieve your symptoms and heal the disorder. The prescriptions filled by your body's internal pharmacy are frequently the safest and most effective treatment. So patience and careful self-observation are often the best choices in self-treatment.

There are many potential benefits of using medical self-test kits. They are usually accurate—about as accurate as professional ones (as required by the FDA)—and many are less expensive than similar tests done by a lab. There is a public health benefit as well: Self-test kits may be used by people who might not get tested otherwise. Self-tests also give individuals a greater sense of control over their health.

However, there are some drawbacks to using home tests. Like all tests, they can give occasional inaccurate results. **False positive** results—in which the test indicates that a person has a disease or condition when he or she really doesn't—can be caused by a variety of unrelated conditions. **False negatives**—in which tests fail to accurately detect a disease or condition—could lead people to think they don't need to see a physician. Home tests are subject to user error; most are fairly simple to use, but be sure to follow the directions carefully.

Results of a home self-test won't answer all your questions. If the result is positive, you'll probably need to visit a physician. Manufacturers of home HIV tests have addressed the need for counseling by having people phone in for test results; callers whose result is positive or inconclusive are routed to a trained HIV counselor.

If you are shopping for a home self-test kit, follow these suggestions for the most accurate result.

- Compare brands before you buy. Some are very simple to use; others are more complex. Some include only one test per package; others have several. Price can vary considerably, and a higher price doesn't necessarily mean a more accurate test.

- Check the expiration date and storage information on the package.

- Read the instructions carefully before you begin, and follow them exactly.

- Be sure to time the test carefully with a watch or clock with a second hand. Don't delay reading the result; it can become inaccurate in as little as 10–20 extra minutes.

- Remember that false negative and false positive results are possible. If you get a negative result from a home test but symptoms persist, see your physician.

- Follow up a positive result with a visit to a physician when appropriate. If you are pregnant or have a medical condition, you'll need to find out the next steps as soon as possible.

Nondrug Options   Nondrug options are often easy, inexpensive, safe, and highly effective. For example, massage, ice packs, and neck exercises may be at times more helpful than drugs in relieving headaches and other pains. Getting adequate rest, increasing exercise, drinking more water, eating more or less of certain foods, using humidifiers, changes in ergonomics when working at desks, and so on are just some of the hundreds of nondrug options for preventing or relieving many common health problems. For a variety of disorders either caused or aggravated by stress, relaxation, visualization, humor, assertive communication, changing negative thoughts, and other stress-management strategies may be the treatment of choice (see the box "Expressive Writing and Chronic Conditions"). Chapter 2 presents a wide variety of stress-management techniques, and Chapter 21 mentions some additional mind-body interventions that consumers may pursue. Before reaching for medications, consider all your self-treatment options.

Self-Medication   Self-treatment with nonprescription medications is an important part of our health care system. Nonprescription or **over-the-counter (OTC) medications** are medicines that the Food and Drug Administration (FDA) has determined are safe for use without a physician's prescription. There are about 100,000 OTC drugs on the market; about 60% of all medications are sold over the counter. Within every 2-week period, nearly 70% of Americans use one or more OTC drugs.

Many OTC drugs are highly effective in relieving symptoms and sometimes in curing illnesses. In fact, many OTC drugs were formerly prescription drugs: More than 600 products sold over the counter today use ingredients or dosage strengths available only by prescription 20 years ago. With this increased consumer choice, however, comes increased consumer responsibility for using OTC drugs safely.

Consumers also need to be aware of the barrage of OTC drug advertising aimed at them. The implication of such advertising is that every symptom can and should be relieved by a drug. Although many OTC products are effective, others are unnecessary or divert attention from better ways of coping. Many ingredients in OTC drugs—perhaps 70%—have not been proven to be effective, a fact the FDA does not dispute. And any drug may have risks and side effects.

Follow these simple guidelines to self-medicate safely:

1. Always read labels, and follow directions carefully. The information on most OTC drug labels now appears in a standard format developed by the FDA (Figure 22-1); ingredients, directions for safe use, and warnings will be clearly indicated. If you have any questions, ask a pharmacist or physician before using a product.

2. Do not exceed the recommended dosage or length of treatment unless you discuss this change with your physician.

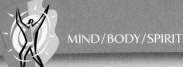
The act of writing down feelings and thoughts about stressful life events has been shown to help people with chronic conditions improve their health. In one recent study, people with asthma or rheumatoid arthritis were asked to write down their feelings about the most stressful event in their lives; they wrote for 20 minutes a day over a three-day period. In follow-up exams four months later, nearly half of the patients who engaged in expressive writing experienced positive changes in their condition such as improved lung function or reduced joint pain. Only about a quarter of the control group, who wrote about their daily plans, experienced a positive change in health.

Investigators remain unsure why writing about one's feelings has beneficial effects. It is possible that expressing feelings about a traumatic event helps people work through the event and put it behind them. The resulting sense of release and control may reduce stress levels and have positive physical effects such as reduced heart rate and blood pressure and improved immune function. Alternatively, expressive writing may change the way people think about previous stressful events in their lives and help them cope with new stressors. Whatever the cause, it's clear that expressive writing can be a safe, inexpensive, and effective supplement to standard treatment of certain chronic illnesses.

What about the effects of expressive writing on otherwise healthy individuals? Other studies have, in fact, found such a benefit: People who wrote about traumatic experiences reported fewer symptoms, fewer days off work, fewer visits to the doctor, improved mood, and a more positive outlook.

If you'd like to try expressive writing to help you deal with a traumatic event, set aside a special time—15 minutes a day for four consecutive days, for example, or one day a week for four weeks. Write in a place where you won't be interrupted or distracted. Explore your very deepest thoughts and feelings and why you feel the way you do. Don't worry about grammar or coherence or about what someone else might think about what you're writing; you are writing just for yourself. You may find the writing exercise to be distressing in the short term—sadness and depression are common when dealing with feelings about a stressful event—but most people report relief and contentment soon after writing for several days.

SOURCES: Smyth, J. M., et al. 1999. Effects of writing about stressful experiences on symptom reduction in patients with asthma or rheumatoid arthritis: A randomized trial. *Journal of the American Medical Association* 281(14): 1304–1309. Spiegel, D. 1999. Healing words: Emotional expression and disease outcome. *Journal of the American Medical Association* 281(14): 1328–1329. Pennebaker, J. 1997. *Opening Up: The Healthy Power of Expressing Emotions.* New York: Guilford Press.

3. Use caution if you are taking other medications, because OTC and prescription drugs and herbs can interact. If you have questions about drug interactions, ask your physician or pharmacist *before* you mix medicines.

4. Try to select medications with one active ingredient rather than combination ("all-in-one") products. A product with multiple ingredients is likely to include drugs for symptoms you don't even have, so why risk the side effects of medications you don't need? Using single-ingredient products also allows you to adjust the dosage of each medication separately for optimal symptom relief with minimal side effects.

5. When choosing medications, try to buy **generic drugs**, which contain the same active ingredient as the brand-name product but generally at a much lower cost. (Brand-name and generic drugs are discussed in more detail later in the chapter.)

6. Never take or give a drug from an unlabeled container or in the dark when you can't read what the label says.

7. If you are pregnant or nursing or have a chronic condition such as kidney disease, consult your physician before self-medicating.

8. The expiration date marked on many medications is an estimate of how long the *unopened* medication is likely to be potent. Once the package is opened, the medication will probably be potent for about a year if stored properly. Mark the date on the package when you open it, and dispose of it safely after a year by taking it to a pharmacy or hospital.

9. Store your medications in a cool, dry place that is out of the reach of children (Figure 22-2).

10. Use special caution with aspirin. Because of an association with a rare but serious problem known as Reye's syndrome, aspirin should not be used by children or adolescents who may have the flu, chicken pox, or any other viral illness.

---

false positive A test result that incorrectly detects a disease or condition in a healthy person.

false negative A test result that fails to correctly detect a disease or condition.

over-the-counter (OTC) medication A medication or product that can be purchased by the consumer without a prescription.

generic drug A drug that is not registered or protected by a trademark; a drug that does not have a brand name.

Terms

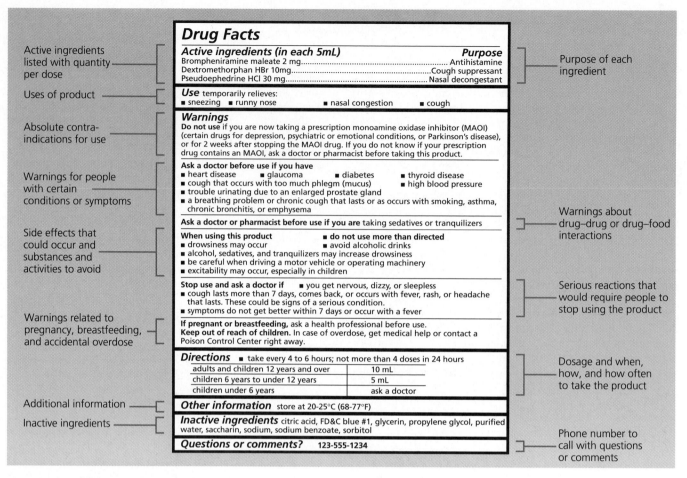

Active ingredients listed with quantity per dose

Uses of product

Absolute contra- indications for use

Warnings for people with certain conditions or symptoms

Side effects that could occur and substances and activities to avoid

Warnings related to pregnancy, breastfeeding, and accidental overdose

Additional information

Inactive ingredients

Drug Facts

Active ingredients (in each 5mL)   **Purpose**
Brompheniramine maleate 2 mg.. Antihistamine
Dextromethorphan HBr 10mg.. Cough suppressant
Pseudoephedrine HCl 30 mg.. Nasal decongestant

Use temporarily relieves:
■ sneezing ■ runny nose   ■ nasal congestion   ■ cough

Warnings
Do not use if you are now taking a prescription monoamine oxidase inhibitor (MAOI) (certain drugs for depression, psychiatric or emotional conditions, or Parkinson's disease), or for 2 weeks after stopping the MAOI drug. If you do not know if your prescription drug contains an MAOI, ask a doctor or pharmacist before taking this product.

Ask a doctor before use if you have
■ heart disease   ■ glaucoma   ■ diabetes   ■ thyroid disease
■ cough that occurs with too much phlegm (mucus)   ■ high blood pressure
■ trouble urinating due to an enlarged prostate gland
■ a breathing problem or chronic cough that lasts or as occurs with smoking, asthma, chronic bronchitis, or emphysema

Ask a doctor or pharmacist before use if you are taking sedatives or tranquilizers

When using this product   ■ do not use more than directed
■ drowsiness may occur   ■ avoid alcoholic drinks
■ alcohol, sedatives, and tranquilizers may increase drowsiness
■ be careful when driving a motor vehicle or operating machinery
■ excitability may occur, especially in children

Stop use and ask a doctor if   ■ you get nervous, dizzy, or sleepless
■ cough lasts more than 7 days, comes back, or occurs with fever, rash, or headache that lasts. These could be signs of a serious condition.
■ symptoms do not get better within 7 days or occur with a fever

If pregnant or breastfeeding, ask a health professional before use.
Keep out of reach of children. In case of overdose, get medical help or contact a Poison Control Center right away.

Directions   ■ take every 4 to 6 hours; not more than 4 doses in 24 hours

adults and children 12 years and over	10 mL
children 6 years to under 12 years	5 mL
children under 6 years	ask a doctor

Other information   store at 20-25°C (68-77°F)

Inactive ingredients citric acid, FD&C blue #1, glycerin, propylene glycol, purified water, saccharin, sodium, sodium benzoate, sorbitol

Questions or comments?   123-555-1234

Purpose of each ingredient

Warnings about drug–drug or drug–food interactions

Serious reactions that would require people to stop using the product

Dosage and when, how, and how often to take the product

Phone number to call with questions or comments

Figure 22-1 Reading and understanding OTC drug labels. SOURCE: Food and Drug Administration. 1999. Over-the-counter human drugs; labeling requirements; final rule. *Federal Register* 64, no. 51(17 March): 13254–13303.

The Home Pharmacy If you were to survey home medicine cabinets, what would you find? On average, there would be 22 medications, including 17 OTC products. You would probably find an oversupply of expired medications and leftover prescription drugs. At the same time, certain essential medications and equipment would be absent. Only a few supplies are actually essential; additional items depend upon the particular health problems you or your family is likely to have (see Figure 22-2). Because many medications deteriorate, buy small quantities of infrequently used medications, and replace them about every 3 years.

GETTING THE MOST OUT OF YOUR MEDICAL CARE

Self-care involves more than self-diagnosis and self-treatment. It includes knowing when to seek professional care and how to get the most out of your medical care. The key to making the health care system work for you lies in good communication with your physician and other members of the health care team. Studies show that patients who are more active in interacting with physicians, who ask more questions, enjoy better health outcomes.

Unfortunately, many people are intimidated by their physicians and afraid to communicate freely. Medical jargon can be very confusing, yet some patients don't ask questions because they fear appearing stupid. Others are afraid to ask why a test or treatment is needed for fear of appearing to challenge the authority of the physician. Patients often conceal personal concerns about sexuality, drug abuse, emotional problems, and cancer. All these fears and others block open communication with the physician.

Physicians share the responsibility for poor communication. They may feel they are too busy or too important to take time to talk with patients. They may ignore questions, use incomprehensible medical jargon, and respond in an unsupportive way to patients' attempts to assert themselves.

Closet

- Analgesic (relieves pain)
- Antacid (relieves upset stomach)
- Antibiotic ointment (reduces risk of infection)
- Antihistamine (relieves allergy symptoms)
- Antiseptic (helps stop infection)
- Fever reducer (adult and child)
- Hydrocortisone (relieves itching and inflammation)
- Decongestant (relieves stuffy nose and other cold symptoms)
- Syrup of ipecac (induces vomiting in case of poisoning)

Medicine Cabinet

- Adhesive bandages
- Adhesive tape
- Alcohol wipes
- Calibrated measuring spoon
- Disinfectant
- Gauze pads
- Thermometer
- Tweezers

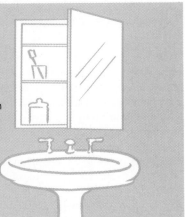

Figure 22-2   Your home medical care kit.   Contrary to tradition, a bathroom medicine cabinet is not a good place to keep medications. Showers and baths create heat and humidity that can cause some drugs to deteriorate rapidly. A cool, dark, and dry place such as the top of a linen closet, preferably in a locked container and out of a child's reach, is best for storing medicines. Use your bathroom medicine cabinet for supplies that aren't affected by heat and humidity.   SOURCE: Lewis, C. 2000. Your medicine cabinet needs an annual checkup, too. *FDA Consumer,* March/April.

The Physician-Patient Partnership

The physician-patient relationship is undergoing an important transformation. The image of the all-knowing physician and the passive patient is slowly fading. What is emerging is more of a physician-patient *partnership,* in which the physician acts more like a consultant and the patient participates more actively. The necessary ingredients in a successful partnership are a sympathetic, caring physician and a prepared, assertive patient. As one observer commented, "It is not enough for the doctor to stop playing God. You've got to get off your knees."

You should try to remember that physicians are human: They have off days, and they make mistakes just as everyone else does. However, you should expect someone who is attentive, caring, able to listen, and able to clearly explain things to you. You also have to do your part. You need to be assertive in a firm but not aggressive manner. You need to express your feelings and concerns, ask questions, and, if necessary, be persistent. If your physician is unable to communicate clearly with you in spite of your best efforts, then you probably need to change physicians.

COMMUNICATE!   To build a partnership with your physician, let him or her know that you want to be an active participant in your health care. One way to do that is to ask questions; another is to ask for written information or literature about your condition or sources where you can read more. Offer information about your personal or family history if you think it's relevant (or remind the physician of such information if it's part of your health record); for example, "I started using a new fabric softener about a month ago—could that be causing this rash?" Discuss your treatment plan with your physician, especially if you're not comfortable with any part of it. For example, "I had a hard time with the side effects of that medication the last time I took it. Is there anything else available?" or "I think I'm mildly depressed, but I don't really want to take an antidepressant. Are there any behavioral things that would help me, like exercise or yoga?"

Your Appointment with Your Physician

Because physicians are often pressed for time, it's a good idea to prepare for your visit ahead of time. Make a written list of your most important concerns and questions, along with notes about your symptoms (when they started, how long they last, what makes them better or worse, what treatments you have already tried, and so on). If there are questions you're uncomfortable about asking, practice discussing them ahead of time. Bring a list of all medications you're taking—prescription, nonprescription, and herbal. Also bring any medical records or test results your physician may not already have.

Present your concerns at the beginning of the visit, to set the agenda. Be specific and concise about your symptoms, and be open and honest about your concerns. Share your hunches with your physician; your guesses can provide vital clues. Ask questions if you don't understand something. Let your physician know if you are taking any drugs, are allergic to any medications, are breastfeeding, or may be pregnant.

There are many potential benefits of e-mail communication with your physician. Both you and your physician may find it more convenient than phone calls or personal appointments because you can send messages briefly, at convenient times. It allows for clarification and advice in writing, which can remove any doubt about what your physician is recommending. Unlike telephone conversations, e-mail is self-documenting, meaning that copies of both your e-mail and those of your physician can be placed in your medical file. For information such as test results, having a written record can be very helpful.

If you like the idea, talk with your physician about the possibility of e-mail communication. If he or she already has a system set up, ask about the policies and procedures. The following guidelines can help you use e-mail with your physician effectively and safely:

- Find out what types of transactions can be carried out over e-mail. For example, can appointment scheduling and prescription refills be handled with e-mail?

- Do not use e-mail communication for emergencies and other time-sensitive issues or for confidential or sensitive information.

- Be concise—to save time for both yourself and your physician.

- Put the type of transaction and your name and medical record number in the appropriate place designated by your physician. She or he may ask that certain information be included in the subject line of your e-mail or at the top of the body of the message.

- If requested, send a reply to the physician's e-mail to acknowledge that you've received and understood the message.

- Keep copies of any e-mail that you send or receive.

- Be aware that your physician may share your e-mail with office staff or other consultants.

SOURCES: American Medical Association. 2000. *Guidelines for Physician-Patient Electronic Communications* (http://www.ama-assn.org/ama/pub/category/2386.html; retrieved December 17, 2000). Sands, D. Z. 2000. *How to Communicate with Your Doctor Using Email* (http://www.healthology.com/focus_article.asp?f=healthcare&c=healthcare_emaildoctor; retrieved October 19, 2000).

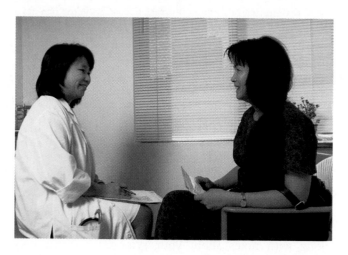

Good communication is a crucial factor in a satisfactory physician-patient partnership.

At the end of the visit, briefly repeat the physician's diagnosis, prognosis, and instructions, and make sure you understand your next steps, such as making another appointment, phoning for test results, watching for new symptoms, and so on. You may also want to ask about the possibility of using e-mail for follow-up (see the box "Communicating with Your Physician via E-Mail").

W. The Diagnostic Process

The first step in the diagnostic process is the medical history, which includes your primary reason for the visit, your current symptoms, your past medical history, and your social history (job, family life, major stressors, living conditions, and health habits). Keeping up-to-date records of your medical history can help you provide your physician with key facts about your health (see the box "Personal Health Profile").

The next step is the physical exam, which usually begins with a review of vital signs: blood pressure, heart rate (pulse), breathing rate, and temperature. Depending on your primary complaint, your physician may give you a complete physical, or the exam may be directed to specific areas, such as your ears, nose, and throat.

Finally, your physician may order medical tests to complete the diagnosis. Diagnostic testing provides a wealth of information to help solve medical problems; such testing now accounts for nearly one-third of our national health bill. Physicians can order X rays, biopsies, blood and urine tests, scans of various types, and a wide array of **endoscopies** to view, probe, or analyze almost any part of the body.

If your physician orders a medical test for you, be sure you know why you need it, what the risks and benefits of the test are for you, how you should prepare for it (for example, by fasting or discontinuing medications or herbal remedies), and what the test will involve. Also ask what the test results mean, since no test is 100% accurate—false positives and false negatives do occur—and interpretation of some procedures is subjective. Sometimes it is important to get an experienced second opinion on a diagnosis.

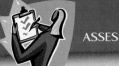

General Information

Age: _____   Total cholesterol: _____   Blood pressure: ___/___

Height: _____   HDL: _____   Other: _____

Weight: _____   LDL: _____   Other: _____

Medical Conditions

Check any of the following that apply to you and add other conditions that might affect your health and well-being.

_____ heart disease   _____ back pain   _____ depression, anxiety, or

_____ lung disease   _____ arthritis   another psychological disorder

_____ diabetes   _____ other injury or joint   _____ eating disorder

_____ allergies   problem   _____ other: _____

_____ asthma   _____ substance abuse problem   _____ other: _____

Medications/Treatments

List any medications or supplements you are taking or any medical treatments you are undergoing. Include the name of the substance or treatment and its purpose. Include both prescription and over-the-counter drugs and any vitamin, mineral, or other dietary supplement you are taking.

_____   _____   _____

_____   _____   _____

_____   _____   _____

Health Care Providers

Primary care physician: name _____   phone _____

Specialist physician: name _____   phone _____

    Condition treated: _____

Other health care provider: name _____   phone _____

    Condition treated: _____

Health insurance provider and policy number: _____

To ensure that you are getting the most out of your medical care, you should also keep a record of your vaccinations and medical screening tests. Chapter 17 provides a list of the currently recommended vaccinations for adults; Chapters 15 and 16 describe screening tests for cardiovascular disease and cancer.

COMMUNICATE!   Sometimes you need someone to go with you to a medical appointment. You may have a serious problem or a worrisome symptom that is causing you undue anxiety; you may be scheduled for an uncomfortable medical procedure, such as an endoscopy; or you may need someone to drive you home. In these situations, don't hesitate to ask a family member or friend to accompany you. Even if you don't think you need it, the support will help relieve your anxiety and make the experience less nerve-wracking. You can say, for example, "I'm sure I'll be okay after this needle biopsy, but I'd find it reassuring to have someone waiting for me when it's done. Would you come with me to my appointment?"

Medical and Surgical Treatments

Once the diagnosis is made, you and your physician can consider treatment options. Many conditions can be treated in a variety of ways; in some cases, lifestyle changes should be considered along with other options.

endoscopy A medical procedure in which a viewing instrument is inserted into a body cavity or opening. Specific procedures are named for the area viewed: inside joints (arthroscopy), inside airways (bronchoscopy), inside the abdominal cavity (laparoscopy), and inside the lower portion of the large intestine, or sigmoid colon (sigmoidoscopy).

Terms

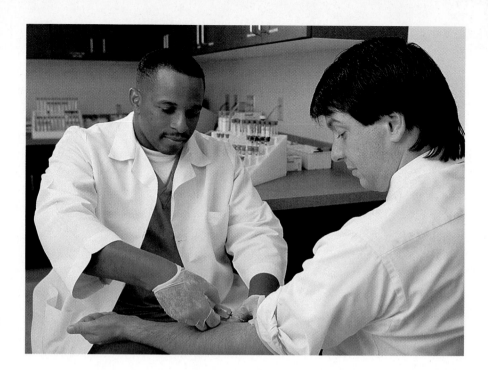

Physicians get information they need from medical tests, but patients have the right to know what the test is for, why they need it, and what the results will indicate. Blood tests are one type of medical test; other tests include X rays, sonograms, urine tests, and endoscopies.

Make sure you know the possible risks and side effects of each treatment option, as well as the likelihood that it will improve your condition.

Prescription Medications Thousands of lives are saved each year by **antibiotics,** heart medications, insulin, and scores of other drugs. But we pay a price for having such powerful tools. A report from the Institute of Medicine (IOM) estimated that preventable medication errors result in more than 7000 deaths each year in hospitals alone, with tens of thousands more in outpatient facilities (see the box "Medical Errors").

Although pharmaceutical companies carry out extensive trials on new drugs, even the most extensive studies involve just a few thousand people. A large natural experiment begins when the drug is approved and physicians start prescribing it to people in the general population. Side effects that did not show up in studies often become apparent when more people begin taking a drug. Consumers need to be especially alert for adverse effects if they are taking a drug that is new to the market.

Physicians may overprescribe drugs, sometimes in response to pressure by patients. Consumers are now the target of multibillion-dollar direct-to-consumer (DTC) advertising campaigns for prescription drugs. Proponents of DTC advertising claim that it enhances public health

by providing educational information to consumers (about such underdiagnosed conditions as diabetes, high cholesterol, and depression) and motivating them to seek medical care. Opponents claim that DTC advertising is more promotional than educational; that it is misleading and omits important precautions; that it is designed to create consumer demand by creating problems and needs; and that it causes patients to pressure physicians to prescribe particular drugs. A recent study found that most DTC ads fail to provide information about how a drug works, its success rate, how long it must be taken, alternative treatments, or helpful lifestyle changes.

Adverse effects from prescription drugs can also occur if a physician prescribes the wrong drug or a dangerous combination of drugs. At the pharmacy, patients may receive the wrong drug or may not be given complete information about drug risks, side effects, and interactions. Problems can occur because of a physician's poor handwriting, misinterpretation of an abbreviated drug name, or similarities between the names and packaging of different drugs. One in four prescribing errors is thought to be caused by similar drug names, such as Celebrex (arthritis treatment), Cerebyx (anticonvulsant), and Celexa (antidepressant).

A recent area of concern is the advent of online pharmacies. Although convenient, some online pharmacies may sell products or engage in practices that are illegal in the offline world. The Food and Drug Administration (FDA) recommends that consumers avoid sites that offer to prescribe drugs for the first time without a physical exam, sell prescription drugs without a prescription, or sell drugs not approved by the FDA. You should also

Terms   **antibiotic** A substance derived from a mold or bacterium that inhibits the growth of other microorganisms.

In May 2000, comedian Dana Carvey sued his heart surgeon for performing angioplasty on the wrong artery, necessitating another operation to clear the artery that was actually blocked. Based on a recent report from the National Academy of Science's Institute of Medicine (IOM), Carvey is not alone in his experience—and may have been one of the lucky ones to survive a serious medical error. The IOM report found that between 44,000 and 98,000 people may be killed each year in hospitals due to medical errors—with many more people affected in outpatient settings. These statistics place medical errors in the top ten leading causes of death among Americans. Although these figures are controversial, no one argues that medical errors are a serious problem that needs to be addressed.

According to the IOM report, medical errors can occur because a health care provider chooses an inappropriate method of care or carries out an appropriate course of care incorrectly. Errors can occur at all stages of the process of care, from diagnosis to treatment to preventive care. Examples of preventable medical errors include prescribing a drug for which a patient has a known allergy, administering an excessively high dose of a medication, administering a drug or treatment to the wrong patient, and passing an infection to a patient because of poor hand washing.

The IOM report made several recommendations for reducing medical errors, including mandatory reporting of serious mistakes to make hospitals more accountable. Strategies for reducing medication errors include having pharmacists accompany doctors on their rounds and having all prescriptions entered into a computerized screening system. Such a system could help eliminate problems stemming from poor handwriting, mix-ups between drugs with similar names, and the prescribing of dangerous combinations of drugs.

What can consumers do to protect themselves from preventable medical errors? The Agency for Healthcare Research and Quality recommends the following:

1. Be an active member of your health care team, and take part in every decision about your health care.

Medications

2. Make sure that all of your physicians know about every medication you are taking, including prescription and over-the-counter drugs and dietary supplements such as vitamins and herbs.

3. Make sure that your physician knows about any allergies or adverse reactions you have had to medications.

4. When your physician writes you a prescription, make sure you can read it.

5. Ask for information about your medications in terms you can understand—both when your medicines are prescribed and when you receive them (see the list of questions on pp. 636).

6. When you pick up your medicine from the pharmacy, ask, "Is this the medicine that my physician prescribed?"

7. If you have any questions about the instructions on a medicine label, ask.

8. Ask your pharmacist for the best device to measure your liquid medication, and ask questions if you're not sure how to use it.

9. Ask for written information about the side effects your medication could cause.

Hospital Stays

10. If you have a choice, choose a hospital at which many patients have the procedure or surgery you need.

11. If you are in a hospital, consider asking all health care workers who have direct contact with you whether they have washed their hands. Hand washing is an important way to prevent the spread of infections in hospitals, but it is not done regularly or thoroughly enough.

12. When you are being discharged from the hospital, ask your physician to explain the treatment plan you will use at home.

Surgery

13. If you are having surgery, make sure that you, your physician, and your surgeon all agree and are clear on exactly what will be done. (Some surgeons will initial the surgery site beforehand.)

Other Steps You Can Take

14. Speak up if you have questions or concerns.

15. Make sure that someone, such as your personal physician, is in charge of your care. This is especially important if you have many health problems or are in a hospital.

16. Make sure that all health professionals involved in your care have important health information about you. Do not assume that all of them know everything they need to.

17. Ask a family member or friend to be there with you and to be your advocate.

18. Know that "more" is not always better when it comes to tests and treatments.

19. If you have a test, don't assume that no news is good news. Ask about the results.

20. Learn about your conditions and treatments by asking your physician and other health care professionals and by using other reliable resources.

SOURCES: Agency for Healthcare Research and Quality. 2000. *20 Tips to Help Prevent Medical Errors*. AHRQ Publication No. 00-PO38. Nordenberg, T. 2000. Make no mistake: Medical errors can be deadly serious. *FDA Consumer*, September–October. Institute of Medicine. 1999. *To Err Is Human: Building a Safer Health System*. Washington, D.C.: National Academy Press.

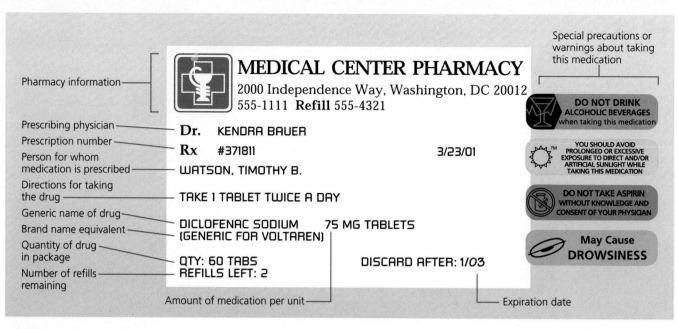

Pharmacy information

MEDICAL CENTER PHARMACY
2000 Independence Way, Washington, DC 20012
555-1111 **Refill** 555-4321

Special precautions or warnings about taking this medication

Prescribing physician

Dr. KENDRA BAUER

Prescription number

Rx #371811   3/23/01

Person for whom medication is prescribed

WATSON, TIMOTHY B.

Directions for taking the drug

TAKE 1 TABLET TWICE A DAY

Generic name of drug

DICLOFENAC SODIUM   75 MG TABLETS

Brand name equivalent

(GENERIC FOR VOLTAREN)

Quantity of drug in package

QTY: 60 TABS   DISCARD AFTER: 1/03

Number of refills remaining

REFILLS LEFT: 2

Amount of medication per unit

Expiration date

DO NOT DRINK ALCOHOLIC BEVERAGES when taking this medication

YOU SHOULD AVOID PROLONGED OR EXCESSIVE EXPOSURE TO DIRECT AND/OR ARTIFICIAL SUNLIGHT WHILE TAKING THIS MEDICATION

DO NOT TAKE ASPIRIN WITHOUT KNOWLEDGE AND CONSENT OF YOUR PHYSICIAN

May Cause DROWSINESS

Figure 22-3   Reading and understanding prescription medication labels.

avoid sites that do not provide access to a registered pharmacist to answer questions or that do not provide a U.S. address and phone number to contact if there's a problem. The National Association of Boards of Pharmacy sponsors a voluntary certification program for Internet pharmacies; to be certified, a pharmacy must have a state license in good standing and allow regular inspections.

Patients also share some responsibility for problems with prescription drugs. Many people don't take their medications properly, skipping doses, taking incorrect doses, stopping too soon, or not taking the medication at all. An estimated 30–50% of the more than 3 billion prescriptions dispensed annually in the United States are not taken correctly and thus do not produce the desired results. Consumers can increase the effectiveness of their treatment and decrease the chances of adverse effects by asking the following questions:

- *Do I really need this prescription, or are there nondrug alternatives?*
- *What is the name of the medication, and what is it supposed to do, within what period of time?*
- *How and when do I take the medication, how much do I take, and for how long? What should I do if I miss a dose?*
- *What other medications, foods, drinks, or activities should I avoid?* Other drugs, including alcohol, herbs, and OTC drugs, can interact with medications, diminishing or increasing their effect (Figure 22-3). For example, certain antibiotics, including ampicillin and tetracycline, may prevent oral contraceptives from working. Others may increase the effects of sunlight on the skin.

- *What are the side effects, and what do I do if they occur?* If you have a drug allergy or other medical condition, such as epilepsy or diabetes, that may require special attention in case of an emergency, wear a medical ID necklace or bracelet or carry a medical ID card. For comprehensive emergency medical service, consider joining Medic Alert; call 1-800-ID-ALERT for more information.
- *Can I take a generic drug rather than a brand-name one?* Generic drugs contain the same ingredients as the original brand-name drug, but they may contain different inactive ingredients. They are usually substantially less expensive, but sometimes physicians have reasons for preferring a particular brand.
- *Is there written information about the medication?* There are many sources of information, including the FDA-approved inserts in drug packaging and books and pamphlets (see Appendix C, Resources for Self-Care).

Remember to store your medications in a cool, dry place, out of direct light. Never share your prescription medications with anyone else, and never use an old prescription for a new ailment.

COMMUNICATE!   Advertisements for prescription drugs used to appear only in medical journals, where they reached physicians who were responsible for selecting and prescribing drugs for their patients. Now that these drugs are being marketed to the public in direct-to-consumer ads, individuals have a role in evaluating the manufacturer's health claims

Surgery Surgical procedures are performed more often in the United States than anywhere else in the world. Each year, more than 70 million operations and related procedures are performed. About 20% are in response to an emergency such as a severe injury, and 80% are **elective surgeries,** meaning the patient can generally choose when and where to have the operation, if at all. Some important questions to ask include the following:

• *Why do I need surgery at this time?* Your physician should be able to explain the reason for the surgery and what is likely to happen if you don't have it. Getting a second opinion about surgery is recommended and may be required by your health insurance plan.

• *What are the risks and complications of the surgery?* Overall risk depends on the type of operation performed, the surgeon, and your general state of health. Ask about the **mortality rate** (risk of death) and the **morbidity rate** (risk of nonlethal complications).

• *Can the operation be performed on an outpatient basis?* **Outpatient** (ambulatory) surgery has many advantages, including lower costs and fewer opportunities for hospital-associated complications.

• *What can I expect before, during, and after surgery?* Knowing what to expect can help you prepare for the surgery and speed your recovery.

PAYING FOR HEALTH CARE

The American health care system is one of the most advanced and comprehensive in the world, but it is also the most expensive (see the box "How Does the U.S. Health Care System Rate?"). In 1999, the nation spent more than $1.2 trillion on health care, or $4300 per person. Health care costs are expected to nearly double in the first decade of the twenty-first century, reaching $2.6 trillion, or about $8700 per person, by 2010. Numerous factors contribute to the high cost of health care in the United States, including the cost of advanced equipment and new technology; expensive treatments for some illnesses and conditions, such as cancer, heart disease, HIV infection, injuries, and low birth weight in infants; the aging of the population; and high earnings by some people in the health care industry and, in some cases, the demand for profits by investors.

The Current System

Health care is currently financed by a combination of private and public insurance plans, patient out-of-pocket payments, and government assistance (Figure 22-4). In 1999, private insurance and individual patients paid about 55% of the total; the government paid the remaining 45%, mainly through Medicare and Medicaid (discussed below). Most nonelderly Americans receive their health insurance through their employers.

Despite high spending, not everyone is included in this financing system. More than 48 million people (17% of the population), the vast majority of them employed, have no health care insurance at all. Many more are underinsured and thus either pay for medical services out of pocket or forgo medical care altogether. The uninsured include almost 11 million children—15% of all American children—most in working, low-income families.

Lack of insurance affects both access to care and quality of care. People without insurance use health services less often and receive poorer care when they do use the services. Children without insurance are less likely to have screening tests and immunizations. They have fewer checkups, are less likely to be treated for injuries and for chronic conditions such as asthma, and are more likely to go without eyeglasses and prescribed drugs.

Another problem is that national health spending is growing faster than the rest of the economy, consuming an ever-increasing share of the U.S. gross domestic product (GDP). Health care spending represented 13.1% of the GDP in 2000 and is projected to reach 15.9% by 2010. Health care costs soared in the 1980s and then were contained to some extent in the 1990s by a large-scale switch from private insurance to managed care (discussed below), which is designed to achieve cost economies. But the savings from this switch were likely a one-time phenomenon, since more than 80% of working Americans are now covered by managed-care plans. Experts predict that health costs will increase drastically in the near future, with much of the increase borne by private insurers and individuals. They also predict trends in reaction to the cost cutting of the 1990s, including greater demands for physician autonomy, more interest in consumer choice, and a renewed focus on quality of care.

elective surgery A nonemergency operation that the patient can choose to schedule.

mortality rate The number of deaths occurring in a population of a given size in a given time period.

morbidity rate The number of illnesses or injuries occurring in a population of a given size in a given time period.

outpatient A person receiving medical attention without being admitted to the hospital.

Terms

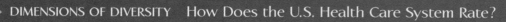

The United States spends more money per capita on health care than any other country. But does this more expensive health care lead to better health among Americans? By some measures, the answer would appear to be no.

The *World Health Report 2000*, prepared by the World Health Organization (WHO), focused on health systems around the world. The criteria used by WHO to evaluate the performance of health systems included the following:

- *Overall level of health:* What is the life expectancy (adjusted for disability) in a country?

- *Distribution of health in the population:* How large a difference in health is seen among individuals and groups? How great are the inequalities?

- *Responsiveness to people's expectations:* Does the health system respect people (maintain dignity, confidentiality, and autonomy) and have a client orientation (provide prompt attention, access to support networks during care, choice of provider, and so on)?

- *Distribution of financing:* How fairly is the financial burden shared among individuals?

Based on the WHO criteria, the United States ranks 37th out of 191 countries overall, and 15th among 25 industrialized countries. The top-ranking countries are France, Italy, Spain, Oman, Austria, and Japan. The U.S. health system ranks first in per capita health expenditures and in its responsiveness to expectations; it ranks much lower in terms of fairness in financial contribution and on how much it achieves given the level of economic resources put toward health care in the United States. Other studies have also rated the U.S. health system poorly on such factors as infant mortality, low birth weight, and life expectancy at 1 year of age.

What is responsible for the relatively poor rating of the United States health system? There is no definitive explanation, but several factors have been proposed, including the lack of a strong primary care infrastructure. Studies have shown that strong and widespread use of primary care benefits health, a fact often cited by supporters of universal health insurance for Americans. Another possible contributor to the poor U.S. performance on health indicators is the high degree of income inequality. Researchers have linked low relative social and economic position in industrialized countries with a significant adverse effect on health. Areas with more equitable distributions of income are also more likely to have better primary care resources available. Finally, as described earlier, health care interventions can also have harmful effects, including those resulting from medical errors. The United States has very high rates of treatment and accompanying adverse effects.

SOURCES: World Health Organization. 2000. *World Health Report 2000—Health Systems: Improving Performance.* Geneva: World Health Organization. Starfield, B. 2000. Is U.S. health really the best in the world? *Journal of the American Medical Association* 284(4): 483–485.

Health Insurance

Health insurance enables people to receive health care they might not otherwise be able to afford. Hospital care costs hundreds of dollars a day, and surgical fees can cost thousands. Health insurance is important for everyone, especially as health care costs continue to rise.

Health insurance plans are either fee-for-service (or indemnity) or managed care. With both types the individual or the employer pays a basic premium, usually on a monthly basis; there are often other payments as well. Insurance policies are sold to both groups and individuals; group plans tend to cover more services and cost less. Group coverage is often available through employers to workers and their families. People who are self-employed or whose employers don't offer group policies may need to buy individual plans. Americans who are 65 or older, have disabilities, or have a low income may receive health insurance through government programs.

Traditional Fee-for-Service (Indemnity) Plans
In a fee-for-service, or indemnity, plan, you can use any medical provider (such as a physician or a hospital) you choose. You or the provider sends the bill to your insurance company, which pays part of it. Usually you have to pay a "deductible" amount each year, ranging from $100 up to several hundred dollars, before the insurer starts covering your expenses. Once you meet the deductible, most plans pay a percentage—often 80%—of what they consider the "usual and customary" charge for covered services. You pay the remaining 20%, which is known as coinsurance. Most indemnity plans cover hospital, surgical, and many medical services, but coverage varies widely from one plan to another.

Freedom of choice is a major benefit of indemnity plans: You can see any physician you choose, including specialists. Your physician is paid based on the services he or she provides. Critics point to the fee-for-service payment system as a contributing factor in the rapid growth of U.S. health care costs because physicians have a financial incentive to order more tests and treatments for their patients.

Managed-Care Plans
Managed-care plans have agreements with certain physicians, hospitals, and health care providers to give a range of services to plan members at reduced cost. In general, you have lower out-of-pocket costs and less paperwork with a managed-care plan than with an indemnity plan, but you also have less freedom in choosing health care providers. Most Americans with job-

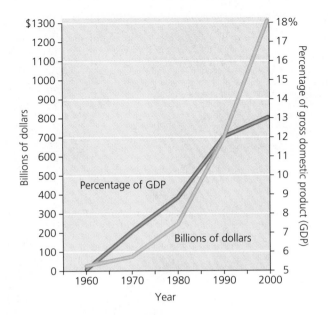

(a) National health care expenditures

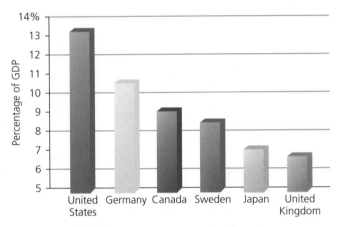

(b) Health care expenditure as a percentage of GDP

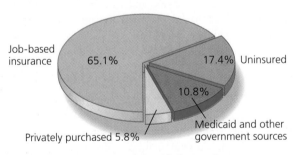

Job-based insurance 65.1%

17.4% Uninsured

10.8%

Privately purchased 5.8%

Medicaid and other government sources

(c) Health insurance coverage of nonelderly Americans (age 0–64)

W. VITAL STATISTICS

Figure 22-4 A statistical look at health care expenditures and health insurance. SOURCES: National Center for Health Statistics. 2000. *Health, United States, 2000.* Hyattsville, Md.: U.S. Public Health Service. Health Care Financing Administration (http://www.hcfa.gov).

based insurance are covered by managed-care plans, which may follow several different models:

• **Health maintenance organizations (HMOs)** offer members a range of services for a set monthly fee. You choose a primary care physician who manages your care and refers you to specialists if you need them. If you go outside the HMO, you have to pay for the service yourself. Physicians in the HMO agree to accept a monthly per-patient fee, or **capitation**, or to charge less than standard fees for services.

• **Preferred provider organizations (PPOs)** are plans that have arrangements with physicians and other providers who have agreed to accept lower fees. If you go outside the PPO, you have to pay more.

• **Point-of-service (POS) plans** are options offered by many HMOs, in which you can see a physician outside the plan and still be partially covered (for example, for a specialist outside the network).

Many managed-care plans try to reduce costs over the long term by paying for routine preventive care, such as regular checkups and screening tests and prenatal care; they may also encourage prevention by offering health education and lifestyle modification programs for members. Other cost-cutting measures are less consumer-oriented. Consumers' choice of physicians is limited, and they may have to wait longer for appointments and travel farther to see participating doctors. Managed-care plans may also try to discourage overtreatment through the use of "gatekeepers." In many plans, patients must get preapproval from their primary care physician or a plan representative for diagnostic tests, referrals to specialists, or hospital treatments. If a patient violates the rules for obtaining services, the plan typically will not cover the cost of the services in question. Nonemergency visits to emergency rooms are also frequently not covered.

Plans based on a capitation system give physicians a financial incentive to limit the number of tests and treatments they offer patients, the reverse of the financial

Terms

managed-care plan A health care program that integrates the financing and delivery of services by using designated providers, utilization review, and financial incentives for following the plan's policies; HMO, PPO, and POS are examples of managed-care plans.

health maintenance organization (HMO) A prepaid health insurance plan in which patients receive health care from designated providers.

capitation A payment to health care providers according to the number of patients they agree to serve, rather than the amount of service rendered.

preferred provider organization (PPO) A prepaid health insurance plan in which providers agree to deliver services for discounted fees; patients can go to any provider, but using nonparticipating providers results in higher costs to the patient.

point-of-service (POS) plan A managed-care plan that covers treatment by an HMO physician but permits patients to seek treatment elsewhere with a higher copayment.

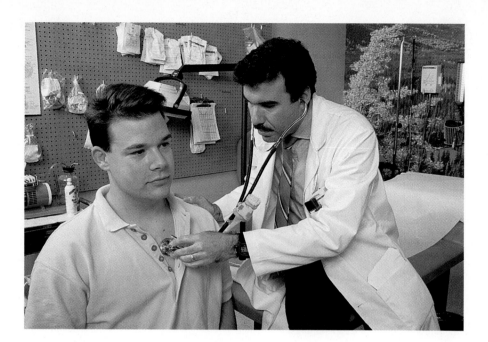

Physicians who work for a health maintenance organization usually receive a salary or monthly payment rather than fees from patients. The advantage of HMOs for patients is that their medical care is prepaid; the disadvantage is that the choice of physicians is narrowed.

incentive in indemnity plans. Critics claim that physicians in managed-care plans deny patients needed services in their efforts to keep costs down.

Government Programs Americans who are 65 or older and younger people with certain disabilities can be covered by **Medicare,** a federal health insurance program that helps pay for both hospitalization and physician services. As a result of limits placed on payments, however, some physicians and managed-care programs have stopped accepting Medicare patients. **Medicaid** is a joint federal-state health insurance program that covers some low-income people, especially children, pregnant women, and people with certain disabilities.

Choosing a Policy

Choosing health insurance can be complicated; it's important to evaluate the coverage provided by different plans and decide which one is best for you (see the box "Choosing a Health Care Plan"). Colleges typically provide medical services through a student health center; some require students to purchase additional insurance if they are not covered by family policies. It's usually economical to remain on a family policy as long as possible.

After college, most people secure group coverage through their place of employment or through membership in an organization. If group coverage is not available, individuals should contact several different insurance

companies for information about policies. Managed-care plans tend to have lower premiums and fewer out-of-pocket costs, an advantage for young adults and families with young children. Traditional fee-for-service plans tend to cost more and involve more paperwork, but they offer a wider choice of providers. If you are choosing insurance, consider a number of different plans and use your critical thinking skills to find the one that best suits your needs.

Tips for Today

Most of the time, you can take care of yourself without consulting a health care provider. You can eat sensibly, get enough exercise, manage stress, minimize your chances of getting an infection, and so on. When you do need professional care, you can continue to take responsibility for yourself by making informed, reasoned decisions about the care and health insurance you obtain.

Right now you can

- Make sure you have enough on hand of any prescription medication that you take and that your prescription is up to date.

- Make sure you have basic first aid supplies at home and prepare or buy a small first aid kit for your car or office.

- Post emergency, poison control, pharmacy, and physicians' phone numbers near the phone and go over them with your family or roommates.

- Following the guidelines in the box "Expressive Writing and Chronic Conditions," write down your thoughts and feelings about a recent stressful or traumatic life event.

Terms   **Medicare** A federal health insurance program for people 65 or older and for younger people with certain disabilities.

Medicaid A federally subsidized state-run plan of health care for people of low income.

Before you choose a health plan, it's important that you understand your options and how they affect your choice of providers and services, costs, and quality of care. The following questions can help guide you in evaluating each of the health plans you are considering:

• *How is the plan rated for quality?* Find out if consumer ratings or consumer satisfaction information is available. Possible sources include the Consumer Assessment of Health Plans (CAHPS), the Health Plan Employer Data and Information Set (HEDIS), or your state health insurance commissioner (check the phone book for contact information).

• *Is the plan accredited?* Many health plans choose to be reviewed and accredited (given a "seal of approval") by the National Committee for Quality Assurance (NCQA), the Joint Commission on Accreditation of Healthcare Organizations (JCAHO), or the American Accreditation HealthCare Commission/URAC.

• *Does the plan include the doctors and hospitals you want?* If you are happy with your current physician, find out which plans he or she is in. If going to a certain hospital is important to you, investigate where a particular physician has privileges and whether a hospital is covered by the plan.

• *Does the plan provide the benefits you need?* Determine which health care services are most important to you and your family and then check to see if the plan covers them. Possible services to consider include the following:

physician office visits

preventive services

diagnostic tests and X rays

outpatient prescription medications

inpatient medical and hospital costs

physical therapy

drug and alcohol counseling

prenatal and well baby care

eye exams and glasses or contact lenses

mental health services

complementary therapies such as acupuncture

home health care

care for preexisting or chronic conditions

• *Do the doctors, pharmacies, and other services in the plan have convenient times and locations?* Find out about such things as after-hours care and parking as well.

• *Does the plan fit your budget?* Consider all the applicable costs of a plan: monthly premiums, annual deductibles, and copayments for doctor and hospital visits and prescription drugs. Also find out about how much more you will need to pay if you go outside the health plan's network of physicians, hospitals, and other providers to obtain services.

SOURCE: Agency for Health Care Policy and Research. 1998. *Your Guide to Choosing Quality Health Care*. AHCPR Pub. No. 99-0012. Washington, D.C.: U.S. Department of Health and Human Services.

SUMMARY

• Self-care involves assessing the body for significant symptoms, which may indicate the need for professional assistance.

• Home medical tests allow cost savings, convenience, privacy, an increased sense of control, and sometimes more comprehensive information.

• Informed self-care requires knowing how to evaluate symptoms so that you don't go to a physician too soon or too late. It's necessary to see a physician if symptoms are severe, unusual, persistent, or recurrent.

• Self-treatment doesn't necessarily require medication, but OTC drugs can be a helpful part of self-care.

• Good communication with the physician and other members of the health care team is essential.

• Preparation for a visit to a physician should include making a written list of questions or concerns and bringing a list of all medications. During the visit, it's important to be open, to ask questions, and to request clarification.

• The diagnostic process involves a medical history, a physical exam, and medical tests. Patients should ask questions about medical tests and treatments recommended by their physicians.

• Safe use of prescription drugs requires knowledge of what the medication is supposed to do, how and when to take it, and what the side effects are.

• All surgical procedures carry risk; patients should ask about alternatives and get a second opinion.

• Health insurance plans are usually described as either fee-for-service (indemnity) or managed-care plans. Indemnity plans allow consumers more choice in medical providers, but managed-care plans are less expensive.

• Government programs include Medicaid, for the poor, and Medicare, for those who are 65 and over or chronically disabled.

Even though we sometimes have to entrust ourselves to the care of medical professionals, that doesn't mean we give up responsibility for our own behavior. Following medical instructions and advice often requires the same kind of behavioral self-management that's involved in quitting smoking, losing weight, or changing eating patterns. For example, if you have an illness or injury, you may be told to take medication at certain times of the day, do special exercises or movements, or change your diet.

The medical profession recognizes the importance of patient adherence, or compliance, and encourages different strategies to support it, such as the following:

1. Use reminders placed at home, in the car, at work, on your computer screensaver, or elsewhere that improve follow-through in taking medication and keeping scheduled appointments. To help you remember to take medications:

    • Link taking the medication with some well-established routine, like brushing your teeth or eating breakfast.

    • Use a medication calendar, and check off each pill.

    • Use a medication organizer or pill dispenser.

    • Plan ahead; don't wait until the last pill to get a prescription refilled.

2. Use a journal and other forms of self-monitoring to keep a detailed account of health-related behaviors, such as pill taking, diet, exercise, and so on.

3. Use self-reward systems so that desired behavior changes are encouraged, with a focus on short-term rewards.

If these strategies don't help you stick with your treatment plan, you may need to consider other possible explanations for your lack of adherence. For example, are you confused about some aspect of the treatment? Do you find the schedule for taking your medications too complicated, or do the drugs have bothersome side effects that you'd rather avoid? Do you feel that the recommended treatment is unnecessary or unlikely to help? Are you afraid of becoming dependent on a medication or that you'll be judged negatively if people know about your condition and treatment? An examination of your attitudes and beliefs about your condition and treatment plan can also help improve your compliance.

TAKE ACTION

1. Examine all the medications in your medicine cabinet. Discard any that have expired or are unlabeled. Ask your physician or pharmacist whether you should keep any medications you are uncertain about. Compare the contents of your medicine cabinet with the list of medications in Figure 22-2, and expand your supplies if you need to.

2. Before your next visit to your physician, prepare a written list of your concerns. Be prepared to ask questions. After the visit, review how it went. Were your concerns satisfactorily addressed? Were you able to communicate your needs? Did you feel involved and in control? What aspects would you like to handle better the next time?

3. Ask your physician whether you have any medical condition that may require special attention in an emergency. If you do, complete a medical ID card for your wallet, or obtain a medical ID bracelet or necklace. More complete emergency service can be obtained by joining Medic Alert (call 1-800-ID-ALERT for information).

JOURNAL ENTRY

1. ***Critical Thinking*** Studies have shown that people often ignore the warnings and instructions on labels for OTC drugs; for example, they drive after taking an antihistamine that causes drowsiness or take more than the recommended dosage of a cold remedy or a stimulant. Do people have a responsibility to use medications as directed, or do they have the right to choose any course of action affecting their own bodies or health, even if their choices have potential negative consequences for others, such as an automobile crash? In your health journal, write a brief essay outlining your opinion about individual responsibility for the correct use of medications. Explain your reasoning.

2. Using the insurance guidelines in the chapter, evaluate your current coverage. In your health journal, make a list of the services it covers and does not cover; put a check mark next to the services you are most likely to need. Examine the cost of the policy, including the deductibles and copayments and the maximum limits on coverage. Also look at the rules governing your choice of physicians. Does your current plan meet your needs? Does it lack any services that are important for you or cover any unnecessary ones?

See Appendix C for self-care resources.

SELECTED BIBLIOGRAPHY

Ayanian, J. Z., et al. 2000. Unmet health needs of uninsured adults in the United States. *Journal of the American Medical Association* 284(16): 2061–2069.

Bell, R. A., R. L. Kravitz, and M. S. Wilkes. 2000. Direct-to-consumer prescription drug advertising, 1989–1998. A content analysis of conditions, targets, inducements, and appeals. *Journal of Family Practice* 49(4): 329–335.

Bell, R. A., M. S. Wilkes, and R. L. Kravitz. 2000. The educational value of consumer-targeted prescription drug print advertising. *Journal of Family Practice* 49(12): 1092–1098.

Blendon, R. J., et al. 2001. Health policy 2001: The implications of the 2000 election. *New England Journal of Medicine* 344(9): 679–684.

Blumenthal, D. 2001. Controlling health care expenditures. *New England Journal of Medicine* 344(10): 766–769.

Charles, C., A. Gafni, and T. Whelan. 2000. How to improve communication between doctors and patients. Learning more about the decision making context is important. *British Medical Journal* 320(7244): 1220–1221.

Coughlin, A. M., et al. 2000. Multidisciplinary treatment of chronic pain patients: Its efficacy in changing patient locus of control. *Archives of Physical Medicine and Rehabilitation* 81(6): 739–740.

Dudley, R. A., and H. S. Luft. 2001. Managed care in transition. *New England Journal of Medicine* 344(14): 1087–1092.

Greene, H. L. 2001. The pros and cons and home testing. *HealthNews*, January.

Health Care Financing Administration. 2001. *National Health Expenditures Aggregate and per Capita Amounts, Percent Distribution, and Average Annual Percent Growth, by Sources of Funds: Selected Calendar Years 1960–1999* (http://www.hcfa.gov/stats/nhe-oact/tables/t1.htm; retrieved May 2, 2001).

Health Care Financing Administration. 2001. *National Health Expenditures and Selected Economic Indicators, Levels and Average Annual Percent Change: Selected Calendar Years 1980–2010* (http://www.hcfa.gov/stats/NHE-Proj/proj2000/tables/1.htm; retrieved May 2, 2001).

Henkel, J. 2000. Buying drugs online: It's convenient and private, but beware of "rogue sites." *FDA Consumer*, January–February.

Hogan, C., P. B. Ginsburg, and J. R. Gabel. 2000. Tracking health care costs: Inflation returns. *Health Affairs* 19: 217–223.

Hollon, M. F. 1999. Direct-to-consumer marketing of prescription drugs: Creating consumer demand. *Journal of the American Medical Association* 281: 382–384.

Holmes, A. F. 1999. Direct-to-consumer prescription drug advertising builds bridges between patients and physicians. *Journal of the American Medical Association* 281: 380–382.

How to talk with your doctor. 1999. *Journal of the American Medical Association* 282(24): 2422.

Iglehart, J. K. 1999. The American health care system: Expenditures. *New England Journal of Medicine* 340(1): 70–76.

Iglehart, J. K. 2000. Revisiting the Canadian health care system. *New England Journal of Medicine* 342(26): 2007–2012.

Institute of Medicine Committee on Quality of Health Care in America. 2001. *Crossing the Quality Chasm: A New Health System for the 21st Century.* Washington, D.C.: National Academy Press.

Kuttner, R. 1999. The American health care system: Health insurance coverage. *New England Journal of Medicine* 340(2): 163–168.

Leape, L. L. 2000. Institute of Medicine medical error figures are not exaggerated. *Journal of the American Medical Association* 284(1): 95–97.

Lipman, M. M. 2000. Should you take health advice from drug ads? *Consumer Reports on Health*, October.

Lorig, K., et al. 1999. Evidence suggesting that a chronic disease self-management program can improve health status while reducing hospitalization: A randomized trial. *Medical Care* 37: 5–14.

McDonald, C. J., M. Weiner, and S. L. Hui. 2000. Deaths due to medical errors are exaggerated in Institute of Medicine report. *Journal of the American Medical Association* 284(1): 93–95.

Mechanic, D., D. D. McAlpine, and M. Rosenthal. 2001. Are patients' office visits with physicians getting shorter? *New England Journal of Medicine* 344(3): 198–204.

Moynihan, R., et al. 2000. Coverage by the news media of the benefits and risks of medications. *New England Journal of Medicine* 342(22): 1645–1650.

Prescription for trouble. 2001. *Consumer Reports*, February.

Rodriguez, I., et al. 2001. Drug-induced QT prolongation in women during the menstrual cycle. *Journal of the American Medical Association* 285(10): 1322–1326.

Schroeder, S. A. 2001. Prospects for expanding health insurance coverage. *New England Journal of Medicine* 344(11): 847–852.

Sobel, D. 2000. The cost-effectiveness of mind-body medicine interventions. *Progress in Brain Research* 122: 393–412.

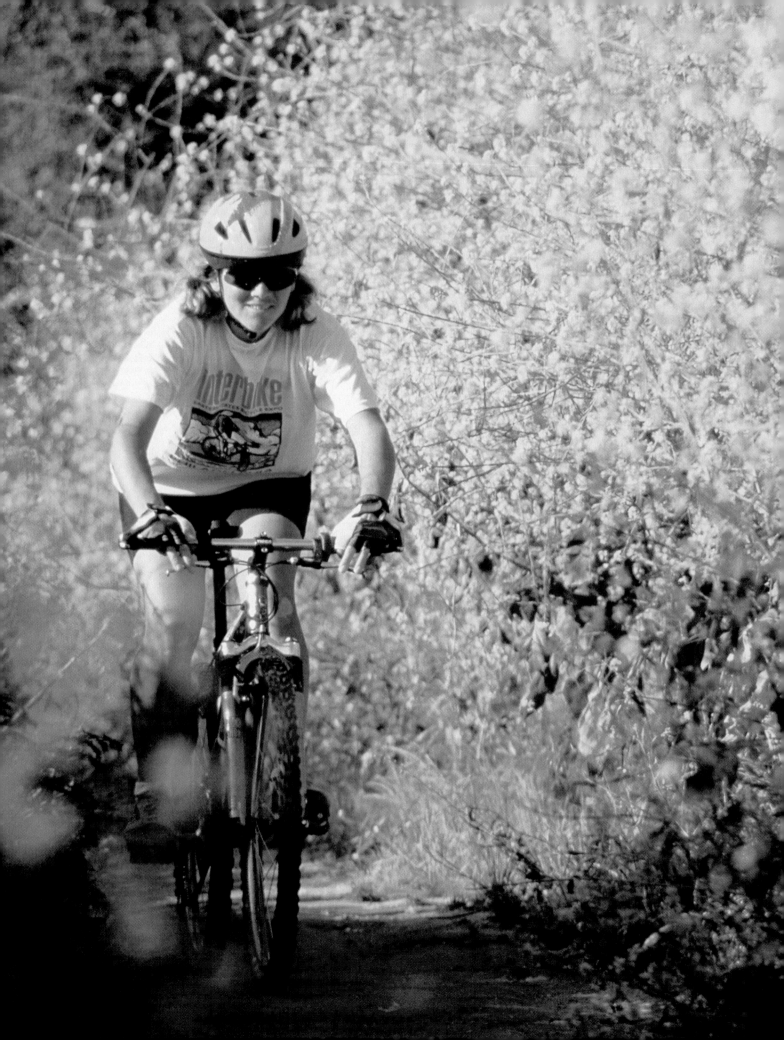

After reading this chapter, you should be able to

- Discuss factors that contribute to unintentional injuries.

- List the most common types of unintentional injuries and strategies for preventing them

- Describe factors that contribute to violence and intentional injuries

- Discuss different forms of violence and how to protect yourself from intentional injuries

- List strategies for helping others in an emergency situation

Personal Safety: Protecting Yourself from Unintentional Injuries and Violence

23

TEST YOUR KNOWLEDGE

1. More people are injured each year through intentional acts of violence than through unintentional injuries (accidents).
    True or false?

2. It is dangerous to be wearing a safety belt if your car catches on fire or is submerged in water.
    True or false?

3. Unintentional injuries at home (from causes such as falls and fires) cause three deaths every
    a. hour
    b. day
    c. week

4. By what percentage does wearing a bicycle helmet reduce your risk of head injury in a crash?
    a. 35%
    b. 65%
    c. 85%

5. About what percentage of sexual assaults against women are committed by strangers?
    a. 20%
    b. 40%
    c. 80%

ANSWERS

1. FALSE. Far more people are injured and killed each year through unintentional injuries than through violence. Your lifetime odds of dying from an unintentional injury are 1 in 37, while the odds of your being murdered are 1 in 169.

2. FALSE. Safety belts will help prevent you from being knocked unconscious, so you'll have a better chance of escaping the car. (Only 0.5–1% of motor vehicle crashes involve fire or submersion.)

3. A. Home injuries cause a death every 19 minutes; overall, unintentional injuries are the leading cause of death for people under the age of 35.

4. C. Despite the safety benefits of helmet use, less than 50% of cyclists wear head protection regularly.

5. A. The vast majority of sexual assaults against women are committed by friends, acquaintances, or intimate partners.

E ach year, about 150,000 Americans die from injuries, and many more are temporarily or permanently disabled. Injuries can be intentional or unintentional. An **intentional injury** is one that is purposely inflicted, by either oneself or another person; examples are homicide, suicide, and assault. If an injury occurs when no harm is intended, it is considered an **unintentional injury.** Motor vehicle crashes, falls, and fires often result in unintentional injuries. (The word *accidents* was formerly used to describe unintentional injuries, but it is now considered inaccurate because it suggests events beyond human control. *Injuries* are predictable outcomes of factors that can be controlled or prevented.) Although Americans tend to express more concern about intentional injuries, unintentional injuries are actually more common. The following occurs on an average day in the United States:

- 58 homicides
- 85 suicides
- 265 deaths from unintentional injuries
- 3200 suicide attempts
- 20,400 interpersonal assaults
- 100,000 unintentional injury–related emergency room visits

Unintentional injuries are the fifth leading cause of death among all Americans and the leading cause of death and disability among children and young adults. Heart disease, cancer, and stroke are responsible for more deaths each year than injuries, but because unintentional injuries are so common among people, they account for more **years of potential life lost** than any other cause of death. Suicide and homicide rank eighth and thirteenth respectively on the list of leading causes of death among Americans; because they often affect young people, they also account for many years of potential life lost. Injuries affect all segments of the population, but they are particularly common among men, minorities, and people with low incomes, primarily due to social, environmental, and economic factors. Although rates of both unintentional and intentional injuries have fallen in recent years, they remain a major area of concern.

The economic cost of injuries is high, with more than $500 billion spent each year for medical care and rehabilitation of injured people. But injuries also cause emotional suffering for injured people and their families, friends, and colleagues. Luckily, there are many steps that can be taken to reduce the risk of injuries. Engineering strategies such as safety belts can help lower injury rates, as can the passage and enforcement of safety-related laws, such as those requiring tamper-proof containers for OTC medications. Public education campaigns about risky behaviors such as driving under the influence of alcohol or smoking in bed can also help prevent injuries.

Ultimately, though, it is up to each individual to take responsibility for his or her actions and make wise choices about safety behaviors. Many of the same sensible attitudes, responsible behaviors, and informed decisions that optimize your wellness can improve your chances of avoiding injuries. This chapter explains how you can protect yourself and those around you from becoming the victims of unintentional and intentional injuries.

UNINTENTIONAL INJURIES

Unintentional injuries are the leading cause of death in the United States for people under age 35. Injury situations are generally categorized into four general classes, based on where they occur: motor vehicle injuries, home injuries, leisure injuries, and work injuries. The greatest number of deaths occur in motor vehicle crashes, but the greatest number of disabling injuries occur in the home (Table 23-1). In all of these arenas, the action you take can mean the difference between injury or death and no injury at all.

What Causes an Injury?

Most injuries are caused by a combination of human and environmental factors. Human factors are inner conditions or attitudes that lead to an unsafe state, whether physical, emotional, or psychological. Environmental factors are external conditions and circumstances, such as poor road conditions, a slippery surface, or the undertow of the ocean at the beach.

A common human factor that leads to injuries is risk-taking behavior. People vary in the amount of risk they tend to take in life; young men are especially prone to taking risks. Some people take risks to win the admiration of their peers; other people simply overestimate their physical abilities. Using alcohol or drugs is another common risk factor that leads to many injuries and deaths.

Psychological and emotional factors can also play a role in injuries. People sometimes act on the basis of inadequate or inaccurate beliefs about what is safe or unsafe. For example, a person who believes that safety belts trap people in cars when a crash occurs and who therefore decides not to wear a safety belt is acting on an inaccurate belief. Young people often have unsafe attitudes, such as "I won't get hurt." Attitudes like this can lead to risk taking and ultimately to injuries.

Environmental factors leading to injury may be natural (weather conditions), social (a drunk driver), work-related (defective equipment), or home-related (faulty wiring). Making the environment safer is an important aspect of safety. Laws are often passed to try to make our environment safer; examples include speed limits on roads and highways and workplace safety requirements.

When unsafe human states and unsafe environmental factors interact, an injury is often the result. A good example might be an inexperienced person borrowing a rifle to go hunting with his friends on a cold, rainy afternoon. Those in the group drink alcohol because they mistakenly believe it will keep them warmer. It is not difficult to imagine how the interaction of these human and environmental factors could lead to an injury. Again, it is important to realize that injuries do not "just happen." With hindsight, we can almost always pinpoint the internal and external factors that combined to cause an injury situation.

W. Motor Vehicle Injuries

Motor vehicle crashes are the leading cause of death for Americans between the ages of 1 and 29. The groups most affected by motor vehicle crashes are people age 15–24 and over 75. It is more likely that your death will be caused by a motor vehicle crash than by any other type of unintentional or intentional injury (Table 23-2). **Motor vehicle injuries** also result in the majority of cases of paralysis due to spinal injuries, and they are the leading cause of severe brain injury in the United States.

Factors Contributing to Motor Vehicle Injuries

Common causes of motor vehicle injuries are speeding, aggressive driving, fatigue, cell phones and other distractions, the use of alcohol and other drugs, and the incorrect use of safety belts and other safety devices.

SPEEDING   Nearly two-thirds of all motor vehicle crashes are caused by bad driving, especially speeding. As speed increases, momentum and the force of impact increase, and the time allowed for the driver to react (reaction time) decreases. Speed limits are posted to establish the safest maximum speed limit for a given area under ideal condi-

tions; if visibility is limited or the road is wet, the safe maximum speed may be considerably lower. Many states have raised their highway speed limits since the 1995 repeal of the National Maximum Speed Limit, and overall motor vehicle fatalities have since increased by 6%.

AGGRESSIVE DRIVING   Speeding is also a hallmark of aggressive drivers—those who operate a motor vehicle in an unsafe and hostile manner. Aggressive driving, also known as "road rage," has increased more than 50% since 1990, and one in four U.S. drivers admits to driving aggressively at least some of the time. Other characteristics of aggressive driving include frequent, erratic, and abrupt lane changes; tailgating; running red lights or stop signs;

intentional injury An injury that is purposely inflicted, by either oneself or another person.

unintentional injury An injury that occurs without harm being intended.

years of potential life lost The difference between an individual's life expectancy and his or her age at death.

motor vehicle injuries Unintentional injuries and deaths involving motor vehicles in motion, both on and off the highway or street; incidents causing motor vehicle injuries include collisions between vehicles and collisions with objects or pedestrians.

Terms

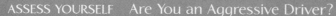
To find out if you are an aggressive driver, check any of the following statements that are true for you:

_____ I consistently exceed the speed limit; I'm often unaware of both my speed and the speed limit.

_____ I frequently follow closely behind the car in front of me.

_____ If I feel the car in front of me is going too slowly, I tailgate.

_____ I change lanes frequently to pass people.

_____ I seldom use my turn signal when changing lanes or turning.

_____ I often run red lights or roll through stop signs.

_____ I react to what I feel is another driver's mistake by cursing, shouting, or making rude gestures; by blocking a car from passing or changing lanes; by using high beams; or by braking suddenly in front of a tailgater.

_____ My personality changes and I become more competitive when I get behind the wheel.

_____ I often get angry or impatient with other drivers and with pedestrians.

_____ I would consider pulling over for a personal encounter with a bad driver.

Each of these statements is characteristic of aggressive drivers; the more items you checked, the greater your road rage. If you checked even one statement, consider taking some of the following steps to reduce your hostility behind the wheel:

- Allow enough time for your trip to reach your destination without speeding.

- Avoid driving during periods of heavy traffic.

- Don't drive when you are angry, tired, or intoxicated.

- Imagine that the other drivers are all people that you know and like. Be courteous and forgiving.

- Listen to soothing music or a book on tape, or practice a relaxation technique such as deep breathing (see Chapter 2).

- Take a course in anger management.

Even if you are successful at controlling your own aggressive driving inpulses, you may still encounter an aggressive driver on the road. The AAA Foundation for Traffic Safety recommends the following strategies to avoid being victim of an aggressive driver.

- Avoid behaviors that may enrage an aggressive driver; these include cutting cars off when merging, driving slowly in the left lane, tailgating, and making rude gestures.

- If you make a mistake while driving, apologize. In surveys, the most popular and widely understood gestures for apologies include raising or waving a hand and touching or knocking the head with the palm of your hand (to indicate "What was I thinking?").

- Refuse to join in a fight. Avoid eye contact with an angry driver, and put distance between your car and his or her vehicle. If you think another driver is following you or trying to start a fight, call the police on a cellular phone or drive to a public place.

SOURCES: New York State Department of Motor Vehicles. 2000. *Aggressive Driving* (http://www.nysgtsc.state.ny.us/aggr-ndx.htm; retrieved December 27, 2000). AAA Foundation for Traffic Safety. 1997. *Road Rage: How to Avoid Aggressive Driving.* Washington, D.C.: AAA Foundation for Traffic Safety.

passing on the shoulder; and blocking other cars trying to change lanes or pass. Aggressive drivers increase the risk of crashes for themselves and others; injuries may also occur if aggressive drivers stop their vehicles and confront each other following an incident. For more on aggressive driving, take the quiz and review the strategies in the box "Are You an Aggressive Driver?"

FATIGUE AND SLEEPINESS   Driving requires mental alertness and attentiveness. Studies have shown that sleepiness causes slower reaction time, reduced vigilance, and delayed information processing. Drowsiness can be caused by not getting enough hours of sleep, by sleep disorders that prevent sleep from being refreshing, or by disruptions caused by shift work that force people to sleep at odd hours. Research shows that even mild sleep deprivation causes a deterioration in driving ability comparable to that caused by a 0.05% blood alcohol concentration—a level considered hazardous when driving.

CELL PHONES AND OTHER DISTRACTIONS   Anything that distracts a driver—a bad mood, pets or children in the car—can increase the risk of a motor vehicle injury. Several common causes of crashes, including failing to yield and disregarding traffic signals and stop signs, have been linked to driver distraction, and it is estimated that distraction is a contributing factor in 25–50% of all crashes. As the use of cell phones has spread, their potential to distract drivers has been recognized. Studies have documented a higher rate of crashes among cell phone users compared to nonusers; see the box "Cellular Phones and Distracted Driving" for strategies on using a phone more safely.

ALCOHOL AND OTHER DRUGS   Alcohol is involved in about half of all fatal crashes. Alcohol-impaired driving is illegal in all states; the legal blood alcohol concentration (BAC) varies by state from 0.08% to 0.10%, but people are impaired at much lower BACs. A driver with a BAC between 0.05% and 0.09% is nine times more likely to

On January 1, 2001, a law banning the use of handheld cellular phones while driving went into effect in Suffolk County, New York. Officials in New York City have proposed a similar ban that would require drivers to use headsets, earpieces, or voice-activated devices or face fines of up to $150. If the ban is passed, New York will join Suffolk County and cities including Brooklyn Heights, Ohio, and Brookline, Massachusetts, in prohibiting the use of a phone while driving unless both hands are on the steering wheel.

Although research findings have been mixed, the available evidence suggests that use of a cell phone while driving can, indeed, increase the risk of motor vehicle crashes. One study found that motorists who talk on the phone face a fourfold increase in their risk of a collision; the risk of a fatal crash is also higher. It is unclear, however, if bans such as those in Suffolk County will help reduce the risk: Studies have not found much benefit in the use of headsets, perhaps because it is the mental distraction of talking that is a factor in crashes rather than one hand holding the phone.

The safest strategy is not to use your phone while driving. For people who live in areas where cell phone use is legal while driving and who choose to use a phone, the following strategies may help increase safety:

- Be very familiar with your phone and its functions, especially speed dial and redial.

- Store frequently called numbers on speed dial so you can place calls without looking at the phone.

- Use a hands-free device so that you can keep both hands on the steering wheel.

- Let the person you are speaking to know you are driving and be prepared to end the call at any time.

- Don't place or answer calls in heavy traffic and hazardous weather conditions.

- Don't take notes or look up phone numbers while driving.

- Time calls so that you can place them when you are at a stop.

- Never engage in stressful or emotional conversations while on the road. If you are discussing a complicated or emotional matter, pull over to the side of the road or into a parking lot to complete your conversation.

Remember, as a driver, your primary obligation is to pay attention to the road—for your own safety and the safety of others.

SOURCES: Lueck, T. J. 2000. Giuliani and Vallone call for limits on use of cell phones by drivers. *New York Times,* December 20. World of Wireless Communications. 2000. *Consumer Resources: Driving Safety Tips* (http://www.wow-com/consumer/driving/safetyold.cfm; retrieved December 16, 2000). Redelmeier, D. A., and R. J. Tibshirani. 1997. Association between cellular-telephone calls and motor vehicle collisions. *New England Journal of Medicine* 336(7): 453–458.

---

have a crash than a person who has not been drinking. The combination of fatigue and alcohol use increases the risk even further. Because alcohol affects reason and judgment as well as the ability to make fast, accurate, and coordinated movements, a person who has been drinking will be less likely to recognize that he or she is impaired.

Other substances also affect judgment and driving ability. A recent study found that hay fever sufferers who had taken diphenhydramine (an antihistamine found in over-the-counter allergy medications such as Benadryl) were as impaired as if they were legally drunk. Use of many over-the-counter and all psychoactive drugs is potentially dangerous if you plan to drive. (For a full discussion of the effects of alcohol and other drugs on users, refer to Chapters 9 and 10.)

SAFETY BELTS, AIR BAGS, AND CHILD SAFETY SEATS   The improper use of safety belts, air bags, and child safety seats contributes to injuries and deaths in motor vehicle crashes. Only 68% of motor vehicle occupants use safety belts, even though you are twice as likely to be injured in a crash if you do not wear one. Of drivers not wearing a safety belt who have been killed in automobile crashes, an estimated 60–70% would have survived if they had been wearing one. If you wear a combination lap and shoulder belt, your chances of surviving a crash are three to four times better than those of a person who doesn't wear one.

Some people think that if they are involved in a crash, they are better off being thrown free of their vehicle. In fact, the chances of being killed are 25 times greater if you are thrown from a vehicle, whether it is due to injuries caused by hitting a tree or the pavement or by being hit by another vehicle. Safety belts not only prevent you from being thrown from the car at the time of the crash but also provide protection from the "second collision." If a car is traveling at 65 mph and hits another vehicle, the car stops first; then the occupants stop because they are traveling at the same speed. The second collision occurs when the occupants of the car hit something inside the car, such as the steering column, dashboard, or windshield. The safety belt stops the second collision from occurring and spreads the stopping force of the collision over the body.

Since 1998, all new cars have been equipped with dual air bags—one for the driver and one for the front passenger. Although air bags provide supplementary protection in the event of a collision, most are useful only in head-on collisions. They also deflate immediately after inflating and therefore do not provide protection in collisions involving multiple impacts.

Air bags deploy forcefully and can injure a child or short adult who is improperly restrained or sitting too close to the dashboard. To ensure that air bags work safely, always follow these basic guidelines: Place infants in rear-facing infant seats in the back seat; transport children age 12 and under in the back seat; always use safety belts or appropriate safety seats; and keep 10 inches between the air bag cover and the breastbone of the driver or passenger. If necessary, adjust the steering wheel or use seat cushions to ensure that an inflating air bag will hit a person in the chest and not in the face. Another adjustment should be made for children who have outgrown child safety seats but are still too small for adult safety belts alone (usually ages 4 to 8). These children should be secured using booster seats that ensure that the safety belt is positioned low across their waist.

In the rare event that a person cannot comply with air bag guidelines, permission to install an on-off switch that temporarily disables the air bag can be applied for from the National Highway Traffic Safety Administration (NHTSA). Air bags currently prevent far more injuries than they cause and are expected to save at least 3200 lives each year once they are installed in all vehicles. Advanced air bag systems are slowly being introduced that include such risk-reduction technologies as sensors to detect and respond to crash severity, seat position, passenger size, and whether a passenger is wearing a safety belt.

Preventing Motor Vehicle Injuries

About 75% of all motor vehicle collisions occur within 25 miles of home and at speeds lower than 40 mph. Strategies for preventing motor vehicle injuries include the following:

- Obey the speed limit. If you have to speed to get there on time, you're not allowing enough time.

- Always wear a safety belt. Fasten the lap belt, even if the vehicle has automatic shoulder belts. The shoulder strap should cross the collarbone and the lap belt should fit low and snug across the hips and pelvic area. The shoulder strap should never be slipped under the arm or behind the back. Pregnant women should position the lap belt as low as possible on the pelvic area.

- Never drive under the influence of alcohol or other drugs. Never ride with a driver who has been drinking or using drugs.

- Keep your car in good working order. Regularly inspect the tires, oil and fluid levels, windshield wipers, spare tire, and so on.

- Always allow enough following distance. Use the "3-second rule": When the vehicle ahead passes a reference point, count out 3 seconds. If you pass the reference point before you finish counting, drop back and allow more following distance.

- Always increase your following distance and slow down if weather or road conditions are poor.

- Choose interstate highways rather than rural roads. Highways are much safer because of better visibility, wider lanes, fewer surprises, and other factors.

- Always signal when turning or changing lanes.

- Stop completely at stop signs. Follow all traffic laws.

- Take special care at intersections. Always look left, right, and then left again. Make sure you have plenty of time to complete your maneuver in the intersection.

- Don't pass on two-lane roads unless you're in a designated passing area and have a clear view ahead.

- Children under the age of 12 should ride in the back seat of a motor vehicle. Young children and infants should ride in approved child safety seats appropriate for their age and size.

Motorcycles and Mopeds

About one out of every ten traffic fatalities among people age 15–34 involves someone riding a motorcycle. In more than two-thirds of crashes involving a car and a motorcycle, the driver of the car is at fault. Injuries from motorcycle collisions are generally more severe than those involving automobiles because motorcycles provide little, if any, protection. Because head injuries are the major cause of death, the use of a helmet is critical for rider safety. Learning the skills to operate the motorcycle safely is another key injury-prevention strategy; operator error is a factor in 75% of fatal crashes involving motorcycles.

Moped riders face additional challenges. Mopeds usually have a maximum speed of 30–35 mph and have less power for maneuverability, especially in an emergency. Moped riders should use caution and take the time to develop the skills needed to handle the vehicle in traffic.

Additional strategies for preventing motorcycle and moped injuries include the following:

- Maximize your visibility by wearing light-colored clothing, driving with your headlights on, and correctly positioning yourself in traffic.

- Develop the necessary skills. Lack of skill, especially when evasive action is needed to avoid a collision, is a major factor in motorcycle and moped injuries. Skidding from improper braking is the most common cause of loss of control.

- Wear a helmet. Helmets should be marked with the symbol DOT, certifying that they conform to federal safety standards established by the Department of Transportation.

- Protect your eyes with goggles, a face shield, or a windshield.

Wearing a bicycle helmet can help you avoid serious head injury, brain damage, or even death in the event of a collision or fall. Helmets have a layer of stiff foam, which absorbs shock and cushions a blow to your head, covered by a thin plastic shell that will "skid" along the ground. For maximum protection, it's important to select a correctly fitting helmet. When you go shopping, remember the four S's: size, strap, straight, and sticker.

• *Size:* Try on several different sizes before making your selection; it may take several tries before you find the most comfortable fit. The helmet should be very snug but not overly tight on your head. Pads are usually provided to help adjust the fit. A good salesperson can also help you get the right fit. When the helmet is strapped onto your head, it should not move more than an inch in any direction, and you should not be able to pull or twist it off no matter how hard you try.

• *Strap:* Be sure that the chin strap fits snugly under your chin and that the V in the strap meets under your ear. Avoid

thin straps, which can be uncomfortable. Check to be sure that the buckle is strong and won't pop open and that the straps are sturdy.

• *Straight:* The helmet should sit straight on your head, not tilted back or forward (see the figure). A rule of thumb is that the rim should be about two finger widths above your eyebrows (depending on the height of your forehead).

• *Sticker:* Since March 1999, helmets sold in the United States must meet uniform safety standards established by the U.S. Consumer Product Safety Commission (CPSC). Look for a sticker or label that says the helmet meets the CPSC standard. If a helmet does not have one, it does not meet federal safety standards and should not be used.

You are more likely to wear your helmet if it is comfortable, so be sure that vents on the helmet provide airflow to promote cooling and sweat control. You will be safer with a brightly colored helmet that makes you more visible to drivers, especially in rainy, foggy, or dark conditions. Reflective tape will also increase your visibility. Finally, a helmet is a good place to put emergency information (your name, address, and phone number, plus any emergency medical conditions and an emergency contact). Tape change inside the helmet for a phone call.

If you are involved in a crash, replace your helmet. Even if the helmet doesn't have any visible signs of damage, its ability to protect your head may be compromised. As the Bicycle Helmet Safety Institute says, "No one ever complains about the cost of their second bike helmet."

SOURCES: Bicycle Helmet Safety Institute. 2000. *A Consumer's Guide to Bicycle Helmets* (http://www.helmets.org/webdocs/guide.htm; retrieved July 26, 2000). National Safety Council. 2000. *Choose the Right Helmet for Your Favorite Summer Sport* (http://www.nsc.org/pubs/fsh/archive/summr00/helmet.htm; retrieved July 26, 2000).

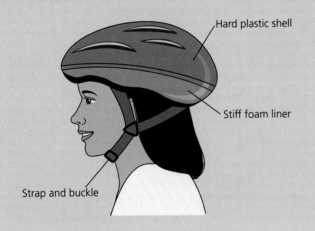

Hard plastic shell

Stiff foam liner

Strap and buckle

• Drive defensively, particularly when changing lanes and at intersections, and never assume that you've been seen by other drivers.

Bicycles   Injuries to bicyclists and pedestrians are considered motor-vehicle-related because they are usually caused by motor vehicles. Bicycle injuries result primarily from riders not knowing or understanding the rules of the road, failing to follow traffic laws, not having sufficient skill or experience to handle traffic conditions, or being intoxicated. Bicycles are considered vehicles; bicyclists must obey all traffic laws that apply to automobile drivers, including stopping at traffic lights and stop signs.

Head injuries are involved in about two-thirds of all bicycle-related deaths. Wearing a helmet reduces the risk of head injury by 85%, but fewer than 50% of cyclists wear helmets (see the box "Choosing a Bicycle Helmet"). Safe cycling strategies include the following:

• Wear safety equipment, including a helmet, eye protection, gloves, and proper footwear. Secure the bottom of your pant legs with clips, and secure your shoelaces so they don't get tangled in the chain.

• Maximize your visibility by wearing light-colored, reflective clothing. Equip your bike with reflectors, and use lights, especially at night or when riding in wooded or other dark areas.

• Ride with the flow of traffic, not against it, and follow all traffic laws. Use bike paths when they are available.

• Ride defensively; never assume that drivers have seen you. Be especially careful when turning or crossing at corners and intersections. Watch for cars turning right.

• Stop at all traffic lights and stop signs. Know and use hand signals.

- Continue pedaling at all times when moving (no coasting) to help keep the bike stable and to maintain your balance.
- Properly maintain the working condition of your bike.

Pedestrians

Pedestrians Pedestrians are no match for the speed, size, and weight of motor vehicles, particularly the popular sport utility vehicles. About one in seven motor vehicle deaths involves pedestrians, and more than 90,000 pedestrians are injured each year. The highest rates of death and injury occur among the very young and the elderly. Nearly one-third of all pedestrian deaths occur when people cross or enter the roadway between intersections. Alcohol intoxication plays a significant role in up to half of all adult pedestrian fatalities.

The following strategies can help prevent injuries when you're walking or jogging:

- Walk or jog in daylight.
- Maximize your visibility by wearing light-colored, reflective clothing.
- Face traffic when walking or jogging along a road, and follow traffic laws.
- Avoid busy roads or roads with poor visibility.
- Cross only at marked crosswalks and intersections.
- Don't listen to a radio, tape, or CD on headphones while walking.
- Don't hitchhike; it places you in a potentially dangerous situation.

COMMUNICATE! If you have a problem managing your anger, especially when you're driving, you can help yourself by making changes in how you listen and talk to yourself internally. Learn to recognize what makes you angry and how anger feels to you. Physiologically, anger causes a rush of adrenaline, producing a variety of physical symptoms that may include a faster heartbeat, faster breathing, muscle tension, a knot in the stomach, and trembling. Learn to calm yourself by taking slow, deep breaths; imagining a calm, peaceful place; or using other techniques that have relaxed you in the past. Think through the consequences of losing your temper and the benefits of maintaining control. Talk to yourself about the situation, looking for a neutral explanation, deciding you're not going to let someone get to you, or realizing you don't need to prove yourself. In short, stay in control of yourself by stopping to breathe, relax, and think.

Home Injuries

A person's place of residence, whether it be a house, an apartment, a trailer, or a dormitory, is considered home. People spend a great deal of time at home and feel that they are safe and secure there. However, home can be a dangerous place. The most common fatal **home injuries** are falls, fires, poisoning, suffocation, and unintentional firearm injuries.

Falls About 85% of fatal falls involve people age 45 and over, but falls are the fifth leading cause of unintentional death for all people under 25. Most deaths occurring from falls involve falling on stairs or steps or from one level to another. Falls also occur on the same level, from tripping, slipping, or stumbling. Alcohol is a contributing factor in many falls. Strategies for preventing falls include the following:

- Install handrails and nonslip applications in the shower and bathtub.
- Keep floors, stairs, and outside areas clear of objects or conditions that could cause slipping or tripping, such as ice, snow, electrical cords, and toys.
- Put a light switch by the door of every room so no one has to walk across a room to turn on a light. Use night lights in bedrooms, halls, stairs, and bathrooms.
- When climbing a ladder, use both hands. Never stand higher than the third step from the top. When using a stepladder, make sure the spreader brace is in the locked position. With straight ladders, set the base out 1 foot for every 4 feet of height.
- Don't use chairs to reach things; they are meant to be sat on, not stood on.
- If there are small children in the home, place gates at the top and bottom of stairs. Never leave a baby unattended on a bed or table. Install window guards to prevent children from falling out of windows.

Fires Each year in the United States, approximately 80% of fire deaths and 65% of fire injuries occur in the home; a death caused by a residential fire occurs every 2 hours. Most fires begin in the kitchen, living room, or bedroom. Cooking is now the leading cause of home fire injuries; careless smoking is the leading cause of fire deaths, followed by problems with heating equipment and arson. To prevent fires, it's important to dispose of all cigarettes in ashtrays and to never smoke in bed. Other strategies include proper maintenance of fireplaces, furnaces, heaters, chimneys, and electrical outlets, cords, and appliances. If you use a portable heater, keep it at least 3 feet away from curtains, bedding, or anything else that might catch fire. Never leave heaters on unattended.

It's important to be adequately prepared to handle fire-related situations. Plan at least two escape routes out of each room, and designate a location outside the home as a meeting place. For practice, stage a home fire drill; do it at night, since that's when most deadly fires occur.

Install smoke detectors on every level of your home. Your risk of dying in a fire is almost twice as high if you do not use them. Clean the detectors and check the batteries once a month, and replace the batteries at least once a year. (More than 90% of U.S. homes have at least one smoke alarm, but about half are no longer functioning a year after installation, most commonly because batteries need to be replaced or dust and debris need to be cleaned out of the unit.) Be sure that all residents are familiar with the sound of the smoke detector's alarm; when it goes off, take it seriously.

If a fire does occur, following these strategies can help prevent injuries:

- Get out as quickly as possible, and go to the designated meeting place. Don't stop for a keepsake or a pet. Never hide in a closet or under a bed. Once outside, count heads to see if everyone is out. If you think someone is still inside the burning building, tell the firefighters. Never go back inside a burning building.

- If you're trapped in a room, feel the door. If it is hot, or if smoke is coming in through the cracks, don't open it; use the alternative escape route. If you can't get out of a room, go to the window and shout or wave for help.

- Smoke inhalation is the largest cause of death and injury in fires. To avoid inhaling smoke, crawl along the floor away from the heat and smoke. Cover your mouth and nose, ideally with a wet cloth, and take short, shallow breaths.

- If your clothes catch fire, don't run. Drop to the ground, cover your face, and roll back and forth to smother the flames. Remember: stop-drop-roll.

Although house fires cause the most deaths, hot water causes the most nonfatal burns. Young children are particularly at risk. Place barriers around stoves and radiators, and keep young children out of the kitchen, where they might be burned by spills. Put pans on rear burners, and turn pot handles toward the back of the stove. Keep hot foods away from the edge of counters and tables, and don't put them on a tablecloth that a small child can pull. Set your water heater no higher than 120°F. Always test the contents of a baby bottle; when bottles are heated in microwave ovens, the liquid can become scalding before the outside of the bottle gets very hot.

Poisoning   More than 2 million poisonings and over 9000 poison-related deaths occur every year in the United States. Poisons come in many forms, some of which are not typically considered poisons. For example, medications are safe when used as prescribed, but overdosing and incorrectly combining medications with another substance may result in poisoning. Other poisonous substances in the home include cleaning agents, petroleum-based products, insecticides and herbicides, cosmetics, nail polish and remover, and many houseplants. All potentially poisonous substances should be

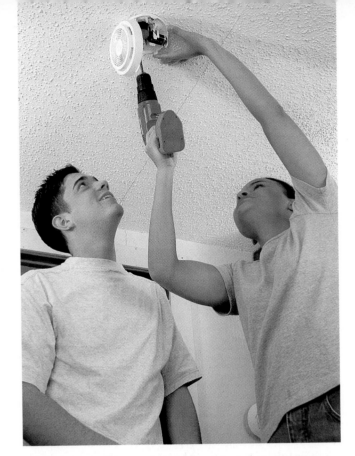

The risk of dying in a fire is reduced by half if you use a smoke detector. Install detectors on every floor, check them monthly, and replace the batteries at least once a year.

used only as directed and stored carefully, out of the reach of children.

The most common type of poisoning by gases is carbon monoxide poisoning. Carbon monoxide gas is emitted by motor vehicle exhaust and some types of heating equipment. The effects of exposure to this colorless, odorless gas include headache, blurred vision, and shortness of breath, followed by dizziness, vomiting, and unconsciousness. Carbon monoxide detectors similar to smoke detectors are available for home use; they should be used according to the manufacturer's instructions. To prevent poisoning by gases, never operate a vehicle in an enclosed space, have your furnace inspected yearly, and use caution with any substance that produces potentially toxic fumes.

A key strategy for preventing serious poisoning injuries is to look up the phone number for the nearest

home injuries Unintentional injuries and deaths that occur in the home and on home premises to occupants, guests, domestic servants, and trespassers; falls, burns, poisonings, suffocations, unintentional shootings, drownings, and electrical shocks are examples.

Terms

Poison Control Center and post it in a convenient location. A Poison Control Center offers expert emergency advice 24 hours a day. It is also a good idea to keep syrup of ipecac on hand. This nonprescription plant extract can be used to induce vomiting, but *it should be used only on the advice of the Poison Control Center or your physician.*

If a poisoning does occur, it's important that you act quickly. Remove the poison from contact with the victim's eyes, skin, or mouth, or move the victim away from contact with poisonous gases. Call the Poison Control Center immediately for instructions; do not follow the emergency instructions on product labels because they may be incorrect. Depending on the situation, you may be instructed to give the victim water to drink, to flood affected parts of the skin or eyes with water, or to induce vomiting. If you are advised to go to an emergency room, take the poisonous substance or container with you.

Suffocation and Choking   Suffocation and choking account for nearly 4000 deaths annually in the United States. Young children account for nearly half of these deaths. Children can suffocate if they put small items in their mouths, get tangled in their crib bedding, or get trapped in airtight appliances like old refrigerators. Keep small objects out of reach of children under age 3, and don't give them raw carrots, hot dogs, popcorn, or hard candy. Examine toys carefully for small parts that could come loose; don't give plastic bags or balloons to small children.

Adults can also become choking victims, especially if they fail to chew food properly, eat hurriedly, or try to talk and eat at the same time. Many choking victims can be saved with the **Heimlich maneuver** (Figure 23-1). The American Red Cross recommends the Heimlich maneuver (also called "abdominal thrusts") as the easiest and safest thing to do when an adult is choking. Back blows administered in conjunction with abdominal thrusts are an acceptable procedure for dislodging an object from the throat of an infant.

Firearms   More than half of all unintended firearm deaths occur to people age 10–29. People who use firearms should remember the following:

- Never point a loaded gun at something you do not intend to shoot.

- Store unloaded firearms under lock and key, in a place separate from the ammunition.
- Always inspect firearms carefully before handling.
- Behave in the safe and responsible manner advocated in firearms safety courses.

Proper storage is critical. Do not assume that young children cannot fire a gun: About 25% of 3–4-year-olds and 70% of 5–6-year-olds have enough finger strength to pull a trigger. Every year, about 120 Americans are unintentionally shot to death by children under 6. An estimated 8.3 million children live in households with unlocked guns, including 2.6 million who live in households where guns are stored loaded or with ammunition nearby.

Probably the best advice for anyone who picks up a gun is to assume it is loaded. Too many deaths and injuries occur when someone unintentionally shoots a friend while under the impression that the gun he or she is handling is not loaded. In addition, if you plan to handle a gun, you should avoid the use of alcohol and drugs, which may affect your judgment and coordination. (Firearms and intentional injuries are discussed later in the chapter.)

Leisure Injuries

Leisure activities encompass a large part of our free time, so it is not surprising that **leisure injuries** are a significant health-related problem in the United States. Key factors in leisure injuries include misuse of equipment, lack of experience and skill, use of alcohol or other drugs, and failure to use appropriate safety equipment. Specific safety strategies for activities associated with leisure injuries include the following:

- Don't swim alone, in unsupervised places, under the influence of alcohol, or for an unusual length of time; use caution when swimming in unfamiliar surroundings or in water colder than 70°F. Check the depth of water before diving. Make sure residential pools are fenced and that children are never allowed to swim unsupervised.

- Always use a **personal flotation device** (life jacket) when on a boat.

- For all sports and recreational activities, make sure facilities are safe, follow the rules, and practice good sportsmanship. Develop adequate skill in the activity, and use proper safety equipment, including, where appropriate, helmets, eye protection, correct footwear, and knee, elbow, and wrist pads.

- If using equipment such as skateboards, mountain bikes, or all-terrain vehicles, wear a helmet and other safety equipment, and avoid excessive speeds and unsafe stunts. Playground equipment should

Terms

Heimlich maneuver A maneuver developed by Henry J. Heimlich, M.D., to help force an obstruction from the airway.

leisure injuries Unintentional injuries and deaths that occur in public places or places used in a public way, not involving motor vehicles; includes most sports and recreation deaths and injuries; falls, drownings, burns, and heat and cold stress are examples.

personal flotation device A device designed to save a person from drowning by buoying up the body while in the water; also called a *life jacket.*

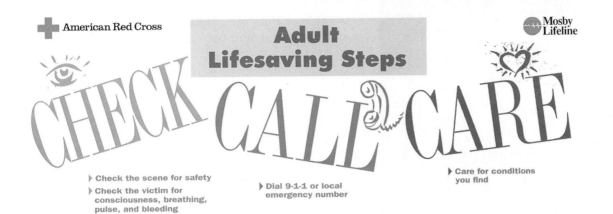

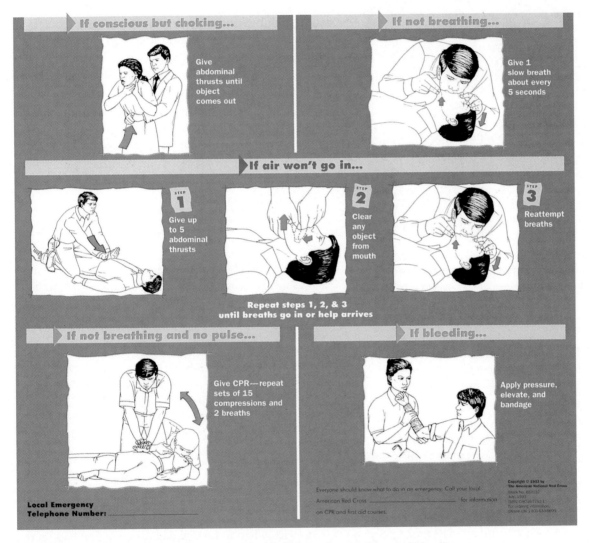

Figure 23-1 **Rescue breathing, first aid for choking, and ways to control bleeding; procedures recommended by the American Red Cross.** SOURCE: Courtesy of the American Red Cross. All rights reserved in all countries.

be used only for those activities for which it is designed.

- If you are active in excessively hot and humid weather, drink plenty of fluids, rest frequently in the shade, and slow down or stop if you feel uncomfortable. Danger signals of heat stress include excessive perspiration, dizziness, headache, muscle cramps, nausea, weakness, rapid pulse, and disorientation.

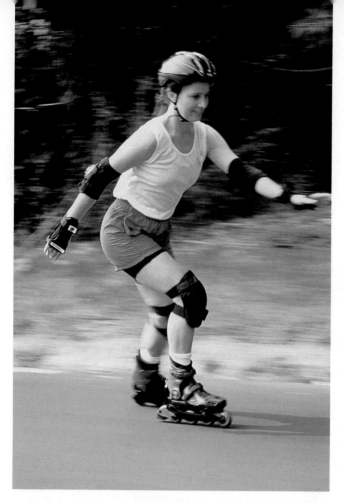

Leisure activities injure more than 6 million people each year, including 250,000 in-line skaters. The use of proper safety equipment—helmet, wrist guards, and elbow and knee pads—is critical for injury prevention.

- Do not use alcohol or other drugs during recreational activities—such activities require coordination and sound judgment. Don't chew gum or eat while active to avoid choking.

For more on exercise safety, refer to Chapter 13. Two activities that have recently become popular and that are associated with many leisure injuries are in-line skating and the use of nonmotorized scooters.

In-Line Skating Injuries More than 26 million Americans use in-line skates, and more than 250,000 are injured badly enough each year to wind up in an emergency room. Injuries to the wrist and head are most common; many occur because users do not wear appropriate safety gear. Researchers estimate that more than one-third of all serious injuries could be prevented if all skaters wore helmets and wrist and elbow protection.

To reduce your risk of being injured while rollerblading, wear a helmet, elbow and knee pads, wrist guards, a long-sleeved shirt, and long pants. Alcohol use appears to be a significant factor in in-line skating injuries that occur on college campuses. Because in-line skating involves skill, judgment, and coordination, it makes sense not to mix skating and drinking.

Scooter Injuries Some 5 million scooters were sold in 2000, up from almost zero in 1999. These newly popular scooters are lightweight and have low-friction wheels for quickness and portability. Along with their skyrocketing popularity have come scooter-related injuries. Over 27,000 people were treated for scooter-related injuries in hospital emergency rooms in 2000, and two deaths related to scooter use have been reported. The most common injuries are arm or hand fractures and dislocations, cuts and bruises, and sprains; 85% of injuries have involved children under the age of 15. Viewing scooters as toys more than transportation may lead riders to ignore important safety precautions:

- Wear a helmet that meets bicycle helmet standards, along with knee and elbow pads.
- Be sure that handlebars, the steering column, and all nuts and bolts are securely fastened.
- Ride on smooth, paved surfaces away from motor vehicle traffic. Avoid streets and surfaces with water, sand, gravel, or dirt.
- Don't ride after dark.
- Closely supervise young children.

COMMUNICATE! It takes extra time and effort to be safe, and sometimes people don't want to be bothered with taking necessary precautions. If you have a friend or family member who resists safety measures—whether it's wearing a safety belt in a car, a helmet on a bike, a personal flotation device on a boat, or safety equipment while in-line skating, skateboarding, or riding a scooter—you can do him or her a favor by insisting that the safety measures be taken. You may make some impression on the person by quoting the kind of statistics mentioned in this chapter, but your best argument may simply be, "I care about you and I don't want you to get hurt."

Work Injuries

Since 1912, when industrial records were first kept in the United States, the work site has become a much safer place, as evidenced by a reduction in the unintentional death rate of nearly 76%. That figure becomes even more impressive when one realizes that the size of the labor force has more than doubled and production has increased more than tenfold. One very significant factor to account for such a marked decline in **work injuries** has been the Occupational Safety and Health Act of 1970. As a result of that act, the Occupational Safety and Health

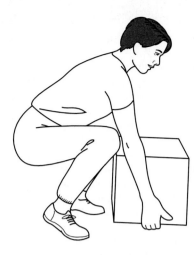

Figure 23-2 Correct lifting technique. Stay upright, bending at the knees and hips.

Repetitive Strain Injuries Musculoskeletal injuries and disorders in the workplace include **repetitive strain injuries (RSIs)**. RSIs are caused by repeated strain on a particular part of the body. Twisting, vibrations, awkward postures, and other stressors may contribute to RSIs. **Carpal tunnel syndrome** is one type of RSI that has increased in recent years due to increased use of computers, both at work and in the home (see the box "Carpal Tunnel Syndrome" for more information).

General strategies for preventing work-related injuries include following the safety instructions associated with the job, finding out where first aid equipment is located and knowing how to use it, watching for and reporting safety hazards, and using any safety equipment that is provided by the employer. Whatever the working conditions, employees should make a conscious effort to avoid hazardous situations.

VIOLENCE AND INTENTIONAL INJURIES

Administration (OSHA) was created within the U.S. Department of Labor to ensure a safer and healthier environment for workers.

Despite improvements, nearly 4 million Americans suffer disabling injuries on the job each year. Although laborers make up less than half of the workforce, they account for more than 75% of all work-related injuries and illnesses. Such jobs usually involve extensive manual labor and lifting, neither of which is addressed in OSHA safety standards. Skin disorders account for nearly 40% of reported occupational illnesses; the introduction of more hazardous chemicals at the work site means that these disorders are of increasing concern. Most fatal occupational injuries involve crushing injuries, severe lacerations, burns, and electrocutions; among women, the leading cause of workplace injury deaths is homicide.

Back Injuries Back problems account for more than 20% of work injuries; many of these could be prevented through proper lifting technique (Figure 23-2):

- Avoid bending at the waist. Remain in an upright position and crouch down if you need to lower yourself to grasp the object. Bend at the knees and hips.
- Place feet securely about shoulder-width apart; grip the object firmly.
- Lift gradually, with straight arms. Avoid quick, jerky motions. Lift by standing up or pushing with your leg muscles. Keep the object close to your body.
- If you have to turn, change the position of your feet. Twisting is a common and dangerous cause of injury. Plan ahead so that your pathway is clear and turning can be minimized.
- Put the object down gently, reversing the rules for lifting.

Violence—the use of physical force with the intent to inflict harm, injury, or death upon oneself or another—is a major public health concern in the United States. More than 2 million Americans are victims of violent injury each year; about three violent crimes occur every minute. Worldwide, interpersonal violence is the third leading cause of death among people age 15–44. Examples of types of violence are assault, homicide, sexual assault, domestic violence, suicide, and child abuse.

It is difficult to determine the overall level of violence in our society because the major sources of data, which are police reports and victim surveys, are often at odds. In general, the overall violent crime rate increased between the 1950s and 1970s and then leveled off until the mid-1980s, when it again began to rise. Since 1993, however, the rate of violent crime has declined by over 20%; the homicide rate in 1999 was at its lowest level since 1966.

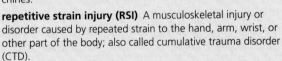

work injuries Unintentional injuries and deaths that arise out of and in the course of gainful work, such as falls, electrical shocks, exposure to radiation and toxic chemicals, burns, cuts, back sprains, and loss of fingers or other body parts in machines.

repetitive strain injury (RSI) A musculoskeletal injury or disorder caused by repeated strain to the hand, arm, wrist, or other part of the body; also called cumulative trauma disorder (CTD).

carpal tunnel syndrome Compression of the median nerve in the wrist, often caused by repetitive use of the hands, such as in computer use; characterized by numbness, tingling, and pain in the hands and fingers; can cause nerve damage.

Terms

Carpal tunnel syndrome (CTS) is a repetitive strain injury characterized by pressure on the median nerve in the wrist. The median nerve travels from the forearm to the hand through a tunnel in the wrist formed by the wrist bones (carpals) and associated tendons and covered by a ligament (see the figure). The median nerve can become compressed for a variety of reasons, including swelling of the surrounding tendons caused by pregnancy, diabetes, arthritis, or repetitive wrist motions during activities such as typing, cutting, or carpentry work. Symptoms of CTS include numbness, tingling, burning, and/or aching in the hand, particularly in the thumb and the first three fingers. The pain may worsen at night and may shoot up from the hand as far as the shoulder.

Many cases of carpal tunnel syndrome clear up on their own or with minimal treatment. Modification of the movement that is causing the problem is critically important. For example, adjusting the height of a computer keyboard so that the wrists can be held straight during typing can help relieve pressure on the wrists. CTS is often first treated by immobilizing the wrist with a splint during the night. People may also be given anti-inflammatory drugs or injections of cortisone in the wrist to reduce swelling. In a small percentage of severe cases, surgery to cut the ligament and reduce the pressure on the nerve may be recommended.

If you engage in activities like typing or cutting that involve repetitive motions, there are some strategies you can try to reduce your risk of developing carpal tunnel syndrome. Begin by modifying your work environment to reduce the stress on your wrists. Alternate activities to avoid spending long stretches of time engaged in the same motion. Warm up your wrists before you begin any repetitive motion activity, and take frequent breaks to stretch and flex your wrists and hands:

- Extend your arms out in front of you and stretch your wrists by pointing your fingers to the ceiling; hold for a count of five. Then straighten your wrists and relax your fingers for a count of five.

- With arms extended, make a tight fist with both hands and then bend your wrists so your knuckles are pointed toward the floor; hold for a count of five. Then straighten your wrists and relax your fingers for a count of five.

Repeat these stretches several times, and finish by letting your arms hang loosely at your sides and shaking them gently for several seconds.

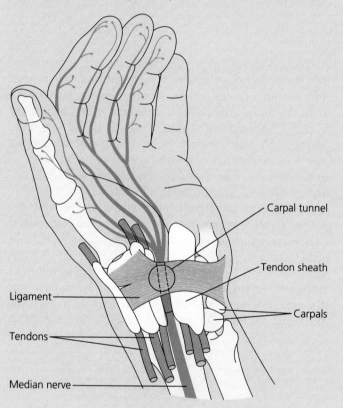

Carpal tunnel

Tendon sheath

Ligament

Carpals

Tendons

Median nerve

SOURCES: American Academy of Orthopaedic Surgeons. 2000. *Exercises to Do at Work to Prevent Carpal Tunnel Syndrome* (http://orthoinfo.aaos. org/fact/thr_report.cfm?Thread_ID=15&topcategory=Hand; retrieved March 11, 2001). National Institute of Neurological Disorders and Stroke. 2000. *Carpal Tunnel Syndrome* (http://www.ninds.nih.gov/health_and_ medical/disorders/carpal_doc.htm; retrieved March 11, 2001). Detecting carpal tunnel syndrome. 1999. *Journal of the American Medical Association* 282(2): 206.

Possible factors cited for this decline include the aging of the population, reduced unemployment, the decline of the crack cocaine trade, law enforcement strategies to get guns off the street, violence prevention programs for youth, and longer prison sentences. In comparison to other industrialized countries, U.S. rates of of violence are abnormally high in only two areas—homicide and firearm-related deaths. The U.S. homicide death rate is four to ten times that of similar countries, and the firearm death rate in the United States exceeds that of other developed countries eightfold.

Factors Contributing to Violence

Everyone gets angry sometimes, but few people translate their angry and aggressive impulses into action. Most in-

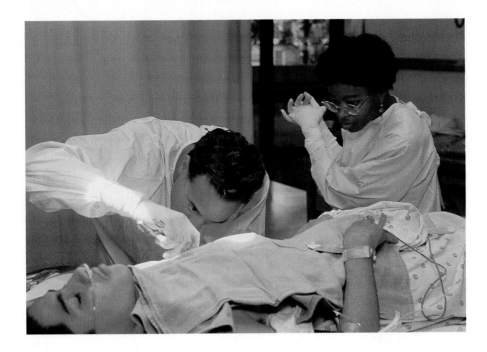

For every violent death that occurs in the United States, there are at least 100 nonfatal injuries caused by violence. The victims of most types of violence are statistically likely to be young (under 25 years), poor, in a minority, urban, and—except for rape and domestic violence—male.

tentional injuries and deaths are associated with an argument or the committing of another crime. However, there are a great many forms of violence, and no single factor can explain all of them.

Social Factors   Rates of violence are not the same throughout society; they vary by geographic region, neighborhood, socioeconomic level, and many other factors. In the United States, violence is highest in the West, followed by the South, and among those who are disadvantaged in some way. Neighborhoods that are disadvantaged in status, power, and economic resources are typically the ones with the most violence. Rates of violence are highest among young people and minorities, groups that have relatively little power. People under age 25 account for nearly half the arrests for violent crimes in the United States and about 40% of the arrests for homicide.

People who feel a part of society (have strong family and social ties), who are economically integrated (have a reasonable chance at getting a decent job), and who grow up in areas where there is a feeling of community (good schools, parks, and neighborhoods) are significantly less likely to engage in violence. American society, where more than one-third of all children live in poverty and where the gap between rich and poor keeps growing, should be expected to breed violence. Many criminologists feel we have a growing underclass of people who cannot expect to have even the worst permanent jobs. That absence of hopes and dreams, when combined with family devastation and poverty, certainly contributes to violent behavior.

Studies have shown that the environment on college campuses can contribute to violence. The nature of college campuses—transitory communities rather than permanent places where people work and live together over the long term—means that there is less incentive for people to cooperate and coexist amicably. Some campus groups even promote the ideas of bigotry and bias toward others, particularly toward individuals about whom they know little or with whom they have had little contact. Ignorance and insensitivity to differences can be precursors to acts of violence. College students must become more familiar with concepts like inclusion, tolerance, and diversity if the problem is to be addressed.

Violence in the Media   The mass media play a major role in exposing audiences of all ages to violence as an acceptable and effective means of solving problems. Children may view as many as 10,000 violent acts on television and in movies each year. The consequences of violence, on both perpetrator and victim, are shown much less frequently.

The role of media violence on violent behavior is an area of controversy. However, it makes sense for parents to be aware of the potential influence of the media on their children. A child may not clearly understand the distinctions between the fantasy world portrayed in the media and the complexities of the real world. Parents should consider monitoring the TV shows, movies, video games, music, and other forms of media to which children are exposed. Watching programs with children gives parents the opportunity to talk to children about violence and its consequences, to explain that violence is not the best way to resolve conflicts or solve problems, and to point out examples of positive behaviors such as kindness and cooperation.

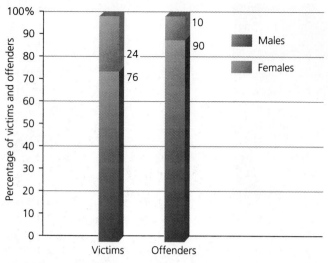

(a) Homicide victims and offenders by sex

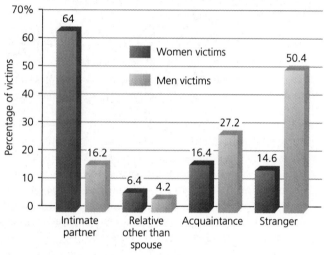

(b) Adult victims of violence by victim-offender relationship and sex of victim

W. VITAL STATISTICS

Figure 23-3   Facts about violence in the United States.
SOURCES: Federal Bureau of Investigation. 2000. *Crime in the United States. Uniform Crime Reports, 1999.* Washington, D.C.: U.S. Department of Justice. Tjaden, P., and N. Thoennes. 2000. *Full Report of the Prevalence, Incidence, and Consequences of Violence Against Women.* Washington, D.C.: U.S. Department of Justice.

Gender   In most cases, violence is committed by men (Figure 23-3). Males are more than nine times more likely than females to commit murder, and three times more likely than females to be murdered. Some researchers have suggested that the male hormone testosterone is in some way linked to aggressive behavior. Others point to prevailing cultural attitudes about male roles (men as dominant and controlling) as an explanation for the high rate of violence among men. However, these theories do not explain just why it is that violent men are more likely

to live in the West, belong to minorities, be poor, and be young.

Women do commit acts of violence, including a small but substantial proportion of murders of spouses. This fact has been used to argue that women have the same capacity to commit violence as men, but most researchers feel that there are substantial differences. Men often kill their wives as the culmination of years of violence or after stalking them; they may kill the entire family and themselves at the same time. Women virtually never kill in these circumstances; rather, they kill their husbands after repeated victimization or while being beaten.

Interpersonal Factors   Although most people fear attack from strangers, the majority of victims are acquainted with their attacker (see Figure 23-3). Approximately 60% of murders of women and 80% of sexual assaults are committed by someone the woman knows. In many cases, the people we need to fear the most live in our own household. Crime victims and violent criminals tend to share many characteristics—that is, they are likely to be young, male, in a minority, and poor.

Alcohol and Other Drugs   Substance abuse and dependence are consistently associated with interpersonal violence and suicide. Intoxication affects judgment and may increase aggression in some people, causing a small argument to escalate into a serious physical confrontation. On college campuses, alcohol is involved in about 95% of all violent crimes.

Firearms   Many criminologists feel that the high rate of homicide in the United States is directly related to the fact that we are the only industrialized country in which handguns are widespread and easily available. Simply put, most victims of assaults with other weapons don't die, but the death rate from assault by handgun is extremely high. The possession of a handgun can change a suicide attempt to a completed suicide and a violent assault to a murder. Every hour, guns are used to kill four people in the United States.

Over 100,000 deaths and injuries occur in the United States each year as a result of the use of firearms. Firearms are used in more than two-thirds of homicides, and studies reveal a strong correlation between the incidence of gun ownership and homicide rates for a given area of the country. Over half of all suicides involve a firearm, and people living in households in which guns are kept have a risk of suicide that is five or more times greater than that of people living in households without guns. Men between the ages of 15 and 34 have the highest risk of death from homicide and suicide when guns are the weapon used.

Research indicates that of all firearms, handguns are the murder weapon of choice, used in about 80% of homicides involving firearms. People at particularly high risk for being murdered by handguns are teenagers and young adults.

Assault

Assault is the use of physical force by a person or persons to inflict injury or death on another; homicide, aggravated assault, and robbery are examples of assault. Research indicates that the victims of assaultive injuries and their perpetrators tend to resemble one another in terms of ethnicity, educational background, psychological profile, and reliance on weapons. In many cases, the victim actually magnifies the confrontation through the use of a weapon.

Homicide

Men, teenagers, young adults, and members of minority groups, particularly African Americans and Latinos, are most likely to be murder victims. Although homicide rates for African Americans have declined dramatically in the past 25 years, no other cause of death so greatly differentiates African Americans from other Americans: Among black males, the rate of death from homicide is about six times higher than the rate for the U.S. population as a whole. Poverty and unemployment have been identified as key factors in homicide, and this may account for the high rates of homicide among blacks and other minority groups.

Most homicides are committed with a firearm, occur during an argument, and occur among people who know one another. Intrafamilial homicide, where the perpetrator and victim are related, accounts for about one out of every eight homicides. About 40% of family homicides are committed by spouses, usually following a history of physical and emotional abuse directed at the woman. Wives are more likely to be murdered than husbands, and when a wife kills her husband, it is usually in self-defense.

Gang-Related Violence

Violence results from more than just individual acts, as evidenced by the number of injuries and deaths resulting from gang activities. Gangs are most frequently associated with large cities, but gang activity also extends to the suburbs and even to rural areas. It is estimated that more than 800,000 Americans belong to gangs; the average age for joining a gang is 14. Most gangs control a particular territory and will oppose other gangs, as well as police and community efforts to eliminate them. Gangs may be involved in illegal drug trade, extortion, and "protection" schemes. Gang members are more likely than non–gang members to possess weapons, and violence may result from conflicts over territory or illegal activities.

Gangs are more common in areas that are poor and suffer from high unemployment, population density, and crime. In these areas, an individual may feel that his or her chance of legitimate success in life is out of reach and know that involvement in the drug market makes some gang members rich. Often, gangs also serve as a mechanism for companionship, self-esteem, support, and security; indeed, in some areas, gang membership may be viewed as the only possible means of survival.

To prevent gang violence, individuals, communities, and lawmakers must work together to address factors linked to gang membership and activities. A successful program for combating gangs in Los Angeles includes mediators to help handle disputes or negotiate truces between gangs, job skill development for ex–gang members, and programs for at-risk youths that incorporate tutoring, counseling, and recreational activities. The program helps create an anti-gang community infrastructure by promoting neighborhood watch groups, community-based anti-gang activities, and economic development.

Hate Crimes

When bias against another person's race or ethnicity, national origin, religion, sexual orientation, or disability motivates a criminal act, the offense is classified as a hate crime. Hate crimes may be committed against people or property; those against people may include intimidation, assault, and even rape or murder. Crimes against property most frequently involve graffiti, the desecration of churches or synagogues, cross burnings, and other acts of vandalism or property damage.

About 10,000 hate crimes are reported every year; many more go unreported. Crimes against people make up about 70% of all incidents; intimidation and assault are the most common offenses. Racial or ethnic bias was cited as the motivating bias in 55% of the hate crimes reported in 1999; religion was cited in 18% of the cases, sexual orientation in 17%, and national origin in 11%.

Hate crimes may be extremely brutal acts perpetrated at random on total strangers by multiple offenders. Suspects are frequently not identified, but research indicates that a substantial number of hate crimes are committed by males under age 20. Hate crimes are frequently, but not always, associated with fringe groups that have extremist ideologies, such as the Ku Klux Klan and neo-Nazi groups. The Southern Poverty Law Center tracks more than 450 hate groups and group chapters currently active in the United States; the rapid growth of hate sites on the Internet is another area of concern.

A variety of factors lead to the prejudice and intolerance that is a major force behind hate crimes. A social context of unemployment and hard economic times, an influx of immigrants, and the growth of visible minority rights movements have been associated with the recent increases in hate crimes in the United States. To combat hate crimes, individuals and communities must foster tolerance, understanding, and an appreciation of differences among people.

School Violence

Tragedies like the shootings at Columbine High School in Colorado have brought national attention to the problem of school violence. According to the National School Safety Center, more than 275 school-associated violent deaths of students, faculty, and administrators have occurred since 1992. A majority of these deaths occurred in urban areas and involved use of a firearm; as with other types of violence, both victims and offenders were predominantly young men. Homicide and suicide are the most serious and least common types of violence in schools; an estimated 400,000 less serious incidents of violence and crime occur each year, including theft, vandalism, and fights not involving weapons.

How risky is the school environment for students? Research indicates that children are actually much safer at school than away from it. Less than 1% of all homicides among youths age 5–19 occur at school, and 90% of schools report no incidents of serious violence. Children and adolescents are far more likely to be killed by an adult in their own home or away from school than they are to die as a result of school-associated violence. According to the CDC, the overall number of violent incidents has decreased steadily since 1992; however, the number of multiple-victim events may have increased. Recent school shootings received so much attention in part because they were unusual—they took place in predominantly white suburban or rural schools and involved multiple victims.

Although schools are basically safe places overall, there are steps that can be taken to identify at-risk youths and improve safety for all students. Characteristics associated with youths who have caused school-associated violent deaths include a history of uncontrollable angry outbursts, violent and abusive language and behavior, isolation from peers, depression and irritability, access to and preoccupation with weapons, and lack of support and supervision from adults. Recommendations for reducing school violence include offering classroom training in anger management and improved self-control, providing mental health and social services for students in need, developing after-school programs that help students build self-esteem and make friends, and keeping guns out of the hands of children and out of schools.

Workplace Violence

Each year U.S. workers experience an average of 1.5 million minor assaults, 400,000 serious assaults, 85,000 robberies, 50,000 sexual assaults, and 1000 homicides. In about 60% of cases, workplace violence is committed by strangers; acquaintances account for nearly 40% of cases, and intimates for 1%. Police and corrections officers have the most dangerous jobs, followed by taxi drivers, security guards, bartenders, mental health professionals, and workers at gas stations and convenience and liquor stores. Middle school teachers are nearly three times more likely than high school teachers and twenty times more likely than college or university teachers to experience workplace violence.

Most of the perpetrators of workplace violence are white males over 21 years of age. Firearms are used in more than 80% of workplace homicides, and the majority of these homicides occur during the commission of a robbery or other crime. General crime prevention strategies, including controls on firearms, may help reduce the rate of workplace violence injuries and deaths.

Family and Intimate Violence

Violence in families challenges some of our most basic assumptions about the family. Family violence generally refers to any rough and illegitimate use of physical force, aggression, or verbal abuse by one family member toward another. Such abuse may be physical and/or psychological in nature. Based on reported cases each year, an estimated 5–7 million women and children are abused in the United States.

Battering Studies reveal than 95% of domestic violence victims are women; 20–35% of women who visit medical emergency rooms are there for injuries related to ongoing abuse. Violence against wives/intimate partners, or battering, occurs at every level of society but is more common at lower socioeconomic levels. It occurs more frequently in relationships with a high degree of conflict—an apparent inability to resolve arguments through negotiation and compromise. About 25% of women report having been physically assaulted or raped by an intimate partner and more than 50% report having experienced some type of abuse—physical or psychological—in a relationship.

At the root of much of this abusive behavior is the need to control another person: Abusive partners are controlling partners. They not only want to have power over another person, but also believe they are entitled to it, no matter what the cost to the other person. Abuse includes behavior that physically harms, arouses fear, prevents a person from doing what she wants, or compels her to behave in ways she does not freely choose. Controlling people use a variety of psychological, emotional, and physical tactics to keep their partners bound to them. Early in a relationship, a person's tendency to be controlling may not be obvious. If you are concerned about whether a person you are dating has the potential to be abusive, review the guidelines in the box "Recognizing the Potential for Abusiveness in a Partner."

In abusive relationships, the abuser (in most cases a man) usually has a history of violent behavior, traditional beliefs about gender roles, and problems with alcohol abuse. He has low self-esteem and seeks to raise it by dominating and imposing his will on another person. Re-

There are no sure ways to tell whether someone will become abusive or violent toward an intimate partner, but there are warning signs that you can look for. (Remember that, although most abusive relationships involve male violence directed at a woman, women can also be abusive, as can partners in a same-sex relationship. Because most abusers are male, the following material refers to the abuser as "he.") If you are concerned that a person you are involved with has the potential for violence, observe his or her behavior, and ask yourself these questions:

- What is this person's attitude toward women? How does he treat his mother and his sister? How does he work with female students, female colleagues, or a female boss? How does he treat your women friends?

- What is his attitude toward your autonomy? Does he respect the work you do and the way you do it? Or does he put it down, or tell you how to do it better, or encourage you to give it up? Does he tell you he'll take care of you?

- How self-centered is he? Does he want to spend leisure time on your interests or his? Does he listen to you? Does he remember what you say?

- Is he possessive or jealous? Does he want to spend every minute with you? Does he cross-examine you about things you do when you're not with him?

- What happens when things don't go the way he wants them to? Does he blow up? Does he always have to get his way?

- Is he moody, mocking, critical, or bossy? Do you feel as if you're "walking on eggshells" when you're with him?

- Do you feel you have to avoid arguing with him?

- Does he drink too much or use drugs?

- Does he refuse to use condoms or take other precautions for safer sex?

Listen to your own uneasiness, and stay away from any man who disrespects women, who wants or needs you intensely and exclusively, and who has a knack for getting his own way almost all the time.

If you are in a serious relationship with a controlling person, you may already have experienced abuse. Consider the questions on the following list:

- Does your partner constantly criticize you, blame you for things that are not your fault, or verbally degrade you?

- Does he humiliate you in front of others?

- Is he suspicious or jealous? Does he accuse you of being unfaithful or monitor your mail or phone calls?

- Does he "track" all your time? Does he discourage you from seeing friends and family?

- Does he prevent you from getting or keeping a job or attending school? Does he control your shared resources or restrict your access to money?

- Has he ever pushed, slapped, hit, kicked, bitten, or restrained you? Thrown an object at you? Used a weapon on you?

- Has he ever destroyed or damaged your personal property or sentimental items?

- Has he ever forced you to have sex or to do something sexually you didn't want to do?

- Does he anger easily when drinking or taking drugs?

- Has he ever threatened to harm you or your children, friends, pets, or property?

- Has he ever threatened to blackmail you if you leave?

If you answered yes to one or more of these questions, you may be experiencing domestic abuse. If you believe you or your children are in imminent danger, look in your local telephone directory for a women's shelter, or call 9-1-1. If you want information, referrals to a program in your area, or assistance, contact one of the organizations listed in For More Information at the end of the chapter.

SOURCES: Family Violence Prevention Fund. 1996. *Take Action Against Domestic Violence.* San Francisco, Calif.: Family Violence Prevention Fund. How to tell if you're in an abusive situation. 1994. *San Francisco Chronicle,* 24 June. Jones, A. 1994. *Next Time She'll Be Dead.* Boston: Beacon Press.

search has revealed a three-phase cycle of battering, consisting of a period of increasing tension, a violent explosion and loss of control, and a period of contriteness, in which the man begs forgiveness and promises it will never happen again. The batterer is drawn back to this cycle over and over again, but he never succeeds in changing his feelings about himself.

Battered women often stay in violent relationships for years. They may be economically dependent on their partners, believe their children need a father, or have low self-esteem themselves. They may love or pity their husbands, or they may believe they'll eventually be able to stop the violence. They usually leave the relationship only when they become determined that the violence must end. Battered women's shelters offer physical protection, counseling, support, and other assistance.

Many batterers are arrested, prosecuted, and imprisoned. Treatment programs are helpful in some cases, but not all. Programs focus on stress management, communication and conflict-resolution skills, behavior change, and individual and group therapy. A crucial factor in changing violent behavior seems to be a partner's adamant insistence that the abuse stop.

Stalking and Cyberstalking   Battering is closely associated with **stalking**, characterized by harassing behaviors such as following or spying on a person and making verbal, written, or implied threats. In the United States, it is estimated that 1 million women and 400,000 men are stalked each year; about 87% of stalkers are men. About half of female victims are stalked by current or former intimate partners; of these, 80% had been physically or sexually assaulted by that partner during the relationship. A stalker's goal may be to control or scare the victim or to keep her or him in a relationship. Most stalking episodes last a year or less, but victims may experience social and psychological effects long after the stalking ends.

The use of the Internet, e-mail, chat rooms, and other electronic communications devices to stalk another person is known as **cyberstalking**. As with offline stalking, the majority of stalkers are men, and the majority of victims are women, although there have been same-sex cyberstalking incidents. Online incidents of harassment or abuse are becoming more common and more serious, and the U.S. Department of Justice estimates that nearly one-half million people each year experience cyberstalking. As the seriousness of the crime is being recognized, several states have passed cyberstalking or related laws and a federal law is under consideration. There is concern that the impersonal nature of electronic communication may lower the barriers to harassment and threats because a cyberstalker does not have to physically confront the victim, thus making stalking more common.

Cyberstalkers may send harassing or threatening e-mails or chat room messages to the victim, or they may encourage others to harass the victim—for example, by impersonating the victim and posting inflammatory messages and personal information on bulletin boards or in chat rooms. Guidelines for staying safe online include

- Never use your real name as an e-mail username or chat room nickname. Select an age- and gender-neutral identity.

- Avoid filling out profiles for accounts related to e-mail use or chat room activities with information that could be used to identify you.

- Do not share personal information in public spaces anywhere online or give it to strangers.

- Learn how to filter unwanted e-mail messages.

- If you do experience harassment online, do not respond to the harasser. Log off or surf elsewhere.

If you receive unwanted online contact, make it clear to that person that you want all contact to stop. If harassment continues, contact the harasser's Internet service provider (ISP) by identifying the domain of the stalker's account (after the "@" sign); most ISPs have an e-mail address for complaints. Often, an ISP can try to stop the conduct by direct contact with the harasser or by closing his or her account. Save all communications for evidence, and contact your ISP and your local police department. (See Chapter 4 for more on safely interacting with people online.)

Violence Against Children Violence is also directed against children. At least 1 million American children are physically abused by their parents and another 1 to 2 million are victims of neglect every year. Parental violence is one of the five leading causes of death for children age 1–18. Parents who abuse children tend to have low self-esteem, to believe in physical punishment, to have a poor marital relationship, and to have been abused themselves (although many people who were abused as children do not grow up to abuse their own children). Poverty, unemployment, and social isolation are characteristics of families in which children are abused. Single parents, both men and women, are at especially high risk for abusing their children. Very often one child, whom the parents consider different in some way, is singled out for violent treatment.

When government agencies intervene in child-abuse situations, their goals are to protect the victims and to assist and strengthen the families. The most successful programs are those that emphasize education and early intervention, such as home visits to high-risk first-time mothers. Educational efforts focus on stress management, money management, job-finding skills, and information about child behavior and development. Parents may also receive counseling and be referred to substance-abuse treatment programs. Support groups like Parents Anonymous are effective for parents committed to changing their behavior.

Elder Abuse Each year, at least 500,000 older persons are abused; only one in six incidents is reported. Most abusers are family members who are serving as caregivers. Elder abuse can take different forms: physical, sexual, or emotional abuse, financial exploitation, neglect, or abandonment. Neglect is the most common form of abuse, accounting for about 55% of reported cases. Elders who have lost some mental or physical functions and must rely on others for care are most at risk and may suffer malnutrition, dehydration, mismanaged medication, or infection due to poor hygiene. Physical abuse accounts for about 15% of reported cases and financial exploitation for about 13%.

Abuse often occurs when caring for a dependent adult becomes too stressful for the caregiver, especially if the elder is incontinent, has suffered mental deterioration, or is violent. Abuse may become an outlet for frustration. Many believe that the solution to elder abuse is support in the form of greater social and financial assistance, such as adult day-care centers and education and public care programs.

COMMUNICATE! It's normal to feel angry when someone you love or trust lets you down, but don't let your anger hurt you or anyone else. Learn to talk about your feelings and to express yourself calmly, describing your disappointment, frustration, anger, or displeasure without losing your temper. For example, you might say, "I am so disappointed and angry that you repeated what I told you in confidence." Learn to listen to others without getting upset if they give you negative feedback; try to see the situation from the other person's point of view. Look for creative ways to negotiate difficult problems and find compromises. Anger is part of life, but it shouldn't control you or your relationships.

WWW. Sexual Violence

The use of force and coercion in sexual relationships is one of the most serious problems in human interactions. The most extreme manifestation of sexual coercion—forcing a person to submit to another's sexual desires—is rape, but sexual coercion occurs in many more subtle forms, including sexual harassment.

Sexual Assault: Rape Sexual coercion that relies on the threat and use of physical force or takes advantage of circumstances that render a person incapable of giving consent (such as when drunk) constitutes **sexual assault** or **rape**. When the victim is younger than the legally defined "age of consent," the act constitutes **statutory rape**, whether or not coercion is involved. Coerced sexual activity in which the victim knows or is dating the rapist is often referred to as **date rape** (or acquaintance rape).

Any woman—or man—can be a rape victim. It is conservatively estimated that at least 3.5 million females are raped annually in the United States. According to the U.S. Department of Justice, a woman is sexually assaulted in the United States every two minutes. Some men are raped by other men, perhaps 10,000 annually; the majority of male victims are not in prison and most know their assailant. It is estimated that less than one-third of all sexual crimes are reported.

WHO COMMITS RAPE? Men who commit rape may be any age and come from any socioeconomic group. Some rapists are exploiters in the sense that they rape on the spur of the moment and mainly want immediate gratification. Some attempt to compensate for feelings of sexual inadequacy and an inability to obtain satisfaction otherwise. Others are more hostile and sadistic and are primarily interested not in sex but in hurting and humiliating a particular woman or women in general.

Most women are in much less danger of being raped by a stranger than of being sexually assaulted by a man they know or date. Surveys suggest that as many as 25% of women have had experiences in which the men they were dating persisted in trying to force sex despite pleading, crying, screaming, or resisting. Surveys have also found that more than 60% of all rape victims were raped by a current or former spouse, boyfriend, or date.

Most cases of date rape are never reported to the police, partly because of the subtlety of the crime. Usually no weapons are involved, and direct verbal threats may not have been made. Rather than being terrorized, the victim usually is attracted to the man at first. Victims of date rape tend to shoulder much of the responsibility for the incident, questioning their own judgment and behavior rather than blaming the aggressor.

Sometimes husbands rape their wives. Strong evidence suggests that 15% of American women who have ever married have been raped by their husbands or ex-husbands; as many as 60% of battered women may have been raped by their husbands. A charge of mate rape can now be taken to court in nearly all states.

FACTORS CONTRIBUTING TO DATE RAPE One factor in date rape appears to be the double standard about appropriate sexual behavior for men and women. Although the general status of women in society has improved, it is still a commonly held cultural belief that nice women don't say yes to sex (even when they want to) and that real men don't take no for an answer.

There are also widespread differences between men and women in how they perceive romantic encounters and signals. In one study, researchers found that men tend to interpret women's actions on dates, such as smiling or talking in a low voice, as indicating an interest in having sex, while the women interpreted the same actions as just being "friendly." Men's thinking about forceful sex also tends to be unclear. One psychologist reports that men find "forcing a woman to have sex against her will" more acceptable than "raping a woman," even though the former description is the definition of rape.

Aside from the double standard and unclear perceptions and thinking about sex, men who rape their dates tend to have certain attributes, including hostility toward women, a belief that dominance alone is a valid motive for sex, and an acceptance of sexual violence. They may feel that force is justified in certain circumstances, such as if they are sexually involved with a woman and she refuses to "go all the way," if the woman is known to have slept with other men, or if the woman shows up at a party where people are drinking and taking drugs. The man often primes himself to force himself sexually on his date by drinking, which lowers his ordinary social inhibitions. Many college men who have committed date rape tried to seduce their dates by plying them with alcohol first.

DATE-RAPE DRUGS   Recently there has been an increase in the reported use of "date-rape drugs" besides alcohol. Drugs used in date-rape situations include flunitrazepam (Rohypnol), gamma hydroxybutyrate (GHB), and ketamine hydrochloride ("Special K"). As described in Chapter 9, these drugs have a variety of effects, including sedation; if slipped surreptitiously into a drink, they can incapacitate a person within about 20 minutes and make her or him more vulnerable to assault. Rohypnol, GHB, and other drugs also often cause anterograde amnesia, meaning victims have little memory of what happens while they are under the influence of the drug. (See Chapter 9 for more on the effects of these and other psychoactive drugs.)

The Drug-Induced Rape Prevention and Punishment Act of 1996 adds up to 20 years to the prison sentence of any rapist who uses a drug to incapacitate a victim. Supporters of the law likened dropping a drug in a victim's drink to putting a knife to her throat. The makers of Rohypnol are modifying the pills so they will be a more noticeable color and will dissolve more slowly, thereby reducing the likelihood that Rohypnol can be used as a date-rape drug; however, other drugs in powdered or liquid form can be slipped into drinks unnoticed. Strategies such as the following can help ensure that your drink is not tampered with at a bar or party:

- Check with campus or local police to find out if drug-facilitated sexual assault has occurred in your area and, if so, where.
- Drink moderately and responsibly. Avoid group drinking and drinking games.
- Be wary of opened beverages—alcoholic or nonalcoholic—offered by strangers. When at an unfamiliar bar, watch the bartender pour your drink.
- Let your date be the first to drink from the punchbowl at a bar, club, or rave.
- If an opened beverage tastes, looks, or smells strange, do not drink it. If you leave your drink unattended, such as when you dance or use the restroom, obtain a fresh drink when you return to your table.
- If you go to a party, club, or bar, go with friends. Have a prearranged plan for checking on each other

visually and verbally. If you feel giddy or lightheaded, get assistance.

Date rape is largely a result of sexual socialization in which the man develops an exaggerated sexual impulse and puts a premium on sexual conquests. Sex and violence are linked in our society, and coercion is accepted by some adolescents as an appropriate form of sexual expression. Both males and females can take actions that will reduce the incidence of acquaintance rape; see the box "Preventing Date Rape" for specific suggestions.

DEALING WITH A SEXUAL ASSAULT   Experts disagree about whether a woman who is faced with a rapist should fight back or give in quietly to avoid being injured or gain time in the hope of escaping. Some rapists say that if a woman had screamed or resisted loudly, they would have run; others report they would have injured or killed her. (If a rapist is carrying a weapon, most experts advise against fighting unless absolutely necessary.) A woman who is raped by a stranger is more likely to be physically injured than a woman raped by someone she knows. Each situation is unique, and a woman should respond in whatever way she thinks best. If a woman chooses not to resist, it does not mean that she has not been raped.

If you are threatened by a rapist and decide to fight back, here is what Women Organized Against Rape (WOAR) recommends:

- Trust your gut feeling. If you feel you are in danger, don't hesitate to run and scream. It is better to feel foolish than to be raped.
- Yell—and keep yelling. It will clear your head and start your adrenaline going; it may scare your attacker and also bring help. Don't forget that a rapist is also afraid of pain and afraid of getting caught.
- If an attacker grabs you from behind, use your elbows for striking the neck, his sides, or his stomach.
- Try kicking. Your legs are the strongest part of your body, and your kick is longer than his reach. Kick with your rear foot and with the toe of your shoe. Aim low to avoid losing your balance.
- His most vulnerable spot is his knee; it's low, difficult to protect, and easily knocked out of place. Don't try to kick a rapist in the crotch; he has been protecting this area all his life and will have better protective reflexes there than at his knees.
- Once you start fighting, keep it up. Your objective is to get away as soon as you can.
- Remember that ordinary rules of behavior don't apply. It's OK to vomit, act "crazy," or claim to have a sexually transmitted disease.

If you are raped, tell what happened to the first friendly person you meet. Call the police, tell them you were raped, and give your location. Try to remember as many facts as you can about your attacker; write down a

Terms   **incest** Sexual activity between close relatives, such as siblings or parents and their children.

Guidelines for Women

- Believe in your right to control what you do. Set limits, and communicate these limits clearly, firmly, and early. Say "no" when you mean "no."

- Be assertive with someone who is sexually pressuring you. Men often interpret passivity as permission.

- If you are unsure of a new acquaintance, go on a group date or double date. If possible, provide your own transportation.

- Remember that some men assume sexy dress and a flirtatious manner mean a desire for sex.

- Remember that alcohol and drugs interfere with clear communication about sex.

- Use the statement that has proven most effective in stopping date rape: "This is rape, and I'm calling the police."

Guidelines for Men

- Be aware of social pressure. It's OK not to "score."

- Understand that "no" means "no." Don't continue making advances when your date resists or tells you she wants to stop. Remember that she has the right to refuse sex.

- Don't assume sexy dress and a flirtatious manner are invitations to sex, that previous permission for sex applies to the current situation, or that your date's relationships with other men constitute sexual permission for you.

- Remember that alcohol and drugs interfere with clear communication about sex.

---

description as soon as possible. Don't wash or change your clothes, or you may destroy important evidence. The police will take you to a hospital for a complete exam; show the physician any injuries. Tell the police simply, but exactly, what happened. Be honest, and stick to your story.

If you decide that you don't want to report the rape to the police, be sure to see a physician as soon as possible. You need to be checked for pregnancy and STDs.

THE EFFECTS OF RAPE   Rape victims suffer both physical and psychological injury. For most, physical wounds heal within a few weeks. Psychological pain may endure and be substantial. Even the most physically and mentally strong are likely to experience shock, anxiety, depression, shame, and a host of psychosomatic symptoms after being victimized. These psychological reactions following rape are called rape trauma syndrome, which is characterized by fear, nightmares, fatigue, crying spells, and digestive upset. (Rape trauma syndrome is a form of post-traumatic stress disorder; see Chapter 3.) Self-blame is very likely; society has contributed to this tendency by perpetuating the myths that woman can actually defend themselves and that no one can be raped if she doesn't want to be. Fortunately, these false beliefs are dissolving in the face of evidence to the contrary.

Many organizations offer counseling and support to rape victims. Look in the telephone directory under Rape or Rape Crisis Center for a hotline number to call. Your campus may have counseling services or a support group.

Child Sexual Abuse   Child sexual abuse is a sexual act imposed on a minor. Adults and older adolescents are able to coerce children into sexual activity because of their authority and power over them. Threats, force, or the promise of friendship or material rewards may be used to manipulate a child. Sexual contacts are typically brief and consist of genital manipulation; genital intercourse is much less common.

Sexual abusers are usually male, heterosexual, and known to the victim. The abuser may be a relative, a friend, a neighbor, or another trusted adult acquaintance. Child abusers are often pedophiles, people who are sexually attracted to children. With other adults, they may have poor interpersonal and sexual relationships and feel socially inadequate and inferior.

One highly traumatic form of sexual abuse is **incest,** sexual activity between people too closely related to legally marry. The most common forms of incest are father-daughter (which includes stepfather-stepdaughter) abuse, brother-sister abuse (usually an adolescent boy abusing a preadolescent girl), and uncle-niece abuse; mother-son sexual activity is rare. Adults who commit incest may be pedophiles, but very often they are simply sexual opportunists or people with poor impulse control and emotional problems.

Most sexually abused children are between ages 8 and 12 when the abuse first occurs. More girls are sexually abused than boys. The degree of trauma for the child can be very serious, but it varies with the types of encounters, their frequency, the child's age and relationship to the abuser, and the parents' response. Father-daughter abuse may be the most traumatic form, in part because it is a violation of the basic parent-child relationship and because the abuse tends to be more frequent. Abused children may be depressed or moody, exhibit hyperactivity, play violently with others or with inanimate objects, talk nonsense, or unintentionally injure themselves.

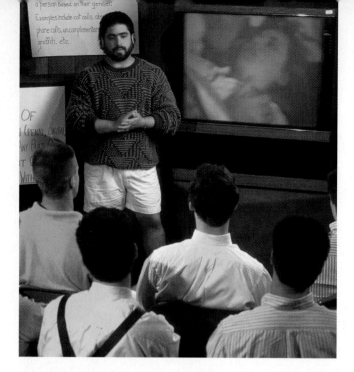

Date rape and sexual harassment are important issues for college students. The goals of this college workshop are to raise men's awareness of the double standard about appropriate sexual behavior for men and women and to examine the differences in how men and women may perceive each other's comments and actions.

Sexual abuse is often unreported. Surveys suggest that as many as 27% of women and 16% of men were sexually abused as children. An estimated 150,000–200,000 new cases of child sexual abuse occur each year. It can leave lasting scars, and adults who were abused as children are more likely to suffer from low self-esteem, depression, anxiety, eating disorders, self-destructive tendencies, sexual problems, and difficulties in intimate relationships.

If you were a victim of sexual abuse as a child and feel it may be interfering with your functioning today, you may want to address the problem. A variety of approaches may help, such as joining a support group of people who have had similar experiences, confiding in a partner or friend, or seeking professional help.

Sexual Harassment Unwelcome sexual advances, requests for sexual favors, and other verbal, visual, or physical conduct of a sexual nature constitute **sexual harassment** if such conduct explicitly or implicitly does any of the following:

- Affects academic or employment decisions or evaluations
- Interferes with an individual's academic or work performance
- Creates an intimidating, hostile, or offensive academic, work, or student living environment

Extreme cases of sexual harassment occur when a manager, professor, or other person in authority uses his or her ability to control or influence jobs or grades to coerce people into having sex or to punish them if they refuse. A hostile environment can be created by such conduct as sexual gestures, displaying of sexually suggestive objects or pictures, derogatory comments and jokes, sexual remarks about clothing or appearance, obscene letters, and unnecessary touching or pinching. Sexual harassment can occur between people of the same or opposite sex. Although sexual harassment is forbidden by law, many cases go unreported. In a survey of 17,000 federal employees, 42% of women and 15% of men reported having been sexually harassed.

If you have been the victim of sexual harassment, you can take action to stop it. Be assertive with anyone who uses language or actions you find inappropriate. If possible, confront your harasser either in writing, over the telephone, or in person, informing him or her that the situation is unacceptable to you and you want the harassment to stop. Be clear: "Do not *ever* make sexual remarks to me" is an unequivocal statement. If assertive communication doesn't work, assemble a file or log documenting the harassment, noting the details of each incident and information about any witnesses who may be able to support your claims. You may discover others who have been harassed by the same person, which will strengthen your case. Then file a grievance with the harasser's supervisor or employer, such as someone in the dean's office if you are a student or someone in the human resources office if you are an employee.

If your attempts to deal with the harassment internally are not successful, you can file an official complaint with your city or state Human Rights Commission or Fair Employment Practices Agency, or with the federal Equal Employment Opportunity Commission. You may also wish to pursue legal action under the Civil Rights Act or under local laws prohibiting employment discrimination. Very often, the threat of a lawsuit or other legal action is enough to stop the harasser.

What You Can Do About Violence

It is obvious that violence in our society is not disappearing and that it is a serious threat to our collective health and well-being. This is especially true on college campuses, which in a sense are communities in themselves but which sometimes lack the authority or guidance to tackle the issue of violence directly (see the box "Staying Safe on Campus"). Although government and law enforcement agencies are working to address the problem of violence, individuals must take on a greater responsibility to bring about change. New programs are being developed at the grass-roots level to deal with problems of violence directly. Schools are now providing training for conflict resolution and are educating people about the diverse

College campuses can be the site of criminal activity and violence just as any other environment or living situation can be—and so they require the same level of caution and awareness that you would use in other situations. Two key points to remember: 80% of campus crimes are committed by a student against a fellow student, and alcohol or drug use is involved in 90% of campus felonies. Drinking or drug use can affect judgment and lower inhibitions, so be aware if you or another person is under the influence. Here are some suggestions for keeping yourself safe on campus:

- Don't travel alone after dark. Many campuses have shuttle buses that run from spots on campus such as the library and the dining hall to residence halls and other locations. Escorts are often available to walk with you at night.

- Be familiar with well-lit and frequently traveled routes around campus if you do need to walk alone.

- If you have a car, follow the usual precautions about parking in well-lit areas, keeping the doors locked while you are driving, and never picking up hitchhikers.

- Always have your keys ready as you approach your residence hall, room, and car. Don't lend your keys to others.

- Let friends and family members know your schedule of classes and activities to create a sort of buddy system.

- Be sure the doors and windows of your dorm room have sturdy locks, and use them.

- Don't prop open doors or hold doors open for nonstudents or nonresidents trying to enter your dorm. Be aware of nonresidents around your dorm. If someone says that he or she is meeting a friend inside, that person should be able to call the friend from outside the building.

- Keep valuables and anything containing personal information—credit cards, wallets, jewelry, and so on—hidden. Secure expensive computer and stereo equipment with cables so that it can't be easily stolen. Use a quality U-shaped lock whenever you leave a bicycle unattended.

- Be alert when using an ATM and don't display large amounts of cash.

- Stay alert and trust your instincts. Don't hesitate to call the police or campus security if something doesn't seem or feel right.

The Jeanne Clery Disclosure of Campus Security Policy and Campus Crime Statistics Act, named for a Lehigh University student who was murdered in her residence hall in 1986, requires colleges and universities to collect and report campus crime statistics. You can now review this information online at the Crime Statistics Web site of the U.S. Department of Education's Office of Postsecondary Education (http://ope.ed.gov/security/Search.asp).

SOURCES: U.S. Department of Education, Office of Postsecondary Education. 2000. *Campus Security* (http://www.ed.gov/offices/OPE/PPI/security.html; retrieved December 16, 2000). Security on Campus, Inc. 2000. *Campus Safety: Tips and Evaluation Brochure* (http://www.soconline.org/information/tips/index.html; retrieved December 16, 2000).

---

nature of our society, thereby encouraging tolerance and understanding.

Looking at the problem of violence from a public health perspective points to the importance of the social environment. As with any public health problem, one potential approach is to identify and target high-risk groups for intervention. Violence prevention programs currently focus on conflict-resolution training and the development of social skills. These measures have proven effective, but for behavior change to be lasting, the focus of such programs must expand beyond individual intervention to include social and environmental factors.

Reducing gun-related injuries may require changes in the availability, possession, and lethality of the 12 million firearms sold in the United States each year. As part of the Brady gun control law, computerized instant background checks are performed for most gun sales to prevent purchases by convicted felons, people with a history of mental instability, and certain other groups. In some states, waiting periods are required in addition to the background checks. Some groups advocate a complete and universal federal ban on the sale of all handguns.

Safety experts also advocate the adoption of consumer safety standards for guns, including features such as childproofing and indicators to show if a gun is loaded. Technologies are now available to personalize handguns to help prevent unauthorized use. Magnetic encoding, touch memory, radio frequency, and fingerprint reading are ways to identify the owner and prevent use by others. Although surveys indicate that the public may be willing to pay the increased costs for personalizing a handgun, firearms manufacturers have been hesitant to redesign their products for safety purposes. Education about proper storage is also important: Surveys indicate that more than 40% of homes with children contain guns; in about 23% of gun-owning households, the weapon is

sexual harassment Unwelcome sexual advances, requests for sexual favors, and other conduct of a sexual nature that affects academic or employment decisions or evaluations; interferes with an individual's academic or work performance, or creates an intimidating, hostile, or offensive academic, work, or student living environment.

Terms

stored loaded, and in 28% the gun is kept hidden but not locked. To be effective, any approach to firearm injury prevention must have the support of law enforcement and the community as a whole.

PROVIDING EMERGENCY CARE

By following the safety guidelines described in this chapter and being aware of the potential risks associated with different activities, you can avoid many injuries on the road, at home, at work, and in public places. However, some injuries will inevitably occur. Therefore, it is also important to prepare for situations when you may need to provide emergency care for yourself or others. If you are prepared to help, you can improve someone else's chances of surviving or of avoiding permanent disability.

A course in **first aid** can help you respond appropriately when someone is injured. One important benefit of first aid training is learning what *not* to do in certain situations. For example, a person with a suspected neck or back injury should not be moved unless other life-threatening conditions exist. A trained person can assess emergency situations accurately before acting. An emergency first aid guide is provided inside the back cover of this book.

Emergency rescue techniques can save the lives of people who are choking, who have stopped breathing, or whose hearts have stopped beating. As described earlier, the Heimlich maneuver is used when a victim is choking. Pulmonary resuscitation (also known as rescue breathing, artificial respiration, or mouth-to-mouth resuscitation) is used when a person is not breathing (see Figure 23-1). **Cardiopulmonary resuscitation (CPR)** is used when a pulse cannot be found. Training is required before a person can perform CPR. Courses are offered by the American Red Cross and the American Heart Association. A new feature of some of these courses is training in the use of automatic external defibrillators (AEDs), which monitor the heart's rhythm and, if appropriate, deliver an electrical shock to restart the heart. Because of the importance of early use of defibrillators in saving heart attack victims, these devices are being installed in public places, including casinos, airports, and certain office buildings.

As a person providing assistance, you are the first link in the **emergency medical services (EMS) system.** Your responsibility may be to render first aid, provide emotional support for the victim, or just call for help. It is important to remain calm and act sensibly. The basic pattern for providing emergency care is check-call-care:

- *Check the situation:* Make sure the scene is safe for both you and the injured person. Don't put yourself in danger; if you get hurt too, you will be of little help to the injured person.

- *Check the victim:* Conduct a quick head-to-toe examination. Assess the victim's signs and symptoms, such as level of responsiveness, pulse, and breathing rate. Look for bleeding and any indications of broken bones or paralysis.

- *Call for help:* Call 9-1-1 or a local emergency number. Identify yourself and give as much information as you can about the condition of the victim and what happened.

- *Care for the victim:* If the situation requires immediate action (no pulse, shock, etc.), provide first aid if you are trained to do so (see Figure 23-1).

Like other kinds of behavior, avoiding and preventing injuries and acting safely involve choices you make every day. If you perceive something to be a serious personal threat, you tend to take action to protect yourself. Ultimately, your goal is healthy, safe behavior. You can motivate yourself to act in the safest way possible by increasing your knowledge and level of awareness, by examining your attitudes to see if they're realistic, by knowing your capacities and limitations, by adjusting your responses when environmental hazards exist, and, in general, by taking responsibility for your actions. You can't eliminate all risks and dangers from your life—no one can do that—but you can improve your chances of avoiding injuries and living to a healthy, ripe old age.

Tips for Today

Although people worry about violence, unintentional injuries—such as those resulting from car crashes, falls, and fires—are much more common. In fact, unintentional injuries are the leading cause of death for people under the age of 35. To protect yourself from injuries, learn to incorporate sensible safety precautions into your daily life.

Right now you can

- Pick up anything on the floor of your home that could cause tripping or slipping.

- Make sure the electrical outlets in your home are not overloaded and that extension cords do not run under rugs or where people walk.

- Test the batteries in the smoke detectors in your home and replace them if they aren't working.

- Check your bike helmet to make sure it fits properly and meets the requirements described in the box "Choosing a Bicycle Helmet." Wear it the next time you go for a ride.

Terms
first aid Emergency care given to an ill or injured person until medical care can be obtained.

cardiopulmonary resuscitation (CPR) An emergency first aid procedure that combines artificial respiration and artificial circulation; used in first aid emergencies where breathing and blood circulation have stopped.

emergency medical services (EMS) system A system designed to network community resources for providing emergency care.

Why do you get injured? What human and environmental factors contribute to injuries? Identifying those factors is one step toward making your lifestyle safer. Changing unsafe behaviors *before* they lead to injuries is an even better way of improving your chances.

For the next 7–10 days, keep track of any mishaps you are involved in or injuries you receive, recording them on a daily behavior record like the one shown in Chapter 1. Count each time you cut, burn, or injure yourself, fall down, run into someone, or have any other potentially injury-causing mishap, no matter how trivial. Also record any risk-taking behaviors, such as failing to wear your safety belt or bicycle helmet, drinking and driving, exceeding the speed limit, putting off home or bicycle repairs, and so on. For each entry (injury or incidence of unsafe behavior), record the date, time, what you were doing, who else was there and how you were influenced by him or her, what your motivations were, and what you were thinking and feeling at the time.

At the end of the monitoring period, examine your data. For each incident, determine both the human factors and the environmental factors that contributed to the injury or unsafe behavior. Were you tired? Distracted? Did you not realize this situation was dangerous? Did you take a chance? Did you think this incident couldn't happen to you? Was visibility poor? Were you using defective equipment? Then consider each contributing factor carefully, determining why it existed and how it could

have been avoided or changed. Finally, consider what preventive actions you could take to avoid such incidents or change your behaviors in the future.

As an example, let's say that you usually don't use a safety belt when you run local errands in your car and that several factors contribute to this behavior: You don't really think you could be involved in a crash so close to home, you only go on short trips, you just never think to use it, and so on. One of the contributing factors to your unsafe behavior is inadequate knowledge. You can change this factor by obtaining accurate information about auto crashes (and their usual proximity to a victim's home) from this chapter and from library or Internet research. Just acquiring information about auto crashes and safety belt use may lead you to examine your beliefs and attitudes about safety belts and motivate you to change your behavior.

Once you're committed, you can use behavior change techniques described in Chapter 1, such as completing a contract, asking family and friends for support, and so on, to build a new habit. Put a note or picture reminding you to buckle up in your car where you can see it clearly. Recruit a friend to run errands with you and to remind you about using your safety belt. Once your habit is established, you may influence other people—especially people who ride in your car—to use safety belts all the time. By changing this behavior, you have reduced the chances that you or your passengers will suffer a serious injury or even die in a vehicle crash.

SUMMARY

- Injuries are caused by a dynamic interaction of human and environmental factors. Risk-taking behavior is associated with a high rate of injury.

- Key factors in motor vehicle injuries include aggressive driving, speeding, a failure to wear safety belts, alcohol and drug intoxication, fatigue, and distraction.

- Motorcycle, moped, and bicycle injuries can be prevented by developing appropriate skills, driving or riding defensively, and wearing proper safety equipment, especially a helmet.

- Most fall-related injuries are a result of falls at floor level, but stairs, chairs, and ladders are also involved in a significant number of falls.

- Careless smoking and problems with cooking or heating equipment are common causes of home fires. Being prepared for fire emergencies means planning escape routes and installing smoke detectors.

- The home can contain many poisonous substances, including medications, cleaning agents, plants, and fumes from cars and appliances.

- Performing the Heimlich maneuver can prevent someone from dying from choking.

- The proper storage and handling of firearms can help prevent injuries; assume that a gun is loaded.

- Many injuries during leisure activities result from the misuse of equipment, lack of experience, use of alcohol, and a failure to wear proper safety equipment.

- Most work-related injuries involve extensive manual labor when lifting. Back problems are most common; newer problems include repetitive strain injuries.

- Factors contributing to violence include poverty, the absence of strong social ties, the influence of the mass media, cultural attitudes about gender roles, problems in interpersonal relationships, abuse of alcohol and other drugs, and the widespread availability of firearms.

- Types of violence include assault, homicide, gang-related violence, hate crimes, school violence, and workplace violence.

- Battering and child abuse occur at every socioeconomic level. The core issue is the abuser's need to control other people.

- Elder abuse is often a result of stress on a caregiver.
- Most rape victims are women, and most know their attackers. Factors in date rape include different standards of appropriate sexual behavior for men and women and different perceptions of actions.
- Child sexual abuse often results in serious trauma; usually the abuser is a trusted adult.
- Sexual harassment is unwelcome sexual advances or other conduct of a sexual nature that affects academic or employment performance or evaluations or

that creates an intimidating, hostile, or offensive academic, work, or student living environment.
- Strategies for reducing violence include conflict-resolution training, social skills development, and education programs that foster tolerance and understanding among diverse groups.
- Steps in giving emergency care include making sure the scene is safe for you and the injured person, conducting a quick examination of the victim, calling for help, and providing emergency first aid.

TAKE ACTION

1. Contact the American Red Cross or American Heart Association in your area, and ask about first aid and CPR classes. These courses are usually given frequently and at a variety of times and locations. They can be invaluable in saving lives. Consider taking one or both of the courses.

2. Find out what resources are available on your campus or in your community for victims of rape, hate crimes, or other types of violence. Does your campus sponsor any violence prevention programs or activities? If so, consider participating in one.

3. Contact your local fire department and obtain a checklist for fire safety procedures. What would you do if a fire started in your home? What types of evacuation procedures would be necessary? Do a practice fire drill at home to see what problems might arise in a real emergency.

4. Look up the nearest Poison Control Center in your telephone book, and post the number near your telephone. Contact the center, and ask them to send you information on poisonings. Read it carefully so you know what to do in case of poisoning.

WW. JOURNAL ENTRY

1. In your health journal, list the positive behaviors that help you avoid injuries and keep you safe. What can you do to reinforce and support these behaviors? Then list the behaviors that keep you from following safety guidelines or that put you at risk for being injured. How can you change one or more of them?

2. *Critical Thinking* Federal, state, and local governments have passed many regulations and laws to enforce a certain level of safety among citizens,

such as laws regulating safety belts, helmets, and firearms. Some people believe that government should not be involved in issues of individual safety and injury prevention; others feel the government has a right to demand certain behaviors for the public good. How do you feel about this issue? Write a brief essay outlining your opinion; be sure to explain your reasoning.

FOR MORE INFORMATION

Books

Henderson, H., ed. 2001. *Domestic Violence and Child Abuse Sourcebook.* Detroit, Mich.: Omnigraphics. *Provides comprehensive, up-to-date information about domestic violence, including community and national sources of assistance.*

James, L., and D. Nahl. 2000. *Road Rage and Aggressive Driving: Steering Clear of Highway Warfare.* Amherst, N.Y.: Prometheus Books. *How to control your temper behind the wheel or understand the rage of a loved one. Also looks at other dangerous driving habits such as cell phone use.*

Kelly, K., and R. C. Duncan. 2000. *Living Safe in an Unsafe World: The Complete Guide to Family Preparedness.* New York: New American Library. *Simple advice on being prepared for emergencies, from fires to safe traveling.*

Kiphuth, D., A. S. Jagoda, and E. Levine. 2000. *The Good Housekeeping Family First Aid Book.* New York: Hearst Books. *Easy and comprehensive guide to first aid.*

Lindquist, S. 2000. *The Date Rape Prevention Book: The Essential Guide for Girls and Women.* Naperville, Ill.: Sourcebooks. *How to avoid problem situations and what to do when confronted with danger.*

WW. Organizations, Hotlines, and Web Sites

American Automobile Association Foundation for Traffic Safety. Provides consumer information about all aspects of traffic safety; Web site has online quizzes and extensive links.
800-305-SAFE
http://www.aaafts.org

American Bar Association: Domestic Violence. Provides information on statistics, research, and laws relating to domestic violence.

http://www.abanet.org/domviol/home.html

American Red Cross Disaster Services. Find out what you can do to prepare for disasters or become involved in disaster services.

http://www.redcross.org/services/disaster

Consumer Product Safety Commission. Provides information and advice about safety issues relating to consumer products.

http://www.cpsc.gov

CyberAngels. Provides information on online safety and help and advice for victims of cyberstalking.

http://www.cyberangels.org

National Center for Injury Prevention and Control. Provides consumer-oriented information about preventing unintentional injuries and violence.

770-488-1506

http://www.cdc.gov/ncipc

http://www.cdc.gov/safeusa

National Center for Victims of Crime. An advocacy group for crime victims; provides statistics, news, safety strategies, tips on finding local assistance, and links to related sites.

800-FYI-CALL

http://www.nvc.org

National Highway Traffic Safety Administration. Supplies materials about reducing deaths, injuries, and economic losses from motor vehicle crashes.

800-424-9393

http://www.nhtsa.dot.gov

National Safety Council. Provides information and statistics about preventing unintentional injuries.

630-285-1121

http://www.nsc.org

National Violence Hotlines. Provide information, referral services, and crisis intervention.

800-799-SAFE (domestic violence); 800-422-4453 (child abuse); 800-656-HOPE (sexual assault)

Prevent Child Abuse America. Provides statistics, information, and publications relating to child abuse, including parenting tips.

312-663-3520

http://www.preventchildabuse.org

Sexual Assault Information Page. Provides information on a wide variety of topics relating to sexual violence.

http://www.cs.utk.edu/~bartley/saInfoPage.html

World Health Organization: Violence and Injury Prevention. Provides statistics and information about the consequences of intentional and unintentional injuries worldwide.

http://www.who.int/violence_injury_prevention

The following sites provide statistics and background information on violence and crime in the United States:

Bureau of Justice Statistics: http://www.ojp.usdoj.gov/bjs

Federal Bureau of Investigation: http://www.fbi.gov

Justice Information Center: http://www.ncjrs.org

SELECTED BIBLIOGRAPHY

Burt, C. W., and M. D. Overpeck. 2001. Emergency visits for sports-related injuries. *Annals of Emergency Medicine* 37(3): 301–308.

Centers for Disease Control and Prevention. 2000. Intimate partner violence among men and women. *Morbidity and Mortality Weekly Report* 49(30): 691–694.

Centers for Disease Control and Prevention. 2000. Prevalence and health consequences of stalking. *Morbidity and Mortality Weekly Report* 49(29): 653–655.

Centers for Disease Control and Prevention. 2001. Surveillance for fatal and nonfatal firearm-related injuries. *CDC Surveillance Summaries* 50(SS2)

Centers for Disease Control and Prevention. 2000. Unpowered scooter-related injuries—United States, 1998–2000. *Morbidity and Mortality Weekly Report* 49(49): 1108–1110.

Coker, A. L., et al. 2000. Frequency and correlates of intimate partner violence by type: Physical, sexual, and psychological battering. *American Journal of Public Health* 90(4): 553–559.

Cole, T. B. 2001. Complementary strategies to prevent firearm injury. *Journal of the American Medical Association* 285(8): 1071–1072.

Federal Bureau of Investigation. 2000. *Crime in the United States. Uniform Crime Reports, 1999.* Washington, D.C.: U.S. Department of Justice.

Krug, E. G., G. K. Sharma, and R. Lozano. 2000. The global burden of injuries. *American Journal of Public Health* 90(4): 253–256.

Li, G., et al. 2001. Use of alcohol as a risk factor for bicycling injury. *Journal of the American Medical Association* 285(7): 893–896.

Marenco, J. P., et al. 2001. Improving survival from sudden cardiac arrest. The role of the automatic external defibrillator. *Journal of the American Medical Association* 285(9): 1193–1200.

National Highway Traffic Safety Administration, Expert Panel on Driver Fatigue and Sleepiness. 2000. *Drowsy Driving and Automobile Crashes* (http://www.nhtsa.dot.gov/people/injury/drowsy_driving1/drowsy.html; retrieved December 16, 2000).

National Safety Council. 2000. *Injury Facts.* Itasca, Ill.: National Safety Council.

National School Safety Center. 2001. *Report on School Associated Violent Deaths* (http://nssc1.org/savd/savd.pdf; retrieved March 11, 2001).

Philip, P., et al. 2001. Fatigue, alcohol, and serious road crashes in France. *British Medical Journal* 322(7290): 829–830.

Rivara, F. P., et al. 2000. Effectiveness of automatic shoulder belt systems in motor vehicle crashes. *Journal of the American Medical Association* 283(21): 2826–2828.

Schuster, M. A., et al. 2000. Firearm storage patterns in U.S. homes with children. *American Journal of Public Health* 90(4): 588–594.

United Nations Children's Fund. 2000. Domestic violence against women and girls. *Innocenti Digest* No. 6.

U.S. Department of Justice. 1999. *1999 Report on Cyberstalking: A New Challenge for Law Enforcement and Industry* (http://www.usdoj.gov:80/criminal/cybercrime/cyberstalking.htm; retrieved December 27, 2000).

Violence in the media. 2000. *Journal of the American Medical Association* 283(20): 2748.

Weiler, J. M., et al. 2000. Effects of fexofenadine, diphenhydramine, and alcohol on driving performance. A randomized, placebo-controlled trial in the Iowa driving simulator. *Annals of Internal Medicine* 132(5): 354–363.

Williamson, A. M., and A. M. Feyer. 2000. Moderate sleep deprivation produces impairments in cognitive and motor performance equivalent to legally prescribed levels of alcohol intoxication. *Occupational and Environmental Medicine* 57(10): 649–655.

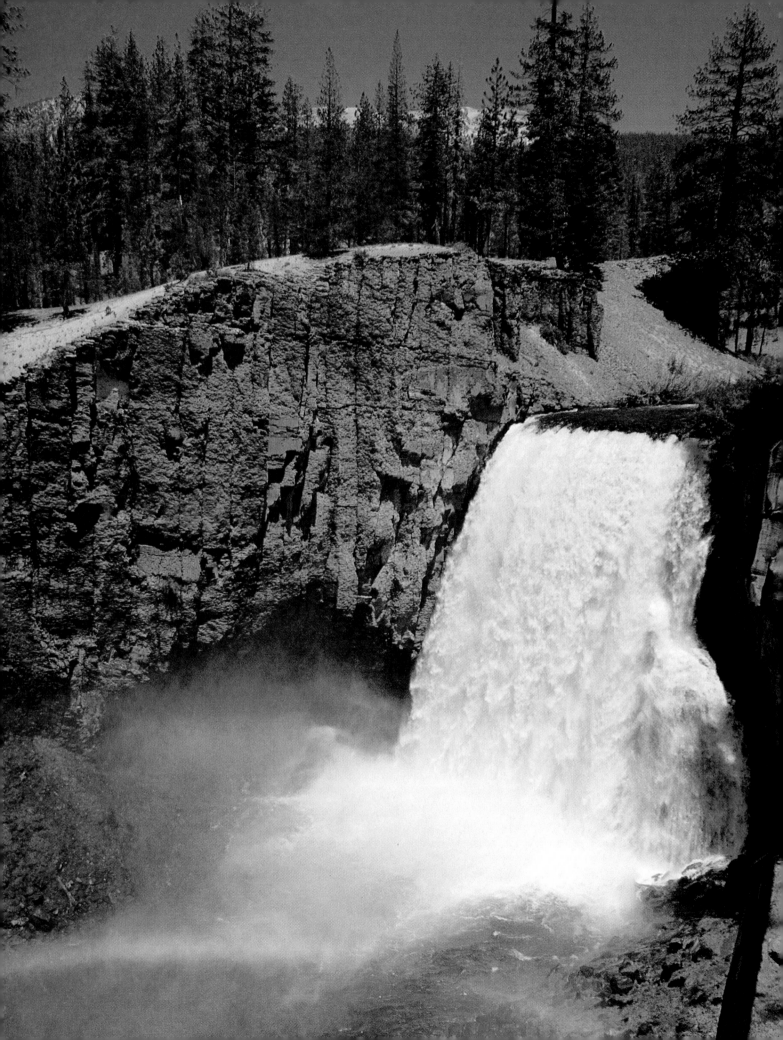

After reading this chapter, you should be able to

- Describe the methods used to deal with the classic environmental concerns of clean water and waste disposal

- Discuss the effects of rapid increases in human population and list factors that may limit or slow world population growth

- Describe the short- and long-term effects of air, chemical, and noise pollution and exposure to radiation

- Outline strategies that individuals, communities, and nations can take to preserve and restore the environment

Environmental Health

24

TEST YOUR KNOWLEDGE

1. The world's population, currently at about 6.1 billion, is increasing by about _____ people every minute?
   a. 50
   b. 100
   c. 150

2. Where ozone gas occurs naturally in the upper atmosphere, it benefits human health by protecting earth from harmful UV radiation; when created from pollutants released at ground level, ozone gas harms human health by negatively affecting respiratory function.
   True or false?

3. Which of the following statements about sport utility vehicles is true?
   a. They currently account for about half of all new vehicles sold.
   b. They get relatively poor gas mileage.
   c. They currently have weaker pollution standards than regular cars and so pollute more.

4. Most oil pollution comes from large spills that occur when tankers run aground or ships clean out their holds at sea.
   True or false?

5. Most of the energy used by a standard incandescent light bulb is converted into light.
   True or false?

W e are constantly reminded of our intimate relationship with all that surrounds us—our environment. Although the planet supplies us with food, water, air, and everything else that sustains life, it also presents us with natural occurrences—earthquakes, hurricanes, drought, climate changes—that destroy life and disrupt society. In the past, humans have frequently had to struggle against the environment to survive. Today, in addition to dealing with natural disasters, we also have to find ways to protect the environment from the by-products of our way of life.

Environmental health has historically focused on preventing infectious diseases spread by water, waste, food, rodents, and insects. Although these problems still exist, the focus of environmental health has expanded and become more complex, for several reasons. First, we now recognize that environmental pollutants contribute not only to infectious diseases but to many chronic diseases as well. In addition, technological advances have increased our ability to affect and damage the environment. And finally, rapid population growth, which has resulted partly from past environmental improvements, means that far more people are consuming and competing for resources than ever before, magnifying the effect of humans on the environment.

Environmental health is therefore seen as encompassing all the interactions of humans with their environment and the health consequences of these interactions. Fundamental to this definition is a recognition that we hold the world in trust for future generations and for other forms of life. Our responsibility is to pass on to the next generation an environment no worse, and preferably better, than the one we enjoy today (see the box "Nature and the Human Spirit"). Although many environmental problems are complex and seem beyond the control of the individual, there are ways that people can make a difference in the future of the planet.

CLASSIC ENVIRONMENTAL HEALTH CONCERNS

The field of environmental health originally grew out of efforts to control communicable diseases. When certain insects and rodents were found to carry microorganisms that cause disease in humans, campaigns were undertaken to eradicate or control these animal vectors. It was also recognized that pathogens could live and be transmitted in sewage, drinking water, and food. These discoveries led to the development of such practices as systematic garbage collection, sewage treatment, filtration and chlorination of drinking water, food inspection, and the establishment of public health enforcement agencies.

These successful efforts to control and prevent communicable diseases changed the health profile of the developed world (see Chapter 1). Although Americans rarely contract cholera, typhoid fever, plague, diphtheria, or other diseases that once killed entire populations, it doesn't mean these diseases have been eradicated worldwide. For example, there are over 250,000 cases of cholera each year.

In the United States, a huge, complex health system is constantly at work behind the scenes attending to the details of these concerns. Every time this system is disrupted, danger recurs. Every time a flood, a hurricane, an earthquake, a tornado, or some other natural disaster damages a community, these areas again become of prime importance. And every time we venture beyond the boundaries of our everyday world, whether traveling to a less-developed country or camping in a wilderness area, we are reminded of the importance of these basics: clean water, sanitary waste disposal, safe food, and insect and rodent control.

WWW. Clean Water

Few parts of the world have adequate quantities of safe, clean drinking water, and yet few things are as important to human health.

Water Contamination and Treatment Many cities rely at least in part on wells that tap local groundwater, but often it is necessary to find lakes and rivers to supplement wells. Because such surface water is more likely to be contaminated with both organic matter and pathogenic microorganisms, it is purified in water-treatment plants before being piped into the community. At treatment facilities, the water is subjected to various physical and chemical processes, including screening, filtration, and disinfection (often with chlorine), before it is introduced into the water supply system. **Fluoridation,** a water-treatment process that reduces tooth decay by 15–40%, has been used successfully in the United States for more than 50 years.

In most areas of the United States, water systems have adequate, dependable supplies, are able to control waterborne disease, and provide water without unacceptable color, odor, or taste. However, problems do occur. In 1993, more than 400,000 people became ill and 100 died when Milwaukee's drinking water was contaminated with the bacterium *Cryptosporidium*. The Centers for Disease Control and Prevention (CDC) estimate that 1 million Americans become ill and 900–1000 die each year from microbial illnesses from drinking water. Pollution by hazardous chemicals from manufacturing, agriculture, and

In this excerpt from her book *The Sense of Wonder*, noted scientist and author Rachel Carson affirms the nurturing power of the natural world and urges us to appreciate the deep relationship between nature and the human spirit.

> What is the value of preserving and strengthening this sense of awe and wonder, this recognition of something beyond the boundaries of human existence? Is the exploration of the natural world just a pleasant way to pass the golden hours of childhood or is there something deeper?
>
> I am sure there is something much deeper, something lasting and significant. Those who dwell, as scientists or laymen, among the beauties and mysteries of the earth are never alone or weary of life. Whatever the vexations or concerns of their personal lives, their thoughts can find paths that lead to inner contentment and to renewed excitement in living. Those who contemplate the beauty of the earth find reserves of strength that will endure as long as life lasts. There is symbolic as well as actual beauty in the migration of the birds, the ebb and flow of the tides, the folded bud ready for spring. There is something infinitely healing in the repeated refrains of nature—the assurance that dawn comes after night, and spring after the winter.

SOURCE: Carson, R. 1956. *The Sense of Wonder.* New York: Harper & Row. Copyright © 1956 by Rachel Carson. Copyright © renewed 1984 by Roger Christie.

household wastes is another concern. (Chemical pollution is discussed later in the chapter.) The *Healthy People 2010* report sets the goal of increasing from 85% to 95% the proportion of Americans with drinking water that meets standards set by the U.S. Environmental Protection Agency (EPA).

Water Shortages   Water shortages are also a growing concern. Some parts of the United States are experiencing rapid population growth that outstrips the ability of local systems to provide adequate water to all. Many proposals are being discussed to relieve these shortages, including long-distance transfers, conservation, the recycling of some water, such as the water in office-building air conditioners, and the sale of water by regions with large supplies to areas with less available water.

According to the World Health Organization (WHO), only about 35% of the world's people have an adequate water supply. Less than 1% of the world's fresh water—about 0.007% of all the water on earth—is readily accessible for direct human use. Groundwater pumping and the diversion of water from lakes and rivers for irrigation are further reducing the amount of water available to local communities. In some areas, groundwater is being removed at twice the rate at which it is replaced. The Aral Sea, located in Kazakhstan and Uzbekistan, was once one of the world's largest inland seas. Since the 1960s, it has lost two-thirds of its volume to irrigation, and the exposed seabed is now as big as the Netherlands. People living in the area have experienced severe water and food shortages and increased rates of respiratory disease and throat cancer linked to dust storms from the dry seabed. Due to agricultural diversions, the Yellow River ran dry for the first time in China's 3000-year history in 1972, failing to reach the sea for 15 days that year; by 1998, this period had grown to 226 days. In the United States, the Colorado River is now diverted to the extent that it no longer flows into the ocean.

What You Can Do to Protect the Water Supply

- Take showers, not baths, to minimize your water consumption. Don't let water run when you're not actively using it while brushing your teeth, shaving, or hand-washing clothes. Don't run a dishwasher or washing machine until you have a full load.

- Install sink faucet aerators and water-efficient shower heads, which use two to five times less water with no noticeable decrease in performance.

- Purchase a water-saver toilet, or put a displacement device in your toilet tank to reduce the amount of water used with each flush.

- Fix any leaky faucets in your house. Leaks can waste thousands of gallons of water per year.

- Use organic rather than chemical fertilizers, and don't overfertilize your lawn or garden; the extra could end up in the groundwater.

- Don't pour toxic materials such as cleaning solvents, bleach, or motor oil down the drain. Store them until you can take them to a hazardous waste collection center.

- Replant your lawn and garden with plants requiring less water. Avoid watering your lawn during the hottest part of the day in order to minimize evaporation.

Waste Disposal

Humans generate large amounts of waste, which must be handled in an appropriate manner if the environment is to be safe and sanitary.

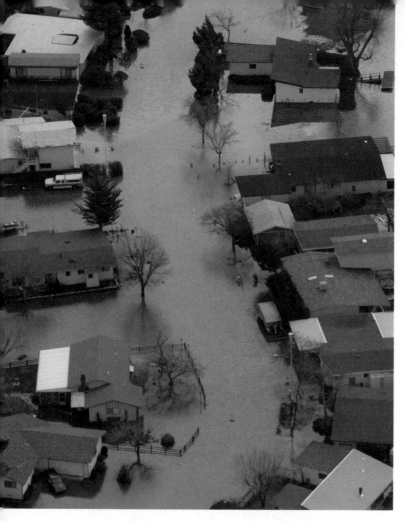

We often take for granted the well-organized system responsible for environmental health in our society, but natural disasters remind us of its fragility. In addition to forcing people from their homes, flooding can cause widespread disruption in essential services such as the delivery of electricity, gas, and clean drinking water, which increases the probability of disease transmission.

Sewage   Prior to the mid-nineteenth century, many people contracted diseases such as typhoid, cholera, and hepatitis A by direct contact with human feces, which were simply disposed of at random. Once the links between sewage and disease were discovered, practices began to change. People learned how to build sanitary outhouses and how to locate them so they would not contaminate water sources. As plumbing moved indoors, sewage disposal became more complicated. In rural areas, the **septic system,** a self-contained sewage disposal system, worked quite well; today, many rural homes still rely on septic systems.

Different approaches became necessary as urban areas developed. Most cities have sewage-treatment systems that separate fecal matter from water in huge tanks and ponds and stabilize it so that it cannot transmit infectious diseases. Once treated and biologically safe, the water is released back into the environment. The sludge that remains behind may be spread on fields as fertilizer if it is free from **heavy metal** contamination, or it may be burned or buried. If incorporated into the food chain, heavy metals, such as lead, cadmium, copper, and tin, can cause illness or death; therefore, these chemicals must be prevented from being released into the environment when sludge is burned or buried.

In addition to regulating industrial discharge, many cities have now begun expanded sewage-treatment measures to remove heavy metals and other hazardous chemicals. This action has resulted from many studies linking exposure to such chemicals as mercury, lead, and **polychlorinated biphenyls (PCBs)** with long-term health consequences, including cancer and damage to the central nervous system. The technology to effectively remove heavy metals and chemicals from sewage is still developing, and the costs involved are immense.

Solid Waste   The bulk of the organic food garbage produced in American kitchens is now dumped in the sewage system by way of the mechanical garbage disposal. The garbage that remains is not very hazardous from the standpoint of infectious disease because there is very little food waste in it, but it does represent an enormous disposal and contamination problem.

WHAT'S IN OUR GARBAGE?   The biggest single component of household trash (38.2% by weight) is paper products, including junk mail, glossy mail-order catalogs, and computer printouts. Yard waste is the next biggest source by weight (12.6% before recycling). Plastics make up 10.2% of all trash by weight but take up about 18% of landfill space. Most of this plastic waste is in the form of packaging, which accounts for about one-third of the 6 million tons of plastics produced each year in the United States. Other significant sources of trash include metals (7.6% by weight), glass (5.7%), and wood (5.4%). About 1% of the solid waste is toxic; a new source of toxic waste is the disposal of computer components in both household and commercial waste. Burning, as opposed to burial, reduces the bulk of solid waste, but it may release hazardous material into the air.

Solid waste is not limited to household products. Manufacturing, mining, and other industries all produce large amounts of potentially dangerous materials that cannot

Terms

septic system A self-contained sewage disposal system, often used in rural areas, in which waste material is decomposed by bacteria.

heavy metal A metal with a high specific gravity, such as lead, copper, or tin.

polychlorinated biphenyl (PCB) An industrial chemical used as an insulator in electrical transformers and linked to certain human cancers.

sanitary landfill A disposal site where solid wastes are buried.

simply be dumped. The experiences of communities like Love Canal near Buffalo, New York, and Times Beach, Missouri, clearly demonstrated the dangers of the careless disposal of toxic wastes. At Love Canal, toxic industrial wastes had been dumped into a waterway for years until, in the 1970s, nearby residents began to suffer from associated birth defects and cancers. Human health was affected, the government had to step in, people had to move from homes, and huge costs were incurred.

DISPOSING OF SOLID WASTE   Since the 1960s, much solid waste has been buried in **sanitary landfill** disposal sites. Careful site selection and daily management are an essential part of this approach to disposal. First, the site is thoroughly studied to ensure that it is not near groundwater, streams, or any other source of water that could be contaminated by leakage from the landfill. Sometimes protective liners are used around the site, and nearby monitoring wells are now required in most states. Layers of solid waste are regularly covered with thin layers of dirt until the site is filled. Some communities then plant grass and trees and convert the site into a park. Landfill is relatively stable; almost no decomposition occurs in the solidly packed waste.

Burying solid waste in sanitary landfills has several disadvantages. Much of this waste contains chemicals, ranging from leftover pesticides to nail polish remover to paints and oils, which should not be released indiscriminately into the environment. Despite precautions, buried contaminants do leak into the surrounding soil and groundwater. Burial is also expensive and requires huge amounts of space.

Industrial toxic waste poses an even greater disposal problem. In 1980, Congress enacted the Superfund program to clean up inactive hazardous waste sites that are a threat to human health and the environment. Because many such sites are in areas with high population density, 60 million Americans live within 4 miles of a priority Superfund site. By 2000, cleanup was complete at 50% of priority sites, but further action was still needed at about 750 priority sites and nearly 10,000 other sites.

Because of the expense and potential chemical hazards of any form of solid waste disposal, many communities today encourage individuals and businesses to recycle their trash. Some cities offer curbside pickup of recyclables; others have recycling centers to which people can bring their waste. These materials are not limited to paper, glass, and cans but also include such things as discarded tires and used oils. Recycling programs have been successful in reducing the proportion of solid waste sent to landfills: in 1980, 81% went to landfills; in 2000, about 55%. (Currently, about 28% of solid waste is recycled and 17% is burned.) However, the total amount of garbage Americans generate will probably continue to rise as the population increases, and researchers estimate that 80% of the nation's landfills will be closed within 20 years.

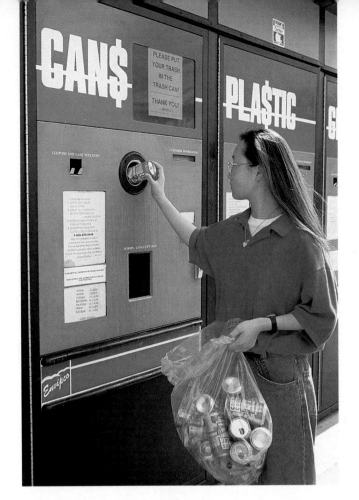

Recycling paper, cans, bottles, and plastics conserves resources, saves energy, and keeps large amounts of solid wastes out of landfills. Some communities have curbside pickup recycling, while others have drop-off sites. Manufacturers and researchers are looking at new ways to use recycled materials.

What You Can Do to Reduce Garbage

- Buy products with the least amount of packaging you can, or buy products in bulk (see the box "How to Be a Green Consumer"). For example, buy large jars of juice, not individually packaged juice drinks. Buy products packaged in glass, paper, or metal containers; avoid plastic and aluminum (unless it's recycled). Reuse glass containers to store products bought in bulk or other household items.

- Buy recycled or recyclable products. Avoid disposables; instead, use long-lasting or reusable products such as refillable pens and rechargeable batteries.

- Avoid using foam or paper cups and plastic stirrers by bringing your own china coffee mug and metal spoon to work or wherever you drink coffee or tea. Pack your lunch in reusable containers, and use a cloth or plastic lunch sack or a lunch box.

- To store food, use glass jars and reusable plastic containers rather than foil and plastic wrap.

It may seem like a hassle to consider the environmental impact of the things you buy, but a few simple choices can make a big difference without compromising your lifestyle. You can quickly and easily develop habits that direct your consumer dollar toward environmentally friendly products and companies.

- Remember the three Rs of green consumerism:
  Reduce the amount of trash and pollution you generate by consuming and throwing away less.
  Reuse as many products as possible—either yourself or by selling them or donating them to charity.
  Recycle all appropriate materials and buy recycled products whenever possible.

- Choose products packaged in refillable, recycled, reusable containers or in readily recyclable materials, such as paper, cardboard, aluminum, or glass. Don't buy products that are excessively packaged or wrapped; for specific guidelines, see the section "What You Can Do to Reduce Garbage."

- Look for products made with the highest possible content of recycled paper, metal, glass, plastic, and other materials.

- Choose simple products containing the lowest amounts of bleaches, dyes, and fragrances. Look for organically grown foods and clothes made from organically grown cotton or Fox Fibre or another naturally colored type of cotton.

- Buy high-quality appliances that have an Energy Star seal from the EPA or some other type of certification indicating that they are energy- and water-efficient.

- Get a reusable cloth shopping bag. Don't bag items that don't need to be bagged. If you forget to bring your bag to the store, it doesn't matter much if you use a paper or plastic bag to carry your purchases home. What's important is that you reuse whatever bag you get.

- Don't buy what you don't need—borrow, rent, or share. Take good care of the things you own, repair items when they break, and replace them with used rather than new items, whenever possible. Sell or donate used items rather than throwing them out.

- Walk or bike to the store. If you must drive, do several errands at once to save energy and cut down on pollution.

- Look beyond the products to the companies that make them. Support those with good environmental records. If some of your favorite products are overpackaged or contain harmful ingredients, write to the manufacturer.

- Keep in mind that doing something is better than doing nothing. Even if you can't be a perfectly green consumer, doing your best on any purchase *will* make a difference.

SOURCES: U.S. Environmental Protection Agency. 2000. *Reduce, Reuse, and Recycle* (http://www.epa.gov/epaoswer/non-hw/muncpl/reduce.htm; retrieved January 11, 2001). Makower, J., J. Elkington, and J. Hailes. 1993. *The Green Consumer.* New York: Penguin Books. Madigan, C. O., and A. Elwood. 1995. *Life's Big Instruction Book.* New York: Warner Books.

- Recycle your newspapers, glass, cans, paper, and other recyclables. If your sanitation department doesn't pick up recyclables, take them to a local recycling center. If you receive something packaged with foam pellets, take them to a commercial mailing center that accepts them for recycling.

- Start a compost pile for your organic garbage (non-animal food and yard waste) if you have a yard. If you live in an apartment, you can create a small composting system using earthworms, or take your organic wastes to a community composting center.

- Stop junk mail. To cancel your junk mail, send a request to Mail Preference Service, Direct Marketing Association, P.O. Box 9008, Farmingdale, NY 11735.

COMMUNICATE!   When it comes to protecting the environment, we have opportunities every day to influence our friends, colleagues, and neighbors. You can use the information and ideas in this chapter not only to make changes in your own behavior but also to help others do the same. For example, you might say, "Even though our curbside recycling program takes only newspapers and cans, I found out that the county recycling center takes all kinds of other things—cardboard, paper, plastic, magazines. I've been going every month or so. Do you want to join me next month?"

Food Inspection

Diseases and death associated with foodborne illnesses and toxic food additives have decreased substantially ever since the passage of the Pure Food and Drug Act of 1906. Many agencies inspect food at various points in production. On the federal level, the U.S. Department of Agriculture (USDA) inspects grains and meats, and the U.S. Food and Drug Administration (FDA) is responsible for ensuring the wholesomeness of foods and regulating the chemicals that can be used in foods, drugs, and cosmetics. On the state level, public health departments inspect dairy herds, milking barns, storage tanks, tankers that transport milk, and processing plants. Local health departments inspect and license restaurants.

Overall, the food distribution system in the United States is safe and efficient, but cases of foodborne illness do occur. It is estimated that every American suffers an average of two or three episodes of foodborne illness

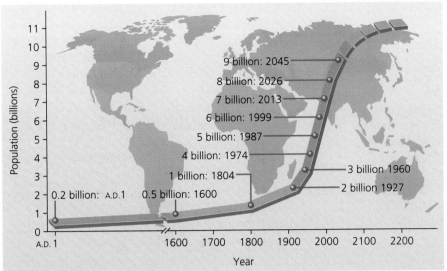

W_W VITAL STATISTICS

Figure 24-1 World population growth.
The United Nations estimates that the world's population will continue to increase dramatically until it stabilizes at about 11 billion people in 2200. SOURCE: United Nations Population Division. 2001. *World Population Prospects: The 2000 Revision.* New York: United Nations.

every year. Recent outbreaks of serious illness have been traced to contaminated and undercooked fast-food hamburgers, unpasteurized juice, and imported produce. Many cases of foodborne illness can be prevented through the proper storage and preparation of food. (For guidelines on avoiding foodborne illness, see Chapter 12.)

Insect and Rodent Control

A great number of illnesses can be transmitted to humans by animal and insect vectors. In recent years, we have seen outbreaks of encephalitis transmitted by mosquitoes; Lyme disease from ticks in the Northeast, Midwest, and West; Rocky Mountain spotted fever from another type of tick in the Southeast; bubonic plague from fleas on wild mammals in the West; and West Nile virus transmitted by mosquitoes. Rodents carry forms of hantavirus, tapeworms, and *Salmonella*.

Disability and death from these diseases can be prevented by spraying insecticides when necessary, wearing protective clothing, and exercising reasonable caution in infested areas. Individuals should be concerned about possible exposure to rodent-borne illnesses if they see rodents or rodent droppings in the home. In public facilities, such sightings should be reported to the local or state health department. Children should be warned to never play with sick animals. Travelers should be careful about mosquito bites, especially in developing countries and where disease warnings have been posted. For tips on avoiding tickborne illnesses, see Chapter 17.

POPULATION GROWTH

Throughout most of history, humans have been a minor pressure on the planet. About 200 million people were alive in the year A.D. 1; by the time Europeans were settling in the United States 1600 years later, the world population had increased gradually to 500 million. But then it began rising exponentially—zooming to 1 billion by about 1830, more than doubling by 1950, and then doubling again in just 40 years (Figure 24-1).

The world's population, currently about 6.1 billion, is increasing at a rate of about 78 million per year—150 people every minute. The United Nations projects that world population will exceed 9 billion by 2050 and will continue to increase until it levels off at about 11 billion in 2200. Nearly all of this increase takes place in less-developed regions; each year, the population of Asia increases by 50 million, that of Africa by 17 million, and that of Latin America by nearly 8 million. In 1950, the more developed regions accounted for 32% of the world's population; their share dropped to 20% in 2000 and is expected to further decline to 13% in 2050. Changes are also projected for the world's age distribution: The proportion of people age 60 and over will increase from 10% in 2000 to about 21% in 2050, and by 2050, there will be more older persons than children.

This rapid expansion of population, particularly in the past 50 years, is generally believed to be responsible for most of the stress humans put on the environment. A large and rapidly growing population makes it more difficult to provide the basic components of environmental health discussed earlier, including clean and disease-free food and water. It is also a driving force behind many of the newer environmental health concerns, including chemical pollution, global warming, and the thinning of the atmosphere's ozone layer.

How Many People Can the World Hold?

No one knows how many people the world can support, but most scientists agree that there is a limit. The primary factors that may eventually put a cap on human population are the following:

- *Food.* Enough food is currently produced to feed the world's entire population, but economic and sociopolitical factors have led to food shortages and famine. Food production can be expanded in the future, but better distribution of food will be needed to prevent even more widespread famine, as the world's population continues to grow. For all people to receive adequate nutrition, the makeup of the world's diet may also need to change. Because animal products require more resources to produce, the world could support nearly twice as many vegetarians as people eating a typical American diet, which is based heavily on animal products.

- *Available land and water.* Rural populations rely on trees, soil, and water for their direct sustenance, and a growing population puts a strain on these resources—forests are cut for wood, soil is depleted, and water is withdrawn at ever-rising rates. These trends contribute to local hardships and to many global environmental problems, including habitat destruction and species extinction (see the box "Natural Ecosystems and Biodiversity").

- *Energy.* Currently, most of the world's energy comes from nonrenewable sources: oil, coal, natural gas, and nuclear power. As nonrenewable sources are depleted, the world will have to shift to renewable energy sources, such as hydropower, solar, geothermal, wind, biomass, and ocean power. Supporting a growing population, maintaining economic productivity, and preventing further environmental degradation will require greater energy efficiency and an increased use of renewable energy sources.

- *Minimum acceptable standard of living.* The mass media have exposed the entire world to the American lifestyle and raised people's expectations of living at a comparable level. But such a lifestyle is supported by levels of energy consumption that the earth cannot support worldwide. The United States has 5% of the world's population but uses 25% of the world's energy. By contrast, India has 16% of the population but uses only 3% of the energy. An average American consumes 280 times the amount of energy that the average Ethiopian does. If *all* people are to enjoy a minimally acceptable standard of living, the population must be limited to a number that the available resources can support.

Factors That Contribute to Population Growth

Although it is apparent that population growth must be controlled, population trends are difficult to influence and manage. A variety of interconnecting factors fuel the current population explosion:

- *High fertility rates.* The combination of poverty, very high child mortality rates, and a lack of social provisions of every type is associated with high fertility rates in the developing world. Perhaps families have to have more children to ensure that enough survive childhood to work for the household and to care for parents in old age.

- *Lack of family planning resources.* Half the world's couples don't use any form of family planning, and 300 million couples worldwide say they want family planning services but cannot get them.

- *Lower death rates.* Although death rates remain relatively high in the developing world, they have decreased in recent years because of public health measures and improved medical care.

Changes in any of these factors can affect population growth, but the issues are complex. Increasing death rates through disease, famine, or war might slow population growth, but few people would argue in favor of these as methods of population control. Although the increased availability of family planning services is a crucial part of population management, cultural, political, and religious factors also need to be considered.

To be successful, population management must change the condition of people's lives, especially poverty, to remove the pressures for having large families. Research indicates that the combination of improved health, better education, and increased literacy and employment opportunities for women works together with family planning to decrease fertility rates. Unfortunately, in the fastest-growing countries, the needs of a rapidly increasing population use up financial resources that might otherwise be used to improve lives and ultimately slow population growth.

WWW. POLLUTION

As mentioned earlier, the classic environmental health concerns are not just historical. They still have the potential to cause serious problems today under certain circumstances, and they take on added significance as our population grows. At the same time, new problems are arising, and some long-standing problems are gaining increased public attention. Many of these modern problems are problems of pollution. The term *pollution* refers to any unwanted contaminant in the environment that may pose a health risk.

WWW. Air Pollution

Air pollution is not a human invention or even a new problem. The air is "polluted" naturally with every forest fire, pollen bloom, and dust storm, as well as with

Our world supports an abundant variety of life. Scientists have identified some 1.75 million species, but they suspect that there are probably 10–80 million more. Different environments generate diverse life strategies, so that each **ecosystem**—from desert to tropical rainforest—contains a unique, close-knit community of organisms, linked together in a **food chain** or web. Plants use sunlight and soil for their needs. In turn, they sustain herbivores (plant eaters), which may themselves succumb to predators. When predators and surviving herbivores die, they become food for scavengers, then insect larvae, and finally bacteria, which break them down into organic substances. These, drawn from the soil by plants, help maintain the cycle. A similar system, based on plankton, exists in the oceans. Disruption at any point in this intricate, balanced cycle can alter or destroy an entire ecosystem.

Natural ecosystems provide humans with a wide variety of essential services. They maintain the climate and the composition of the atmosphere, cycle water and nutrients, produce food, dispose of organic wastes, generate and maintain soils, control pests, and pollinate crops; in addition, ecosystems support biological diversity, or **biodiversity,** represented by both the millions of different species on the earth and the genetic diversity within these species.

Biodiversity is critical, as the basis for the future evolution of new species and as a genetic bank from which humans can draw useful genetic material and compounds. Although thus far we have examined few of these resources, the ones we have used provide many benefits, including medicines and pest and disease resistance for crops. For example, many children with leukemia can now be saved by drugs developed from the rosy periwinkle plant, and species of wild rice in India and wild tomato in Peru have provided domestic species with the disease resistance they need to be productive.

Human activity—driven by poverty and population growth in the developing world and excessive consumerism in the industrial nations—threatens biodiversity. Some species and populations are being lost through direct action, such as the overharvesting of whales, elephants, and certain fish; the overexploitation of musk deer, turtles, black bears, and certain plants has been linked to a growing worldwide demand for traditional Chinese medicines. But the major danger comes indirectly, from habitat destruction: We are paving over, chopping down, digging up, draining, and poisoning many areas. The destruction of tropical rainforests, which are disappearing at the rate of an acre every second, is of particular concern. Rainforests cover only about 7% of the planet but are thought to harbor more than half the world's species.

Extinction is irreversible, and species are disappearing far faster (50–100 a day) than they can be identified and assessed for useful properties. The current extinction rate is nearly 1000 times higher than the rate over the past 65 million years. Some scientists fear that humans are precipitating a wave of mass extinction so great that the diminished stock of species will not be an adequate base on which natural selection can work to rebuild biodiversity. Even if adequate, it could take more than 10 million years for biodiversity to "bounce back." And because of the many ties between organisms and the physical environment, mass extinction could also threaten the functioning of the entire biological world.

What can be done to maintain biodiversity? The United States has laws that protect specific endangered species, which by indirectly preserving natural communities help maintain biodiversity. International laws and conventions also protect certain rare species, although enforcement continues to be a problem. The Convention on Biological Diversity, signed by more than 175 countries (but *not* the United States) since the 1992 Earth Summit in Rio de Janeiro, deals specifically with the issue of biodiversity. It commits countries to preserving and managing biological resources and to integrating plant and animal preservation into economic planning. It also allows countries that are rich in species but poor in cash to share in the profits from the sale of medicines or other products derived from their biological resources. Although much still needs to be done to protect the biodiversity of our world, these actions are a step in the right direction.

---

countless other natural pollutants. To these natural sources, humans have always contributed the by-products of their activities. During the Industrial Revolution, English cities had far more daily air pollution than we can observe or even imagine today. However, we now live long enough to experience both the short-term and the long-term consequences of air pollution. Also, increased population growth, combined with more industrialization using old technologies, concentrates the problems and makes them more visible to the public—and possibly more dangerous.

Air Quality and Smog   Air pollution can cause illness and death if pollutant levels are high; young children,

older adults, and people with chronic health conditions are particularly at risk. The EPA uses a measure called the

Terms

ecosystem The community of organisms (plants and animals) in an area, and the nonliving physical factors with which they interact.

food chain The transfers of food energy and other substances in which one type of organism consumes another.

biodiversity The variety of living things on the earth, including all the different species of flora and fauna and the genetic diversity among individuals of the same species.

Air Quality Index (AQI) to indicate whether air pollution levels pose a health concern. The AQI is used for five major air pollutants:

• Carbon monoxide (CO): An odorless, colorless gas, CO forms when the carbon in **fossil fuels** does not completely burn. The primary sources of CO are vehicle exhaust and fuel combustion in industrial processes. CO deprives body cells of oxygen, causing headaches, fatigue, and impaired vision and judgment; it also aggravates cardiovascular diseases.

• Sulfur dioxide (SO_2): SO_2 is produced by the burning of sulfur-containing fuels such as coal and oil, during metal smelting, and by other industrial processes; power plants are a major source. SO_2 narrows the airways, which may cause wheezing, chest tightness, and shortness of breath, particularly in people with asthma; it may also aggravate symptoms of CVD.

• Nitrogen dioxide (NO_2): NO_2 is a reddish-brown, highly reactive gas formed when nitric oxide combines with oxygen in the atmosphere; major sources include motor vehicles and power plants. In people with respiratory diseases such as asthma, NO_2 affects lung function and causes symptoms such as wheezing and shortness of breath; NO_2 exposure may also increase the risk of respiratory infections.

• Particulate matter (PM): Particles of different sizes are released into the atmosphere from a variety of sources, including combustion of fossil fuels, crushing or grinding operations, industrial processes, and dust from roadways. PM can accumulate in the respiratory system and aggravate cardiovascular and lung diseases and increase the risk of respiratory infections. PM exposure is associated with increased rates of hospital admissions, physician visits, and premature death.

• Ground-level ozone: At ground level, ozone is a harmful pollutant; where it occurs naturally in the upper atmosphere, it shields the earth from the sun's harmful ultraviolet rays. (The health impact of the thinning of this protective ozone layer is discussed later in the chapter.) Ground-level ozone is formed when pollutants emitted by cars, power plants, industrial boilers, refineries, chemical plants, and other sources react chemically in the presence of sunlight (photochemical reactions). Ozone can irritate the respiratory system, reduce lung function, aggravate asthma, increase susceptibility to respiratory infections, and inflame and damage the lining of the lungs.

AQI values run from 0 to 500; the higher the AQI, the greater the level of pollution and associated health danger. When the AQI exceeds 100, air quality is considered unhealthy, at first for certain sensitive groups of people and then for everyone as AQI values get higher. For local areas, AQI values are calculated for each of the five pollutants listed above; the highest value becomes the AQI rating for that day. Depending on the AQI value, precautionary health advice may be provided; for example, see the AQI chart for ozone shown in Figure 24-2. Information on the AQI in your area is often available in newspapers, on television and radio, on the Internet, and from state and local telephone hotlines.

The term **smog** was first used in the early 1900s in London to describe the combination of smoke and fog. What we typically call smog today is a mixture of pollutants, with ground-level ozone being the key ingredient. Major smog occurrences are linked to the combination of several factors. Heavy motor vehicle traffic, high temperatures, and sunny weather can increase the production of ozone. Pollutants are also more likely to build up in areas with little wind and/or where a topographic feature such as a mountain range or valley prevents the wind from pushing out stagnant air.

A weather event called a **temperature inversion** also contributes to smog buildup. A temperature inversion occurs when there is little or no wind and a layer of warm air traps a layer of cold air next to the ground. Normally, the sun heats the earth, making the air closest to the ground warmer than that just above it. Warm air rises and is replaced by cooler air, which in turn is warmed and rises, thereby producing a natural circulation. This circulation, combined with horizontal wind circulation, prevents pollutants from reaching dangerous levels of concentration.

Terms

Air Quality Index (AQI) A measure of local air quality and what it means for health. Concentrations of five major pollutants are measured and assigned index values between 0 and 500, with values above 100 considered unhealthy; the highest of the five values becomes the overall AQI for the day. Health warnings and recommendations may be issued when AQI values exceed 100.

fossil fuels Buried deposits of decayed animals and plants that are converted into carbon-rich fuels by exposure to heat and pressure over millions of years; oil, coal, and natural gas are fossil fuels.

smog Hazy atmospheric conditions resulting from increased concentrations of ground-level ozone and other pollutants. Smog most commonly occurs when oxides of nitrogen and hydrocarbons, primarily from motor vehicle exhaust, react in the presence of sunlight; also known as *photochemical smog*. (The term was first used to describe the combination of smoke and fog in early-twentieth-century London.)

temperature inversion A weather condition in which a cold layer of air is trapped by a warm layer so that pollutants cannot be dispersed.

greenhouse effect A warming of the earth due to a buildup of carbon dioxide and certain other gases.

global warming An increase in the earth's atmospheric temperature when averaged across seasons and geographical regions.

Index Values	Levels of Health Concern	Cautionary Statements
0–50	Good	None
51–100*	Moderate	Unusually sensitive people should consider limiting prolonged outdoor exertion.
101–150	Unhealthy for sensitive groups	Active children and adults, and people with respiratory disease, such as asthma, should limit prolonged outdoor exertion.
151–200	Unhealthy	Active children and adults, and people with respiratory disease, such as asthma, should avoid prolonged outdoor exertion; everyone else, especially children, should limit prolonged outdoor exertion.
201–300	Very unhealthy	Active children and adults, and people with respiratory disease, such as asthma, should avoid all outdoor exertion; everyone else, especially children, should limit outdoor exertion.
301–500	Hazardous	Everyone should avoid all outdoor exertion.

*Generally, an AQI of 100 for ozone corresponds to an ozone level of 0.08 parts per million (averaged over 8 hours).

Figure 24-2   Air Quality Index (AQI) for ozone.   SOURCE: U.S. Environmental Protection Agency. 2000. *Air Quality Index: A Guide to Air Quality and Your Health.* Pub. no. EPA-454/R-00-005.

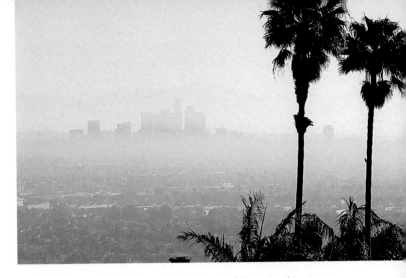

Smog tends to form over Los Angeles because of the natural geographical features of the area and because of the tremendous amount of motor vehicle exhaust in the air. The health effects of smog are most noticeable in people who already have some respiratory impairment.

When there is a temperature inversion, this replacement and cleansing action cannot occur. The effect is like covering an area with a dome that traps all the pollutants and prevents vertical dispersion. If this condition persists for several days, the buildup of pollutants may reach dangerous levels and threaten people's health. Many cities have plans for shutting down certain industries and even curtailing transportation if unsafe levels are approached. States and federal governments have "clean air" legislation that has helped improve U.S. air quality in the past 20 years. However, it is estimated that 60–130 million people in the United States still live in areas with unhealthy air.

The Greenhouse Effect and Global Warming   The temperature of the earth's atmosphere depends on the balance between the amount of energy the planet absorbs from the sun (mainly as high-energy ultraviolet radiation) and the amount of energy radiated back into space as lower-energy infrared radiation. Key components of temperature regulation are carbon dioxide, water vapor, methane, and other "greenhouse gases"—so named because, like a pane of glass in a greenhouse, they let through visible light from the sun but trap some of the resulting infrared radiation and reradiate it back to the earth's surface. This reradiation causes a buildup of heat that raises the temperature of the lower atmosphere, a natural process known as the **greenhouse effect.** Without it, the atmosphere would be far cooler and much more hostile to life.

Human activity may be tipping this balance toward **global warming** (Figure 24-3). The concentration of greenhouse gases is increasing because of human activity, especially the combustion of fossil fuels. Carbon dioxide levels in the atmosphere have increased rapidly since the onset of the Industrial Revolution, and current levels are higher than at any time in the past 160,000 years. Deforestation, often by burning, also sends carbon dioxide into the atmosphere and reduces the number of trees available to convert carbon dioxide into oxygen. But energy use in the developed world is the primary cause of increases in the concentrations of greenhouse gases (Table 24-1). The United States alone is responsible for one-third of the world's total emissions of carbon dioxide.

According to a 2001 report from the United Nations–sponsored Intergovernmental Panel on Climate Change, the average global temperature will likely increase by about 2.5–10.4°F (1.4–5.8°C) by 2100, with a corresponding significant rise in sea level. Although the full implications of climate change are unknown, possible consequences include the following:

- Increased rainfall and flooding in some regions, increased drought in others. Coastal zones, where half the world's people live, would be severely affected.

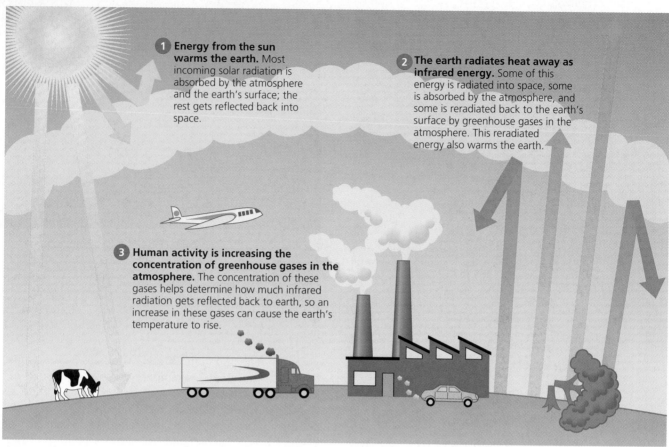

1. **Energy from the sun warms the earth.** Most incoming solar radiation is absorbed by the atmosphere and the earth's surface; the rest gets reflected back into space.

2. **The earth radiates heat away as infrared energy.** Some of this energy is radiated into space, some is absorbed by the atmosphere, and some is reradiated back to the earth's surface by greenhouse gases in the atmosphere. This reradiated energy also warms the earth.

3. **Human activity is increasing the concentration of greenhouse gases in the atmosphere.** The concentration of these gases helps determine how much infrared radiation gets reflected back to earth, so an increase in these gases can cause the earth's temperature to rise.

Figure 24-3   The greenhouse effect.

- Increased mortality from heat stress, urban air pollution, and tropical diseases (due to the spread of disease-carrying organisms like mosquitoes). Severe weather events such as hurricanes and tornadoes may also increase, along with associated deaths.

- A poleward shift of about 50–350 miles (150–550 km) in the location of vegetation zones, affecting crop yields, irrigation demands, and forest productivity.

Since record-keeping began in the mid-1800s, 8 of the 10 hottest years have occurred since 1990. Data from tree rings and other sources suggest that recent temperatures are the warmest in 1000 years. What can be done? The Kyoto Protocol to the UN Convention on Climate Change calls for industrialized countries to cut greenhouse gas emissions to about 5.2% below 1990 levels by 2008–2012; U.S. emissions, however, have actually increased by more than 10% since 1990.

Thinning of the Ozone Layer   A second air pollution problem is the thinning of the **ozone layer** of the atmosphere, a fragile, invisible layer about 10–30 miles above the earth's surface, shielding the planet from the sun's hazardous ultraviolet (UV) rays. Since the mid-1980s, scientists have observed the seasonal appearance and growth of a "hole" in the ozone layer over Antarctica. More recently, thinning over other areas—including Canada, Scandinavia, the northern United States, Russia, Australia, and New Zealand—has been noted.

The ozone layer is being destroyed primarily by **chlorofluorocarbons (CFCs)**, industrial chemicals used as coolants in refrigerators and in home and automobile air conditioners; as foaming agents in some rigid foam products, including insulation; as propellants in some kinds of aerosol sprays (most such sprays were banned in 1978); and as solvents. When CFCs rise into the atmosphere,

Terms

ozone layer A layer of ozone molecules (O_3) in the upper atmosphere that screens out UV rays from the sun.

chlorofluorocarbons (CFCs) Chemicals used as spray-can propellants, refrigerants, and industrial solvents, implicated in the destruction of the ozone layer.

acid precipitation Rain, snow, sleet, or hail with a low pH (acid), caused by atmospheric moisture combining with products of industrial combustion to form acids such as sulfur dioxide; harmful to forests and lakes, which cannot tolerate changes in acidity/alkalinity.

Table 24-1	Sources of Greenhouse Gases
Greenhouse Gas	**Sources**
Carbon dioxide	Fossil fuel and wood burning, factory emissions, car exhaust, deforestation
Chlorofluorocarbons (CFCs)	Refrigeration and air conditioning, aerosols, foam products, solvents
Methane	Cattle, wetlands, rice paddies, landfills, gas leaks, coal and gas industries
Nitrous oxide	Fertilizers, soil cultivation, deforestation, animal feedlots and wastes
Ozone and other trace gases	Photochemical reactions, car exhaust, power plant emissions, solvents

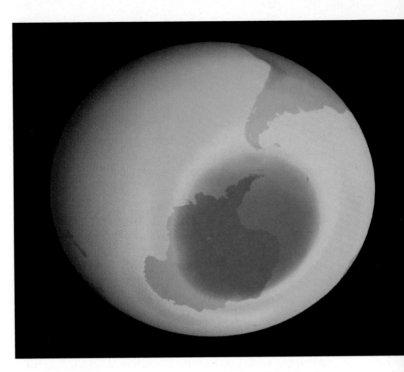

The thinning of the ozone layer is of concern because ozone absorbs ultraviolet radiation from the sun. This image from October 2000 shows the hole extending over Antarctica and the tip of South America.

winds carry them toward the polar regions. During winter, circular winds form a vortex that keeps the air over Antarctica from mixing with air from elsewhere. Ice crystals form in the Antarctic clouds during the cold, sunless months; chemical reactions taking place on these crystals, which wouldn't take place in air, free chlorine atoms from CFCs. When stimulated by the reappearance of the sun, the chlorine atoms begin destroying ozone. When the polar vortex weakens in the summer, winds richer in ozone from the north replenish the lost Antarctic ozone, but the ozone hole's growth each year may be contributing to the general thinning of the global ozone layer.

Since 1979, about 15% of Antarctic ozone has been destroyed, although locally and seasonally up to 95% of the ozone disappears (forming the "hole"). The hole above Antarctica in late 2000 was larger and deeper than any previous ozone hole. Spreading over 11 million square miles, an area three times larger than the land mass of the United States, the 2000 ozone hole extended over populated areas of South America, where residents were advised to stay indoors and take other measures to avoid UV exposure. (UV radiation levels under the hole were high enough to cause sunburn within 7 minutes.) In the Northern Hemisphere, ozone levels have declined by about 10% since 1980, and certain areas may be temporarily depleted in late winter and early spring by as much as 40%.

The loss of ozone is of concern because without the ozone layer to absorb the sun's UV radiation, life on earth would be impossible. The potential effects of increased long-term exposure to UV light for humans include skin cancer, wrinkling and aging of the skin, cataracts and blindness, and reduced immune response. The United

Nations Environment Programme predicts that a drop of 10% in overall ozone levels would cause a 26% rise in the incidence of nonmelanoma skin cancer. Some scientists blame ozone loss over Australia for a recent rise in melanoma cases there.

UV light may interfere with photosynthesis and cause lower crop yields; it may also kill phytoplankton and krill, the basis of the ocean food chain. And because heat generated by the absorption of UV rays in the ozone layer helps create stratospheric winds, the driving force behind weather patterns, a drop in the concentration of ozone could potentially alter the earth's climate systems.

Worldwide production and use of CFCs has declined rapidly since the danger to the ozone layer was recognized. Industrialized nations agreed to eliminate CFC production and use by 2000, and limits have also been placed on other agents that destroy ozone. By 2000, metered-dose inhalers for conditions like asthma were the only significant commercial product to contain CFCs, and CFC-free inhalers are already available for some medications. However, use of some ozone-depleting agents, including bromine and halon-1211, is still increasing. In addition, future ozone losses are inevitable because CFCs persist in the atmosphere for 50–150 years.

Acid Precipitation   A by-product of many industrial processes, **acid precipitation** occurs when atmospheric pollutants combine with moisture in the air and fall to earth as highly acidic rain, snow, sleet, or hail. It occurs especially when coal containing large amounts of sulfur is burned and sulfur dioxide, sulfur trioxide, nitrogen dioxide, nitric acid, and other chemicals are released into the atmosphere. These concentrations can be carried great distances by the prevailing winds and form a highly acidic mixture containing sulfuric acid and nitric acid. Most of the pollutants in acid precipitation are produced by coal-burning electric power plants. Other sources are motor vehicles and certain industrial activities, such as smelting.

Acidification of lakes and streams due to acid precipitation has completely eradicated fish and other aquatic species in some areas. Trees are also affected because acid precipitation damages leaves, strips the soil of key nutrients, and releases toxic substances such as heavy metals from the soil; in some areas of central Europe, entire forests are dying. The air pollutants that cause acid precipitation reduce visibility and cause respiratory problems in some people. Acid precipitation also corrodes metals and damages stone and paint on buildings, monuments, and cars; repairs can cost billions of dollars. Acid precipitation appears to be causing the most damage in Canada, the northeastern United States, Scandinavia, and parts of central Europe. In the United States, the areas most affected are the Adirondacks, the mid-Appalachian highlands, the upper Midwest, and high elevations in the West.

Energy Use and Air Pollution

Americans are the biggest energy consumers in the world (see the box "Environmental Health: Good News and Bad News). We use energy to create electricity, transport us, power our industries, and run our homes. About 75% of the energy we use comes from fossil fuels—oil, coal, and natural gas; the remainder comes from nuclear power and renewable energy sources (such as hydroelectric, wind, and solar power).

Energy consumption is at the root of many environmental problems, especially those relating to air pollution. Automobile exhaust and the burning of oil and coal by industry and by electricity-generating plants are primary causes of smog, acid precipitation, and the greenhouse effect. The mining of coal and the extraction and transportation of oil cause pollution on land and in the water; coal miners often suffer from serious health problems related to their jobs. Nuclear power generation creates hazardous wastes and carries the risk of dangerous releases of radiation.

Two key strategies for controlling energy use are conservation and the development of nonpolluting, renewable sources of energy. Although the use of renewable energy sources has increased in recent years, renewables still supply only a small proportion of our energy, in part because of their cost. Some countries have chosen to promote energy efficiency by removing subsidies or adding taxes on the use of fossil fuels. This strategy is reflected in the varying prices drivers pay for gasoline. According to a 2000 report from the U.S. Energy Information Agency, the average per gallon price of unleaded gasoline is about $1.70 in the United States. While U.S. gas prices are at a record high, they are still several dollars a gallon lower than in many European and Asian countries. It is not surprising that per-capita energy use in the United States is twice that of many European countries. The International Center for Technology Assessment estimates that the actual price of gasoline—including tax breaks, government subsidies, and environmental, health, and social costs of gas usage—is as high as $15.14 per gallon.

Actions that individuals can take to promote energy efficiency and cut their use of energy are listed in the section "What You Can Do to Prevent Air Pollution."

Indoor Air Pollution

Although most people associate air pollution with the outdoors, your home may also harbor potentially dangerous pollutants. Some of these compounds trigger allergic responses, and others have been linked to cancer. Common indoor pollutants include the following:

- *Environmental tobacco smoke (ETS),* a human carcinogen that also increases the risk of asthma, bronchitis, and cardiovascular disease (see Chapter 11). Several states and cities have passed legislation known as Clean Indoor Air Acts, which state that any enclosed, indoor areas used by the public shall be smoke-free except for certain designated areas.

- *Carbon monoxide and other combustion by-products,* which can cause chronic bronchitis, headaches, dizziness, nausea, fatigue, and even death. Common sources in the home are wood stoves, fireplaces, kerosene heaters and lamps, and gas ranges.

- *Formaldehyde gas,* which can cause eye, nose, and throat irritation; shortness of breath; headaches; nausea; lethargy; and, over the long term, cancer. This gas can seep from resins used in particle board, plywood paneling, and some carpeting and upholstery; it is also emitted by certain paints and floor finishes, permanent press clothing, and nail polish.

- *Biological pollutants,* including bacteria, dust mites, mold, and animal dander, which can cause allergic reactions and other health problems. These allergens need nutrients and moisture to survive and are typically found in bathrooms, damp or flooded basements, humidifiers, air conditioners, and even some carpets and furniture.

Asbestos and radon, two other dangerous indoor pollutants, are discussed later in the chapter.

What You Can Do to Prevent Air Pollution

- Cut back on driving. Ride your bike, walk, use public transportation, or carpool in a fuel-efficient vehicle.

Recent years have seen both progress and setbacks on environmental issues, and new problems continue to be recognized. The following are just a few issues of current concern.

More and More Consumers

Birth rates are dropping worldwide, from an average of 3.7 children per woman in 1980 to 3.2 in 1990 and 2.7 in 2000. Despite this trend, world population continues to skyrocket, increasing by about 9000 people every hour. It's estimated that world population will grow by more than a billion people between 2000 and 2013. A larger population puts an even greater strain on the earth's resources. Although much of this increase is occurring in the developing countries, people in industrialized countries consume the bulk of the energy and resources. The World Wildlife Fund estimates that if people in the developing world consumed as much as those living in the richest countries, humans would need another two planets to cope.

Waiting for the Ozone Layer to Heal

Since the chemicals responsible for the thinning of the ozone layer were identified, the production and use of most of these compounds have greatly declined. Unfortunately, the thinning of the ozone layer is likely to continue for some time because CFCs and other ozone-destroying agents persist in the atmosphere for decades. The "hole" in the ozone layer over Antarctica has continued to grow, both in size and depth, and now extends over populated areas during part of the year. Thinning in the ozone layer over the Arctic, northern Europe, and North America has also been noted. People in many parts of the world may soon be subject to periodic UV alerts and advised to stay indoors or wear complete sun protection.

Rising Temperatures and Severe Weather

Scientists continue to debate the extent of global warming and degree to which human activities are contributing to it. Another area of debate, one in which the public has a great deal of interest, is whether global warming could be responsible for the apparent recent increase in severe weather events—hurricanes, droughts, floods, tornadoes, and other catastrophes. In the past 20 years, the United States has been hit with $170 billion worth of weather-related damage; to date, 1998 was both the hottest year on record in the United States and the year with the greatest number of severe weather events. Worldwide, the number of natural disasters has increased more than fourfold since the 1950s.

Researchers cannot conclusively link global warming to extreme weather at this time, but answers may begin to emerge as more data are collected and better computer models are created. One intriguing new area of study is the question of whether global warming is increasing the frequency and severity of El Niño, a periodic disruption of the ocean-atmosphere system in the tropical Pacific that has important consequences for weather around the world. El Niño is characterized by a weakening of the trade winds and a warming of the eastern and central equatorial Pacific Ocean; these changes bring increased rainfall to some areas and drought to others, along with secondary effects such as floods and fires. Recent data suggest in the past 20 years, El Niños have been longer, stronger, and more frequent than in the previous 120 years.

Transportation: SUVs and HEVs

Despite recent increases in gas prices in the United States, more than 70% of American commuters drive alone to work, and low-fuel-economy sport utility vehicles (SUVs) remain popular. Every gallon of gas burned puts about 20 pounds of carbon dioxide into the atmosphere, contributing to global warming; motor vehicles are also key sources of ozone and other pollutants. Some SUVs average fewer than 10 miles per gallon, and the largest SUVs increase greenhouse gas emissions by 6 or more tons per year compared to an average car.

On the bright side, 2000 saw the introduction of a new class of car, the hybrid electric vehicle (HEV). HEVs combine a conventional internal combustion engine with an electric motor, resulting in about twice the fuel economy of conventional vehicles. The combination allows for the extended range and rapid refueling that consumers are accustomed to from conventional cars. The HEVs currently for sale are priced competitively and can travel 500–700 miles on a single tank of gas. Researchers hope that hybrid technology can be extended to all classes of vehicles and that Americans can be convinced to use more-fuel-efficient vehicles and to travel more frequently on public transportation, in carpools, or on foot.

- Keep your car tuned up and well maintained. Use only unleaded gas, and keep your tires inflated at recommended pressures. To save energy when driving, avoid quick starts, stay within the speed limit, limit the use of air conditioning, and don't let your car idle unless absolutely necessary. Have your car's air conditioner checked and serviced by a station that uses environmentally friendly refrigerants (car air conditioners made before 1994 are a major source of CFCs).

- Buy energy-efficient appliances, and use them only when necessary. Run the washing machine, dryer, and dishwasher only when you have full loads, and do laundry in warm or cold water instead of hot; don't overdry your clothes. Clean refrigerator coils and clothes dryer lint screens frequently. Towel or air-dry your hair rather than using an electric dryer.
- Replace incandescent bulbs with compact fluorescent bulbs (not fluorescent tubes). Although they cost more initially, they'll save you money over the

life of the bulb. They produce a comparable light, last longer, and use only 25–35% of the energy of a regular bulb, thereby lowering carbon dioxide emissions from electric power plants.

- Make sure your home is well-insulated with ozone-safe agents; use insulating shades and curtains to keep heat in during winter and out during summer. Seal any openings that produce drafts. In cold weather, put on a sweater and turn down the thermostat. In hot weather, wear lightweight clothing and, whenever possible, use a fan instead of an air conditioner to cool yourself.

- Plant and care for trees in your own yard and neighborhood. Because they recycle carbon dioxide, trees work against global warming. They also provide shade and cool the air, so less air conditioning is needed.

- Before discarding a refrigerator, air conditioner, or humidifier, check with the waste hauler or your local government to ensure that ozone-depleting refrigerants will be removed prior to disposal. If you use a metered-dose inhaler, ask your physician if an ozone-safe inhaler is available for your medication.

- To prevent indoor air pollution, keep your house adequately ventilated, and buy some houseplants; they have a natural ability to rid the air of harmful pollutants.

- Keep paints, cleaning agents, and other chemical products in their original, tightly sealed containers.

- Don't smoke, and don't allow others to smoke in your room, apartment, or home. If these rules are too strict for your situation, limit smoking to a single, well-ventilated room.

- Clean and inspect chimneys, furnaces, and other appliances regularly. Install carbon monoxide detectors.

COMMUNICATE! Many people resist the idea of carpooling, even though it's an excellent way to lower the number of cars on the road and thus reduce the amount of motor vehicle exhaust entering the air. If you find you have classmates or colleagues traveling to school or work at about the same time as you, see if you can set up a carpool with them. You might say, "I notice that we come to work from the same neighborhood every day. Would you be interested in carpooling? We'd be able to use the carpool lane on the highway, so we'd avoid some of the traffic slowdowns, and we'd both save on gas and mileage—to say nothing of helping the environment a little."

Chemical Pollution

Chemical pollution is by no means a new problem. The ancient Romans were plagued by lead poisoning, and over 200 years ago in Europe, the phrase "mad as a hatter" came from the hatters' practice of preparing felt hats with mercury, which destroyed the central nervous system.

The difference today is that new chemical substances are constantly being created and introduced into the environment—as pesticides, herbicides, solvents, cleaning fluids, flame retardants, and hundreds of other products. We have many more chemicals, in more concentrated forms and in wider use, and larger numbers of people are exposed and potentially exposed to them than ever before.

Chemical pollutants have been responsible for several environmental disasters, including thousands of deaths and injuries among people in Bhopal, India, that occurred when a powerful chemical used in manufacturing the insecticide Sevin was released from a plant. Catastrophes illustrate the short-term potential for disaster, but the long-term health consequences may be just as deadly. The following are brief descriptions of just a few current problems.

Asbestos A mineral-based compound, asbestos was widely used for fire protection and insulation in buildings until the late 1960s. Microscopic asbestos fibers can be released into the air when this material is applied or when it later deteriorates or is damaged. These fibers can lodge in the lungs, causing **asbestosis,** lung cancer, and other serious lung diseases. Similar conditions are risks in the coal mining industry, from exposure to coal and silica dust (black lung disease), and in the textile industry, from exposure to cotton fibers (brown lung disease).

Asbestos can pose a danger in homes and apartment buildings, about 25% of which are thought to contain some asbestos. Areas where it is most likely to be found are insulation around water and steam pipes, ducts, and furnaces; boiler wraps; vinyl flooring; floor, wall, and ceiling insulation; roofing and siding; and fireproof board. An experienced contractor can pinpoint asbestos-containing materials in a home, which can then be analyzed by a laboratory. If any of these materials begin to release asbestos fibers, the asbestos must be sealed off, encapsulated, or removed by a professional.

Lead Lead poisoning continues to be a serious problem, particularly among children living in older buildings

Terms

asbestosis A lung condition caused by inhalation of microscopic asbestos fibers, which inflame the lung and can lead to lung cancer.

pesticides Chemicals used to prevent the spread of diseases transmitted by insects and to maximize food production by killing insects that eat crops.

biomagnification The accumulation of a substance in a food chain.

Residents of poor and minority communities are often exposed to more environmental toxins than residents of wealthier communities, and they are more likely to suffer from health problems caused or aggravated by pollutants. Poor neighborhoods are often located near highways and industrial areas that have high levels of air pollution; they are also common sites for hazardous waste production and disposal. Residents of substandard housing are more likely to come into contact with lead, asbestos, carbon monoxide, pesticides, and other hazardous pollutants associated with peeling paint, old plumbing, poorly maintained insulation and heating equipment, and attempts to control high levels of pests such as cockroaches and rodents. Poor people are more likely to have jobs that expose them to asbestos, silica dust, and pesticides, and they are more likely to catch and consume fish contaminated with PCBs, mercury, and other toxins.

The most thoroughly researched and documented link among poverty, the environment, and health is lead poisoning in children. Many studies have shown that children of low-income black families are much more likely to have elevated levels of lead in their blood than white children. One survey found that two-thirds of urban African American children from

families earning less than $6000 a year had elevated lead levels. The CDC and the American Academy of Pediatrics recommend annual testing of blood lead levels for all children under age 6, with more frequent testing for children at special risk.

Asthma is another health threat that appears to be linked with both environmental and socioeconomic factors. The number of Americans with asthma has grown dramatically in the past 20 years; most of the increase has occurred in children, with African Americans and the poor hardest hit. Researchers are not sure what accounts for this increase, but suspects include household pollutants, pesticides, air pollution, cigarette smoke, and allergens like cockroaches. These risk factors are likely to cluster in poor urban areas where inadequate health care may worsen asthma's effects.

A new push for research on the health effects of exposure to toxins on low-income communities is being called for by the environmental justice movement. New studies are investigating the links between environmental factors and respiratory problems, skin diseases, and cancer. While health researchers seek to quantify the health impacts, neighborhood activists continue to fight against the "dumping" of pollution in poor communities.

and adults who are exposed to lead in the workplace. When lead is ingested or inhaled, it can damage the central nervous system, cause mental impairment, hinder oxygen transport in the blood, and create digestive problems. Severe lead poisoning may cause coma or even death. Some symptoms of lead poisoning, including anemia, headaches, and abdominal pain, may cease if exposure stops, but neurological damage can be permanent. Lead damage to the brain can start even before birth if a pregnant woman has elevated levels of lead in her body.

The CDC estimates that as many as 1.2 million children under age 6 may have unsafe lead levels in their blood. Many of these children live in poor, inner-city areas (see the box "Poverty and Environmental Health"). Long-term exposure to low levels of lead may cause kidney disease; it can also cause lead to build up in bones, where it may be released into the bloodstream during pregnancy or when bone mass is lost from osteoporosis. Little is known about the effect of lead stored in or freed from bone.

Young children can easily ingest lead from their environment by picking up dust and dirt on their hands and then putting their fingers in their mouth. Lead-based paints are believed to be the chief culprit in lead poisoning of children. They were banned from residential use in 1978, but as many as 57 million American homes still contain lead paint. The use of lead in plumbing is now also banned, but some old pipes and faucets contain lead that can leach into drinking water.

Lead gets into the air from industrial and vehicle emissions, from tobacco smoke and paint dust, and from the burning of solid wastes that contain lead. Levels of lead in the air have dropped sharply as leaded gas use has declined, but many vehicles still use leaded fuel. Lead occurs naturally in soil, which also collects lead from the air and other sources. Other sources of lead are foods stored or served in lead-glazed pottery or lead crystal and processed foods sold in lead-soldered cans.

Pesticides   Pesticides are used primarily for two purposes: to prevent the spread of insect-borne diseases and to maximize food production by killing insects that eat crops. Both uses have risks as well as benefits. Take, for example, the pesticide DDT. Recognized as a powerful pesticide in 1939, DDT was extremely important in efforts to control widespread insect-borne diseases in tropical countries and increase crop yields throughout the world. But in 1962, biologist Rachel Carson questioned the safety of DDT in her book *Silent Spring,* pointing out that the pesticide disrupts the life cycles of birds, fish, and reptiles. DDT also builds up in the food chain, increasing in concentration as larger animals eat smaller ones, a process known as **biomagnification.** Despite its effectiveness as a pesticide, DDT was banned in the United States in 1972 because the costs associated with its use—to wildlife and potentially to humans—were too high. Most pesticide hazards to date have been a result of overuse, but there are concerns about the health effects of long-term exposure to small amounts of pesticide residues in foods, especially for children.

Mercury A naturally occurring metal, mercury is a toxin that affects the nervous system and may damage the brain, kidneys, and gastrointestinal tract; increase blood pressure and heart rate; and cause cancer. Mercury slows fetal and child development and causes irreversible deficits in brain function. The EPA estimates that tens of thousands of babies are born each year after being exposed to levels of mercury at which some studies have shown adverse health effects. Coal-fired power plants are the largest producers of mercury; other sources include mining and smelting operations and the disposal of consumer products containing mercury.

Mercury persists in the environment, and, like pesticides, it is bioaccumulative. In particular, large, long-lived fish may carry high levels of mercury. The FDA recommends that pregnant women, women of childbearing age who may become pregnant, women who are breastfeeding, and young children not consume shark, swordfish, king mackerel, and tilefish. Because of health concerns, some cities and stores have banned the sale of mercury fever thermometers, a small but significant source of mercury. If a thermometer breaks or is disposed of improperly, mercury can enter the environment; if it vaporizes into the atmosphere, it can be hazardous to health. To safely clean up mercury from a broken thermometer, increase ventilation in the room and pick up the mercury with an eyedropper or scoop up the beads with a piece of heavy paper. Dispose of it and any contaminated instruments by placing them in a plastic bag and taking them to an appropriate hazardous waste disposal site. Replace mercury thermometers with one of the many mercury-free alternatives.

The list of real and potential chemical pollution problems may well be as long as the list of known chemicals. To the preceding list we can add recent concern about arsenic in drinking water, formaldehyde in synthetic building materials, and other by-products of our industrial age. As mentioned earlier, hazardous wastes are also found in the home and should be handled and disposed of properly. They include automotive supplies (motor oil, antifreeze, transmission fluid), paint supplies (turpentine, paint thinner, mineral spirits), art and hobby supplies (oil-based paint, solvents, acids and alkalis, aerosol sprays), insecticides, batteries, computer and electronic components, and household cleaners containing sodium hydroxide (lye) or ammonia. These chemicals are dangerous when inhaled or ingested, when they contact the skin or the eyes, or when they are burned or dumped. Many cities provide guidelines about approved disposal methods and have hazardous waste collection days. Look in the government pages of your phone book under Environmental Health or Hazardous Waste.

What You Can Do to Prevent Chemical Pollution

- When buying products, read the labels, and try to buy the least toxic ones available. Choose nontoxic nonpetrochemical cleansers, disinfectants, polishes, and other personal and household products.

- Dispose of your household hazardous wastes properly. If you are not sure whether something is hazardous or don't know how to dispose of it, contact your local environmental health office or health department. Don't burn trash.

- Buy organic produce or produce that has been grown locally. Wash, scrub, and, if appropriate, peel fruits and vegetables. Consider eating less meat; animal products require more pesticides, fertilizer, water, and energy to produce.

- If you must use pesticides or toxic household products, store them in a locked place where children and pets can't get to them. Don't measure chemicals with food-preparation utensils, and wear gloves whenever handling them.

- If you have your house fumigated for pest control, be sure to hire a licensed exterminator. Keep everyone, including pets, out of the house while the crew works and, if possible, for a few days after.

Radiation

Many people are afraid of **radiation**, in part because they don't understand what it is. Basically, radiation is energy. It can come in different forms, such as ultraviolet rays, microwaves, or X rays, and from different sources, such as the sun, uranium, and nuclear weapons (Figure 24-4). These forms of electromagnetic radiation differ in wavelength and energy, with shorter waves having the highest energy levels. Of most concern to health are gamma rays produced by radioactive sources such as nuclear weapons, nuclear energy plants, and radon gas; these high-energy waves are powerful enough to penetrate objects and break molecular bonds. Although gamma radiation cannot be seen or felt, its effects at high doses can include **radiation sickness** and death; at lower doses, chromosome damage, sterility, tissue damage, cataracts,

Terms

radiation Energy transmitted in the form of rays, waves, or particles.

radiation sickness An illness caused by excess radiation exposure, marked by low white blood cell counts and nausea; possibly fatal.

nuclear power The use of controlled nuclear reactions to produce steam, which in turn drives turbines to produce electricity.

radon A naturally occurring radioactive gas emitted from rocks and natural building materials that can become concentrated in insulated homes, causing lung cancer.

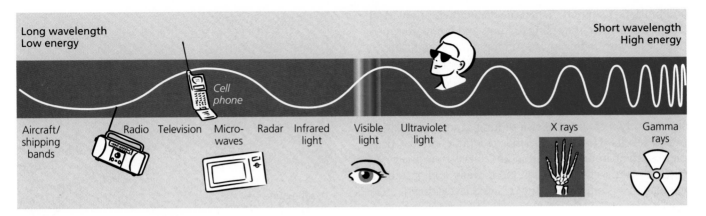

Long wavelength
Low energy

Short wavelength
High energy

Aircraft/shipping bands Radio Television Micro-waves Radar Infrared light Visible light Ultraviolet light X rays Gamma rays

Cell phone

Figure 24-4 Electromagnetic radiation. Electromagnetic radiation takes the form of waves that travel through space. The length of the wave determines the type of radiation: The shortest waves are high-energy gamma rays; the longest are radio waves and extremely low-frequency waves used for communication between aircraft, ships, and submarines. Different types of electromagnetic radiation have different effects on health.

and cancer can occur. Other types of radiation can also affect health; for example, exposure to UV radiation from the sun or from tanning salons can increase the risk of skin cancer. The effects of some sources of radiation, such as cell phones, remain controversial.

Nuclear Weapons and Nuclear Energy Nuclear weapons pose a health risk of the most serious kind to all species. Public health associations have stated that in the event of an intentional or unintentional discharge of these weapons, the casualties would run into the hundreds of thousands or millions. Reducing these stockpiles is a challenge and a goal for the twenty-first century.

Power-generating plants that use nuclear fuel also pose health problems. When **nuclear power** was first developed as an alternative to oil and coal, it was promoted as clean, efficient, inexpensive, and safe. In general, this has proven to be the case. Power systems in several parts of the world rely on nuclear-generating plants. However, despite all the built-in safeguards and regulating agencies, accidents in nuclear power plants do happen, many due to human error (as at Three Mile Island in the United States and Tokaimura in Japan), and the consequences of such accidents are far more serious than those of similar accidents in other types of power-generating plants. The 1986 fire and explosion at the Chernobyl nuclear power station in Ukraine caused hundreds of deaths and increased rates of genetic mutation and cancer; the long-term effects are not yet clear. The zone around Chernobyl has been sealed off to human habitation and could be unsafe for the next 24,000 years.

An additional, enormous problem is disposing of the radioactive wastes these plants generate. They cannot be dumped in a sanitary landfill because the amount and type of soil used to cap a sanitary landfill is not sufficient to prevent radiation exposure. Deposit sites have to be developed that will be secure not just for a few years but for tens of thousands of years—longer than the total recorded history of human beings on this planet. To date, no storage method has been devised that can provide infallible, infinitely durable shielding for nuclear waste.

Medical Uses of Radiation Another area of concern is the use of radiation in medicine, primarily the X ray. The development of machines that could produce images of internal bone structures was a major advance in medicine, and applications abounded. Chest X rays were routinely given to screen for tuberculosis, and children's feet were even X rayed in shoe stores to make sure their new shoes fit properly. But, as is often the case, this new technology had disadvantages. As time passed, studies revealed that X ray exposure is cumulative and that no exposure is absolutely safe.

Early X ray machines are no longer used because of the high amounts of radiation they give off. Each "generation" of X ray machines has used less radiation more effectively. From a personal health point of view, individuals should never have a "routine" X ray examination; each such exam should have a definite purpose, and its benefits and risks should be carefully weighed.

Radiation in the Home and Workplace Recently, there has been concern about electromagnetic radiation associated with such common modern devices as microwave ovens, computer monitors, cellular telephones, and even high-voltage power lines. These forms of radiation do have effects on health, but research results are inconclusive.

Another recent area of concern is **radon,** a naturally occurring radioactive gas found in certain soils, rocks, and building materials. When the breakdown products of radon are inhaled, they cling to lungs and bombard sensitive tissue with radioactivity. Among miners, exposure to high levels of radon has been shown to cause lung cancer. Radon can enter a home by rising though the soil into the basement through dirt floors, cracks, and other openings. Research into whether exposure to low levels of radon significantly increases the risk of lung cancer has yielded mixed results. However, the EPA recommends that people test their homes for radon and take appropriate actions—sealing cracks in basement walls and installing ventilation systems—to bring elevated levels down.

What You Can Do to Avoid Radiation

- If your physician orders an X ray, ask why it is necessary. Only get X rays that you need, and keep a record of the date and location of every X ray exam.

- Check with your local or state health department to find out if there are radon problems in your area. If there are, consider buying a home radon testing kit.

- Find out if there are radioactive sites in your area. If you live or work near such a site, form or join a community action group to get the site cleaned up.

Noise Pollution

We are increasingly aware of the health effects of loud or persistent noise in the environment. Concerns focus on two areas: hearing loss and stress. Prolonged exposure to sounds above 80–85 **decibels** (a measure of the intensity of a sound wave) can cause permanent hearing loss (Figure 24-5). The scream of an infant, the noise in a machine shop, and freeway traffic sounds can all exceed the safe range. Two common potential sources of excessive noise are (1) the workplace and (2) large gatherings of people at sporting events and rock concerts. The Occupational Safety and Health Administration (OSHA) sets legal standards for noise in the workplace, but no laws exist regulating noise levels at rock concerts, which often exceed OSHA standards for the workplace.

Most hearing loss occurs in the first 2 hours of exposure, and hearing usually recovers within 2 hours after the noise stops. But if exposure continues or is repeated frequently, hearing loss may be permanent. The employees of a club where rock music is played loudly are at greater risk than the patrons of the club, who might be exposed for only 2 hours at a time. Another possible effect of exposure to excessive noise is **tinnitus,** a condition of more or less continuous ringing or buzzing in the ears.

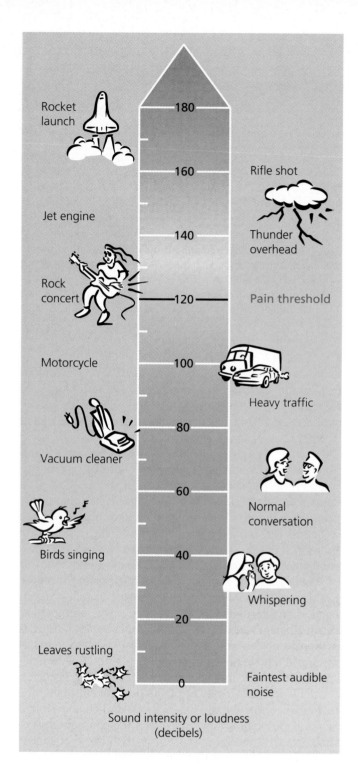

Figure 24-5 The intensity of selected sounds. Hearing damage can occur after 8 hours of exposure to sounds louder than 80 decibels; regular exposure to more than 100 decibels for longer than 1 minute can cause permanent hearing loss. Children may suffer damage to their hearing at lower levels of sound than adults.

Terms   **decibel** A unit for expressing the relative intensity of sounds on a scale from 0 for the average least perceptible sound to about 120 for the average pain threshold.

tinnitus Ringing in the ears, a condition that can be caused by excessive noise exposure.

Excessive noise is also an environmental stressor, producing the typical stress response described in Chapter 2: faster heart rate, increased respiration, higher blood pres-

The following list of statements relates to your impact on the environment. Put a check mark next to the statements that are true for you.

_____ I ride my bike, walk, carpool, or use public transportation whenever possible.

_____ I keep my car tuned up and well maintained.

_____ My residence is well insulated.

_____ Where possible, I use compact fluorescent bulbs instead of incandescent bulbs.

_____ I turn off lights and appliances when they are not in use.

_____ I avoid turning on heat or air conditioning whenever possible.

_____ I run the washing machine, dryer, and dishwasher only when they have full loads.

_____ I run the clothes dryer only as long as it takes my clothes to dry.

_____ I dry my hair with a towel rather than a hair dryer.

_____ I keep my car's air conditioner in good working order and have it serviced by a service station that recycles CFCs.

_____ When shopping, I choose products with the least amount of packaging.

_____ I choose recycled and recyclable products.

_____ I avoid products packaged in plastic and unrecycled aluminum.

_____ I store food in glass jars and waxed paper rather than plastic wrap.

_____ I take my own bag along when I go shopping.

_____ I recycle newspapers, glass, cans, and other recyclables.

_____ When shopping, I read labels and try to buy the least toxic products available.

_____ I dispose of household hazardous wastes properly.

_____ I take showers instead of baths.

_____ I take short showers and switch off the water when I'm not actively using it.

_____ I do not run the water while brushing my teeth, shaving, or hand-washing clothes.

_____ My sinks have aerators installed in them.

_____ My shower has a low-flow showerhead.

_____ I have a water-saver toilet or a water displacement device in my toilet.

_____ I snip or rip plastic six-pack rings before I throw them out.

_____ When hiking or camping, I never leave anything behind.

Statements you have not checked can help you identify behaviors you can change to improve environmental health.

---

sure, and so on. A chronic and prolonged stress response can have serious effects on health.

What You Can Do to Avoid Noise Pollution

- Wear ear protectors when working around noisy machinery.

- When listening to music on a headset with a volume range of 1–10, keep the volume no louder than 4; your headset is too loud if you are unable to hear people around you speaking in a normal tone of voice.

- Avoid loud music. Don't sit or stand near speakers or amplifiers at a rock concert, and don't play a car radio or stereo so high that you can't hear the traffic.

- Avoid exposure to painfully loud sounds, and avoid repeated exposure to any sounds above 80 decibels.

HEALING THE ENVIRONMENT

Faced with a vast array of confusing and complex environmental issues, you may feel overwhelmed and conclude that there isn't anything you can do about global problems. But this is not true. If everyone made individual changes in his or her life, the impact would be tremendous. (To assess your current lifestyle, refer to the box "Environmental Health Checklist.")

At the same time, it is important to recognize that large corporations and manufacturers are the ones primarily responsible for environmental degradation. Many of them have jumped on the "environmental bandwagon" with public relations and advertising campaigns designed to make them look good, but they haven't changed their practices nearly enough to make a difference. To influence them, people have to become educated, demand changes in production methods, and elect people to office who consider environmental concerns along with sound business incentives.

Large-scale changes and individual actions complement each other. What you do every day *does* count. Following the suggestions in the What You Can Do sections throughout this chapter will help you make a difference in the environment. In addition, you can become a part of larger community actions to work for a healthier world:

- Share what you learn about environmental issues with your friends and family.

- Join, support, or volunteer your time to organizations working on environmental causes that are important to you.

- Contact your elected representatives and communicate your concerns. For guidelines on how to be heard, see the box "Making Your Letters Count."

It takes only a few minutes to write to an elected official, but it can make a difference on an environmental issue you care about. When elected officials receive enough letters or e-mails on an issue, it does influence their vote—they want to be re-elected, and your vote counts! To give your letter the greatest possible impact, use these guidelines:

• Use your own words and your own stationery.

• Be clear and concise. Keep your letter to one or two paragraphs, never more than one page.

• Focus on only one subject in each letter, and identify it clearly. Refer to legislation by its name or number.

• Request a specific action—vote a particular way on a piece of legislation, request hearings, cosponsor a bill—and state your reasons for your position.

• If you live or work in the legislator's district, say so.

• Courteous letters work best. Don't be insulting or unnecessarily critical.

Your phone book has addresses of all state and local representatives. You can write to the president or vice president at the White House:

President (Vice President) _____
White House
Washington, D.C. 20500
president@whitehouse.gov
vice.president@whitehouse.gov

United States senators and representatives can be reached at the following addresses:

The Honorable _____   The Honorable _____
U.S. Senate   U.S. House of Representatives
Washington, D.C. 20510   Washington, D.C. 20515

Members of Congress also have e-mail addresses and many have Web sites; you can find a directory of this information at http://lcweb.loc.gov/global/legislative/email.html.

Tips for Today

Environmental health involves protecting ourselves from environmental dangers and protecting the environment from the dangers we ourselves create. The two are intimately connected, and both require that we take responsibility for our actions every day.

Right now you can

• Turn the lights off in any unoccupied rooms.

• Plan to buy compact fluorescent light bulbs to replace your incandescent ones.

• Turn the heat down a few degrees and put on a sweater, or turn the air conditioner off and change into shorts.

• Make an appointment to have your car checked if it's not running well or needs a tune-up.

• Check your trash can for recyclable items—soda cans, plastic water bottles, white paper, magazines—and put aside any you find for recycling or take them to your recycling bins.

SUMMARY

• Environmental health encompasses all the interactions of humans with their environment and the health consequences of those interactions.

• Concerns with water quality focus on pathogenic organisms and hazardous chemicals from industry and households, as well as on water shortages.

• Sewage treatment prevents pathogens from contaminating drinking water; it must also often deal with heavy metals and hazardous chemicals.

• The amount of garbage is growing all the time; paper is the biggest component. Recycling can help solid waste disposal problems.

• The world's population is increasing rapidly, especially in the developing world. Factors that may eventually limit human population are food, availability of land and water, energy, and minimum acceptable standard of living.

• Increased amounts of air pollutants are especially dangerous for children, older adults, and people with chronic health problems.

• Factors contributing to the development of smog include heavy motor vehicle traffic, hot weather, stagnant air, and temperature inversion.

• Carbon dioxide and other natural gases act as a "greenhouse" around the earth, increasing the temperature of the atmosphere. Levels of these gases are rising through human activity; as a result, the world's climate could change.

• The ozone layer that shields the earth's surface from the sun's UV rays has thinned and developed holes in certain regions.

• Acid precipitation occurs when certain atmospheric pollutants combine with moisture in the air.

• Environmental damage from energy use can be limited through energy conservation and the development of nonpolluting, renewable sources of energy.

- Indoor pollutants can trigger allergies and illness in the short term and cancer in the long term.
- Potentially hazardous chemical pollutants include asbestos, lead, pesticides, mercury, and many household products. Proper handling and disposal are critical.
- Radiation can cause radiation sickness, chromosome damage, and cancer, among other health problems.

- Loud or persistent noise can lead to hearing loss and/or stress; two common sources of excessive noise are the workplace and rock concerts.
- Most health advances today must come from lifestyle changes and improvements in the global environment. The impact of personal changes made by every concerned individual could be tremendous.

TAKE ACTION

1. Prepare an inventory to find out what hazardous chemicals you have in your household. Read the labels for disposal instructions. If there aren't any instructions, call your local health department and ask how to dispose of specific chemicals. Also ask if there are hazardous waste disposal sites in your community or special pickup days. If possible, get rid of some or all of the hazardous wastes in your home.

2. Investigate the recycling facilities in your community. Find out how materials are recycled and what they are used for in their recycled state. If recycling isn't available in your community, contact your local city hall to find out how a recycling program can be started.

3. Keep track of exactly how many bags (or gallons) of trash your household produces per week. Is it more or less than the national weekly average of 6.73 bags (87.5 gallons) per three-person household? In either case, try to reduce it by recycling, composting, and buying and using fewer disposable products.

Ww. JOURNAL ENTRY

1. In your health journal, list the positive behaviors that help you protect the environment. What can you do to reinforce and support these behaviors? Then list the behaviors that may harm the environment. How can you change one or more of them?

2. *Critical Thinking* Some developing nations want to "catch up" with the West in terms of economic development and standard of living by using the same kinds of industrial practices that developed nations have used to get where they are. They are cutting down forests to raise cattle for beef, using pesticides that have been banned in the developed nations, and polluting their water and air with industrial and agricultural wastes. Do you think it's fair to expect them to be environmentally conscious when the developed nations were not? Do they have a right to the same standard of living that Americans have, no matter what the environmental costs? Write a short essay that makes a case for or against their continuing use of these practices.

FOR MORE INFORMATION

Books

Athanasiou. 1998. *Divided Planet: The Ecology of Rich and Poor.* Athens: University of Georgia Press. *Discusses environmental issues in the context of the economic inequality between developed and developing nations.*

Getis, J. 1999. *You Can Make a Difference: Be Environmentally Responsible,* 2nd ed. New York: McGraw-Hill. *Describes environmental problems and suggestions for individual action.*

Nadakavukaren, A. 2000. *Our Global Environment: A Health Perspective,* 5th ed. Prospect Heights, Ill.: Waveland Press. *A broad survey of major environmental issues and their effects on personal and community health.*

Stevens, W. K. 2001. *The Change in the Weather: People, Weather, and the Science of Climate.* New York: Delacorte. *Describes the scientific debate about global warming and severe weather events and what might be done to reverse current trends.*

Yassi, A. 2001. *Basic Environmental Health.* New York: Oxford University Press. *A comprehensive introduction to environmental health concerns.*

Useful annual or biennial publications include the following:
Brown, L., et al. 2001. *State of the World 2001.* New York: Norton.
National Wildlife Federation. 2001. *2001 Conservation Directory.* Washington D.C.: National Wildlife Federation.
World Resources Institute. 2000. *World Resources 2000–2001.* New York: Oxford University Press.

Ww. Organizations, Hotlines, and Web Sites

The Earth Times. An international online newspaper devoted to global environmental issues.
http://www.earthtimes.org

Energy Efficiency and Renewable Energy Network (EREN). U.S. Department of Energy. Provides information about alternative fuels and tips for saving energy at home and in your car.

http://www.eren.doe.gov

Environmental News Network. Provides daily environmental news and special reports in print, audio, and video.

http://www.enn.com

Environmental Organization Web Directory. An environmental search engine with an extensive and well-organized collection of links.

http://www.webdirectory.com/

Fuel Economy. Provides information on the fuel economy of cars made since 1985 and tips on improving gas mileage.

http://www.fueleconomy.gov

Garbage. Provides information and links about ways to reduce solid and hazardous waste.

http://www.learner.org/exhibits/garbage

Indoor Air Quality Information Hotline. Answers questions, provides publications, and makes referrals.

800-438-4318

National Lead Information Center. Provides information packets and specialist advice.

800-LEAD-FYI

National Safety Council Environmental Health Center. Provides information on lead, radon, indoor air quality, hazardous chemicals, and other environmental issues.

800-55-RADON (Radon Hotline)

http://www.nsc.org/ehc.htm

Ozone Hole Tour. An illustrated look at the science behind the Antarctic ozone hole.

http://www.atm.ch.cam.ac.uk/tour

Student Environmental Action Coalition (SEAC). A coalition of student and youth environmental groups; Web site has contact information for local groups.

215-222-4711

http://www.seac.org

United Nations. Several UN programs are devoted to environmental problems on a global scale; the Web sites provide information on current and projected trends and on international treaties developed to deal with environmental issues.

http://www.undp.org/popin (Population Division)

http://www.unep.org (Environment Programme)

U.S. Environmental Protection Agency (EPA). Provides information about EPA activities and many consumer-oriented materials. The Web site includes special sites devoted to global warming, ozone loss, pesticides, and other areas of concern.

http://www.epa.gov

Worldwatch Institute. A public policy research organization focusing on emerging global environmental problems and the links between the world economy and the environment.

http://www.worldwatch.org

There are many national and international organizations working on environmental health problems. A few of the largest and best known are listed below:

Greenpeace: 800-326-0959; http://www.greenpeace.org

National Audubon Society: 212-979-3000; http://www.audubon.org

National Wildlife Federation: 202-797-6800; http://www.nwf.org

Nature Conservancy: 703-841-5300; http://www.tnc.org

Sierra Club: 415-977-5500; http://www.sierraclub.org

SELECTED BIBLIOGRAPHY

American Council for an Energy-Efficient Economy. 2000. *Green Book: Market Trends* (http://www.greenercars.org/gctext.html; retrieved January 13, 2001).

Centers for Disease Control and Prevention. 2000. Recommendations for blood lead screening of young children enrolled in Medicaid: Targeting a group at high risk. *MMWR Recommendations and Reports* 49(RR14): 1–13.

Centers for Disease Control and Prevention 2001. Blood and hair mercury levels in young children and women of childbearing age—United States, 1999. *Morbidity and Mortality Weekly Report* 50(8): 140–143.

D'Agnese, J. 2000. Why has our weather gone wild? *Discover,* June, 72.

Epstein, P. R. 2000. Is global warming harmful to health? *Scientific American,* August, 50–57.

Friedrich, M. J. 2000. Poor children subject to "environmental injustice." *Journal of the American Medical Association* 283(23): 3057–3058.

Gleick, P. H. 2001. Safeguarding our water: Making every drop count. *Scientific American,* February.

International Center for Technology Assessment. 1998. *The Real Price of Gas* (http://www.icta.org/projects/trans/rlprexsm.htm; retrieved March 3, 1999).

Intergovernmental Panel on Climate Change. 2001. *Climate Change 2001: Impacts, Adaptation and Vulnerability.* Geneva: Intergovernmental Panel on Climate Change.

Karl, T. R., and K. E. Trenberth. 1999. The human impact on climate. *Scientific American,* December, 100–105.

National Oceanic and Atmospheric Administration. 2000. *2000 Southern Hemisphere Ozone Hole Area* (http://www.cpc.ncep.noaa.gov/products/stratosphere/sbuv2to/ozone_hole_plot.gif; retrieved January 12, 2001).

National Oceanic and Atmospheric Administration. 2000. *What Is an El Niño?* (http://www.pmel.noaa.gov/toga-tao/el-nino-story.html; retrieved January 12, 2001).

National Research Council. 2000. *Toxicological Effects of Methylmercury.* Washington, D.C.: National Academy Press.

Raven, P. H. 1999. Remarks at the XVI International Botanical Congress. Plants in peril: What should we do? *Journal of International Wildlife Law and Policy* 2(2).

Sala, O. E., et al. 2000. Global biodiversity scenarios for the year 2100. *Science* 287(5459): 1770–1774.

Samet, J. M., et al. 2000. Fine particulate air pollution and mortality in 20 U.S. cities, 1987–1994. *New England Journal of Medicine* 343(24): 1742–1749.

United Nations Population Division. 2001. *World Population Prospects: The 2000 Revision.* New York: United Nations.

U.S. Department of Energy, Hybrid Electric Vehicle Program. 2000. *What Is an HEV?* (http://www.ott.doe.gov/hev/what.html; retrieved January 13, 2001).

U.S. Environmental Protection Agency. 1999. *Smog—Who Does It Hurt? What You Need to Know About Ozone and Your Health.* Pub. no. EPA-452/K-99-001.

U.S. Environmental Protection Agency. 2000. *Air Quality Index: A Guide to Air Quality and Your Health.* Pub. no. EPA-454/R-00-005.

U.S. Environmental Protection Agency. 2000. *Municipal Solid Waste Generation, Recycling, and Disposal in the United States.* Pub. no. EPA-530/F-00-024.

U.S. Environmental Protection Agency. 2001. *America's Children and the Environment.* Washington, D.C.: U.S. Environmental Protection Agency.

U.S. Environmental Protection Agency, Superfund Program. 2000. *Superfund Cleanup Figures* (http://www.epa.gov/superfund/actin/process/mgmtrpt.htm; retrieved January 11, 2001).

U.S. Global Change Research Project. 2000. *Climate Change Impacts on the United States.* Washington, D.C.: U.S. Global Change Research Project.

Nutritional Content of Popular Items from Fast-Food Restaurants

Arby's

	Serving size g	Calories	Protein g	Total fat g	Saturated fat g	Total carbohydrate g	Sugars g	Fiber g	Cholesterol mg	Sodium mg	Vitamin A	Vitamin C	Calcium	Iron	% calories from fat
												% Daily Value			
Regular roast beef	154	388	23	19	7	33	N/A	3	43	1009	N/A	N/A	N/A	N/A	44
Super roast beef	247	523	25	27	9	50	N/A	5	43	1189	N/A	N/A	N/A	N/A	46
French dip	195	475	30	22	8	40	N/A	3	55	1411	N/A	N/A	N/A	N/A	41
Junior roast beef	126	324	17	14	5	35	N/A	2	30	779	N/A	N/A	N/A	N/A	39
Roast chicken Caesar sandwich	300	660	41	24	5	70	N/A	N/A	80	1900	N/A	N/A	N/A	N/A	33
Roast turkey & swiss	327	630	42	30	8	52	N/A	N/A	80	1670	N/A	N/A	N/A	N/A	43
Breaded chicken fillet	240	623	28	28	5	46	N/A	5	45	1016	N/A	N/A	N/A	N/A	40
Han 'n cheese	169	359	24	14	5	34	N/A	2	53	1283	N/A	N/A	N/A	N/A	35
Jalapeño bites	110	330	7	21	9	29	N/A	2	40	670	N/A	N/A	N/A	N/A	57
Cheddar curly fries	120	333	5	18	4	40	N/A	0	3	1016	N/A	N/A	N/A	N/A	49
Potato cakes	85	204	2	12	2	20	N/A	0	0	397	N/A	N/A	N/A	N/A	53
Red ranch dressing	14	75	0	6	1	5	N/A	0	0	115	N/A	N/A	N/A	N/A	72
French-toastix	124	430	10	21	5	52	N/A	3	0	550	N/A	N/A	N/A	N/A	44
Jamocha shake	340	384	15	10	3	62	N/A	0	36	262	N/A	N/A	N/A	N/A	23

N/A: not available.

SOURCE: Triare Restaurant Group, 1998–2000, http://www.arbysrestaurant.com. Permission pending.

Burger King

	Serving size g	Calories	Protein g	Total fat g	Saturated fat g	Total carbohydrate g	Sugars g	Fiber g	Cholesterol mg	Sodium mg	Vitamin A	Vitamin C	Calcium	Iron	% calories from fat
												% Daily Value			
Whopper®	278	680	29	39	12	53	9	4	80	940	10	15	10	30	52
Whopper Jr.®	172	420	20	24	8	32	6	2	55	520	4	8	8	20	51
Double Whopper® w/cheese	387	1020	53	65	25	55	9	4	170	1460	15	15	30	40	57
BK Big Fish™ sandwich	263	710	24	38	14	67	4	4	50	1200	2	0	8	20	48
BK Broiler® chicken sandwich	258	550	30	25	5	52	5	3	105	1110	6	10	6	20	41
Chicken Tenders® (8 pieces)	123	340	22	19	5	20	0	<1	50	840	0	0	0	4	50
Ranch dipping sauce	28	120	1	13	2	1	N/A	N/A	5	85	N/A	N/A	N/A	N/A	98
Barbecue dipping sauce	28	35	0	0	0	9	N/A	N/A	0	400	N/A	N/A	N/A	N/A	0
French fries, medium	116	370	4	17	5	49	0	4	0	760	0	2	0	6	41
Onion rings, medium	94	330	5	16	4	41	5	3	0	470	0	0	10	0	44
Chocolate shake, medium	397	440	12	10	6	75	67	4	30	330	8	0	30	15	21
Croissan'wich® w/sausage, egg & cheese	153	500	19	36	13	26	5	1	190	1020	8	0	15	15	65
French toast sticks	112	390	6	20	4.5	46	11	2	0	440	0	0	6	10	46
Dutch apple pie	113	340	2	14	3	15	23	1	0	470	2	0	0	8	37
Chicken club sandwich	242	620	30	32	8	54	6	4	75	1460	6	10	8	20	47

N/A: not available.

SOURCE: Burger King Corporation, 2001, http://www.burgerking.com. Burger King® trademarks, trade name, and Nutritional Guide are reproduced with permission from Burger King Brands, Inc.

Domino's Pizza

(1 serving = 2 of 8 slices or ¼ of 14-inch pizza; 2 of 8 slices or ¼ of 12-inch pizza; 1 6-inch pizza)

	Serving size	Calories	Protein	Total fat	Saturated fat	Total carbohydrate	Sugars	Fiber	Cholesterol	Sodium	Vitamin A	Vitamin C	Calcium	Iron	% calories from fat
	g		g	g	g	g	g	g	mg	mg	\% Daily Value				
14-inch lg. hand-tossed cheese	219	516	21	15	7	75	6	4	32	1080	18	0	26	23	26
14-inch lg. thin crust cheese	148	382	17	17	7	43	6	2	32	1172	18	0	32	8	40
14-inch lg. deep dish cheese	257	677	26	30	11	80	9	5	41	1575	21	<1	33	31	40
12-inch med. hand-tossed cheese	159	375	15	11	5	55	5	3	23	776	13	0	19	17	26
12-inch med. thin crust cheese	106	273	12	12	5	31	4	2	23	835	13	0	23	5	40
12-inch med. deep dish cheese	181	482	19	22	8	56	6	3	30	1123	15	<1	24	22	41
6-inch deep dish cheese	216	598	23	28	10	68	7	4	36	1341	17	<1	30	30	42
Toppings: pepperoni	*	98	5	9	3	<1	<1	<1	20	364	†	†	†	†	83
ham	*	31	5	2	<1	<1	<1	<1	12	292	†	†	†	†	58
Italian sausage	*	110	5	9	3	3	<1	<1	22	342	†	†	†	†	74
bacon	*	153	8	13	4	<1	<1	<1	22	424	†	†	†	†	77
beef	*	111	6	10	4	<1	<1	<1	21	309	†	†	†	†	81
anchovies	*	45	9	2	<1	<1	<1	<1	18	791	†	†	5	6	40
extra cheese	*	68	7	6	3	<1	<1	<1	15	228	11	†	12	†	79
cheddar cheese	*	71	5	6	3	<1	<1	<1	18	110	4	†	13	†	76
Barbeque buffalo wings	25	50	5	2	<1	2	1	<1	26	175	†	†	†	†	36
Breadsticks (1 piece)	37	116	3	4	<1	16	<1	<1	0	152	†	†	†	†	31
Double cheesy bread	43	142	4	6	2	18	<1	<1	6	183	†	†	†	†	38

* Topping information is based on minimal portioning requirements for one serving of a 14-inch large pizza; add the values for toppings to the values for a cheese pizza. The following toppings supply fewer than 15 calories per serving: green and yellow peppers, onion, olives, mushrooms, pineapple.
† Contains less than 2% of the Daily Value of these nutrients.

SOURCE: Domino's Pizza, 2001, http://www.dominos.com. Reproduced with permission from Domino's Pizza LLC.

Jack in the Box

	Serving size	Calories	Protein	Total fat	Saturated fat	Total carbohydrate	Sugars	Fiber	Cholesterol	Sodium	Vitamin A	Vitamin C	Calcium	Iron	% calories from fat
	g		g	g	g	g	g	g	mg	mg	\% Daily Value				
Breakfast Jack®	126	280	17	12	5	28	3	1	190	750	8	6	15	20	39
Supreme croissant	164	530	21	34	10	37	6	0	225	1060	8	6	10	10	58
Hamburger	104	250	12	9	3.5	30	5	2	30	610	0	0	10	20	32
Jumbo Jack®	271	550	27	30	10	43	12	2	75	880	10	15	15	25	49
Sourdough Jack®	233	690	34	45	15	37	3	2	105	1180	15	15	20	25	59
Chicken fajita pita	230	320	24	10	4.5	34	6	3	55	850	20	25	20	15	28
Grilled chicken fillet	242	480	27	24	6	39	6	4	65	1110	8	15	20	25	45
Chicken supreme	305	830	33	49	7	66	5	3	65	2140	10	15	20	20	53
Jack Spicy Chicken®	252	570	24	29	2.5	52	9	2	50	1020	8	15	15	10	46
Garden chicken salad	253	200	23	9	4	8	4	3	65	420	70	20	20	4	41
Blue cheese dressing	57	210	1	15	2.5	11	4	0	25	750	0	0	2	0	64
Chicken teriyaki bowl	502	670	26	4	1	128	27	3	15	1730	130	40	10	25	5
Monster taco	138	270	12	17	6	19	2	4	30	630	10	4	20	8	57
Egg rolls (3 pieces)	170	440	15	24	6	40	5	4	30	1020	15	20	8	25	49
Chicken breast pieces (5)	150	360	27	17	3	24	0	1	80	970	4	2	2	10	43
Stuffed jalapeños (7 pieces)	168	530	16	31	12	46	5	4	60	1730	20	35	30	8	53
Barbeque dipping sauce	28	45	1	0	0	11	7	0	0	310	0	4	0	0	0
Seasoned curly fries	125	410	6	23	5	45	0	4	0	1010	6	0	4	10	51
Onion rings	120	450	7	25	5	50	3	3	0	780	4	30	4	15	50
Cappuccino classic ice cream shake	16 oz	630	11	29	17	80	58	0	90	320	15	0	35	0	41

SOURCE: Jack's Nutrition Facts, Rev. 2000. The following trademarks are owned by Jack in the Box, Inc.: Breakfast Jack,® Jumbo Jack,® Sourdough Jack,® Jack in the Box.® Reproduced with permission from Jack in the Box Inc.

KFC

	Serving size	Calories	Protein	Total fat	Saturated fat	Total carbohydrate	Sugars	Fiber	Cholesterol	Sodium	Vitamin A	Vitamin C	Calcium	Iron	% calories from fat
	g		g	g	g	g	g	g	mg	mg	% Daily Value				
Original Recipe® breast	153	400	29	24	6	16	0	1	135	1116	*	*	4	6	54
Original Recipe® thigh	91	250	16	18	4.5	6	0	1	95	747	*	*	2	4	65
Extra crispy chicken breast	168	470	39	28	8	17	0	<1	160	874	*	*	2	6	54
Extra crispy chicken thigh	118	380	21	27	7	14	0	<1	118	625	*	*	2	6	64
Hot & spicy breast	180	505	38	29	8	23	9	1	162	1170	*	*	6	6	52
Hot & spicy thigh	107	355	19	26	7	13	0	1	126	630	*	*	2	4	66
Tender Roast sandwich w/sauce	211	350	32	15	3	26	1	1	75	880	4	*	4	10	39
Tender Roast sandwich w/o sauce	177	270	31	5	1.5	23	<1	1	65	690	*	*	4	10	17
Hot wings (6 pieces)	135	471	27	33	8	18	0	2	150	1230	*	*	4	8	63
Colonel's Crispy Strips™ (3)	115	300	26	16	4	18	1	1	56	1165	2	*	*	6	48
Chunky chicken pot pie	368	770	29	42	13	69	8	5	70	2160	80	2	10	10	49
Corn on the cob	162	150	5	1.5	0	35	8	2	0	20	2	6	*	*	9
Mashed potatoes w/gravy	136	120	1	6	1	17	0	2	,1	440	*	*	*	2	45
BBQ baked beans	156	190	6	3	1	33	13	6	5	760	8	*	8	10	14
Cole slaw	142	232	2	13.5	2	26	20	3	8	284	9	58	3	*	52
Biscuit (1)	56	180	4	10	2.5	20	2	<1	0	560	*	*	2	6	50
Potato salad	160	230	4	14	2	23	9	3	15	540	10	*	2	15	55

*Contains less than 2% of the Daily Value of these nutrients.

SOURCE: KFC Corporation, 2001, http://www.kfc.com. Reproduced with permission from Kentucky Fried Chicken Corporation.

Taco Bell

	Serving size	Calories	Protein	Total fat	Saturated fat	Total carbohydrate	Sugars	Fiber	Cholesterol	Sodium	Vitamin A	Vitamin C	Calcium	Iron	% calories from fat
	g		g	g	g	g	g	g	mg	mg	% Daily Value				
Taco	86	170	9	10	4	12	<1	3	30	330	8	0	8	4	53
Taco Supreme®	124	210	9	14	6	14	2	3	40	350	8	6	10	6	60
Double Decker Taco Supreme®	109	380	15	18	7	39	3	9	40	760	8	6	15	10	43
Beef soft taco	109	210	11	10	4	20	1	3	30	570	8	0	8	6	43
Chicken soft taco	109	190	13	7	2.5	19	1	2	35	480	4	2	8	4	33
Chicken Burrito Supreme	117	410	20	16	6	49	4	8	45	1120	45	8	15	10	35
Beef Double Burrito Supreme	319	510	23	23	9	52	4	11	60	1500	50	8	15	15	41
Chili cheese burrito	156	330	13	13	5	40	2	4	25	900	20	0	15	6	35
Bean burrito	218	370	13	12	3.5	54	3	12	10	1080	45	0	15	15	29
Nachos Supreme	218	440	14	24	7	44	3	9	35	800	0	6	15	15	49
Nachos BellGrande®	342	760	20	39	11	83	4	17	35	1300	10	8	20	20	46
Pintos 'n cheese	140	180	9	8	4	18	1	10	15	640	45	0	15	10	40
Mexican rice	148	190	5	9	3.5	23	,1	,1	15	750	100	2	15	8	43
Beef Fiesto Burrito	202	370	14	15	5	49	3	4	30	1110	30	0	10	10	36
Meximelt®	148	290	15	15	7	22	2	4	45	830	8	0	20	6	47
Chalupa Supreme,® beef	171	380	14	23	8	29	3	3	40	580	6	8	15	10	55
Chalupa nacho cheese, chicken	171	350	16	19	4.5	29	3	2	25	640	6	8	8	10	49
Gordita Supreme,® beef	171	300	17	14	5	27	4	3	35	550	2	6	15	10	42
Gordita Santa Fe,® chicken	171	370	17	20	4	30	3	3	40	610	4	6	15	10	49

SOURCE: Taco Bell Corporation, 2001, http;://www.tacobell.com. Reproduced with permission from the Taco Bell Corporation.

	Serving size	Calories	Protein	Total fat	Saturated fat	Total carbohydrate	Sugars	Fiber	Cholesterol	Sodium	Vitamin A	Vitamin C	Calcium	Iron	% calories from fat
	g		g	g	g	g	g	g	mg	mg	% Daily Value				
Single w/everything	219	420	25	20	7	37	8	3	70	930	6	10	15	25	43
Big Bacon Classic	282	580	33	31	12	45	11	3	95	1500	15	20	25	30	48
Jr. hamburger	118	280	15	10	3.5	34	7	2	30	610	2	2	10	20	32
Jr. bacon cheeseburger	166	390	20	20	8	34	7	2	55	870	8	10	15	20	46
Grilled chicken sandwich	189	300	24	8	1.5	36	8	2	55	730	4	10	10	15	24
Caesar side salad (no dressing)	92	110	9	6	2.5	6	1	1	15	600	35	25	15	6	49
Grilled chicken salad (no dressing)	338	190	22	8	1.5	10	5	4	45	680	120	60	20	10	38
Taco salad (no dressing)	468	380	26	19	10	28	8	8	65	1040	45	45	35	25	45
Blue cheese dressing (2T)	28	180	1	19	3.5	0	0	0	15	170	0	0	2	0	95
Ranch dressing, reduced fat, calories (2T)	28	60	1	5	1	2	1	0	10	240	0	0	2	0	75
Soft breadstick	44	130	4	3	.5	23	N/A	1	5	250	0	0	4	9	21
Biggie fries	159	470	7	23	3.5	61	0	6	0	150	0	15	3	7	44
Baked potato w/broccoli & cheese	411	470	9	14	2.5	80	6	9	5	470	35	120	20	25	27
Baked potato w/chili & cheese	439	620	20	24	9	83	7	9	40	780	20	60	35	30	35
Chili, small, plain	227	210	15	7	2.5	21	5	5	30	800	8	6	8	6	30
Chili, large w/cheese & crackers	363	405	28	16.5	7	37	8	7	60	1380	14	10	22	26	37
Chicken nuggets (5)	75	230	11	16	3	11	0	0	30	470	0	2	2	2	63
Barbeque sauce	28	45	1	0	0	10	7	0	0	160	0	0	0	4	0
Frosty dairy dessert, medium	298	440	11	11	7	73	56	0	50	260	20	0	41	8	23
Chicken club sandwich	216	480	30	21	5	44	6	2	65	1000	4	10	10	15	39

N/A: not available.

SOURCE: Wendy's International, Inf., 2001, http://www.wendys.com. Reproduced with permission from Wendy's International, Inc.

Information on additional foods and restaurants is available online:

Arby's: http://www.arbysrestaurant.com

Burger King: http://www.burgerking.com

Domino's Pizza: http://www.dominos.com

Hardees: http://www.hardees.com

Jack in the Box: http://www.jackinthebox.com

KFC: http://www.kfc.com

McDonald's: http://www.mcdonalds.com

Subway: http://www.subway.com

Taco Bell: http://www.tacobell.com

Wendy's: http://www.wendys.com

White Castle: http://www.whitecastle.com

This self-care guide will help you manage some of the most common symptoms and medical problems:

- Fever
- Sore throat
- Cough
- Nasal congestion
- Ear problems
- Nausea, vomiting, or diarrhea
- Heartburn and indigestion
- Headache
- Low-back pain
- Strains and sprains
- Cuts and scrapes

Each symptom is described here in terms of what is going on in your body. Most symptoms are part of the body's natural healing response and reflect your body's wisdom in attempting to correct disease. Self-care advice is also given, along with some guidelines about when to seek professional advice. In most cases, the symptoms are self-limiting; that is, they will resolve on their own with time and simple self-care strategies.

No medical advice is perfect. You will always have to make the decision about whether to self-treat or get professional help. This guide is intended to provide you with more information so you can make better, more informed decisions. If the advice here differs from that of your physician, discuss the differences with him or her. In most cases, your physician will be able to customize the advice to your individual medical situation.

The guidelines given here apply to *generally healthy adults*. If you are pregnant or nursing, or if you have a chronic disease, particularly one that requires medication, check with your physician for appropriate self-care advice. Additionally, if you have an allergy or suspected allergy to any recommended medication, check with your physician before using it.

If you have several symptoms, read about your primary symptom first, and then proceed to secondary symptoms. Use your common sense when determining self-care. If you are particularly concerned about a symptom or confused about how to manage it, call your physician to get more information.

FEVER

A fever is an abnormally high body temperature, usually over 100°F (37.7°C). It is most commonly a sign that your body is fighting an infection. Fever may also be due to an inflammation, an injury, or a drug reaction. Chemicals released into your bloodstream during an infection reset the thermostat in the hypothalamus of your brain. The message goes out to your body to turn up the heat. The blood vessels in your skin constrict, and you curl up and throw on extra blankets to reduce heat loss. Meanwhile, your muscles begin to shiver to generate additional body heat. The resulting rise in body temperature is a fever. Later, when your brain senses that the temperature is too high, the signal goes out to increase sweating. As the sweat evaporates, it carries heat away from the body surface.

A fever may not be all bad; it may even help you fight infections by making the body less hospitable to bacteria and viruses. A high body temperature appears to bolster the immune system and may inhibit the growth of infectious microorganisms.

Most generally healthy people can tolerate a fever as high as 103–104°F (39.5–40°C) without problems. Therefore, if you are essentially healthy, there is little need to reduce a fever unless you are very uncomfortable. Older adults and those with chronic health problems such as heart disease may not tolerate the increased metabolic demand of a high fever, and fever reduction may be advised.

Most problems with fevers are due to the excessive loss of fluids from evaporation and sweating, which may cause dehydration.

Self-Assessment

1. If you are sick, take your temperature several times throughout the day. Oral temperatures should not be measured for at least 10 minutes after smoking, eating, or drinking a hot or cold liquid. When using an oral glass thermometer, first clean it with rubbing alcohol or cool soapy water (hot water may break it). Then shake it down until it reads 95°F or lower. Place the thermometer under your tongue, and leave it in place for a *full 3 minutes*. (If you leave it in for only 2 minutes, the temperature reading will be off by at least half a degree.) To read the thermometer, notice where the colored column ends, and compare it with the degrees marked in lines on the thermometer. If you are using an electronic digital thermometer, follow the directions that came with it.

"Normal" temperature varies from person to person, so it is important to know what is normal for you. Your normal temperature will also vary throughout the day, being lowest in the early evening. If you exercise or if it is a hot day, your temperature may normally rise. Women's body temperature typically varies by a degree or more through the menstrual cycle, peaking around the time of ovulation. Rectal temperatures normally run about 0.5–1.0°F higher than oral temperatures. If your recorded temperature is more than 1.0–1.5°F above your normal baseline temperature, you have a fever.

2. Watch for signs of dehydration: excessive thirst; very dry mouth; infrequent urination with dark, concentrated urine; and light-headedness.

Self-Care

1. Drink plenty of fluids to prevent dehydration—at least 8 ounces of water, juice, or broth every 2 hours.

2. Take a sponge bath using lukewarm water; this will increase evaporation and help reduce body temperature naturally.

3. Don't bundle up. This decreases the body's ability to lose excess heat.

4. Take aspirin substitute (acetaminophen, ibuprofen, or naproxen sodium). For adults, two standard-size tablets every 4–6 hours can be used to reduce the fever and the associated headache and achiness. Do not use aspirin in anyone younger than age 20 because some younger people with chicken pox, influenza, or other viral infections have developed a life-threatening complication, Reye's syndrome, after taking aspirin.

When to Call the Physician

1. Fever over 104°F (40°C), or 102°F (38.8°C) if over 60 years old

2. Persistent fever: 102° (38.8°C) or higher for 2 full days; 101° (38.3°C) or higher for 3 full days; or 100° or higher for 4 full days

3. Recurrent unexplained fevers

4. Fever accompanied by a rash, stiff neck, severe headache, difficulty breathing, cough with brown sputum, severe pain in the side or abdomen, painful urination, convulsions, or mental confusion

5. Fever with signs of dehydration

6. Fever after starting a new medication

SORE THROAT

A sore throat is caused by inflammation of the throat lining resulting from an infection, allergy, or irritation (especially from cigarette smoke). If you have an infection, you may also notice some hoarseness from swelling of the vocal cords and "swollen glands," which are enlarged lymph nodes that produce white blood cells to help fight the infection. The lymph nodes, part of your body's defense system, may remain swollen for weeks after the infection subsides.

Most throat infections are caused by viruses, so antibiotics are not effective against them. However, about 20–30% of throat infections are due to streptococcal bacteria. This type of microbe can cause complications such as rheumatic fever and rheumatic heart disease and therefore should be diagnosed by a physician and treated with antibiotics. Strep throat is usually characterized by very sore throat, high fever, swollen lymph nodes, a whitish discharge at the back of the throat, and the absence of other cold symptoms such as a cough and runny nose (which suggest a viral infection). Allergy-related sore throats are usually accompanied by running nose, sneezing, and watery, itchy eyes.

Self-Assessment

1. Take your temperature.

2. Look at the back of your throat in a mirror. Is there a whitish, puslike discharge on the tonsils or in the back of the throat?

3. Feel the front and back of your neck. Do you feel enlarged, tender lymph nodes?

Self-Care

1. If you smoke, stop smoking to avoid further irritation of your throat.

2. Drink plenty of liquids to soothe your inflamed throat.

3. Gargle with warm salt water (1/4 tsp salt in 4 oz water) every 1–2 hours to help reduce swelling and discomfort.

4. Suck on throat lozenges, cough drops, or hard candies to keep your throat moist.

5. Use throat lozenges, sprays, or gargles that contain an anesthetic to temporarily numb your throat and make swallowing less painful.

6. Try aspirin substitute to ease throat pain.

7. For an allergy-related sore throat, try an antihistamine such as chlorpheniramine.

When to Call the Physician

1. Great difficulty swallowing saliva or breathing

2. Sore throat with fever over 101°F (38.3°C), especially if you do not have other cold symptoms such as nasal congestion or a cough

3. Sore throat with a skin rash

4. Sore throat with whitish pus on the tonsils

5. Sore throat and recent contact with a person who has had a positive throat culture for strep

6. Enlarged lymph nodes lasting longer than 3 weeks

7. Hoarseness lasting longer than 3 weeks

COUGH

A cough is a protective mechanism of the body to help keep the airways clear. There are two types of cough: a dry cough (without mucus) and a productive cough (with mucus). Common causes of cough include infection (viral or bacterial), allergies, and irritation from smoking and pollutants. If you have a cold, the cough may be the last symptom to improve, because the airways may remain irritated for several weeks after the infection has resolved.

Your airways are lined with hairlike projections called cilia, which move back and forth to help clear the airways of mucus, germs, and dust. Infections and cigarette smoking paralyze and damage this vital defensive mechanism.

Self-Assessment

1. Take your temperature.

2. Observe your mucus. Thick brown or bloody mucus suggests a bacterial infection.

Self-Care

1. If you are a smoker, stop smoking. Smoking irritates the airways and undermines your body's immune defenses, leading to more serious infections and longer-lasting symptoms. Most people do not feel like smoking when they have a cold with a cough. If you want to quit, a cold may provide an excellent opportunity to do so.

2. Drink plenty of liquids (at least six 8-ounce glasses a day) to help thin mucus and loosen chest congestion.

3. Use moist heat from a hot shower or vaporizer to help loosen chest congestion.

4. Suck on cough drops, throat lozenges, or hard candy to keep your throat moist and help relieve a dry, tickling cough.

5. If you have a dry, nonproductive cough or the cough keeps you from sleeping, you can use a cough syrup or lozenge that contains the nonprescription cough suppressant dextromethorphan. Because a cough that produces mucus is protective, it is generally not advisable to suppress a productive cough.

When to Call the Physician

1. Cough with thick brown or bloody sputum

2. Cough with high fever—above 102°F (38.8°C)—and shaking chills

3. Severe chest pains, wheezing, or shortness of breath

4. Cough that lasts longer than 4 weeks

NASAL CONGESTION

Nasal congestion is most commonly caused by infection or allergies. With infection, the nasal passages become congested because of increased blood flow and mucus production. This congestion is actually part of the body's defense to fight infection. The increased blood flow raises the temperature of the nasal passages, making them less hospitable to germs. The nasal secretions are rich in white blood cells and antibodies to help fight and neutralize the invading organisms and flush them away. Nasal congestion associated with sore throat, cough, and fever usually indicates a viral infection. Green nasal discharge is common with viral infections; it does not mean you need an antibiotic.

Nasal congestion caused by allergies is often accompanied by a thin, watery discharge, sneezing, and itchy eyes; it is sometimes associated with a seasonal pattern. In an allergic reaction, the offending allergen (such as pollen, dust, mold, or dander) triggers the release of histamine and other chemicals from the cells lining the nose, throat, and eyes. These chemicals cause swelling, discharge, and itching. Antihistamine drugs block the release of these irritating chemicals.

Self-Assessment

1. Take your temperature.

2. Observe the color and consistency of your nasal secretions. A thick brown or bloody discharge suggests a bacterial sinus infection.

3. Tap with your fingers over the sinus cavities above and below the eyes. If the tapping causes increased pain, you may have a bacterial sinus infection.

Self-Care

1. If you smoke, stop smoking to prevent continuing irritation of the nasal passages.

2. Use moist heat from a hot shower or vaporizer to help liquefy congested mucus.

3. Use a decongestant nasal spray or drops to temporarily relieve congestion. However, if these decongestants are used for more than 3 days, they can cause "rebound congestion" that actually creates more nasal congestion. As an alternative, use saltwater nose drops (¼ tsp salt in ½ cup of boiled water, cooled before using).

4. Try an oral decongestant such as pseudoephedrine (60 mg every 6 hours) to help shrink swollen mucous membranes and open nasal passages. In some people, these medications can cause nervousness, sleeplessness, or heart palpitations. If you have uncontrolled high blood pressure, heart disease, or diabetes, check with your physician before using decongestants.

When to Call the Physician

1. Nasal congestion with severe pain and tenderness in the forehead, cheeks, or upper teeth and a high fever (above 102°F or 38.8°C)

2. Thick brown or bloody nasal discharge

3. Nasal congestion and discharge unresponsive to self-care treatment and lasting longer than 3 weeks

EAR PROBLEMS

Ear symptoms include earache, discharge, itching, stuffiness, and hearing loss. They may be caused by problems in the external ear canal, eardrum, middle ear, or eustachian tube (the passageway that connects the middle ear space to the back of the throat). The ear canal can become blocked by excess wax, producing hearing loss and a sense that the ear is plugged. An infection of the external ear canal due to excessive moisture and trauma is often referred to as "swimmer's ear." It can cause pain, a sense of fullness, discharge, and itching. Congestion and blockage of the eustachian tube by a cold or allergy can result in pain, a sense of fullness, and hearing loss. A middle ear infection often produces severe pain, hearing loss, and fever.

Self-Assessment

1. Take your temperature. A fever may be a sign of infection.

2. Have someone look into the ear canal with a flashlight or otoscope. Look for wax blockage or a red, swollen canal indicating an external ear infection.

3. Wiggle the outer part of the ear. If this increases the pain, an infection or inflammation of the external canal is the likely cause.

Self-Care

1. If blockage of the ear canal with wax is the problem, first try a hot shower to liquefy the wax, and use a wash cloth to wipe out the ear canal. You can also use a few drops of an over-the-counter wax softener and then flush the canal gently with warm water in a bulb syringe. Do not use sharp objects or cotton swabs; they can scratch the canal or push the wax in deeper.

2. To treat mild infections of the external ear canal, you must thoroughly dry the ear canal. A few drops of a drying agent (Burrow's solution) on a piece of cotton gently inserted into the canal can act as a wick to dry the canal.

3. To relieve congestion and blockage of the eustachian tube, try a decongestant like pseudoephedrine, a nasal spray (but for no longer than 3 days), or an antihistamine. Hot showers or a vaporizer may help loosen secretions, and yawning or swallowing may help open the eustachian tube. For a mild plugging sensation without fever or pain, pinch your nostrils and blow gently to force air up the eustachian tube and "pop" your ears.

When to Call the Physician

1. Severe earache with fever
2. Puslike or bloody discharge from the ear
3. Sudden hearing loss, especially if accompanied by ear pain or recent trauma to the ear
4. Ringing in the ears or dizziness
5. Any ear symptom lasting longer than 2 weeks

NAUSEA, VOMITING, OR DIARRHEA

Nausea, vomiting, and diarrhea usually are defensive reactions of your body to rapidly clear your digestive tract of irritants. These symptoms may be caused by a viral infection, foodborne illness, medications, or other types of infection. Vomiting dramatically ejects irritants from your stomach, and nausea discourages eating to allow the stomach to rest. With diarrhea, overstimulated intestines flush out the offending irritants.

The major complications of vomiting and diarrhea are dehydration from fluid losses and decreased fluid intake and a risk of bleeding from irritation of the digestive tract.

Self-Assessment

1. Take your temperature. A fever is often a clue that an infection is causing the symptoms.

2. Note the color and frequency of vomiting and diarrhea. This will help you estimate the severity of fluid losses and check for bleeding (red, black, or "coffee grounds" material in the stool or vomit; iron tablets and Pepto-Bismol can also cause black stools).

3. Watch for signs of dehydration: very dry mouth; excessive thirst; infrequent urination with dark, concentrated urine; and light-headedness.

4. Look for signs of hepatitis, an infection of the liver: a yellow color in the skin and the white parts of the eyes.

Self-Care

1. To replace fluids, take frequent, small sips of clear liquids such as water, noncitrus juice, broths, flat ginger ale, or ice chips.

2. When the vomiting and diarrhea have subsided, try nonirritating, constipating foods like the BRAT diet: bananas, rice, applesauce, and toast.

3. For several days, avoid alcohol, milk products, fatty foods, aspirin, and other medications that might irritate the stomach. Do not stop taking regularly prescribed medications without discussing this change with your physician.

4. Medications are not usually advised for vomiting. For diarrhea, over-the-counter medications containing kaolin, pectin, or attapulgite may help thicken the stool. Loperamide, now available without a prescription, can be used to ease diarrhea.

When to Call the Physician

1. Inability to retain any fluids for 12 hours or signs of dehydration
2. Severe abdominal pains not relieved by the vomiting or diarrhea
3. Blood in the vomit (red or "coffee grounds" material) or in the stool (red or black tarlike material)
4. Vomiting or diarrhea with a high fever (above 102°F or 38.8°C)
5. Yellow color in skin or white parts of the eyes
6. Vomiting with severe headache and a history of a recent head injury
7. Vomiting or diarrhea that lasts 3 days without improvement
8. If you are pregnant or have diabetes
9. Recurrent vomiting and/or diarrhea

HEARTBURN AND INDIGESTION

Indigestion and heartburn are usually a result of irritation of the stomach or the esophagus, the tube that connects the mouth to the stomach. The stomach lining is usually protected from stomach acids, but the esophagus is not. Therefore, if stomach acids "reflux," or back up into the esophagus, the result is usually a burning discomfort beneath the breastbone. The esophagus is normally protected by a muscular valve that allows food to enter the stomach but prevents stomach contents from flowing upward into the esophagus. Certain foods (such as chocolate), medications, and smoking can loosen and open this protective sphincter valve. Overeating, lying down, or bending over can also cause the stomach acids to gain access to the sensitive lining of the esophagus.

Self-Assessment

1. Look for a pattern in the symptoms. Do they occur after eating certain foods, taking certain medications, or when you bend over or lie down? Do certain foods or an antacid relieve the symptoms?

2. Observe your bowel movements. Black tarlike stools may indicate bleeding in the stomach (iron tablets and Pepto-Bismol can also cause black stools).

Self-Care

1. Avoid irritants such as smoking, aspirin, ibuprofen, naproxen sodium, alcohol, caffeine (coffee, tea, cola), chocolate, onions, carbonated beverages, spicy or fatty foods, acidic foods (vinegar, citrus fruits, tomatoes), or any other foods that seem to make your symptoms worse.

2. Take nonabsorbable antacids such as Maalox, Mylanta, or Gelusil every 1–2 hours and especially before bedtime, or try an acid reducer, now available without a prescription (Pepcid, Tagamet, or Zantac).

3. Avoid tight clothing.

4. Avoid overeating; eat smaller, more frequent meals.

5. Don't lie down for 1–2 hours after a meal. Elevate the head of your bed with 4- to 6-inch blocks of wood or bricks. Adding extra pillows usually makes things worse by creating a posture that increases pressure on the stomach. Using a waterbed also usually makes reflux worse. Try sleeping on your left side, which may reduce reflux compared to sleeping on your back or right side.

6. If you are overweight in the abdominal area, weight loss may help. Abdominal obesity can increase pressure on the stomach when you are lying down.

When to Call the Physician

1. Stools that are black and tarlike or vomit that is bloody or contains material that looks like coffee grounds

2. Severe abdominal or chest pain

3. Pain that goes through to the back

4. No relief from antacids

5. Symptoms lasting longer than 3 days

Recurrent or persistent abdominal pain may be a symptom of an ulcer, a raw area in the lining of the stomach or duodenum (the first part of the small intestine). About 1 in 5 men and 1 in 10 women develop an ulcer at some time in their lives. Most ulcers are linked to infection with the bacterium *Helicobacter pylori*; people who regularly take nonsteroidal anti-inflammatory drugs like aspirin or ibuprofen are also at risk for ulcers because these drugs irritate the lining of the stomach. *H. pylori* infection is relatively easy to diagnose and treat, and other medications are available to treat ulcers linked to other causes. Many of the

self-care measures described above are also frequently recommended for people with ulcers.

HEADACHE

Headache is one of the most common symptoms. There are four major types of headache: tension, migraine, cluster, and sinus. Tension headaches, migraines, and cluster headaches are described in Chapter 2 (p. 39). Sinus headaches are caused by blockage of the sinus cavities with resulting pressure and pain in the cheeks, forehead, and upper teeth. Headache caused by elevated blood pressure is very uncommon and occurs only with very high pressures.

Self-Assessment

1. Take your temperature. The presence of fever may indicate a sinus infection. Fever, severe headache, and a very stiff neck suggest meningitis, a rare but serious infection around the brain and spinal cord.

2. Tap with your fingers over the sinus cavities in your cheeks and forehead. If this causes increased pain, it may indicate a sinus infection.

3. For recurrent headaches, keep a headache journal. Record how often and when your headaches occur, associated symptoms, activities that precede the headache, and your food and beverage intake. Look for patterns that may provide clues to the cause(s) of your headaches.

Self-Care

1. Try applying ice packs or heat on your neck and head.

2. Gently massage the muscles of your neck and scalp.

3. Try deep relaxation or breathing exercises.

4. Take aspirin or aspirin substitute for pain relief. Over-the-counter products containing a combination of aspirin, acetaminophen, and caffeine are approved by the FDA for treating migraines.

5. If pain is associated with nasal congestion, try a decongestant medication like pseudoephedrine.

6. Try to avoid emotional and physical stressors (like poor posture and eyestrain).

7. Try avoiding foods that may trigger headaches, such as aged cheeses, chocolate, nuts, red wine, alcohol, avocados, figs, raisins, and any fermented or pickled foods.

When to Call the Physician

1. Unusually severe headache

2. Headache accompanied by fever and a very stiff neck

3. Headache with sinus pain, tenderness, and fever

4. Severe headache following a recent head injury

5. Headache associated with slurred speech, visual disturbance, or numbness or weakness in the face, arms, or legs

6. Headache persisting longer than 3 days

7. Recurrent unexplained headaches

8. Increasing severity or frequency of headaches

9. Severe migraine headaches. In recent years, many new prescription medications have been approved for the prevention and treatment of migraines.

LOW-BACK PAIN

Pain in the lower back is a very common condition; it is most often due to a strain of the muscles and ligaments along the spine, often triggered by bending, lifting, or other activity. Low-back pain can also result from bone growths (spurs) irritating the nerves along the spine or pressure from ruptured or protruding discs, the "shock absorbers" between the vertebrae. Sometimes back pain is caused by an infection or stone in the kidney. Fortunately, however, simple muscular strain is the most common cause of low-back pain and can usually be effectively self-treated.

Self-Assessment

1. Take your temperature. Back pain with high fever may indicate a kidney or other infection.

2. Check for blood in your urine or frequent, painful urination, which may also indicate a kidney problem.

3. Observe for tingling or pain traveling down one or both legs *below* the knee with bending, coughing, or sneezing. These symptoms suggest a disc problem.

Self-Care

1. Lie on your back or in any comfortable position on the floor or a firm mattress, with knees slightly bent and supported by a pillow. Rest for 1–3 days if the pain persists.

2. Use ice packs on the painful area for the first 3 days, and then continue with cold or change to heat, whichever gives more relief.

3. Take aspirin or aspirin substitute for pain relief as needed.

4. After the acute pain has subsided, begin gentle back and stomach exercises. Practice good posture and lifting techniques to protect your back. Try to resume gentle, everyday activities like walking as soon as possible. Bed rest beyond 3 days is no longer advised. To learn more about proper back exercises and use of your back, consult a physical therapist or your physician.

When to Call the Physician

1. Back pain following a severe injury such as a car crash or fall

2. Back pain radiating down the leg *below* the knee on one or both sides

3. Persistent numbness, tingling, or weakness in the legs or feet

4. Loss of bladder or bowel control

5. Back pain associated with high fever (above 101°F or 38.3°C), frequent or painful urination, blood in the urine, or severe abdominal pain

6. Back pain that does not improve after 2 weeks of self-care

STRAINS AND SPRAINS

Missteps, slips, falls, and athletic misadventures can result in a variety of strains, sprains, and fractures. A strain occurs when you overstretch a muscle or tendon (the connective tissue that attaches muscle to bone). Sprains are caused by overstretching or tearing ligaments (the tough fibrous bands that connect bone to bone). Depending on the severity and location, a sprain may actually be more serious than a fracture, because bones generally heal very strongly while ligaments may remain stretched and lax after healing. After a sprain, it may take 6 weeks for the ligament to heal.

After most injuries, you can expect pain and swelling. This is the body's way of immobilizing and protecting the injured part so that healing can take place. The goal of self-assessment is to determine whether you have a minor injury that you can safely self-treat or a more serious injury to an artery, nerve, or bone that should be treated by your physician.

Self-Assessment

1. Watch for coldness, blue color, or numbness in the limb beyond the injury. These may be signs of damage to an artery or a nerve.

2. Look for signs of a possible fracture, which would include a misshapen limb, reduced length of the limb on the injured side compared to the uninjured side, an inability to move or bear weight, a grating sound with movement of the injured area, extreme tenderness at one point along the injured bone as you press with your fingers, or a sensation of snapping at the time of the injury.

3. Gently move the injured area through its full range of motion. Immobility or instability suggests a more serious injury.

Self-Care

1. Immediately immobilize, protect, and rest the injured area until you can bear weight on it or move it without pain. Remember: If it hurts, don't do it.

2. To decrease pain and swelling, immediately apply ice (a cold pack or ice wrapped in a cloth) for 15 minutes every hour for the first 24–48 hours. Then apply ice or heat as needed for comfort.

3. Immediately elevate the injured limb above the level of your heart for the first 24 hours to decrease swelling.

4. Immobilize and support the injured area with an elastic wrap or splint. Be careful not to wrap so tightly as to cause blueness, coldness, or numbness.

5. Take aspirin or aspirin substitute for pain as needed.

When to Call the Physician

1. An injury that occurred with great force such as a high fall or motor vehicle crash

2. Hearing or feeling a snap at the time of the injury

3. A limb that is blue, cold, or numb

4. A limb that is bent, twisted, or crooked

5. Tenderness at specific points along a bone

6. Inability to move the injured area

7. A wobbly, unstable joint

8. Marked swelling of the injured area

9. Inability to bear weight after 24 hours

10. Pain that increases or lasts longer than 4 days

CUTS AND SCRAPES

Cuts and scrapes are common disruptions of the body's skin. Fortunately, the vast majority of these wounds are minor and don't require stitches, antibiotics, or a physician's care. An abrasion involves a scraping away of the superficial layers of skin. Abrasions, though less serious, are often more painful than cuts because they disrupt more skin nerves. There are two types of cuts: lacerations (narrow slices of the skin) and puncture wounds (stabs into deeper tissues).

Normal healing of a cut or abrasion is a remarkable process. After the bleeding stops, small amounts of serum, a clear yellowish fluid, may leak from the wound. This fluid is rich in antibodies to help prevent an infection. Redness and swelling may normally occur as more blood is shunted to the area, bringing white blood cells and nutrients to speed healing. There may also be some swelling of nearby lymph nodes, which are another part of your body's defense against infection. Finally, a scab forms. This is "nature's bandage," which protects the area while it heals.

The main concerns about cuts are the possibilities of damage to deeper tissues and the risk of infection. Damage to underlying blood vessels may lead to severe bleeding as well as blueness and coldness in areas beyond the wound. Injured nerves may produce numbness and a loss of the ability to move parts of the body beyond the injured area. Damaged muscles, tendons, and ligaments can also result in inability to move areas beyond the cut.

Wound infection usually does not take place until 24–48 hours after an injury. Signs of infection include increasing redness, swelling, pain, pus, and fever. One of the most serious, though fortunately uncommon, complications of puncture wounds is tetanus ("lockjaw"). This bacterial infection thrives in areas not exposed to oxygen, so it is more likely to develop in deep puncture wounds or dirty wounds. Tetanus is not likely to develop in minor cuts or wounds caused by clean objects like knives. You need a tetanus immunization shot following a cut under the following conditions:

- If you have never had the basic series of three tetanus immunization injections

- If you have a dirty or contaminated wound and it has been longer than 5 years since your last injection

- If you have a clean, minor wound and it has been longer than 10 years since your last injection

Self-Assessment

1. Look for warning signs of complications: persistent bleeding, numbness, an inability to move the injured area, or the later development of pus, increasing redness, and fever.

2. Measure the size of the cut. If your cut is shallow, less than ¼ inch deep, less than an inch long, and not in a high-stress area (such as a joint, which bends) and you can easily hold the edges of the wound closed, it probably won't need stitches.

Self-Care

1. Apply direct pressure over the wound until the bleeding stops. The only exception is puncture wounds, which should be encouraged to bleed freely (unless spurting a large amount of blood) for a few minutes to flush out bacteria and debris.

2. Try to remove any dirt, gravel, glass, or foreign material from the wound with tweezers or by gentle scrubbing.

3. Wash the wound vigorously with soap and water, followed by an application of hydrogen peroxide solution as an antiseptic.

4. If it is an abrasion, cover the area with a sterile adhesive bandage until a scab forms. For minor lacerations, close the cut with a butterfly bandage or a sterile adhesive tape, drawing the edges close together but not overlapping. If there is an extra flap of clean skin, leave it in place for extra protection. Do not attempt to close a puncture wound. Instead, soak the wound in warm water for 15 minutes several times a day for several days. Soaking helps keep the wound open and thus prevents infection.

When to Call the Physician

1. Bleeding that can't be controlled with direct pressure

2. Numbness, weakness, or an inability to move the injured area

3. Any large, deep wound

4. A cut in an area that bends and with edges that cannot easily be held together

5. Cuts on the hands or face unless clean and shallow

6. A contaminated wound from which you cannot remove the foreign material

7. Any human or animal bite

8. If you need a tetanus immunization (see indications noted earlier)

9. Development of increasing redness, swelling, pain, pus, or fever 24 hours or more after the injury

10. If the wound is not healing well after 3 weeks

BOOKS AND AUDIOTAPES

American College of Obstetricians and Gynecologists. 2000. *Encyclopedia of Women's Health and Wellness*. Washington, D.C.: American College of Obstetricians and Gynecologists. *A comprehensive look at women's health that includes checklists, questionnaires, and many other helpful tools.*

American Medical Women Association. 2001. *Complete Family Health Book*. New York: Golden Books. *A comprehensive guide to family health.*

Ammer, C. 2000. *The New A to Z of Women's Health: A Concise Encyclopedia*, 4th ed. New York: Facts on File. *An easy-to-use reference covering a wide variety of women's health topics.*

Brubaker, M., et al. 1999. *Surgery: A Patient's Guide from Diagnosis to Recovery*. San Francisco: UCSF Nursing Press. *A comprehensive look at surgery from diagnosis to the postsurgery recovery process at home.*

Griffith, H. W. 2000. *Complete Guide to Prescription and Nonprescription Drugs, 2001 Edition*. New York: Perigee. *A comprehensive guide to side effects, warnings, and precautions for the safe use of over 4000 brand-name and generic drugs.*

Griffith, H. W. 2000. *The Complete Guide to Symptoms, Illness, and Surgery*, 4th rev. ed. New York: Perigee. *An up-to-date reference covering signs and symptoms, illnesses and disorders, and surgeries.*

Hogan, R. W. 2000. *The PDR Pocket Guide to Prescription Drugs*, 4th ed. New York: Pocket Books. *An easy-to-use reference to over 1000 prescription drugs.*

Inlander, C. B., K. Morales, and the People's Medical Society. 2000. *Family Health for Dummies*. Foster City, Calif.: IDG Books. *Addresses a wide range of health topics.*

Kemper, D. W. 1999. *Healthwise Handbook: A Self-Care Manual for You*. Boise, Id.: Healthwise. *Practical guidelines for home care of common medical problems in adults and children.*

Komaroff, A. L., ed. 1999. *Harvard Medical School Family Health Guide*. New York: Simon & Schuster. *A comprehensive, easy-to-use guide to symptoms, disorders, treatments, medical emergencies, and the health care system.*

Lerner, P., and J. Lerner. 2000. *Lerner's Consumer Guide to Health Care*. Seattle, Wash.: Lerner Communications. *Presents advice on how to obtain quality medical care and to negotiate the bureaucracy of the health care system.*

Lorig, K. et al. 2000. *Living a Healthy Life with Chronic Conditions*. Palo Alto, Calif.: Bull. *A helpful guide to dealing with chronic illness.*

Medical Economics Staff, ed. 2001. *PDR Family Guide to Prescription Drugs*, 8th ed. New York: Three Rivers Press. *A comprehensive guide to prescription drugs.*

Medical Economics Staff, ed. 2001. *PDR for Nonprescription Drugs and Dietary Supplements*, 22nd ed. Montvale, N.J.: Medical Economics. *A clinical reference covering food and drug interactions, side effects, contraindications, costs, and other information on over-the-counter drugs and supplements.*

Men's Health Books, ed. 2000. *The Complete Book of Men's Health*. Emmaus, Pa.: Rodale Press. *An illustrated guide to men's health, with an emphasis on prevention.*

Muth, A. S. 2001. *Surgery Sourcebook: Basic Consumer Health Information About Major Surgery and Outpatient Surgeries*. Detroit: Omnigraphics. *A comprehensive, consumer-oriented look at surgery.*

Naparastek, B. *Health Journeys*. Akron, Ohio: Image Paths (800-800-8661; http://www.healthjourneys.com). *A selection of high-quality audiotapes for imagery for relaxation, mental health, illness management, and preparation for surgery.*

Pryor, J. L., and S. Glass. 2000. *It's in the Male: Everyone's Guide to Men's Health*. Minnetonka, Minn.: Appladay Press. *A concise guide to key men's health concerns.*

Rothenberg, M. A., and C. F. Chapman. 2000. *Dictionary of Medical Terms: For the Nonmedical Person*, 4th ed. Hauppauge, N. Y.: Barrons Educational Series. *Includes basic definitions of many medical terms.*

Rybacki, J. J., and J. W. Long. 2001. *The Essential Guide to Prescription Drugs*. New York: HarperResource. *A comprehensive drug reference that includes descriptions of how each drug works, possible side effects, and other precautions.*

Self-Care Advisor: The Essential Home Health Guide for You and Your Family. 2000. Alexandria, Va.: Time-Life. *Provides advice on more than 300 common health problems, including symptoms, suggestions for home care, advice on when to call the doctor, and tips for prevention.*

Shannon, J. B., ed. 1999. *Medical Tests Sourcebook*. Detroit: Omnigraphics. *Provides basic consumer information on a wide variety of medical tests.*

Silverman, H., ed. 2000. *The Pill Book*, 9th rev. ed. New York: Bantam. *Provides descriptions and illustrations of more than 1500 of the most commonly prescribed drugs.*

Sobel, D., and R. Ornstein. 1998. *Mind and Body Health Handbook*. Los Altos, Calif.: DRx. *Presents step-by-step instructions for how to use your mind to relieve stress, boost immunity, improve mood, and manage illness.*

See Chapter 1 for a list of general health-related newsletters and magazines.

HEALTH INFORMATION CENTERS

Consumer Information Center (Pueblo, CO 81009, 888-8PUEBLO; http://www.pueblo.gsa.gov).

National Health Information Center (P.O. Box 1133, Washington, DC 20013, 800-336-4797); http://www.health.gov/nhic).

Office of Minority Health Resource Center (P.O. Box 37337, Washington, DC 20013, 800-444-6472; http://www.omhrc.gov).

SELF-HELP AND MUTUAL AID GROUPS

Self-help groups provide information and peer support for nearly every conceivable medical condition or problem. Look in the telephone book for a local chapter, or contact one of the following self-help clearinghouses for the names of self-help groups in your community.

American Self-Help Clearinghouse (St. Clare's Health Services, 25 Pocono Road, Denville, NJ 07834, 973-326-8853; http://www.mentalhelp.net/selfhelp).

National Self-Help Clearinghouse (365 5th Avenue, Suite 3300, New York, NY 10016, 212-817-1822; http://www.selfhelpweb.org).

TELEPHONE HOTLINES

For hotlines relating to the main topics of this text, see the For More Information sections at the end of each chapter. Additional hotlines are listed below. Extensive lists of health-related hotlines and clearinghouses are available from the National Health Information Center (800-336-4797; http://www.health.gov/nhic), the American Self-Help Clearinghouse (973-326-8853; http://www.mentalhelp.net/selfhelp/fonenums/helpline.htm), and Johns Hopkins Info-Net (http://infonet.welch.jhu.edu/advocacy.html).

Blindness: American Foundation for the Blind, 800-232-5463; National Library Service for the Blind and Physically Handicapped, 800-424-8567; Recording for the Blind and Dyslexic, 800-221-4792.

Chronic fatigue syndrome: CFIDS Association, 800-442-3437.

Consumer products: U.S. Consumer Product Safety Commission, 800-638-2772: FDA National Hotline, 888-463-6332.

Deafness/hearing problems: American Speech Language and Hearing Association, 800-638-8255; Dial-a-Hearing Screening Test, 800-222-EARS: National Institute on Deafness and Other Communication Disorders, 800-241-1044, 800-241-1055 (TTY)

Disabling conditions: Americans with Disabilities Act Hotline, 800-949-4232 (Voice/TTY); Job Accommodation Network, 800-232-9675 (Voice/TDD).

Down syndrome: National Down Syndrome Society, 800-221-4602.

Endometriosis: Endometriosis Association, 800-992-3636.

Epilepsy: Epilepsy Foundation of America, 800-EFA-1000; Epilepsy Information Service, 800-642-0500

Gambling: National Council on Compulsive Gambling, 800-522-4700.

Headache: National Headache Foundation, 800-843-2256; American Council for Headache Education, 800-255-ACHE.

Hemophilia: National Hemophilia Foundation, 888-463-6643.

Irritable bowel syndrome: International Foundation for Functional Gastrointestinal Disorders, 888-964-2001.

Kidney disease: American Kidney Fund, 800-638-8299; National Kidney Foundation, 800-622-9010.

Lung disease/respiratory disorders: Lung Line, sponsored by the National Jewish Medical and Research Center, 800-222-LUNG, 800-552-LUNG (recorded information, 24 hours); American Lung Association, 800-LUNG-USA.

Lupus: Lupus Foundation of America, 800-558-0121.

Multiple sclerosis: Multiple Sclerosis Foundation, 800-441-7055.

Parkinson's disease: American Parkinson's Disease Association, 800-223-2732; National Parkinson Foundation, 800-327-4545.

Rare disorders: National Organization for Rare Disorders, 800-999-6673.

Self-abuse and self-mutilation: SAFE (Self-Abuse Finally Ends), 800-DONT-CUT.

Sickle-cell disease: Sickle Cell Disease Association of America, 800-421-8453.

Spina bifida: Spina Bifida Association of America, 800-621-3141.

Spinal cord injury: Christopher Reeve Paralysis Association, 800-225-0292.

Sports and sports injuries: Women's Sports Foundation, 800-227-3988.

Sudden infant death: American SIDS Institute, 800-232-SIDS.

THE INTERNET

The Internet is a global network of computers that links together commercial online communication services, such as America Online and CompuServe, with tens of thousands of university, government, and corporate networks. The Internet is composed of many parts, including World Wide Web documents, e-mail, newsgroups, mailing lists, and chat rooms. With access to the Internet, you can obtain in-depth information about hundreds of wellness topics and keep up with the latest research; you can also connect with people worldwide who share a medical problem or another challenge to wellness.

To reach the Internet, you need a computer, a modem, access to the network through a provider, and browser software, which allows you to navigate. Internet access is often available to students at little or no cost through college computer centers. If you have to obtain access through a commercial Internet service provider, choose one that suits your needs and your budget. Bare-bones access is available at low cost, but you may need to obtain additional software, including a browser such as Netscape Navigator or Microsoft Internet Explorer. Online services such as America Online, CompuServe, and Microsoft Network are often more expensive, but they provide all the necessary software and offer many features, including e-mail, newsgroups, and Web browsers.

The World Wide Web

The World Wide Web is made up of computer files called Web pages or Web sites that have been created by individuals, companies, and organizations. The Web is considered a user-friendly part of the Internet because it offers easy access and navigation and has media capabilities, such as audio, video, and animation.

Each Web site is identified by an address or uniform resource locator (URL), such as http://www.healthfinder.gov. To access a site, you can type the URL into the appropriate screen of your browser or you can click on a *hyperlink*, a shortcut to another Web page or to a different part of the current page. When you view a Web page, hyperlinks may appear as images or as text that is a different color and/or is underlined. By clicking on links, you can jump quickly from one Web site to related sites, even if they are located on the other side of the world.

To search out information on a particular topic, you need to use a search engine or directory, such as one of the following:

AltaVista	http://www.altavista.com
Ask Jeeves	http://www.askjeeves.com
Excite	http://www.excite.com
Fast Search	http://www.alltheweb.com
Go/Infoseek	http://www.go.com
Google	http://www.google.com
Hotbot	http://www.hotbot.com
Lycos	http://www.lycos.com
Northern Light	http://www.northernlight.com
Yahoo!	http://www.yahoo.com

These search engines search a unique database of Web pages, so you will obtain different results from different search engines. A meta–search engine like the two listed below simultaneously submits your search to multiple search engines:

Dogpile	http://www.dogpile.com
MetaCrawler	http://www.go2net.com/search.html

To use a search engine, you may need to enter key words or navigate through a series of increasingly more specific directories; some search engines offer both key word and directory searches. Within seconds, the search engine will generate a list of sites (with hyperlinks) that match your search parameters, often with a brief description of each site.

When you are searching, it's best to make your searches as specific as possible. Searching for key words such as "AIDS" or "cancer" will yield thousands or even millions of matches. Use more specific phrases, such as "HIV vaccine" or "cervical cancer treatment." If the search engine has a help section, take a look at it. Different engines have different rules for how best to enter key words. For example, you may need to enclose phrases in quotation marks or put plus or minus signs between words to obtain an appropriate result. If you don't find the information you are looking for using one search engine, try another. In addition, there are search engines and directories that specialize in health and medicine:

Achoo	http://www.achoo.com
Health A to Z	http://www.healthatoz.com
Health on the Net	http://www.hon.ch
HealthWeb	http://healthweb.org
Karolinska Institutet	http://micf.mic.ki.se/Diseases
Medical Matrix	http://www.medmatrix.org
MedWeb	http://www.medweb.emory.edu/MedWeb
MedWorld: Medbot	http://www-med.stanford.edu/medworld/medbot

Listed below is a sampling of Web sites that contain information on a variety of wellness topics and/or links to many other appropriate sites. For Web sites dealing with a specific health topic, refer to the For More Information section in the appropriate chapter. Hyperlinks to all the sites in this text can be accessed from the *Core Concepts in Health* Online Learning Center (http://www.mhhe.com/insel9).

American Academy of Family Physicians
http://aafp.org
http://www.familydoctor.org

CDC Health Information A to Z
http://www.cdc.gov/health/diseases.htm

Dr. Koop's Community
http://www.drkoop.com

Duke University Healthy Devil On-Line
http://gilligan.mc.duke.edu/h-devil

Go Ask Alice
http://www.goaskalice.columbia.edu

Healthfinder
http://www.healthfinder.gov

HealthTouch Online
http://www.healthtouch.com

InteliHealth
http://www.intelihealth.com

Mayo Health Oasis
http://www.mayohealth.org

Medem
http://www.medem.com

MedicineNet
http://www.medicinenet.com

Merck
http://www.merck.com

National Center for Health Statistics
http://www.cdc.gov/nchs

National Women's Health Resource Center
http://www.healthywomen.org

NetWellness
http://www.netwellness.org

New York Online Access to Health
http://www.noah-health.org

NIH Health Information Index
http://www.nih.gov/health

NLM Medline Plus
http://www.nlm.nih.gov/medlineplus

Thrive Online
http://thriveonline.oxygen.com

U.S. Consumer Gateway: Health
http://www.consumer.gov/health.htm

WebMD
http://webmd.com

WellnessWeb
http://wellweb.com

Usenet Newsgroups

Newsgroups consist of archived messages, articles, and postings about a particular topic; they are similar to bulletin boards. Commercial online services maintain members-only newsgroups, but many more are available on the Internet. To locate a newsgroup on a particular topic, use a search engine or visit a site devoted to newsgroups, such as Deja.com (http://www.deja.com).

You are free to browse any newsgroup's articles. Postings on related topics are often grouped together in a "thread," consisting of an original message that began a discussion and all the replies to that message. A busy newsgroup can receive thousands of postings a day, and older articles are deleted to make room for new ones. If you find an article of interest, print it or save it to your computer—it may be deleted from the newsgroup by your next visit.

In addition to browsing, reading, and saving newsgroup postings, you can also be an active participant. You can reply to a message, either to the person who posted it or to the entire newsgroup, or you can post a new message that starts a new thread of discussion. To ensure that your postings are appropriate, it's often a good idea to observe a newsgroup for a while or look at its "frequently asked questions" page prior to becoming an active member.

Listserv Mailing Lists

Listservs are similar to newsgroups, except that messages are delivered by e-mail to all subscribers to the mailing list rather than posted at a public site. Once you subscribe to a mailing list, you receive messages posted by other subscribers and you can post your own messages. As with newsgroups, it's a good idea to read messages for a while before joining the discussion. You can stop subscribing to a mailing list at any time.

To locate listservs for a particular topic, do a key word search using a search engine by entering the topic and the word *listserv.* Or try the extensive mailing list directory at Liszt (http://www.liszt.com).

Real-Time Communication: Chat Rooms

With access to the Internet, you may also have the opportunity to participate in real-time communication with people from around the world. You can sign on to a particular chat group and communicate with others who are signed on to the same group at that time. You can have a "public" conversation, in which everyone in the chat room is included, or a "private" conversation between you and one other person. Many chat groups have a moderator who can kick people off and/or refuse them further access if they don't behave appropriately. For reasons of privacy and security, many people suggest that chat room participants avoid divulging too much personal information. See the sections on online relationships (p. 101) and cyberstalking (p. 664) for specific guidelines.

Evaluating Information from the Internet

Anyone can post information and advice on the Internet—true or false, good or bad. When evaluating information from the Internet, ask the following questions:

• *What is the source of the information? Who is the author or sponsor of the Web page?* Web sites maintained by government agencies, professional organizations, or established academic or medical institutions are likely to present trustworthy information. Many other groups and individuals post accurate information, but it is important to watch your sources carefully.

Many sites will describe their sponsor on the home page; alternatively, they may have an "about us" or "who we are" link that provides this information. Take a look at the backgrounds, qualifications, and credentials of the people who are behind the information at the site. Beware of sites that don't indicate the sources of the information they post; if you don't know where it comes from, you can't assess it's validity.

As you click on links and move from page to page, also pay attention to where you are. Even if you start out at a trustworthy site, the click of a button can catapult you into a completely different site. Learn how to read your current Web address so that you know when you've left one site and entered another. Look at the abbreviation in the server name in the URL, which will change according to the sponsor's purpose—for example, "org" for organizational, "gov" for governmental, "edu" for educational, and "com" for commercial.

• *How often is the site updated?* Most Web pages will indicate the date of their most recent modifications. Major organizations may update their Web sites on a daily or weekly basis. Look for sites that are updated frequently.

• *What is the purpose of the page? Does the site promote particular products or procedures? Are there obvious reasons for bias?* The same common sense you'd use to evaluate any factual claim applies to the Internet. Be wary of sites that sell specific products, use testimonials as evidence, appear to have a social or political agenda, or ask for money. Many sites sponsored by commercial companies and lay organizations do provide sound, useful information; however, it's a good idea to consider possible sources of bias in the information they present.

• *What do other sources say about a topic?* To get a broad perspective on a piece of information, check out other online sources or ask a professional. You are more likely to obtain and recognize quality information if you use several different sources. Be wary of claims that appear at only one site.

• *Does the site conform to any set of guidelines or criteria for quality and accuracy?* A number of organizations have developed codes of conduct or ethical standards for health-related sites; these codes include criteria such as use of information from respected sources and disclosure of the site's sponsors. These organizations include the following:

American Accreditation HealthCare Commission
    http://www.urac.org

American Medical Association
    http://www.ama-assn.org

Health Internet Ethics
    http://www.hiethics.com

Health on the Net Foundation
    http://www.hon.ch

Internet Healthcare Coalition
    http://www.ihealthcoalition.org

Look for sites that identify themselves as conforming to some code or set of principles.

• *Is the site easy to use? Does it have links to other sites?* In addition to strong content, good Web pages should be easy to use, be clearly organized, and have a good search capability.

For more on finding and evaluating online wellness-related information, check out the following Web sites:

California Medical Association (select Health Care Links)
http://www.cmanet.org

CDC: Internet Health Related Hoaxes and Rumors
http://www.cdc.gov/hoax_rumors.htm

Oncolink Source Reliability Information
http://www.oncolink.upenn.edu/resources/reliability

Science Panel on Interactive Communication and Health
http://www.scipich.org

Search Engine Watch
http://www.searchenginewatch.com

UC Berkeley Library Internet Tutorial
http://www.lib.berkeley.edu/TeachingLib/Guides/
Internet/FindInfo.html

Credits

Photos

Chapter 1 p. 0, © Rudi Von Briel/PhotoEdit; p. 3, © David Young-Wolff/PhotoEdit; p. 13, © Spencer Grant/PhotoEdit; p. 21, © Richard Lord/PhotoEdit; p. 24, © Bob Collins/The Image Works; p. 25, © Kent Meireis/The Image Works

Chapter 2 p. 28, © Bob Daemmrich/Stock Boston; p. 35, © David Young-Wolff/PhotoEdit; p. 44, © Clive Bryant/PhotoEdit; p. 46, © David Young-Wolff/PhotoEdit; p. 51, © Jim Cummins/FPG International

Chapter 3 p. 58, © Bob Daemmrich/Stock Boston; p. 61, © Rhoda Sidney/Stock Boston; p. 62, © Gary A. Conner/PhotoEdit; p. 69, © David Young-Wolff/PhotoEdit; p. 81, © N. Rowan/The Image Works; p. 82, © J. Pickerell/The Image Works

Chapter 4 p. 88, © Michael Schwarz/The Image Works; p. 91, © Myrleen Cate/PhotoEdit; p. 99, © R. Lord/The Image Works; p. 100, © David Young-Wolff/PhotoEdit; p. 102, © Amy C. Etra/PhotoEdit; p. 107, © Laura Dwight/PhotoEdit

Chapter 5 p. 112, © David Young-Wolff/PhotoEdit; p. 118, © Bob Daemmrich/Stock Boston; p. 122, © Paul Conklin/PhotoEdit; p. 127, © Cleo Photography/Jeroboam; p. 132, © David Young-Wolff/PhotoEdit; p. 136, © Michelle Bridwell/PhotoEdit

Chapter 6 p. 140, © Joel Gordon; p. 143, © Joel Gordon; p. 145, © Dion Ogust/The Image Works; p. 147, © Joel Gordon; p. 149, © Joel Gordon; p. 151, © Sonda Dawes/The Image Works; p. 155, © Joel Gordon; p. 164, © Jeff Greenberg/The Image Works

Chapter 7 p. 172, © Crandall/The Image Works; p. 175, © Bob Daemmrich/Stock Boston; p. 178T, © Andrew Holbrooke/ The Image Works; p. 178B, © A. Ramey/Stock Boston; p. 189, © Mary Kate Denny/PhotoEdit

Chapter 8 p. 192, © Richard Hutching/PhotoEdit; p. 195, © Amy Ramey/PhotoEdit; p. 206, © Petit Format/Nestle/Science Source/Photo Researchers, Inc.; p. 208, © Joel Gordon; p. 214, © David J. Sams/Stock Boston/PictureQuest; p. 218, © Owen Franken/Stock Boston

Chapter 9 p. 224, © Bonnie Kamin; p. 228, © Myrleen Cate/PhotoEdit; p. 237, © Will Hart/PhotoEdit; p. 243, © Richard Hutchings/PhotoEdit; p. 245, © James Marshall/The Image Works; p. 248, © Gary Wagner/Stock Boston

Chapter 10 p. 256, © Bonnie Kamin/PhotoEdit; p. 258, © David Young-Wolff/PhotoEdit; p. 261, © Akos Szilvasi/Stock Boston; p. 263, © Amy Ramey/PhotoEdit; p. 267, © David Young-Wolff/PhotoEdit; p. 279, © Bonnie Kamin

Chapter 11 p. 284, © Joel Gordon; p. 290, © Spencer Grant/Stock Boston; p. 293, © Michael Newman/PhotoEdit; p. 298, © Joel Gordon; p. 300, © Stephanie Rausser/FPG International; p. 306, © Karim Shamsi-Basha/The Image Works

Chapter 12 p. 312, © N. Richmond/The Image Works; p. 314, © Joel Gordon; p. 327, © Myrleen Cate/PhotoEdit; p. 336, © Bob Daemmrich/Stock Boston; p. 345, © Michael Newman/PhotoEdit

Chapter 13 p. 360, © Collins/The Image Works; p. 363, © David Young-Wolff/PhotoEdit; p. 376, © David Davis/Photo Researchers, Inc.; p. 379, © David Madison Photography; p. 386, © David Young-Wolff/PhotoEdit

Chapter 14 p. 392, © Willie L. Hill, Jr./The Image Works; p. 398, © David Young-Wolff/PhotoEdit; p. 404, © Richard B. Levine; p. 406, © Tony Freeman/PhotoEdit/PictureQuest; p. 412, © Aaron Haupt/Photo Researchers, Inc.; p. 415, © Fred Gebhart

Chapter 15 p. 424, © Spencer Grant/PhotoEdit; p. 429, © Lawrence Migdale/Stock Boston; p. 433, © Gary Conner/PhotoEdit; p. 441, © Steven Rubin/The Image Works; p. 444, © Joel Gordon

Chapter 16 p. 456, © Moredun Animal Health, Ltd/Science Photo Library/Photo Researchers, Inc.; p. 461, © Tony Freeman/PhotoEdit; p. 467, © Jeff Greenberg/PhotoEdit; p. 476, © Michael Newman/PhotoEdit/PictureQuest; p. 483, © Amy C. Etra/PhotoEdit

Chapter 17 p. 491, © Bob Daemmrich/The Image Works; p. 497, © Prof. P. Motta/Dept. of Anatomy. University "La Sapienza," Rome/Science Photo Library/Photo Researchers, Inc.; p. 506, © John Durham/Photo Researchers, Inc.; p. 510, © Alán Gallegos/AG Photograph

Chapter 18 p. 520, © Sonda Dawes/The Image Works; p. 532, © Mark Richards/PhotoEdit; p. 534, © Joel Gordon; p. 538, © N. Richmond/The Image Works; p. 549, © Phillip Hayson/Photo Researchers, Inc.

Chapter 19 p. 552, © Woinarowicz/The Image Works; p. 554, © Esbin-Anderson/The Image Works; p. 557, © Myrleen Cate/PhotoEdit; p. 558, © M. Greenlar/The Image Works; p. 571, Everett Collection

Chapter 20 p. 574, © Joel Gordon; p. 576, © Steve Martson/The Image Works; p. 578, © Mark Godfrey/The Image Works;

p. 587, © Bob Daemmrich/Stock Boston/PictureQuest; p. 592, © Paul Conklin/PhotoEdit

Chapter 21 p. 600, © Bonnie Kamin; p. 604, © David K. Crow/PhotoEdit; p. 612, © W. Hill, Jr./The Image Works; p. 618, © Dick Blume/The Image Works; p. 619, © Bob Daemmrich/Stock Boston

Chapter 22 p. 624, © Tony Freeman/PhotoEdit; p. 627, © Myrleen Cate/PhotoEdit; p. 632, © Cindy Charles/ PhotoEdit/PictureQuest; p. 634, © Charles Gupton/Stock Boston; p. 640, © Crandall/The Image Works

Chapter 23 p. 645, © Jonathan Nourouk/PhotoEdit; p. 653, © Bob Daemmrich/Stock Boston; p. 656, © Tom McCarthy/ PhotoEdit; p. 659, © Jonathan Nourok/PhotoEdit; p. 668, © Bob Mahoney/The Image Works

Chapter 24 p. 674, © Tony Prettyman/PhotoEdit; p. 678, © Sean Ramsay/The Image Works; p. 679, © David Young-Wolff/PhotoEdit; p. 685, © A. Ramey/PhotoEdit; p. 687, Courtesy NASA

Index

mucus production, 498
multi-infarct dementia, 562
·multiple myeloma (MM), 473
multiple sclerosis (MS), 511, 515
mumps, 499, 508–509
murder, 647, 658, 660–662
muscle mass, 364–365, 377
muscular endurance, **362–363**
muscular strength, **362**–363, 377. *See also* strength
　　training
music therapy, 51, 56
mutagens, **472**, 473
mutations, 473–474
mycardium, 294
Mycobacterium tuberculosis, 502, 504
mycoplasmas, 502–**503**
myocardial infarction, 294–**295**, 439. *See also* heart
　　attacks
myotonia, **123**, 125

naltrexone, 274
Narcotics Anonymous (NA), 248–249
National Center for Complementary and Alterna-
　　tive Medicine (NCCAM), 603, 609, 619, 622
National Cholesterol Education Program (NCEP),
　　319, 429, 446–447
National Health Information Center (NHIC), 27
National Institute of Mental Health (NIMH), 57, 86
National Institutes of Health (NIH), 612, 614
National Nutritional Foods Association (NNFA), 343
National Nutrition Summit 2000, 395
National Sleep Foundation, 57
National Women's Health Information Center, 27
Native Americans. *See* American Indians
Nature Hawaiians, 8
natural killer cells, 494, **495–496**
nature and the human spirit, 677, 683
Necator americanus, 502
necrotizing fascitis, 503, 514
needle exchange programs, 235
neglect, 664
Neisseria, 502
Neisseria gonorrhoeae, 523, 537
Neisseria meningitidis, 503
neoplasms, 458–459. *See also* cancer
Nepal, 183
nervous system. *See* central nervous system
Netherlands, 167
neurology, 607
neurotransmitters, 76, 365, **366**–367
neutrophils, **494–495**
Newman, Paul, 571
niacin, 323, 356, 358
nickel intake, 358
nicotine
　　addiction to, 225, 286–288, 299
　　in clove cigarettes and bidis, 299
　　definition, **287**
　　heart disease, 428
　　immediate effects of, 293–294
　　insomnia, 45
　　poisoning by, 292
　　potential for dependence, 232
　　replacement therapy, 307
　　in spit tobacco, 297
　　substitutes, 307
Nigeria, 183
Nipah virus, 514
nitrates and nitrites, 336, 348, 471, 476–478
nitrogen dioxide, 684
nitrosamines, **478**
nitrous oxide, 687
NOAH: New York Online Access to Health, 27
nocturnal emissions, **128**

No-Doz. *See* caffeine
noise pollution, 694–695
noncorporeal continuity, **577**
nonessential (storage) fat, **394**
non-Hodgkin's lymphoma (NHL), 472–473
nonnutritive sweeteners, 393
nonoxynol-9, 151, 525
nonsteroidal anti-inflammatory drugs (NSAIDs),
　　560–561, 563
nonverbal communication, 96–97
norepinephrine, 32–**33**, 76, 367
normality, 58, **60**
Norplant implants, 147–148, 161
nortriptyline, 307
Norwalk viruses, 346
Novartis Pharmaceutical Corporation, 79
NSAIDs (nonsteroidal anti-inflammatory drugs),
　　560–561, 563
nuclear power, **692**–693
nuclear weapons, 693
nucleotide bases, 473
nurse-midwives, 215–216
nurses, 607–608
nursing homes, 568
nutrition, 313–359
　　additives and residues, 345–346, 348
　　aging and, 556–557
　　alcohol and, 265
　　antioxidants, 322, 325–327, 476–477, 563, 565
　　assessment, 333
　　average American diet, 332
　　behavior change strategy, 452–453
　　beverages, 336–337, 352
　　caloric intake, 403
　　cancer prevention and, 457, 462–463, 465,
　　　475–477
　　carbohydrate craving, 403
　　carbohydrates, 121, 320–322, 334–336, 342,
　　　350, 407
　　cardiovascular health and, 434–435, 446–449
　　college students, 340
　　commitment to a healthy diet, 349–350
　　daily menu example, 359
　　definition, **315**
　　dietary fiber (*See* fiber, dietary)
　　essential nutrients, 314
　　ethnic foods, 351
　　exercise programs, 383
　　fats (*See* fats, dietary)
　　food labels, 340–343
　　food safety, 211
　　low-calorie sweeteners, 393, 408
　　minerals, 324–325
　　organic foods, 346–348
　　phytochemicals, 327
　　preconception, 196–197
　　during pregnancy, 210–211
　　premenstrual problems and, 120–121
　　proteins, 315–316
　　recipes, 354
　　safe food handling, 346–347
　　stress and, 44
　　supplements, 121, 211, 378
　　vitamins and minerals, 322–325
　　water, 324–326
　　Web sites and organizations, 354
　　See also dietary recommendations; dietary
　　　supplements
nuts, 331

obesity
　　cancer and, 462–463, 477–478, 484
　　definition, **394**–397
　　ethnicity and, 8

　　genetic factors, 393, 401–402
　　health risks of, 364, 397–398, 431
　　kidney cancer, 471
　　prevalence of, 393–395
　　socioeconomic status and, 404
　　See also weight; weight management
obituaries, 589
obsessions, 72–**73**
obsessive-compulsive disorder (OCD), 72, **73**, 81,
　　511
obstetrics, 607
occupational exposure, 478
Occupational Safety and Health Administration
　　(OSHA), 656–657, 694
Oenothera biennis L., 615
oil pollution, 675
oils, 331, 437. *See also* fats, dietary
older adults. *See* aging
olestra, 414
olive oil, 437, 446, 449
Olympic games, drug testing at, 378
omega-3 fatty acids
　　Alzheimer's disease, 563
　　colon cancer, 476
　　in eggs, 344
　　heart health, 317–318, 435, 437, 448
omega-6 fatty acids, 318, 476
oncogenes, **474–475**
oncologists, 460–**461**
On Death and Dying, 588
ophthalmology, 607
opioids, 52, **238**, 252
opportunistic infections, **522–523**, 531
optimism, 34, 47–48, 58, 66–67
optometrists, **607**
oral cancer, 298, 470, 476
oral contraceptives (OC)
　　advantages, 145
　　costs, 161
　　definition, **142**
　　disadvantages, 145–147
　　effectiveness, 147, 160
　　as emergency contraceptives, 147–148
　　interference by antibiotics, 636
　　lupus, 515
　　nutrition and, 357
　　smoking and, 302, 428, 434
　　St. John's wort and, 616
　　types of, 142–147
oral-genital stimulation, 132–133
oral sex, 132–133, 525, 533–534
Orasure test, 529
Oregon, physician-assisted suicide in, 582–583
organ donors, 575, 584–586
organic foods, **346–348**
organ transplants, 586, 616
orgasm, **123**
orgasmic dysfunction, **125**–126
oriental traditional medicine, 609–611, 616–617
orlistat (Xenical), 414
OSHA (Occupational Safety and Health Adminis-
　　tration), 656–657, 694
osteoarthritis (OA), 560–561
osteopaths, 605
osteoporosis
　　aging, 560–562
　　calcium intake, 324–326
　　definition, **324, 562**
　　ethnicity, 197
　　exercise and, 366
　　injectable contraceptives, 148
　　prevention, 553
　　smoking, 302
other-directed, **60**, 61